A tailored education experience —
Sherpath book-organized collections

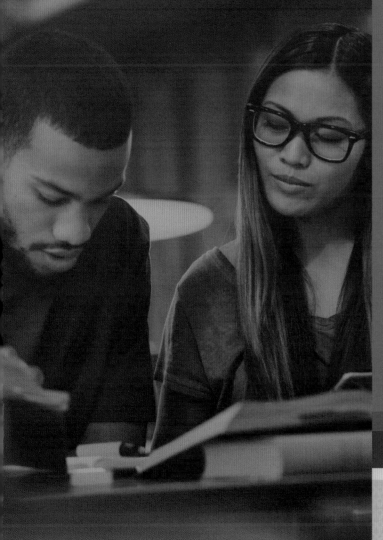

Sherpath is the digital teaching and learning technology designed specifically for healthcare education.

Sherpath book-organized collections offer:

Objective-based, digital lessons, mapped chapter-by-chapter to the textbook, that make it easy to find applicable digital assignment content.

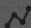

Adaptive quizzing with personalized questions that correlate directly to textbook content.

Teaching materials that align to the text and are organized by chapter for quick and easy access to invaluable class activities and resources.

Elsevier ebooks that provide convenient access to textbook content, even offline.

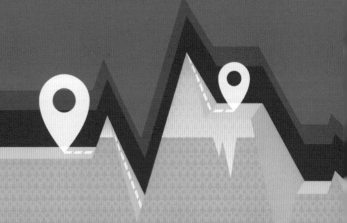

VISIT
myevolve.us/sherpath
today to learn more!

21-CS-0280 TM/AF 6/21

Keltner's

Psychiatric Nursing

Ninth Edition

Debbie Steele, PhD, RN, LMFT

Professor
Christian Counseling
Gateway Seminary
Ontario, California

ELSEVIER

Elsevier
3251 Riverport Lane
St. Louis, Missouri 63043

KELTNER'S PSYCHIATRIC NURSING, NINTH EDITION   ISBN: 978-0-323-79196-0

Notice

Previous editions copyrighted 2019, 2015, 2011, 2007, 2003, 1999, 1995, and 1991.

Senior Content Strategist: Yvonne Alexopoulos
Senior Content Development Manager: Lisa P. Newton
Publishing Services Manager: Julie Eddy
Senior Project Manager: Rachel E. McMullen
Design Direction: Bridget Hoette

Printed in India

Last digit is the print number: 9 8 7 6 5 4 3 2 1

Working together
to grow libraries in
developing countries

www.elsevier.com • www.bookaid.org

CONTRIBUTORS

Nanci A. Swan Claus, DNP, CRNP, NP-C
Assistant Professor
Acute, Chronic and Continuing Care
    Department
University of Alabama at Birmingham
Birmingham, Alabama

Marcus Otavio Guimaraes Debiasi, DDS, MS-BMS, BSN, MSN, PMHNP-BC
Student Health and Wellness Center
University of Alabama at Birmingham
Birmingham, Alabama

Jonathan S. Dowben, MD
Senior Staff Child Psychiatrist
Child and Family Behavioral Health
    Service
Brooke Army Medical Center
Fort Sam Houston, Texas

Susanne A. Fogger, DNP, PMHNP-BC, CARN-AP, FAANP
Professor
Community, Systems and Family
University of Alabama at Birmingham
Birmingham, Alabama

Karmie M. Johnson, DNP, RN, PMHNP-BC, CNE
Assistant Professor
School of Nursing
University of Alabama at Birmingham
Birmingham, Alabama

Joan Grant Keltner, PhD, RN
Professor
School of Nursing
University of Alabama at Birmingham
Birmingham, Alabama

Norman L. Keltner, EdD, RN, CRNP
Professor (Retired)
School of Nursing
University of Alabama at Birmingham
Birmingham, Alabama

Peter C. Kowalski, MD
Chief Medical Officer
Physician Services
NorthCare of Oklahoma
Oklahoma City, Oklahoma

Randy L. Moore, DNP, RN
Program Director, VA Nursing Academic
    Partnership
Nursing
VA Medical Center
Birmingham, Alabama
Assistant Professor
Adult Health Nursing
University of Alabama School of Nursing
Birmingham, Alabama

W. Chance Nicholson, PhD, MS, PMHNP-BC
Assistant Research Professor
Nell Hodgson Woodruff School of Nursing
Emory University
Atlanta, Georgia

Kate Pfeiffer, MS, APRN, PMHNP-BC, PMHCNS-BC
Instructor
Nell Hodgson Woodruff School of Nursing
Emory University
Atlanta, Georgia

Marie Smith-East, PhD, DNP, PMHNP-BC
Director of the Psychiatric Mental Health
    Nurse Practitioner Program and
    Clinical Assistant Professor
School of Nursing
Duquesne University
Pittsburgh, Pennsylvania

Debbie Steele, PhD, RN, LMFT
Professor
Christian Counseling
Gateway Seminary
Ontario, California

Helene Vossos, DNP, MSN, APRN, PMHNP-BC, ANP-BC
Director of PMHNP-DNP Program and
    Assistant Professor
School of Nursing
University of North Florida
Jacksonville, Florida
Psychiatric Mental Health Nurse
    Practitioner, Primary Care NP
Heroes Mile, Veterans for Veterans
Daytona, Florida

Barbara Jones Warren, PhD, RN, APRN, PMHCNS-BC, FNAP, FAAN
Professor and Director, Psychiatric Mental
    Health Nurse Practitioner Specialty
College of Nursing
The Ohio State University
Columbus, Ohio

ANCILLARY WRITERS

Charla K. Hollin, RN, BSN
Allied Health Division Chair, University of
    Arkansas Rich Mountain, Mena, Arkansas
TEACH for Nurses, PowerPoint Slides

Linda Turchin, RN, MSN, CNE
Professor Emeritus of Nursing
Fairmont State University
School of Nursing
Fairmont, West Virginia
*Test Bank; NCLEX® Examination-Style
    Questions*

REVIEWERS

Megan E. Gross, PhD, MPH, RN
Assistant Professor of Nursing
Department of Nursing
Messiah University
Mechanicsburg, Pennsylvania

Jennifer Lynn Guzman, DNP, MSN-Ed, RN
Professor of Nursing
Department of Health Sciences
Citrus College
Glendora, California

David Murray Meston Sharp, RN, RMN, RGN, RNT, MA, MSNED, PhD, MS
Professor of Nursing
School of Nursing
Mississippi College
Clinton, Mississippi

"*Of making many books there is no end, and much study is a weariness to the flesh.*" Solomon said this way back around 950 BC. How did he know? I mean, he got it right on both ends. There are millions of books out there, and studying is hard, tiring work. With King Solomon in mind, we have attempted to write a book that you will enjoy reading—at least for a textbook. We have tried to write in a clear, concise style. We deliver a *psychotherapeutic management* approach consisting of three interlinking parts described as *Me, Meds, and Milieu*. We have tried to write from a holistic perspective including important concepts such as "caring," "adverse childhood events/trauma," "DSM-5 nosology," "psychopharmacology," "neurobiology," and "family systems." We emphasize how you will interact with psychiatric patients, the medications you will give to your patients, and how you will assist in making their environment more therapeutic.

In this newest edition, we have added Next-Generation NCLEX™ (NGN) Examination-Style Questions to assist you in preparing for licensure. You also have access to case studies to help you in developing care plans during your clinical experiences. In the midst of much study and weariness, our hope is that you will understand more about what happens to people throughout the life span that promotes your ability to connect with them in a caring and compassionate manner.

TEACHING AND LEARNING RESOURCES

FOR INSTRUCTORS

Instructor Resources on Evolve, available at http://evolve. elsevier.com/Keltner/, provides a wealth of material to help you make your psychiatric nursing instruction a success. In addition to all of the Student Resources, the following are provided for instructors:
- *TEACH for Nurses* **Lesson Plans**, based on the chapter Learning Objectives in the textbook, serve as ready-made, modifiable lesson plans and a complete roadmap to link all parts of the educational package. These concise and straightforward lesson plans can be modified or combined to meet your particular scheduling and teaching needs.
- **PowerPoint Presentations** are organized by chapter with approximately 400 slides for in-class lectures. These are detailed and include customizable text and image lecture slides to enhance learning in the classroom or in Web-based course modules. If you share them with students, they can use the note feature to help them with your lectures.
- **Audience Response Questions for i > clicker and other systems** are provided with one to three multiple-answer questions per chapter to stimulate class discussion and assess student understanding of key concepts.
- *New* **Next-Generation NCLEX™ (NGN)-Style Case Studies** for Psychiatric Nursing: Six NGN-style case studies focused on Psychiatric-Mental Health Nursing.
- The **Test Bank** has more than 900 test items, complete with the correct answer, rationale, cognitive level of each question, corresponding step of the nursing process, appropriate NCLEX format, Client Needs label, and text page reference(s).

FOR STUDENTS

Student Resources on Evolve, available at http://evolve. elsevier.com/Keltner/, provides a wealth of valuable learning resources for students.
- An updated **Evolve website for students** includes NCLEX® Examination-Style Questions, Answer Key for NGN case studies, answers to Chapter Critical Thinking Questions, Psychotropic Drug Monographs, and Video Lectures.

As is true of all nursing text authors, our goal is to present accurate and meaningful information to the student without the distraction of sexist language. Where possible, we have made every attempt to avoid the use of sexist pronouns by using plural nouns and pronouns or "his or her" rather than risk stigmatizing by gender. To avoid awkwardness of style, we have sometimes referred to the nurse as "she" and the patient as "he."

ACKNOWLEDGMENTS

The fact that *Psychiatric Nursing* warrants a ninth edition speaks of the vision and acumen of Dr. Norman Keltner. He is especially renowned in the world of nursing as an expert in the field of psychopharmacology. He was a pioneer in pushing nurses to have an in-depth understanding of the holistic nature of nursing care for those experiencing mental disorders. He developed a philosophy and approach to psychiatric nursing care with three interlinking parts described as *Me, Meds, and Milieu*. Dr. Keltner is known as an excellent clinician who loved consulting and working with veterans during his tenure at the University of Alabama at Birmingham.

I am deeply grateful and humbled that Dr. Keltner provided me the opportunity of a lifetime to collaborate on the seventh and eighth editions of his nursing textbook and trusted me with carrying out his legacy in this ninth edition. I also want to acknowledge the extraordinary work of researchers, educators, and practitioners who have contributed to the development of his *Keltner's Psychiatric Nursing* textbook.

DS

CONTENTS

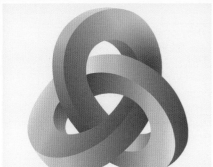

Me, Meds, Milieu

Norman L. Keltner and Debbie Steele

We dare not lengthen this book much, lest it be out of moderation and should stir men's antipathy because of its size.

Aelfric, Abbot of Eynsham (955–1020)

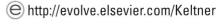
http://evolve.elsevier.com/Keltner

LEARNING OBJECTIVES

- Describe the components of psychotherapeutic management.
- Explain the way in which the balancing of psychotherapeutic management components forms a powerful therapeutic model of care.

- Recognize the relationship between the continuum of care and the psychotherapeutic management model.
- Identify the various levels of care within the continuum of care.

Where to start? You start with basics—the basic tools you need to work with people who have mental health problems. Whether as a student or as a seasoned psychiatric nurse, when you look in the mirror and ask yourself, "What are my tools?," the answer will be: "I have Me, Meds, and the Milieu." (*Milieu* is a French word for environment, but because it is/was commonly used in psychiatry, we will use it too.) This text consistently advances this simplistic model and calls the model *psychotherapeutic management*. Most often, instead of "Me," we use the term *nurse-patient relationship*, but because you are the nurse in the nurse-patient relationship, the use of "Me" just helps to make the point. The psychiatric nurse has three ways to work with patients: interpersonal skills, medication skills, and the ability to enhance (or create or construct) a safe and therapeutic environment. Thus we delightedly use the attention-grabbing chapter title, "Me, Meds, Milieu" to introduce the psychotherapeutic management model.

Although we admit the model is simplistic, we do not believe it is easy to master. Learning to communicate therapeutically is a continuous process. Understanding psychiatric medicines is far from simple. It not only takes a lot of work, but it also hinges on how well you learned anatomy, physiology, and pharmacology. Anybody can give a pill, but a competent nurse understands the many dimensions of the drugs

given. Finally, modifying an environment to make it both safe and therapeutic takes tremendous skill and consistency. The rest of this chapter explores the concept of psychotherapeutic management—a unifying model of organizing your thinking and your care. This chapter also provides an overview of various sources of mental health care and support—the so-called *continuum of care*.

PSYCHOTHERAPEUTIC MANAGEMENT

Psychiatric nurses need models of care that are effective for patient care, as well as capitalize on the uniqueness of the discipline. Psychotherapeutic management offers a real-world approach to psychiatric nursing care that recognizes the interdependence of the mental health profession while emphasizing the unique strengths of psychiatric nursing. It seeks to answer the question, "*What do psychiatric nurses do that is different from other mental health professionals, particularly social workers, psychiatrists, and psychologists?*" Psychiatric treatment can be divided into four basic categories: (1) use of words, (2) use of drugs, (3) use of environment, and (4) use of therapies. Psychotherapeutic management emphasizes the first three of these categories: (1) *words* from which nurses develop and maintain the nurse-patient relationship, (2) *drugs*, specifically psychotropic drugs, and (3) *environment*

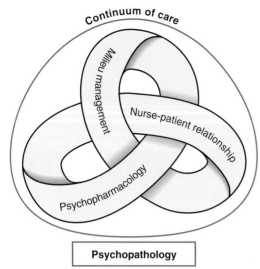

FIG. 1.1 Psychotherapeutic management in the continuum of care is based on an understanding of psychopathology.

NORM'S NOTES STOP!! Take a good look at this chapter. It will make a lot of sense because it gives you a practical approach for conceptualizing what you are doing with patients. When you work with patients, you need to focus on three things: (1) ME: how *you* will interact with them, (2) MEDS: the *medications* they need, and (3) MILIEU: how you can affect their *environment*. This approach arms you with a strategy. Now, although the framework is simple, the basics of the psychotherapeutic management approach are not simple—far from it. You will spend the entire term understanding what goes into fleshing out this model.

or *milieu*. However, the nurse cannot effectively use these interventions unless she has a sound understanding of psychopathology (Fig. 1.1).

Stated another way, the psychiatric nurse has three intervention tools to rely on:
1. Me (nurse)
2. Meds
3. Milieu (or environment)

One Size Does Not Fit All!

The authors want to encourage you to embrace the power of psychotherapeutic management paradigm and approach every patient with this model in mind. Simply (there's that word again), you can approach every patient by asking the following questions: "How should I interact with this patient?," "What kind of medicine should he be taking?," and "What are the environmental issues that will promote health and safety?"

One type of intervention might take priority over another depending on the situation. The particular approach depends on the patient's diagnosis (i.e., psychopathology) and level of functioning. For example, the nurse learns to use *different words* when speaking with a patient with a diagnosis of schizophrenia as opposed to a patient with a diagnosis of depression. More than likely, the patient with schizophrenia requires antipsychotic medications, whereas the depressed patient receives antidepressant drugs—hence drug management is different. Finally, the patient with schizophrenia might need an environment that reduces stressors, whereas a key environmental concern for the patient with depression or bipolar disorder might be safety (e.g., suicide prevention). In other words, the psychotherapeutic management model recognizes that one size does not fit all.

Application of Psychotherapeutic Management Interventions

The application of psychopathology and the knowledgeable use of psychotherapeutic management skills extend beyond inpatient settings into various care settings, such as outpatient programs, residential services, and home care. The needs of the individual and the setting in which care is delivered influence the degree to which each component of psychotherapeutic management is provided within the continuum of care (Fig. 1.2).

For example, individuals with depression in an inpatient setting benefit most when a therapeutic nurse-patient relationship, an antidepressant, and a well-managed milieu are available. When one component is missing from the equation, treatment is compromised. Just think about the possibilities when one part is missing. For example, what if the psychiatrist orders the right antidepressant (say, Lexapro), but the nursing staff does not carefully observe a potentially suicidal patient? The results could be disastrous! This abbreviated example demonstrates that all components of the psychotherapeutic management equation should be present for patients to realize maximum benefit from nursing care.

PSYCHOTHERAPEUTIC MANAGEMENT: THREE INTERVENTIONS

Therapeutic Nurse-Patient Relationship

Distinguishing therapy from being therapeutic is crucial for the student of psychiatric nursing. Therapy is the focus of graduate-level psychiatric nursing training, as well as the graduate programs in other disciplines. It is not taught at the basic nursing program level. What you will be taught is how to be therapeutic. Think about the difference, and savor it. You can learn to be a therapeutic nurse in the short time you are taking this course. When this course is completed, the student is *not a therapist* but should possess *therapeutic skills*.

Unit II of this book is devoted to the "Me" dimension of psychotherapeutic management. A new vocabulary of words and concepts are discussed within a relationship context. Specifically, general communication skills, the nature of the nurse-patient relationship, working with groups of patients,

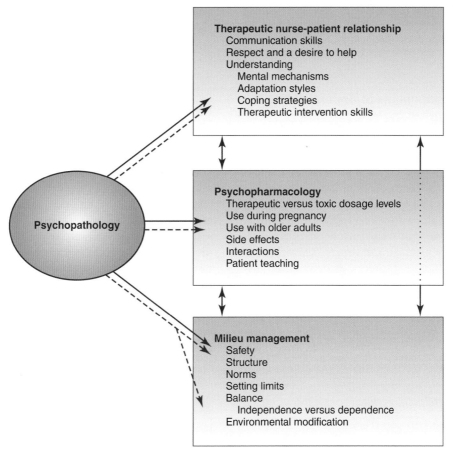

FIG. 1.2 Psychotherapeutic management model.

working with the families of patients, and other related concepts are discussed.

Psychopharmacology

Unit III of this book is devoted to the contribution of psychotropic drugs to psychiatric care, the responsibilities of the nurse, and essential information about these drugs. Most other textbooks do not provide a separate unit for psychotropic drugs, preferring to integrate the information into the presentation of specific psychiatric disorders and issues. We would argue that the role of psychiatric medicines is so significant that a thorough treatment becomes necessary.

Psychopharmacology is an important dimension of psychotherapeutic management because psychotropic drugs have enabled millions of people to live increasingly independent lives. However, *drug intervention is neither always desirable nor appropriate*, but, when drug therapy is indicated, patients may respond more rapidly than they would without drugs.

The nurse who uses the nursing process model can assess patients' responses to medication, plan to respond to side effects should they occur, implement those plans, and evaluate for desired results. The nurse's pivotal role, particularly in an inpatient setting, allows intervention before serious drug-related problems occur. In addition, the nurse administers medications and makes decisions regarding as-needed (prn)

medications. Finally, the nurse needs a sound foundation in psychopharmacology to teach patients about drugs. For these and other reasons, the nurse must have immediate access to information about psychotropic drugs.

Milieu Management

Milieu (or environmental) management is a proactive approach to care that forges therapeutic benefits from patients' surroundings, whether in the hospital, outpatient setting, or home. The five environmental elements that nurses must consider in creating a therapeutic milieu are the following:
1. Safety: keeping the patient free from danger or harm
2. Structure: the physical environment, regulations, and schedules
3. Norms: specific expectations of behavior (e.g., acceptance, nonviolence, privacy)
4. Limit setting: clear and enforceable limitations on behaviors
5. Balance: negotiating the line between dependence and independence.

Some of these elements might overlap; for example, safety is a component of all the dimensions of milieu. Voogt and colleagues (2016) suggest that by providing and structuring the therapeutic milieu, patients' capabilities are maximized. More details regarding milieu management are discussed in Unit IV.

Other Important Components of Understanding Psychiatric Nursing

Psychopathology: The Key to Psychotherapeutic Management

Unit V discusses psychopathology and provides the foundation on which the three components of psychotherapeutic management rest. It lays the groundwork for an understanding of psychopharmacology, the nurse-patient relationship, and milieu management. Unit V also includes detailed information about the major psychiatric disorders. Schizophrenia, depressive disorders, bipolar disorders, anxiety-related disorders, cognitive disorders, personality disorders, sexual disorders, substance-related disorders, and eating disorders are considered in separate chapters of Unit V.

 CRITICAL THINKING QUESTION

1. If you or a family member were to develop a mental health problem, which aspect of psychotherapeutic management would be most important to you?

Special Populations

In Unit VI, the problems and needs of special populations are discussed. Unit VI contains chapters on survivors of violent behavior, children and adolescents, older adults, and soldiers and veterans.

 CRITICAL THINKING QUESTION

2. Based on your clinical setting, what is your evaluation of the components of the psychotherapeutic management model that you have observed?

CONTINUUM OF CARE: ALL THE PLACES TO IMPLEMENT ME, MEDS, AND MILIEU

The continuum of care provides individuals with a wide range of treatment options. Not everyone needs admission to a hospital, and our economy cannot afford this level of care for the large number of people with mental health problems. The hope is to have an integrated approach that provides the most appropriate care within a seamless continuum. Fig. 1.3 illustrates a decision tree for the continuum of care. The first step after a mental health problem is suspected is to confirm its existence. You would do the same thing if you heard a knocking sound in your car. Is there really anything wrong here? The next step is to ask this question: *Does this person require hospitalization?*

If the answer is *yes*, then appropriate treatment should happen even though it can be expensive. In addition, to establish credibility, we have to admit that the bar is pretty high for admitting someone to a hospital—particularly against the will of the person. On the other extreme, homeless persons with mental illness, when seeking psychiatric hospitalization, may do so more as a short-term housing arrangement than for apparent psychiatric reasons. Either way, medical necessity has to be established by hospitals based on the individual's ability to function.

If the answer is *no*, hospitalization is not needed, then several treatment alternatives are available. Fig. 1.3 identifies residential services, traditional outpatient services, day treatment programs, self-help resources, and telehealth. There are many other options as well. When hospitalization is necessary, discharge planning is started soon after admission, and on discharge the same continuum of treatment options is considered for the released individual.

The role of nurses and other professionals is to assess the individual's current level of functioning and direct the individual to appropriate resources. Coordination of services for the individual necessitates multidisciplinary collaboration. Without this coordination, the continuum of care will not be seamless and may hinder the very thing it purports to help. Multidisciplinary care has been expanded to include not only professional staff but also nonprofessionals, patients (many treatment environments prefer the term *consumer*), family, peers, and various nonpsychiatric resources (e.g., representatives from Medicare, Medicaid, nursing homes, group homes, and medical clinics).

The decision tree in Fig. 1.3 may seem tedious to review but is very helpful once grasped. It is helpful in matching the needs of the individual with appropriate services based on safety requirements, intensity of supervision needed, severity of symptoms, level of functioning, and type of treatment needed. Following are some great examples:

1. A mother with auditory hallucinations telling her to kill her newborn infant needs inpatient hospitalization with 24-hour nursing care and supervision in a safe environment.
2. A teenager with thoughts of suicide but without a plan might be managed effectively by attending a day treatment program 5 days a week for 2 weeks.
3. A middle-aged man with a diagnosis of schizophrenia and a history of not regularly taking his antipsychotic medication and who needs a place to live might be appropriately placed in a group home with 24-hour supervision.
4. An elderly woman with chronic alcoholism who has completed acute detoxification might need referral to outpatient counseling or a self-help group such as Alcoholics Anonymous.
5. A retired military family in rural Minnesota may need therapy via telepsychiatry (TP) on a weekly basis.

For any individual, additional referrals along the continuum of care should be made as needs change. An individual might be referred to mental health services at the suggestion of a family physician, minister, police officer, family member, friend, or staff from any of the programs within the

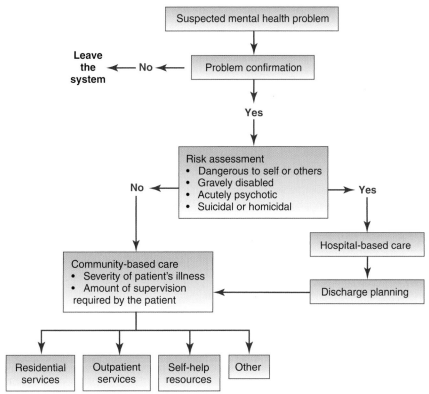

FIG. 1.3 Decision tree for continuum of care.

continuum. Self-referral is also a means whereby individuals can gain entry into the mental health system.

NORM'S NOTES The idea of a "continuum of care" might not grab you like a chapter titled "Schizophrenia." However, this concept is very important. There must be different options and different levels of care for everyone. As said earlier in the chapter, one size does not fit all. Furthermore, people cannot just be dropped out of one program with nowhere to turn. People with mental disorders should not have to fend for themselves. There needs to be a system in place, and, in most places in the United States, there is. The continuum of care provides resources for the neediest among us all the way to those who are almost ready to embrace all aspects of their lives.

Hospital-Based Care

For many people hospitals are the point of entry into the health care system. Patients admitted to acute psychiatric hospitals 20 to 30 years ago stayed about 4 to 6 weeks. If you go back even further, patients admitted to large state hospitals could be hospitalized for 20 to 30 years. Currently, length of stay is typically 3 to 5 days, which is largely driven by economic decisions. As reimbursement has decreased, the goals, staffing patterns, acuity of patients, and discharge planning of hospitalization have also changed.

- The goals are crisis intervention and safety.
- Staffing must be cost-effective while maintaining quality of service.

- Acuity of patients has increased.
- Discharge planning begins immediately after admission.

The highest priority for admission to hospital-based care is safety for self and others. When a patient is deemed a danger to himself (suicidal) or to others (homicidal), 24-hour supervision in a secure environment is required. Often these individuals are first seen in an emergency department. Other individuals who require hospitalization include those who are at risk for accidental harm to self (i.e., individuals who are gravely disabled). For example, individuals who are acutely psychotic or who are confused and disoriented might not function well enough to meet their basic needs for food, clothing, shelter, medical care, or physical safety. In addition to safety and protection, hospitalization provides thorough medical and psychiatric evaluation to identify the underlying cause of presenting symptoms.

Another group that are admitted for acute psychiatric hospitalization includes individuals who are withdrawing from addictive substances that may produce life-threatening conditions. Some individuals are admitted for a medical evaluation or because a medical illness produces or complicates a psychiatric disorder. Types of hospital-based care include:

- Locked units (individuals cannot enter or leave without a key or key card)
- Open or unlocked units
- Psychiatric intensive care units for high-acuity patients
- Specialty units (e.g., adult, geriatric, child and adolescent, substance abuse)

Long-Term Care (Residential Services)

Residential services are available to help individuals who need long-term care. Most states have long-term care facilities for individuals needing prolonged 24-hour supervision. The length of stay is variable, from 3 months to years. There are more than 8 million people in approximately 30,000 nursing homes or residential care communities in the United States (Deardorff & Grossberg, 2016).

Nursing homes are available for people who require 24-hour supervision and medical nursing care. This level of care is often required for individuals with severe developmental disabilities, dementia, or acute and chronic medical illnesses.

Group homes might provide temporary or permanent housing for individuals with chronic mental disorders. Depending on the needs of the residents, staff might be present for 24 hours a day or less. Some group homes provide group therapy and structured activities, whereas others might provide only meals, a bed, and laundry facilities.

Traditionally, *halfway houses* were available for individuals recovering from substance use and abuse. Residents were expected to seek employment and participate in cooking and cleaning chores. Residents also attended self-help groups that meet on site, such as Alcoholics Anonymous. Some halfway houses are open to individuals with other mental health problems.

Apartment living programs provide varying degrees of supervision and programming. Staff might be on site on a daily basis, offering group sessions and activities, or they visit periodically to provide medication assistance and facilitate attendance to various appointments.

Boarding homes are generally staffed by nonprofessionals but have professional supervision available on an intermittent basis. *Shelters* provide room and board to homeless people. Some homes might provide services for specific populations, such as victims of violence (e.g., abused women and their families) or individuals with addictions.

Jail is also a major facility for "housing" the mentally ill. Although we do not mean to trivialize this reality by including its mention here, it is a fact. Nasrallah (2016) refers to society's lack of understanding or perhaps even denial of this issue, as *societal anosognosia*. Chapter 2 discusses the issue of transinstitutionalization in more detail.

Traditional Outpatient Services

Outpatient treatment traditionally has occurred in mental health clinics and private offices. The person providing treatment might be a psychiatrist, psychologist, social worker, marriage and family therapist, psychiatric nurse practitioner, nurse, or other professional. The number of visits per week or month varies according to the individual's needs. The typical pattern for an individual with a chronic mental illness might be a visit once a month with a counselor or case manager and periodic appointments with a psychiatrist for medication review. During these visits, an assessment of needs for additional services is made to determine whether the individual requires more intensive treatment or a different type of treatment.

Clinical Example: Loss of self-care abilities

Larry, a 31-year-old man with a diagnosis of chronic schizophrenia, attends a community support program. He meets with his case manager every other week after he receives his haloperidol decanoate injection (a long-acting form of the drug that is given once every 2–4 weeks) from the nurse. The nurse assesses for effectiveness of the medication and for side effects. Larry also participates in a social club, which offers lunch and social activities twice weekly. The psychiatrist meets with him every 3 months for medication evaluation.

Day Treatment Programs

Individuals who need minimal supervision, structured activities, and focused treatment may benefit from a day treatment program. These programs vary in length from 4 to 8 hours per day and 1 to 5 days per week. Programming can occur during the day, evening, and night. Depending on the community, these programs might provide treatment for specific populations based on age (child, adolescent, adult, or older adult) or type of problem (addiction or chronic mental illness).

Clinical Example: Loss of a life partner

John, a 52-year-old man with severe depression resulting from the unexpected death of his wife, is discharged from the hospital but is unable to return to work. He attends a partial program for 2 weeks that meets from 10 A.M. to 3 P.M., Monday through Friday. He attends groups that focus on exercise, spirituality, coping with loss, and emotional support. Lunchtime provides an opportunity for socialization with program members.

Self-Help Groups

Self-help groups are another source of support on the continuum of care (Table 1.1). Self-help group meetings are conducted by members, not professionals, and may take place on a weekly basis.

Telepsychiatry

Telehealth facilitates integrated, patient-centered care via synchronous video, telephone, email, text, and e-consults. TP has been found to be comparable to in-person care as it facilitates access to care and leverages expertise at a distance (Hilty, Sunderji, Suo, Chan, & McCarron, 2018). It can also be more convenient and cost-effective for patients and healthcare providers.

TABLE 1.1	Self-Help Groups
Type of Group	**Examples**
Addiction-based	Alcoholics Anonymous
	Narcotics Anonymous
	Overeaters Anonymous
Survivor-based	Survivors of Suicide
	Incest Survivors Anonymous
	Adult Children of Alcoholics
Disorder-based	Eating disorders
	Bipolar disorder
	Family and caregiver support groups
	National Alliance for the Mentally III
Loss-based	Grief, divorce, bereavement support groups
Medically based	Lupus, cancer, chronic fatigue syndrome, AIDS support groups
Prevention-based	Parenting, boundaries in relationships

AIDS, Acquired immunodeficiency virus.

Other Outpatient Programs

As noted in Fig. 1.3, the previously described outpatient programs do not constitute an exhaustive list of treatment options available. Other programs commonly available include *psychiatric home care*, which provides mental health services to people who are homebound because of their illness or disability. Many areas also provide *community outreach programs*, which reach individuals in places where there is a lack of traditional medical and social services. Sometimes these programs comprise *mobile crisis teams*, treating individuals who are homeless or transient. An even more aggressive approach to supporting those in need of mental health services is the *Assertive Community Treatment (ACT)* model, which mobilizes interprofessional teams (e.g., nurses, physicians, social workers) that are responsible for providing services 24 hours a day, 7 days a week. The team can go anywhere and provide mental health care or provide services as mundane (yet monumental for some patients) as helping with shopping, laundry, or transportation.

Clinical Example: Loss of cognition
Joe, an 80-year-old man with Alzheimer disease, lives at home with his wife. The nurse assesses Joe's mental status and level of functioning. Assistance is given to Joe's wife in implementing safety measures in the home because of Joe's wandering behavior. The nurse assists with arranging respite care so that Joe's wife can go shopping and attend a weekly caregivers' support group.

PRIMARY CARE

We would be remiss if we did not acknowledge the role that primary care physicians and nurse practitioners play in treating individuals with mental health problems. General practitioners prescribe 65% of antianxiety medications, 60% of antidepressants, 50% of stimulants, and 35% of antipsychotic drugs (Mark, 2010; Mark et al., 2009). Individuals with mental

health problems such as anxiety disorders, depression, and addictions seek help in primary care offices and clinics. Three reasons for this are:
1. Stigma of mental health care (no one will know)
2. Lack of knowledge about who to see and where to get help
3. Reduced access to care

Psychiatric medications are sometimes prescribed by primary care providers without a comprehensive history and assessment of the patient. The patient's immediate need might be addressed, but other modes of treatment that could benefit the patient might not be provided. The nurse working in primary care areas will be in contact with individuals with mental health needs and should be prepared to provide appropriate interventions (i.e., self, drugs, milieu). Thus, psychotherapeutic management is relevant in the primary care setting too.

⃝ CRITICAL THINKING QUESTION

4. During one of your visits to a homeless shelter, you meet Ann, who is 19 years old. Ann has been homeless for 2 months and until recently had been living with friends. Ann has bipolar disorder, which was diagnosed 5 months ago. She lost her job as a waitress and quickly emptied her small savings account to pay rent and buy food. She has not been taking her medication because of lack of money. Ann is motivated to work but is having difficulty finding a job and housing. She is feeling overwhelmed, alone, and afraid. What community resources in your area would be helpful to Ann?

Use of the Nursing Process in the Community

The nursing process is the foundation of case management. Effective use of the nursing process in the areas of psychiatric rehabilitation, crisis intervention, home care, therapy, consultation and liaison, resource linkage, and advocacy enhances these services to psychiatric patients (Fig. 1.4). The nurse should be skilled in synthesizing and communicating these resources in an understandable and useful manner to patients. The nursing process and the psychotherapeutic management model are readily adapted to outpatient psychiatric care.

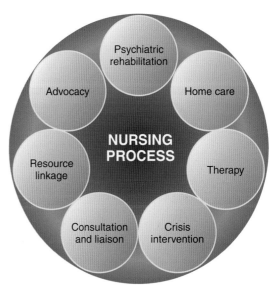

FIG. 1.4 Case management components.

STUDY NOTES

1. Your tools as a psychiatric nurse are Me, Meds, and Milieu.
2. Psychotherapeutic management is a model of care that clarifies the nature of psychiatric nursing and distinguishes psychiatric nursing practice from the practice of other disciplines.
3. The components of psychotherapeutic management include a therapeutic nurse-patient relationship (Me), psychopharmacology (Meds), and Milieu or "environment" management, all of which are supported by a basic understanding of psychopathology.
4. Psychopharmacologic understanding is important because nurses administer medication, make decisions about as-needed (prn) medication, and evaluate for therapeutic and adverse responses to medication.
5. Because humans are incapable of not interacting with their environment, milieu management is an important nursing consideration. Nurses are uniquely responsible for developing the patient's treatment environment.
6. An understanding of psychopathology facilitates the nurse-patient relationship, lays the groundwork for understanding psychopharmacology, and provides a theoretical structure for milieu management.
7. In the continuum of care, the individual is guided to services based on specific needs at a given point in time.
8. Assessment of the individual's needs, their level of functioning, and the level of supervision required determines referral to hospital-based or community-based care.
9. Most acute psychiatric hospital-based care is now provided on a short-term basis, focusing on crisis intervention and safety.
10. Discharge planning begins at the time of admission and continues throughout hospitalization.
11. The psychotherapeutic management model is a comprehensive approach to short-term hospitalization.
12. Continuum of care includes inpatient hospitalization, outpatient services, residential care, self-help activities, and other resources.
13. The nursing process and the psychotherapeutic management approach can be adapted in any setting along the continuum of care.

REFERENCES

Deardorff, J. W., & Grossberg, G. T. (2016). Psychiatric consultations in long-term care: An evidence-based practical guide. *Current Psychiatry*, *15*(11), 39.

Hilty, D., Sunderji, N., Suo, S., Chan, S., & McCarron, R. (2018). Telepsychiatry and other technologies for integrated care: Evidence base, best practice models and competencies. *International Review of Psychiatry*, *30*(6), 292–309. https://doi.org/10.1080/09540261.2019.1571483.

Mark, T. L. (2010). For what diagnoses are psychotropic medications being prescribed? A nationally representative survey of physicians. *CNS Drugs*, *24*, 319–326.

Mark, T. L., Levit, K. R., & Buck, J. A. (2009). Datapoints: Psychotropic drug prescriptions by medical specialty. *Psychiatric Services*, *60*(9), 1167. https://doi.org/10.1176/ps.2009.60.9.1167.

Nasrallah, H. A. (2016). The scourge of societal anosognosia about the mentally ill. *Current Psychiatry*, *15*(8), 19.

Voogt, L. A., Nugter, A., Goossens, P. J. J., & van Achterberg, T. (2016). An interview study on "Providing Structure" as an intervention in psychiatric inpatient care: The nursing perspective. *Perspectives in Psychiatric Care*, *52*, 208. https://doi.org/10.1111/ppc.12119.

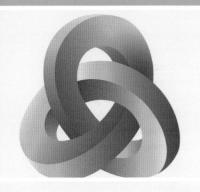

2

Historical Issues

Norman L. Keltner and Helene Vossos

Nescire autem quid ante quam natus sis acciderit, id est semper esse puerum.

Marcus Tullius Cicero (106–43 BC)

ⓔ http://evolve.elsevier.com/Keltner

LEARNING OBJECTIVES

- Describe the enormity of mental health concerns in both human and financial contexts.
- Explain the history of psychiatry as a foundation for current psychiatric nursing practice.
- Identify the significant changes that occurred during the period of the Enlightenment.
- Relate the contributions of early scientists to the current understanding of mental illness.

- Explain the impact of psychotropic medications on psychiatric care.
- Analyze the immediate and long-term effects of the community mental health movement.
- Describe the impact of the Decade of the Brain on psychiatric care.
- Identify the specific strengths that enable psychiatric nurses to become effective in the new continuum of care.

Epidemiologic evidence indicates that 51.5 million American adults (>18 years old) meet the criteria for a mental disorder during any 12-month period, with about 21% having a diagnosable mental illness at any given time (National Institute of Mental Health, 2020). Many of these disorders are considered mild in nature with many sufferers going untreated. However, many are not mild: four of the top medical disorders causing disability are psychiatric disorders (i.e., major depression, schizophrenia, bipolar spectrum disorder, and

NORM'S NOTES Read Cicero's statement again. Oh, you didn't take Latin, either. Well, let's put it in English—"*Not to know what happened before you were born, that is to be always a boy, to be forever a child.*" Besides perhaps being a little sexist, Cicero makes a strong point. This chapter discusses history, and when you understand history, you understand context. Without an understanding of history, many things do not and cannot make sense. More than that, this chapter describes where we have been, and how we got to where we are now. History can help you to understand things better, such as the homeless man sitting on the sidewalk who is acting strangely or the incessant ads for antidepressants in the media. It provides a foundation for the rest of the book. Now if Cicero and I have not convinced you of the importance of history, read the summary of Rosenhan's study in Box 2.1. If it doesn't get you fired up, check your pulse!

alcohol use disorder) (Nasrallah, 2012a). Approximately half of all mental disorders start by the midteens. Table 2.1 provides a breakdown by diagnosis of the disorders prevalent over the course of 12 months in American society. The pervasiveness of these maladies includes approximately 13.1 million American adults who have a serious mental disorder with 8.6 million (65.1%) receiving treatment (Moller, 2017). There is tremendous cost associated with disability, including issues from invisible barriers for treatment such as stigma. The prevalence of mental disorders signifies that there is a great need for psychiatric health care professionals, especially nurses, currently and in the foreseeable future.

BENCHMARKS IN PSYCHIATRIC HISTORY

And a certain woman had suffered many things of many physicians, and had spent all that she had, and was nothing bettered, but rather grew worse.

Mark 5:25–26, King James Version (1611)

The modern era of psychiatric care can be traced from events that occurred in England and France near the end of the 18th century, a time referred to as *the Enlightenment*. Before this time (or *Preenlightenment*), mentally ill people were often regarded as no better than wild animals. Confinement was the most restrictive method of coping with the mentally ill,

TABLE 2.1 Twelve-Month Prevalence Rate of Mental Disorders in the United States		
Mental Disorders	Approximate Percentage >17 Years Old (%) (Unless Noted for Children)	Gender Representation
Anxiety disorders	19% overall	Female
Agoraphobia	1.3%	Female
Bipolar spectrum disorders	2.8%	Equal
Panic disorder	2.7%	Female
Social anxiety disorder	7.1%	Female
Specific phobia	9.1%	Female
Separation anxiety	1.2%	Equal
Generalized anxiety disorder	2.7%	Female
Posttraumatic stress disorder	3.6%	Female
Obsessive compulsive disorder	1.2%	Equal
Suicide attempts	0.4%–.0.7%	Male

This information has been derived from the National Institute of Mental Health (2018). Twelve-month and lifetime prevalence and lifetime morbid risk of anxiety and mood disorders in the United States. https://www.nimh.nih.gov/health/statistics/index.shtml. American Psychiatric Association. (2013). *Diagnostic and statistical manual of mental disorders* (5th ed.). APA.

who were often chained. The mentally ill were thought to be immune to normal biologic stressors such as cold, heat, and hunger. Mentally ill individuals were often placed on display for the amusement of their caretakers and the paying public. For example, until 1770, a small fee was charged to visitors of St. Mary of Bethlem Hospital (aka "Bedlam") in England. At Bicêtre in France, the attendants served as "ringmasters," using whips to "encourage" their patients to perform. These warehouses for the tormented discouraged outside intrusion and attracted employees who were at the bottom levels of society, both socially and morally.

As the late 1700s approached, a day of enlightenment dawned: the establishment of the asylum. Five periods stand out as benchmarks in the evolution of modern psychiatric care (Table 2.2):

Benchmark I: approximately 1790s
Benchmark II: mid to late 1800s
Benchmark III: 1950s
Benchmark IV: 1960s
Benchmark V: 1990s

During each of these periods, the way of thinking about the mentally ill underwent significant changes.

Benchmark I: Period of Enlightenment

To consider madness incurable … is constantly refuted by the most authentic facts.

Philippe Pinel, December 11, 1794
(cited in Weiner, 1992)

Pinel's comment captured a new way of thinking (people could get better) and launched a new era. The modern age of psychiatric care began with Philippe Pinel in France and another visionary, William Tuke, in England. In 1793 Pinel became the superintendent of the French institution

BOX 2.1 On Being Sane in Insane Places

Rosenhan wondered whether the "sane" could be distinguished from the "insane." He selected eight pseudopatients (people who pretended to be mentally ill) and instructed them to attempt to gain admission to public mental hospitals. The task was much easier than anyone had anticipated. Twelve hospitals in five states were used. The pseudopatient group consisted of a graduate student in psychology, three psychologists (including Rosenhan himself), a pediatrician, a psychiatrist, a painter, and a housewife; three were women, and five were men. No one in the hospital knew of the deception. The pseudopatients were trained to do the following:

1. Call the hospital, and make an appointment.
2. On arriving at the hospital, tell the psychiatrist that they had been hearing voices.
3. On being asked to describe the voices, say that they were not sure but remembered the words *empty, hollow,* and *thud.*
4. Other than giving this false information and false information about their names, occupations, and employers, they were to be truthful and "normal" from that point forward.
5. Immediately on admission, they were to cease simulating abnormal behavior and behave "normally."
6. When asked how they were doing, they were told to respond "fine" and to inform the staff that they were no longer experiencing problems.

Despite behaving normally, none of the pseudopatients were discovered by the staff. However, approximately 25% of the other patients made comments about the pseudopatients' "sanity," and a few even guessed that the pseudopatients were doing some type of undercover work. Rosenhan noted reluctance by the staff to recognize mental health in their patients. He stated, "Having once been labeled schizophrenic, there is nothing the pseudopatients can do to overcome the tag." Pseudopatient histories were written to support their diagnoses. In other words, psychiatrists saw problems that had never existed.

The pseudopatients were also asked to write down their observations. At first, they followed elaborate precautions to avoid detection; however, they were soon jotting down

Continued

BOX 2.1   On Being Sane in Insane Places—cont'd

observations in front of the staff. The pseudopatients discovered that no one was paying attention to them.

Another part of the experiment was to determine the amount of time spent with patients. This amount was difficult to measure; thus a proxy behavior was substituted—time that the nurses spent outside the nurses' station. Nursing attendants had the highest percentage of time spent outside the station (11.3%). Rosenhan found that measuring registered nurse time outside the nurses' station was impossible because it occurred so infrequently. Psychiatrists were even worse because they hid behind their closed office doors; at least the patients were able to see the nurses. Rosenhan concluded, "Those with the most power have least to do with patients, and those with the least power are most involved with them."

Rosenhan decried the powerlessness and the depersonalization experienced by the pseudopatients. He remembered how he was frequently awakened in the hospital to which he had been admitted: "Come on you m----f----s, out of bed."

The pseudopatients were hospitalized on average for 19 days before they were deemed well enough for discharge. The range of stay was from 7 to 52 days.

On the flip side, individuals with mental illness or mental disorders are very vulnerable patients. This population may be unaware that they are mentally ill. Individuals with mood disorders such as major depressive disorder and thought disorders such as schizophrenia may experience suicidal ideation and require psychiatric hospitalization for stabilization. Psychiatric

nurses are heroes caring for these individuals when the patients are at the lowest points in their lives.

In addition, 75% of chronic seriously mentally ill (SMI) symptoms begin by age 24. Significantly, it may be 10 years that pass until these individuals seek mental health services. Imagine the silent suffering these people are going through. Nurses make a huge difference. According to the American Psychiatric Nurses Association (2017), individuals living with a SMI carry a higher mortality rate, cost Americans $193 billion in lost earnings annually, and 75% of all counties in America have a shortage of mental healthcare professionals. Nurses, psychiatric mental health nurses, and healthcare professionals have a pivotal role in providing services for this population. Mental health nurses assess with intake screenings, evaluations, triage, administer lifesaving medication, and provide crisis intervention and stabilization services. The nursing role encompasses coordinating care and educating patients and their families within their communities. The opportunities in psychiatric mental health nursing are boundless, and using the art and science of nursing to provide expert evidence-based interventions produces positive outcomes. In the next chapter, continue to expand on the knowledge of working to reduce stigma for these patients while learning about assessment, treatment, and how to effectively make a difference in the lives of these patients. It is gratifying to be able to provide care for these individuals as they ride the wave of crisis to stabilization, to outpatient coordinated care. When nurses provide inspiration and compassionate care, patients flourish.

From Rosenhan, D. L. (1973). On being sane in insane places. *Science, 179*, 250.

Bicêtre (for men) and, later, the Salpêtrière (for women). Pinel was dismayed by the conditions that he found and wrote of the patients, "They were abandoned to the incompetence of a callous director and to the cold brutality of servants …" (Weiner, 1992). Soon after assuming leadership, Pinel unchained the shackled, clothed the naked, fed the hungry, and abolished whips and other tools of abuse. Simultaneously, in England, Tuke was planning a private facility that would ensure moral treatment for the mentally ill after he witnessed the deplorable conditions in public facilities. In 1796, based on Quaker teachings, his York Retreat opened for patients, providing "a place in which the unhappy might obtain refuge—a quiet haven in which the shattered bark might find a means of reparation or safety" (Charland, 2007; Gollaher, 1995). Pinel and Tuke crafted this first benchmark of modern psychiatric care.

Asylum

The concept of the asylum developed from the humane efforts of Pinel and Tuke. The term *asylum* can mean protection, social support, or sanctuary from the stresses of life. A touring Cuban gymnast pleading for asylum is a good example of this definition. However, asylum more often provokes an image of mistreatment and neglect. It was the first definition that motivated Pinel, Tuke, and other similarly minded individuals. Understanding that

mental illness worsened with deplorable conditions, these individuals sought to provide an environment relatively free from stressors. Their language is inappropriate today—"madness," "lunacy," "insanity," "idiocy," "feeblemindedness"—but these were the accepted terms of their day. These early reformers were driven by a desire to improve the lot of abandoned, mentally ill persons and to provide asylum or sanctuary.

Dorothea Dix (1802–1887), one of the first major reformers in the United States, was instrumental in developing the concept of asylum; she played a direct role in opening 32 state hospitals. Her efforts have been described as a crusade. Several years before launching her crusade, she visited Tuke's York Retreat. Undoubtedly, Tuke's moral treatment influenced her to confront the pain and suffering that she had witnessed in the United States. Dix came to believe that the people of America had an obligation to their mentally ill brothers and sisters. She proposed to alleviate suffering with adequate shelter, nutritious food, and warm clothing. In Gollaher's biography of Dix (1995), he quotes from one of her Memorials, the documents that she wrote to expose the terrible plight of the insane. From her Massachusetts Memorial, he notes: "*Concord*: A woman from the [Worcester] hospital in a cage in the almshouse. *Lincoln*: A woman in a cage. *Medford*: One idiotic subject chained, and one in a close [or narrow] stall for 17 years ….

TABLE 2.2   Benchmark Periods in Psychiatric History

Period	Key People or Developments	Significant Change in Thinking	Result(s)
Enlightenment, ~1790s	Pinel (1745–1826) Tuke (1732–1822)	Human dignity upheld.	Asylum movement developed.
Scientific Study, ~1870s	Freud (1856–1939): Emphasized the importance of early life experiences	Mental illness could be studied.	Study of the mind and treatment approaches to psychiatric conditions flourished.
Scientific Study	Kraepelin (1856–1926): Studied the brain	Classification of mental disorders	
Psychotropic Drugs, ~1950s	1949: Lithium 1950: Thorazine 1952: MAOIs 1958: TCAs 1960: Benzodiazepines	If some mental disorders are caused by chemical imbalances, then chemicals could restore the balance: people would no longer need to be confined.	Destigmatization of mental illness occurred; parents and others not to blame.
Community Mental Health, 1960s	Community Mental Health Centers Act (1963)	People have the right to be treated in their own community.	*Advantage*: Intervention in familiar surroundings has helped many people and is less expensive. *Disadvantage*: Homelessness linked to deinstitutionalization; many people "slip through the cracks" of the system.
Decade of the Brain, 1990s	Congressional mandate	If we can understand the brain, we can help millions of people with mental disorders.	Increase in funding for brain research, leading to new treatment strategies
National Institute of Mental Illness, 2000s	Hillary Clinton	Outreach for children and safe use of medication to treat young children.	Collaboration programs under the Surgeon General outlining goals and strategies to improve services for children and adolescents with mental disorders along with federal agencies.
Research was furthered for The Adolescents Depression Study, (TADS), Clinical Antipsychotic Trials of Intervention Effectiveness (CATIE), National Alliance for Research on Schizophrenia and Depression (NARSAD) became one of the largest doner organizations to fund brain research.		The first meeting in Chicago about minority youth, emotional and behavioral disorders impacting violence Meeting in schools and general public was initiated to discuss prevention programs. Recovery program is adopted. Theory of Attachment in psychotherapy.	
Results from research studies promoted effective medication treatment options and psychotherapy (Dr. Beck).	Dr. Linda Brady	The memorandum of agreement (MOA) between the Army and NIMH invested $50 million into research to reduce Army/Veteran suicides.	Research led to executive order to expand suicide prevention programs, develop Veteran programs to improve early diagnosis and treatment of posttraumatic stress disorder, traumatic brain injury and reduce suicide risks. Aimed to implement better treatment options and prevention programs.
2008 New Veteran Strategic Program			
2013–2015 Mapping of the brain, genetic and neurotransmitter research make gains.	Dr. T. Sudhof, MD mapped the molecular mechanisms of neurotransmitter release and chemical messaging.	Early identification of first episodes of psychosis in schizophrenia	
In 2021, on the horizon, genomic testing for psychotropic medications, substance use disordered treatment, recovery programs, telepsychiatry and community-based programs.	National Institute of Mental Health, Centers for Medicare and Medicaid Services, Substance Abuse and Mental Health Services Administration.	Four objectives, 1. define mechanisms of complex behaviors, 2. how, when, where to intervene, 3. aim for cures and prevention, and 4. strengthen the public health	Findings are significant in a team-based community care model exploring a diverse variety of treatments to reduce symptoms aimed at preventing fast deterioration in this disorder. Coordinated and integrated care.

MAOIs, Monoamine oxidase inhibitors (which are antidepressants); *TCAs*, tricyclic antidepressants. National Institutes of Health (NIH). (2017). The NIH almanac: National Institute of Mental Illness (NIMH). https://www.nih.gov/about-nih/what-we-do/nih-almanac/national-institute-mental-health-nimh

Granville: One often closely confined … now losing the use of his limbs from want of exercise."

Although Dix is rightfully credited with being the first reformer to have a nationwide perspective, other, more regional sanctuaries had been established before she began her crusade. The first asylum in the United States was the Eastern Lunatic Asylum in Williamsburg, Virginia, founded in 1773. Other institutions followed, such as the Frankford Asylum near Philadelphia (1813), the Bloomingdale Asylum in New York (1818), and the Hartford Retreat in Connecticut (1824). The Philadelphia and New York asylums were established under Quaker influence and thus can be traced to Tuke.

The period of Enlightenment was relatively short-lived. Within 100 years of the establishment of the first asylum, the reformers were being charged with misuse and abuse of their charges. State hospitals were beset with problems. The first definition of asylum *(sanctuary)* had materialized in the form of hospitals built in rural settings. Patients were isolated geographically and socially and, after release, from follow-up care. Patients were also isolated from public scrutiny, which enabled many large institutions to become closed systems. As might be guessed, the beneficence of the reformers was not shared by the many caretakers who followed. Within this relatively brief period, the meaning of asylum changed; it evolved from a *place of refuge* to a *place of torment*.

Currently a renewed interest in asylum, which is considered a place of rest and restoration, exists (Nasrallah, 2015). This concept can be considered in terms of the four *P*s: parents, professionals, patients, and public, each of which has a stake in the discussion of asylum. Wasow (1993) has written persuasively of the need for asylum: "Some people's illnesses are so severe that they will always need asylum." Individuals who struggle with complex treatment-resistant thought (psychotic) disorders may become a danger to themselves or others and may require psychiatric institutionalization, known as an asylum (or psychiatric inpatient admission). A call to action for compassionate access to psychiatric services, medication, and a continuum of care is needed. The concepts of total freedom to total hospitalization should reflect on the diverse needs of serious mentally ill people who can practice self-care with minimal oversight. Healthcare reform has placed community mental health-based agencies in communities aimed to provide services with the least restrictive environment. Nurses are essential in assisting these vulnerable individuals with presence, education, and resources.

❓ CRITICAL THINKING QUESTIONS

1. Which of the two definitions of *asylum* do you believe is more prevalent currently in psychiatric nursing?
2. What are some negative outcomes of hospitalization that you have witnessed or with which you have been personally involved?

Benchmark II: Period of Scientific Study

Around 1850, however, a great transformation began as medicine moved from the clinic into the laboratory, and doctors increasingly shifted their interest from prognosis and care to diagnosis and cure.

George Makari (2009)

The shift in focus from sanctuary to treatment is linked to the second benchmark in psychiatric care, personified by Sigmund Freud (1856–1939). Toward the last third of the 19th century, several scientists devoted themselves to understanding the mind and mental illness. The fruits of their labor held great promise, some of which is still unfulfilled. Nonetheless, the efforts forever changed the world's view: mental illness need not be suffered (however humanely patients were treated) but might be alleviated. In a sense, psychiatric care was popularized, and specialty training was more sought out.

Early Scientists

Although Freud had the greatest impact on the world's view of mental illness, he neither thought nor worked in a vacuum. Other men and women had tremendous influence on this newly enthusiastic and optimistic approach to mental illness. Emil Kraepelin (1856–1926) made tremendous contributions to the classification of mental disorders. He was a true scientist whose classic descriptions of schizophrenia are valuable reading. Eugen Bleuler (1857–1939) coined the term *schizophrenia* and added a note of optimism to its treatment. Others, many of whom were colleagues or disciples of Freud, made significant contributions to the emerging field of psychiatry.

Freud's contributions still influence psychiatric care, although for a number of years belittling his thinking has been popular, with some of the criticisms quite convincing. Nonetheless, paraphrasing a statement made by Sir Isaac Newton (1642–1727): If we see far today, it is because we stand on the shoulders of giants. Freud was a giant because he believed that people could get better.

Freud described human behavior in psychological terms. He developed a theory of motivation, established the usefulness of talking (catharsis), explained the importance of dreams, and proposed to unlock the hidden parts of the mind. He introduced terms that have become part of our language—*psychoanalysis*, *defense mechanisms*, and *free association*. The work of others evolved from Freud's studies. Alfred Adler, Carl Jung, Ernest Jones, Otto Rank, Helene Deutsch, Karen Horney, and Anna Freud (Freud's youngest child) all made significant and, in most cases, lasting contributions to the field of modern psychiatry.

However, Freud's inspiration reached far beyond the people with whom he worked personally. Society in general is indebted to him, even though conflicting opinions about his ideas have emerged. Freud challenged society to look at human beings objectively and fostered a milieu of thinking about the mind and mental disorders. Unit II builds on these concepts and is devoted to the implementation of strategies for working with psychiatric patients.

Benchmark III: Period of Psychotropic Drugs

From this milieu of theory and scientific thought came the third benchmark, which began around 1950 with the discovery of psychotropic drugs. Chlorpromazine (Thorazine), haloperidol (Haldol), both antipsychotic medications, and lithium, an antimanic agent, were introduced first, and imipramine (Tofranil), a tricyclic antidepressant, was introduced a few years later. The impact of these drugs has been powerful. Patients who appeared beyond reach became less agitated and experienced a reduction in psychotic thinking. Depressed patients regained the ability to function. Hospital stays were shortened, and hospital environments improved. Psychotropic drugs have allowed many patients to be treated in less restrictive environments; however, ethical, moral, and legal questions have arisen with this treatment modality. Unit III is devoted to an understanding of the role of psychotropic drugs in the treatment of mental disorders.

Benchmark IV: Period of Community Mental Health

If the foregoing suggests the notion that one benchmark period ended entirely before the next one began, then we will clarify that misunderstanding. Trends tend to overlap as advocates of one view struggle to defend existing strategies while more dynamic forces emerge elsewhere. As the various treatment approaches were being developed in the milieu derived from Freud's theories, criticism grew, and the state hospital system continued its plunge into "psychiatric Siberia." In 1948 the popular movie *The Snake Pit* portrayed a mindless, ineffective, and at times cruel system of care. In an even more devastating exposé, the book *The Shame of the States*, by Albert Deutsch (1948), vividly revealed with words and photographs the deplorable conditions in several large state hospitals in the United States.

Legislators were watching, reading, and listening; legislation was passed that would change the approach to psychiatric care. In 1946, President Truman signed the National Mental Health Act, enabling the establishment of the National Institute of Mental Health a few years later (in 1949). In 1947, the Hill-Burton Act legislated funds to build general hospitals that included psychiatric units (Table 2.3). This initiative began the effort for early intervention and helped shorten the length of hospitalization for psychiatric patients.

In 1961, the Joint Commission on Mental Illness and Health, appointed by President Kennedy, published a report entitled *Action for Mental Health*. Kennedy urged increased support for the state hospital system in recognition of the need for improved treatment of the mentally ill population. Opponents of the state hospital system overwhelmed supporters of this report. The more outspoken critics of state hospitals declared that these hospitals were actually the cause of mental illness. The era of the large state hospitals was over.

Rather than increasing monetary support for the state hospital system, a convergence of forces set the stage for this fourth benchmark period in psychiatric history:

TABLE 2.3	Legislative Events That Changed Psychiatric Care in the United States
Year	**Legislative Act**
1946	President Truman signed the National Mental Health Act.
1947	Hill-Burton Act allocated funds for general hospitals to develop psychiatric units.
1949	National Institute of Mental Health established
1961	President Kennedy established Joint Commission on Mental Illness and Health.
1963	Community Mental Health Centers Act

1. The public's declining confidence in the state hospital system
2. The failure of various treatment approaches to eradicate mental illness
3. The legislative climate that had begun in the 1940s, emphasizing the civil rights of mentally ill people
4. The newfound faith in psychotropic drugs

These factors led to the enactment of the Community Mental Health Centers Act in 1963, which virtually destroyed the state hospital system. A deliberate shift was made from institutional to extrainstitutional care; the goal was deinstitutionalization of the state hospital system population. The problem of geographic isolation was addressed with the establishment of community treatment centers and community living arrangements. Keeping the individual closer to the family addressed issues of isolation from family members. Isolation from follow-up care was remedied because various levels of care were available locally in the continuum of care (see Chapter 1). Eventually, community mental health programs were developed to meet the needs of all those living within the boundaries of a designated area.

Deinstitutionalization

The practice, over the past four decades, of releasing people with severe mental illnesses from institutions has been one of the largest social experiments in twentieth century America.

E. Fuller Torrey (1997)

Deinstitutionalization refers to the depopulating of state mental hospitals. State hospitals reached their peak population in 1955 and then slowly began the process of trimming their census rolls. This process began with growing concern about hospital "asylums" (i.e., a place of poor treatment or no treatment) and was nurtured by some of the negative events discussed earlier in the chapter. A more subtle influence was the growing disillusionment of psychiatry and psychiatric nursing with the chronically mentally ill and a turning to the *worried well*. Lest the importance of this statement escape the reader, the concept will be reworded. Nurses and physicians gravitated toward people with whom they could identify. *It is much easier to counsel and medicate a woman going through the crisis of divorce than to attempt to understand the babblings of a person with schizophrenia.*

These factors clearly laid the groundwork for deinstitutionalization; however, federal actions helped fully ignite the process. The first, as noted, was the Community Mental Health Centers Act of 1963. The second federal action was legislation that provided mentally disabled persons with an income while living in the community. This legislation was named Aid to the Disabled and is now called Supplemental Security Income and Social Security Disability Insurance. The number of individuals with mental disorders receiving these benefits has increased dramatically in recent years.

Shifting the Cost of Mental Illness or "Follow the Money"

State governments soon found that Aid to the Disabled, even when supplemented by the state, was less expensive than public hospitalization because the federal government paid most of the costs. The federal share grew by 3100% between 1963 and 1994 (Torrey, 1997). Naturally, state financial incentives declined as the involvement of the federal government increased.

Perhaps the final event in the deinstitutionalization movement was the change in commitment laws. Out of concern for the civil rights of mental patients, involuntary commitment of individuals to a state hospital became difficult. The state had to demonstrate that individuals brought for involuntary commitment were a clear danger to themselves or to others. These sweeping changes were reactions to years of injustice during which persons said to be mentally ill could be detained and involuntarily committed, with little recourse, for long periods. Rosenhan's (1973) classic study, summarized in Box 2.1, illustrates how difficult it was for a sane person to be discharged from a mental hospital. The stage was set for the rapid depopulation of state hospitals. Currently, for many patients and families, getting into a state hospital can be extremely difficult. (Think of recent tragedies in which the families of perpetrators of horrendous crimes lament that they could not "get any help.")

Depopulation of State Hospitals

The state hospital population reached its peak in 1955, with 558,922 patients. Stated another way, in 1955, there was 1 psychiatric bed for every 300 Americans, but by 2010, there was only 1 bed for every 3000 Americans (Nasrallah, 2012b). Currently, the state hospital population is approximately 70,000 patients, a decline of more than 85%. Perhaps 1 million people would currently be in state hospitals if the proportions of 1955 were in effect. If this projection is correct, greater than 900,000 individuals who might have been hospitalized years ago are currently living outside such institutions. This decline has resulted in the closing of many state hospitals. Patients hospitalized today require a high level of care, have few social relationships, are often psychotic, and are typically acutely ill young men. Table 2.4 provides insights into where mentally ill people outside of institutions might be living. Prisons and

TABLE 2.4 Where Individuals With Severe Mental Illness Live

Nursing homes
Prisons/jails
State hospitals
Homeless
Home with families, group or board-and-care structured homes, or on their own

jails provide a significant amount of the mental health "care" in the United States. In fact, there are 300% more patients with severe mental illness in jails and prisons than in hospitals in the United States (Torrey, 2010). Ellis and Alexander (2017) note that 29% of jails hold psychiatric patients without charges while awaiting evaluation.

Community Effects: From Deinstitutionalization to Transinstitutionalization

There are some ideas so absurd that only an intellectual could believe them.

George Orwell

The effects of deinstitutionalization are also evident in community agencies. For example, emergency department use by acutely disturbed individuals has increased dramatically in the absence of the previous system. Emergency psychiatric services are sagging from the load they now carry. Some general hospital psychiatric units are overwhelmed at times with a continuous flow of patients being admitted and discharged. Many professionals believe that the typical patient is also different. Compared with the patients of the 1960s and 1970s, patients now are more aggressive, and many are armed when first seen in the emergency department. Puffenberger (2007) suggests that the term *deinstitutionalization* no longer captures what we are witnessing. The term *transinstitutionalization* more aptly depicts reality. The Los Angeles County Jail has been described as the largest mental health system in the world.

? CRITICAL THINKING QUESTION

3. It has been stated that the fields of psychiatry and psychiatric nursing lost interest in the seriously mentally ill and became more interested in working with the worried well. Do you believe that this is still true in psychiatric nursing? Support your answer.

Benchmark V: Decade of the Brain

I would argue that psychiatric care in America, as a whole, is much worse now than when I finished training in 1990, primarily because of changes in healthcare reimbursement.

Jule P. Miller III, MD (2015)

The 1990s were declared the Decade of the Brain by the U.S. Congress. During this decade, a steep increase in brain research occurred that coincided with an increased interest in biologic explanations for mental disorders. That interest continues to the present moment. President Obama's *Brain Initiative* was launched with $110 million of federal funds earmarked for the year 2014 alone.

The impetus in 1990 for this benchmark was the significant changes in the *Diagnostic and Statistical Manual (DSM)-III* (published in 1980). However, in many ways, the emphasis on brain biology represented a completion of the circle started by Kraepelin 100 years before. Kraepelin believed that brain pathology was at the root of serious mental disorders.

Significant changes in public awareness occurred because of the Decade of the Brain, which enabled clinicians to address complex topics with patients and families. Nursing responded to this challenge with a significant augmentation of psychobiologic content in academic nursing programs and a torrent of continuing education programs. In fact, psychiatric nursing textbooks published before 1990 provided very little, if any, information about psychobiology and psychopharmacology, leaving many nursing graduates of that period inadequately prepared. All psychiatric nursing textbooks now provide this information. In addition, psychiatric mental health nurse practitioners are experts as psychotropic providers.

The Decade of the Brain brought many challenges, but the benefits have been tremendous in terms of making psychiatric nursing a more viable specialty. It crystallized the fact that mental disorders are caused by a host of factors: biologic, neurologic, adverse childhood events, developmental, and sociocultural. The various factors associated with mental disorders enables individuals to move beyond blaming toward a focus on what can be done to ameliorate the pain and suffering. The Decade of the Brain brought nursing back into the mainstream of psychiatric care. Neuroscience is of interest to nurses and other healthcare professionals.

Can Brain Biology be Overemphasized?

The answer is YES! Many times psychiatrists and psychiatric nurse practitioners are seen and hired almost exclusively to prescribe pills. Much is lost of their great skill when this occurs. Although thinking that serious mental illness is an accumulation of "bad" experiences/choices led to lengthy, costly, and mostly ineffective treatments, reducing people to biological systems in need of chemical tuning-up fails as well, with many unintended consequences. The famous quote by Pogo fits, "We have met the enemy and he is us!"

The last decade of neuroscience research has been vast and yet exciting. Neuroimaging research has provided knowledge to quantify the brain's anatomical structures and functionality within a highly complex conceptual framework. There is ongoing interest in the field of neuroimaging, and much research is currently in process. In addition, research in understanding the brain from a biopsychosocial perspective is ongoing and informing psychiatric providers with theory and tools to help patients and their families. Nurses are in a unique position to provide holistic care as they will gain knowledge about the intrapsychic and interpersonal dynamics of mental health and mental disorders.

ISSUES THAT AFFECT THE DELIVERY OF PSYCHIATRIC CARE

Several important issues affecting the delivery of psychiatric care remain for discussion:
1. Although briefly discussed earlier in this chapter, the *paradigm shift* that has occurred in the way we think about and treat mental disorders is very important. The way we conceptualize a disorder informs all decisions about that disorder.
2. *Homelessness* is a problem that also influences psychiatric care. Vast numbers of individuals are standing on street corners with signs pleading for money, and studies have indicated that many of these people have a serious mental disorder.
3. The need for and the reality of *community-based care* is another issue. What mechanisms are in place to fortify the continuum of care?
4. Finally, we have developed a system of care that is driven by carefully described signs and symptoms. This *bible of diagnoses* (DSM-5) is indispensable in our psychiatric care delivery system.

Paradigm Shift in Psychiatric Care

Psychiatry generally lost interest in the seriously mentally ill (SMI) as a result of the influx of psychoanalysts in the 1930s and 1940s. As Freud himself had discovered, his analytic approach was most helpful to persons with less severe problems and was not particularly helpful to psychotic patients. Thus, as Freudian thinking influenced more psychiatrists and psychiatric nurses, a natural withdrawal from the SMI and a refocusing on individuals more amenable to treatment occurred. "Asylum psychiatry, and the Kraepelinian model on which it was based, fell into relative decline" (Wilson, 1993).

Public mental hospitals lost prestige, as did the physicians and nurses working in them. Within the psychiatric nursing fraternity, staff nurses were not as highly valued as nurses who worked in the role of therapist. In many cases, as participants in a self-fulfilling prophecy, the devalued inpatient psychiatric nurses in public hospitals became what they were perceived to be. They were often derisively referred to as either *crazy or lazy.*

The mainstream of psychiatry and psychiatric nursing turned from chronically disturbed patients to individuals with lowered self-esteem, individuals who were striving to reach their potential, and individuals who were existentially unhappy (Detre, 1987). Psychiatry changed its focus from one extreme of the psychiatric care continuum (the SMI) to the other (the worried well) over a few decades. Social issues started to emerge as legitimate professional concerns. Psychiatry and psychiatric nursing became interested in issues such as homelessness, poverty, racism, alternative lifestyles, and sexism on a professional level.

Homelessness

Many psychiatric professionals believe that homelessness can be directly linked to benchmark IV. The most popular view 30 years ago was that homeless people (mostly white men) were skid row bums, alcoholics, and hobos who chose to be homeless. The current belief is that the homeless are people who have been displaced by social policies over which they have no control. It has been estimated that 2.5 million children are now homeless in the United States, representing 1 out of 30 children (Broman, 2018). It was estimated that 18% of these children have a learning disability or mental health disorder.

Estimates concerning the prevalence of mental illness among this population vary. The consensus is that 25% of the adult homeless population have a severe mental illness and that approximately 54% (women) to 84% (men) suffer from alcohol abuse (Gerber, 2013). In addition, many suffer from other substance use disorders (drug abuse); 21% of veterans who are homeless have a substance use disorder (SAMHSA, 2016). Seventy percent of homeless individuals have received mental healthcare services in the past, and 28% had at least one psychiatric hospitalization (SAMHSA, 2016).

People who are homeless and mentally ill present a challenge to the mental health and political systems in the United States; these individuals are usually single or divorced and have a weak social support system. The homeless who experience SMI are found in parks, in downtown areas, soup kitchens, jails, and general hospitals and often present a troubling appearance. Furthermore, the economic turmoil experienced by most Americans in recent years has filtered down to the streets. Many homeless mentally ill persons have become bold in their efforts to survive, assaulting the sensitivities of passersby. From aggressive panhandling to embarrassing public elimination of bodily wastes, societal standards are being affronted. Although much of this alienating behavior is required for survival on the "mean" streets, it is behavior that offends mainstream America. The dilemma is real, and mental health professionals are searching for answers.

As mentioned, homeless people may live exclusively on the streets (so-called *street people*), or they may live in homeless communities, shelters, halfway houses, or board-and-care homes. A possible third group includes individuals who are able to stay for short periods in cheap hotels or with friends ("couch surfers"), alternating between this and nights in less accommodating surroundings. Another significant group moves among homeless shelters, rehabilitation programs, jails, and prisons.

Homelessness is an end product of chronic mental illness and probably exacerbates it as well. Stated another way, many chronically ill persons end up on the streets because of their inability to succeed in a competitive society, and once they are on the streets, the stresses of the homeless life compound their mental health problems; they are in a no-win situation. Proponents of deinstitutionalization argue that these particular problems are not inherently a part of depopulating state hospitals but have resulted instead because money has not followed patients into the community. They attempt to make the case that community mental health has never been allocated the resources necessary to realize its promise. Traditionalists point to the homeless and the disproportionate effect experienced by some minority groups as evidence of the need for change. These critics maintain that homelessness is more than a lack of shelter—it is a lack of support systems available in the public mental health system.

Community-Based Care

The future of psychiatric care and psychiatric nursing will be linked to continuing efforts to prevent mental health problems and to treat existing disorders more effectively. Because of economic realities, much of that will be a community-based effort as part of the continuum of care. Specific problems associated with community mental health were the liberalization of commitment laws, which allowed SMI patients to go untreated, and restrictive confidentiality rulings, which made discussing the difficult issues of treatment with family members a legal concern. As newspaper editorials, grassroots mental health organizations, and families have clamored about the obvious unmet needs of the SMI, the mental health and legal communities have rallied to respond. This insistence has culminated in thoughtful and deliberate dialogue among mental health professionals, with the objective of making the mental health system work. The Recovery Model, which is discussed in Chapter 7, is an outcome of these discussions.

To make the system work, a seamless continuum of care that coordinates the activities of diverse treatment sources and facilitates movement between and among its entities is needed. Until this seamless continuum is developed, many patients will slip through the cracks of the system as both bureaucratic dysfunction and corporate self-interest drain energy away from programs. Box 2.2 suggests how the system is changing to develop this seamless continuum of care. Box 2.3 presents typical individual movement through the continuum of care, from the most restrictive to a less restrictive environment.

Diagnostic Bible of Psychiatry

Labels provide a usually false yet comforting sense of being able to control the uncontrollable.
    Allen J. Frances and Helen Link Egger (1999)

BOX 2.2 Systemic Changes in Providing Nursing Care for the Mentally Ill

In the new health care reality, community mental health must move rapidly away from some practices and toward new ways of conceptualizing the system:

Away from	Toward
Symptom stabilization	Recovery and reintegration
Professionals having all the answers	Including consumers and families
Medication management	Holistic thinking (e.g., therapy, housing, finances)

BOX 2.3   Example of a Continuum[a] of Care in Seriously Mentally Ill Patients

1. Commitment to a state hospital
2. Day treatment (five times per week) while living at a state- or county-licensed residential facility
3. Day treatment (1–3 days per week); seeking or beginning gainful employment
4. Scheduled follow-up with therapist and prescribing clinician; living in the community

[a]From *most* restrictive to *least* restrictive for a patient with a severe mental illness.

The *Diagnostic and Statistical Manual of Mental Disorders (DSM-5)* (APA, 2013) outlines the signs and symptoms required for clinicians to assign a specific diagnosis to a patient. Not only are diagnoses based on these criteria, but also all third-party payers insist on a *DSM* diagnosis before considering reimbursement payments. The *DSM* has been published in seven editions since its inception in 1952:

DSM-I	1952	106 diagnoses
DSM-II	1968	185 diagnoses
DSM-III	1980	265 diagnoses
DSM-III-R (Revised)	1987	292 diagnoses
DSM-IV	1994	361 diagnoses
DSM-IV-TR (Text Revision)	2000	361 diagnoses
DSM-5	2013	~376 diagnoses

The first edition was published in a spiral-bound notebook, cost only a few dollars, and described approximately 106 disorders. It was heavily influenced by Freudian or psychoanalytic thinking. As Grob (1987) has noted, the *DSM* relied on and reflected "… an extraordinary broadening of psychiatric boundaries and a rejection of the traditional distinction between mental health and mental abnormality. To move from a concern with illness in institutional populations to the incidence in the general population represented an extraordinary intellectual leap."

The development of the third edition was turned over to Robert Spitzer, a psychiatrist in his mid-40s. Working for 6 years on the new manual, he finally pulled together a document that improved the reliability of psychiatric diagnosis (Spiegel, 2005). Historically, this was a watershed moment. As one Freudian psychiatrist was heard to say, "The biologists have stolen psychiatry from us."

There are significant changes of format and thinking in the new *DSM-5*. The first noticeable change is the switch from Roman numerals (IV) to Arabic numerals (5). In addition, it is the first major rewrite of the manual in more than 20 years. More than 130 people worked on it, with an advisory group of 400 available as backup resources. The *DSM-5* represents a paradigm shift toward an "etiopathophysiologic" classification of psychiatric disorders that is, it is hoped, more clinically useful (Tandon, 2012). The researchers and authors of the DSM-5 introduced "cultural issues" to assist the clinician in differentiating between a mental disorder and a cultural syndrome,

cultural idiom of distress, or cultural explanation in a construct of identifying culture-bound syndromes. This was aimed at reducing misdiagnosis and promoting the understanding of cultural meaning, habits, and behaviors that are not associated with a mental disorder. Nonetheless, there is much discussion among leaders in psychiatry in terms of how best to classify mental disorders as intellectual concepts moving forward toward the future of the DSM. A description of these changes and potential challenges is provided in Chapter 23.

Psychiatric Nursing Education: Three Firsts
First Psychiatric Nurse

The official history of psychiatric nursing in the United States began more than 130 years ago. Linda Richards, the first American psychiatric nurse, was a graduate of the New England Hospital for Women. Richards spent much of her professional career developing nursing care in psychiatric hospitals and directed a school of psychiatric nursing in 1880 at the McLean Psychiatric Asylum in Waverly, Massachusetts. Because of her efforts, more than 30 asylums had developed schools for psychiatric nurses by 1890.

First Psychiatric Nursing Textbook

In 1920 Harriet Bailey wrote the first psychiatric nursing textbook. The title of the book, *Nursing Mental Diseases*, reflects the appropriate terminology of the day. An important distinction for psychiatric nursing is that it was not brought into the greater nursing fold until the 1940s. Because psychiatric nurses were trained in state hospitals, they were allowed to work only in state hospitals. In 1937, the National League for Nursing (then called the National League for Nursing Education) recommended that psychiatric nursing be made part of the curriculum of general nursing programs.

First Psychiatric Nursing Theorist

In the 1950s the views of Hildegard Peplau, an important figure in psychiatric nursing, shaped and gave direction and a theoretical framework to psychiatric nursing practice and contributed to the development of a professional climate. Peplau (1952, 1959) developed a model for psychiatric nursing practice. Her book, *Interpersonal Relations in Nursing* (1952), influences practice to this day; her approach, heavily influenced by Dr. Harry Stack Sullivan, emphasizes the interpersonal dimension of practice. Peplau also wrote a history of psychiatric nursing that carefully traced the unfolding of the profession. She might be the most important historical figure in psychiatric nursing.

CURRENT AND FUTURE HISTORICAL ISSUES

Although there are many future trends already underway, perhaps two bear a brief mention: telepsychiatry and pharmacogenetic (PG) testing. Telepsychiatry is a relatively recent trend in psychiatric care. Psychiatrists and psychiatric nurse practitioners are using this technology to treat patients at a distance. In October 2020, President Donald Trump signed an executive order to expand availability of telepsychiatry and telehealth technology. This included online mental health and substance use disorder tools and services. As the Covid-19 pandemic in 2020 struck, the implementation of expanded online technology aimed to reduce suicides, drug-related opioid overdose deaths, and overall poor behavioral-health outcomes. Online telepsychiatry (telehealth) is a methodology that reduces social isolation and opens up access to behavioral health care and psychiatric nursing services. Telepsychiatry will continue to grow as a viable option after the Covid-19 pandemic. According to Mary Moller (2017), there are 25,000 active psychiatrists and 19,000 active psychiatric advanced practice registered nurses (APRNs). That yields a ratio of 986 patients per licensed prescriber. Telepsychiatry is a major force in making these numbers more manageable, providing treatment accessibility, and reducing barriers to psychiatric care.

PG testing allows prescribers to better understand the pharmacokinetic profile of phenotyping and genotyping of their patients (Preskorn, 2016). This knowledge, of course, allows for more precise prescribing practices. More will be said of this matter in Unit III.

? CRITICAL THINKING QUESTION

4. If it is the patient who truly counts, why get caught up in *DSM* terminology? Doesn't this serve to distance the nurse from the patient?

SUMMARY

Even if we wanted to, we could not get away from psychiatric concerns. Our daily newspapers and television jog us from any indifference we might have with accounts of mentally disordered individuals committing crimes or suicide. Furthermore, the selective serotonin reuptake inhibitors/serotonin-norepinephrine reuptake inhibitors (SSRIs; e.g., Prozac, Paxil, and Zoloft/SNRIs; Cymbalta, Effexor, Fetzima) are ubiquitous. Tens of millions of Americans are taking these medications.

Humane psychiatric care started to develop in the late 1700s and has evolved through at least five distinct periods: Enlightenment, Scientific Study, Psychotropic Drugs, Community Mental Health, and Decade of the Brain. Viewed another way, the biologic aspect of mental illness was embraced, but this understanding gave way to a Freudian or psychoanalytic view, which directed the clinician to search for what was behind the symptoms. Many patients are living out a dark drama from childhood (psychosocial stressors), while others are suffering from present-day biologic disturbances (e.g., a neurotransmitter disturbance) and other brain events. Currently, psychiatric nursing acknowledges that mental health problems are caused by a mixture of biologic imbalances and psychosocial stressors.

The *DSM*, sometimes referred to as the bible of psychiatric diagnosis, is the *lingua franca* (i.e., unifying language) of psychiatry. To participate fully in clinical discussions, nurses need a basic understanding of its concepts.

STUDY NOTES

1. Understanding the principles of psychiatric nursing is important because mental health problems affect approximately 25% of the population over a year's time.
2. Modern psychiatry can be traced through five benchmark periods: Enlightenment, Scientific Study, Psychotropic Drugs, Community Mental Health, and Decade of the Brain.
3. Historically, mentally ill people were often confined, but the period of Enlightenment ushered in an era in which the mentally ill were treated humanely.
4. The asylum movement (providing sanctuary from the hostile world) grew out of the humane emphasis of the period of Enlightenment and resulted in the development of state hospital systems.
5. During the period of scientific study, men such as Freud, Kraepelin, and Bleuler studied people objectively; this effort resulted in both psychodynamic and biologic understanding of mental disorders.
6. During the period of psychotropic drugs, antipsychotic drugs (early 1950s), antidepressant drugs (late 1950s),

and other drugs were developed and greatly contributed to the treatment of specific mental disorders.
7. The period of community mental health began as a result of several converging factors, including:
   - Hostility toward state hospitals (sometimes warranted)
   - Psychotropic drugs
   - Civil rights
   - Financial incentives (which did not always materialize)
8. Deinstitutionalization, which changed the locus of treatment from large public hospitals to the community, is a product of the community mental health movement.
9. In 1955 more than a half-million patients were in state hospitals; currently, approximately 70,000 are in these hospitals.
10. A large percentage of the homeless in the United States has a diagnosable mental disorder. Critics of deinstitutionalization place some of the blame for homelessness on the community mental health movement.
11. Community mental health nurses have a major role in the continuum of care because of their specialized

training in patient care, comprehensive services, patient education, and case management.

12. Psychiatric care and psychiatric nursing have evolved during the 20th century. At one time, psychiatric nursing was closely associated with the care of the SMI, but, similar to psychiatrists, nurses in the field became professionally interested in the worried well. Currently, psychiatric nurses are interested in understanding the multiple variables affecting patients with mental disorders.

13. The *DSM* is the bible of psychiatric diagnoses. Nurses who seek to provide the best care and who want to advocate for patients must effectively learn these concepts.

REFERENCES

American Psychiatric Association (2013). *Diagnostic and statistical manual of mental disorders* (5th Ed.). APA.

American Psychiatric Nurses Association (2017). Expanding mental health services in American. https://www.apna.org/files/public/Resources/Expanding_Mental_Health_Care_Services_in_America-The_Pivotal_Role_of_Psychiatric-Mental_Health_Nurses_04_19.pdf

Broman, B. (2018). American Institutes for Research (AIR). National Center on Family Homelessness. https://www.air.org/center/national-center-family-homelessness

Charland, L. C. (2007). Benevolent theory: Moral treatment at the York retreat. *History of Psychiatry, 18*, 61–80. https://doi.org/10.1177/0957154X07070320.

Detre, T. (1987). The future of psychiatry. *The American Journal of Psychiatry, 5*(144), 621–625. https://doi.org/10.1176/ajp.144.5.621.

Deutsch, A. (1948). *The shame of the states.* Harcourt Brace. https://doi.org/10.1177/000271624926200181.

Ellis, H., & Alexander, V. (2017). The mentally ill in jail: Contemporary clinical and practice perspectives for psychiatric-mental health nursing. *Archives of Psychiatric Nursing, 31*, 217.

Frances, A. J., & Egger, H. L. (1999). Whither psychiatric diagnosis. *The Australian and New Zealand Journal of Psychiatry, 33*, 161.

Gerber, L. (2013). Bringing home effective nursing care for the homeless. *Nursing, 43*, 32.

Gollaher, D. (1995). *Voice for the mad: The life of Dorothea Dix.* Free Press.

Grob, G. (1987). The forging of mental health policy in America: World War II to the new frontier. *Journal of the History of Medicine and Allied Sciences, 42*, 410.

Makari, G. (2009). On the shifting boundaries of medicine. *The Lancet, 373*, 206.

Miller, J. P. (2015). 30 Years of psychiatry, with no fundamental progress. *Current Psychiatry, 14*, 45.

Moller, M. (2017). Advancing the role of advanced practice psychiatric nurses in today's psychiatric workforce. *Current Psychiatry, 16*, 15.

Nasrallah, H. (2015). A biopsychosocial 'therapeutic placenta' for people with schizophrenia. *Current Psychiatry, 14*, 16.

Nasrallah, H. (2012a). The hazards of serendipity. *Current Psychiatry, 11*, 14.

Nasrallah, H. (2012b). Psychiatry and the politics of incarceration. *Current Psychiatry, 11*, 4.

National Institutes of Health (NIH). (2017). The NIH almanac: National Institute of Mental Illness (NIMH). https://www.nih.gov/about-nih/what-we-do/nih-almanac/national-institute-mental-health-nimh

National Institute of Mental Health (NIMH). (2020). Any mental illness (AMI) among U. S. adults. https://www.nimh.nih.gov/health/statistics/mental-illness.shtml

Peplau, H. (1952). *Interpersonal Relations in Nursing.* Putnam.

Peplau, H. (1959). Principles of psychiatric nursing. In S. Arieti (Ed.), *American Handbook of Psychiatry* (pp. 1840–1856). Basic Books.

Preskorn, S. H. (2016). Genetic and related laboratory tests in psychiatry: What mental health practitioners need to know. *Current Psychiatry, 15*, 19.

Puffenberger, G. (2007). Pharmacy orientation (slide presentation for new pharmacists). MHM Services, used with permission.

Rosenhan, D. L. (1973). On being sane in insane places. *Science, 179*, 250.

Spiegel, A. (2005). The dictionary of disorder. *The New Yorker, 56*, 56.

Substance Abuse and Mental Health Services Administration (SAMHSA) (2016). Ending homelessness. https://www.samhsa.gov/homelessness-programs-resources/hpr-resources/ending-veteran-homelessness

Tandon, R. (2012). Getting ready for DSM-5: Part 1. *Current Psychiatry, 11*, 33.

Torrey, E. F., et al. (2010). *More mentally ill persons are in jails and prisons than hospitals: A survey of the states.* Treatment Advisory Center.

Torrey, E. F. (1997). The release of the mentally ill from institutions: A well-intentioned disaster. *The Chronicle of Higher Education, 43*, B4.

Wasow, M. (1993). The need for asylum revisited. *Hospital & Community Psychiatry, 44*, 207.

Weiner, D. B. (1992). Philippe Pinel's "memoir on madness" of December 11, 1794: A fundamental text of modern psychiatry. *American Journal of Psychiatry, 149*, 725.

Wilson, M. (1993). DSM-III and the transformation of American psychiatry: A history. *American Journal of Psychiatry, 150*, 399.

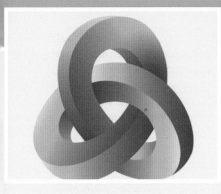

Legal Issues

Kate Pfeiffer and W. Chance Nicholson

 http://evolve.elsevier.com/Keltner

LEARNING OBJECTIVES

1. Define terms that apply to legal issues in psychiatric care.
2. Define self-determinism and discuss its impact on patient rights in mental health care.
3. Discuss legal protections and legal rights for persons living with mental disorders.
4. Delineate the differences between voluntary and involuntary psychiatric treatment.
5. Define HIPAA, confidentiality, mandates to inform, and implications of these in provision of mental health care.

INTRODUCTION

Understanding legal issues in healthcare settings is vitally important. Caring for patients with mental disorders requires a high level of expertise in understanding their legal rights. Many of these individuals experience alterations in mood, cognition, and behavior that influence decision-making ability, especially during times of increased stress. Additionally, individuals with mental disorders are often mischaracterized due to stigma, and as a result, patients' rights and legal issues may become issues of concern.

The legal rights and ethical considerations for healthcare decision-making can be complex and individuals living with mental disorders are often vulnerable to mistreatment, abuse, and neglect of their rights. Nurses must commit to legal and ethical accountability to their patients in professional nursing practice. The evolution of these rights guaranteeing legal protection for this population approximately parallels the advances made in jurisprudence and social systems.

Governmental systems and regulatory bodies thoughtfully attempt to achieve balance between the rights of individuals and the rights of society at large. This chapter begins with a brief review of basic legal principles and sources of law that inform mental health delivery and serve as the basis for legally sound psychiatric nursing practice (Box 3.1).

In addition, the nurse's role in these and other legal issues are presented throughout the chapter to understand and apply legal, regulatory, and compliance issues.

> **NORM'S NOTES** Legal stuff has a reputation for seeming boring, and can put most of us to sleep, but people who live with mental health problems have extremely important rights. One of the most important things you can do is understand the rights of people with mental health problems, whether it is your patient, a friend, a classmate, or a family member.

SOURCES OF LAW

Understanding sources of law and legal limits that influence nursing practice are fundamentally important to safe patient care. There are three basic sources of law: (1) statutory law; (2) common law; (3) administrative law.

Statutory Law

Statutory law follows a chain of legislative command, with the Constitution of the United States being the highest in the hierarchy of enacted written law. Statutory laws are enacted by federal, state, and local legislative bodies, such as the Nurse Practice Acts that define the scope of nursing practice for each state. **Statutory laws are either civil or criminal, designed to protect individual rights.**

BOX 3.1 Sources of Laws Affecting Psychiatric Nursing

1. U.S. Constitution
2. Individual federal and state statutes
3. Precedent-setting legal cases
4. The Joint Commission
5. Centers for Medicare and Medicaid Services

Common Law

Common law results from legal principles applied to cases based on evolving reasons, opinions, and precedents cited in previous court cases. Judges create or abide common law with each ruling or court decision. The judicial system serves as a mechanism for reviewing legal disputes where conflict exists between any laws. Importantly, common law is subject to jurisdiction rulings, which inform variations in laws from state to state. Moreover, this allows greater flexibility in meeting evolving social or public needs. Many of these rulings have influenced the current legal view of mental illness, ultimately shaping treatment and social norms to simultaneously protect the public and the rights of the individual. Examples of these laws include informed consent and the patient's right to refuse treatment, which will be explored later in this chapter.

Administrative Law

A third source of law is *administrative law*. These are public laws issued by administrative or government agencies authorized by statute to administer the enacted laws of federal and state governments, such as the State Boards of Nursing, which issue standards for nursing practice, licensure, and compliance monitoring in the interest of public safety. Monitoring and implementing laws for federal and state legislative bodies is difficult because congress cannot legislate every action. This branch of law controls the administrative operations of government and regulates the social, political, and economic domains of human collaboration.

TORTS (CIVIL LAW)

Reasonable Care (Standard of Care)

Health care liability to meet the standard of care encourages appropriate professional conduct and protects the public (Appel, 2019). A nurse assumes a standard of care (both medical and psychological) in patients under the imposition of a duty to care. A nurse must always exercise expected professional judgments and actions within their scope of practice in the context of care provided. These are the minimum necessary requirements for acceptable nursing care. In other words, a nurse must exercise a standard of prudence and caution defined by the degree of skill and knowledge expected by reasonable nurses in the care and treatment of patients, as described specifically in their state's Nurse Practice Act, federal and state laws, and policies of their healthcare institution. In court cases in which nurses are sued for negligence, the question is always the following: "Did the nurse meet the standard of care?"

Duty to Care

Duty to care is a legal obligation imposed on a person who is in a position to perform an action that could potentially harm others (by acting or not acting). This duty can arise between a nurse and a patient or via a statute or contract between physician and patient. The duty to care can arise from a telephone conversation, or it can arise out of a voluntary act of assuming the care of a patient.

Breach of Duty

Breach of duty is the failure to provide a reasonable standard of care owed to a person. This failure includes either doing or refraining from doing a particular act in a circumstance where the risk of harm exists.

Negligence

Negligence is personal wrongdoing described as the failure to perform care that is ethically expected or what a reasonably careful person would do under the same circumstances. Unlike a criminal law violation, negligence is conduct considered below reasonable care (or ethics) when the conduct accounts for the potential harm that could be brought to another person.

All four of the following elements must be present for a plaintiff to recover damages caused by negligence:
1. Duty to care
2. An obligation of reasonable care (i.e., standard of care)
3. Breach of duty
4. Injury proximately caused by a breach of duty

If proof of violation is present in all four elements, then the plaintiffs are said to have presented a *prima facie* (proven) case of negligence.

Clinical Example: Nurses fail their duty

A patient was admitted to a psychiatric facility late at night from a general hospital emergency department ½ hour away. The patient overdosed on a long-acting opioid drug. Although the patient was pronounced medically stable by the first hospital, the admission assessment upon arrival to the psychiatric facility noted that the patient was somnolent with an irregular respiration rate of 12 breaths/min. The patient's respiratory irregularity did not improve, but neither the physician on call nor the paramedics were called. The patient died of respiratory arrest overnight. The nurses did not meet their obligation to meet the standard of care.

Proximate Cause or Causation

The fourth element necessary to establish negligence requires that a direct relationship exists between the negligent conduct and the resulting harm suffered by the patient. The mere departure from a standard of care is insufficient to enable a patient to recover damages, unless the patient demonstrates that the departure was unreasonable and the direct cause of the patient's injuries. Foreseeability, as an element of negligence, is the reasonable anticipation that harm or injury is likely to result from an act or an omission to act. The test for foreseeability is whether anyone of reasonable prudence and intelligence would incur the same harm against another in the same circumstance.

Malpractice

A form of professional negligence is called *malpractice*. Malpractice claims can be brought against various professions, including nurses. These claims against nurses are often the result of the nurse's failure to maintain a standard of care in their professional setting (e.g., hospital). Implementing evidence-based care consistent with current practice policies and procedures helps protect against malpractice. Areas of concern that can lead to suits in nursing care include inappropriate dissemination of confidential information, illegal confinement, failure to obtain consent for medication and other treatments, inadequate treatment, medication errors, and the breach of duty to warn of threatened suicide or harm to others.

A nurse who exceeds clinical boundaries or fails to act as a reasonable and prudent nurse would, in the same or similar circumstances, incurs liability to the employer.

Nursing Implications

Nurses often have job responsibilities that include delegating tasks to unlicensed assistive personnel (UAP) on their healthcare team. It is critical to understand that UAP who exceed their clinical scope of authority and are under the direction or supervision of a nurse may cause liability to be incurred on the nurse. When a nurse delegates this authority to the assistant, the nurse remains accountable for the consequences of the act *and* for the adequate supervision of the assistant. When delegating, the nurse, at a minimum, should:

1. Know and follow institutional policies and procedures of scope and authority.
2. Ensure that UAP assigned are qualified to carry out the tasks that they are expected to perform.
3. Know the state limitations and responsibilities of nursing practice and scope.

Clinical Example: If you're in charge, it's on you!

Clara Meyers, a 40-year-old woman with a history of recent depression with sleep deprivation and suicidal ideation, is admitted to your unit, sedated, and placed on suicide precautions. The nurse assigns a new nursing assistant to check on the patient every 15 min for the entire shift. The nursing assistant, having checked the patient every 15 min for 2 h and finding her asleep, decides that every 30 min is sufficient. The nurse who delegated this task was unaware that the new assistant had only general nursing assistant training and had never been oriented on a psychiatric unit. During the 30-min period when the patient was left alone, she managed to get out of bed and go to the bathroom, where she fell and fractured her pelvis. In the subsequent lawsuit, the nurse was identified as liable for the decision of the assistant that resulted in the fall.

Mental Health Laws

Federal and state legislatures have enacted many laws to protect the welfare and rights of individuals with mental illness. Statutes vary among states; nurses must be aware of their state's laws.

TREATMENT AND PATIENT RIGHTS

In addition to the information discussed in the following section, the Centers for Medicare and Medicaid Services (CMS) publication *Federal Register* and the American Hospital Association (AHA) Patient's Bill of Rights are important sources on patient rights and regulations, shaping institutional policy. Aside from legal and ethical patient care issues, these rights must be ensured for eligibility and reimbursement with Medicare and Medicaid programs.

Right to Self-Determine, Give Consent, or Refuse Treatment

Fundamental to many issues in healthcare is an individual's right to make their own health care choices for treatment. *Self-determinism* has its roots in principles of individual autonomy and independence. All individuals living with mental illness may consent or refuse treatment based on *self-determinism*; this is essential to management of one's day-to-day wellbeing. *Self-determinism* is protected by *The Patient Self-Determination Act (PDSA)*, passed by the U.S. Congress in 1990 (Murray & Wortzel, 2019). This law is designed to protect individuals against mistreatment and discrimination by guaranteeing the right to make healthcare choices and receive information regarding advanced care options to ensure continuity of decision-making during times of incapacitation. We will discuss advanced care directives later in this chapter.

One of the most important concepts underlying a patient's right to self-determine is an individual's ability to consent or refuse treatment. Legally, all patients have the right to refuse treatment unless immediate intervention is required, such as in a psychiatric emergency with imminent risk of harm to the patient or another person. These are rights protected under the U.S. Constitution, and many of its amendments, such as the right to equal protection.

Clinical Example: I want what I didn't have

Ned Little-Moore, a 65-year-old, well-nourished but unkempt man, was brought to the hospital by a social worker for psychiatric evaluation. Since his wife's death 3 years earlier, neighbors report suspicion that his house has been taken over by drug dealers. He is often seen outside at night, sleeping on the porch, despite cold weather. Furthermore, Mr. Little-Moore has approached neighbors for food and has told them that the drug dealers have taken his social security check. During the evaluation, Mr. Little-Moore insists that he willingly allows others to live in his home. He is alert and oriented, and no evidence of psychiatric disorder is found during evaluation. He declines offers of assistance to find other housing.

Capacity and Competency

In mental health treatment, exacerbations of illness may complicate factors of consent and decision-making. An individual must display capacity for understanding to make an informed decision. *Capacity* is the ability to make an informed decision and is assessed by a physician or psychologist (Muller, 2019). Adherence to infection prevention protocols to mitigate spread of Covid-19 is an application of these principles to an ethical dilemma. How does the nurse maintain patient autonomy and support capacity in a patient who refuses to socially distance, take a Covid test, or wear a mask? Understanding the patient's capacity to refuse these measures with regards to legal and ethical guidelines is critically important to protection of both the patient and the community (Russ et al., 2020).

Competency for decision-making is closely related but is a legal determination. Competency differs in scope between states and is generally based on the following ideas: ability to communicate choices, understand information relevant to the situation and its consequences, and compare risks and benefits of treatment decisions (Jeste et al., 2018; Lamont et al., 2019). Individuals are competent to make their own treatment decisions unless a judge has evidence to decide otherwise. This holds true regardless of treatment setting or legal status of the admission. Only after a court decides that a person is not competent to understand the need for treatment or act in their own best interest, can medications or other treatments be imposed on that person (Box 3.2). Once an individual is judged *incompetent* by the court, there may be an appointment of a conservator or legal guardian to assume some or many responsibilities, such as entering contracts, financial management, and other personal affairs. The individual may lose rights such as the right to marry, vote, drive a car, and make day-to-day decisions. The reach

---

BOX 3.2   A Precedent-Setting Case

Eleanor Riese, a 44-year-old woman, was first hospitalized at age 25 (in 1968) when she was given a diagnosis of schizophrenia. She was prescribed thioridazine (Mellaril), which brought her psychosis under control. After treatment, she was able to live alone for many years. Riese stopped taking her medication, and speculation asserted it was because of Mellaril-related bladder infections. Her psychosis returned, and she was in and out of psychiatric hospitals as a voluntary patient.

In 1985 Riese was admitted to Saint Mary's Hospital and Medical Center, San Francisco, California. Her status was eventually changed from voluntary to involuntary because she refused to take her medications. The American Civil Liberties Union (ACLU) sued on behalf of the rights of Riese and other involuntary patients to refuse medications.

The ACLU prevailed in the case, and it was determined that patients have the right to refuse treatment. If a mentally ill patient refuses to take medications, a court hearing must be scheduled to determine whether medications would benefit the patient in getting better. The hearing is called a Riese Hearing, and the judge determines if the patient would benefit from medications. This decision is based on input from the psychiatrist regarding treatment of the patient with psychotropic medications. Once the determination has been made, if the patient refuses oral medications, a substitute suitable injectable is given.

Modified from *Riese v. St. Mary's Hospital and Medical Center, 259 Cal. Rptr. 669, 774 P.2d 698.* (1989). https://www.apa.org/about/offices/ogc/amicus/riese.

---

of legal guardians over the gravely disabled person (the conservatee) varies by need and state.

Nursing Implications

During the course of medication administration, nurses may find themselves coaxing a patient into taking it. The nurse must always ensure that coercion is not forced or ethically misleading to the patient. Actions such as placing refused medications in food or liquid are considered forcing. The deception is also counterproductive to the ethical foundation of the therapeutic nurse-patient relationship. Sometimes, it is not clear what constitutes a psychiatric emergency. Nurses might be held liable if their interpretation of a psychiatric emergency differs from that of another professional or a judge (reasonable standard of care).

Suspension of Patient Rights

Hospitals and other health care settings use privilege systems to protect patients and reinforce unit policy and appropriate behavior. Based on an individual's ability to follow unit rules and risk to self or others, privileges on and off the unit may be awarded or restricted, such as access to group sessions, gym, and phone.

Nursing Implications

Restricting or suspending a patient's rights requires the nurse to document clearly that allowing the patient to continue to exercise the specific right might result in harm to the patient or others and must be supported by institutional policy. For example, a suicidal patient's right to access personal belongings might be suspended because it is believed that the patient might attempt to harm themselves with those objects. The nurse must document this concern and suspension of this right in the nurse's notes.

Right to Treatment in the Least Restrictive Environment

The right to self-determinism with regard to psychiatric care choices and refusal includes the right to utilize the least restrictive environment and means of treatment. An individual has the right to freedom from unnecessary restriction when less restrictive, appropriate interventions are available in the community. This right is central to the ideology of the deinstitutionalization movement of the 1960s, and extends to excessive interventions, including unnecessary hospitalizations, medication administration, and physical restraint.

Nursing Implications

The nurse has treatment responsibilities and can be held liable if the patient does not receive adequate treatment with the appropriate level of care. The following clinical example illustrates the issue of the right to treatment using the least restrictive alternative.

Clinical Example: He ain't heavy

Hef Tee is a 69-year-old Vietnam veteran who has comorbid dementia and posttraumatic stress disorder characterized by periods of flashbacks and depression. After a flashback, Mr. Tee is often confused and wanders about for days looking for friends he lost in the war. He poses no obvious danger to others or himself. His family is deceased, and he lives alone. When he is picked up by the police for loitering and evaluated by the social worker, Mr. Tee insists on going home. His case is heard before the court, which rules that he does not need commitment to a psychiatric unit but does need a structured environment such as assisted living. The social worker finds placement in the community, and Mr. Tee agrees.

Rights Regarding Seclusion and Restraint

Throughout history, restraints and segregation interventions have been used for behavioral management and the promotion of safety in medical and psychiatric settings. *Restraint* is a broad term characterizing *any form* of limitation of a person's movement or access to his or her own body and/or restriction of freedom of movement. These include physical holds, bed rails, lap trays, restraint devices, or medications. *Seclusion* is the process of involuntarily confining a person alone.

The use of restraint and seclusion techniques has come under scrutiny due to injuries and deaths associated with their use. No longer viewed as therapeutic, these methods are now considered potentially traumatizing (U.S. Department of Health and Human Services, Substance Abuse and Mental Health Services Administration [SAMHSA], 2019a, b). Strategies to prevent harm and protect the patient's right to autonomy are balanced carefully against the nurse's obligation to provide safe and ethical care.

Restraints and seclusion have been replaced with more appropriate individual and milieu interventions, and many inpatient facilities have shifted toward restraint-free policies.

The Joint Commission has developed standards to guide efforts to reduce the use of restraints in both medical and psychiatric facilities. The CMS has also published within their Patient's Rights document strict rules for restraint and seclusion use in hospitals that receive Medicare and Medicaid funds, resulting in lower rates of both seclusion and restraint practices (Staggs, 2020).

Clinical Example: Somebody needs to be fired!

Mr. Buck Tindal is a 75-year-old man admitted to the psychiatric unit of a large teaching hospital for observation and treatment related to recent behaviors suggestive of dementia. Mr. Tindal, although confused at times, is able to feed himself, bathe without assistance, and self-manage toileting needs on admission. Mr. Tindal experiences nocturia most nights. Because the staff is concerned about falling related to multiple bathroom trips, Mr. Tindal has been "legally" physically restrained. Immediately, he begins wetting the bed, something he had not done since childhood. Within 2 weeks, Mr. Tindal becomes increasingly confused, with difficulty feeding and bathing. A note in his chart describes urinary incontinence.

Nursing Implications

Nurses who understand the potential negative physical, psychological, and legal consequences associated with restraint and seclusion are more apt to look for alternative strategies. The most valuable interventions aim to prevent escalation in behavior and loss of control. Attention to the nurse-patient relationship, therapeutic milieu, and principles of pharmacologic management can all reduce the need for restrictive measures. Guidelines issued by CMS for the use of seclusion and restraints are substantially different in medically and behaviorally necessary situations. Although laws differ from state to state, general guidelines for use in psychiatric settings include multiple elements important for the nurse to document, as follows:

1. Staff members involved in decisions to restrain or seclude and staff who apply or remove restraints must receive special training and demonstrate competency.
2. Alternatives must be considered before the use of restraint and seclusion.
3. Although nurses might be allowed to implement restraint or seclusion in emergent situations, a physician's order is required within 1 hour. Physician assistants and advanced practice nurses can also write restraint and seclusion orders.
4. The least restrictive method or device possible must be chosen.
5. Nurses should carefully document events leading to the intervention and justification for use.
6. Orders must contain the type of restraint, rationale for use, and time limitations.
7. As-needed (prn) orders are not permitted. Each episode must be based on imminent risk.
8. Restraint and seclusion are used for the shortest possible time. The nurse must tell the patients what behaviors are expected before release and reevaluate the patients at least every 2 hours for continued need of restraint and seclusion.
9. Patients must be observed constantly during restraint and seclusion, with documentation of safety and comfort interventions at least every 15 minutes.
10. Patients must be debriefed after restrictive interventions.
11. Patients have the right to request notification of a family member or other person in the event that restraints or seclusion are implemented.
12. Death of any patient while in restraints, even when restraints did not contribute to death in the judgment of the health care provider, is required to be reported to the US Food and Drug Administration (FDA).

❓ CRITICAL THINKING QUESTION

1. Some psychiatric professionals believe that the courts have gone too far in protecting the rights of patients and have actually set up barriers to effective mental health care. What do you think?

Clinical Example: Give me that old time religion

Kim Young is a 28-year-old married nonbinary person. Mx. Young is very committed to their community and church, having committed to countless hours of volunteer work. Friends and family describe them as a person with boundless energy who never appears to stop. Their volunteer hours continue to increase, and Mx. Young begins to preach outside local bars and restaurants without consent from establishment managers. Their behavior becomes increasingly erratic and paranoid. When the owner of a local tavern calls the police after they refuse to leave, Mx. Young begins to curse him and becomes highly agitated. Their speech is disorganized, with loose associations between topics. The police de-escalate the situation and transport them to a psychiatric unit, where Mx. Young is involuntarily committed. When approached by the staff, they remain agitated, confused, and restless. They shout and scream related to fear and confusion. Mx. Young is not oriented to place or time. Four-point physical restraint is ordered. Mx. Young experiences seclusion and restraint thereafter for the aggressive behavior secondary to psychosis before stabilization with treatment. The nursing progress record (Box 3.3) and the restraint and seclusion nursing notes provide a record of the behavior and the nursing responses to that behavior.

BOX 3.3	**Nursing Progress Record for Kim Young (Case Example)**

Time	Format
0210	Patient continues to pace hallway, dayroom, and room; at 0235, asks for sleep medications; patient states that walking is the best way to get well.
0315	Patient refuses to go to room and tries to resist; paces dayroom and at times kneels as if in prayer.
0430	Patient is asleep on top of bed, naked; door is open.
0830	Patient refuses medication; appears very agitated.
0930	Patient is very agitated; tears up another patient's magazine and throws it into the trash; patient is placed in seclusion.
0945	Patient paces in room while praying loudly.
1000	Patient increases pacing and intermittently hits walls.
1015	Patient's agitation is escalated; when staff goes into room to check on patient, swings at staff; patient is placed in four-point restraint by four female and two male staff members; patient states that "Christ lives in me"; Haldol 5 mg IM and Cogentin 2 mg IM are given.

IM, Intramuscular.

Assault, Battery, and False Imprisonment

Assault

Assault is the apprehension of physical contact or the person's mental security, or the deliberate threat coupled with the apparent ability to do physical harm to another. In assault, no actual contact is necessary. Making verbal threats in an attempt to force a patient to take medication against their will (without reasonable cause) constitutes an assault.

Battery

A battery is an intentional touching of another's person, in a socially impermissible manner, without that person's consent. Battery is intentional conduct that violates the physical security of another. The recipient of the battery does not have to be aware that a battery has occurred. Clinically relevant examples of battery are: force used in unlawful detention of a patient, or if a nurse physically apprehended and forced a patient (without reasonable cause) to move, such as to a room.

False Imprisonment

False imprisonment is the unlawful *restraint* of an individual's personal liberty or the unlawful confinement of an individual. The only necessity is that an individual who is physically confined to a given area experiences a reasonable fear that force, which may be implied by words, threats, or gestures, will be used to detain or intimidate him or her *without legal justification.* Examples include the following:

1. Excessive force used to restrain a patient constitutes false imprisonment and battery.
2. Preventing a patient from leaving a health care facility constitutes false imprisonment.
3. Wrongfully committing a patient to a psychiatric facility constitutes false imprisonment.

A psychiatric facility should have a policy that defines the parameters of confinement, and the nurse must follow the policy guidelines. Please note that in example 2 in the list, a patient committed by a court order or petition can be prevented from leaving a facility, and doing so is legal—thus not false imprisonment. In addition, if a person is considered a danger to self or others, they can be held for safety reasons; however, even then, for extended confinement a court order is often pursued. Most facilities and states have a 72-hour hold policy on such individuals, which prevents them from leaving or allows the facility to confine them for up to 3 days.

COMMITMENT ISSUES

Similar to medically focused care, the vast majority of psychiatric care occurs in outpatient, community settings. The decision to receive treatment in a psychiatric facility is important, and generally reserved for acute crisis, and self-management at home is no longer a healthy option for mental health stability, or for a forensic commitment, discussed later in this chapter.

TABLE 3.1 Types of Behaviors Susceptible to Involuntary Commitment

All States	Some States
Risk of harm through self-neglect, grave disability, or failure to meet basic needs	Risk of physical deterioration without commitment
Risk that a person might physically injure or kill himself	Potential danger to property
Risk that a person might physically harm other persons	Risk of relapse or mental deterioration

From Mossman, D. L. (2013). Psychiatric "holds" for nonpsychiatric patients. *Current Psychiatry*, 12, 34.

Voluntary Inpatient Care

If inpatient hospitalization is required, most people with mental health problems enter of their own volition. This is called a *voluntary admission* or *voluntary commitment*. Each state has laws for observation, evaluation, and treatment for mental illness. Although specific state and institutional policies vary, in a voluntary admission the patient consents to treatment and is free to leave at any time, maintaining their civil rights. After individuals are assessed and stabilized via their course of treatment, they may discharge. Voluntary patients who want to sign themselves out may do so, even against medical advice, unless the psychiatric care provider determines that the patient is at imminent risk to self or others and should be placed on an involuntary commitment status.

Involuntary Inpatient Care

At times, an individual may enter a mental health care facility through *involuntary admission* or *involuntary commitment*. Involuntary treatment means that an individual who has the legal capacity to consent to mental health treatment refuses to do so. All states allow emergency commitment of individuals with acute mental illness crises who pose a danger to themselves or others, and the process must be conducted consistent with respect to state and federal statutes (Table 3.1). There are also ethical considerations for the nurse and for the patient who is being held against their will and vulnerable to these circumstances (Nussbaum, 2020).

This commitment process must demonstrate probable cause under the Fourth Amendment of the U.S. Constitution. The U.S. Supreme Court has repeatedly held that the civil commitment process is also subject to the restraints of the Fourteenth Amendment of the U.S. Constitution. The state must produce clear and convincing evidence to prove that a person is experiencing severe mental illness and imminently dangerous. Failure to comply with these guidelines can render a commitment illegal.

While these vary by state, in general, there are three common elements to involuntary hospitalization.

- The person is imminently dangerous to themselves (i.e., experiencing suicidal intent)
- The person is imminently dangerous to another person (i.e., experiencing homicidal intent)
- The person is unable to care for their own essential human needs of health or safety, such as food, clothing, and shelter because of a mental illness. This is also sometimes called *"gravely disabled"* (i.e., cannot distinguish between food and non-food items secondary to psychosis).

Commitment Timelines and Status

Involuntary treatment is divided into three common categories:
1. Emergency care (acute stabilization)
2. Short-term observation and treatment
3. Long-term commitment (3, 6, or 12 months)

Involuntary treatment is the area of psychiatric care from which most legal issues arise. Although involuntary commitment usually implies inpatient care, it can also be applied to outpatient treatment, known as *outpatient commitment* (e.g., residential treatment for substance use) (Evans, Harrington, Roose, Lemere, & Buchanan, 2020).

Emergency Care (Acute Stabilization)

An involuntary emergency hold may be utilized in patients who lack capacity for healthcare decision-making due to severe mental illness. An authorized person such as a police officer signs documents to place an individual under involuntary care for short-term emergency evaluation for observation and acute stabilization treatment. The length of the involuntary status varies from state to state; typically, 48 to 72 hours is the average (SAMHSA, 2019a, b).

Short-Term Observation and Treatment

During the emergency evaluation period, if it is suspected that further hospitalization is needed, a certification hearing takes place. A complaint or probable cause statement is written, indicating that the person is a danger to self or others or remains gravely disabled. In this context, probable cause under the Fourth Amendment means that known facts would lead an ordinary person to believe that the person detained is mentally disordered and is a danger to self or others or is gravely disabled. The probable cause hearing is held to determine not whether the person is mentally ill, but whether just cause exists to keep the person for treatment against his or her will. If probable cause exists, individuals can be detained for observation and treatment. These individuals must be informed of their rights on being certified for this level of involuntary care.

Long-Term Commitment

Long-term commitment is reserved for persons who require prolonged psychiatric care but refuse to seek such help voluntarily. These hospitalizations can last from approximately 90 days to much longer and are usually conducted at state hospitals. Often, an individual will receive acute stabilization at a local or regional hospital before they transfer to the long-term facility. Individuals are usually brought before a hearing officer, which is a major part of the system of checks and balances that decreases the possibility of someone being railroaded into a mental hospital.

Nursing Implications

The paradox for individuals who require inpatient care is that the process of becoming a patient can itself cause trauma and related anxiety and/or depression while also violating human rights. The psychiatric nurse should be aware of these important considerations in addition to the ethical and legal implications that accompany psychiatric hospitalizations in the pursuit of balancing non-maleficence with patient autonomy.

Additionally, because the law determines the length of this involuntary treatment period, staff must scrupulously adhere to legal time constraints. The nursing staff must remain aware of the exact point at which the emergency treatment elapses and prepare the patient for discharge at that time. Patients might be asked to remain voluntarily in the facility, and if they refuse, they might be asked to sign out against medical advice. Patients must be released when no legal basis exists for continued confinement in the hospital. The hospital staff might suggest voluntary admission and might require patients to sign out against medical advice if voluntary admission is refused. The staff cannot hold someone simply because they believe that the individual needs to be protected from herself or himself.

 CRITICAL THINKING QUESTION

2. What if a patient, who will die without treatment, wants to leave the hospital? Does she have the right to refuse treatment and go home? Is wanting to go home to die a sign of mental illness?

ADVANCED CARE DIRECTIVES AND MENTAL HEALTH

All health care facilities that serve Medicare or Medicaid patients must provide each of their adult patients with written information regarding their right to make decisions about their medical care, consistent with federal and state laws, including the right to choose the healthcare they receive during a period of crisis or if they are unable to make a decision regarding their treatment. This is accomplished through the utilization of written instructions called *advanced care directives*. A *living will* states what treatment should (or should not) be provided. These may list specific actions that the patient can choose to implement under a life-threatening condition, such as mechanical ventilator support or artificial nutrition. A durable power of attorney is a written document in which one person authorizes another person as a proxy to make health care decisions as directed by the advanced care directive if needed. Since the passage of the Patient Self-Determination Act, all states have endorsed laws addressing advanced directives.

Psychiatric advanced care directives are comparatively new legal protections designed to maintain patient autonomy by directing the course of a psychiatric treatment, and are authorized by law in many, but not all, states. These are made in advance of a mental health crisis with the individual and their healthcare provider regarding treatment preferences, visitors, and decision-making proxies (Sofer, 2019). Directives about treatment can be disclosed in many areas, including, but not limited to:

(1) the use of specific medications, including dose and route
(2) the use of specific treatment options, such as ECT
(3) the use of behavior management including restraint, seclusion, and sedation
(4) a list of the individuals who are to be notified and allowed to visit
(5) a consent to contact health care providers and obtain treatment records
(6) a willingness to participate in research studies (Murray & Wortzel, 2019).

Unfortunately, issues of decision-making, capacity, competency, and safety can all arise and complicate the execution of such directives. A compelling example is the case of Nancy Hargrove, a woman who lived in Vermont (where there is no separate psychiatric advance directive) and who was diagnosed with schizophrenia. In her durable power of attorney, she did clearly refuse all psychiatric treatment. When she needed hospitalization, the big question was whether it was legal to administer involuntary medications to this patient. The court ruled that the ability to override the treatment wishes of someone with mental illness is discriminatory, and in violation of the Americans with Disabilities Act. It should be noted that this judgment may not be rendered in all states (Murray & Wortzel, 2019). The National Resource Center on Psychiatric Advance Directives provides resources and guidance by state: https://www.nrc-pad.org/states/.

 CRITICAL THINKING QUESTION

3. What if you learned from a patient during an individual session that his company was getting ready to launch a product that would cause the value of the company's stock to soar. Could you ethically use this information to enhance your investment savings?

Nursing Implications

Nurses should be aware of the patient's right to establish advance directives for both physical and mental health care in the form of a written statement of preference or by legal documentation of a durable power of attorney. Nurses should also be familiar with and follow employer procedures and laws that govern how the patient is made aware of this right. The following actions are also important to ensure that the patient's right to self-determination is exercised:

1. Documentation in the medical record of either properly executed forms or a statement or signed waiver must be made indicating that the patient chooses not to exercise his or her right to provide advance directives.

2. The attorney in fact chosen by the patient is consulted before making decisions regarding the patient in areas specified by the document.
3. All members of the health care team are made aware of advance directives and that they are considered in treatment planning.

PRIVACY AND CONFIDENTIALITY

Right to Confidentiality of Records

In addition to matters related to the right to self-determine one's treatment, and the right to refuse it altogether, privacy and *patient confidentiality* are enormously important rights. Patient information is privileged material and should be protected for all patient populations, regardless of admission status or setting. Confidentiality is essential in the nurse-patient therapeutic relationship. However, maintaining confidentiality is not always as easy as it might appear; hence professional judgment is required. The guidelines in Box 3.4 provide a framework for appropriate monitoring to ensure confidentiality. As straightforward as these guidelines are, they do not cover every situation or address exceptions. The rule of confidentiality is not absolute and cannot always be guaranteed. For example, information about a patient at risk for self-harm must be made available to appropriate individuals. Keeping this type of information confidential constitutes professional malpractice.

Health Insurance Portability and Accountability Act

The Health Insurance Portability and Accountability Act (HIPAA) took effect in April 2003. This provides legal protection of patient rights in several areas, including privacy and confidentiality of patient information. To keep pace with emerging electronic medical records technology, the Health Information Technology for Economic and Clinical Health Act of 2009 (HITECH) extended from HIPAA, was passed, protecting who can view and receive electronic patient records, and mandate security for health records (Rosenbloom et al., 2019).

For example, even though computer technology speeds the transfer and storage of personal medical information, it has also proven to be a venue for invasion of privacy. HIPAA gives patients more control over their medical records and ensures penalties for individuals who handle a patient's medical record inappropriately. The following are five rights that patients have under HIPAA legislation (U.S. Department of Health and Human Services, 2020):

1. Right to be educated about HIPAA privacy regulations
2. Right to access their own medical records
3. Right to correct or add to their medical records
4. Right to demand their authorization before their medical records are disclosed to others and right to request an accounting of everyone their information has been disclosed to
5. Right to request a preferred method of communication (e.g., do not leave appointment reminders on voicemail, send medical bill to brother's address).

Nursing Implications

The nurse should document all confidential information that is released in the nursing notes, including the date and circumstances under which disclosure was made, the names of the individuals or agencies receiving the disclosure and their relationships to the patient, and the specific information disclosed. To release information about patients, a consent form must be signed first. Most states provide legal redress for patients if a nurse willfully discloses confidential information without the proper signature.

The therapeutic modality of group therapy, which nurses often lead, is particularly vulnerable to violations of confidentiality. The group leader should always address this issue when starting a group or when a new member is introduced to the group. Nurses who lead group sessions must acknowledge the limitations to confidentiality that exist in the group format. After such a proclamation is made, forthrightness by group members concerning their thoughts, feelings, and behaviors might decline.

It is critical that staff discuss patient information only in private or authorized settings. *For example, several nursing students went to lunch and started discussing a patient. The patient's family was in the adjoining booth. The family heard the conversation and reported it back to the hospital. The students were reprimanded but were given a "second chance."*

BOX 3.4 Tips for Monitoring Confidentiality

1. Keep all patient records secure by closing charts and locking screens.
2. Carefully consider the content of all written entries.
3. Release information only with written consent.
4. Disguise any identifying clinical material when it is used for educational purposes.
5. Share information only with people who need to know, not with friends, or in public areas.
6. Guard written material taken outside the clinical area.
7. Do not access written or electronic information out of curiosity.
8. Note that fax transmissions to unsecured areas in which a receipt error is a possibility might be prohibited.
9. Know to whom you are talking when relaying patient information on the phone; "family" might be a reporter, boss, or insurance attorney.

? CRITICAL THINKING QUESTION

4. Confidentiality is stressed in nursing school, but it might be violated. What should you do when one of your classmates is discussing a patient inappropriately? Is it a violation of confidentiality to discuss a patient by name in a clinical conference?

Breaching Confidentiality

A *breach of confidentiality* is third-party disclosure of private information without authorized consent from the patient or legal compulsion to do so. For example, disclosing health care information with a family member of a patient who has not consented to share this information is a breach of confidentiality. Unauthorized breaches of confidentiality can incur liability for the nurse and healthcare organization.

Clinical Example: You are so special!

Students frequently find themselves in the following situation. After developing a relationship with a patient, the student might hear, "I want to tell you something, but I don't want anyone else to know." What is the proper response? Is it a breach of the patient's right to confidentiality to tell others or to record what is said in the patient's chart? The student must let the patient know that anything said within the context of the nurse-patient relationship will be shared with other team members when appropriate.

Duty to Warn Third Parties

An exception to the patient's right to confidentiality is the *duty to warn*, based on the landmark case *Tarasoff v. The Regents of the University of California*, 17 Cal 3rd 425 (1976). Here, a graduate student at the University of California, Prosenjit Poddar, dated a young woman named Tatiana Tarasoff briefly in 1969. After their brief relationship ended, Poddar became distraught and confided in a psychologist his intent to kill his former girlfriend. The psychologist notified campus police to request their assistance in detaining the man. The police detained, questioned, and released Poddar. A few months later, he killed Tatiana Tarasoff on October 27, 1969. Her parents brought a successful suit against the University of California, claiming that the therapist had a duty to warn their daughter of Poddar's threats and that he should have been hospitalized. The court initially dismissed the claims, but in 1974 the California supreme court ruled that therapists must warn all foreseeable victims of their patients' potentially violent actions. Because of the outcry from privacy advocates and mental health providers, the ruling was revised, and in 1976, it was found that therapists *have a duty to exercise reasonable care* in protecting foreseeable victims of patients' violent actions (Piel & Opara, 2018).

Following this case, most states adopted their own statutes to detail when a mental health clinician can or must notify police or victims in an attempt to prevent harm. The duty to protect endangered third parties is now a national standard of practice, although some jurisdictions still hold that any disclosure of confidential information is a violation of patient rights (see Box 3.4).

Confidentiality in the nurse-patient relationship is both an ethical duty and a legal issue. The psychiatric nurse must balance a duty to protect confidentiality with a responsibility to warn society of possible danger.

Nursing Implications

A nurse who is aware of a patient's intention to cause harm to self or others must communicate this information to other professionals and take steps to protect the potential recipient of harm. Not all comments or vague threats should be reported. The Tarasoff ruling specifies that a specific threat to a readily identifiable person or persons must be made. Whenever possible, a decision to communicate confidential patient communications should be discussed with the clinical team (or ethics committee) before taking action to ensure that patients' rights are balanced with rights of third parties. Documentation in the patient's record is crucial for effective communication of this information. The nurse who fails to take prudent action can be held liable. See the following example.

Clinical Example: Better warn somebody!

Warren Sumbodee is a 36-year-old man with a history of physical abuse toward his wife for the last 7 years. Six months ago, his wife left the marriage with the support of a domestic violence program. Mr. Sumbodee grows progressively more agitated at the thought of being unable to contact her. When he fails to find her at her place of employment, he tells her fellow employees that when he finds her, he intends to kill her. The police are called, and Mr. Sumbodee is arrested. He is involuntarily admitted to a psychiatric hospital for a 72-hour emergency evaluation. During the course of admission, Mr. Sumbodee specifically tells the therapist of a specific plan to harm his wife. On review, the police and Mrs. Sumbodee are warned of his threats.

Patient Rights and the Local, State, and Federal Justice System

Mental illness and the justice system collide in many ways. Since the deinstitutionalization movement of the 1960s, the U.S. incarceration rate has more than tripled to one of the largest populations of prisoners in the world (U.S. Department of Justice [USBJ], 2018). Thirty-seven percent of people currently residing in state and federal prisons have been diagnosed with a mental illness (USBJ, 2017). Jails and prisons have become de facto psychiatric institutions, yet the justice system is unable to adequately meet the needs of persons impacted by the justice system who experience mental illness. Despite societal advances in mental health treatment and advocacy, major challenges remain.

STUDY NOTES

1. The understanding of the rights of mentally ill persons has evolved over the centuries. Currently, based on several precedent-setting legal decisions and laws, protection of the mentally ill person's rights has been established.

2. Three categories of commitment include:
   a. Voluntary patient: the person requests hospitalization and voluntarily agrees to be admitted.
   b. Involuntary commitment: a person with the legal capacity to consent refuses to do so and is treated against his will.
   c. Commitment of an incapacitated person: treatment of a person who does not have the legal capacity to consent to treatment.

3. Patients under psychiatric care have many rights guaranteed by the US Constitution and the constitutions of individual states.

4. Seclusion and restraint are special procedures for coping with assaultive and dangerous patients; these patients can be isolated or mechanically restrained to prevent injury to the patient, other patients, or staff.

5. Patients, including involuntarily admitted patients, must give informed consent before they are given psychotropic drugs and retain the right to refuse medication. Except for emergency situations, involuntarily admitted patients cannot be given medication against their will without judicial approval.

6. Psychiatric patients have the right to be treated in the least restrictive alternative or least restrictive environment. In other words, if patients can receive appropriate care close to home in a community agency, they cannot be forced to go to a public mental hospital, far away from family and friends.

REFERENCES

Appel, J. M. (2019). When liability and ethics diverge. *Focus, 4*(17), 382–386. https://doi.org/10.1176/appi.focus.20190031.

Evans, E. A., Harrington, C., Roose, R., Lemere, S., & Buchanan, D. (2020). Perceived benefits and harms of involuntary civil commitment for opioid use disorder. *The Journal of Law, Medicine & Ethics, 48*(4), 718–734. https://doi.org/10.1177/1073110520979382.

Jeste, D. V., Eglit, G. M. L., Palmer, B. W., Martinis, J. G., Blanck, P., & Saks, E. R. (2018). Supported decision making in serious mental illness. *Psychiatry, 81*(1), 28–40. https://doi.org/10.1080/00332747.2017.1324697.

Lamont, S., Stewart, C., & Chiarella, M. (2019). Capacity and consent: Knowledge and practice of legal and healthcare standards. *Nursing Ethics, 26*(1), 71–83. https://doi.org/10.1177/0969733016687162.

Muller, L (2019). Competency versus capacity. *Professional Case Management, 24*(20), 95–98. https://doi:10.1097/NCM.0000000000000348.

Murray, H., & Wortzel, H. S. (2019). Psychiatric advance directives: Origins, benefits, challenges, and future directions. *Journal of Psychiatric Practice®, 25*(4), 303–307. https://doi.org/10.1097/PRA.0000000000000401.

Nussbaum, A. M. (2020). Held against our wills: Reimagining involuntary commitment: Involuntary psychiatric treatment for people with serious mental illness should focus on returning to health rather than reducing danger. *Health Affairs, 39*(5), 898–901. https://doi.org/10.1377/hlthaff.2019.00765.

Piel, J. L., & Opara, R. (2018). Does *Volk v DeMerleer* conflict with the AMA *Code of Medical Ethics* on breaching patient confidentiality to protect third parties? *American Medical Association Journal of Ethics, 20*(1), 10–18.

Rosenbloom, S. T., Smith, J. R. L., Bowen, R., Burns, J., Riplinger, L., & Payne, T. H. (2019). Updating HIPAA for the electronic medical record era. *Journal of the American Medical Informatics Association, 26*(10), 1115–1119. https://doi.org/10.1093/jamia/ocz090.

Russ, M. J., Sisti, D., & Wilner, P. J. (2020). When patients refuse COVID-19 testing, quarantine, and social distancing in inpatient psychiatry: Clinical and ethical challenges. *Journal of Medical Ethics, 46*, 579–580. https://doi.org/10.1136/medethics-2020-106613.

Sofer, D (2019). Psychiatric advanced directives. *American Journal of Nursing, 119*(5), 16–17. https://doi.101097/01.NAJ.0000557905.82033.d4.

Staggs, V. S. (2020). Variability in psychiatric facility seclusion and restraint rates as reported on hospital compare site. *Psychiatric Services, 71*(9), 893–898. https://doi.org/10.1176/appi.ps.202000011.

U.S. Department of Health and Human Services. (2020). *Your rights under HIPAA*. https://www.hhs.gov/hipaa/for-individuals/guidance-materials-for-consumers/index.html.

U.S. Department of Health and Human Services, Substance Abuse and Mental Health Services Administration [SAMHSA]. (2019a). *Civil commitment and the mental health care continuum: Historical trends and principles for law and practice*. https://www.samhsa.gov/ebp-resource-center.

U.S. Department of Health and Human Services, Substance Abuse and Mental Health Services Administration. [SAMHSA] (2019b). *Trauma and violence*. https://www.samhsa.gov/trauma-violence.

U.S. Department of Justice, Bureau of Justice Statistics. (2017, June) *Indicators of mental health problems reported by prisoners and jail inmates, 2011-2012*. https://www.bjs.gov/content/pub/pdf/imhprpji1112.pdf.

U.S. Department of Justice, Bureau of Justice Statistics. (2018, April) *Correctional populations in the United States, 2016*. https://www.bjs.gov/content/pub/pdf/cpus16.pdf.

4

Psychobiologic Bases of Behavior

Peter C. Kowalski and Jonathan S. Dowben[a]

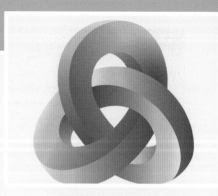

 http://evolve.elsevier.com/Keltner

LEARNING OBJECTIVES

- Describe the importance of the psychiatric nurse's understanding of brain biology.
- Identify and describe gross neuroanatomical structures.
- Differentiate the functions of the sympathetic and parasympathetic nervous systems.

- Describe the function and localization of the nervous system.
- Identify the role of specific neurotransmitters in schizophrenia, depression, anxiety, and dementia.

NEUROANATOMY REVIEW

The nervous system is composed of nerve cells, or *neurons*, and other cell types that serve as neuron supporters and play critical roles in neurotransmission. The human brain contains 100 billion neurons that can be classified into at least 1000 different types and each neuron connects to other neurons with up to 10,000 synapses (Kandel, Schwartz, Jessell, Siegelbaum, & Hudspeth, 2013).

The brain and spinal cord form the *central nervous system* (CNS). Nerves and their accompanying structures that exist outside of the CNS form the *peripheral nervous system* (PNS). The brain consists of the cerebrum, cerebellum, and brainstem. In proportion to its significance, the adult brain consists of 2% of overall body weight, but it accounts for 20% of the body's energy consumption.

Physical observation of the brain shows a distinction between gray matter, which is composed of dendrites and nerve cell bodies, and white matter, made of axons, which are surrounded by sheaths of myelin. Both areas are named for the colors that they display on gross examination. Observation also reveals many grooves and convoluted, raised areas on the cerebral surface, referred to respectively as gyri (singular: gyrus) and sulci (singular: sulcus).

Neurons

Neurons are the basic subunit of the nervous system. A neuron is composed of a cell body with a large nucleus, an axon, and dendrites. The cell body and dendrites of the neuron make up the gray matter of the cortex and brain nuclei. The myelinated axons make up the white matter. Neurons transmit information by sending action potentials, or waves of electric depolarization, down their axon processes to other neurons. Two processes project from the cell body: *dendrites* and *axons*. The dendrites receive impulses from other neurons and transmit these impulses to the cell body. Interesting facts concerning axons include:

- Some axons are 3 feet long but invisible to the naked eye.
- Some axons synapse with thousands of dendrites and receive impulses from thousands of other neurons.

In spite of the huge numbers and types of neurons, among them there is remarkable consistency of components, internal signaling mechanisms, patterns of connections between nerve cells and their targets (e.g., muscles, glands), and how they are shaped and modified by their environment. Some basic principles of nerve functioning include dynamic polarization, meaning that electrical signals within a nerve cell flow in only one direction:

1. From several dendrites, the short processes that extend and branch out from the main body of the cell and that receive incoming signals from another nerve cell
2. To the cell body which contains the nucleus of the cell
3. To the axon, a single tubular process that extends from the cell body to send signals to other nerve cells

The sequence of nervous electrical impulses can be remembered by the mnemonic "D-N-A," representing Dendrite → Nucleus (cell body) → Axon. To increase the speed of transmission, axons are wrapped in a lipid sheath called myelin (which is white), like electrical wires are coated with plastic polymers for insulation. Nerves do not connect randomly with each other but make specific connections with others to form networks. Axons end mostly on dendrites and cell bodies of other nerve cells and (less often) other axons. The space from the axon to the nearby neuron is called a synapse; electrical signals cause the release of chemical messengers or neurotransmitters from the presynaptic axon. These

[a]The authors would like to thank Richard A. Sugerman for his previous contribution to this chapter.

TABLE 4.1 Classification of Selected Neurotransmitters and Pathways

Category	Neurotransmitter	Location in Central Nervous System	Major Pathways
Cholinergic	Acetylcholine	Basal nucleus of Meynert and in the pons	Basal nucleus of Meynert to cerebral cortex; septal area to hippocampus
Monoamines	Dopamine	Substantia nigra	Nigrostriatal
		VTA	Mesolimbic
		VTA	Mesocortical
		Hypothalamus	Tuberoinfundibular
	Norepinephrine	Locus ceruleus	Locus ceruleus (in pons) to thalamus, cerebral cortex, cerebellum, and spinal cord
	Serotonin	Raphe nuclei	Rostral (i.e., going upward) raphe nuclei to thalamus, striatum, hypothalamus, hippocampus, nucleus accumbens, and prefrontal cortex. Caudal (i.e., going downward) raphe nuclei to cerebellum and spinal cord
Amino acids	GABA	Most common inhibitory transmitter in brain	Purkinje cells to deep cerebellar nuclei; striatonigral
	Glutamate	Most common excitatory transmitter in brain	Widely distributed in central nervous system

Note: This table presents a simplified summary of many of the better-known neurotransmitters and the general location where they are produced and released in the nervous system.
GABA, γ-Aminobutyric acid; *VTA*, ventral tegmental area.
From Keltner, N. L., & Folks, D. (2005). *Psychotropic drugs* (4th ed.). Mosby.

neurotransmitters diffuse over the gap (only 20 nm) between the cells (i.e., the synaptic cleft) and bind onto neurotransmitter receptors on the post-synaptic cell, which then causes signal propagation of electrical impulses in that cell. That signal propagation, or depolarization, is caused by:

1. A rapid change in the electrical properties of the nerve cell membrane
2. Produced by influx of positive charged ions from outside of the cell
3. Which neutralizes the negatively charged interior of the nerve cells
4. Thus generating an action potential that spreads downstream, ultimately toward the axon, where the process starts again

Neurons release neurotransmitters. Neurotransmitters are divided into four major groups or systems: cholinergics, monoamines, neuropeptides, and amino acids (Table 4.1). Specific examples for each group, where these specific transmitters are concentrated in the brain, and major brain pathways that use these neurotransmitters are indicated in Table 4.2. Neurotransmitters are thought to play major roles in some mental disorders (see Table 4.2). These concepts will be presented in detail in the disorders and pharmacology chapters.

Glia

Although glia were previously overlooked in favor of nerve cells, there is growing recognition of the role that glia serve to support and maintain nerve cells and assist in availability of chemical messengers in the nervous system. Glial cells are more abundant than neurons. Unlike neurons, they do not generate action potentials, which occur when cell membranes depolarize to propagate a nervous impulse that travels rapidly

TABLE 4.2 Neurotransmitters and Related Mental Disorders

Neurotransmitter	Mental Disorder
Increase (↑) in dopamine	Schizophrenia
Decrease (↓) in norepinephrine	Depression
Decrease (↓) in serotonin	Depression
Decrease (↓) in acetylcholine	Alzheimer disease
Decrease (↓) in GABA	Anxiety

Note: This table is a simplified explanation. A more detailed explanation is offered in appropriate chapters. GABA, γ-Aminobutyric acid.

along the axons of neurons to carry information between them. They are classified in three general groups with subtypes: oligodendrocytes, astrocytes, and microglia. A rough estimate of the composition of human brain is: 50% neurons, 20% astrocytes, 20% oligodendrocytes, and 10% microglia (Nestler, Kenny, Russo, & Schaefer, 2020).

Oligodendrocytes are cells that form myelin around axons to speed conductions of nervous impulses traveling through the cell membrane of the neuron. Their membranes wrap around the axon many times and can form the myelin sheath for several neurons at a time. They may also help provide trophic support to neurons by providing lactate to the neuron. In the PNS, these are termed Schwann cells.

Astrocytes form a bridge between capillaries and neurons. Their end feet attach to the basement membrane of endothelial cells and provide the blood-brain barrier that controls the entry of molecules and foreign bodies into the CNS. This blood-brain barrier keeps out water-soluble molecules, proteins, and ions but allows passage of fat-soluble moieties like gasses and alcohol. Astrocytes provide nutrients, maintain ion balance in CSF, help regulate blood flow, and form scar tissue in response to neural injury. They also play a role in storing and releasing glutamate, an excitatory neurotransmitter.

Microglia are similar to macrophages and monocytes and provide an important immune defense for the brain. They are wandering cells that remove cellular debris from injured and dying cells. They also release growth-promoting molecules to assist in nerve regeneration. Microglia help form and develop neuronal circuits through formation and pruning of synapse connections which are necessary for learning and memory, and by producing growth factors to support nerve cell maturation and survival (Vecchiarelli et al., 2021).

Cerebrum

The cerebrum constitutes the bulk of the nervous system. It has four divisions, or lobes. From front to back, these are the frontal, temporal, parietal, and occipital lobes. These subdivisions and their various functions are described shortly. The cerebrum is physically divided in half, or into hemispheres. Its hemispheres are spatially distinguished as right- or left-sided and are connected by bundles of nerve fibers, which allow for cross-communication between the two sides. The largest bundle is called the corpus callosum, but there are many other smaller pathways between the hemispheres. Because there may be several equivalent terms in neuroanatomy, pathways are also called tracts, fasciculi, peduncles, or lemnisci. When the corpus callosum is severed, as has been done in several instances for treatment of intractable seizures, a phenomenon known as "split brain syndrome" develops, confirming the lateralization of functions between the hemispheres. The dominant hemisphere (usually the left side) specializes in written language, syntax, and analytic functions, whereas the nondominant hemisphere (usually the right side) processes nonverbal functions such as visual-spatial tasks, music, and facial recognition. After the procedure, actions performed by one side are incomprehensible to the other. Although old memories and skills are preserved by each side, new tasks requiring communication between the sides, like learning to play a musical instrument, are impossible to learn.

The four cerebral lobes are separated by three deep grooves/sulci: the central sulcus, the lateral sulcus (or the lateral fissures of Sylvius), and the postcentral gyrus. After birth, the smooth surface of the cerebrum forms folds and grooves, which reflect nerve cell growth, until brain maturation is complete in adulthood. The reshaping of the cortical surface area is a function of increased neural volume. A comparison can be made to the coastline of Norway. If it did not have its many fjords, it would stretch to 1600 miles; but with them, it stretches to over 15,000 miles!

Nervous System Pathways

Every part of the cerebrum receives afferent "entering" pathways from cortical or subcortical areas and projects efferent "leaving" pathways to these locations. The cortex has primary association areas supplied by afferents from sensory organs, with secondary association areas dedicated to refinements of those signals. Similarly, it has primary association areas for movement to supply efferent signals for muscles, with secondary association areas for refinement of those signals. A sensory pathway typically consists of a relay of three neurons, starting with a nerve cell in a sensory ganglion located outside the spinal cord. This neuron projects to the second neuron in the spinal cord or brainstem, which then "hands off" the signal to the third neuron in the thalamus. The thalamus is a kind of central warehouse for the CNS that ships and receives signals to the upper and lower brain areas. A motor pathway typically originates in the motor cortex and projects to neurons in the spinal cord or brainstem to supply its muscular target. These pathways are influenced at all levels by interneurons, which can dampen or enhance signals in these pathways.

> The terms *anterior* or *ventral* as opposed to *posterior* or *dorsal* are the same. This direction occurs on the axial plane, from front to back, or nose to occiput. The terms *superior* or *rostral* are opposed to their respective terms *inferior* or *caudal*, from head to tail, in the coronal plane. *Lateral* as opposed to *medial* refers to outer versus inner direction on the sagittal plane. Imagine viewing a patient face to face. You would be looking at him from the coronal plane. A view of him from the side is the sagittal view. Looking down on the top of his head is the axial view. However, radiographic convention (such as computed axial tomography [i.e., CAT scan]) dictates that the axial view should be represented from the bottom up, like viewing his head when standing at his feet as he is lying down.

Four Lobes of the Cerebrum: Frontal, Temporal, Parietal, Occipital

Frontal: thinking and moving. The frontal lobes are divided into motor and prefrontal areas. The motor area is divided into the primary motor cortex and the premotor cortex. Lying rostral (see the box on neuroanatomical directions) to the central sulcus, the primary motor cortex or "motor strip" generates descending signals to lower brain areas to control voluntary muscle activity. Nerve cells in the motor strip are topographically organized in a map, or homunculus, of the human body, with certain areas disproportionate to their body size (Fig. 4.1).

In front of the motor strip lies the premotor cortex, which prepares, guides, and sequences muscle movement and suppresses motor activity from lower brain areas. The corticospinal tract is a two-neuron pathway descending from the motor cortex (Fig. 4.2A). It descends through the corona radiata, and 80% of these neurons cross an area of the medulla called the pyramids to continue descending on the opposite side of the spinal cord (Fig. 4.2B). There, it terminates on the second nerve cell in the sequence, the lower motor neuron, which then innervates the muscles of the body. The remaining 20%

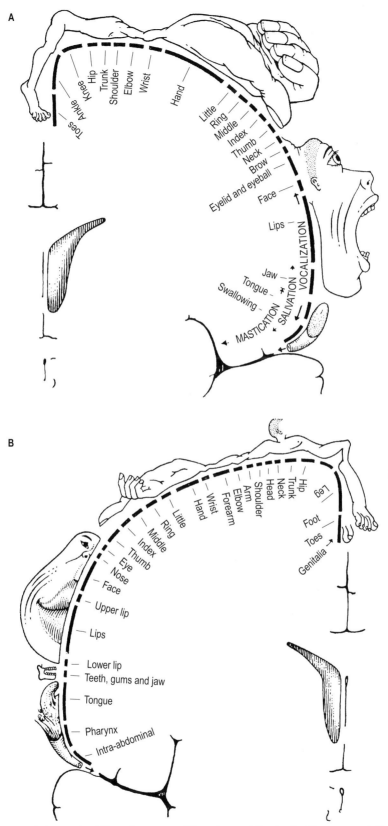

FIG. 4.1 Homunculus diagram of the motor (A) and sensory (B) regions of the brain. Sizes are relative to the amount of cortex dedicated to the body part. (From Standring, S. [2004]. *Gray's anatomy: The anatomical basis of clinical practice* [39th ed.]. Elsevier.)

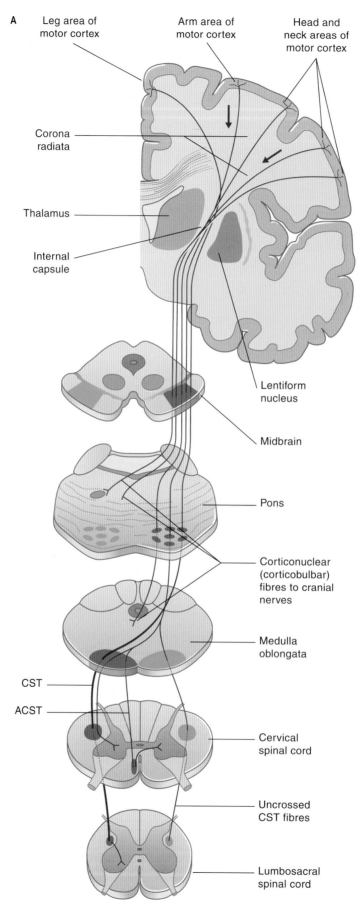

A

Leg area of motor cortex

Arm area of motor cortex

Head and neck areas of motor cortex

Corona radiata

Thalamus

Internal capsule

Lentiform nucleus

Midbrain

Pons

Corticonuclear (corticobulbar) fibres to cranial nerves

Medulla oblongata

CST

ACST

Cervical spinal cord

Uncrossed CST fibres

Lumbosacral spinal cord

FIG. 4.2 (A) Distribution of the corticospinal tract.

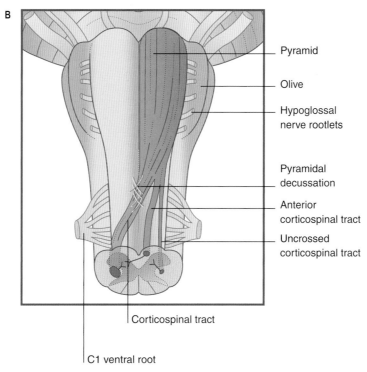

Pyramid

Olive

Hypoglossal
nerve rootlets

Pyramidal
decussation

Anterior
corticospinal tract

Uncrossed
corticospinal tract

Corticospinal tract

C1 ventral root

FIG. 4.2, cont'd   (B) Crossing or decussation of the pyramids. *CST,* Corticospinal tract; *ACST,* anterior corticospinal tract. (From Mtui, E., Gruener, G., & Dockery, P. [2015]. *Fitzgerald's clinical neuroanatomy and neuroscience* [7th ed.]. Elsevier.)

of the corticospinal tract theoretically might be responsible for some limited motor recovery in patients with hemisected spinal cords; however, any significant long-term recovery is rare at best. The term pyramidal is used because most neurons pass through the pyramids of the medulla. The term extrapyramidal refers to nerves that do not pass through this area and that control involuntary movements and reflexes. These include the basal ganglia, cerebellum, and other brain areas that indirectly influence motor activity. Disturbances in the extrapyramidal system (EPS) are marked by abnormal involuntary movements, hypokinesis, alterations in muscle tone, and postural disturbances. Disturbances of this functional network are manifested in conditions such as Parkinson disease (PD) and Huntington disease, as well as with adverse effects of antipsychotic medications (i.e., extrapyramidal side effects [EPSEs]). More about this system is covered later in the section "Movement" and in Chapter 14.

The lower posterior frontal lobes also contain an area that is responsible for expressive speech and language (the Broca area). The prefrontal cortex, which comprises the anterior two-thirds of the frontal lobes, is the center of executive functions, conscious thought, and regulation of emotions (see the sections "Attention," "Memory," "Cognition," and "Emotions").

Temporal: Smelling, Hearing, Speaking

The temporal lobes are divided into (1) pre-olfactory and olfactory areas for odor detection and processing, with connections to the limbic system for corresponding emotional responses; (2) primary and secondary auditory association

areas (unlike the other sensory modalities, these areas are highly interconnected between hemispheres for receiving and localizing sounds in space); (3) a speech receptive area (the Wernicke area, which also includes part of the inferior parietal lobe); (4) areas involved in complex visual processing, such as facial recognition (fusiform gyrus); and (5) areas critical for memory encoding, retrieval, integration with emotional states, and consolidation into other brain areas for long-term storage (see later in the section "Memory").

Parietal: sensing. The parietal lobes contain the primary somatosensory cortex posterior to the central gyrus, which is so interconnected with the motor strip that it is sometimes referred to as the sensorimotor strip, and behind that, posterior portions essential for performance of complicated motor tasks, tactile discrimination, right-left distinction, spatial orientation, number and letter recognition, and many others. The somatosensory areas also have a sensory representation of the body surface, a homunculus, similar to that of the motor strip. For example, the area for hand movement on the motor strip is roughly equal to the area of hand sensation on the somatosensory strip.

Occipital: seeing. The occipital lobes at the back of the brain include the primary visual cortex. This cortex is innervated by thalamic nuclei, which are in turn supplied by the optic nerve. Optic nerve fibers form binocular vision by uncrossed fibers from the medial or nasal visual field with crossed fibers from the lateral visual field. In other words, binocular vision is dependent on sensory input from both eyes. The occipital cortex also includes the visual association cortex, which includes all of the occipital lobes and portions of the parietal and temporal lobes. It enables visual recognition and analysis; perception of depth, color, and movement; and recall of images. In contrast to temporal lobe lesions, which can produce various types of visual aphasias (e.g., inability to understand written language or recognize familiar faces), lesions in the primary visual cortex of the occipital lobe result in loss of vision (blindness) from the contralateral visual field; that is, damage to the left side of the primary visual cortex results in loss of vision from the right visual field.

Cerebellum

The cerebellum consists of two hemispheres separated by a central portion called the vermis. It receives sensory input and motor signals from the cerebral cortex. It is supplied by afferents from the spinocerebellar tracts, which carry input from touch and pressure receptors and proprioceptive endings, and interconnective pathways from the basal ganglia and the vestibular system. Communicating mostly through the thalamus, it coordinates sensory input from somatosensory cortices and primary and secondary motor areas for the overall purpose of allowing a movement to be executed the way it is intended. The three divisions of the cerebellum regulate balance, stabilize the eyes during movement, and influence muscle tone and coordination of the extremities and skilled voluntary movements and speech. The cerebellum also plays a role in learning and regulation of other behaviors in ways that continue to be discovered. Differences between movement disorders associated with cerebellar dysfunction and movement disorders associated with basal ganglia dysfunction are presented in Box 4.1.

Cerebellar dysfunction can produce intention tremors on the same side of the body as the lesion. In contrast to basal ganglia resting tremors, which occur at rest, intention tremors occur when a person is asked to touch something, such as his or her own nose or a physician's moving finger. Such individuals have tremors when they attempt to concentrate on moving a limb. Basal ganglia disorders involve hypokinesis, impairment in postural reflexes, and, as mentioned above, resting tremor.

Brainstem

The brainstem is one of the oldest regions in the human brain. Its structure resembles the entire brain of present-day reptiles. It is the origin of all motor cranial nerves and the termination of all sensory cranial nerves except for the olfactory (smell) and optic (sight) nerves. Nerve cell bodies in the brainstem are necessary for respiration, cardiac output, and other vital functions. The brainstem is divided into the midbrain, pons, and medulla oblongata, and it connects the cerebrum to the spinal cord. The midbrain contains the substantia nigra, which is pigmented black from neuromelanin, and the ventral tegmental area (VTA). Both are adjacent to each other and supply dopamine to higher brain areas. The substantia nigra projects a bundle of dopamine fibers through the nigrostriatal pathway to the striatum, which consists of the caudate nucleus and putamen. Dopamine afferents from the substantia nigra assist voluntary movement commands

---

BOX 4.1   Differences Between Basal Ganglia and Cerebellar Movement Disorders

General Difference
- Cerebellar dysfunction: Awkwardness of intentional movement
- Basal ganglia dysfunction: Meaningless, unintentional movement that occurs unexpectedly

Cerebellar Disorders
- Ataxia: Awkwardness of posture and gait; lack of coordination; overshooting the goal when reaching for an object; inability to perform rapid, alternating movements, such as finger tapping; awkward use of speech muscles, resulting in irregularly spaced sounds
- Decreased tendon reflexes on affected side
- Asthenia: Muscles tiring easily
- Intention tremor: Noticed when intending to do something, such as reaching for a pencil
- Adiadochokinesia: Inability to perform fine, rapidly repeated coordinated movements

Basal Ganglia Disorders
- Parkinsonism: Rigidity, bradykinesia, resting tremor, mask-like face, shuffling gait
- Chorea: Sudden, jerky, and purposeless movements (e.g., Huntington disease, Sydenham chorea)
- Athetosis: Slow, writhing, snakelike movements, especially of fingers and wrists
- Hemiballismus: Sudden, wild flailing of one arm
- Nystagmus: Involuntary rapid eye movements

Modified from Goldberg, S. (2003). *Clinical neuroanatomy* (3rd ed.). MedMaster.

---

from the corticospinal tract to modulate movement, maintain appropriate muscle tone, and adjust posture. The VTA projects pathways through the mesolimbic and mesocortical pathways to limbic and cortical areas, respectively. The limbic target of the mesolimbic pathway is the nucleus accumbens, which integrates dopamine input from the VTA and glutamate input from the prefrontal cortex to determine motivational response to environmental stimuli. It is the center of the brain's reward system and is the primary mediator for substance abuse and addictions. The mesocortical pathway assists the prefrontal cortical areas with cognition and attention, and lower dopamine activity in this area is associated with attention-deficit/hyperactivity disorder. The pons, which means "bridge," connects the cerebellum and cerebrum. It has nuclei that regulate breathing and rapid eye movement (REM) sleep, or dream states, and sleep paralysis. It contains parts of the trigeminal (cranial nerve V) motor and sensory nuclei and the abducens, facial, and vestibulocochlear (cranial nerves VI, VII, and VIII) nuclei. The medulla is the site of the decussation, or crossing over, of the pyramidal corticospinal tract, and it is the site of other cranial nerve nuclei and autonomic (involuntary) nerve groups that regulate respiration, digestion, cardiac functions, and other automated functions of the body.

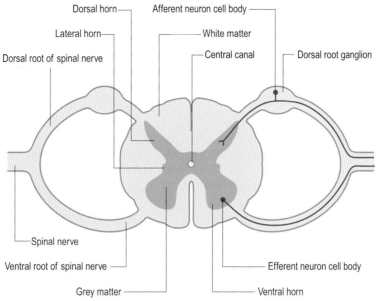

FIG. 4.3 Transverse section through the spinal cord illustrating the disposition of gray and white matter and the attachment of dorsal and ventral spinal nerve roots. (From Standring, S. [2004]. *Gray's anatomy: The anatomical basis of clinical practice* [39th ed.]. Elsevier.)

Spinal Cord

The spinal cord forms an interface between the CNS and the rest of the body. It consists of ascending and descending pathways to and from higher areas in the brain, and the segmentally localized nerve clusters that link these areas with spinal nerves, which innervate the rest of the body and form the PNS. Spinal nerves are divided into sensory, motor, and autonomic components. Sensory nerves from the periphery, whose cell bodies lie in the dorsal root ganglia (a specialized nerve cluster that runs outside of and parallel to the spinal cord), comprise the somatic division of the PNS. They innervate the skin, muscle, and joints of the body and relay information about touch, proprioception (the location of one part of the body in relation to other parts), pain, and temperature to the dorsal column of the spinal cord. Nerve clusters in the dorsal column interface with the endings of the sensory nerves and relay information upward to higher levels of the CNS. Motor nerve clusters in the ventral horn of the spinal cord receive information from the corticospinal tract descending from the brainstem and cortex, leave the spinal cord through spinal nerves, and innervate skeletal muscles (Fig. 4.3).

Autonomic Nervous System

The autonomic component of the PNS supplies the viscera, or internal organs of the body, and is divided into the parasympathetic and the sympathetic nervous systems; the former is usually involved in inhibiting body processes or generating energy, and the latter is associated with stimulating body processes or expending energy. The autonomic pathways are usually composed of a sequence of two nerve cells, and the cell body of the first neuron, or *preganglionic*

neuron, resides in the spinal cord. Its axon connects to a *postganglionic* nerve cell outside of the CNS in a clump of neurons called an *autonomic ganglion*. Most parasympathetic ganglia are located near the organs to which they connect, and most sympathetic ganglia reside close to and on either side of the spinal cord. Parasympathetic nerves project from cranial nerves III, VII, IX, and X and from sacral regions S2 to S4. They mediate pupillary and ciliary body constriction (III); lacrimation or tearing (VII); salivation (IX); and respiration, digestion, cardiac function, and many body functions from the neck down to the second segment of the transverse colon (cranial nerve X). Parasympathetic nerves from below the second, third, and fourth sacral bodies, known as pelvic splanchnic nerves, innervate the bladder, urethral sphincter, rectum, and sexual organs. Sympathetic nerves extend from below the first thoracic vertebra and extend to the second or third lumbar vertebrae. They mobilize the body's "fight-or-flight" responses to threats via pupillary dilation, enhancing the heart rate and forcing cardiac contractions, bronchodilation, breakdown of glucose reserves in the liver, increasing muscular contractility, decreasing gut motility, perspiration, piloerection, and shunting blood flow away from organs that are not necessary for immediate survival to those that are. It also mediates ejaculation in sexual functioning. The sympathetic nerves are responsible for balancing the effects of the parasympathetic nervous system, for example, by maintaining blood pressure and body temperature in a balanced process called *homeostasis*, which causes the body to "feed and breed" and then "rest and digest."

Ventricular System

The brain floats in approximately 140 mL (about the volume of a small cup of coffee) of cerebrospinal fluid (CSF);

however, the CNS produces approximately 800 mL of fluid per day. CSF circulates around the brain in the subarachnoid space and inside ventricles in the brain. CSF bathes the brain and spinal cord for nutrient support and shock absorption. Certain drugs cross the blood-brain barrier and others do not. For those that do (psychoactive agents), CNS clearance times are different from plasma clearance times in the systemic circulation. This can affect dosing times and frequencies if the CNS is the intended pharmacological target.

Three connective tissue layers, known as meninges, cover the brain. The subarachnoid space is a narrow space that is located between the middle meningeal layer (arachnoid) and innermost layer (pia mater) and adheres to the brain. The thick outer layer, the dura mater, attaches to the inner surface of many bones of the skull.

FUNCTIONAL LOCALIZATION OF THE NERVOUS SYSTEM

Movement

The basal ganglia are groups of nerve cells that lie beneath the cortical layers. Unlike the cerebellum, which affects dynamic movements, the basal ganglia influence static muscular activities like posture and stabilization of limbs. The basal ganglia include the caudate nucleus and the putamen (both collectively termed the *striatum*) as well as the globus pallidus. Because of connections with the frontal cortex, the caudate is also involved in cognitive and emotional processes. The putamen receives excitatory input from the sensorimotor strip. In turn, nerve pathways from the inhibitory cells of the caudate and putamen project to the internal and external divisions of the globus pallidus. Dopamine tracts from the substantia nigra excite the caudate and putamen, thereby inducing inhibitory effects from these two nuclei. The external globus pallidus projects inhibition to the subthalamic nucleus, which in turn excites the internal globus pallidus. The net effect of these three nerve groups is to return inhibitory effects to the thalamus, which reduces its inhibitory effects on the cortex and results in cortical activation. This system of neural circuitry is called the cortico-striatal-thalamic loop, or CSTC loop, and plays a sentinel role in understanding PD, the adverse effects of antipsychotics, and possibly obsessive-compulsive disorder and other psychiatric conditions. A reduction of dopamine influence on the caudate and putamen causes less inhibition to the globus pallidus, with the downstream effect of less cortical excitation. In PD, the death of dopamine-releasing cells in the substantia nigra reduces dopamine. Without the excitatory effect of dopamine to the striatum, more pallidal firing reduces thalamic activity. Cortical activating effects are reduced, and there is a decline in initiation and execution of motor activity, causing bradykinesia; disinhibition of muscular control causes resting tremor, rigidity, and loss of postural reflexes. Treatment efforts in PD are directed at resupplying dopamine to the CNS via L-dopa or providing dopamine agonists. Because the effectiveness of these medications declines due to a declining cell population

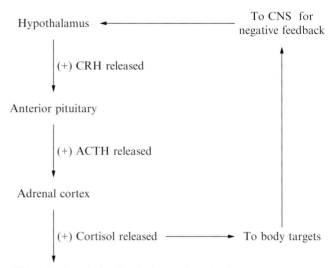

FIG. 4.4 Hypothalamic-pituitary-adrenal axis.

in the substantia nigra, some cases are treated with surgical implantation of a pacemaker near the subthalamic nucleus, which increases pallidal inhibition and results in cortical activation. Similar problems emerge when dopamine is blocked by neuroleptics; this effect is countered with anticholinergic agents, which reduce the cholinergic activity in the striatum, thus enhancing dopamine.

Hormonal Regulation

In addition to controlling the autonomic nervous system and regulating sleep and wakefulness (see the sections "Sleep" and "Level of Consciousness" below), the hypothalamus controls the body's homeostasis by hormonal release. It monitors sodium and water balances, levels of oxygen in the bloodstream, body temperature, feeding and appetite, thirst and fluid intake, growth, sexual development, thyroid and adrenal gland functioning, lactation, rage, and emotional arousal.

The hypothalamus has two types of connections to the pituitary for hormonal release. A portal system of blood vessels carries released hormones to the anterior pituitary, where the circulating factor is taken up to stimulate a cascade of stimulating hormones that target an endocrine gland in the periphery. In response to the pituitary stimulating hormone, the endocrine organ releases its physiologic hormone to cause its intended biologic effects; this hormone also circulates back to the hypothalamus to cut off a further hormonal cascade via negative feedback. For example, corticotropin-releasing hormone (CRH), which is released by the hypothalamus, stimulates the release of adrenocorticotropic hormone (ACTH). ACTH then stimulates the release of cortisol from the adrenal gland. Cortisol inhibits further release of CRH from the hypothalamus (Fig. 4.4). Similar cascades exist for thyroid hormone, sex hormones, growth hormone, and prolactin (Table 4.3).

The posterior pituitary (Fig. 4.5) is directly innervated by the hypothalamus and releases vasopressin, or antidiuretic hormone (ADH), to stimulate water resorption by the kidneys, or oxytocin to stimulate uterine contractions during

TABLE 4.3 Hormonal Cascade From the Hypothalamus to Behavioral Effects

Hypothalamus-Made Hormones	Pituitary Gland	Target Gland or Hormone	Possible Behavioral Effect
Corticotropin-releasing hormone (CRH)	Stimulates production of two hormones: 1. ACTH 2. β-Endorphin	Adrenal gland—produces cortisol and cortisol-related hormones ACTH drives cortisol production	1. Stress causes release of cortisol 2. Depressed children have decreased diurnal cortisol secretory pattern 3. Depressed adolescents have increased cortisol around sleep onset 4. CRH increases in patients with PTSD 5. Patients with PTSD have a blunted ACTH response to CRH 6. β-Endorphin is involved in endorphin pleasure pathway and feeling good
Thyroid-releasing hormone (TRH)	Stimulates production of TSH	Thyroid gland produces T_4 and T_3	1. Adding T_3 or T_4 to an antidepressant regimen may potentiate medication's response 2. In PTSD, T_3 level may be increased
Prolactin-releasing factor (PRF)	Stimulates production of prolactin	Mammary glands—produce milk	No significant effects; feminizing effect

Note: This table lists the following: (1) hypothalamic hormones—states whether they are releasing or inhibiting; (2) the specific hormones that they affect in the anterior pituitary gland (Griffin & Ojeda, 2004); (3) the way in which they affect hormone production; (4) the target glands or body cells affected; and (5) the proposed effects of the hormones on behavior (Charney, Nestler, & Bunney, 2008). *ACTH,* Adrenocorticotropic hormone; *PTSD,* posttraumatic stress disorder; *TSH,* thyroid-stimulating hormone; T_3, triiodothyronine; T_4, thyroxine.

childbirth. Other hypothalamic functions are integral to fear and rage displays, sexual arousal, and memory, by way of connections to the limbic circuit and thalamus.

Sleep

The need to sleep is universal, but a definite answer as to why we need sleep remains elusive (Nestler, Kenny, Russo, & Schaefer, 2020). Sleep is important for the consolidation of memory into long-term storage. But as a general restorative period for the body, sleep and quiet wakefulness expend about the same amount of energy. Sleep also has the disadvantage of reducing vigilance against threat. But it is prevalent in all animal species and therefore has a fundamental function which lacks a full explanation. Lack of sleep has profound consequences on emotional and physical health. The invention of the lightbulb has disrupted a finely tuned physiologic orchestration of several processes. A more complete explanation of sleep can be found in many references and what follows is a basic description of sleep and wakefulness.

There is a reciprocal inhibitory exchange between the major ascending arousal pathways and sleep-inducing areas of the brain. The three arousal pathways are:
1. *cholinergic* cell groups in the pons which provide input to the relay and reticular nuclei of the thalamus, known as the pedunculopontine and laterodorsal tegmental (PPT/LDT) nuclei,
2. *monoaminergic* circuits: noradrenergic neurons of the locus coeruleus, serotoninergic dorsal and median raphe nuclei, dopaminergic neurons of the ventral periaqueductal grey matter, and the histaminergic tuberomammilary nucleus (TMN), all collectively known as the ascending reticular activating system (ARAS), and

3. *orexin*-containing cell groups in the lateral hypothalamus, which promote wakefulness by up-regulating monoaminergic neuronal populations (Schwartz & Roth, 2008).

Sleep is initiated by the inhibitory GABA-ergic and galaninergic neurons of the ventrolateral preoptic nucleus (VLPO). They quiet the ascending monoaminergic arousal system during sleep.

The interaction between arousal and sleep systems function to suppress the activity of one system while the other is in operation. This provides stability to each system, while providing a rapid transition from one state to another, thereby enhancing survival. Intrusion of sleep states into periods of arousal can have drastic consequences (e.g., driving a motor vehicle and falling asleep).

There is a homeostatic sleep drive that builds the longer a person stays awake. Adenosine accumulates in the cholinergic pathway of the basal forebrain while awake. Recovery sleep leads to a decline in adenosine. Caffeine antagonizes adenosine receptors, temporarily attenuating the effects of sleep deprivation.

A circadian rhythm which is regulated by environmental cues like light exposure entrains the sleep cycle. This rhythm is controlled by the supra-chiasmatic nucleus (SCN). With exposure to light, retinal ganglion cells relay input to the SCN which inhibits the pineal gland via a complex circuit. The absence of light causes the synthesis and release of melatonin. Melatonin receptors MT1 and MT2 have sleep-promoting effects and reduce body temperature, which enhances sleep continuity.

Sleep exists in two phases which alternate along with brief periods of wakefulness: non-rapid eye movement (NREM)

Two hypothalamic neurons

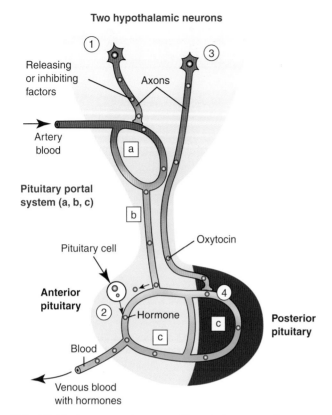

FIG. 4.5 Pituitary portal system. The pituitary portal system has a capillary bed (a) at the base of the hypothalamus, a capillary bed (c) in the pituitary gland, and a portal vein (b) in between. Hypothalamic neurons (1, 3) make hormones (i.e., neurotransmitters). The neuron (1) releases its hormone into the capillary bed (a), and the hormone descends through the portal vessel (b) into the pituitary gland capillary bed (c). The hormone leaves the capillary bed and causes anterior pituitary gland cells to release specific hormones back into the capillary (2) for transport to glands or cells elsewhere in the body. A few hormones from the hypothalamus inhibit the production of pituitary gland cell hormones. The neuron (3) directly releases its hormone (e.g., oxytocin) into the posterior pituitary portion of the capillary bed (c). The hormone again leaves the blood (4) and travels to glands or cells elsewhere in the body.

and REM. NREM typically progresses from drowsiness or stage N1 to deeper stages N2 and N3. This phase is characterized by reduced body temperature and metabolism. Lighter phases predominate in the early portion of sleep and deeper phases occur later in the cycle. In the later portion of the cycle, REM sleep increases in frequency and duration. The brain is active in REM sleep, similar to wakefulness. But the body is generally paralyzed except for eye muscles. Dreaming occurs in all stages of sleep, but is most vivid during REM sleep.

Level of Consciousness

Consciousness is the "property of being aware of oneself and one's place in the environment" (Kandel, Schwartz, Jessell, Siegelbaum, & Hudspeth, 2013). This can be observed by watching an individual respond appropriately to his or her environment. The basis of responsive control is a consistent state of global alertness, which is subtended by *the ascending arousal system*, a network extending from the brainstem and hypothalamus to the thalamus and cerebral cortex. Full self-awareness can be compromised by defective communication between the two cerebral hemispheres; for example, hemi-agnosia, or neglect syndrome, is the inability to recognize stimulation on one side after a cerebral injury on the opposite side. Changes or aberrations in the level of consciousness can reflect injury to the brainstem, which produces waves of excitatory input to higher brain areas by thalamic and hypothalamic pathways. Higher-level injuries, such as bilateral frontal cerebral hemorrhage, can induce coma by increasing intracranial pressure, and metabolic states like hepatic encephalopathy can induce generalized brainwave slowing with associated reduction or impaired level of consciousness. To assess focal brainstem structural injury, patterns of respiration (Cheyne-Stokes breathing), asymmetric responses to pain or motor reflexes, loss of pupillary response to light or unilateral pupil dilation, loss of conjugate eye gaze or combined movement of both eyes in the direction when the head is moved or when cool or warm water is poured into the ear, and patterns of limb posturing (decerebrate = both arms and legs extended, decorticate = arms flexed, legs extended) can indicate this important and emergent state for immediate intervention.

Sensation

Information from the periphery to higher brain areas must pass through several nerve relays and undergo processing before the brain can integrate and act adaptively to this information. Different sensations are conducted by different nerve types. Stubbing one's toe can elicit an initial sensation, followed by a distinctly different and even more unpleasant sensation, created by different nerve pathways traveling at different speeds from toe to brain. Spinal nerves transmit sensations from areas close to the level at which they are located, because of their embryological formation in common with other structures they supply, such as bone and muscle. Dermatomes are skin areas innervated by a single dorsal root and can help correlate the site of injury to damage at a specific level of the spinal cord.

The somatosensory system refers to pathways carrying touch, pressure, pain, temperature, position, movement, and vibration from peripheral areas into conscious awareness of these sensations. A three-neuron circuit from the spinal cord, brainstem, and thalamus shunts information into a part of the parietal cortex (postcentral gyrus) termed the somatosensory cortex. Information from the thalamus and primary somatosensory cortex is relayed for further processing to the secondary somatosensory cortex, then to other brain areas such as the motor cortex for initiation of responses.

In the spinothalamic pathway, the axons of second-order nerves (those nerves second in a multiple-nerve chain), which convey pain, temperature, light touch, and firm pressure, cross the midline of the body at the level at which they reside in the spinal cord, then ascend to the thalamus to terminate on the third neuron in the sequence. The posterior column pathway consists of second-order axons that convey discriminative touch, awareness of position, tactile movement across the skin, textures, shapes, and vibration. They ascend on the same side of the body until they reach the medulla and then terminate on another group of neurons. This additional third-order neuronal relay ascends to the thalamus to synapse on the somatosensory cortex.

This distinction can be clinically significant because a unilateral spinal cord injury may damage the sensation for pain and temperature on the opposite side of the body, as well as proprioception (awareness of joint position) and touch localization on the same side of the body at the level below the injury. This is called Brown-Séquard syndrome and illustrates the different locations of sensory pathways and where they cross the midline.

Pain

Sensations can be altered by normal and pathological states at the spinal cord level. Diversion of afferent pain stimuli can be accomplished by affecting the "gates" of pain processing by transdermal electrical nerve stimulation, known as TENS. Chronic, repeated pain stimuli can cause a process called *central sensitization*, an inflammatory soup of neurokinins, substance P, and other pain-inducing neurotransmitters and neuropeptides that attenuates pain control and creates painful responses to sensations that normally do not cause pain (technically called allodynia). Phantom limb pain, the persistence of pain perceived as emanating from a previously amputated limb, is an example of this phenomenon.

Pain contributes to heightened alertness, avoidance, distress, increased motion even to agitation, and many physiological responses associated with sympathetic overarousal. Pain can mobilize adaptive responses to reduce pain, which, when employed over time, may lead to maladaptive responses (e.g., chronic dependence on opioid analgesia). Pain can also be reduced by the descending spinal pathways, which reduce the upward flow of pain-inducing stimuli.

Perception

Perception is the integration of sensory input for purposes of interpreting the environment in a two-step process. First, recognition of sensation occurs at higher brain areas; elaboration and attention to sensation follows, based on the individual's experience and expectations. A blindfolded person can distinguish a coin from a piece of ice placed in his hand because of aggregated information streams of size, weight, temperature, texture, and pain information, which are compared with past experiences and exposure to these objects. Inputs from each location and sensory modality are represented in the somatosensory cortex in a map-like representation of a little human, or *homunculus*, which is disproportionate to the actual human body because it exaggerates sensory input from the face. Your face is more sensitive than your elbow because sensory input from the face (as with input from mouth, hands, and feet) is more greatly represented in the homunculus than other areas like the limbs and trunk. Sensory information from this area is routed to memory traces residing in the association cortices to form a mental representation of any given experience to provide context and meaning for that experience. This stream of sensation, combined with association links with contextual memory systems in the temporal and frontal lobes, reacts to and monitors whatever is objectively observable by sensory modalities.

Reward

The ventral striatum contains the nucleus accumbens, the central mediator of sensations of reward and pleasure. This area is innervated by dopamine-releasing neurons from a brainstem area called the ventral tegmentum. Pleasure-inducing activities and euphoric drugs activate this area. It has connections with association areas and memory systems that can induce cravings with environmental cues and memories. Instabilities in the availability of responses of dopamine receptors may predispose certain individuals to addictions. Reward also plays a part in sustaining activities that require ongoing attention and concentration, which may be deficient in individuals with attention-deficit/hyperactivity disorder.

Attention

Intentional processing of internal and external stimuli is a hallmark of consciousness. Adaptive responses mandate flexible shifting between these inputs. Attention is the selection of relevant information over irrelevant information. Attention consists of the interworking of brain areas dedicated to arousal, orientation, and detection. Motivation for these activities is provided by brain areas involved in both pleasure and pain, the latter providing more valence and reinforcement. Touching a hot stove leaves a more memorable impression than tasting candy. The prefrontal regions of the frontal lobe modulate information streams from deeper brain areas, such as the ascending arousal system; impulses that drive hunger, aggression, and sexual arousal; stress signals from the amygdala, which cause unpleasant emotional states; memory retrieval from the hippocampus and entorhinal cortex in the temporal lobe; and pain and other body signals from the somatosensory cortex. The prefrontal cortex (PFC) can also connect with other specialized brain regions that identify aspects of the environment such as facial recognition, colors, shapes, and locations. Sustaining attention involves coordination among several brain regions.

The collective experience of attention involves:
1. Arousal, or maintenance of alertness
2. Salience, or the screening out of irrelevant sensory input
3. Focusing, or the ability to shift attention away from one thing to another and to select competing inputs
4. Concentration, or the ability to sustain purposeful allocation to a selected input (for example, a college student blocking out noise in the dorm and focusing on his or her studies)

Because it is a finite cellular entity, attention is necessarily limited, providing a "spotlight" of immediate attention, with many other stimuli filtered out in the process. Because other areas are reengaged in shifts of attention (retrieval of

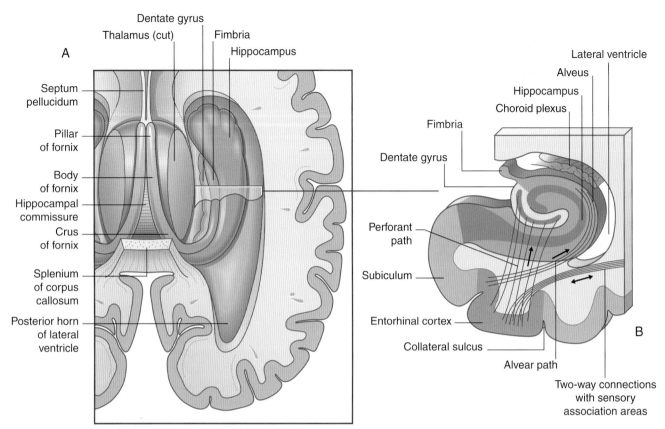

FIG. 4.6 Hippocampal complex. (A) View from above. (B) Enlargement from (A) showing the entorhinal cortex and the three component parts of the hippocampal complex. (From Mtui, E., Gruener, G., & Dockery, P. [2015]. *Fitzgerald's clinical neuroanatomy and neuroscience* [7th ed.]. Elsevier.)

memories and associations), a delay in attentional awareness accompanies such a change, to the delight of illusionists and pickpockets.

When the brain goes "offline"—that is, when daydreaming or when withdrawn from focusing on the external environment—brain activity intensifies in the medial and lateral parietal, medial prefrontal, and medial and lateral temporal cortices. Although widely debated, this "default network" appears to support consolidation of memories, emotional processing, self-evaluation and reference, and even story comprehension.

When an individual observes another's movement, nerve cells ("mirror neurons") respond in that individual's brain as if they were actually performing that action. Mirroring may occur not only in motor brain areas, but in wider areas such as language comprehension and emotional relatedness, helping to negotiate a socially complex environment. Dysfunction in this system may serve as a partial explanation for autism.

Memory

Memory is not a solitary system but involves several capacities performed by widely spread brain areas. As currently conceived, working memory is stored in frontal cortical areas and involves the encoding, storage, and retrieval of information, which degrades after a few minutes. A "visual-spatial scratchpad" stores images and action; a "phonological loop" records language and sounds for temporary use in the immediate environment, with the possibility of transfer into longer-term storage. Working memory occurs in the association cortices of the prefrontal cortex.

Episodic or contextual memory is mediated by the hippocampus from information acquired through one of the senses. This information is processed by the association cortices of that particular modality and then conveyed through the perirhinal, parahippocampal, and entorhinal cortices to the hippocampus. There, information follows a tri-synaptic pathway, which binds and organizes it for return to the association cortices. Memory traces linked to cues from the environment are combined with other memory traces that are temporally related to an event to form a more complete memory of that event. One remembers an event based on the retrieval and consolidation of partial memories occurring within the context of that event. The hippocampus and its affiliated structures permit the retrieval of associational cues, links them, and delivers them, like an air traffic controller directs a jet onto a runway (Fig. 4.6).

Semantic memory, occurring in the parietal lobes, is involved with the retrieval of memories that do not have contextual cues. Remembering the address where you grew up does not need a cue or context to retrieve it; it is simply there in permanent storage to recover when needed. It is a more stable neural formation, and information may be available for much longer periods than in the previously described memory systems.

Motor skills or habits, like riding a bicycle, are encoded in the basal ganglia, do not involve reflection or conscious awareness, and closely resemble the motor activities occurring during the time when learning first occurred. A patient with Alzheimer disease (AD) who learned a skill before the onset of dementia may be able to continue that procedure well past the decline in episodic memory, which is the first manifestation of that disease. The patient may be able to drive a car well, but because of hippocampal degeneration with the loss of navigational skills, he or she may soon become easily lost!

Memory Review

- Episodic/contextual memory—Hippocampus
- Semantic memory—Parietal lobe
- Motor skills memory—Basal ganglia

Cognition

Cogito ergo sum (I think, therefore I am)

—Descartes

Effective higher cognition includes integrating and effectively applying the summation of many areas of brain functioning, including judgment, volition, adaptive switching between concrete and abstract thinking, and suppressing unwanted, undesirable, or habitual responses. It includes (but is not limited to) the following processes:

- Attention and vigilance: Responding correctly to stimuli and not responding to distractions (e.g., reading an article or watching a show)
- Working memory: Maintaining and using information just received (e.g., remembering and entering a pass code as it is being communicated)
- Verbal learning: Remembering verbal information over longer periods of time (e.g., remembering what somebody was told to do in the immediate future)
- Visual learning: Remembering visual information over longer periods of time (e.g., remembering where you left your keys)
- Problem-solving and reasoning: Applying strategies to new or changed circumstances (e.g., learning to use a tool or instrument for the first time)
- Processing speed: Responding efficiently with accurate responses (e.g., braking when an animal darts in front of a car)
- Social cognition: Recognizing and responding to social cues and signals, like emotional responses, facial expressions, and significance of social interactions (e.g., recognizing another's emotional state and responding in kind)

These processes are implemented by the executive functions of the prefrontal cortex, which can do the following:
1. Monitor the environment.

2. Identify relevant stimuli.
3. Devise plans of action to engage the environment:
   a. Select an option
   b. Implement it
   c. Monitor it on the basis of an anticipated result
   d. Modify it as needed to achieve the intended result
4. Remember the experience.

Areas involved in reasoning and cognition include the dorsolateral prefrontal cortex, the ventrolateral prefrontal cortex, the anterior cingulate cortex, the hippocampus, the basal ganglia (caudate nucleus), and the cerebellum.

Emotions

Emotions are the culmination of body feedback ("gut feelings"), regulation and integration of such activated body states by the hypothalamus, the recruitment of hippocampal and semantic memory processes, the enlistment of pain and pleasure centers in the amygdala and nucleus accumbens, and the conscious representation of this processing in the prefrontal areas. Prefrontal areas, such as the orbitofrontal cortex and cingulate gyrus, modulate emotional responses by inhibiting socially inappropriate impulses, promoting empathy, and monitoring the environment for salient cues and stimuli. Our skeletal muscles (e.g., facial expressions) allow us to communicate our emotions and be understood by others. The concept and terrain of the limbic system has expanded and shifted over the 80 years since it was first conceptualized. States of unpleasant feelings, under normal circumstances, are reset by inhibitory relays from the medial prefrontal cortex to the amygdala. These dysphoric states can be reduced directly by biofeedback or meditation, interpersonal relatedness, methods of cognitive and emotional expression (e.g., writing, art, physical activities, psychotherapy, vulnerability), and certain CNS inhibitory agents such as benzodiazepines. Indirect reduction is possible via serotonergic and/or noradrenergic supplementation to the medial prefrontal cortex via antidepressants to reduce the "inhibition of return to normal" mood. Widespread activation and underactivation of normally cross-synchronous brain areas involved in mood, cognition, sleep, arousal, perceptual, and association areas may result in mood lability, euphoria, excitement, and depressed states in varying combinations. These unsteady waves can be diminished by mood-stabilizing agents, which appear to balance inhibitory and excitatory influences contributing to such extremes. To paraphrase Sigmund Freud, a reasonable goal of mental health treatment is not to numb or subvert emotional expression, but to transform the misery of psychological disorders into the common unhappiness of everyday life (Fig. 4.7).

CLINICAL APPLICATION

As explained throughout this text, many mental disorders have biologic bases. A brief overview of these biologic influences is presented here, but more thorough discussions of these issues are presented in the chapters dealing with each respective disorder. This approach is consistent with our

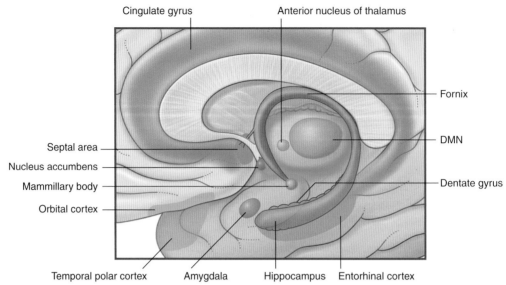

FIG. 4.7 Medial view of cortical and subcortical limbic areas. *DMN*, Dorsal medial nucleus of the thalamus. (From Mtui, E., Gruener, G., & Dockery, P. [2015]. *Fitzgerald's clinical neuroanatomy and neuroscience* [7th ed.]. Elsevier.)

belief that the biologic context of mental disorders is inextricably linked to symptoms and behaviors and is part of a holistic approach to understanding patients with psychiatric disorders. The student is urged to use this chapter as a foundation to the understanding of brain anatomy and physiology and to build on this foundation by applying this information to other chapters.

Schizophrenia

Several psychobiologic influences on schizophrenia have been proposed. First, some researchers have noted that an increase in ventricular size is apparent in many people with schizophrenia. In schizophrenia, increased ventricle size is likely related to neurodevelopmental factors; that is, the brain around the ventricles has failed to develop, and the ventricles have enlarged to fill the empty space. This phenomenon is referred to as an increase in *ventricular brain ratios*. In addition, in many individuals with schizophrenia, a decrease in the gray matter and white matter of the cortex and in the major subcortical nuclei is evident.

Other biologic differences found in people with schizophrenia include a decrease in cerebral blood flow, particularly in the prefrontal areas of the cortex. The term used to describe this condition is *hypofrontality*. Imaging technology that tracks blood flow and glucose metabolism has substantiated this physiologic change. These brain changes result in a decline in frontal cognitive functions, such as organizing, planning, learning, problem solving, and critical thinking.

The most celebrated and widely known biologic theory for schizophrenia is the dopamine hypothesis. According to this theory, schizophrenia is caused by alterations of dopamine levels in the brain. Chapter 24 elaborates on this theory and the biologically related genetic theory of schizophrenia. Antipsychotic medications are discussed in Chapter 14.

CASE STUDY

Schizophrenia

R. W., a 35-year-old divorced Native American female with a history of past episodic alcohol abuse, began feeling rage and distress after the birth of her fourth child. She was assessed at the emergency department, prescribed anxiolytics, and referred to an outpatient counselor at a mental health agency. She returned to the emergency room several months later with similar feelings of greater intensity and was treated with intravenous lorazepam for a presumed manic episode. She became calmer there and again was referred back for outpatient behavioral management. A month later, she began hearing voices, seeing indistinct but threatening figures outside of her home, and having persecutory delusions. She was admitted to an inpatient psychiatric unit in an agitated and resistant state. She believed the voices she was hearing were part of a government program to scan and insert thoughts into her brain. She avoided windows, fearing that someone might shoot her from outside. She was guarded and evasive during her clinical interview. She refused a physical examination, but urinalysis showed a urinary tract infection. Other laboratory investigations were unremarkable. Her appearance, speech, and thought rate were appropriate, her mood was anxious, her affect was mildly blunted, and her thought content was markedly illogical with referential ideation and bizarre and persecutory delusions.

She requested a discharge from the hospital but was held for an involuntary admission and released by an independent examiner. She was later hospitalized on several occasions and repeated a cycle of stabilization with antipsychotics and referrals to psychiatrists for follow-up. She would attend these for a few visits, then terminate her care with these psychiatrists. Her primary care physician would then maintain her antipsychotic medication until she would stop them, decompensate, and be readmitted for psychotic decompensations. Negative symptoms such as withdrawal, negativism, and decline in executive functions followed and began to predominate her clinical presentation progressively following each decompensation.

Depression

Mood disorders are also thought to have a biologic basis. Decreased amounts of norepinephrine and serotonin, two important brain neurotransmitters, are thought to play

CASE STUDY

Depression with Posttraumatic Stress Disorder Associated with Rape and Assault

V. H., a 28-year-old married housewife, was admitted to a psychiatric hospital for the first time for increasing depression with suicidal ideation. She had become increasingly hopeless and suicidal for the previous 2 months. She delivered her third child 3 months earlier and experienced postpartum depression, as she had with her two previous pregnancies. After this last delivery, she separated from her husband and began a relationship with a male acquaintance. She later said she sought support and affirmation from this relationship, but he pressed her for sex beyond her consent, then physically threatened and raped her. She reported this to the authorities. She reconciled with her husband, who was supportive of her. She had flashbacks and routine nightmares of the rape and wanted to move away from where she lived to avoid the perpetrator.

She had been taking sertraline 100 mg daily, which had lately become ineffective for her depression. She had insomnia and was treated with diphenhydramine. She made some superficial lacerations on her arms with a dull razor, then wrote several suicide notes. The discovery of these notes by her husband led to her assessment and admission. Her mother, who had bipolar disorder with several psychiatric hospitalizations, helped take her to the hospital but berated her and threatened a relational cut-off because of her condition. She reported past neglect from her family of origin for her depression, denial of her feelings, and even (when younger) physical assaults by her mother whenever she expressed depressive or unhappy states.

Her marriage had been rocky, with frequent separations, a divorce, and a subsequent remarriage. She reported that her husband drank when they were separated and was unavailable to help with their children. They had some marital counseling, but she felt they needed more. She had a counselor and had her antidepressants prescribed by her primary care physician. She had not consulted a psychiatrist previously. She reported past ineffective trials of citalopram and bupropion. She denied previous symptoms suggestive of paranoia, mania, or psychosis. She drank two to four alcoholic beverages per sitting twice a month and denied the use of other substances.

Her physical examination was remarkable only for breast lactation, and her medical and surgical history were notable for nephrolithiasis, peptic ulcer disease, preeclampsia, chronic sinusitis, tonsillectomy, cholecystectomy, and knee arthroscopy. She was diagnosed with recurrent severe major depressive disorder and posttraumatic stress disorder. Sertraline was increased to 200 mg daily, with augmentation with aripiprazole 2.5 mg at night; prazosin was initiated up to 2 mg at night for nightmares; and she used triazolam 0.125 mg at bedtime as needed for insomnia. Her nightmares diminished, her mood improved as she participated in hospital therapy, she and her husband worked on their issues in marital therapy, and she was able to transition in a few days to an intensive outpatient program for continued care.

a role in depression. Apparently, an overall deficiency exists in the concentration of these neurotransmitters, and psychopharmacologic treatment is based on restoring them to optimal levels. Other neurotransmitters, such as γ-aminobutyric acid (GABA), dopamine, and acetylcholine may also be factors in the development of depression. Chapter 25 discusses these neurotransmitters and the roles of cell receptor, thyroid, hypothalamic, and pituitary function in depression.

Anxiety Disorders

Anxiety disorders appear to have a biologic basis. Research has indicated that drugs that activate GABA receptors, causing an inhibitory effect, can calm anxious patients. Other neurotransmitters, such as norepinephrine, dopamine, and serotonin, might also have roles in anxiety. When the sympathetic system is stimulated by epinephrine, norepinephrine, and dopamine, an anxiety-like reaction occurs. Anxiety disorders are discussed in Chapter 27.

Dementias

Dementias are directly related to brain pathology. Alzheimer disease (AD), the leading cause of dementia in the United States, is caused by brain atrophy, which has been demonstrated microscopically by the presence of neurofibrillary tangles and amyloid plaques. Patients with AD tend to have enlarged ventricles, narrowing of the cortical ribbon (gray matter), widening of the sulci, and decreases in the width of the gyri. A loss of cholinergic pathways is also found in patients with AD, contributing to memory problems. Patients with AD forget recent events, facts, how to use words, and how to use common objects. AD and other dementias are discussed in Chapter 28.

Degenerative Diseases

PD is a degenerative disease that affects motor function and emotional stability. In patients with parkinsonism, microscopic examination of the basal ganglia, specifically the caudate nucleus and globus pallidus, reveals degenerative changes. The most significant change is the deterioration of the substantia nigra, the primary site of synthesis of dopamine in the brain. The decreased availability of dopamine in the EPS leads to resting tremors, bradykinesia, and rigidity. Parkinsonism is discussed in greater detail in Chapters 13 and 28.

Demyelinating Diseases

Multiple sclerosis is a demyelinating disease. In this disorder, the myelin and eventually the axons are attacked and gradually broken down by the body's own immune system. This degeneration of myelin typically causes various problems, including loss of sensation, muscle weakness, fatigue, double vision, and tingling in the extremities. People with multiple sclerosis also experience psychological symptoms, undoubtedly related to demyelinization that occurs in the brain.

Anorexia Nervosa

Anorexia, a disorder characterized by the refusal to eat and various emotional problems, appears to be associated with hypothalamic dysfunction. Anorexia is discussed in more detail in Chapter 32.

Trauma

Individuals who have experienced CNS trauma can have brain insults similar to the lesions found in dementia or parkinsonism. Victims of head trauma from automobile accidents and sport injuries (e.g., football) can exhibit symptoms based on the site, severity, and frequency of the trauma. Individuals with an injury to the temporal lobe might experience memory loss or aphasia; individuals with a prefrontal lobe injury might experience personality changes or psychosis. Dementia pugilistica (i.e., punch drunk syndrome, boxer's disease), a dementia syndrome with the same molecular pathology as AD, can result from repeated blows to the head such as those occurring in the sport of boxing.

Chemical Dependency

The biologic pathways that might be responsible for the control of addictive substances are important avenues to explore due to the tremendous cost in human lives and productivity that drug abuse extracts from society. Research studies indicate that the nucleus accumbens is an important piece of the addiction puzzle. Chapter 31 addresses substance abuse.

Early Life Stress and Trauma

Another psychobiologic issue worth contemplating is the developmental impact of early life trauma or significant stress. As noted, the brain continues to develop after birth and becomes larger, more sophisticated, and more efficient. One aspect of this continued development is ongoing myelination. As individuals age, myelin thickens around axons, improving the precision and efficacy of connections among neurons. Myelination continues throughout the teenage years, while pruning eliminates about 40% of synapses. Even during late adolescence, parents and others should be aware of the good and bad possibilities of dynamic brain processes. Some of the very last connections to develop are connections that help individuals use good judgment, solve problems, and self-regulate. Prolonged stress or significant trauma can compromise these processes.

At an even earlier age, stress and trauma increase cortisol levels. Excessive cortisol levels can cause atrophy of the hippocampus, impairing hippocampal activities such as memory and learning. Attachment theory consistently demonstrates that maternal deprivation or rejection causes profound behavioral changes in the child's later life. Children nurtured in good environments have lifelong advantages over deprived ones. Sustained or overwhelming early life stressors can lead to an increase in hypothalamic-pituitary-adrenal activity. Increased hypothalamic release of corticotropin-releasing factor causes increased release of ACTH from the anterior pituitary gland and results in a subsequent elevation of systemic cortisol. An elevated cortisol level is associated with increased heart rate, muscle tension, anger, anxiety, fear, and depression. When adulthood is reached, an individual who has experienced years of elevated cortisol is likely to be burdened with a hypersensitive hypothalamic-pituitary-adrenal system that overreacts to stress and often leads to a life of depression and anxiety. Significant stress, trauma, maternal behavior, and maltreatment during childhood and adolescence are mental health issues because they have the potential to alter the structure and chemistry of the brain permanently.

CASE STUDY

An Unusual Case: Hysterical Blindness Associated with Migraine

The patient is a 24-year-old male who has had chronic migraine headaches for 6 years after sustaining a whiplash injury from a roller-coaster ride. He subsequently developed bilateral transient complete visual loss, occurring only after the onset of migraine, which persists for hours to weeks after such episodes. He has had noncontributory ophthalmic, neurologic examinations, neuroimaging, and other studies at an academic hospital, and he has undertaken various migraine treatments, including triptans, verapamil, topiramate, lamotrigine, and hydrocodone. Only the last medication has resulted in some reduction in migraine pain, with shortened duration of blindness. His migraines were typically preceded by sharp frontal and periorbital pain radiating to the occiput, followed by a visual aura of wavy lines, then dots, then photophobia and sensitivity to sounds, then the full expression of headache pain and loss of vision. The resolution of his blindness occurred in reverse fashion to its onset, with gradual central clearing, followed by the appearance of small dots on the peripheral vision, then restoration of full vision. The patient started escitalopram 6 months before a psychiatric consultation, which helped ease stress and depression associated with his condition.

He is highly disabled by his visual loss, having to rely on his parents for his daily care. He has chronic continuous daily tension-type headaches in between migraine attacks, which can occur three to five times per week. His longest bout of continuous blindness has lasted 4 months, with migraines occurring within this period at the same frequency. There appears to be no discernible pattern or associated or contributing factors to the blindness.

Multiple MRIs, both when symptomatic and asymptomatic, were normal. CT brain scan showed tonsillar enlargement and Chiari malformation but no obstruction of cerebrospinal fluid. He had repair of atrial septal defect 6 weeks before the onset of visual disturbances associated with migraines. His medical history is otherwise unremarkable.

Mental status indicated reddened eyes and exhausted facial expression; depressed and anxious mood; and unremarkable speech, memory, concentration, attention, perceptions, insight, judgment, thought form, rate, and content. There did not appear to be identifiable secondary gain or indifference associated with his blindness, and he was quite bothered by it.

Conversion hysteria did not seem to explain the presence of visual loss, and understanding this symptom as part of a larger, complex pain syndrome seemed more acceptable to the patient. Combinations of nortriptyline, escitalopram, tramadol, and pregabalin resulted in less migraine pain and shorter periods of visual loss (2 to 3 hours per episode). The frequency of migraine was three to four times per week at last reporting.

STUDY NOTES

1. The brain is a complex organ composed of 100 billion neurons, and changes in its anatomy or physiology affect behavior. Holistic nursing care requires an understanding of the impact of brain dysfunction on behavior.

2. Neurons are the basic subunits of the nervous system. A neuron consists of a cell body; *dendrites* that transmit information to the cell body; and a process called an *axon*, which transmits impulses away from the cell body.

3. Impulses travel from one neuron to another by sending a chemical called a *neurotransmitter* across a microscopic gap, known as a *synaptic cleft*.

4. Many mental disorders that were formerly thought to have psychological etiologic factors are now known to be influenced by brain dysfunction.

5. The nervous system is divided into the CNS and the PNS.

6. The nervous pathways in the brain are composed of myelinated axons (white matter) that connect and communicate among brain nuclei (gray matter).

7. The two major neurotransmitters in the EPS are dopamine (inhibitory and excitatory) and acetylcholine (excitatory).

8. The dopamine hypothesis postulates that schizophrenia results from alterations of levels of dopamine in the brain.

9. The neurotransmitter theory of depression states that depression is related to decreased levels of norepinephrine, serotonin, or both.

10. Anxiety disorders might be related to alterations in GABA levels.

REFERENCES

Charney, D. S., Nestler, E. J., & Bunney, B. S. (2008). *Neurobiology of mental illness* (3rd ed.). Oxford University Press.

Goldberg. S. (2003). *Clinical neuroanatomy made ridiculously simple* (3rd ed.). MedMaster.

Griffin, J. E., & Ojeda, S. R. (2004). *Textbook of endocrine physiology* (5th ed.). Oxford University Press.

Kandel, E. R., Schwartz, J. H., Jessell, T. M., Siegelbaum, S. A., & Hudspeth, A. J. (2013). *Principles of neural science* (5th ed.). McGraw-Hill.

Keltner, N. L., & Folks, D. (2005). *Psychotropic drugs* (4th ed.). Mosby.

Mtui, E., Gruener, G., & Dockery, P. (2015). *Fitzgerald's clinical neuroanatomy and neuroscience* (7th ed.). Elsevier.

Nestler, J., Kenny, P., Russo, S., & Schaefer, A. (2020). *Nestler, hyman, & malenka's molecular neuropharmacology: A Foundation for Clinical Neuroscience* (4th ed). McGraw Hill.

Schwartz, J., & Roth, T. (2008). Neurophysiology of sleep and wakefulness: Basic science and clinical implications. *Neuropharmacology, 6*(4), 367–378. https://doi.org/10.2174/157015908787386050.

Standring. S. (2004). *Gray's anatomy: the anatomical Basis of clinical practice* (39th ed.). Elsevier.

Vecchiarelli, H., Šimončičová, E., & Tremblay, M. (2021). Microglial involvement with psychiatric diseases. *Psychiatric Times, 38*(1), 32–36.

5

Cultural Issues

Barbara Jones Warren

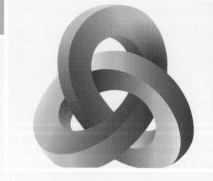

ⓔ http://evolve.elsevier.com/Keltner

LEARNING OBJECTIVES

- Understand the importance of the effect of cultural variables on health and health care.
- Describe the components of cultural competence.
- Describe the factors involved in patients' and nurses' cultural perspectives.
- Articulate the differences in and the importance of worldview perspectives.

- Explain how incorporation of cultural competence can enhance psychiatric nursing clinical excellence.
- Analyze the symptoms suggestive of culture-bound syndromes.
- Apply understanding of ethnopharmacology as it might relate to a specific drug and a specific ethnic group.

Culture is a critical component of patients' lives that affects their health care attitudes and actions as well as their ability to understand and use the interventions that psychiatric nurses develop (Campinha-Bacote, 2007; Warren, 2020). *Culture* is the internal and external manifestation of learned and shared values, beliefs, and norms of a person, group, or community used to help individuals function in life and understand and interpret life occurrences (McFarland & Wehbe-Alamah, 2018). The cultural perspectives and patterns of both the nurse and the patient influence the nurse-patient interaction. These perspectives and patterns also affect a patient's level of mental health. For example, a patient's behaviors might be labeled as *pathologic* if a nurse misinterprets the patient's normal and/or culturally relevant beliefs and health care actions (Warren, 2020). A patient labeled as noncompliant or nonadherent might not be receiving culturally competent care (Purnell & Fenkl, 2019). The purpose of this chapter is to explain the role of the nurse and the connection between culture and cultural competence as they relate to psychiatric nursing.

BASIC CONCEPTS

Importance of Cultural Competence

Cultural competence is the process whereby the nurse develops ongoing expertise and understanding in the areas of cultural awareness, knowledge, and skills to promote effective health care. The term *competence* does not imply that the process ends but that the nurse is always learning about the phenomenon of culture related to patients (Campinha-Bacote, 2007; Warren, 2020; Warren, Campinha-Bacote, & Munoz, 1994). A culturally competent psychiatric nurse not only possesses

knowledge about the process of cultural competence but also incorporates cultural competence into interactions with peers, students, patients, families, and communities. The use of cultural competence in conjunction with the psychotherapeutic management model serves as an evidenced-based health care approach that can enhance clinical excellence and promote recovery of psychiatric patients. Research on the use of culturally competent mental health strategies indicates that cultural competence is key to patients' recovery process (Andrews & Boyle, 2016; Anthony, 1993; Felix et al., 2018; Warren, 2020). A psychiatric nurse does not need to know everything about every patient's culture. The key is knowing how to assess culture and incorporate knowledge from the assessment into a shared decision-making process regarding patient plans (McFarland & Wehbe-Alanah, 2018).

NORM'S NOTES Nurses must be culturally relevant. In many parts of the United States, nurses might work with five or more distinct cultural groups on an ongoing basis. How can you do this and provide the type of nursing care that takes into account the various cultural backgrounds? Dr. Warren has spent many years helping nurses learn this. This chapter outlines some basic nursing behaviors to help you help all patients.

Culture and Psychiatric Nursing

The US Surgeon General's seminal report on mental health has emphasized the need for culturally competent mental health care (US Surgeon General, 2001). Nurses provide services to a multitude of patients from diverse cultures. The term *cultural diversity* might encompass areas such as age, gender, socioeconomic status, religion, race, ethnicity, mental illness, and physically challenging conditions (Campinha-Bacote, 2007; Institute of Medicine, 2003; McFarland & Wehbe-Alamah, 2018; Munoz et al., 2007; Spector, 2017). Nurses need to be aware that patients define their own cultural perspectives (citation). The *Diagnostic and Statistical Manual of Mental Disorders, Fifth Edition (DSM-5)* has incorporated additional information regarding specific cultural features for each diagnostic category and a chapter on cultural formulation that includes specific assessment forms for the interviewer and the informant (American Psychiatric Association, 2013; Warren, 2013a). It is important to note that information included in the DSM-5 chapter on cultural formulation is not a disorder category (Warren, 2020). It is a brief summary of persons' interpretation and explanation of how they describe symptoms related to stress (APA, 2013).

Barriers to Culturally Competent Care

A growing knowledge and research base indicates that patients' adherence to treatment increases when cultural needs are incorporated into health care planning (American Psychiatric Association, 2013; US Surgeon General, 2001; Carbray, Cacchione, Limandri, & Warren, 2016). Because nurses are often the gatekeepers for health care systems, knowledge of cultural factors related to psychiatric care is important. The most common barrier to the delivery of culturally competent nursing care involves miscommunication between nurses and patients. A nurse might lack knowledge and sensitivity regarding a patient's cultural beliefs and practices; the nurse might not recognize the importance and value of these beliefs to the patient as they relate to health care practices. Similarly, patients might be unaware of the nurse's cultural perspectives and misinterpret health care recommendations from the nurse (Carbray, Kaas, Limandri, & Warren, 2016). Consequently, to facilitate successful relationships with their patients, nurses must understand their own cultural beliefs and values and how these beliefs and values influence patient care. This cultural awareness facilitates the psychotherapeutic relationship and the nursing process (Warren, 2020).

? CRITICAL THINKING QUESTION

1. How would a nurse use the best evidence therapeutically and in a culturally competent manner in his care of a patient who is refusing to follow a nursing care plan because it does not align with the patient's cultural belief system?

Another barrier to culturally competent care results from failure to assess the patient's cultural perspective. A variety of clinical cultural assessment tools and models are available for assessing cultural perspectives (Warren, 2015). Finally, barriers to culturally competent nursing care are primarily grounded in differences between nurses' and patients' cultural worldviews (Tables 5.1–5.4). These differences can increase miscommunication and negatively affect the

TABLE 5.1 European-American Worldview

Component	Perspective
Cultural value	Value is placed on the member or object or on the attainment of the object.
Knowledge	Knowledge is acquired according to proof of the existence of anything—that is, the ability of an individual to see, hear, touch, taste, or smell it.
Logic	Dichotomous mode of reasoning is used.
Relationship	Relationships are developed based on the perceived need for them.

TABLE 5.2 African, African American, Hispanic, and Arabic Worldview

Component	Perspective
Cultural value	Value is placed on the development and maintenance of interpersonal relationships.
Knowledge	Knowledge bases are developed through the use of the affective or feeling senses.
Logic	Reasoning ability is based on the union of opposites.
Relationship	Development of interpersonal relationships is based on the fact that all relationships are interrelated across all continua.

TABLE 5.3 Asian, Asian American, and Polynesian Worldview

Component	Perspective
Cultural value	Value is placed on the balance between member and group interactions.
Knowledge	Knowledge bases are developed in striving for transcendence of the mind and body.
Logic	Reasoning ability is based on the belief that the mind and body can exist independently of the physical world.
Relationship	Development of relationships is grounded in the belief that everyone and everything in the physical and spiritual worlds are related.

nurse-patient relationship and interaction. Nurses may state that a patient is "noncompliant" if the patient does not follow the nurse's plan of care. The patient may simply not understand what the nurse is suggesting because the plan does not include the patient's cultural needs. Noncompliance indicates "refusal, denial, disobedience, not following directions of the nurse" (Warren, 2020). A more culturally competent approach intimates that the patient is an advocate for change and understands and supports a plan that includes his culturally competent healthcare strategy.

TABLE 5.4	**Native American Worldview**
Component	**Perspective**
Cultural value	Value is placed in the context of a person's relationship to a Greater or Supreme Being.
Knowledge	Knowledge bases are developed on the basis of a person's understanding of an individual's relationship with the Greater or Supreme Being.
Logic	Reasoning ability is grounded in the belief that every person is innately good and has no evil within.
Relationship	Development of relationships with another person, group, or community is grounded in the idea that the Greater or Supreme Being is in every person; hence, all persons should be valued.

Cultural Etiology of Illness and Disease

Nurses' and patients' health care actions and beliefs are generally formulated by three factors: (1) their definition of health, (2) their perception of how illness occurs, and (3) their cultural worldview (Luckmann, 2017; Spector, 2017). Nurses and patients might define *health* quite differently.

Closely connected to a nurse's or patient's definition of health is his or her belief of how illness and disease occur. The nurse or patient might believe that illness and disease are created by natural, unnatural, or scientific causes. A person who believes in the concept of *natural* cause of illness or disease believes that everyone and everything in the world is interrelated, and that a disruption of this connectedness (e.g., a tornado) causes an illness or disease (L. Purnell, 2019; L.D. Purnell & Fenkl, 2019; Spector, 2017). Conversely, nurses or patients might believe that *unnatural* or outside forces create illness and disease. An individual might believe that another person enlists the services of a magician, witch, ghost, or supernatural being to cast a spell or hex on him or her. Finally, nurses or patients might believe in the *scientific* cause of illness—specific, concrete explanations exist for every illness and disease (i.e., the entrance of pathogens such as viruses, bacteria, and germs into the body) (Campinha-Bacote, 2007; Warren, 2013a, 2013b). The scientific model is the typical model taught in most Western culture schools of nursing. However, many non-Western cultures acknowledge and teach health care providers the importance of natural and unnatural causes of illness.

Patients' health care beliefs and actions are related not only to the way in which health, illness, and the cause of illness are defined but also to individual worldviews. There are four primary worldviews: (1) analytic, (2) relational, (3) community, and (4) ecologic. The primary worldview is often the one that individuals express or are comfortable with when they are with family or significant others or during stressful times. Many individuals use a mixture of the four worldviews or adopt another worldview when they are in another environment, such as a work or business setting. The nurse's failure to

understand the patient's primary worldview might negatively affect the nurse-patient relationship and impede successful interventions and mental health outcomes. Overarching worldviews that may be associated with ethnic populations are presented in Tables 5.1 to 5.4. One caveat to remember is that nurses and patients may use components from more than one world view that they value and incorporate into their everyday interactions with others (Warren, 2020).

> **? CRITICAL THINKING QUESTION**
>
> 2. A nurse enters a patient's room and is ready to do the daily morning assessment. However, the patient is not responsive to the nurse's immediate need to conduct the assessment. The nurse complains that the patient is "non-compliant." The patient says "the nurse is always in a hurry and never listens to me." Are the worldviews of the patient and nurse in conflict? What are two suggestions you can make that would help the situation between the nurse and the patient?

Four Worldviews

A person who expresses the analytic worldview values detail to time (e.g., being on time, starting on time, ending on time), individuality, and possessions. A person with this view prefers to learn through written, hands-on, and visual resources. The relational worldview is grounded in a belief in spirituality and the significance of relationships and interactions between and among individuals. The preferred learning style is through verbal communication. An individual who expresses the community worldview believes that community needs and concerns are more important than individual ones. The valued learning style includes quiet, respectful communication as well as meditation and reading. The ecologic worldview is based on a belief that a form of interconnectedness exists between human beings and the earth and that individuals have a responsibility to take care of the earth. Learning is accomplished through quiet observation and contemplation, and verbal communication is minimized.

Worldviews form the basis for the expression of culturally bound mental health and wellness issues. For example, a patient or nurse using an analytic worldview perspective might espouse specific detail to time, calculations, individuality, and the importance of acquiring material objects. Being on time for appointments, immediately getting to the purpose of a health visit, and using printed pamphlets and books for health education are valued. Nurses and other health care professionals must be extremely accurate and precise when providing care for these patients. The components of the analytic worldview, including individuality and valuing material goods, are often embodied in traditional values, beliefs, and actions of American society.

An individual with a relational worldview values the development of interactions and relationships, usually prefers learning through verbal communication, and views spirituality as an important context for living life. These individuals might want to chat for a moment before getting to the heart of the health visit. They might desire the involvement of relatives, friends, or spiritual and religious advisors during the health visit or during the nurse's development of the nursing process. Individuals from African American or Hispanic cultures often possess the relational worldview (Anderson et al., 2019; Warren, 2013a, 2015).

Individuals with a community worldview value the importance and needs of the community over the individual. People with this perspective often use meditation and contemplation techniques. A patient with this view is respectful and polite regarding health care advice and might not want to question a nurse or physician. This reticence might occur even if the patient does not understand the nurse's recommendation. People from some Asian cultural groups often embody these philosophies (Warren, 2015).

Finally, a patient or nurse with an ecologic worldview values interconnectedness with other people and the universe, takes responsibility for others and the world, and feels a need to maintain peace and tranquility. These individuals prefer a quiet, restful approach in interactions with others. Conversation is respectful, concise, and often kept to a minimum. Individuals from some of the indigenous or Native American cultures might embrace this worldview.

 CRITICAL THINKING QUESTION

3. How can a nurse form a therapeutic relationship with a patient who is from Navajo culture and lives life using an ecologic worldview?

CULTURE-BOUND MENTAL HEALTH ISSUES

Culture-bound syndromes are recurring patterns of behavior that create disturbing experiences for individuals (American Psychiatric Association, 2013). These behaviors might or might not be congruent with symptoms presented in *DSM-5* for various diagnostic categories. However, because these behaviors can be culture-based, nurses must be aware of the symptoms to accurately assess patients who are from racially and ethnically diverse cultures. The Cultural Formulation Tool from *DSM-5* is a valuable assessment tool for nurses because it can assess both the nurse and the patient.

People from racially and ethnically diverse cultures often use culturally specific language to describe mental distress that they experience. One example involves the description of depressive symptoms and the actual symptomatology. Native Americans might state that they are "having heart pain" or are "heartbroken" when they experience depressive symptoms (Warren, 2015). A person of Hispanic descent might say that her "soul was lost" *(susto)* because of another person's ability to cause a frightening experience or to place an "evil eye" *(mal ojo)* on her (American Psychiatric Association, 2013). Someone who is experiencing a lost soul might be lethargic, have appetite and sleep changes, and have multiple physical complaints. Because good health is contingent on the restoration of a person's equilibrium, an ill person might initially

consult a healer or "root doctor" to help break the spell of the evil eye and return the lost soul (Purnell & Kenkl, 2019). Traditional Western health care might be the last resource that the person contacts regarding their symptoms. Nurses must be knowledgeable about and sensitive to these beliefs.

People from diverse cultural groups often describe psychotic symptoms differently. Individuals from Malaya and Laos use the term *running amok*. People from certain Native American nations might use the term *ghost sickness*. African American and Appalachian American individuals might say a *spell* has been cast on them. A more inclusive description of culture-bound syndromes can be found in *DSM-5* (American Psychiatric Association, 2013).

Clinical Example

A 33-year-old woman who is from Appalachian culture is worried because she is sure that her illness is due to a hex placed on her by another woman in the community. How would you, as a nurse, provide care for her? Do you attempt to convince her that her ideas are wrong and there is no such thing as a hex?

The assessment of possible culture-bound syndromes and the cultural expression of psychiatric symptoms must be part of the psychotherapeutic and nursing processes. This additional assessment can provide important information that the nurse needs to provide culturally competent services for patients.

ALTERNATIVE THERAPIES

People from racially and ethnically diverse groups often may prefer to use alternative therapies. These treatments might include the use of acupuncture, acupressure, nutritional therapies, skin scraping, moxibustion, and cupping. Acupressure and acupuncture restore balance by stimulating linear and circular lines throughout the body, known as meridians, with the use of needles *(acupuncture)* or pressure *(acupressure)* (McFarland & Wehbe-Alaneah, 2018; Luckmann, 2017; Warren, 2015). *Nutritional therapies* might include the use of certain foods or herbs. *Skin scraping* or *coining, moxibustion,* and *cupping* are used to restore balance by bringing heat to the skin surface, which allows the release of the toxin or evil spirit from the affected body area (Purnell & Fenkl, 2019; Spector, 2017). In the case of skin scraping or coining, a person (generally a healer in the community) uses a coin and briskly rubs or scrapes the skin surface. In moxibustion, a cotton ball containing a substance known as *moxa* is ignited with a match in a small glass or cup, which is then placed on the skin above a meridian. The belief is that the illness or evil is released from a person's body when heat is generated within the meridians. However, skin abrasions and contusions, often occurring on the skin as a result of skin scraping or coining, moxibustion, or cupping, might provide a climate for infection.

Certain cultural groups (e.g., Hispanic, South American) believe that certain liquids, foods, or medicines must be taken in balance to restore health (Spector, 2017; Warren, 2020). A medicine might be labeled as being *hot* and might need to be taken in conjunction with a *cold* liquid or food to be effective. The terms *hot* and *cold* do not refer to temperature but instead indicate how the substance reacts within the body to restore equilibrium.

ETHNOPHARMACOLOGY

Ethnopharmacology is the study of pharmacogenetic, pharmacodynamic, and pharmacokinetic influences based on different ethnic, racial, and cultural groups (Carbray et al., 2016a). Culturally competent care is enhanced when this type of cultural knowledge is incorporated into patient care.

Individuals react to pharmacologic interventions based on their normal biologic makeup, environmental influences, and cultural influences (Carbray et al., 2016a). Specific ethnic, racial, and cultural differences affect a patient's medication options and dose requirements (Carbray et al., 2016b).

Variation in metabolism is most often cited as the cause of cross-ethnic differences in response to medications. Carbray et al. (2016a) indicated that individuals from certain racial and ethnic groups have a genetically based pharmacokinetic variation that causes them to be fast or slow metabolizers. Drugs might accumulate in a patient's body when medications are metabolized too slowly. For example, people of Asian (about 50%) and Native American descent are more sensitive to the effects of alcohol than people from other ethnic and racial backgrounds. This sensitivity is based on their relative deficiency of aldehyde dehydrogenase, resulting in slowed metabolism of the highly toxic intermediate product, acetaldehyde. Symptoms include a reddened flush to the neck and face, tachycardia, and a burning sensation in the stomach.

Most psychotropic drugs are metabolized by the cytochrome P-450 system (Carbray et al., 2016a). Basically, only two cytochrome P-450 enzymes (see Chapter 12 for this discussion), 2D6 and 2C19, appear to have extensive cross-ethnic variability. Substrates of these enzymes are metabolized more slowly (poor metabolizers) in a certain percentage

TABLE 5.5 Metabolism by 2D6 and 2C19 Enzymes: Cross-Ethnic Variability

Ethnic Group	2D6-Poor Metabolizers (%)	2C19-Poor Metabolizers (%)
African Americans	~2	~19
Whites	3–9	2.5–6.7
Hispanics	1–4.5	~5
Native Americans	0–5.2	0
East Asians	0–2.5	17–22

Modified from Keltner, N. L., & Steele, D. (2019). *Psychiatric nursing* (7th ed.). Elsevier.

of each of these cultural groups (Warren, 2015). This cross-ethnic variability is shown in Table 5.5.

NURSE'S ROLE IN CULTURAL ASSESSMENT

Nurses should not only use the process of cultural competence in their practice settings but should also help others understand the need for culturally competent health care. One skill that every nurse must develop is the ability to integrate cultural factors into the health assessment (Spector, 2017).

Cultural Assessment Issues

Nurses must include some basic elements within their cultural assessments of patients, including communication, orientation, nutrition, family relationships, health beliefs, education, spiritual or religious views, and biologic or physiologic elements. Table 5.6 provides a handy assessment sheet to consider when evaluating culturally relevant information.

Questions and observations relative to cultural issues must be smoothly and sensitively incorporated into the nursing assessment process to ensure that the nurse does not appear rude or intrusive. Including someone from the patient's community or from the same cultural background during the assessment interview might be appropriate. Cultural preservation, cultural negotiation, and cultural repatterning are

TABLE 5.6 Cultural Assessment Worksheet

Assessment Area	Questions or Areas of Inquiry
Communication	1. Do you speak any foreign languages? 2. Is English your first language? 3. Does the patient speak English fluently? 4. Does the patient prefer an interpreter? 5. Does the patient believe that appropriate touching is acceptable? 6. Does the patient use ethnic behaviors?
Orientation	1. How long have you lived where you now live? 2. Where were you born? 3. With which ethnic, racial, or cultural group do you identify yourself? 4. How closely do you follow the traditional values, beliefs, and practices of your self-identified group? 5. What are the patient's thoughts on the following: human nature, development of knowledge, work ethic, relationship with nature?

TABLE 5.6	Cultural Assessment Worksheet—cont'd
Assessment Area	**Questions or Areas of Inquiry**
Nutrition	1. Do you have certain foods you prefer? 2. What kind of foods do you eat when you are ill? 3. Do you avoid certain foods because of your beliefs?
Significant others and family	1. Whom do you consider as important to you? 2. Is there anyone that you would like me to contact or not contact while you are here for treatment? 3. How are decisions made in your home environment? 4. In your home, what are the roles for children, women, and men? 5. What are some of the social customs or practices that you do at home? 6. Share with me three of your most important values.
Health	1. What brought you here for treatment today? 2. What do you think will help you feel better or get well? 3. Have you used treatments in the past that were helpful for you? 4. What type of treatments do you not like or feel uncomfortable receiving? 5. Is there something you think I can assist you with to help you improve? 6. Who do you usually go to for help or treatment when you are ill? 7. What do you think causes physical and mental problems?
Education	1. How do you prefer to learn new things and tasks (e.g., reading, watching television or videos, talking with someone)? 2. How have you received your education (e.g., in school, by self-instruction)? 3. How would you prefer to pay for your treatment?
Spirituality and religion	1. Do you consider yourself spiritual or religious? If so, what does that mean to you? 2. Do you have a religious preference? 3. Are there certain individuals you like to talk with regarding your spiritual views, religious beliefs, or health care? Are there certain practices in which you like to participate?
Biology and physiology	1. Do you have any specific health problems or disease conditions in your family of origin? 2. Are there certain medications, herbs, or therapies that you avoid because they make you ill? 3. Are there specific skin, hair, grooming, or health care needs that you prefer? 4. Are you taking any medications now? (Include an examination of vitamin, nutritional, and herbal approaches.) 5. How many cigarettes do you smoke every day? 6. How many glasses of wine do you drink per week? 7. How many cans or bottles of Coke, root beer, or beer do you drink per week? 8. How many cups of tea or coffee, or both, do you drink every day? 9. Are there any other beverages that you drink every day? 10. How many bars or pieces of chocolate do you eat every day?

From Warren, B. J., Campinha-Bacote, J., & Munoz, C. (1994). *Cultural assessment worksheet.* Authors.

other culturally competent techniques that nurses might use during assessment and care planning.

Cultural preservation is the nurse's ability to acknowledge, value, and accept a patient's cultural beliefs. *Cultural negotiation* is the nurse's ability to work within a patient's cultural belief system to develop culturally appropriate interventions. *Cultural repatterning* is the nurse's ability to incorporate cultural preservation and negotiation to identify patient needs, develop expected outcomes, and evaluate outcome plans (Andrews & Boyle, 2016; McFarland & Wehbe-Alamah, 2018). The Critical Thinking Questions and Clinical Example

in this chapter provide examples of how these three techniques might be incorporated into the care of a patient.

SUMMARY

Cultural competence is an important part of effective psychiatric nursing. Important components for the development of culturally competent nursing care include the nurse's understanding of the concepts of a worldview, culture-bound syndromes, and ethnopharmacology and the nurse's role in assessing patients for cultural variables that might affect patient care.

STUDY NOTES

1. Culture is the manifestation of beliefs, values, and norms of an individual, group, or community used for daily life functioning.
2. Cultural competence is the process whereby the nurse develops cultural awareness, knowledge, and skills to promote effective health care for patients.
3. Cultural diversity refers to unique differences in areas such as age, gender, socioeconomic status, religion, race, and ethnicity.
4. A person's worldview is a perspective reflecting what the person values in how she functions and interacts with others on a daily basis.
5. Barriers to culturally competent care include miscommunication, failure to assess for a cultural perspective, and differences in worldview.
6. Illness can be viewed as resulting from natural, unnatural, or scientific (i.e., explainable) causes.
7. Four worldviews are analytic, relational, community, and ecologic.
8. Culture-bound syndromes are recurring patterns of behavior that create disturbing experiences for people.
9. Patients from non-Western cultures might use acupuncture, acupressure, nutritional therapies (e.g., herbal remedies), skin scraping, moxibustion, and cupping to treat illness.
10. Ethnopharmacology involves the study of genetic and culture-related factors that can affect metabolism of medications.
11. An important nursing role is the incorporation of cultural knowledge into addressing health and health care.

REFERENCES

American Psychiatric Association. (2013). *Diagnostic and statistical manual of mental disorders* (5th ed.). APA.

Anderson, C., Cene, C., Warren, B. J., Jackson, R., & Williams, K. P. (2019). Stress, resilience, and cardiovascular disease risk among African-American women: Results from the Women's Health Initiative. *Circulation: Cardiovascular Quality and Outcomes, 12*(4), e005284. https://doi.org/10.1161/CIRCOUTCOMES.118.005284.

Andrews, M. M., & Boyle, J. S. (2016). *Transcultural concepts in nursing care* (7th ed.). Wolters Klower.

Anthony, W. A. (1993). Recovery from mental illness: The guiding vision of the mental health services in the 1990s. *Psychiatric Rehabilitation Journal, 2*, 17. https://doi.org/10.1037/h0095655.

Campinha-Bacote, J. (2007). *The process of cultural competence in the delivery of healthcare services: The journey continues* (5th ed.). Transcultural C.A.R.E. Associates.

Carbray, J. C., Cacchione, P. Z., Limandri, B. J., & Warren, B. J. (2016). Assessment, diagnosis, and epidemiology using a recovery paradigm. *APNA e-series, Bipolar Spectrum Disorders*, issue 1 of 3, 1–25.

Carbray, J. C., Kaas, M., Limandri, B. J., & Warren, B. J. (2016a). Biological interventions for bipolar disorder across the lifespan. *APNA e-series, Bipolar Spectrum Disorders*, issue 2 of 3.

Carbray, J. C., Kaas, M., Limandri, B. J., & Warren, B. J. (2016b). Psychoeducation, counseling and psychotherapy: Evidence-based components in the therapeutic relationship. *APNA e-series, Bipolar Spectrum Disorders*, issue 3 of 3.

Felix, A. S., Shisler, R., Nolan, T. S., Warren, B. J., Rhoades, J., Barnett, K. S., & Williams, K. P. (2018). High-effort coping and cardiovascular disease among women: A systematic review of the John Henryism hypothesis. *J Urban Health: Bulletin of the New York Academy of Medicine, 96*(Suppl 1), 12–22. https://doi.org/10.1007/s11524-018-00333-1.

Institute of Medicine (2003). Unequal treatment: Confronting racial and ethnic disparities in healthcare. Washington, D.C.: National Academy Press.

Keltner, N., & Steele, D. (2019). *Psychiatric nursing.* Elsevier.

Luckmann, J. (2017). *Transcultural communication in nursing (Kindle).* Centage.

McFarland, M, & Wehbe-Alamah, H. (2018). Leininger's transcultural nursing: Concepts, theories, research & practice (4th ed.). New York: McGraw-Hill.

Munoz, R, & Prim, A. Ananth, J., & Ruiz, P. (2007). Life in color: Culture in American psychiatry. Chicago: Hilton Publishing.

Purnell, L. (2019). Update: The Purnell theory and model for culturally competent health care. *Journal of Transcultural Nursing, 30*(2), 98–105. https://doi.org/10.1177/1043659618817587.

Purnell, L. D., & Fenkl, E. A. (2019). *Handbook for culturally competent care.* Nature Switzerland.

Spector, R. (2017). *Cultural diversity in health and illness* (8th ed., Kindle). Pearson.

US Surgeon General. (2001). *Mental health: Culture, race, and ethnicity, a supplement to mental health: A report of the Surgeon General.* US Department of Health and Human Services.

Warren, B. J. (2020). The synergistic influence of life experiences and cultural nuances on development of depression: A cognitive behavioral perspective. *Issues in Mental Health Nursing, 41*(1), 3–6. https://DOI:10,1080/01612840.2019.1675828.

Warren, B.J., & Campinha-Bacote, J., & Munoz, C. (1994). Cultural assessment worksheet. Columbus, Ohio: Authors.

Warren, B. J. (2013a). How culture is assessed in the DSM-5. *Journal of Psychosocial Nursing, 51*, 40–45.

Warren, B. J. (2013b). Culturally sensitive psychopharmacology. In L. G. Leahy & C. G. Kohler (Eds.), *Clinical manual of psychopharmacology for nurses* (pp. 379–402). Washington, D.C: American Psychiatric Publishing, Inc.

Warren, B. J. (2015). Cultural issues. In N. L. Keltner & D. Steele (Eds.), *Psychiatric nursing* (pp. 50–56). Elsevier.

Warren, B. J., Campinha-Bacote, J., & Munoz, C. (1994). *Cultural assessment worksheet.* Authors.

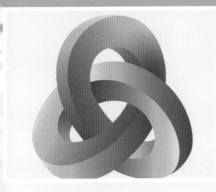

6

Spirituality Issues

Debbie Steele[a]

http://evolve.elsevier.com/Keltner

LEARNING OBJECTIVES

- Define the term *spirituality*. Differentiate between spirituality and religion.
- Explain two helpful theoretical constructs regarding spirituality.
- Discuss and evaluate benefits and concerns of addressing spiritual care in patients' treatment.
- Be familiar with the *Diagnostic and Statistical Manual of Mental Disorders*, *Fifth Edition (DSM-5)* and the International Classification of Nursing Practice diagnoses related to spiritual care.

- Know two pieces of practical advice from psychiatric patients themselves regarding communication about spiritual concerns.
- Identify how the nurse can intervene, including using the HOPE or FICA questions.
- Know how and when to make a referral to a spiritual care professional.

One criticism of some psychological theories is that they are psychology without the psyche, and this suits people who think they have no spiritual needs or aspirations. But here, both doctor and patient deceive themselves.... In a word, they do not give enough meaning to life, and it is only meaning that liberates. (Jung, 1984, p. 198)

How does nursing address, or even approach, concepts such as forgiveness, peace, trust, belief, doubt, fear, alienation, hope, joy, love, grief, transcendence, discovery, mystery, meaning, purpose, relationship, or gratitude? These notions fall within the concept of spirituality. The purpose of this chapter is to give nurses some ways to help patients identify their spiritual needs and access appropriate spiritual resources.

Individuals have religious and spiritual needs which are directly linked with their physical and emotional health and well-being. Nurses are in a unique position to support patients and their family's spiritual needs in their delivery of care, particularly in a hospital setting. Assessing and caring for the spiritual needs of patients is part of providing holistic nursing care (Vogel & Schep-Akkerman, 2018). Spirituality in psychiatric nursing has recently been defined as a search for life meaning, purpose, and connectedness based on one's values and capacity to interact with others (Clark & Emerson, 2021).

Within the nursing context, we want to be sure that we understand what a patient means when talking of spiritual

concerns or needs. It is helpful to ascertain what patients use to cope (or what is a source of distress) by asking whether they are a part of a supportive community, identifying spiritual needs, and supporting the patient's beliefs. "If patients indicate from the start that they are not religious or spiritual, then questions should be re-directed to asking about what gives life meaning and purpose and how this can be addressed in their health care" (Koenig, 2008).

People hold strong opinions about spirituality and religion, but a significant percentage—39%—of young Americans aged 18 to 29 are religiously unaffiliated, four times as many as a generation ago (Cooper et al., 2016). More than 70% of adults in the United States identify as Christian (Pew Research Center, 2015). However, almost 23% of American adults of all ages identify themselves as "unaffiliated" with any particular religion (Table 6.1). One could say, then, that the second largest "religious group" in the United States is those with no religious affiliation (Pew Research Center, 2015).

Researchers have devoted considerable effort to understand the difference between being spiritual and being religious. Spirituality involves a journey of personal transcendence and awareness for the purpose of making sense of life and coping in times of adversity or illness. Spirituality does not require an institutional framework. In contrast, a religious person is typically involved with a religious tradition and attends a religious institution. Religion often focuses on meeting the spiritual needs of members, as well as providing a sense of belonging and identity (Krause, Pargament, Hill, & Ironson, 2019). Spirituality and religion are both known

[a]The author would like to thank Gordon I.G. Pugh for his previous contribution to this chapter.

TABLE 6.1   Changes in Major Religious Traditions in the United States

	2007	2014	Change[a]
	%	%	%
Christian	78.4	70.6	−7.8
Protestant	51.3	46.5	−4.8
Evangelical	*26.3*	*25.4*	*−0.9*
Mainline	*18.1*	*14.7*	*−3.4*
Historically black	*6.9*	*6.5*	*−*
Catholic	23.9	20.8	−3.1
Orthodox Christian	0.6	0.5	−
Mormon	1.7	1.6	−
Jehovah's Witness	0.7	0.8	−
Other Christian	0.3	0.4	−
Non-Christian faiths	4.7	5.9	+1.2
Jewish	1.7	1.9	−
Muslim	0.4	0.9	+0.5
Buddhist	0.7	0.7	−
Hindu	0.4	0.7	+0.3
Other world religions[b]	<0.3	0.3	−
Other faiths[b]	1.2	1.5	+0.3
Unaffiliated	16.1	22.8	+6.7
Atheist	1.6	3.1	+1.5
Agnostic	2.4	4.0	+1.6
Nothing in particular	12.1	15.8	+3.7
Don't know/refused	0.8	0.6	−0.2
	100.0	100.0	

[a]The "change" column displays only statistically significant changes; blank cells indicate that the difference between 2007 and 2014 is within the margin of error.
[b]The "other world religions" category includes Sikhs, Baha'is, Taoists, Jains, and a variety of other world religions. The "other faiths" category includes Unitarians, New Age religions, Native American religions, and a number of other non-Christian faiths. From Pew Research Center. (2015, May 12). *America's changing religious landscape.* http://www.pewforum.org/2015/05/12/americas-changing-religious-landscape/.

to mitigate or reduce the emotional distress associated with mental and physical distress.

It is hoped that this chapter will help you understand how to consider the spiritual concerns of patients and families. First, we discuss understandings and uses of spirituality. Next, we examine how spiritual concerns can look within different nursing contexts. Finally, we look at specific ways for you as a nurse to help with spiritual concerns.

NORM'S NOTES Spiritual care—what is it? We all have a spirit, and we can feel it. Spiritual care attempts to go beyond the facts of psychiatry and brain biology and deal with that intangible part of our being that we call a spirit, but it can get tricky. You cannot impose your spiritual worldview on a patient, but how can you talk about spiritual issues without bringing your own values to the discussion? This chapter attempts to show how to deal with these competing forces—without reducing spiritual care to a meaningless behavior.

TOWARD AN UNDERSTANDING OF SPIRITUALITY

Psychiatry Based on Greek *Psyche* (The Soul)

The word *psychiatry* comes from two Greek words, *psyche* (soul) and *iatreia* (healing)—"healing of the soul." *Psyche* has a variety of meanings—the breath of life, the seat of feelings and emotions, and the part of human beings that transcends the earthly. The term *spirituality* is used to describe things beyond mere biologic existence.

Common Understandings of Spirituality

Spirit refers to something not strictly physical, which gives life, depth, and meaning to existence (Jung, 1980). Common understandings of spirituality have to do with making sense of life or searching for the ultimate meaning and purpose in life, often involving a relationship with the transcendent and seeking to be at peace. Spirituality is a natural part of human existence, and all people have spiritual needs regardless of their religious beliefs. Spiritual needs may consist of talking to a counselor, prayer, being with family and friends, singing, listening to music, attending a religious service, or participating in a religious ritual (Noome, Kilmer, Leeuwen, Dijkstra, & Vloet, 2017). The word *spirituality* is generally used in two ways. The first way sees the human spirit as inextricably connected to a transcendent source (God or a higher power or a universal spirit) and is often expressed within an individual's faith or religious community. The second way seeks to distinguish spirituality from a religious perspective by emphasizing aspects of the human spirit and its relationship to other human spirits in ways that are not dependent on the notion of a higher power but rather have faith in human beings' goodness and its possibilities to cure the ills of humankind (de Botton, 2013).

Spirituality in Relation to a Transcendent Spirit (Theistic View)

The theistic view is exemplified in the creation story of the world's three largest monotheistic religions (Christianity, Islam, and Judaism). God created the world, including human beings. God "breathed life" into a human being, who becomes a living soul. According to this view, human lives are inspired (literally, breathed into) by a Supreme Being. Therefore, one's existence is rooted in having ultimate meaning in a God who helps people make sense of evil, calamity, and disease.

Spirituality in Relation to Human Spirit (Humanistic View)

The humanistic view explains how people attempt to bring meaning and purpose into their lives apart from a religious community or an understanding of God. The material world is all there is, so meaning is created within the individual who is free to choose his or her life meaning (Hall & Hill, 2019). According to this view, spiritual fulfillment equates with feeling fully alive and connected to others, as well as to the broader environment. The emphasis is on the human spirit, both individually and collectively. The two understandings (theistic and humanistic) are not mutually exclusive; however, the latter understanding deemphasizes (and sometimes completely rejects) the theistic approach.

Other Helpful Perspectives for the Psychiatric Nurse

Spiritual Use and Abuse

A client's spiritual and/or religious perspectives can be either positive or negative based on prior experiences when (a) well-being was enhanced or (b) the client's problems and symptoms were exacerbated (Cashwell & Swindle, 2018). Religious and spiritual practices have been found to play a significant role in coping with distressful and challenging circumstances in life. It can also stimulate peace, optimism, meaning in suffering, forgiveness, and reconciliation to oneself and others (George & Bance, 2020). On the other hand, some individuals have had negative experiences at the hands of those who claim religion. Religious abuse comes in many forms, including emotional, sexual, physical and/or mental betrayal that occurs within a religious context or setting, with results that are traumatizing. The power differential present in every type of abuse may be even stronger in religious abuse, particularly when the abuse is at the hands of spiritual authorities in their religious community. It is important for nurses to create safety around discussions of spirituality, providing space in case patients have experienced spiritual trauma in the past (Cashwell & Swindle, 2018).

Making Meaning in Suffering by Finding Hope

People who are suffering are naturally driven to find a sense of meaning in their lives (Hall & Hill, 2019). Viktor Frankl was a psychiatrist who experienced intense suffering as a prisoner in Nazi concentration camps during World War II. He recognized that although individuals cannot always choose their circumstances, they always have a choice about their attitudes toward their experiences. He witnessed overwhelming helplessness at the death camps. He noticed that prisoners who had no desire to live first gave up hope, then life. For example, prisoners who did not exchange their cigarettes for food "were those who had lost the will to live and wanted to 'enjoy' their last days." Many of the prisoners who found a reason to live maintained hope and were able to survive (Frankl, 1984).

Trust and the Spirituality of Human Development

Bowlby (1988) recognized the crucial role of early childhood relationships on human development. Attachment Theory helps us understand our need to develop and maintain intimate emotional bonds with specific individuals, which is assumed to be a fundamental requirement of human nature. During infancy and childhood, bonds will develop with parents or primary caregivers who are the providers of comfort, support, and protection. Patterns of attachment operate most efficiently in interactions when two people respond promptly and lovingly when called upon for support and emotional security. When faced with distress or challenges, individuals'

attachment styles have been shown to influence the types of strategies that they use to regulate their anxiety. When caregivers are able to function as a secure base and a safe haven, their children are able to develop a secure attachment bond. When caregivers are unable to provide these key interactions, an insecure attachment bond develops. Children with insecure attachment often adopt one of two strategies to get their needs met: (a) minimizing or disregarding their emotional needs or (b) anxiously amplifying their emotional needs (Bock et al., 2018). The quality of early childhood attachment towards parents/caregivers will determine individuals' enduring style of relating to others, particularly their ability to trust. A chronic failure to attach leading to feelings of rejection and threats of abandonment will cause stress and oftentimes will be experienced as traumatic.

During difficult life circumstances, many people will attempt to make sense of their experiences. The majority of people will possess beliefs about themselves and the world as being safe, predictable, and just. However, individuals with insecure attachment generally do not possess beliefs that the world is safe, that God and others are reliable, or that they are valuable in others' eyes. Thus, these individuals may seek assistance with making sense of their suffering with trusted others, including healthcare workers (see Chapters 7 and 33 for more information on Attachment Theory and trauma).

Importance of Spiritual Care

People often look for meaning when they are in a situation that requires nursing care. Nursing, medical, and accrediting groups have recognized this importance. The International Classification of Nursing Practice or ICNP (2016) provides the nursing diagnoses of Impaired Spiritual Status and Spiritual Distress under the category of Coping Component: Cluster of elements that involve the ability to deal with responsibilities, problems, or difficulties.

The *DSM-5* (American Psychiatric Association, 2013) has a diagnostic category dedicated to a "Religious or Spiritual Problem" (see *DSM-5* box). The Joint Commission (Ehman, 2013) has maintained that patients have a basic right to care that respects their cultural factors, religious beliefs, and spiritual values. For this accreditation body, the spiritual aspect is viewed as unique and separate from the cultural, mental, emotional, psychosocial, and religious aspects.

DSM-5 DIAGNOSES OF SPIRITUAL PROBLEMS

DSM-5

Religious or Spiritual Problem

This category can be used when the focus of clinical attention is a religious or spiritual problem. Examples include distressing experiences that involve loss or questioning of faith, problems associated with conversion to a new faith, or questioning of spiritual values that might not necessarily be related to an organized church or religious institution.

From American Psychiatric Association. (2013). *Diagnostic and statistical manual of mental disorders (5th ed.)*. APA.

INTERSECTION OF SPIRITUALITY AND MENTAL OR EMOTIONAL DISTRESS

Mental illness is a distressing situation that can give rise to important spiritual questions. Oates (1978) identified how aspects of schizophrenia affect the patient's spiritual perspective. The incapacity to symbolize—that is, the patient's concrete thinking—can cause special problems because religious language is symbolic by nature. Oates related the story of a schizophrenic patient who decompensated while at a Pentecostal religious gathering: she was terrified at the thought of Jesus "entering her heart." To her, this was a literal invasion of her body.

Oates (1978) stated that although religion can be a common theme in hallucinations and delusions and that these vary among cultures, the diminished capacity for trust tends to be consistent cross-culturally. Peteet, Lu, & Narrow, 2011 noted that it is important to ask, "What about this disorder is important to understand in order to distinguish religious/spiritual experiences from psychopathology?" Trust is built on consistently demonstrating genuinely compassionate behavior on the part of the caregiver. The most practical advice comes from patients themselves, who reported that they want most of all for their spiritual care provider to (1) be authentic, caring, and respectful and (2) speak slowly and in concrete terms.

> **? CRITICAL THINKING QUESTION**
>
> 1. Psychiatric patients describe concrete thinking during a psychotic episode. How can these patients be open to spiritual care when spiritual language is by nature symbolic?

HEALTH CARE APPLICATIONS

Suffering and Illness Elicit Crises

We recognize that not everyone who reads this textbook will become a psychiatric nurse and that there are a variety of situations in which nurses will encounter patients who express spiritual needs. These issues are important in psychiatric settings, but patients with chronic medical conditions, patients with acute disease, and patients needing end-of-life care, whether in an outpatient or inpatient setting, are also likely to have spiritual concerns, as are their loved ones. Even during a patient's "routine" visits to a health care provider, the nurse can encounter some level of spiritual concern.

A major life crisis, such as facing one's own mortality (e.g., with a life-altering diagnosis), is among the most difficult points in a person's life. Suffering, distress, illness, death, and grief can induce an existential urgency that causes people to consider their own mortality and their sense of belonging. Although this type of crisis might be common, it almost always comes unexpectedly. At these critical life junctures, people have the opportunity to become more acutely aware of and interested in issues of meaning and their place in the world. These concerns can provide an opportunity for people to evaluate what is important to them.

Clinical Attention to Spiritual Concerns

Talking about religion and spirituality is powerful and personal. Bringing up the topic can be difficult for both patients and nurses for a number of reasons. Patients may be reticent to discuss their religious beliefs and experiences out of fear of negative or inappropriate responses from nurses. For example, some individuals who are experiencing serious mental illness may exhibit religious convictions that are deemed delusional (pathological) by professionals. On the other side, nurses may be reluctant to broach or assess for religion or spirituality due to a fear of imposing their values on patients or simply because they feel uneasy addressing religion/spirituality with patients (Cashwell & Swindle, 2018). Current research suggests that therapists, psychiatrists, and physicians in the United States and Western Europe tend to be less often religiously affiliated in comparison with consumers of mental health care. The presence of this "religiosity gap" may be one of the factors that prevent mental health carers from focusing their attention on the spiritual concerns of patients and their families. In essence, a professional's worldview will influence the assessment, diagnosis, and treatment of mental illness. Mental health professionals who consider themselves religious or spiritual will tend to inquire more readily about patient's religion/spirituality (Amerongen-Meese et al., 2018).

Patients are predominantly referred to chaplains by nurses for emotional issues such as anxiety, pain, depression, grief, and end-of-life support (Poncin et al., 2020). Amerongen-Meeuse and colleagues (2018) suggest that many patients appreciate it when health professionals initiate spiritual conversations and appear to be interested in that part of their lives. It is also important to consider that patients and family members may feel vulnerable and need safety to share their spiritual distress and concerns. As nurses attend and attune to the patient's narrative, nonverbal behaviors, and emotions, they can more effectively discern and respond to their spiritual issues.

How Can the Nurse Assess and Intervene in a Realistic Way?

The trust that many nurses naturally demonstrate is at the core of providing quality spiritual care. The discussion in this chapter can help you to identify spiritual strengths and concerns. Patients express a strong preference for the basic spiritual care provided by nurses as spiritual care generalists "including listening, communicating and expressing compassion," but they recommend that board-certified chaplains—spiritual care specialists—be involved when more in-depth spiritual care is appropriate to address complex needs (Health Care Chaplaincy Network, 2016). The Health Care Chaplaincy Network (2017) reminds nurses that spiritual care also includes empathy, being non-judgmental, and conveying that the patient is not alone.

Koenig (2008) reminded nurses that they should do five things regarding spiritual care: (1) take a spiritual history; (2) support and show respect for the patient's beliefs; (3) pray with the patient if the nurse is comfortable doing so *and* if the patient wants *and* requests it; (4) provide spiritual care by being kind, gentle, sensitive, and compassionate; and (5) refer to pastoral care. Koenig (2008) stated that nurses and chaplains are "natural allies," not competitors in providing spiritual care.

Whether in a psychiatric setting or in an acute medical situation, taking note of the patient's spiritual concerns is important. A simple spiritual history should be taken. Many spiritual screening tools of different lengths and complexity are available from various disciplines. Among the simplest and easiest to use is the HOPE screening tool. Two physicians at Brown University School of Medicine developed a tool that can provide the health care professional with four concepts to discuss with patients, given the mnemonic device, *HOPE* (Anandarajah & Hight, 2001). The answers can be an opportunity for further exploration of the spiritual issues involved.

H: Sources of *hope*, strength, comfort, meaning, peace, love, and connection

O: The role of *organized* religion for the patient

P: *Personal* spirituality and *practices*

E: *Effects* on medical care and *end-of-life* issues

Puchalski's FICA questions are another convenient way for a health care professional to take a spiritual history (Koenig, 2007):

F: Faith—what is your *faith* tradition?

I: Importance—how *important* is your faith to you?

C: Church/Community—what is your *church* or *community* of faith?

A: Address—how might we *address* your spiritual needs?

If you have time for only one simple question that will demonstrate respect for the patient's spiritual concerns, give you valuable information, and allow for future conversations, Koenig (2007) suggested asking: "Do you have any spiritual needs or concerns related to your health?"

CRITICAL THINKING QUESTION

2. What do you see as the similarities and differences of the HOPE and FICA questions?

USING CLERGY RESOURCES

Close collaboration between chaplains and mental healthcare professionals is necessary to ensure holistic care inclusive of patients' spiritual needs (Poncin et al., 2020). Community clergy are usually not specifically trained to address the spiritual needs of psychiatric patients. Given staff concerns about psychiatric patients' religious delusions and patient reports that they desire competent spiritual care, having a clinically trained professional chaplain as an integral component of the mental health care team makes sense. Even so, patients who desire spiritual care will likely request their spiritual leaders and return to their community of faith, where they are involved in an ongoing way. Many individuals with mental health issues and their family members may prefer to interact with religious-based professionals whom they trust rather than mental health professionals.

Patients with spiritual concerns should be referred to a clinically trained spiritual care professional (preferably a board-certified chaplain). Healthcare facilities provide and use chaplains in many different ways, ranging from community clergy to highly trained chaplains who serve on multidisciplinary teams. When referring patients to chaplains, nurses are encouraged to answer the following questions in their requests: (1) What does the patient/patient's relatives need support with? (2) What do I (as a healthcare professional) need support with? (3) Is it relevant to the meaning that this patient gives to her/his experiences, to her/his beliefs, identity, and values? (Poncin et al., 2020). Having a first-hand understanding of what a professional chaplain does can greatly expand your practice and the resources available to help. As a nursing student, you can ask to shadow a chaplain to see what chaplains do and how they fit into the health care team.

CRITICAL THINKING QUESTIONS

3. How can the HOPE or FICA questions provide an opportunity for further exploration of spiritual issues for a patient who is not involved with organized religion?

4. Did any of the following words catch your attention as you read this chapter? How many of these would you identify as spiritual issues as you care for a patient? Why or why not?

   abandonment anxiety belonging compassion faith forgiveness gratitude grief helplessness hope joy love place presence alone relationship trust

5. Why do you think so many people want to draw a distinction between religion and spirituality?

STUDY NOTES

1. Spirituality is generally understood to be a major component of mental health and psychiatric care.

2. Spirituality is more broadly defined today in our postmodern culture than it was in the past.

3. At its most basic, spirituality has to do with making sense of life, with hopes, plans, and fears; with things that people value; with the way in which individuals relate to others; and with issues of meaning and belonging.

4. There are two basic views of spirituality: (1) theistic view, in which life is ordered and given meaning by a source greater than humankind such as God, and (2) humanistic view, in which life is ordered and given meaning by humankind.

5. ICNP, *DSM-5*, and The Joint Commission recognize the importance of and encourage a spiritual component to nursing care.

6. Nurses should be prepared to provide spiritual assessments, interventions, and referrals.

7. Nurses can use a spiritual screening tool to help patients identify spiritual issues. Two brief tools are included in this chapter, and many facilities have their own approach to a spiritual history or screening.

8. Although often discussed by clinicians, spiritual care remains a neglected component of psychiatric care. Nurses should not be afraid of patients' desires to discuss these issues.

9. There is evidence of the clinical benefits of a healthy spirituality.

10. There is evidence of the harmful consequences of past spiritual abuse.

11. A clinically trained spiritual care professional should be part of the health care team.

12. Patients experiencing physical distress and facing death often find comfort in the transcendent view of spirituality, although these issues can arouse a sense of discomfort for health care providers.

13. Patients with psychiatric disorders frequently present with conditions involving spiritual themes.

14. Nurses can provide comfort, companionship, conversation, and compassion.

15. Nurses can take a spiritual history, pray for the patient under certain conditions, provide spiritual care, and refer to a chaplain as needed.

16. Nurses are encouraged by psychiatric patients to be authentic, caring, and respectful and to speak slowly and in concrete terms.

REFERENCES

American Psychiatric Association. (2013). *Diagnostic and statistical manual of mental disorders* (5th ed.) APA.

Amerongen-Meese, J., Schaap-Jonker, H., Schuhmann, C., Anbeek, C., & Braam, A. (2018). The "religiosity gap" in a clinical setting: Experiences of mental health care consumers and professionals. *Mental Health, Religion & Culture, 21*(7), 737–752. https://doi.org/10.1080/13674676.2018.1553029.

Anandarajah, G., & Hight, E. (2001). Spirituality and medical practice: Using the HOPE questions as a practical tool for spiritual assessment. *American Family Physician, 63*, 81.

Bock, N., Hall, E., Wang, D., & Hall, T. (2018). The role of attachment to God and spiritual self-awareness in predicting evangelical Christians' appraisal of suffering. *Mental Health, Religion & Culture, 21*(4), 353–369. https://doi.org/10.1080/13674676.2018.1494706.

Bowlby, J. (1988). *A secure base: Parent-child attachment and healthy human development.* Basic Books.

Cashwell, C., & Swindle, P. (2018). When religion hurts: Supervising cases of religious abuse. *The Clinical Supervisor, 37*(1), 182–203. https://doi.org/10.1080/07325223.2018.1443305.

Clark, M., & Emerson, A. (2021). Spirituality in psychiatric nursing: A concept analysis. *Journal of the American Psychiatric Association, 27*(1), 22–32. https://doi.org/10.1177/1078390320902834.

Cooper, B., et al. (2016). Exodus: Why Americans are leaving religion—And why they're unlikely to come back. http://www.prri.org/research/prri-rns-poll-nones-atheist-leaving-religion/.

de Botton, A. (2013). A school of life for atheists. https://www.onbeing.org/programs/alain-de-botton-a-school-of-life-for-atheists/.

Ehman, J. (2013). References to spirituality, religion, beliefs, and cultural diversity in JCAHO's 2013 comprehensive accreditation manual for hospitals. http://www.uphs.upenn.edu/pastoral/resed/JCAHOrefs.pdf.

Frankl, V. E. (1984). *Man's search for meaning.* Touchstone.

George, N., & Bance, L. (2020). Religious and spiritual coping: A component of post traumatic growth among female young adults with experiences of child sexual abuse. *International Journal of Social Sciences Review, 8*(1-3), 17–20.

Hall, M., & Hill, P. (2019). Meaning-making, suffering, and religion: A worldview conception. *Mental Health, Religion & Culture, 22*(5), 467–479. https://doi.org/10.1080/13674676.2019.1625037.

Health Care Chaplaincy Network. (2016). Spiritual care: What it means, why it matters in health care. https://www.healthcarechaplaincy.org/docs/about/spirituality.pdf.

Health Care Chaplaincy Network. (2017). Spiritual care and nursing: A nurse's contribution and practice. https://healthcarechaplaincy.org/docs/about/nurses_spiritual_care_white_paper_3_3_2017.pdf.

International Council of Nurses. (2016). CCC-ICNP Equivalency Table for Nursing Diagnoses. International Council of Nurses.

Jung, C. G. (1980). *The archetypes and the collective unconscious [R.F.C. Hull, Trans].* Princeton University Press and Bollingen Foundation.

Jung, C. G. (1984). *Psychology and Western religion [R.F.C. Hull, Trans].* Princeton University Press.

Krause, N., Pargament, K., Hill, P., & Ironson, G. (2019). Exploring religious and/or spiritual identities: Part 1 - assessing relationships with health. *Mental Health, Religion & Culture, 22*(9), 877–891. https://doi.org/10.1080/13674676.2019.1710122.

Koenig, H. G. (2007). *Spirituality in patient care: Why, how, when, and what* (2nd ed.). Templeton Foundation Press.

Koenig, H.G. (2008). Religion, spirituality and health: Research and clinical applications. Presented at North American Association of Christians in Social Work, Orlando, Florida, February 5, 2008.

Noome, M., Kilmer, D., Leeuwen, W., Dijkstra, B., & Vloet, L. (2017). The role of ICU nurses in the spiritual aspects of end-of-life care in the ICU: An exploratory study. *Scandinavian Journal of Caring Sciences, 31*, 569–578. https://doi.org/10.1111/scs.12371.

Oates, W. E. (1978). *The religious care of the psychiatric patient.* Westminster Press.

Peteet, J. R., Lu, F. G., & Narrow, W. E. (Eds.), (2011). *Religious and spiritual issues in psychiatric diagnosis: A research agenda for DSM-V.* APA.

Pew Research Center. (2015). America's changing religious landscape. *The Pew Forum on Religion & Public Life.* http://www.pewforum.org/2015/05/12/americas-changing-religious-landscape/.

Poncin, E., Niquille, B., Jobin, G., Benaim, C., & Rochat, E. (2020). What motivates healthcare professionals' referral to chaplains, and how to help formulate referrals that accurately reflect patients' spiritual needs? *Journal of Health Care Chaplaincy, 26,* 1–15. https://doi.org/10.1080/08854726.2019.1582211.

Vogel, A., & Schep-Akkerman, A. (2018). Competence and frequency of provision of spiritual care by nurses in the Netherlands. *Scandinavian Journal of Caring Science, 32,* 1314–1321. https://doi.org/10.1111/scs.12575.

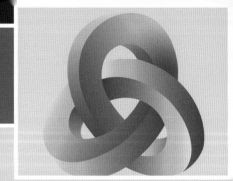

7

Models for Working With Psychiatric Patients

Debbie Steele

 http://evolve.elsevier.com/Keltner

LEARNING OBJECTIVES

- Compare and contrast major therapeutic models that contribute to the understanding of psychiatric patients and their needs.
- Identify key concepts of the major therapeutic models.
- Describe the relevance of each therapeutic model to psychiatric nursing practice.

This chapter provides an overview of some of the mental health models on which psychiatric nursing has been based. A basic knowledge of the following models is essential in guiding the therapeutic relationship and nursing care. The following models have been selected for discussion in this chapter because they provide essential concepts for working with psychiatric patients: recovery, attachment, psychoanalytical, developmental, interpersonal, and cognitive-behavioral. These models are summarized in Table 7.1 and discussed throughout the chapter.

RECOVERY MODEL

The recovery model is well-known among most mental health care professionals. It is paramount that nurses delivering services within the mental health care system have a good working knowledge of this model. To understand the recovery model, nurses must recognize that a paradigm shift is required. In particular, the recovery model moves the mental health care system away from the medical model, which is widely used within the health care industry. The medical model of treatment focuses on a person's disease and dysfunction, whereas the focus of the recovery model is on improving a person's competencies, not simply alleviating symptoms. In general, recovery from a mental disorder does not involve a cure but rather movement toward a meaningful way of life.

Key Concepts

Recovery is defined as "a process of change through which individuals improve their health and wellness, live a self-directed life, and strive to reach their full potential" (Substance Abuse and Mental Health Services Administration [SAMHSA], n.d.). The 10 guiding principles of the recovery model include the following: (1) person-driven, (2) occurs via many pathways, (3) holistic, (4) supported by peers, (5) supported through relationships, (6) culturally based and influenced, (7) supported by addressing trauma, (8) strength-based, (9) based on respect, and (10) emerges from hope.

Recovery-oriented care is person-driven and self-directed, exemplified by mental health professionals collaborating with consumers instead of telling them what to do. Empowerment includes encouraging consumers to try new things, while taking responsibility for their own care as they navigate their unique journey. Recovery is nonlinear, meaning that setbacks are not considered failures. Rather, there is an understanding that symptoms may return, and mental health care services may be necessary for a period of time. During this period, it is important to create an atmosphere of hope, emphasizing consumer strengths and abilities. Respect is demonstrated with mental health care personnel taking care not to identify a person by his diagnosis. The individual is not "bipolar" but is the consumer who is experiencing depressive or manic symptoms.

64

TABLE 7.1   Therapeutic Models

Model	Assumptions	Goals and Approaches	Dialogue
Recovery	Consumers are the experts with identifiable strengths and abilities.	Empowering the consumer and family to define and manage treatment options	*Recovery-oriented responses:* "What are your treatment goals?" "How can I assist you in meeting the goals of your treatment plan?"
Attachment	Emotions shape and organize one's experience.	Developing safe and secure emotional bonds in relationships	*Attachment-oriented response:* "How does that make you feel?" "Of course you would feel sad."
Psychoanalytical (Freud)	Change is a process of *insight*. Personality is developed by early childhood.	Bringing the unconscious into consciousness by enhancing awareness of self and one's effect on others	*Insight-oriented response:* "Tell me about your relationship with your mother."
Developmental (Erikson)	Change involves reexperiencing and resolving developmental crises. Lack of resolution of developmental tasks is related to difficulties in relationships.	Analyzing developmental issues, fears, and barriers to *growth* to facilitate mastery of developmental tasks	*Growth-oriented response:* "I can help you look at ways to develop your ability to trust others."
Interpersonal (Sullivan, Peplau)	Change is a process of relearning interpersonal relationships.	Learning effective interpersonal skills by using the nurse-patient relationship as a vehicle for analyzing interpersonal processes and testing new skills	*Reeducation response:* "Let's talk about what kind of things make you nervous in your relationship with your father."
Cognitive-behavioral (Beck)	Irrational and illogical thoughts, feelings, and behavior are all interrelated. A change in thinking will lead to a change in emotions and actions.	Substituting *rational* beliefs for irrational ones Reducing nonproductive behaviors	*Cognitive-behavioral response:* "Let's make a list of advantages and disadvantages of thinking and acting that way."

Within the recovery model, the goal of treatment is to help consumers develop meaningful roles in their communities, not to develop long-term relationships with the mental health care system. Support systems, including family, peer, and community members, are central to attaining and maintaining recovery. Peer support is an essential element in the recovery process. Peer counselors are individuals who have experience with mental illness within their self-directed journey of recovery. They hold a unique perspective that informs and provides insight for mental health providers, consumers, and their families. After training and certification, peer counselors provide direct support to consumers and educate and provide feedback to mental health care professionals (Ahmed, Mabe, & Buckley, 2012).

Recovery-oriented care is provided in a culturally competent manner that sensitively addresses consumers' race, ethnicity, language preference, age, gender, sexual orientation, religious or spiritual beliefs, and disability. In addition, structural inequities are considered, such as stigmatization, poverty, and homelessness. Recovery-oriented services include social supports, such as housing, income security, employment options, accessible transit systems, paid parental leave, language classes, and educational opportunities.

Relevance to Nursing Practice

Recovery-oriented care is focused on helping consumers achieve a sense of personal autonomy, social connectedness, and community integration. It assumes a sharing of power between the nurse and consumer to facilitate a client-centered vision of recovery (Osborn & Stein, 2017). Nurses play an important role in the process of recovery by examining and deepening their understanding of who the consumer is and how they can help to strengthen their ability to cope, boost confidence, and foster a sense of hope. Ideally, individuals need to be regarded as partners in addressing their own needs. Assessment of the consumer's general perception of his mental health and desire to make changes provides important insights as nurses become partners with the individual in their recovery process. Mental health consumers are active agents in their own recovery as the nurse aids them in exploring personal options and action plans (Jensen et al., 2013).

Psychiatric nurses have become the champions of the recovery movement, which has faced resistance from health care professionals who are accustomed to providing services to patients based on what they think is best for them. When patients do not comply with professional directives, they have been labeled noncompliant, unmotivated, treatment-resistant, and uncooperative. Health care professionals who practice recovery-oriented care understand that a patient's resistance can be a good sign—they have some ideas of their own. Collaboration becomes paramount as nurses learn to listen first and then help patients to move ahead with their preferred plans. Psychiatric nurses best serve consumers by carefully following the recovery model slogan, "Nothing about us without us!" This slogan translates into incorporation of consumers at every level of planning, training, delivery, policy, and evaluation of mental health care services.

ATTACHMENT THEORY

Attachment theory is defined as the natural tendency to develop intimate emotional bonds throughout life, which has been found to be associated with the development of personality and mental disorders. John Bowlby, the founder of attachment theory, theorized that humans are motivated by a need for relationships, focusing his research on children's attachment to primary caregivers. As a trained psychoanalyst in England, Bowlby studied human development and challenged Freud's well-known supposition that humans are compelled by their sexual drives. However, Bowlby (1988) did agree with Freud's emphasis on the importance of early childhood experiences on personality development.

Bowlby hypothesized that early development is determined by how children organize their behavior and thinking to maintain connection with important caregivers. Bowlby (1988) believed that safe emotional caregiving is crucial to children's psychological survival. Moreover, attachment theory asserts that early distortions in children's feeling and thinking occur in response to caregivers' inability to meet children's needs for reassurance and security through emotional support. During infancy and childhood, emotional bonds primarily develop with parents (or primary caregivers) who are looked to for comfort, support, and protection. When these emotional bonds are not created as a result of threatening interactions, the youngster will experience emotional distress, sometimes felt as trauma. There is now strong empirical support for Bowlby's conviction that family dysfunction is related to psychological and emotional disorders in childhood and throughout adulthood. Thus, the development of psychiatric disorders can occur as a result of childhood trauma.

Bowlby based his theory on overwhelming anecdotal evidence compiled over his lifetime. For example, while working with disturbed adolescents at the Child Guidance Clinics in London, Bowlby recognized that conflictual relationships with their parents resulted in emotional symptoms such as misery, callousness, and despair. At times, the boys became overwhelmed with feelings of anger and rage as a result of their distressing relationships with parents and others. These boys were experiencing depression and anxiety, as revealed in their emotional reactions.

In 1951, Bowlby and a young colleague, James Robertson, filmed a young girl's angry protest, despair, and absolute terror being left alone with nurses at a hospital. During this time, parents were not allowed to stay with their children in the hospital. This film was shown to physicians so they could comprehend a child's distress at separation from parents. As the hospital physicians viewed the movie, they were not impressed. They were well aware of the reaction of children handed off to nurses in the hospital. It was normal for children to be upset. Although Robertson was trying to emphasize the child's need for comfort and care by parents and caregivers during times of emotional upset, the message was met with indifference. Inevitably, more convincing was needed to change the practice of parents only being allowed to attend to their hospitalized children for 1 to 2 hours each day.

Up until this point, Bowlby primarily based his theory on anecdotal information. The lack of empirical research led him to work with Ainsworth, 1978, a Canadian researcher who devised a simple experiment known as the Strange Situation. In this experiment, a mother is instructed to go into a lab room with her young child at the invitation of a research assistant. After playing with the child in the lab room, she leaves her child alone with the "strange" research assistant. As would be expected, the child becomes upset when her mother walks away and disappears on the other side of a door. As the child cries, the research assistant tries to offer comfort as needed. Several behaviors were observed when children are left alone with a stranger. Most of the children were visibly distressed when their mothers walk out of the room, resorting to crying, calling for their mothers, and throwing toys. They rejected the contact and comfort of the stranger. The most important part of the experiment focused on how the children responded when their mothers returned to the room. A variety of responses were noted. Although apparently happy to be reunited with their mothers, some of the children had difficulty calming down. They were noted to act aggressively, such as hitting at their mother and throwing down toys that they were handed. Others took a vastly different approach, ignoring their mother and acting in a nonchalant, detached manner. Ainsworth noted three different behavioral responses of the children. It was hypothesized that the children's responses were a reflection of the mother's style of parenting. For example, children who are able to calm down readily have mothers who are consistently warm and comforting. Those children who are anxious and angry tended to have inconsistent and unpredictable mothers; the moms of detached kids tended to be preoccupied and dismissive. There seemed to be a direct correlation of the parenting style and the children's ability to manage their emotional responses, exhibited as anxiety, anger, and even withdrawal.

A researcher at the University of Wisconsin, Harry Harlow et al., (1965), was also discovering the power of parent-child attachment. His studies focused on young monkeys separated from their mother at birth, illustrating what happens to infants and young children in orphanages. Harlow's experiments involved giving isolated infants a choice between a "mother" made out of wire who dispensed food and a soft-cloth mother without food. The young monkeys would run directly to the mother with food to get nourishment and then immediately attach to the cloth mother, spending up to 23 hours a day hugging the soft mother. Harlow coined the term "contact comfort" as a primary need of infants and young monkeys. Harlow's experiments demonstrated the repercussions of early isolation; physically healthy infant primates who were separated from their mothers during the first year of life failed to develop into healthy adults, emotionally, psychologically, and relationally. These monkeys experienced depression, isolation, and erratic behavior as adults. They did not understand the social cues of others and were unable to mate. Ainsworth and Harlow's research provided critical evidence supporting the theory of attachment that helped revolutionize caregiving methods in the Western world (Johnson, 2008).

After Bowlby's death in 1990, a second revolution of the theory of attachment was sparked, maintaining that adults have the same need for attachment and connection as children. Applying the theory of attachment to adults is countercultural to established social and psychological rules of adulthood, namely, that adult maturity is defined by independence and self-sufficiency. In contrast, adult attachment is about being interdependent in relationships, recognizing the importance of being dependent on others for emotional support and comfort.

Research documenting adult attachment was spearheaded by psychologists Cindy Hazan and Phil Shaver (1987). In their studies, they questioned adults about their love relationships to see if they exhibited the same attachment patterns as mothers and children. Their research found that both men and women expressed the need for emotional closeness from their partner and the need that their partner would be there for them when they were upset. In addition, these adults expressed distress when they felt emotionally distant from their partner. These findings provide evidence that adult attachment patterns were uncannily similar to those of children. When adults feel a secure bond with their loved one, they have more confidence and feel empowered to explore the world. When they feel insecure, they become angry and anxious, or they withdraw and stay distant. These two types of attachment styles are developed in childhood and persist into adulthood.

In the past 30 years, hundreds of studies have applied the theory of attachment to adults.

This theory teaches us that we go to our loved ones for comfort when we experience distressing emotions such as anger, sadness, or fear. When the need for comfort and care is not met, a pattern of protesting ensues, characterized by such actions as attacking, defending, demanding, and withdrawing. Unfortunately, such harmful interactions set up vicious cycles that only compound the insecurity as each person is left feeling uncared for and unloved. Isolation and loneliness ensue as the individual struggles through life feeling alone, exasperated by feelings of depression and anxiety.

Relevance to Nursing Practice

A nurse who understands the theory of attachment will be better prepared to provide sensitive and age-appropriate care to clients with mental health symptoms. The nurse should be attuned to the distinct emotional needs of the client, with recognition that the therapeutic relationship serves as a primary change agent in the healing process. The nurse plays the role of creating a safe emotional environment, allowing the individual to achieve the goals of (1) expressing emotions without fear, and (2) developing a deeper awareness of self and others. Given the importance of past relational experiences, care plans should be guided by an assessment of the client's negative patterns of interacting with others, with special attention to the emotions that are triggered by particular situations. The empathic nurse will need to identify the ways in which

the client's relational needs are expressed and work to facilitate healthy expression of these longings through emotionally focused interventions. These interventions are transformative because they provide consistency, responsiveness, and sensitivity in the nurse-client dialogue. This occurs as the nurse gains an understanding of the client's experience through empathic acceptance and reflective curiosity. Nurses who care for clients with understanding, acceptance, and validation will promote healing through the therapeutic relationship.

NORM'S NOTES The recovery model highlights the importance of understanding the meaning individuals have of their health and treatment choices. The Psychiatric-Mental Health Nursing: Scope and Standards of Practice adopted the recovery model, whose slogan is "Nothing about us without us!" I, for one, appreciate this approach and find the slogan refreshing.

Psychoanalytic Theory

Freud's concepts of the levels of consciousness (1936) are central to understanding problems of the personality and behavior. *Consciousness*, or material within an individual's awareness, is only one small part of the mind. The unconscious is a larger area and consists of memories, conflicts, experiences, and material that have been repressed and cannot be recalled at will. Preconscious material refers to memories that can be recalled to consciousness with some effort. Freud believed that uncovering unconscious material generates an understanding of behavior that enables individuals to make choices about behavior and improve their mental health.

Defense Mechanisms

Sigmund Freud and his daughter, Anna, proposed a set of defense mechanisms that has long been influential and accepted by mental health care professionals. Defense mechanisms are activated when an individual's view of self is threatened. This occurs during times of stress when the anxiety is too painful and the person needs to protect himself. When these mechanisms are used excessively, individuals will tend to respond in irrational and illogical ways that do not solve their problems. Defense mechanisms are primarily unconscious behaviors; however, the goal is to bring them into conscious awareness. Common defense mechanisms are described in Table 7.2.

Relevance to Nursing Practice

Psychoanalytic approaches focus on the development of insight, also known as self and other awareness, that facilitates emotional, cognitive, and behavioral change in the individual experiencing psychiatric symptoms. The goals of psychoanalytical and other psychodynamic models are to bring the unconscious into consciousness, enabling individuals to make sense of their past in order to better understand their present behaviors. These approaches underscore the therapeutic significance of processing and transforming

TABLE 7.2 Defense Mechanisms

Defense Mechanism	Definition	Patient Example
Denial	*Unconscious* refusal to admit an unacceptable idea or behavior	Mac, who is alcohol-dependent, believes that he can control his drinking if he so desires.
Repression	*Unconscious* and involuntary forgetting of painful ideas, events, and conflicts	Anna, a victim of incest, has limited memory of her childhood.
Suppression	*Conscious* exclusion from awareness anxiety-producing feelings, ideas, and situations	Aaron states to the nurse that his recent divorce is no big deal.
Rationalization	*Conscious* or *unconscious* attempts to make or prove that one's feelings or behaviors are justifiable	John tells his mom that he bit his sister because she pushed him first.
Intellectualization	*Consciously* or *unconsciously* using only logical explanations without feelings or an affective component	Rene talks about her son's death from cancer as being merciful and shows no signs of her sadness or anger.
Dissociation	The *unconscious* separation of painful feelings and emotions from an unacceptable idea, situation, or object	Mrs. Adams recalls that when her husband was yelling at her, she didn't feel anything inside, she just went numb.
Identification	*Conscious* or *unconscious* attempt to model oneself after a respected person	Kelly states to her nurse, "When I get out of the hospital, I want to be a nurse just like you."
Introjection	*Unconsciously* incorporating values and attitudes of others as if they were your own	Without realizing it, Marie talks and acts similarly to her therapist, analyzing other patients.
Compensation	*Consciously* covering up for a weakness by overemphasizing or making up a desirable trait	Malcolm, who is depressed and unable to share his feelings with others, writes and becomes known for his expressive poetry.
Sublimation	*Consciously* or *unconsciously* channeling instinctual drives into acceptable activities	Guy, a former heroin addict, starts a local Narcotics Anonymous meeting.
Reaction formation	A *conscious* behavior that is the exact opposite of an *unconscious* feeling	Wren, whose parents are divorcing, tells her mother that she doesn't want to spend time with her dad (so her mother doesn't get mad), even though she really misses him.
Undoing	*Consciously* doing something to counteract or make up for a transgression or wrongdoing	After accidentally eating another patient's cookies, Donnelly apologizes to his peer, cleans the refrigerator, and labels everyone's snack with their names.
Displacement	*Unconsciously* discharging pent-up feelings to a less threatening object	A husband comes home after a hard day at work and yells at his wife and kids.
Projection	*Unconsciously* or *consciously* attributing one's own repressed thoughts to someone else	Connie blames her husband for the fight last night, unable to recognize that she was the one who started it.
Conversion	*Unconscious* expression of intrapsychic conflict symbolically through physical symptoms	A student awakens with a migraine headache the morning of a final examination and feels too ill to take the test. If she doesn't pass the exam, she will flunk out of nursing school.
Regression	*Unconscious* return to an earlier and more comfortable developmental level	A 5-year-old child has been wetting the bed at night since the birth of his baby sister.

repressed, disowned, conflicted, or painful emotions (Beutel et al., 2019).

In brief therapeutic encounters, it is helpful for the nurse to recognize and understand the maladaptive defense mechanisms that patients use. The nurse carefully shares observations regarding these mechanisms and works with patients to increase awareness about maladaptive patterns to enhance more productive behaviors. For example, an individual who previously denied a problem with alcohol may be ready to recognize that an arrest for public intoxication, a pending divorce, and three job losses are related to drinking and that a partial day detox facility can be discussed. The nurse is guided by the patient's values, beliefs, and needs as they are discovered.

In traditional long-term psychoanalysis, the advanced practice nurse therapist uses free association (allowing the patient to say everything that comes to mind) so that repressed material can be identified and interpreted for patients. Dream analysis helps patients uncover the meaning of their dreams, which serves to increase awareness about present behavior. Patients' inconsistencies and resistance to therapy are confronted. Transference (an unconscious emotional reaction based on previous experiences) that occurs in the current relationship with the nurse therapist is used to encourage working through feelings that would otherwise remain unconscious.

Not all individuals can tolerate the challenge of confronting intrapsychic conflicts, defenses, and transference issues. Therefore, an integrative approach may be more appropriate for those who cannot tolerate intense probing, especially those who are in crisis. Emotion-focused psychodynamic psychotherapy (EFPP) is an integrative approach that requires emotional attunement by the therapist, who is empathic and provides unconditional positive regard. This is communicated by a warm and gentle engagement and empathic interventions, such as giving words to feelings that a situation may have evoked in the patient. The patient's maladaptive emotional responses are processed in session and transformed into new adaptive emotional experiences (Beutel et al., 2019).

Clinical Example

A college student who is pursuing an engineering degree at the insistence of a domineering parent can be assisted in deciding her career goals, while gaining insight to deal more productively with parental pressures. Patients need support by normalizing their desires and longing, while discovering new and acceptable ways of expressing their needs.

DEVELOPMENTAL MODEL

Erikson's psychosocial theory of development (1950) focuses on the impact of environmental factors, parents, and society on personality development from childhood to adulthood. This theory continues to produce insights into psychosocial development even today. Dunkel and Harbke (2017) make the case that research on Erikson's theory is actually accelerating. According to Erikson's theory, every person must pass through a series of eight interrelated stages over the life cycle from birth to death. Each stage is associated with two possible outcomes. Successful completion of each stage leads to a healthy personality, coupled with successful interactions with others. Failure to complete a stage successfully can result in a reduced ability to grow psychologically and relationally. Table 7.3 outlines adult manifestations of Erikson's eight developmental stages.

TABLE 7.3 Adult Manifestations of Erikson's Stages of Development

Life Stage	Adult Behaviors Reflecting Mastery	Adult Behaviors Reflecting Developmental Problems
I. Trust versus mistrust (0–18 months)	Realistic trust of self and others Confidence in others	Suspiciousness of others Fear of criticism and closeness Withdrawal from others or Overly trusting of others
II. Autonomy versus shame and doubt (18 months–3 years)	Self-control and willpower	Self-doubt Dependence on others for approval or Excessive independence or defiance Impulsiveness and inability to wait
III. Initiative versus guilt (3–5 years)	Curiosity and exploration Initiative balanced with restraint Adequate conscience	Excessive guilt or embarrassment Self-punishment Assuming role as victim or Excessive expression of emotion Little sense of guilt for actions
IV. Industry versus inferiority (6–12 years)	Sense of competence/completion of projects Ability to cooperate and compromise	Feeling unworthy and inadequate Manipulation of others Lack of friends of same gender or Overly high-achieving perfectionistic
V. Identity versus role diffusion (12–20 years)	Confident sense of self in family and among friends Performing adult roles	Feelings of confusion, indecision, and alienation or Acting out behaviors involving alcohol, drugs, or sex
VI. Intimacy versus isolation (18–30 years)	Ability to give and receive love Collaboration and commitment in work and personal relationships	Persistent aloneness or isolation Superficiality in intimate and other relationships Or Possessiveness, jealousy, abusive to loved ones Dependency on others
VII. Generative lifestyle vs. stagnation or self-absorption (30–65 years)	Effectiveness in parental and societal responsibilities Caring guidance of others	Self-centeredness or self-indulgence Lack of interest in welfare of others or Care for others rather than oneself
VIII. Integrity vs. despair (65 years to death)	Feelings of self-acceptance and worth Exploration of philosophy of life and death Valuing one's life	Sense of helplessness, hopelessness, worthlessness, uselessness, meaninglessness/suicide Withdrawal, loneliness, and fear Focusing on past mistakes, failures, and dissatisfactions or Overtaxing strength and abilities

Developed by Schwecke, L., & Wood, S. Indiana University. Revised 2017 by Steele, D., Schwecke, L., & Wood, S.

Key Concepts

Each stage in Erikson's model comprises developmental crises as a result of positive and negative experiences. Mastery of critical tasks in each of the stages affects an individual's ability to master future stages. Erikson believed that the drive of humans to live and grow is opposed by a drive to return to more comfortable earlier states and behaviors, known as regression. Regression is common during times of trauma, prolonged or severe stress, and physiologic or psychiatric illnesses.

Implied *but not clearly described* in Erikson's model is the concept of partial mastery of critical tasks in development. The degree of mastery of each stage is related to the degree of maturity that the adult attains. Deficits in development carried from one stage to the next progressively interfere with functioning until the individual is no longer capable of growing without returning emotionally to an earlier stage to resolve life's crises. For example, a person might develop enough trust in others to engage in superficial relationships but may be unable to maintain intimacy with a spouse. Another person might have enough initiative to secure a job but lack the industry to stay with it. An environmental or social tragedy can shake the early foundations of development, such as when divorce from a spouse threatens the children's sense of trust in others and results in self-doubt.

The regression and lack of mastery of developmental tasks seen throughout the life cycle are not necessarily permanent. Individuals can return to earlier stages to master the missing critical tasks. For example, a young teenage mother may not have developed a healthy sense of identity and intimacy as a result of the responsibilities of caring for a child. This young mother is likely to be drawn back to the issues of identity and intimacy as she relates to her child and others in her new adult world. This crisis creates an inherent conflict in roles, feelings, and behaviors. Mastery of the critical tasks of each stage occurs more easily when it is chronologically appropriate. Overcoming delayed or incomplete development is possible but difficult.

Relevance to Nursing Practice

Most patients with psychiatric disorders demonstrate only partial mastery of the developmental stages consistent with their chronologic age. The nurse conducts an assessment of the patient's level of functioning through the interpretation of verbal and nonverbal behaviors and identifies the degree of mastery of each stage up to the patient's chronologic age. The behavioral manifestations of problems reveal issues to be addressed in working with the patient. For example, patients diagnosed with schizophrenia are often struggling with trust issues, exhibited by suspiciousness and fear of closeness. The nurse must concentrate on trust-building strategies with these patients.

Although Erikson focused on the polarity of each developmental stage (e.g., trust vs. mistrust) as if the positive pole were the desirable task to be accomplished, it is now recognized that the extremes of either pole produce problems in

functioning. For example, being overly trusting can result in being repeatedly taken advantage of by others. Having too much industry might result in working 14 to 16 hours a day without any time for recreation. Nursing interventions involving specific developmental issues are discussed in the chapters on specific disorders.

Clinical Example

A patient was admitted because of multiple cuts on the wrists. She says, "My boyfriend kicked me out. I just want to die. I knew I shouldn't trust anyone, ever!" She later reveals a history of emotional abuse and neglect in her birth family. She admits to a fear of closeness, anger outbursts, and a sense of being out of control in regard to her emotions and her life in general. She acknowledges that she has never really been able to depend on anyone to be there for her emotionally. As she begins to trust the nurse, she experiences the following: (1) unconditional acceptance, (2) normalizing of the anger and sense of being out of control, (3) a safe environment to talk about her past and present pain, and (4) the importance of having a secure support system.

INTERPERSONAL MODEL

Sullivan (1953) developed a comprehensive explanation of interpersonal and intergroup relationships called the *interpersonal theory of psychiatry*, which is consistent with attachment theory. Sullivan, whose background was psychoanalytical, believed that the *interactional* was more important than the *intrapsychic*. Sullivan considered the healthy person a social being with the ability to live effectively in relationships with others. Mental illness was viewed as any degree of lack of awareness or skill in interpersonal relationships. Relationships are viewed as sources of anxiety, maladaptive behaviors, and negative personality formation.

Interpersonal psychotherapy (IPT) focuses on improving mood symptoms while improving relationships, through building adaptive interpersonal skills. Research shows that depressed individuals often exhibit social skills deficits such as hostility and rejection that impair their interpersonal interactions (Berg et al., 2019). Thus, IPT is useful in the treatment of depression and other mood disorders in adolescents and adults (Duffy et al., 2019; Miller et al., 2018).

Key Concepts

IPT addresses the stressful social and interpersonal dynamics associated with the onset of depressive symptoms. IPT does not propose that the only cause of depressive symptoms is interpersonal; rather, depressive symptoms occur within an interpersonal context that is mutually dependent within the illness. The goal of IPT is to improve social functioning by examining interpersonal disputes, role transitions, grief, and interpersonal deficits. Interpersonal disputes and role transitions often occur in family, social, or work settings; there may be differing outlooks and expectations. When patients experience role transitions (e.g., divorce, caring for aging parents, caring for a chronically ill child), IPT teaches that these transitions are seen as losses, may involve a grieving process, and contribute to depressive symptoms. IPT promotes reappraisal of the inevitable stress related to transitions and changing roles. In addition, IPT examines the number and quality of relationships, including the therapeutic relationship with the therapist. Interpersonal difficulties can be identified and addressed within the therapeutic relationship, serving as a model for change (Anderson et al., 2018).

Nurse's Role

The nurse using IPT focuses on a patient's current interpersonal relationships and experiences. The goal of therapy is to develop mature and satisfactory relationships that are relatively free from anxiety. The nurse-patient relationship is a vehicle for analyzing the patient's interpersonal processes and testing new skills in relating. However, the focus of therapy is on the patient's interpersonal issues and distortions created by past experiences. The nurse helps correct these distortions with clear communication, consensual validation, and a warm and collaborative relationship. In challenging a negative self-image, the nurse presents an appraisal of the patient as a worthwhile, respectable individual with rights, dignity, and valuable abilities. The focus of IPT is often on loneliness, fear of rejection, clarifying emotions and their causes, using anxiety for learning about the self and others, managing interpersonal frustrations, and developing self-respect.

Relevance to Nursing Practice

Peplau (1952) played a significant role in applying Sullivan's original concepts regarding interpersonal relationships to nursing practice. Peplau saw a major goal of nursing as helping patients reduce their anxiety and convert it to constructive action. Peplau (1963) elaborated on and applied Sullivan's concept of degrees of anxiety to nursing (pure euphoria, mild anxiety, moderate anxiety, severe anxiety, panic, terror states, and pure anxiety). Peplau described the effects of mild anxiety through panic levels on perception and learning. She saw the nurse's role as helping patients decrease insecurity and improve functioning through interpersonal relationships that can be seen as microcosms of how patients function in other relationships. For example, a patient says, "My wife always knows when I'm upset and wants to help me, but I just say nothing." The nurse might say, "What does that feel like when you think about telling her the truth?" Peplau's focus on emotions, life issues, and interpersonal relationships is relevant for all patients, including those with psychosis dealing with delusions, hallucinations, and distorted thinking. When patients have a sense that the nurse understands what they are saying about themselves and their situations, this allows them to make better sense of their world, making life and relationships more manageable and productive.

Clinical Example

The nurse recognizes that a patient experiences increased anxiety whenever he is beginning a relationship with a woman. The patient complains about not knowing what to say or do when he is alone with a woman (lack of interpersonal skills). "I'm so afraid of acting like an idiot that I get tongue-tied and sweaty (anxiety). It's no wonder that I never see her again." Nursing interventions focus on specific sources of anxiety, overcoming insecurities, rehearsing social conversations with the nurse, and practicing social skills in a small group of patients.

COGNITIVE-BEHAVIORAL MODELS

Cognitive-behavioral therapy (CBT) draws on two theories with significantly different foci: thinking versus behavioralism. Cognitive theory focuses on internal mental processes that affect how one feels and behaves, while behavioral theory concentrates on the effects of the external environment. The CBT model has a person-in-environment perspective in which both the contributions of internal (personal) and external (environmental) phenomena are considered essential to human growth and development (Early & Grady, 2017). Beck's cognitive behavior therapy (2020) focuses on thinking and behavior rather than on expressing feelings. This model uses a cognitive approach based on individuals' abilities to think, analyze, judge, decide, and do. Beck views individuals' present perceptions, thoughts, assumptions, beliefs, values, attitudes, and philosophies as needing modification or change. Individuals' interpretations of events and expectations of themselves and others (not the actual event or people) are seen as causing the maladaptive responses. The goal of therapy is to reevaluate distorted or maladaptive thinking learned in childhood, leading to more productive ways of thinking and behaving.

Key Concepts

Beck believes that individuals think both rationally and irrationally and that irrational or illogical beliefs are responsible for causing problems in a person's life. In theory, irrational thoughts lead to self-defeating behaviors. Individuals are capable of understanding their limitations and can change their values and beliefs while challenging their self-defeating behaviors. The recurrence of irrational thoughts produces emotional disturbances that keep dysfunctional behaviors operant. Cognitive therapy examines the distorted perceptions, erroneous beliefs, self-deceptions, and blind spots that lead to "excessive, inappropriate emotional reactions" to events or stimuli. Reality testing and problem solving are aimed at correcting faulty cognitions and processes; the individual develops "more realistic appraisals of himself and his world" (Beck, 2020).

According to Beck, most individuals subscribe to at least some of the following irrational beliefs and ineffective rules for living:

- One should feel loved and approved by everyone.
- One must be totally competent to be considered worthwhile.

- Individuals have little ability to change or to control their feelings.
- Influences of the past should determine feelings in the present.
- Rejection or unfair treatment has catastrophic consequences.
- One is disliked when a disagreement exists with another.
- One "should" never make mistakes.
- Individuals who are obnoxious "ought" to be judged as rotten or bad.
- Being passive in life is easier than confronting difficulties and responsibilities.

Cognitive therapy has been adapted for individuals who have experienced traumatic events that often undermine basic assumptions about oneself and life, such as a view of the self as weak rather than strong and the world as threatening and fearful rather than benevolent. The focus of therapy is to challenge these latter assumptions and associated automatic thoughts to help individuals develop more logical assumptions, thoughts, feelings, and behaviors.

Both cognitive and behavior theories conceptualize change in terms of new learning. Behavioral therapy (BT) focuses on the learning of new behavior. Resolution of problems happens through the unlearning of old behaviors or of learning new ones (Early & Grady, 2017). BT builds on cognitive therapy by incorporating techniques based on the learning principles of classical and operant conditioning. Behavior therapy techniques include reinforcement, skills training, response prevention, exposure (in vivo or imaginal), and systematic desensitization.

According to CBT, understanding the process of change through new learning is within the control and direction of each individual. CBT assists the client to reinterpret events in a more adaptive manner through a process of recognizing, challenging, and restructuring thinking and behavior (Early & Grady, 2017). It is the most evidence-based therapy used for patients of all ages and diagnoses. CBT involves a variety of techniques and interventions: (1) orientation to the CBT model; (2) identifying automatic thoughts and cognitive errors using thought records; (3) revising automatic thoughts and finding rational alternatives; (4) behavioral methods—scheduling activities and pleasant events; (5) graded task assignments; (6) identifying and modifying core beliefs; and (7) homework, review, and further rehearsal (Beck, 2020). In addition, CBT with seriously ill patients might use a *multicomponent program*, which includes psychoeducation, medication education, problem solving about daily realities, social skills training, and cognitive skill practice.

Motivational enhancement therapy, a variation of CBT, is more widely used in the treatment of individuals with addictions. The goal is to enhance the patient's readiness and willingness to change habits related to the addictions, using *motivational interviewing*. This nonconfrontational approach includes expressing empathy, pointing out discrepancies between current behaviors and future goals, "rolling with resistance," and promoting self-efficacy. Motivational interviewing is a useful technique in the transtheoretical model and stages of change—precontemplation, contemplation,

preparation for action, and maintenance" (Cummins & Tobian, 2018; Krebs et al., 2018; Mallisham & Sherrod, 2017).

Dialectical behavior therapy (DBT) was developed for the treatment of borderline personality disorder, which is viewed as a complex posttraumatic stress disorder (Gorg et al., 2019; Linehan, 1993). The standard model of DBT lasts 12 months and includes individual sessions, skills group, phone coaching, and a therapist consultation team. Interventions include mindfulness techniques to focus attention on bodily sensations, feelings, and conscious thoughts. DBT has been found to reduce self-destructive behavior (e.g., suicidal and self-harm) and aggressive behavior (e.g., anger), as well as enhance coping skills (e.g., distress tolerance and emotion regulation) (McMain et al., 2017).

Relevance to Nursing Practice

The nurse-patient relationship is viewed as a collaborative effort to achieve goals for improved self-esteem, coping, relationships, and lifestyles (Beck, 2020). Because patients have many irrational *shoulds*, *oughts*, and *musts*, the nurse therapist assists the individual in challenging these beliefs and the degree in which they are irrational and illogical. Humor is often used to confront the patient's ineffective thinking. The nurse therapist shares ways to replace irrational thinking with rational thinking to reduce dysfunctional feelings and behaviors. The process of therapy focuses on the present. Patients learn strategies for replacing their irrational thoughts, feelings, and behaviors with more productive ones. The nurse therapist accepts patients as they are and where they are in the healing process. Homework assignments are given to promote focusing on positive statements and behaviors and on skill development. New, positive self-statements are encouraged to enable patients to begin to think, feel, and behave differently. Role playing, modeling, and positive reinforcement are also used.

Clinical Example

A depressed young man says to the nurse, "My friends have stopped coming around to see me. They say I'm always bragging about myself, but I feel like I have to prove myself to them and myself (irrational belief)." Nursing interventions focus on the acceptance of himself as a worthwhile person with a few weaknesses but many positive qualities. Interventions aim to help him process his beliefs that he "must" be totally competent in front of others and never make mistakes.

Clinical Example

A male patient is admitted several weeks after his mother has been diagnosed with terminal cancer. He is exhausted and showing symptoms of misperceptions of reality, delusions, and hallucinations. The patient says, "I can't live without her. I'll lose the house. I can't work if she isn't there to get me up and going in the morning. No one else will help me." The nurse develops a care plan that focuses on (1) offering the patient emotional support, (2) offering stress management strategies, (3) engaging the patient in anticipatory grief work, (4) developing a new support system, and (5) designing specific plans for getting up and being on time for work every day.

INTEGRATIVE APPROACH

Most psychiatric nurses adopt an integrative approach in regard to the therapeutic models presented in this chapter. Concepts from various models that best explain a patient's behavior, problems, and needs are selected. For example, a recently divorced patient states, "I've screwed up my life. All I do is sit at home, cry, and sleep." The nurse might use the attachment theory to identify that the patient is experiencing grief and loss, associated with her tendency to withdraw from others, or the cognitive model to identify the irrational belief that she is a failure in life. In addition, psychiatric nurses recognize that the key component in any therapeutic model is the *patient-nurse relationship*. This important component is discussed in depth in Chapter 9. The *therapeutic alliance* is often the best predictor of the outcome of any treatment approach (Moreno-Poyato et al., 2018).

CRITICAL THINKING QUESTIONS

1. Which concepts and strategies derived from each of the therapeutic models have you observed being used with patients?
2. Read the following case study. Using the models presented in this chapter, name two interventions you would use with this patient.

CASE STUDY

Ms. Levy has been admitted after a suicide attempt. During the admission assessment, she says that she recently began having nightmares about her sexual abuse as a child. She reports a lack of trust in men, yet always seeks their approval. Her interpersonal relationships with women are also stormy. Her anxiety interferes with her work performance. She admits to intense anger about the effect of the abuse on her life but believes that "women shouldn't show their anger." She says that she is afraid to "grow up and be responsible for herself" because she feels overwhelmed by life's stresses.

STUDY NOTES

1. Concepts from various models provide a framework for understanding patients' behaviors and problems.
2. Recovery-oriented care provides a paradigm shift that emphasizes that the nurse must partner with clients to help them achieve their preferred future.
3. Attachment theory helps explain how depression, anxiety, and other mental disorders can begin in childhood as a result of distressing parental interactions, experienced as traumatic for the child.
4. According to Freud, extensive use of defense mechanisms and maladaptive coping behaviors is assessed and understood by the nurse as inhibiting adaptive responses. The nurse helps patients to develop self and other awareness to enhance productive coping mechanisms.
5. Unresolved developmental issues (Erikson) interfere with patients' ability to solve problems and meet their own needs. Those with serious mental illness oftentimes have difficulty with trust issues in relationships.
6. Sullivan developed the interpersonal model to explain how anxiety in childhood is related to a lack of awareness or skill in interpersonal relationships.
7. Peplau used Sullivan's concepts of anxiety as a critical part of her framework in the nurse-patient relationship. Her goal was to help patients manage anxiety and use it for learning interpersonal skills through the nurse-patient relationship.
8. According to the cognitive-behavioral model, replacing irrational beliefs with rational beliefs can reduce stress and anxiety and self-defeating behaviors.
9. An integrative approach allows the use of concepts from many models so that different aspects of patients' thoughts, feelings, behaviors, problems, and needs can be explained more thoroughly. No patient "fits" neatly into just one model.

REFERENCES

Ahmed, A., Mabe, A., & Buckley, P. (2012). Peer specialists as educators for recovery-based systems transformation: The project GREAT experience. http://www.psychiatrictimes.com/addiction/peer-specialists-educators-recovery-based-systems-transformation.

Ainsworth, M., et al. (1978). *Patterns of attachment: A psychological study of the strange situation.* Psychology Press.

Anderson, T., McClintock, A., McCarrick, S., Heckman, T., Heckman, B., Markowitz, J., & Sutton, M. (2018). Working alliance, interpersonal problems, and depressive symptoms in tele-interpersonal psychotherapy for HIV-infected rural persons: Evidence for indirect effects. *Journal of Clinical Psychology, 74*(3), 286–303. https://doi.org/10.1002/jclp.22541.

Beck, J. (2020). *Cognitive behavior therapy: Basics and beyond* (3rd ed.). Guilford Press.

Berg, M., Rogers, E., Liu, W., Mumford, E., & Taylor, B. (2019). The interpersonal context of depression and violent behavior: A social psychological interpretation. *Aggressive Behavior, 45*(4), 437–449. https://doi.org/10.1002/ab.21832.

Beutel, M., Greenberg, L., Lane, R., & Subic-Wrana, C. (2019). Treating anxiety disorders by emotion-focused psychodynamic psychotherapy (EFPP) - An integrative, transdiagnostic approach. *Clinical Psychology & Psychotherapy, 26*, 1–13. https://doi.org/10.1002/cpp.2325.

Bowlby, J. (1988). *A secure base: Parent-child attachment and healthy human development.* Basic Books.

Cummins, D., & Tobian, R. (2018). Motivational enhancement therapy for veterans with chronic pain and substance use.

Health & Social Work, 43(4), 269–273. https://doi.org/10.1093/hsw/hly026.

Duffy, F., Sharpe, H., & Schwannauer, M. (2019). Review: The effectiveness of interpersonal psychotherapy for adolescents with depression - A systematic review and meta-analysis. *Child and Adolescent Mental Health, 24*(4), 307–317. https://doi.org/10.1111/camh.12342.

Dunkel, C., & Harbke, C. (2017). A review of measures of Erikson's stages of psychosocial development: Evidence for a general factor. *Journal of Adult Development, 24*(1), 58–76. https://doi.org/10.1007/s10804-016-9247-4.

Early, B., & Grady, M. (2017). Embracing the contribution of both behavioral and cognitive theories to cognitive-behavioral therapy: Maximizing the richness. *Journal of Clinical Social Work, 45*, 39–48. https://doi.org/10.1007/s10615-016-0590-5.

Freud, S. (1936). *The problem of anxiety.* W.W. Norton.

Gorg, N., Bohnke, J., Priebe, K., Rausch, S., Wekenmann, S., & Ludascher, P. (2019). Changes in trauma-related emotions following treatment with dialectical behavior therapy for postraumatic stress disorder after childhood abuse. *Journal of Traumatic Stress, 32*(5), 764–773. https://doi.org/10.1002/jts.22440.

Harlow, H., Dodsworth, R., & Harlow, M. (1965). Total social isolation in monkeys. *Proceedings of the National Academy of Sciences of the United States of America, 54*, 90–97. https://doi.org/10.1073/pnas.54.1.90.

Hazan, C., & Shaver, P. R. (1987). Romantic love conceptualized as an attachment process. *Journal of Personality and Social Psychology, 52*(2), 511–524. https://doi.org/10.1037/0022-3514.52.3.511.

Jensen, M., Pease, E., Lambert, K., et al. (2013). Championing person-first language: A call to psychiatric mental health nurses. *Journal of American Psychiatric Nurses Association, 19*(3), 146–151. https://doi.org/10.1177/1078390313489729.

Johnson, S. (2008). *Hold me tight: Seven conversations for a lifetime of love.* Little, Brown and Company.

Krebs, P., Norcross, J., Nicholson, J., & Prochaska, J. (2018). Stages of change and psychotherapy outcomes: A review and meta-analysis. *Journal of Clinical Psychology, 74*(11), 1964–1979. https://doi.org/10.1002/jclp.22683.

Linehan, M. M. (1993). *Cognitive behavioral treatment of borderline personality disorder.* Guilford.

Mallisham, S., & Sherrod, B. (2017). The spirit and intent of motivational interviewing. *Perspectives in Psychiatric Care, 53*(4), 226–233. https://doi.org/10.1111/ppc.12161.

Miller, L., Hlastala, S., Mufson, L., Leibenluft, E., Yenokyan, G., & Riddle, M. (2018). Interpersonal psychotherapy for mood and behavior dysregulation: Pilot randomized trial. *Depression and Anxiety, 35*(6), 574–582. https://doi.org/10.1002/da.22761.

Moreno-Poyato, A., Delgado-Hito, P., Suarez-Perez, R., Lluch-Canut, T., Roldan-Merino, J., & Monteso-Curta, P. (2018). Improving the therapeutic relationship in inpatient psychiatric care: Assessment of the therapeutic alliance and empathy after implementing evidence-based practices resulting from participatory action research. *Perspectives in Psychiatric Care, 54*(2), 300–308. https://doi.org/10.1111/ppc.12242.

Osborn, L., & Stein, C. (2017). Community mental health care providers' understanding of recovery principles and accounts of directiveness with consumers. *Psychiatric Quarterly, 88*, 755–767. https://doi.org/10.1007/s11126-017-9495-x.

Peplau, H. E. (1952). *Interpersonal relations in nursing.* Putnam.

Peplau, H. E. (1963). A working definition of anxiety. In S. F. Burd & M. A. Marshall (Eds.), *Some clinical approaches to psychiatric nursing* (pp. 323–327). Macmillan.

Substance Abuse and Mental Health Services Administration [SAMHSA]. (n.d.). SAMHSA's working definition of recovery. http://www.samhsa.gov/recovery.

Sullivan, H. S. (1953). *Interpersonal theory of psychiatry.* Norton.

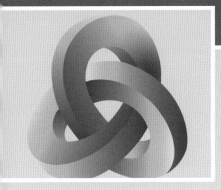

8

Learning to Communicate Professionally

Susanne A. Fogger

http://evolve.elsevier.com/Keltner

LEARNING OBJECTIVES

- Understand major influences on communication.
- Distinguish between social and therapeutic communication.
- Identify goals of therapeutic communication.
- Discuss critical therapeutic communication issues.

- Describe various techniques that facilitate patient-centered communication.
- State common causes of interference with therapeutic communication.

Most communication is a two-way process between two or more individuals. In nursing, this process is focused on patient care and the activities of care. Professional or therapeutic communication is one of the means whereby the nursing process is implemented to achieve quality patient care. In psychiatric nursing, therapeutic communication is one of the most important tools that nurses can use. It is essential to developing the therapeutic relationship, building trust, and providing support and comfort. When working in teams, intraprofessional communication relies on clarity and a common language in communicating patient care issues.

Nurses communicate in a variety of methods to share information, analyze data, collaborate with other disciplines, and deliver services to patients. Nurses must have excellent communication skills to work effectively with patients who have problems processing information because of alterations in function, thinking, feelings, and behaviors. Primary communication goals include ensuring understanding of the patient's meaning, as well as communicating clearly. Nurses coach and support patient communication skill development, which can result in improved self-expression and interpersonal interactions.

CATEGORIES OF COMMUNICATION

Communication between two or more people involves the exchange of information between a sender and a receiver. The product of communication is the message, which is to be interpreted by the receiver. Words (verbal or written)

and behaviors (nonverbal) are the primary channels for communication.

Written Communication

Because written material is a primary means of acquiring and sharing information, all professions require written reports, instructions, or share through the written word their findings and ideas. Mastering vocabulary, grammar, and the organization of ideas is a critical skill that may take time to develop.

NORM'S NOTES How important is clear communication? Well, go visit a divorce court, or human relations department hearing, or a malpractice court. In many of these cases, poor communication can easily be identified and is a major enemy of human happiness and well-being. When you add a person with a mental disorder or an emotional problem to the equation of human interaction, even more "stuff" can be misconstrued.

Health Information Privacy

Whether nurses communicate patient information via written form, telephone, or electronically, all these forms of sharing patient information must comply with the HIPAA. The Standards for Privacy of Individually Identifiable Health Information (U.S. Department of Health and Human

Services, 2013) established a set of national standards for the protection of certain health information. This information is called protected health information by organizations. It is paramount that nurses understand the standards and procedures adopted by their individual work settings for handling patient information.

Telephone Communication

Almost all of the adult population, as well as many teens in the United States, have a cell phone that they carry on their person. Quick phone access can allow patients to "OK Google" to access crisis and suicide services (hotlines). Community mental health centers also might provide phone numbers so that patients can call in-between visits for information or emergencies. Follow-up phone calls from the nurse can help facilitate transitions to new medications or in-home procedures. During the COVID outbreak, phone therapy sessions became a billable item allowing patients to receive care without risk of exposure. The calls may help manage patients' perceived or real emergencies, which can prevent an inpatient admission. Case management for high-risk patients can use phone contact to facilitate discharge planning and increase attendance at follow-up appointments, reducing recidivism. The increased use of smartphones or pay-as-you-go phones decreases feelings of isolation and helps individuals feel connected. In addition, text messages remind patients of upcoming appointments or can be used as check-in reminders.

Electronic Communication

Using secure electronic communication about and to patients requires special attention. E-mail communication or texting is fast and direct, yet it is important to only communicate with patients or other team members on a Health Insurance Portability and Accountability Act (HIPAA)-compliant line. Using social media to "share" photos or identifiable patient experiences is considered a violation of the protection act and may result in job loss and a lawsuit. It is recommended that nurses never post work-related material to avoid crossing the line on social media.

As younger individuals are very comfortable with electronic communication, all must be aware that the ease of communication needs to be balanced with appropriate use. Some practices offer patients the opportunity to communicate directly with their provider if they have questions or concerns about their care on secure portals. Patient satisfaction with services increased when patients were able to contact their providers by e-mail. However, providers are not equally satisfied where security, privacy, legal, ethical, guidelines, standards, and e-mail volume management issues are concerned. Some, but not all, providers prefer to use technology instead of traditional methods of communication (Lee et al., 2021).

Technology also has made therapy available for patients who do not live near a therapist's office. Telepsychiatry allows patients in rural or underserved areas to remain home and interact with the therapist via the Web. Clinicians are able to assess the patient's verbal and nonverbal communication via a HIPPA-secure system. For some adults and adolescents, this

may be their preference, as interactions via the Web may be less threatening than an in-person meeting. Having the availability of telepsychiatry provides services to the individual when travel can be an issue. However, a lack of high-speed internet service may mean that rural patients may be challenged to receive the same services (Raths, 2020).

Electronic Medical Records

Government mandates have increased the number of both inpatient and outpatient facilities using electronic medical records (EMR). Nursing entries may be facilitated by portable tablets with data entry in close proximity to the delivery of patient care. Extra precautions are required to preserve privacy and confidentiality, such as special screens that prevent people passing by from "accidentally viewing" confidential information. The EMR has increased communication among providers caring for the patient. All patients have the right to review their medical records, including reviewing progress notes. With increased patient access to review medical records, nurses must be careful not to include judgmental or negative comments.

The health information available on the Web has exploded in the past 30 years, allowing individuals to easily access health information. Medical reports, self-diagnostic tools, and other "self-help information" present new challenges for nurses as patient educators. Nurses serve as patient advocates to help sift through misinformation, interpret health information, and determine its accuracy based on the best evidence.

Speech and Behavior

In addition to sound, oral communication includes the mannerisms and emotional tone that modify the message. The timbre and tone of voice have meaning. The rate and emphasis of speech affect the message. Body language can enhance or change the meaning of words. Verbal and nonverbal communication must match. Behaviors can negate a verbal message; for example, a patient is not likely to (and should not) believe a nurse who says, "Yes, I will help you," with a frown and an angry tone of voice. Often a confused or delirious patient cannot interpret what the nurse is saying but can be soothed by a gentle smile and pleasant affect.

Dynamics of Therapeutic Communication

Therapeutic communication requires attention to multiple, interacting factors. At the core of therapeutic communication are the words and nonverbal behaviors that relate to patients' health needs and are exchanged between patients and the nurse. Carl Rogers, one of the leaders in psychotherapy of the twentieth century, viewed patients with unconditional positive and nonjudgmental acceptance. Fig. 8.1 illustrates the key variables in communication for the patient and the nurse. Communication is influenced by the following factors: (1) an individual's personal experiences, gender, culture, values, and beliefs; (2) the purpose of the interaction; and (3) the physical and emotional context. The nurse must communicate on the patient's level (according to the individual patient's vocabulary, educational background, and the effects of his or

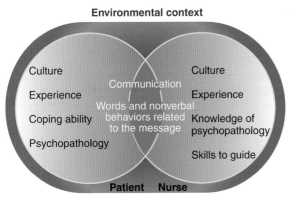

FIG 8.1 Essential and influencing variables of the therapeutic communication environment.

her illnesses) without using a patronizing, condescending, or stigmatizing attitude. Good communication with someone who seems hard of hearing requires assessing the individual's hearing before assuming that the person is deaf. The nurse should speak clearly, enunciate, as well as be visible in front of the patient to assist with conversation.

Interpretation of Communication

Interpretation of a message is filtered through an individual's knowledge, experience, and biases. Some aspects of communication are more commonly understood than others. Words are generally understood more precisely than behaviors. However, anyone who has studied a foreign language appreciates that nuances are often lost in translation because of the limitations of words. The nurse and the patient bring their own experiences to the relationship and have different lenses to understand an event. Having a broad knowledge of the effects of cultures is important if the nurse is to interpret accurately and respond appropriately to patient communications. When the nurse is unclear of the meaning of a statement, it is acceptable to state, "Can you help me understand what you mean? I do not comprehend your meaning when you say…." Clarification can help express meaning that may not be explicit.

Themes in Patient Communications

Patient communications often convey indirect messages or underlying themes about content, mood, or interaction issues. Themes are reflected in patients' thoughts, which engender feelings and then produce behaviors. *Content themes* go beyond the words that the patient is saying and examine underlying messages about patient perceptions of themselves and their problems over time. Their messages relate to beliefs and values, self-concept and self-esteem, a sense of helplessness and hopelessness, suspiciousness, the risk for suicide, and disturbances in thinking or processing of information and beliefs. *Mood themes* relate to affect and the feelings conveyed while patients discuss their issues and concerns. Feelings often reflect shame, guilt, anger, sadness, and fear, which may or may not match the content theme. Their facial expression may be flat, blunted, full-range, euphoric, labile, congruent, or incongruent. Assessing for *interaction themes* involves examining

the ways in which patients relate to family, friends, other patients, and staff. A patient might call the crisis center each time her roommate is out of town to complain about nervousness and loneliness. When the roommate returns, the person quits calling as they are comfortable again. The interaction theme, in this case, might be assessed as one of dependency. The patient who plays one staff member against another and seeks attention by complaining about all the other patients might be showing an interaction theme of manipulation.

In another example, a patient might spend 30 minutes describing his divorce of 3 years ago, two other broken relationships since then, having been laid off from his job, having to sell his house, and feeling as though he is a failure. The underlying *content theme* might be interpreted as a series of major losses. As he describes all these losses, he might convey anger, guilt, or both. These *mood themes* would be congruent with the content theme. However, feelings do not always match the content theme. If the patient were laughing as he described his losses, his jubilant presentation would be considered as an *incongruent mood theme*. The *interaction theme* might be abandonment or social isolation. Themes are frequently an aspect of the patient's care focus, such as a feeling of hopelessness, powerlessness, chronic low self-esteem, or risk for suicide.

Environmental Considerations

The environment can facilitate or impede therapeutic communication. Factors such as noise level, privacy, type of furniture, space, and temperature can affect the quality of communication.

Ensuring privacy for the patient's conversation is important to the communication between the nurse and the patient. Decreasing background noise and ensuring good lighting can provide for clearer communication, especially for individuals who are hard of hearing. *Proxemics* refers to the way in which people perceive and use environmental, social, and personal space during interactions. Typically boundaries of personal space for public and social communication are more distant compared with boundaries for intimate or therapeutic communication. The type of illness; emotional factors such as suspiciousness, anxiety, perceptual distortions, or aggressiveness; the genders of the two parties; and personal comfort also influence the amount of space needed between the patient and the nurse. People generally are more comfortable talking to others when they are speaking on the same eye level, rather than when one person stands over the other. Some patients might require sitting at an angle to the nurse or might need a table or empty chair between themselves and the nurse to feel safe enough to talk.

Physical Considerations

Patients with certain physical problems might experience communication difficulties. Certain sensory limitations, such as hearing loss, might compromise communication, necessitating compensatory measures, such as slow, face-to-face speech for lipreading. During COVID-19, masks are required for safety but hinder communication with the hard of hearing. Nurses can use a mask with a clear panel so the speaker's mouth is visible. Developmental disabilities might seriously limit the ability of patients to comprehend and remember. Simple sentences with a single main idea might have to be repeated several times. Speech impediments or other problems might interfere with the nurse's ability to understand the patient's needs. Asking for repetition, clarification, and validation is important, but this can increase a patient's frustration when the practice becomes excessive. Having patients write their answers is an alternative when they are able to read and write.

Kinesics Considerations

Kinesics is the study of body movements as a form of nonverbal communication. Culturally based body language is another means by which individuals express their emotional state. Avoiding prolonged eye contact is often used to disengage or ignore communication. In some cultures, though, eye contact is avoided, and direct eye contact is considered rude. Crossing the arms over the chest may suggest the individual is feeling defensive. (However, this also might occur when a person is cold.) The nurse must be sensitive to these cues and interpret them in a global context of therapeutic communication. If the message appears inconsistent or confusing, then exploring the meaning of body language might be useful. For example, the nurse might say, "Many times, when people back away from someone, it is because they are afraid. Are you afraid right now?" Body language might communicate feelings or emotions or merely reflect a habit. Ideally, the nurse's behavior communicates caring, confidence, and calmness, as well as conveys hope.

CRITICAL THINKING QUESTION

1. Ann Williams has multiple facial injuries with both eyes patched, is breathing with a ventilator, and has been sedated. In what ways would you modify your techniques to facilitate communication with her?

THERAPEUTIC COMMUNICATION

Social Communication Versus Therapeutic Communication

Social communication involves equal disclosure of personal information and intimacy, and both parties have equal opportunities for spontaneity, with the expectation of mutual confidentiality. Both participants seek to have personal needs met, whereas therapeutic communication focuses on the needs and agenda of the patient only. Therapeutic communication guides the patient to explore current personal issues and occasionally painful feelings. Remaining professional means maintaining a calculated emotional distance, near enough to be involved but objective enough to be helpful. Self-disclosure is inappropriate and may add to the patient's burden. The nurse must refocus the patient's questions about the nurse back to the patient. For example, "You are asking me about my family, but I'm here to talk about you. Can you tell me about your family?" While confidentiality is a "must" to be respected outside the treatment setting, the nurse has a professional obligation to share

patient information with the treatment team with the goal of tailoring treatment to the patient's needs. Clarification of the nurse's role should make it clear that she cannot keep secrets for the patient. The nurse is the patient's advocate, supporter, and teacher, but not a friend. The nurse and the patient must recognize that the role of the nurse is therapeutic. Supervision with more senior nurses can support and model clear communication of boundaries and roles.

Therapeutic Use of Self

In psychiatric nursing, the nurse is the primary therapeutic agent. Using verbal and nonverbal communication, the nurse promotes the individual strengths of the psychiatric patients (compared with treatment procedures and physical interventions used by the medical-surgical nurse). Nursing communication is a major vehicle that helps patients achieve productive thinking and emotional and behavioral outcomes. **The use of self**, **pharmacology, and the environment** are the major components of psychotherapeutic management.

The use of silence and therapeutic listening are important components of the therapeutic use of self and are crucial for getting to know patients as individuals and understand needs and concerns. Therapeutic listening has been described as being composed of the following attributes (Kemper, 1992):

- Being actively alert
- "Hearing" with all the senses
- Using eye contact
- Exhibiting an attending posture
- Ensuring concentration
- Being patient
- Displaying an openness to receive information
- Offering empathy and support
- Asking open-ended questions
- Assimilating verbal and nonverbal information
- Organizing, synthesizing, and interpreting information
- Validating emotional experiences
- Clarifying information
- Responding verbally and nonverbally to encourage patients to continue
- Summarizing important points
- Giving appropriate feedback

CRITICAL THINKING QUESTION

2. Select three or four of the previous behaviors and communicate with a friend. What difference do you see in the way your friend responds?

Therapeutic use of the self requires the nurse to be self-aware and emotionally secure themselves. Facets of important aspects of the use of self include:

Sensitivity to recognize important cues and make decisions about the priority of these cues.

Objectivity is the process of remaining open to as many aspects of patients, their problems, and potential solutions as possible.

Communicating empathy is an essential skill of the psychiatric nurse. Empathy is the ability to recognize and understand the patient's feelings and point of view objectively. Empathy, expressed verbally and nonverbally, conveys caring, compassion, and concern for patients but never implies that the nurse can fully experience patients' feelings. Empathy helps patients to be more accepting of their feelings and express them more readily.

Being therapeutic includes being genuine and sincere, as conveyed by congruent verbal and nonverbal behaviors, authenticity, and honesty (without total self-disclosure by the nurse). Patients must feel respected, valued, and accepted by the nurse, even when some of their behaviors are not tolerated.

The nurse should not evaluate patients' thoughts, feelings, and behaviors judgmentally as being right or wrong; rather, the nurse helps patients evaluate the effects or consequences of these factors.

However, the nurse must also set limits on destructive behaviors to protect the integrity and dignity of the patient, as well as the safety and rights of other patients.

Touch is a complex issue when working with patients who have underlying psychiatric issues. The meaning of touch varies widely among cultures. Touching a patient's hand or shoulder or giving a light hug can convey caring, empathy, support, and acceptance. However, some individuals may have difficulty comprehending the meaning of the nurse's touch. Touching may be misinterpreted as a violation of personal space or privacy or as a sexual gesture or aggressive move. The use of touch with patients must be approached with caution. Patients' behaviors can provide clues as to their ability to tolerate and benefit from touch. For example, a patient who is unable to sit close to the nurse is less likely to want to be touched. A patient who is trusting of the nurse is more likely to accept being touched. A patient who is sexually preoccupied might misinterpret any type of touch. With many patients (particularly patients who have been sexually or physically abused), asking permission before giving a gentle hug is appropriate: "Do you want a hug from me?" If the hug is turned down, the nurse needs to realize that the hesitancy may be based on previous experiences. It is best to ask permission before any touch, such as "May I touch you to check the swelling in your ankles?"

Techniques

Therapeutic techniques are a means of helping patients move toward productive goals but are not goals in themselves. The communication techniques presented in Table 8.1 are arranged in a way that facilitates patients' learning, problem-solving, and change. Interactions with patients do not involve using all these techniques sequentially. Many nurse-patient interactions do not use a complete nursing process in a single session, but they always involve using therapeutic techniques. Occasionally interactions have primarily a social or recreational focus rather than being a problem-solving process, but these still might be beneficial to the patient. Every encounter with a patient can be therapeutic with or without the full use of the nursing process.

TABLE 8.1 **Therapeutic Techniques in Psychiatric Nursing**	
Techniques Fostering Description	
Offering self: Making oneself available and showing interest and concern	"I'll sit with you for a while." "I noticed you have been crying, is there something you would like to talk about?" "I'll stay with you."
Active listening: Paying close attention to verbal and nonverbal communications, patterns of thinking, feelings, and behaviors	Face the patient; maintain eye contact; be open, alert, and patient; respond appropriately.
Silence: Planned absence of verbal remarks to allow patients to think and say more	Maintain eye contact; convey interest and concern in facial expressions.
Empathy: Recognizing and acknowledging patients' feelings	"I can hear how painful it is for you to talk about this."
Questioning: Using open-ended questions to achieve relevance and depth in discussion (not closed yes/no questions)	"Who?" "What?" "Where?" "What did you say?" "What happened?" "Tell me about it."
General leads: Using neutral expressions to encourage patients to continue talking	"Go on; I'm listening." "I hear what you are saying."
Restating: Repeating the exact words of patients to remind them of what they said, to let them know that they are heard	"You say you are going home soon." "Your mother wasn't happy to see you?"
Verbalizing the implied: Rephrasing patients' words to highlight an underlying message	*Patient:* "There is nothing to do at home." *Nurse:* "It sounds as if you might be bored at home."
Clarification: Asking patients to restate, elaborate, or give examples of ideas or feelings	"What do you mean by 'feeling sick inside'?" "Give me an example of feeling 'lost.'"
Techniques Fostering Analysis and Conclusions	
Making observations: Commenting on what is seen or heard to encourage discussion	"You seem restless." "I noticed you had trouble making a decision about..."

Continued

TABLE 8.1   Therapeutic Techniques in Psychiatric Nursing—cont'd

Presenting reality: Offering a view of what is real and what is not without arguing with the patient	"I know the voices are real to you, but I don't hear them." "I don't see it the same way."
Encouraging description of perceptions: Asking for patients' views of their situations	"What do you think is happening to you right now?" "What do you think is the issue with your wife?"
Voicing doubt: Expressing uncertainty about the reality of patients' perceptions and conclusions	"Is that the only way to interpret it?" "What other conclusion could there be?"
Placing an event in time or sequence: Asking for relationships among events	"When did you do this?" "Then what happened?" "What led up to …?" "What is the connection between …?"
Encouraging comparisons: Asking for similarities and differences among feelings, behaviors, and events	"How does this compare with the last time?" "What is different about your feelings today?"
Identifying themes: Asking patients to identify recurrent patterns in thoughts, feelings, and behaviors	"What do you do each time you argue with your wife?" "What feeling do you get when you see your father?"
Summarizing: Reviewing main points and conclusions	"Let's see, so far you have said…"

Techniques Fostering Interpretation of Meaning and Importance

Focusing: Pursuing a topic until its meaning or importance is clear	"Explain more about…" "What bothers you about…?" "What happens when you feel this way?"
Interpreting: Providing a view of the meaning or importance of something	"It sounds as if this is very important to you." "You seem to get in trouble when you…"
Encouraging evaluation: Asking for patients' views of the meaning or importance of something	"So, what does all this mean to you?" "How serious is this for you?" "How important is it to change this behavior?"

Techniques Fostering Problem-Solving and Decision-Making

Suggesting collaboration: Offering to help patients solve problems	"I can help you understand this better." "Let's see if we can find an answer."
Encouraging goal setting: Asking patients to decide on the type of change needed	"What do you think needs to change?" "What do you want to do differently?"
Giving information: Providing information that will help patients make better choices	"I can tell you about your medicines." "There are self-help groups available."
Encouraging consideration of options: Asking patients to consider the pros and cons of possible options	"Which is the best alternative for you?" "What is the good and the not-so-good aspect of that plan? "
Encouraging decisions: Asking patients to make a choice among options	"What would work best?" "What exactly will it take to carry out your plan?"
Encouraging the formulation of a plan: Probing for step-by-step actions that will be needed	"What else do you need to do?"

Techniques Fostering Completion of Plans

Testing New Behaviors and Evaluating Outcomes

Rehearsing: Requesting a verbal description of what will be said or done	"Tell me exactly what you will say to your wife on Friday."
Role-playing: Practicing behaviors; the nurse plays a particular role supporting the patient's efforts to practice their response.	"I'll play your wife. What do you want to say to me?"
Supportive confrontation: Acknowledging the difficulty in changing but push for action	"I know this isn't easy to do, but I believe you can do it." "It's hard, but give it a try."
Limit setting: Discouraging nonproductive feelings and behaviors and encouraging productive ones	"You're slipping into your aggressive tone. Try it again, softening your voice." "That's a negative comment about yourself. Can you tell me something positive?"
Feedback: Pointing out specific behaviors and giving impressions of reactions	"I thought you conveyed anger when you said…" "When you said…, I felt…."
Encouraging evaluation: Asking patients to evaluate their actions and the outcomes	"How well did it work when you tried…?" "What was your husband's reaction?"
Reinforcement: Giving feedback on positive behaviors	"This new approach worked for you. Keep it up!"
Repeating steps of the nursing process if needed: Using the steps of the nursing process to get a description of what happened, the degree of success, and ideas for change	"What would help you do better next time?" "If things didn't go well, what could you do differently next time?"

INTERFERENCE IN THERAPEUTIC COMMUNICATION

In the same manner that therapeutic communication guides the patient toward goals, certain messages and behaviors interfere with reaching these goals. As nurses' skill levels improve, they must identify and work to overcome any habitual communication problems that interfere with effective therapeutic communication.

Nurse's Fears and Feelings

As therapeutic communication involves the use of self, many personal feelings are naturally evoked and may be disturbing. A nurse might easily develop a feeling of fear or anxiety when communicating with individuals who are experiencing psychotic symptoms or physical distress. Fear compromises therapeutic communication. The nurse might have concerns such as, "Could this be me someday?" or "My brother does this sometimes; does that mean he's crazy?" or "What if this patient gets angry with me?" Therapeutic communication relies on coming to terms with these types of issues. People seek help or are forced to seek help because of serious and ongoing difficulties in functioning, not because of an occasional dysfunctional behavior. The nurse should avoid personalizing what patients say and do. Patients who abruptly end a conversation may be responding to their own thoughts or anxieties rather than to something the nurse said. Nurses can benefit from analyzing interactions with patients as well as their own feelings and reactions. Using peers or formal supervision to discuss thoughts and feelings can help prevent nurses from internalizing interactions with patients.

Occasionally a nurse may be afraid of harming patients by saying the wrong thing. Typically patients do not fall apart or act out because of a nurse's single mistake, particularly when there is an overall attitude that is positive and helpful; however, patients are sensitive to malicious intent and rejection. A mistake can become a therapeutic encounter because the nurse can represent a role model for the proper way to admit and apologize for an error. Many people, including patients with mental illness, have trouble recognizing and correcting mistakes with those who are significant to them. In many situations, a sincere apology, when warranted, can strengthen the relationship.

Another concern is the invasion of privacy. Psychiatric nurses investigate personal areas of patients' lives intensely, such as values, beliefs, feelings, intimate relationships, and sexuality, or legally sensitive areas, such as incest, partner abuse, and drug use. Secrets that the patient could not or would not discuss with friends or family are important to explore, especially if shame is an underlying emotion. Although patients may address these issues, they are not easy to discuss. The nurse can enhance patients' abilities to be open and honest by explaining the need to know about a sensitive area, by asking questions in a kind and matter-of-fact manner, by conveying empathy, and by reiterating a desire to help. It is equally important to honor the patient's request to avoid an area of sensitivity. Simply saying, "perhaps you may want to discuss this with me later when you are more comfortable with me," can avoid retraumatizing the patient.

Ineffective Responses

Learning and consistently using effective communication techniques require practice. In particular, the nurse should work toward decreasing the number of yes/no questions (closed-ended questions). Yes/no questions provide little new information and necessitate more questions. However, novice nurses might not always interact as effectively as desired. A nurse might become defensive and withdraw from patients who are cursing angrily rather than discussing the behavior. A patient might pick up on a nurse's anxiety and ask, "Are you scared of us crazies?" There is a tendency to deny this instead of being more truthful and saying, "I am afraid of saying something that might upset you." Nurses might get caught up in the unfounded fears and accusations of paranoid patients and inadvertently reinforce their symptoms.

Distinguishing between fact and distortion in what patients say is often difficult, as the nurse must avoid premature conclusions. For example, staff members did not believe a patient who said he had written the theme song for a popular play. The patient finally brought in his original handwritten sheet music and the list of credits from the play's manuscript for the staff to see. It is helpful to obtain information from family members to validate information or wait until medications and rest help clear delusional thinking.

Nurses might be preoccupied with what to say next rather than with listening, or a nurse might be listening to a patient but not really hearing or understanding what is being said. Nodding one's head as a patient talks might convey, "I hear you" or "I agree with you"—an important difference. Pretending to care is often easily interpreted by the patient as not being genuine and interferes with the healing process.

BOX 8.1   Ineffective or Inappropriate Responses and Behaviors

Asking "why" questions: "Why do you feel that way?"
Looking busy; ignoring the patient, not acknowledging their presence
Seeming uncomfortable with silence; fidgeting
Being opinionated; arguing with the patient
Avoiding sensitive topics; changing the topic
Being superficial or using clichés
Having a closed posture; avoiding eye contact with the patient
Making false promises or reassurances
Giving advice or talking too much
Laughing or smiling inappropriately
Showing disapproval or being judgmental
Using stigmatizing language: "You addicts are all the same"
Belittling feelings or minimizing problems
Being defensive or avoiding the patient
Making flippant or sarcastic remarks
Lying or being insincere
Texting while sitting with the patient

The overuse of one or two therapeutic skills, such as reflecting or restating, can stagnate communication. Giving advice to patients rather than helping them evaluate and choose their own solutions can also impede problem-solving. False reassurances, such as "Everything will be all right" or "Things are bound to get better," are promises that the nurse cannot keep.

Box 8.1 lists other responses and behaviors that are generally ineffective or inappropriate. Mistakes by the nurse generally can be corrected, explanations given, and damage to the relationship reversed. Patients usually evaluate nurses by their overall attitude of caring and concern rather than by a single inappropriate response.

STUDY NOTES

1. Therapeutic techniques are skills to help people communicate better but are not goals in themselves.
2. Therapeutic communication occurs with a plan and a purpose focused on the patient, whereas social communication involves equal levels of intimacy, sharing, and the opportunity for spontaneity.
3. Therapeutic communication differs from social communication because the focus is on the patient's agenda rather than on a give-and-take experience.
4. The goals of psychiatric nursing are to understand the patient's communication, ensure that patients understand the nurse, and support the learning and development of more effective communication skills.
5. Listening is a therapeutic communication technique that requires careful concentration to guide the conversation toward a goal.
6. Nurses are responsible for therapeutic communication and must recognize barriers, including self-awareness of their own limitations.
7. Some common causes of interference with therapeutic communication are fear, lack of knowledge, insecurity, not being genuine, and inappropriate responses.

REFERENCES

Kemper, B. J. (1992). Therapeutic listening: Developing the concept. *Journal of Psychosocial Nursing and Mental Health Services*, *30*, 21.

Lee, K., Ogle, T., Hoberg, H., Linley, L., & Bradford, N. (2021). Patient preference for use of technology in communication about symptoms post hospital discharge. *BMC Health Services*, *21*, 141. https://doi.org/10.1186/s12913-021-06119-7.

Raths, D. (2020, June). Expanding internet access improves health outcomes. Government Technology. https://www.govtech.com/network/Expanding-Internet-Access-Improves-Health-Outcomes.html.

U.S. Department of Health and Human Services. (2013). Standards for privacy of individually identifiable health information. https://www.hhs.gov/sites/default/files/hipaa-simplification-201303.pdf?language=es.

9

Working With an Individual Patient

Debbie Steele

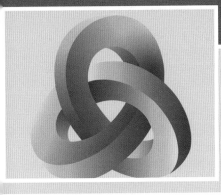

http://evolve.elsevier.com/Keltner

LEARNING OBJECTIVES

- Describe the meaning of being therapeutic.
- Describe the stages of a therapeutic nurse-patient relationship.
- Apply the nursing process to psychiatric nursing practice.
- Identify the components of the mental status examination.

- Describe the importance of a specific nursing diagnosis and care plan.
- Understand the importance of charting, discharge planning, and process recordings.

Peplau (1952) defined nursing as "a significant, therapeutic, interpersonal process. Nursing is an educative instrument, a maturing force, that aims to promote forward movement of personality in the direction of creative, constructive, productive, personal, and community living." The nurse's relationship with patients consists of a series of goal-directed interactions through which the nurse assesses patients' problems, elicits patient input, selects interventions of the patients' choosing (if possible), and evaluates the effectiveness of care. In psychiatric nursing, the nursing process is grounded in the knowledge of the nature of therapeutic relationships, psychopharmacology, and milieu management, all of which are based on an understanding of concepts and processes of human nature and psychopathology. Developing the nurse-patient relationship is the first, and often the most pivotal, step in effective psychotherapeutic management. Building therapeutic alliance is vital through all phases of treatment.

THERAPEUTIC RELATIONSHIPS

Many factors influence the relationship between the nurse and the patient, and various therapeutic activities can be used within the relationship to facilitate successful patient outcomes. Each person is a unique, valuable individual who is struggling with internal needs and external realities; the nurse offers presence and engages in a relationship to support the individual's challenges and recognize unique strengths (McCarthy & Aquino-Russell, 2009). Caring is an essential component of nursing that promotes patients' growth and well-being.

NORM'S NOTES This chapter takes the material presented in Chapter 8 and amplifies it within the context of the nurse-patient relationship. Between your instructor and this textbook, you should learn to be therapeutic—not a therapist, mind you, but therapeutic. Learning to be therapeutic is an enormous gift, and you can use it in all types of situations. For example, how do you react to an angry person or someone who is actively hallucinating? How do you react when a friend learns that her husband is leaving her? This chapter provides some time-tested ideas for common situations that you might face as a nurse or as a friend.

Collaboration

Patients have a right to make decisions about their care. When patients recognize their problems, desire to change, and ask for assistance, the nurse is able to work with them on goals and plans. Collaboration generally produces more effective and enduring change than coercion or simple compliance. However, situations arise during which full collaboration is not possible, such as when patients have an obvious disturbance in their thought processes (e.g., severe hallucinations or delusions). Occasionally, the only goal to which a patient will agree is "to get out of the hospital." However, even this goal provides an opening for discussion of circumstances that are necessary before discharge can occur. Patients with chronic illnesses might be able to agree to only small changes. Unless the nurse is approachable, understanding, and flexible, the patient might feel overwhelmed.

Social Versus Therapeutic Relationships

The importance of recognizing the difference between social and therapeutic communication is crucial. Social communication consists of interactions whereby two individuals are frequently both talking about their own lives, simultaneously. The conversation is related tangentially. For example, a husband might talk about his rough day at work while his wife talks about how hard it was to be home all day with the kids. It would be unusual for the husband to stop talking about his day to focus on his wife's concerns and vice versa. However, in therapeutic communication, the nurse focuses on the patient's agenda and does not share personal information. The nurse's goal is to discover the patient's story and perspective—to be curious about the patient's experience, internally and externally. The gathering of information allows for an ongoing assessment of the patient's needs and goals. The establishment and maintenance of care and connection is crucial in therapeutic relationships.

Some patients may misinterpret the caring communication of the nurse as a social relationship, particularly individuals with a history of unsatisfying relationships. Patients often ask the nurse to be a friend or to go out on a date. In this situation, reminding the patient of the nurse's role and the patient's need for friendship, love, and support becomes necessary—for example, "I realize you would like to date. As a nurse I can help you find ways to form friendships that can offer you emotional support."

BEING THERAPEUTIC VERSUS PROVIDING THERAPY

The nurse's basic education provides the knowledge and skills for being therapeutic in encounters with patients. Psychiatric mental health nurse practitioners receive specialized training in psychopharmacology, advanced studies in mental disorders, and specific therapies and techniques. Advanced practice nurses are trained in how to conduct formalized, ongoing therapy sessions that have a specified time, place, and length, and are process-oriented.

In contrast, nurses who engage in therapeutic activities, in an inpatient setting or outpatient program, recognize that each encounter with patients is part of an overall therapeutic picture—a therapeutic milieu. Patients discuss problems and practical solutions and practice skills needed in real-life situations. Brief encounters offer an opportunity for patients to process feelings and thoughts as they occur. Validation and feedback from the nurse are available quickly. Many patients with severe mental illnesses cannot tolerate intense, ongoing therapy but can benefit from consistent therapeutic encounters with nurses, even when their hospitalization lasts only a few days.

Informal or recreational encounters with patients (e.g., card games, craft classes, holiday parties) might be spontaneous but must be therapeutic. For example, the nurse might observe patients having difficulty in their social skills. Allowing these patients to verbalize their worries and concerns and offering appropriate feedback and support for new thinking and behaviors is appropriate for the nurse. Informal encounters are also opportunities for the nurse to demonstrate ways of handling situations: "Well, we didn't win this hand, but I'm enjoying the game anyway." "I've made that mistake before, too. You're not the only one."

Brief therapeutic relationships are not as formalized as therapy, but are planned, patient-centered, and goal-directed. The nurse purposefully and carefully guides conversations with patients toward the exploration of problems, issues, and needs. The nurse might share some personal data, such as age, marital status, or title, but should rarely disclose personal issues. Occasionally a *brief self-disclosure* might help patients clarify specific issues, feel less vulnerable, or feel more normal: "When I feel depressed, it's usually because I'm angry and not talking about it. What kinds of things do you get angry about?" or "Sometimes I'm afraid to tell my wife something because I don't know how she will react. What is hard for you to talk about with your wife?" Therapeutic self-disclosure facilitates validation, acknowledgement, comfort, honesty, openness, and risk-taking, but never burdens patients with the nurse's problems. To play it safe, it is a good idea for the nurse to ask herself, "Is sharing this information for the patient's benefit or for my benefit?"

STAGES OF DEVELOPMENT OF A THERAPEUTIC RELATIONSHIP

Peplau argued that nursing should be defined as a relationship between two individuals, rather than something that nurses do. For more than half a century, nursing students have been taught about mental health care according to Peplau's theory of nursing. Peplau believed that the nurse and the patient began as strangers and moved in stages to become collaborators in problem-solving. In the *stage of orientation*, patients recognize needs and seek help. The nurse helps patients understand their problems and accept the help that is available. The nurse works actively to foster trust and to develop the relationship. In the *identification and exploration stage*, or *working stage*, clarification of perceptions and expectations about the relationship takes place. Problems and identification of tentative solutions are further defined. Patients become more motivated to take advantage of available resources to resolve problems. Based on the condition of the patients, the therapeutic relationship might fluctuate between dependence and interdependence. Peplau believed that the *resolution stage*, or *termination stage*, needs close attention to avoid destroying the benefits gained from the relationship. The focus in this stage is on the growth that occurred and on helping the patient develop self-responsibility for setting new goals. The entire relationship is viewed as promoting growth and as a learning experience for the nurse and for patients (Peplau, 1952).

Therapeutic relationships vary in depth, length, and focus. A brief therapeutic encounter might last only a few minutes, focusing on patients' *immediate needs, current feelings,* or *observed behaviors.* In a longer-term hospitalization or program, the relationship might last 1 to 3 months, with regular meetings that focus on underlying causes of behaviors, developmental issues, or relationship problems.

In this era of brief hospitalization and time-limited outpatient care, the phases of the nurse-patient relationship are not a sequence of processes; rather, they are a matter of different emphases or goals. The nurse concentrates on nursing approaches in a particular phase, depending on the status and needs of individual patients. For example, approaches used in the orientation phase have priority when a patient is highly suspicious because a need exists to develop trust with the patient. For a patient with good insight and motivation, approaches in the working phase are most important because they concentrate on problem-solving and change. If the patient is to be admitted for only 3 days, approaches used in the termination phase are critical because of the need for formalizing plans for follow-up care and referrals to other services along the continuum of care.

Moving in and out of the three phases might depend on the patient's ability to cope with various issues (Gauthier, 2000). The patient might be ready to work on divorce issues but might be unable to process incest issues until more trust has been established. Regardless of the phase of the relationship that is most appropriate at any given time, events can alter the patient's situation, necessitating a major change in the nurse-patient relationship. For example, if the patient experiences a crisis event, then the nurse must employ crisis intervention strategies.

Stage I: Orientation Stage

The orientation stage involves nurses learning about patients and their initial concerns and needs (Gauthier, 2000). Patients also learn about the roles of the nurse during this first stage. The initial purpose might be stated as broadly as "identifying a problem on which you want to work," or "helping you figure out what has been happening to you lately." After the problems become more evident, the nurse collaborates with patients to define more specific areas to pursue—for example, learning more about appropriate boundaries or processing feelings about a divorce. Nurses also help patients look at realistic options so that patients can make their own decisions.

In a longer-term outpatient relationship between the patient and the nurse, arrangements are made about the time, length, and frequency of meetings. The session might be for 30 to 60 minutes once a week in a clinic or office or in the patient's home. It is helpful for patients to know the length of time the nurse can spend with them and that the relationship will end at the time of discharge or transfer to another level in the continuum of care.

Building Trust

Trustworthiness is built when the nurse is honest regarding intentions, is consistent, and follows through on actions.

Mutual respect and trust are crucial goals. Warmth, interest, and concern are conveyed with words and congruent body language. Clear, specific communications decrease confusion and suspiciousness. Confidentiality is explained in terms of patient information being shared *only* with the immediate unit or program staff and not with anyone outside the treatment setting without the patient's consent, consistent with Health Insurance Portability and Accountability Act (HIPAA) regulations.

Because many patients are afraid or unable to approach the nurse, it is important for the nurse to reach out and initiate conversations. Quiet, withdrawn patients are often overlooked because they do not feel comfortable asking for assistance. An offer to listen and help conveys to patients that they are worthwhile individuals who are respected. Typically, the nurse is nonconfrontational by not openly challenging statements that the patient makes. Such challenges would interfere with trust, resulting in the patient feeling judged or criticized.

Beginning Assessment

The initial interactions provide an opportunity to begin an assessment of patients' needs, coping strategies, defense mechanisms, and adaptation styles. Patients' recurring thoughts, feelings, and behaviors *(themes)* are clues to problem areas. Assessing the degree of a patient's awareness of problems and the ability and motivation to change is important. Although assessment is ongoing and progresses over time, tentative goals are based on the most immediate needs or problems—for example, suicidal or homicidal thoughts, hallucinations, self-mutilation, or acting out.

Managing Emotions

At the time of admission to a unit or a program, patients typically experience painful thoughts and emotions, such as fear, grief, anger, ambivalence, confusion, shame, embarrassment, and guilt. Patients are often afraid of losing control of themselves or of being viewed as weak for expressing their feelings. A way to help patients who are feeling overwhelmed is to talk about their emotions directly. For patients who try to conceal or minimize feelings, the nurse must be alert to indirect references, nonverbal cues, and voice tones. The nurse can then identify the feeling and ask for validation: "Your voice is loud. You seem tense. What are you feeling right now?"

To cope effectively with feelings, particularly anger, nurses should remember that these feelings are not created by their own actions but triggered by situations or significant persons in the patient's history. A patient might displace anger onto the nurse at first. If questioned about the anger, however, the patient is more likely to recognize the real source of his or her emotions. Patients must understand that feelings are natural, but that the way they are expressed can cause a problem. Belittling or minimizing a patient's emotions is inappropriate, as is false reassurance, such as saying "Everything will be all right." Patients might feel worse for a while as they begin to face their problems and feelings, and such reassurance is dishonest as well as inappropriate.

Empathy is expressed as the nurse verbalizes an understanding of the way in which patients see their situation. It can also convey hope for improvement: "I hear how painful this is for you, and it makes sense to me that you would feel that way." Empathetic care is defined as behaviors that support the development of patients' socioemotional capabilities and address their emotional needs (Leana et al., 2018). Empathy is one of the ways that nurses convey emotional support in their relationship with patients. Pejner et al. (2015) propose that emotional support be identified as a priority nursing intervention, as one of the most important components of a therapeutic relationship. After patients are able to talk directly about emotions and understand what they mean, the focus can be on coping more effectively with them. In the orientation stage, resolving the problem situation that created the feelings is not possible, but temporarily reducing the feelings to a tolerable level is possible through explaining the experiences and feelings to an empathic listener.

Providing Emotional Support

Emotional support begins in the orientation stage and continues throughout the nurse-patient relationship. Consistency, respect, affirmation, empathy, and staying with and holding the emotional distress of patients provide an emotional platform conducive to promoting recovery. Such interactions offer a safe place, enabling the patient to overcome emotional resistance, knowing they can discuss anything without the fear of rejection (McAndrews, 2014; Wyder, 2015). Emotional support confirms patients' worth and rights as human beings and involves the nurse avoiding value judgments of patients (e.g., as bad, crazy, lazy), even when patients have made poor choices. Support acknowledges that no one is perfect, that making mistakes is human, and that learning from mistakes is beneficial. Support focuses realistically and concretely on patients' abilities and strengths—for example, the nurse would not say, "You're a good person," but rather, "I'm glad you were able to share your feelings in group today." Patients need recognition of their healthy thoughts, actions, and feelings.

Providing Structure

A major strategy in the orientation stage is to provide structure for patients. When patients experience distress in their thoughts, feelings, or behaviors, it is the nurse's responsibility to provide options for relief. The action might mean offering an as-needed (prn) medication; directing patients to a quieter, less stimulating place; or staying with patients at a comfortable distance. If these measures are ineffective, then seclusion or restraints might be indicated as last-resort strategies. However, providing structure also includes decreasing the withdrawal and isolation of quiet, nonparticipating patients. Spending time with these patients, even in silence, is important. The nurse also can suggest activities, such as watching television or taking a walk with the patient. A major facet of providing structure is *limit setting*. Decreasing or stopping disruptive behaviors is in the best interest of

patients. Limit setting involves explaining facility rules in a calm manner, allowing patients the opportunity to ask questions, provide comments, and discuss alternatives. For example, when a depressed patient is staying in her room for most of the morning, the nurse can gently inform her that the unit rule is that all patients attend lunch together and then participate in groups in the afternoon. The nurse then allows the patient to express her lethargy, avolition, and sadness. Validating the patient's emotional and physical state is important, as the patient feels that the nurse understands her struggle. Then the nurse encourages the patient by asking her if she will agree to attend the afternoon group, offering to sit with her during group time.

Behaviors that typically require immediate intervention are verbal and physical aggression, self-destructive behaviors, setting fires, alcohol or drug abuse, manipulation of others, inappropriate touching of others, indecent exposure, attempts to leave the hospital without permission, and failure to eat or sleep. The nurse first listens to the content and the process of the patients' distressing feelings or thoughts, conveying a calm, open presence. The nurse may also need to provide limit setting in a kind but firm manner: "I know you are angry right now, but I'm having trouble understanding the situation because of all the swearing; if you can slow down, I know I can better understand you" or "I realize that these thoughts are really important to you, but there are other areas I need to know about so I can help you."

The transition from the orientation stage to the working stage is not smooth or firmly defined. Patients' anxiety might increase when they are working on issues, and they might return to more superficial matters for a while. Some patients with chronic illnesses or multiple hospitalizations might need more of a focus on orientation stage interventions because of their difficulty in forming relationships.

Stage II: Working Stage

When patients are ready, the work toward changing their thoughts, feelings, and behaviors can begin. However, drastic changes might not be the goal for some patients, particularly chronically-ill patients. Stabilization, reduction of distressing symptoms, and development of supportive relationships are valid goals. Some patients with chronic, severe symptoms might be hospitalized several times as they navigate through the struggle, the pain, and the limitations resulting from suffering from a mental disorder. Hawamdeh and Fakhry (2014) reported the importance of "being there" for the patient, responsive to their physical and emotional needs. Nurses establish themselves as someone whom the patients can rely on to explore problems, identify possible solutions, and test new behaviors.

In-Depth Data Collection

The nurse facilitates awareness, analysis, and interpretation through in-depth (but selective) exploration and identification of priority issues. Data collection occurs as the nurse takes the time to sit and engage with patients. Pertinent information is shared when patients feel valued and important in their relationship with the nurses (Stewart et al., 2015). During the interview, the nurse inquires about the nature of the problem from the patients' perspective and what can be done to provide relief. The nurse provides reassurance and support using a calm tone of voice with open, friendly body language (Hallett & Dickens, 2015). Strategic interactions increase the nurse's knowledge of patients' strengths, needs, and problems, and of factors that can enhance or interfere with treatment.

Promoting Change

Nurses play an important role in the change process, as they assess a patient's readiness to change and enhance motivation for change. Successful change can be accomplished through the use of motivational interviewing (MI). MI is an evidence-based intervention that is patient-centered, aimed to support motivation for change (Clancy & Taylor, 2016). MI is a semi-directive cognitive-behavioral method that helps patients identify problem behaviors, resolve ambivalence, enhance motivation, and aid in problem-solving and goal setting (Chang et al., 2019). Patient-centered care requires a comprehensive view of patients whose perspectives are focal and whose autonomy is central to care. Care is respectful of and responsive to the patient's preferences, needs, and values. MI encourages patients to explore their personal experiences and recognize how their perceptions and expectations contribute to their readiness to change and confidence. It involves a variety of communication techniques: (1) open-ended questions, (2) reflective listening, and (3) validation. Open-ended questions are used to clarify meaning and elicit the patient's emotion. Reflective listening and validation are used to enhance empathy and respect for the patient's perspective. MI is recovery-oriented, intent on aligning with the patient as an equal partner in care and emphasizing patient strengths to guide care (Hornsten et al., 2014; Mallisham & Sherrod, 2017).

Lasting change is difficult to achieve until the patient endorses the necessity for change. The nurse helps distinguish between the patient's current behavior and his desired goals. The patient reflects on current behaviors and behaviors he would like to adopt. The nurse facilitates the patient's exploration of reasons for change. The struggle to change is called *resistance*, and the nurse's strategy during this phase is supportive. The nurse invites the patient to problem-solve possible solutions to the obstacles involved in change, while instilling hope and avoiding confrontation. Self-efficacy is the patient's own belief and confidence that he or she can make and sustain changes in behavior. The nurse's role is to boost the patient's confidence and provide ongoing encouragement (Clark & Egan, 2015).

Prochaska & Norcross, 2002 describe five stages of the change process: *precontemplation, contemplation, preparation, action*, and *maintenance*. During precontemplation, the patient has yet to acknowledge that there is a problem and does not plan to change any of his or her own behaviors. During early hospitalization, patients are often in this stage. The most successful intervention is to engage the patient and begin to raise his or her awareness of possible issues. The nurse learns the extent to which patients understand their problems by asking for in-depth, detailed descriptions of situations, thoughts, feelings, and behaviors. Once aware of an issue, the patient enters the stage of contemplation. The patient begins to see that there is a problem and thinks about some action but is not committed to any course of action. Ambivalence is the predominant feeling. When the patient is imminently ready to work on change, he or she has entered the preparation stage.

The nurse does not give advice but helps patients solve their own problems. The nurse encourages short-term, realistic, and achievable daily goals. When the patient initiates a change, he or she moves to the action stage. For example, if a patient's goal is to lose weight, he or she may remain in the preparation stage for some time while thinking about and preparing to begin the process of weight loss. The action stage begins when modifications are made to the patient's daily schedule. The maintenance stage is when the patient has met his or her desired goals and can avoid slipping back into familiar patterns or relapsing into the original behavior. Effective behaviors are more likely to continue when the benefits of the behaviors are discussed and reinforcement is given.

Stage III: Termination Stage

In acute inpatient settings and short-term outpatient programs, the patient's work and changes are rarely completed. Patients are discharged or transferred to another level of care. The nurse who is assigned to discharge or transfer the patient will be responsible for discussing and implementing the discharge strategies.

Evaluation and Summary of Progress

The nurse guides discussions to help patients identify *for themselves* the specific changes in thoughts, feelings, and behaviors that have occurred. Even small steps toward long-term goals are discussed. Reinforcing the changes in and strengths of patients is important. Areas or issues that need more work are outlined, while cautioning patients to avoid trying to change everything at once. Patients are encouraged to set priorities for these issues and to establish reasonable time frames for action.

Synthesizing the Outcomes

Synthesizing focuses on the more indirect outcomes of the nurse-patient relationship, such as more open communications or more authentic expression of feelings. As a result of the relationship, patients often feel more comfortable with initiating interactions, making requests, and expressing opinions. As the nurse points out the benefits from the relationship, patients are encouraged to form other relationships with future nurses, counselors, and new friends.

Referrals

For problems that need continuing attention after discharge, referrals to appropriate resources are finalized. Providing a copy of discharge instructions and ensuring patients understand them is a nursing responsibility to help facilitate seamless care. If the patient speaks a language other than English, then the instructions can be translated into the patient's native language.

Discussion of Termination

Regardless of the length, frequency of contact, or intensity of the nurse-patient relationship, discussing the participants' reactions to the relationship is important. Feelings might be positive, ambivalent, or negative, and may vary in degree. Patients might experience anger or fear related to losing the support and acceptance that the nurse provides. Some patients might avoid any discussion of termination. Nonetheless, the nurse should attempt to make it official by saying "good-bye" and stating his or her feelings about the relationship—for example, "I'm glad I had a chance to work with you."

INTERACTIONS WITH SELECTED BEHAVIORS

The purpose of this section is to discuss interventions that are appropriate in brief encounters with patients to address specific troublesome behaviors. The behaviors included here are those the nurse might encounter with any patient, regardless of the patient's diagnosis.

Violent Behavior

Fear of violent behavior and of being injured is a concern with the few patients who do not respond to staff efforts to de-escalate anger. The following are a few precautions that can be taken for protection:

- Stay out of striking distance (this also reduces the threat to the patient).
- Avoid touching patients without approval.
- Change the topic temporarily if a patient's behavior is escalating.
- Suggest time out for the patient in a quiet area with fewer stimuli.
- Avoid entering a room alone with a patient who is not in control of his or her behavior.
- Leave temporarily if the patient is agitated and asking to be left alone.
- Talk to the patient in a measured tone that conveys acceptance and concern.
- Call for staff assistance if the patient's behavior escalates.

Hallucinations

Interventions with a patient with hallucinations generally occur in a sequence with newly admitted patients:

1. The initial approach with patients who appear to be listening to or talking with voices is to comment on their behavior: "You look as if you are listening to something. What do you hear?"
2. If the patient acknowledges hearing something that the nurse cannot hear, then the nurse can say, "Tell me what you hear."

3. The next step is assessment of hallucinations based on the content of the messages, which often reveals the dynamics of the patient's illness and typically revolves around *themes* of powerlessness, hatred, guilt, or loneliness.
4. After the content is known, focusing on how they make the patient feel may be helpful: "I know the voices are important to you; can we talk about how the hallucinations make you feel?"
5. The nurse can also encourage the patient to utilize distraction as a method of dealing with hallucinations. Distraction techniques involve the patient becoming engaged in activities, such as music, art, or physical exercise.

The exception is with hallucinations that command patients to harm themselves or others or to engage in other destructive acts. In such cases, the nurse should contract with patients to avoid acting on the commands they hear and to tell the staff. Another exception is with patients with dementia or severe cognitive impairments. These patients are not likely to be able to process the content or themes of the hallucinations.

Delusions

Patients who are experiencing delusions are encouraged to share the meaning of the delusions with the nurse. For example, "Tell me more about what the delusion means to you." Since the definition of a delusion is a false belief, arguing with a patient about the truthfulness of delusions is ineffective and inappropriate. The underlying *themes* reflected in the delusions can be addressed to help patients share their emotional experiences. For example, "What does it feel like right now as you are telling me about your distressing thoughts?" Careful monitoring is needed if the delusions might lead patients to harm themselves or others; for example, a patient who does not want to eat because he believes that all the food is poisoned needs to be monitored.

Conflicting Values

Occasionally nurses and patients encounter differences in their beliefs or values. Nurses must seek to understand the patient's point of view as the patient sees it. The better the nurse understands the lived experience of the patient, the greater the likelihood that the nurse will provide sensitively attuned quality nursing care. Nurses may assume that those with mental disorders lack insight and therefore may try to argue or convince patients to change their thinking and/or behavior. Concordance refers to the creation of an agreement that respects the beliefs and wishes of the patient, rather than focusing on the patient's ability to follow the nurse's instructions or see their situation from the nurse's perspective (Leibing, 2010). The teaching of health-promoting knowledge and facts is seldom enough to influence the patient to change their behavior (Hornsten et al., 2014). Nurses who display respect and affirm the patient's experience and perspective provide an emotional platform conducive to nurturing trust in the nurse-patient relationship. Such interactions offer a safe place, enabling the patient to overcome emotional resistance, engender sense-making, and move toward a deeper level of self-knowledge, which often precedes change. The goal is to see and care for the patient, not the mental health problem (McAndrews et al., 2014).

Severe Anxiety and Incoherent Speech Patterns

Disturbed thought processes are occasionally evident in speech, especially with patients who are upset, confused, or psychotic. When these processes occur, the typical approach is to clarify the meaning of the communications. However, severely ill or anxious patients might be unable to be clearer, and repeated questions only increase their anxiety. It is more effective to key into their feelings and underlying *themes*, rather than trying to make sense of the content of their speech. Spending frequent, brief time intervals with these patients (without pressuring or frustrating them) offers support and builds trust.

Manipulation

Some patients may behave in a way that appears they are looking for attention, sympathy, or control. It can be difficult for the nurse to properly manage these types of interactions. Understanding what is behind the manipulation can be helpful. Manipulation is a coping strategy that develops typically during childhood or adolescence. It can be viewed as an attempt to overconnect with others. Those who are feeling manipulated will not feel respected. How the nurse responds to these feelings is important for the nurse-patient relationship. It can be helpful for the nurse to approach the patient in a way that focuses on their emotional experience, such as "You seem anxious. Tell me what is going on with you right now?" In addition, the nurse may need to set appropriate limits if the patient's needs seem overwhelming. For example, "I see that you are very anxious. I have about 10 minutes to spend with you; would you like to talk about what is bothering you?"

Crying

Crying is a normal response to sadness and should be allowed and encouraged, verbally and nonverbally. By saying, "It's okay to cry" or quietly offering a tissue, the nurse gives patients permission to cry and relieve tension. Privacy should be provided. The nurse should be as quiet and unobtrusive as possible until the crying has ceased. The nurse should then offer the patient an opportunity to discuss the emotional experience that precipitated the tears.

Sexual Innuendos or Inappropriate Touch

Some patients may verbalize sexual innuendos or try to touch the nurse or other patients inappropriately. Patients should be asked to stop the behavior as a calm request. It may be necessary to communicate to the patient that the nurse or other patients do not feel safe and become afraid when such comments or behavior occurs. Patients generally stop inappropriate behaviors when asked. If the behaviors continue, setting limits will need to be initiated. For example, "I want to talk to you, but I won't be able to do so if you continue to try to touch me." "If you can't stop, I will have to leave and come back later." The nurse is responsible for maintaining professional boundaries in the relationship, especially when the patient is having difficulty with his or her own boundaries.

The nurse should refrain from touching patients who have sexual or boundary issues. It is a good idea for the nurse to ask a patient if she is okay being touched for routine vital signs and other medical procedures. Some patients who have experienced sexual abuse could be triggered when touched. Other patients who are highly sexualized may misinterpret the nurse's touch as perhaps erotic.

Treatment Refusal

Treatment refusal entails an explicit rejection of all or part of a treatment plan by patients. It is important for nurses to realize that treatment refusal and nonadherence/noncompliance are not the same. In nonadherence/noncompliance, the patient agrees to the treatment plan but fails to consistently carry it out. Those patients who are most prone to refuse treatment typically have been diagnosed with the following disorders: bipolar disorder, eating disorders, schizophrenia, substance use disorders, and borderline personality disorder. During exacerbations, prominent symptoms such as hallucinations, delusions, grandiosity, and paranoia may interfere with the patient's insight and judgment. Such symptoms can make it difficult or impossible for patients to know they have a serious problem and are in need of professional care (Gruber, 2010).

In some cases, involuntary hospitalization and other forms of protective, controlling, and coercive measures are utilized in crisis situations. This creates a conflict between patient decision-making and ethical/legal aspects of nursing care (Jansen & Hanssen, 2017).

Occasionally a patient might admit to the need for help but disagrees with the type of treatment offered. Listening, clarifying, and verbalizing thoughts that have been implied are appropriate for identifying the underlying causes of a lack of cooperation. The causes, fears, and outcomes of patients' behaviors are then discussed directly: "What are you afraid will happen in the inpatient unit?" The lack of trust and overwhelming fear are often issues for these patients; measures to assure the patient that she is safe and a great deal of patience from the nurse are needed.

Depressed Affect, Apathy, and Psychomotor Retardation

When patients express sadness, helplessness, hopelessness, lack of energy, or a negative attitude about everything, the nurse uses patience, frequent contact, and empathy as effective methods for dealing with these feelings. Even when patients verbalize their desire for change, they do not always have the energy to make the adjustment quickly. Improvement in personal hygiene, proper nutrition, and a gradual increase in activities are encouraged. Major decisions are postponed until overwhelming emotions have subsided and thinking is more logical and rational.

Suspiciousness

When patients are suspicious, they might be afraid of everyone. The nurse must communicate clearly, simply, and congruently. Misinterpretations by patients should be clarified, but arguments over differences in opinion are to be avoided. Simple rationales or explanations for rules, activities, occurrences, noises, and requests are offered regularly. The participation of patients in unit activities is encouraged but not forced, thus avoiding increasing their fears.

Hyperactivity

Excessive physical and emotional activity of patients is upsetting to other patients, staff, and the hyperactive patients themselves. Patients might unintentionally harm themselves or others. These patients should be in a quiet area, with minimal auditory and visual stimulation. The nurse must remain calm, speak slowly and softly, and respect patients' personal space. Occasionally, prn medications are required, including one to promote sleep.

NURSING PROCESS

The use of the nursing process has the same goal in psychiatric nursing as it has in other areas of nursing: patient-centered, goal-directed action that facilitates health promotion, primary prevention, treatment, and rehabilitation. Nursing care must be adapted to the unique needs of each patient. Individualized care begins with a detailed assessment.

Assessment

Initial Patient Assessment

The assessment begins on admission to a unit or program. Each psychiatric hospital, unit, clinic, and program has its own version of an intake or nursing assessment form. Box 9.1 provides a sample of the type of information included in the initial assessment. Although a newly admitted patient might be "medically cleared," both physical and mental health assessment should be the focus of nursing care. Typically, the term *medical clearance* indicates that a cursory examination was performed.

A multidisciplinary team including at least a nurse, psychiatrist, psychologist, social worker, pharmacist, and dietitian is the foundation for quality care (Zwarenstein, Goldman, & Reeves, 2009). Peer support workers are individuals who have lived experience of mental illness and contribute their knowledge and expertise within multidisciplinary teams (Oborn et al., 2019). A chaplain also might be included on the team to add the component of a spiritual assessment, particularly the guilt and shame associated with trauma and the need for forgiveness (Pyne et al., 2019). Critical facts about the patient should be indicated on intake forms/checklists and summarized in an admission note; the admission note is intended to aid other team members.

Mental Status Examination

The mental status examination (MSE) is a very important component of patient assessment in psychiatric settings. The MSE focuses on the patient's current state in terms of

BOX 9.1   **Initial Patient Assessment**
• **Demographic data:** Full name, gender, age, date of birth, address, marital status, and names and ages of family members, partner, or significant other
• **Admission data:** Date and time of admission and type of admission (voluntary or committed)
• **Reason for admission:** Current problems as perceived by the patient; include stressors, difficulty with coping, developmental issues, "emergency behaviors" (suicidal or homicidal ideas and attempts, aggression, destructive behaviors, risk of escape), and family history
• **Previous psychiatric history:** Dates, inpatient or outpatient, reasons for and types of treatment and their effectiveness, current medications, and compliance
• **Current medical problems and medications:** Allergies, results of laboratory tests, x-rays, and examinations
• **Drug and alcohol use or abuse:** Amount, frequency, duration of past and present use of prescription and illegal substances, date and time of last use, and potential for withdrawal symptoms
• **Disturbances in patterns of daily living:** Sleep, intake, elimination, sexual activity, work, leisure, self-care, and hygiene
• **Culture and spirituality:** Ethnicity, beliefs, practices, and religious preference
• **Support systems:** Amount of contact, nature and quality of relationships, and availability of support

thoughts, feelings, and behaviors. The information related to each of the categories includes the following:

- General appearance: Type, condition, and appropriateness of clothing (for age, season, setting), grooming, cleanliness, physical condition, and posture
- Behaviors during the interview: Degree of cooperation, alliance, and engagement
- Social skills: Friendliness, shyness, or withdrawal
- Amount and type of motor activity: Psychomotor agitation or retardation, restlessness, tics, tremors, hypervigilance, or lack of energy and activity
- Speech patterns: Amount, rate, volume, tone, pressured speech, mutism, slurring, or stuttering
- Degree of concentration and attention span
- Orientation: To time, place, person, and situation and level of consciousness
- Memory: Immediate recall, recent, remote, amnesia, and confabulation
- Intellectual functioning: Educational level, use of language and knowledge, abstract versus concrete thinking (proverbs), and calculations (serial sevens)
- Affect: Labile, blunted, flat, incongruent, or inappropriate
- Mood: Specific moods expressed or observed—euphoria, depression, anxiety, anger, guilt, or fear
- Thought clarity: Coherence, confusion, or vagueness
- Thought content: Helplessness, hopelessness, worthlessness, suicidal thoughts or plans, homicidal thoughts or plans, suspiciousness, phobias, obsessions, compulsions, preoccupations, denial, hallucinations (auditory, visual,

olfactory, gustatory, tactile), or delusions (of reference, influence, persecution, grandeur, religious, nihilistic, somatic)

- Thought processes reflected in speech: Ambivalence, circumstantiality, tangentiality, thought blocking, poverty of thought, loose associations, flight of ideas, perseveration, neologisms, or word salad
- Insight: Degree of awareness of illness, degree of awareness of illness on others
- Judgment: Soundness of problem solving and decisions
- Motivation: Degree of motivation for treatment

Some patients are too ill to participate in or complete the assessment interview. In these cases, objective data, such as patient behaviors and reports by family members, are used. During the initial assessment, behaviors can be described without knowing or identifying their causes—for example, anxiety level, degree of withdrawal, and thought disturbances reflected in speech, voice tone, and general appearance.

Clinical Example

Anita Jarvis, a 46-year-old patient, is separated from her husband, who asked for a divorce and left her 1 week ago. Her son and daughter brought Anita to the hospital after they visited her and found that she had not been getting out of bed to shower or eat. They reported that their mother stated that she wished she were dead. Anita admits to feeling suicidal but denies having any suicide plans. She has no history of medical or psychiatric illnesses and takes no medications. Anita stated that she stopped seeing her friends 1 month ago and does not want to do anything anymore. She is not close to her parents, who live out of state. She called the school in which she teaches 4 days ago and said she was sick. She admits to staying in bed "all the time" but sleeping only 3–4 hr a night. Anita was admitted to the hospital with an initial diagnosis of depression.

Mrs. Jarvis and her situation are used in the chapter examples of a process recording (Table 9.1), MSE (Box 9.2), progress note (Box 9.3), and care plan (at the end of the chapter). The process recording is an example of part of an initial assessment with Mrs. Jarvis.

TABLE 9.1   Sample Process Recording With Mrs. Jarvis

NURSE		PATIENT		ANALYSIS	
Verbal	Nonverbal	Verbal	Nonverbal	Themes	Therapeutic Techniques
What do you prefer to be called, Mrs. Jarvis or Anita?	Has pen in hand, other hand is flat on desk; is looking at patient	(pause) Anita.	Is looking at floor	Content—oriented to person	Questioning, active listening
Anita, we will be better able to help you if we know more about you. What has happened in your life recently?	(Same as above)	(pause) I couldn't get out of bed. (pause) I was so tired.	Is turning head slightly, still looking at the floor; is not smiling or frowning	Content—describes fatigue and effects	Giving information, questioning
				Mood—sadness Interaction—opens up with nurse	
How long have you been feeling so tired?	Is writing, then looking at patient	I don't know. (pause) A week, I guess.	(Same as above)	Content—unsure of time frames, marital separation, possible divorce	Assessing symptoms, active listening
What happened a week ago? I can see this is difficult for you to talk about.	Leans toward patient. Moves tissue box. Looks at patient; both arms are on lap.	(pause) My husband (pause) left.	Tears are in eyes; tries to open purse. Is nodding head; raises eyes slightly; is still not looking at the nurse. Starts to cry; gets tissue. Sobs occasionally.	Mood—sadness, guilt	Focusing, using empathy and silence, questioning
(pause) What did he say when he left?		That he was fed up. (pause) That he wanted a divorce.		Interaction—in conflict with husband, is more trusting of nurse	

Continued

TABLE 9.1   Sample Process Recording With Mrs. Jarvis—cont'd

NURSE		PATIENT		ANALYSIS	
Verbal	Nonverbal	Verbal	Nonverbal	Themes	Therapeutic Techniques
What did you say to him?	Leans slightly toward patient. One arm is on lap, the other is on arm of chair.	I don't know. I don't remember. *(pause)* Maybe I asked him to stay.	Is crying quietly	Content—difficulty describing situation, short-term memory disturbance	Focusing, active listening
Then what happened?	(Same as above)	It's all a blur; I think I cried all day.	(Same as above)	Mood—sadness, guilt Interactions—abandonment, loneliness	Focusing
Who did you talk to?	(Same as above)	No one. *(pause)* My kids are married and gone. I just stayed in bed.	Is the same but crying less often	Content—did not ask for help, avoidance of divorce issue Mood—sadness Interaction—perceived lack of support	Focusing; Assessing support system
When you were feeling so tired, did you have thoughts of killing yourself?	(Same as above)	*(pause)* I was so scared of being alone. I thought I'd rather be dead.	Looks at nurse for the first time; both hands are in lap	Content—aware of fears, suicidal ideation but denies plan, difficulty with problem-solving	Questioning
How did you think about killing yourself?	(Same as above)	I couldn't think of anything. I didn't know what to do.	Looks at floor again; fumbles in purse	Mood—sadness, depression Interaction—abandonment, lack of support, open with nurse	Assessing for safety
Are you still thinking about suicide?	Hands patient a tissue	Not really. But *(pause)* I still wish I were dead. I don't know what to do.	Blows nose and then puts hands in lap; looks at nurse	Content—minimizing suicidal ideation but ambivalent, helpless Mood—sadness	Assessing for safety; Focusing
While you are here, we are going to support you while you consider options about what to do so you won't feel so alone and scared. *(pause)*	Leans forward. Looks at patient. Both hands on lap.	(Silence)	Looks at floor; crying has stopped; looks at nurse	Interaction—asking for help	Suggesting collaboration, verbalizing the implied, active listening
It will help us if I ask you some additional questions.	Turns back to papers. Is ready to write.	Okay.	Looks at nurse		Assessing mental status

Nurse introduces himself to Mrs. Jarvis and leads the way to the office, walking slowly but slightly ahead of the patient. The patient follows without looking at the nurse. In the office, the nurse sits in a chair at a desk and opens a folder of papers. The patient sits in a chair at the side of the desk, holding her purse with both hands on her lap.

BOX 9.2 Mental Status Examination with Mrs. Jarvis

- **General appearance:** Dressed appropriately for season; clothes are clean but wrinkled; hair is unwashed and uncombed; slouched shoulders; pale; blank expression
- **Affect:** Blunted
- **Mood:** Depressed, anxiety level moderate, guilt and covert anger expressed
- **Behaviors during interview:** Slow to respond but cooperative
- **Social skills:** Withdrawn, no unusual habits, reduced socialization, poor eye contact
- **Amount and type of motor activity:** Slowed, crying at times, no tics or tremors noted
- **Speech patterns:** Amount is reduced with slowed rate and soft tone
- **Degree of concentration and attention span:** Decreased concentration, easily distracted by stimuli, slight shortening of attention span
- **Orientation:** Aware of person, place, and time; responsive
- **Memory:**
  - **Immediate recall:** Remembers nurse's name

- **Recent:** Difficulty organizing sequence but mostly complete except for last week
- **Remote:** Good detail on birth of children
- **Thought clarity:** Clear, coherent
- **Thought content:** Expressing helplessness, hopelessness, and suicidal thoughts but denies a plan; fears being alone; no evidence of hallucinations or delusions
- **Thought process:** No disturbances noted
- **Intellectual functioning:** College education evident in vocabulary, abstract thinking evident in discussion of love and fidelity
- **Insight:** Aware of problems in facing divorce but not yet able to describe factors leading to separation from husband
- **Judgment:** No impairment until last 2 weeks, when she became unable to make decisions, take action, or seek support
- **Motivation for treatment:** Wants help with depression, fatigue, and handling divorce; unable to state what type of help she needs

---

BOX 9.3 Progress Note Components

- **Subjective content:** The patient's statements about his or her own thoughts, feelings, behaviors, and problems.
- **Objective data:** The nurse's observations or measurements, such as the patient's appearance, nonverbal behaviors, and vital signs.
- **Analysis or conclusions:** The nurse's impressions of what the patient is experiencing or demonstrating in behavioral or descriptive terms (not medical diagnoses); defenses, mood, and issues are identified; depressed mood and paranoid ideas can be discussed, but "depression" and "paranoia" are not listed as illnesses; conclusions about changes (regression or progression) in the patient and medication responses are described.
- **Plans:** Actions that nurses or other team members can take to intervene with the problems described in the progress note.

Sample Progress Note for Mrs. Jarvis
Date and time: 02/03/2014, 1600.
S: Patient states that she is a little less tired. States she is still unsure of what led to the separation and cannot face living alone. Admits to thoughts of suicide but denies plan:

"I still wish I were dead." Verbalizes a "no-suicide contract." Verbalizes that she still does not know what to do about impending divorce and being alone in the future. Said she called her school to extend her sick leave and called her son and daughter, who will visit this evening.
O: Exhibits blunted affect with depressed mood, slowed motor activity, and slowed speech. Attended one therapeutic group and a craft activity but participated only briefly. Napped for only 2 hours this shift.
A: Patient cannot describe her thoughts and feelings, but sadness, helplessness, and hopelessness are evident. Anger is barely evident at this point. Suicidal but denies plan. Support is available from her adult children.
P:
1. Approach and sit with patient frequently.
2. Encourage verbalization of feelings, especially sadness and fear of being alone.
3. Monitor energy level and suicidal ideation.
4. Continue medications as ordered.
5. Encourage participation in group meetings and activities.

Ongoing Assessments

Even when the initial assessment is complete, each encounter with a patient involves a continuing assessment that may or may not be congruent with the initial assessment. No one acts or feels the same way 24 hours a day, 7 days a week. The ongoing assessment often involves an investigation of patients' statements and actions at the moment: "You have been sitting alone for a while. How are you feeling? What have you been thinking about?" When the nurse decides to investigate

a patient's specific behavior, exploring the following might be valuable:

- Context or situation that precipitated the behavior
- The patient's thoughts at the time
- The patient's feelings then and now
- How the behavior makes sense in that context
- In what way was the behavior adaptive or maladaptive
- How this episode fits with the total picture of the patient
- Whether a change is desired

A sample MSE with Mrs. Jarvis is presented in Box 9.2.

Nursing Diagnosis

A nursing diagnosis is the identification of patient's problems based on conclusions about the dynamics evident in verbalizations and behaviors. It is directly related to the content, mood, and interaction themes. Emergency behaviors (e.g., suicidal or homicidal ideas or attempts, aggression, destructive behaviors, risk of arson or escape) are given priority in establishing nursing diagnoses and in negotiating no-harm agreements with patients. Suicidal ideation should be regularly assessed, even after a patient has verbalized that she has started to feel more hopeful. The diagnosis should be specific and indicate a desired outcome for the patient. NANDA International diagnoses are the most commonly used nursing diagnoses. The International Classification of Diseases (ICD-10) is another accepted classification and diagnostic system useful to nurses. The development of a nursing diagnosis will typically contain the following three components:

1. Risk for actual problems
2. Contributing, causative, or etiologic factors
3. Defining characteristic or behavioral outcome

The statement is typically written as follows: (Problem) related to (contributing factor) as evidenced by (behavioral outcome)—for example, "Anxiety, moderate, related to marital problems as evidenced by ineffective problem solving."

Actual or potential problems are identified from the list by NANDA International or ICD-10. Contributing or causative factors can include stressors, losses, past experiences, developmental issues, environmental circumstances, relationship issues, and self- or other perceptions. Defining characteristics or behavioral outcomes are the verbal and nonverbal cues that reflect the patient's actual or potential problems. These distressing emotions, behaviors, or cues are the focus of the nursing interventions—symptoms and experiences that the patient would find helpful to change. Nursing diagnoses are intended to focus on the patients' human responses to health conditions or life processes (Rubensson & Salzmann-Erikson, 2019).

Outcome Identification

A goal or outcome specifies a desired response to replace one that is unwanted. Expecting patients to change a negative self-image to a more positive view of self during a short inpatient stay or outpatient program is unrealistic. A more realistic goal would be to ask patients to write a list of their strengths, abilities, and positive qualities. This goal is achievable and measurable. Short-term goals or outcomes are those achievable in perhaps 4 to 6 days for hospitalized patients and longer for patients in other settings. Long-term goals or outcomes relate to issues that require follow-up counseling after discharge to another type of service within the continuum of care. For example, a patient's short-term goal might be to identify difficulties in family relationships. The longer-term goal is to identify what happens to the patient emotionally within her family interactions that lead to her depression. By increasing awareness of her emotions, the patient might be better able to address family situations in a way that leads to a desired outcome.

Establishing goals and outcomes *with* a patient requires a high degree of reciprocity and collaboration. The nurse must understand the problems the patient wants to address and the goals the patient wants to achieve. Patient desires and motivation play a major role in attaining outcomes (Sandhu et al., 2015).

Planning and Intervention
Nursing Care Plans

Nursing staff, on units or in programs, often develop standardized care plans with desired outcomes for certain types of patient problems. These care plans might focus on psychiatric diagnoses (e.g., major depression) or more specific problems (e.g., self-mutilation). Standardized care plans are also called *clinical pathways, critical pathways,* or *multidisciplinary care plans.* The initial care plan might be updated at any time but begins with one or two behavior-oriented problems to be addressed immediately (e.g., suicide, aggression, arson, escape, withdrawal or isolation, delusions, hallucinations, impulsive or compulsive acts, suspiciousness, uncooperativeness, or altered thought processes). For example, a patient who has suicidal ideation (problem) would be expected to sign a no-harm agreement (outcome) within 24 hours (time constraint) and to verbalize a plan when experiencing suicidal ideation (outcome) by day 3 of admission (time constraint). Related nursing interventions would include (1) an agreement with the patient for safety, (2) removal of dangerous objects from the patient and the patient's room, and (3) assessment for suicidal ideation during every shift.

Given the current managed care climate, a goal of standardized care plans is to expedite treatment activities to achieve patient outcomes in a cost-effective manner (i.e., quickly). Nursing interventions focus particularly on "safety, structure, support, and symptom management." However, the nurse must remember that each patient is an individual, even when some of the patient's problems fit into a standardized plan. A patient's unique problems and needs must be addressed when formulating the plan of care.

The focus of psychiatric nursing is often on the verbal strategies that are used to guide patients in solving problems for themselves and achieving desired outcomes. Psychiatric nurses are primarily facilitators and educators. Patients might need help with developing specific and concrete plans for reaching their goals. For example, a patient might set a goal of finding a new apartment but needs assistance in locating rental options and evaluating the pros and cons of each option.

Progress Notes and Shift Reports

The style of charting progress notes, be it by written notes or electronic medical record (EMR), varies in each setting, but the components are basically the same: the patient's statements and the nurse's observations, analyses, and plans. Charting and shift reports are important ways of communicating with team members to ensure the continuity of care. These reports are also ways of evaluating the effectiveness of treatment plans and progress toward short-term and long-term patient outcomes. The nurse must remember that the entire chart is a legal document subject to review by peer review agencies, quality improvement staff, and accreditation bodies. Box 9.3 details the components of a progress note and provides a sample note for Mrs. Jarvis. Shift reports are a concise, focused, and abbreviated list of the items included in the progress notes.

Evaluation
Patient Progress

The more specific, realistic, attainable, and measurable the goals are, the greater the likelihood that patients and nurses will have a sense of progress, as evidenced in the evaluation. When the patient or nurse becomes aware of a lack of progress toward goals, this evaluation should lead to reassessment. Evaluating patient progress is important in determining patient referrals to other levels of care and collaboration within the continuum of care. In addition to evaluating the progress of patients, nurses should evaluate the quality of their interventions and their professional activities.

Discharge Summaries

Many facilities and programs expect nurses to participate in writing transfer or discharge summaries and discharge instructions that are discussed with patients. Summaries usually identify outcomes that the patient has achieved and outcomes that patient seeks to address in the future. Medication (including dosages and times), follow-up appointments (with dates and times), and referrals to other services are often included in the discharge instructions. It is important to assess and address the patient's feedback regarding the discharge instructions.

Process Recordings

Peplau (1968) used process recordings in her writings to show applications of concepts and examples of nursing interventions. A process recording is a learning activity that helps students to connect theory with practice, and promote student reflection. The process recording is the written recollection of the interaction between a student and client, a first-person verbatim that recreates the verbal and non-verbal communication that occurred in their interaction. Process recordings are an accessible and inexpensive training tool that develops the students' recalling capacity, offers immediate feedback, facilitates learning, enhances self-awareness and reflection, promotes student satisfaction from learning, and increases self-competence. Through process recordings, students are able to internalize learning over time and apply the insights they gain from their encounters with clients (Karpetis, 2019). Audiotape or videotape recordings are more accurate compared with written reports, but it is not always possible to obtain them in most settings or with many patients, due to confidentiality issues. A sample written process recording with Mrs. Jarvis is presented in Table 9.1.

> **❓ CRITICAL THINKING QUESTION**
>
> 1. For the patient, Mrs. Jarvis, can you identify two additional nursing diagnoses, two additional short-term goals, two additional long-term goals, and four additional nursing interventions?

◎ CARE PLAN

Name: Anita Jarvis   **Admission Date: _____**

DSM-5 Diagnosis: Major Depressive Disorder

Assessment	Areas of strength: Has a supportive family, had good work record, has asked for help, able to think abstractly
	Problems: Lying in bed or the couch most of the day, unable to care for self, has suicidal thoughts but denies having a plan, exhibits decreased socialization, impending divorce
Diagnoses	*Risk for suicide related to impending divorce and suicidal ideation
	*Anxiety related to fear of isolation and living alone, as evidenced by expressed helplessness
	*Hopelessness related to negative self-appraisal, as evidenced by not caring for self
Outcomes	Short-term goals
Date met: _____	Patient will agree to talk with staff when she thinks about wanting to die.
Date met: _____	Patient will verbally express sadness related to divorce situation.
Date met: _____	Patient will participate in two unit activities every day.
	Long-term goals
Date met: _____	Patient will describe options related to living alone after discharge.
Date met: _____	Patient will verbalize confidence in her ability to care for herself.
Date met: _____	Patient will describe resources available to her, especially if she becomes suicidal again.
Planning and Interventions	Nurse-patient relationship: Initiate suicide precautions as a nursing measure, monitor energy level and suicidal ideations, encourage activities of daily living, teach relaxation techniques, offer support as feelings are expressed, reinforce strengths, assist in compiling a list of resources.
	Psychopharmacology: Fluoxetine 20 mg PO every morning.
	Milieu management: Encourage patient to stay out of room; request patient attendance at grief and loss, psychoeducation, community, and recreational groups.
Evaluation	Patient will stay with daughter after discharge; patient called employer and requested extended sick leave.
Referral	Patient made appointment for outpatient counseling; patient has information on divorce recovery group and a 24-hr crisis and suicide hotline.

*International Council of Nurses. (2016). CCC-ICNP Equivalency Table for Nursing Diagnoses.

STUDY NOTES

1. To be therapeutic, the nurse uses verbal and nonverbal communication to convey a willingness to listen, genuine respect, desire to help, and understanding of the patient as a person with unique strengths, problems, and needs.

2. The nurse-patient relationship is a series of purposeful interactions that focus on the patient's thoughts, feelings, and behaviors.

3. The nurse-patient relationship is a tool that the nurse can use to assess the patient's experiences, select and carry out specific interventions, and evaluate the effectiveness of care.

4. Each stage of the nurse-patient relationship (orientation, working, termination) involves specific tasks that are employed according to the strengths, needs, and problems of each patient at a given time.

5. Patient behaviors that interfere with the recovery process must be addressed by the nurse.

6. The nursing process is a tool used by the nurse to assess each patient systematically, select and carry out specific nursing interventions, and evaluate the effectiveness of the interventions on patient outcomes.

7. The initial patient assessment is holistic and includes data from all members of the multidisciplinary team, the patient, and the family.

8. Written patient assessments, care plans, and progress notes provide an important means of ensuring consistency and continuity of care.

9. Evaluation of patient progress is a foundation for discharge planning and for referrals to other services within the continuum of care.

10. Process recordings are learning tools used to clarify communication and facilitate professional growth.

REFERENCES

Chang, Y., Cassilia, J., Warunek, M., & Scherer, Y. (2019). Motivational interviewing training with standardized patient simulation for prescription opioid abuse among older adults. *Perspectives in Psychiatric Care, 55*(4), 681–689. https://doi.org/10.1111/ppc.12402.

Clancy, R., & Taylor, A. (2016). Engaging clinicians in motivational interviewing: Comparing online with face-to-face post-training consolidation. *International Journal of Mental Health Nursing, 25*(1), 51–61. https://doi.org/10.1111/inm.12184.

Clark, G., & Egan, S. (2015). The Socratic method in cognitive behavioural therapy: A narrative review. *Cognitive Therapy & Research, 89*(6), 863–879. https://doi.org/10.1007/s10608-015-9707-3.

Gauthier, P. A. (2000). Use of Peplau's interpersonal relations model to counsel people with AIDS. *Journal of the American Psychiatric Nurses Association, 6*, 119. https://doi.org/10.1067/mpn.2000.108534.

Gruber, J. (2010). Unquiet treatment: Handling treatment refusal in bipolar disorder. *Journal of Cognitive Psychotherapy: An International Quarterly, 24*(1), 16–25.

Hallett, N., & Dickens, G. (2015). De-escalation: A survey of clinical staff in a secure mental health inpatient service. *International Journal of Mental Health Nursing, 24*(4), 324–333. https://doi.org/10.1111/inm.12136.

Hawamdeh, S., & Fakhry, R. (2014). Therapeutic relationships from the psychiatric nurses' perspectives: An interpretative phenomenological study. *Perspectives in Psychiatric Care, 50*, 178–185. https://doi.org/10.1111/ppc.12039.

Hornsten, A., et al. (2014). Strategies in health-promoting dialogues – primary healthcare nurses' perspective—a qualitative study. *Scandinavian Journal of Caring Sciences, 28*, 235–244. https://doi.org/10.1111/scs.12045.

International Council of Nurses. (2016). *CCC-ICNP Equivalency Table for Nursing Diagnoses.* International Council of Nurses.

Jansen, T., & Hanssen, I. (2017). Patient participation: Causing moral stress in psychiatric nursing? *Scandinavian Journal of Caring Sciences, 31*, 388–394. https://doi.org/10.1111/scs.12358.

Karpetis, G. (2019). In-depth learning in field education evaluating the effectiveness of process recordings. *Journal of Social Work Practice, 33*(1), 95–107. https://doi.org/10.1080/02650533.2017.1400956.

Leana, C., Meuris, J., & Lamberton, C. (2018). More than a feeling: The role of empathic care in promoting safety in health care. *ILR Review, 71*(2), 394–425. https://doi.org/10.1177/0019793917720432.

Leibing, A. (2010). Inverting compliance, increasing concerns: Aging, mental health, and caring for a trustful patient. *Anthropology & Medicine, 17*(2), 145–158. https://doi.org/10.1080/13648470.2010.493600.

Mallisham, S., & Sherrod, B. (2017). The spirit and intent of motivational interviewing. *Perspectives in Psychiatric Care, 53*, 226–233. https://doi.org/10.1111/ppc.12161.

McAndrews, S., et al. (2014). Measuring the evidence: Reviewing the literature of the measurements of therapeutic engagement in acute mental health inpatient wards. *International Journal of Mental Health Nursing, 23*, 212–220. https://doi.org/10.1111/inm.12044.

McCarthy, C. T., & Aquino-Russell, C. (2009). A comparison of two nursing theories in practice: Peplau and Parse. *Nursing Science Quarterly, 22*, 34. https://doi.org/10.1177/0894318408329339.

Oborn, E., Barrett, M., Gibson, S., & Gillard, S. (2019). Knowledge and expertise in care practices: The role of the peer worker in mental health teams. *Sociology of Health & Illness, 41*(7), 1305–1322. https://doi.org/10.1111/1467-9566.12944.

Pejner, M., Ziegert, K., & Kihlgren, A. (2015). Older patients' in Sweden and their experience of the emotional support received from the registered nurse—A grounded theory study. *Aging & Mental Health, 19*(1), 79–85. https://doi.org/10.1080/13607863.2014.917605.

Peplau, H. E. (1952). *Interpersonal relations in nursing.* Putnam.

Peplau, H. E. (1968). Psychotherapeutic strategies. *Perspectives in Psychiatric Care, 6*, 264. https://doi.org/10.1111/j.1744-6163.1968.tb01058.x.

Prochaska, J. A., & Norcross, J. C. (2002). Stages of change. In J. C. Norcross (Ed.), *Psychotherapy relationships that work* (pp. 303–313). Oxford University Press.

Pyne, J., Rabalais, A., & Sullivan, S. (2019). Mental health clinician and community clergy collaboration to address moral injury in veterans and the role of the veterans affairs chaplain. *Journal of Health Care Chaplaincy, 25*, 1–19. https://doi.org/10.1080/08854726.2018.1474997.

Rubensson, A., & Salzmann-Erikson, M. (2019). A documentation analysis of how the concept of health is incorporated in care plans when using the nursing diagnosis classification system (NANDA-1) in relation to individuals with bipolar disorder. *Scandinavian Journal of Caring Sciences, 33*, 986–994. https://doi.org/10.1111/scs.12697.

Sandhu, S., et al. (2015). Reciprocity in therapeutic relationships: A conceptual review. *International Journal of Mental Health Nursing, 24*(6), 460–470. https://doi.org/10.1111/inm.12160.

Stewart, D., et al. (2015). Thematic analysis of psychiatric patients' perception of nursing staff. *International Journal of Mental Health Nursing, 24*, 82–90. https://doi.org/10.1111/inm.12107.

Wyder, M., et al. (2015). Therapeutic relationships and involuntary treatment orders: Service users' interactions with health-care professionals on the ward. *International Journal of Mental Health Nursing, 24*(2), 181–189. https://doi.org/10.1111/inm.12121.

Zwarenstein, M., Goldman, J., & Reeves, S. (2009). Interprofessional collaboration: Effects of practice-based interventions on professional practice and healthcare outcomes. *The Cochrane Database of Systematic Reviews, 3*, https://doi.org/10.1002/14651858.CD000072.pub2.

10

Working With Groups of Patients

Susanne A. Fogger

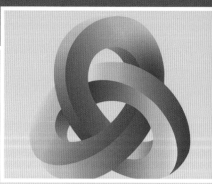

http://evolve.elsevier.com/Keltner

LEARNING OBJECTIVES

- Describe specific therapeutic benefits of groups.
- Recognize new applications for groups.
- Identify the major purpose of each type of group.
- Recognize qualities of a group leader.
- Identify intervention strategies for common management issues in groups.

Working with groups of patients is an integral component of psychiatric care. Nurses have 24-hour accountability for patient care on the inpatient psychiatric unit and often are responsible for leading patient groups. This responsibility dictates economic use of nursing personnel; working with groups of patients addresses staff concerns while providing a proven therapeutic intervention as well as educational activities. Similarly, the need for groups in the community or outpatient arena such as intensive outpatient treatment has increased because of brief psychiatric hospital stays, as well as the demands of managed care for the least expensive, most effective outcomes. In addition, social distancing since COVID-19 has increased the isolation of an already vulnerable population. People with psychiatric illnesses face problems in their daily living similar to anyone else with the additional complications related to the manifestations of their illness. Despite the added burden of unproductive cognitions interfering with how patients manage conflicts and interpersonal relationships, each has the capacity to learn new coping methods and negotiate life's problems. Group therapy provides opportunities to learn new interpersonal skills and practice in a safe environment. Most groups deal with current here-and-now issues and stressors. Patients gain awareness and knowledge about their maladaptive behaviors and thoughts. They learn how these behaviors impede communication and become aware of alternatives that help them make better decisions and choices. On inpatient units and in community settings, nurses lead numerous educational and skill-development groups. Nurses also lead groups for patients' families to teach them about mental illness, self-care, and coping with the behaviors of a mentally ill family member.

This chapter addresses two questions:
1. Given a patient population that has serious interpersonal and cognitive disturbances, how does group work benefit the individual?
2. What can the nurse realistically expect to accomplish through formal and informal group work with patients?

The type of group may be dependent on location, as inpatient units tend to be short-term and problem-focused, whereas intensive outpatient groups may be a cohort configuration and more stable in their membership. COVID-19 has changed the face of many outpatient therapy groups as they have moved to online delivery adding the need for healthcare-compliant and encrypted software. Typically inpatient groups are composed of acutely ill patients or individuals with persistent and severe mental illness. Nurses need solid interpersonal skills with strategies for managing patients at whatever level they may be. Issues regarding benefits, types, leadership, and common group management techniques are addressed. As working effectively

NORM'S NOTES You will frequently work with groups of patients—it is economical, practical, and has therapeutic advantages. Although the traditional group therapy session is rarely seen these days, psychoeducational and support groups are very common. Beyond such relatively formal atmospheres, you will have many opportunities for informal group activities as patients, clients, or consumers congregate in gathering places. A subtle message given in this chapter is that you are always on duty. Wherever patients are mingling casually, your interactions are important and should be therapeutic.

with groups of patients is inextricably related to milieu management, understanding basic principles can enhance the development of group skills.

BENEFITS OF GROUPS

Patients benefit from any group experience in the following ways:

- Decreases isolation and feelings of loneliness.
- Gaining knowledge about ways to relate to and communicate with others.
- Gaining personal acceptance, reassurance, and support from peers as well as observing role modeling from the group leader.
- Gaining feelings of hopefulness and a sense of empowerment regarding their ability to help themselves as well as others in the group.
- Benefiting from supported and coached skill development, with the opportunity to test out new behaviors with others.
- Within a safe, structured environment, learning to trust and share feelings, concerns, and ideas.
- Individuals' strengths are affirmed, enhancing self-esteem.
- Experiencing a sense of importance, belonging, as well as an increased sense of worth.

These benefits can occur for individual patients given a therapeutic group situation. Each group, depending on its goal or purpose, might focus on one particular outcome. For example, an activity group for art might focus on acceptance; no matter what the patient paints or draws, their work will be appreciated with positive regard for their efforts.

THERAPEUTIC FACTORS

Irving Yalom, who is considered the "father of group therapy," described 11 therapeutic factors that help patients feel accepted and heard, regardless of the therapeutic group (Box 10.1) (Behenck, Wesner, Finkler, & Heldt, 2017; Yalom & Leszcz, 2020). Patients experience certain factors or benefits, depending on the type of group in which they participate. Yalom originally related the therapeutic factors to psychotherapy groups but developed its application to brief, one-time-only groups along the continuum of care. It is important for the nurse to understand the meaning of these therapeutic factors and their significance to patients. Understanding how groups help patients can increase the likelihood nurses will initiate, lead, and participate in formal and informal groups. Nurses cannot make therapeutic factors happen, but they facilitate their development and promote the principles.

TYPES OF GROUPS

Creating a positive environment in which an inpatient group can be beneficial is an art form. Each session should be treated as a separate entity, with the patient feeling that something positive has been attained during the group session

---

BOX 10.1   Yalom's Therapeutic Factors

- **Instillation of hope:** Patients receive hope from observing others who have benefited from the group experience.
- **Universality:** Patients experience relief in knowing that they are not alone and unique but that others experience similar problems, feelings, and concerns.
- **Imparting of information:** Patients learn or are provided information about areas related to their needs.
- **Altruism:** Patients experience themselves as helpful or useful to others.
- **Corrective recapitulation of primary family group:** Patients review previous dysfunctional family patterns and learn that these patterns can be changed to meet their present needs effectively.
- **Development of socializing techniques:** Patients are taught appropriate social skills.
- **Imitative behavior:** Patients selectively model healthy behaviors of the leader and other group members.
- **Catharsis:** Patients not only are allowed to express feelings but also are taught ways to express them appropriately.
- **Existential factors:** Patients share feelings about "ultimate concerns" of existence, such as death or isolation, and learn to accept that there is a limit to their control of these issues.
- **Cohesiveness:** Patients experience feelings of being accepted, valued, and part of a group experience.
- **Interpersonal learning:** Patients learn how their behaviors affect others and more appropriate ways of relating in the supportive atmosphere of the group.

From Yalom, I., & Leszcz, M. (2020). *The theory and practice of group psychotherapy* (6th ed.). Basic Books.

(Behenck, Wesner, Finkler, & Heldt, 2017; Yalom & Leszcz, 2020). A positive inpatient group experience favorably predisposes patients to seek treatment on an outpatient basis and remain engaged in their care.

Numerous types of groups can be offered in both inpatient and outpatient settings, including psychoeducational, relapse prevention, and activities to support self-expression and competency building. Cognitive behavior therapy, self-help, special problem groups, and multifamily or couple groups are also available in some treatment settings. Traditional therapy groups, such as psychoanalytic or insight-oriented groups, are seldom offered in an inpatient setting because of the acuity of patients, brief inpatient stays, and reimbursement issues. Frequent patient turnover on inpatient units necessitates focusing on topics that can stand independently and deal with patients' immediate needs.

While support groups used an online format prior to COVID-19, group therapy via the internet often became the only way to safely reach out to people. Facilities adapted by using Zoom for healthcare application software which was HIPAA-compliant and also encrypted to ensure the safety of patient data from hacking. Individuals who had broadband access were able to attend therapy groups from the safety of their homes. This was invaluable as many facilities were closed to in-person visits (Wright et al., 2021). In addition, these groups did not add to the stress of travel, or increase the patients' risk of acquiring an infection. The groups supported interpersonal skill development, decreased social isolation, and provided ongoing care to support recovery.

Psychoeducational Groups

Nurses who work in inpatient or outpatient settings lead groups to offer patients and their families a variety of content and skills. Typically groups deal with medication, the dynamics and management of illness, problem-solving, stress management, anger management, social skills, basic living skills, and relapse prevention (Table 10.1). Groups run by an advanced practice psychiatric nurse may include cognitive behavior therapy, dialectical behavior therapy, or other types of therapy. Patients have expressed increased satisfaction with inpatient care when psychoeducational groups focused on illness management, substance abuse, outpatient treatment, and living skills. The reduction in inpatient stays has increased the need for patients to learn skills that help them manage their illnesses in the community setting.

Group sessions vary in length but typically last 30 to 60 minutes for content presentation and discussion. How long the group meets varies, depending on the patients' level of cognitive and behavioral impairment. An inpatient group might be a 40-minute discussion of medication management while an outpatient group on interpersonal skill development or a supportive group might be 60 to 90 minutes in length. The nurse's expertise, empathy, and support help patients realize that they can successfully learn to manage their illnesses while also improving their ability to cope with their situations.

Nurses also provide psychoeducational programs for families of mentally ill individuals. Families often express interest around content on illnesses, medication benefits and side effects, communication with the ill family member, and ways to manage crisis situations with their family member. In addition, nurses can coach how to negotiate with the mental health system and managed care. Families benefit not only from the information that they receive in groups but also from the high level of support provided. In addition, families experience less anger and have improved relationships with family members as they learn new family communication skills. They also learn about available resources along the continuum of healthcare. Families look to the nurse as an advocate and expert to help them arrange for needed services.

Maintenance Groups

The very nature of nursing implies support through therapeutic interactions. Support means accepting, empathizing, and showing concern while listening to and talking with patients. The nurse's presence, genuine interest, and encouragement facilitate the expression of patients' feelings and concerns. The nurse is instrumental in helping patients cope with their feelings and situations. As such, support is useful in many types of group situations.

This type of group's purpose is to reinforce or maintain existing strengths, rather than to confront or change behaviors or defenses. Patients in a support group can be acutely or chronically ill. Group members might need a great deal of reassurance and emotional support. Patients often need help to reduce their anxiety to mild or moderate levels, and skills to reduce anxiety can be taught during group sessions.

The reality orientation group is an example of a support group frequently found in inpatient settings. Patients who exhibit confusion and short attention spans resulting from some psychopathologic factor can benefit from participation. The professional must provide an atmosphere of safety and security because these patients might be frightened, unsure, anxious, uncomfortable, and isolated. The reality orientation group can assist patients with decreasing isolation and increasing their self-efficacy. Focusing on the "here and now"

TABLE 10.1	**Psychoeducational Groups**	
Type	**Nurse's Purpose or Role**	**Examples**
Illness	Teach patients and families the content related to dynamics of illness, symptoms of illness, signs of relapse, management of illness, and dealing with crises	Addiction processes, coping with symptoms, management of moods, causes and treatments of illnesses, trigger recognition, relapse prevention, community resources
Medication	Administer medications Assess symptoms and side effects Explain type and purpose of medication, dosage, therapeutic effects, and side effects Provide support measures to prevent relapse	Groups based on category of medications (e.g., antipsychotics vs. antidepressants, intramuscular vs. oral)
Problem-solving	Help identify and describe current problems, discuss and develop solutions and their effects, decide on an alternative method and how to try it Evaluate and choose another method, if necessary	Milieu issues, conflict resolution, job concerns, relationship issues, discharge planning, housing issues
Stress management	Teach and facilitate adaptive coping behaviors	Lifestyle balance and management, relaxation training, tension reduction strategies, anger management, mindful meditation, yoga, and tai chi
Social skills	Teach, develop, and practice skills to enhance interactions with others; focus on realistic, day-to-day patient needs	Assertiveness training, handling social interactions (e.g., meeting new people, going on interviews, negotiating the return of a purchase)

(what is going on right now in this environment) provides a framework with structure, social support, and reality testing. The nurse, as leader of this group, facilitates the orientation to time, person, and place; rules and routines of the unit; and behavioral expectations, including some limit setting. Feeling valued, respected, and important as human beings are feelings that these patients might not have experienced for some time.

Activity Groups

The general goals of activity groups are to help patients increase self-esteem, expression of feelings, and social interaction. Withdrawn, depressed, and regressed patients benefit from these groups because these individuals have experienced isolation and have difficulty with interpersonal relationships. The activity is *a vehicle* or means to facilitate (1) self-expression of both positive and negative feelings in a creative way, (2) patient interaction, and (3) enjoyment.

Recreation groups provide the opportunity to have fun and relieve tension. Exercise groups or groups that foster physical activity benefit individuals mentally and physically by improving physical health and reducing psychiatric and social disability. Movement can be a way of helping the individual feel "part of the group." These groups enable patients to experience a sense of participation, acceptance, and accomplishment. Individuals with serious mental illness often have sedentary lifestyles and possibly comorbid physical health problems. Many psychiatric medications can induce weight gain, so diet modification and teaching concerning nutrition coupled with daily exercise can aid in reducing the risk. Integration of a structured program, such as a walking or exercise group, can be helpful. Individuals with serious mental illness value exercise as a component of their treatment.

Self-Help and Special Problem Groups

Many groups focus on helping individuals with special problems; examples are weight loss, child abuse, anorexia and bulimia, anxiety management, or medical issues such as diabetes and heart disease. These groups are homogeneous, meaning that all group members share the same problem. Members feel accepted and understood by the group and are more willing to share concerns and ask questions. Information is shared, in addition to personal feelings and difficulties. Members assist each other with helpful strategies. Members do not feel alone or isolated with their problem. They observe how others with the same problem are coping effectively. The nurse who leads special problem groups is interested, knowledgeable, and skilled in working with patients with specific problems. Weight Watchers (WW)® is an example of this type of support group.

Traditional self-help groups are also homogeneous but are *not* professionally organized or led. Self-help groups are organized and led by members with the same problem, such as in Alcoholics Anonymous (AA). The premise is that an individual with a problem (such as cocaine or alcohol abuse) can be truly understood and helped by others with the same problem who have learned to cope with the illness. Millions of people participate in self-help groups. Some groups, such as AA, have volunteers available for 24-hour support. Members of self-help groups have the lived experience of "having been there, done that" and understand problems, cope with stress, as well as confront each other about dysfunctional behaviors.

Professionals might be invited to a self-help group for a specific purpose, such as providing an educational program. Nurses commonly refer individuals to self-help groups for support and can assist the patient in how to conduct a search for self-help groups in their area. There is a clear separation between the professional and self-help groups. Professionals do not "run" or "manage" AA. However, there are nurses who may attend AA for their own recovery needs. This type of self-help group is anonymous due to the stigma of the illness, so it is important to maintain the anonymity of the members. Should the nurse visit a meeting, it is important to realize that meetings are designated as "open," meaning anyone can attend, or "closed," in which only members (those with the illness) may attend.

In addition, support for families includes ALANON, which is a group just for people affected by those who are addicted to alcohol. Other local mental health organizations such as Mental Health America and the National Alliance for the Mentally Ill (NAMI) can be contacted for further information. NAMI is for families of patients with mental illness and can be very helpful as a support. Their website is a helpful reference for families and can be found at: http://www.nami.org.

GROUP MANAGEMENT ISSUES

Group Leadership

Group leadership functions range from formal to informal. The inpatient psychiatric nurse might engage in spontaneous, informal interactions with a group of patients in a card game or participate formally in a planned, structured group session. An informal card game provides the nurse with an opportunity for therapeutic interpersonal interaction, socialization, and role-modeling behavior. Another example might be responding to medication questions that arise in small informal groups; the nurse reinforces medication benefits, shares helpful management tips, and alleviates anxiety or concerns. These informal, spontaneous interventions with groups of patients occur repeatedly during the course of a day on an inpatient unit.

Although degrees of formality and types of patients vary, the nurse invariably uses group leadership skills to meet patients' interpersonal needs in the therapeutic milieu. As managers and providers of patient care (24 hours a day), nurses intervene with groups of patients in the milieu setting. Consequently, nurses must use effective communication skills to interact with groups of patients (described later in this chapter).

Nurses on inpatient units should be aware of factors that influence the clinical setting. Short-stay inpatient hospitalization affects group work in many ways. For example, short hospitalizations result in a rapid turnover of patients; expecting trust and cohesion to develop in such a group is unrealistic. Patients are admitted with acute symptoms of serious illnesses. The nurse must quickly assess the mental status of patients to determine whether they can tolerate a group session and involve patients based on their level of functioning. Manic, severely depressed, or actively psychotic patients *may not* be appropriate group members. Assessing the patient's ability to tolerate the stimulation and interaction with others may require giving the individual permission to leave the group if necessary. Charting patient progress within the group should address the patient's ability to stay focused on concerns and overall group themes. The group goals may include decreasing social isolation and improving interpersonal skills. Similarly, in the community, nurses must consider realistic factors that impinge on treatment. Patients might be limited to a specific number of visits because of payment providers, or might be limited to a specific number of days during the course of a year. For patients in rural areas, transportation issues may affect the ability of patients to participate.

It is important to explain confidentiality issues to group participants. Patients should understand that what is said or takes place in the group setting should remain private and "stay in group"—put simply, "Do not gossip about group to people outside of the group." However, statements within group sessions might be shared with staff members or the treatment team because of their responsibility for patient care. In reality, group confidentiality can be difficult to ensure because trust and cohesion might not be fully developed. This does not apply to educational content, such as information about medication, which can be shared outside of the treatment setting.

Physical Setting

Physical arrangements are important considerations in creating an atmosphere that is conducive to group work. Finding adequate space or a private room is often difficult but is nevertheless important to ensure privacy and a quiet atmosphere. Adequate lighting, comfortable temperature, ample seating, and proper equipment also contribute to successful group functioning. A box of tissues available at the start can prevent a distracting group scramble looking for tissues when an individual is sharing painful emotions. Forming a circle of chairs allows patients to see each other and indicates an expectation that patients will relate to the leader and other group members. Sitting around a large table is also an option, with the goal being that all members are "equally at the table." Members sitting on the outside of the circle should be invited in. Chairs in rows might be appropriate for a didactic session but does not allow for effective interpersonal communication flow. A blackboard, dry marker board, or other media such as a DVD player can enhance learning if it is to be an

educational group. Handouts or printed materials might be useful for patients and families to take home for future reference. Groups conducted online have to establish expectations unique to this method of delivery. Often technical issues can be a challenge as connectivity can vary, altering the sound and visual quality. Clarification may be required for each session that the line is HIPAA-compliant and is encrypted for the group's safety.

Nurse leaders must be active, empathic, and able to provide structure. Because of time constraints, leaders cannot afford to be nondirective or to allow the group to be free-floating. The nurse must be goal-directed and focus on the here and now in each session. The leader succinctly states the group's purpose at the beginning of the session, and most of the time is spent on the work to be accomplished. Patients generally prefer leaders who provide the group "with an active structure" (Yalom & Leszcz, 2020). The final 5 to 10 minutes are used to summarize and close the session. The summary should have a positive focus and include information that the patients have learned or gained from the group. The leader gives positive feedback to the group regarding progress during the session.

Expectations or group rules must be explicit, such as patients are expected to arrive on time and remain for the entire session, if possible. Cell phones or other devices need to be turned off and the expectation of "no calls during group" should be made explicit. For an inpatient group, the group leader might permit patients to pace or leave the room and then return when they are able. The inability to sit still for an extended period might be the result of anxiety or medication side effects (usually akathisia). The decision to exclude patients from the group should be made carefully. The nurse might exclude patients who are acutely manic, disoriented, and too psychotic to benefit from group. Patients who are hostile and verbally threatening are also inappropriate for group sessions. If the group is in a common area, ensure that there are signs up warning of "group in progress" to avoid interruption during the session.

COMMON MANAGEMENT ISSUES

Interventions for groups are based on facilitative communication techniques (see Chapter 8). Nurses use skills with patients individually and within groups. Nurses who facilitate group interactions on a therapeutic level help enable patients to share thoughts, feelings, and problems. Basic communication skills useful for nurse leaders are detailed in Table 10.2. These skills are not unique to the group setting but can be used on a daily basis. These interventions are therapeutic, regardless of the type of group. The use of positive feedback helps patients to use new skills. For example, to use a particular assertiveness skill, the patient goes off on a tangent. The nurse might say, "You have done well, Sam. When you gave us the example of saying to your boss, 'I need to talk with you about my work schedule,' you used an excellent example of 'I' statements." The nurse chooses to repeat the portion of Sam's statement that is realistic and is a correct example of an

TABLE 10.2 Communication Skills: Eliciting, Qualifying, and Clarifying Communication

Techniques of the Leader(s)	Group Member Response	Outcome
1. **Giving information**: "My purpose in offering this group experience is..."	Further validates his assumptions: "How is this going to happen?"	Leader(s) and member(s) enter into a dialogue in which member(s) get more information that helps them make decisions and build trust in group experience.
2. **Seeking clarification**: "Did you say you were upset with John because he said that?"	Might try to restate his thoughts or feelings: "Yes, I guess I was upset."	Member becomes aware that he was unclear and learns to identify thoughts and feelings more precisely, at the same time taking responsibility for them.
3. **Encouraging description and exploration** (delving further into communication or experiences): "How did you feel when Joann said that to you?"	Elaborates on his message: "I was angry."	Member deals in great depth with an experience in the group and again takes responsibility for his reactions. (This example also places events in time or in sequence, lending further perspective to group events.)
4. **Presenting reality**: "Would other members think Joann was unstable if they interviewed her for a job and she appeared anxious?"	Listens and considers other possibilities.	Member compares perception of self with others' perceptions of him.
5. **Seeking consensual validation** (seeking mutual understanding of what is being communicated): "Did I understand you to say that you feel better now than you did last week?"	Further clarification: "Well, yes, I'm better than last week but not as good as I'd like to be."	Group and leader(s) learn how member views his progress and how they should receive his evaluation of himself.
6. **Focusing** (identifying a single topic to concentrate on): "Could we identify one problem you have and talk more about that?"	Channels thinking: Members might think of the most puzzling problem they have.	Group leader(s) identify specific topics that they can resolve before the meeting ends. They increase their understanding of one problem before jumping to others.
7. **Encouraging comparison** (asking members to compare and contrast their experiences with others in the group): "How did the rest of the group handle this problem?"	Group members share their experiences as they relate to the topic.	Leader(s) and members gain greater insight into their commonalities and differences and learn from one another alternative ways of responding to problems.
8. **Making observations**: "You look more comfortable now, John, than you did at the beginning of the meeting." *or* "The group has been silent for the last 5 minutes."	Group members have something to respond to: "I feel more at ease now." *or* "I think we are quiet because we are bored."	Group members and leader(s) place attention on significant events and can elaborate on their meanings.
9. **Giving recognition or acknowledging**: "John, you are new to the group. Perhaps we can introduce ourselves."	Feels acknowledged and included: "Yes, I'm John, and I came here because..."	Members view specific instances as important, and the leader(s) reinforce the behavior or event that they choose to notice—in this case, the desire to come to group.
10. **Accepting** (not necessarily agreeing with but receiving communication with openness): "Yes, I hear you say that you don't know if you want to be in the group or not."	Feels heard and understood without fear of attack.	Members learn that even "nonacceptable" attitudes can be talked about, and perhaps any thought is not so horrible that they cannot share it.
11. **Encouraging evaluation** (asking the group as a whole or individual members to judge their experiences): "When Marilyn is supportive of you, does that make you feel better?" *or* "How did we do in helping Joann with her problem?"	Member reflects on progress made: "Not exactly, because I don't know if I can trust her to be honest." *or* "It was hard. I'd like to know from her."	The criteria for success become clearer to members, and new directions might be formulated as a result of the discussion.
12. **Summarizing** (encapsulating in a few sentences what has occurred): "The group discussed several issues and problems today. They were..."	Members recall significant points and events and block out consideration of new or extraneous topics.	Members and leader(s) place in perspective and identify salient points of a group session. Such a summary can lead to a better understanding of group process.

From Van Servellen (1983). *Group and family therapy.* Mosby.

"I" statement for emphasis and clarity. As a result, the patient feels a sense of accomplishment and increased self-esteem.

TYPES OF PATIENTS IN GROUPS

Dominant Patient

A dominant patient may monopolize the entire group session to the extent that other patients might believe that they do not have the opportunity to participate. The nurse uses gatekeeping techniques to offer all patients the opportunity to contribute to the group. For example, the nurse can say, "Cathy, you are doing well in contributing to our session today, but I would like to hear what others are thinking." This intervention can forestall monopolization of the group by a single patient without putting her down, while providing others with the opportunity to express themselves. Anticipate that other patients in the group will be unable to handle this patient as they will be overly polite, or might be shy. If the group leader is intimidated or cannot control the patient, the integrity of the group is compromised.

Uninvolved Patient

The uninvolved patient presents another challenge to the nurse leader. The patient might be quiet because of anxiety or fear of saying the wrong thing. Patients with chronic schizophrenia find relating in group sessions to be difficult and threatening. The nurse can say, "It's hard to talk about ourselves in the group, but I know that everyone here has something important to share." The nurse recognizes that patients are mistrustful and anxious but can relate the message that each individual is important and capable of helping another. Periodically asking the person "What are your thoughts on this?" can help them feel part of the group.

Some patients who are uninvolved in the group might believe themselves to be at a higher level of functioning than the other members. These patients might believe that they are not as sick as the others, or do not belong in the group, and would not benefit from the session. The nurse leader might give attention to these members by giving them a job to perform for the group—for example, arranging chairs for the session or calling other group members to remind them of the group. Respect and recognition by the nurse are therapeutic for these patients, as they come to recognize that they can contribute and benefit.

❓ CRITICAL THINKING QUESTIONS

1. During a group session on medication management, a patient states, "I learn more by listening." How would you involve this patient in the group discussion?
2. During a group session, the nurse observes two patients whispering and snickering to each other. How would you handle this situation?

Hostile Patient

Hostility might mask a patient's fear, unresolved anger, or even hurt toward others. To help this patient verbalize feelings of anger appropriately, the nurse can say, "Melody, you sound angry today. What happened?" or "Tell us about it." The nurse directly confronts this patient in a supportive manner and attempts to help the patient deal with her thoughts and feelings. Allowing verbal or nonverbal hostility to continue jeopardizes the progress of the group session. Unchecked hostility causes discomfort and uneasiness and impairs the ability of other patients to attend, as they may not feel safe. Patients might also mistakenly interpret anger as being directed toward them. It may be helpful to ask, "Is your irritability with someone in the group?" This will help the group understand if the person's mood is about them or not. This can be an opportunity to focus on interpersonal skills such as "What was your perception of what just occurred?" In addition, the group leader can encourage patients to talk about feelings and gain confidence in speaking about their perceptions.

Distracting Patient

Some patients' behaviors and verbalizations can be very distracting to other members of the group. The group may become distracted when inappropriate comments are made and when delusions or hallucinations are voiced in the group. For the patient who has verbalized a delusion, the nurse could use empathy, focus on the underlying need, present reality, and refocus the group. For example, the patient might state, "Everyone here is against me." The nurse could reply, "It must upset you to feel that way. I want to assure you that you are safe with me." The nurse ultimately brings the group members back to the topic that they were discussing. For the patient who is hallucinating, the nurse reassures the patient's emotion, and then returns to the topic of discussion. A simple statement to the group such as, "We are talking about side-effect management of atypical antipsychotics. Let's review what we've talked about so far." The nurse does not confront the individual in group but may meet with the patient after group for one-to-one interaction.

The patient who verbalizes a sexually inappropriate comment can be handled by the nurse using limit setting. For example, the nurse could state, "Jim, that comment is inappropriate. We are discussing symptoms that could indicate relapse."

These group interventions help the nurse develop as a group leader. Patients quickly recognize the group leader's empathy, understanding, and respect for each patient as caring behaviors. Even though some patients make only minimal progress toward their individual treatment goals, interacting with the nurse who possesses and exhibits these traits can increase the patients' feelings of worth as human beings. The nurse's tactful method of managing these behaviors can role-model adaptive ways of behaving in the future.

▮ STUDY NOTES

1. The psychiatric nurse interacts and intervenes with patients and families in informal groups as well as in formally-structured sessions in inpatient and community settings.

2. Patients benefit from group experiences by gaining acceptance, hopefulness, and support from others. Through mutual sharing of feelings and problems, patients learn how their communication methods and behaviors interfere with relationships. Their strengths are reinforced and accumulated.

3. Families of mentally ill patients benefit from the information and support that they receive in a group.

4. Nurse leaders must be active, empathic, goal-directed, and comfortable keeping in the "here and now" for each group session.

5. Various types of groups exist in inpatient and outpatient settings that can benefit patients with acute and chronic illnesses. Typical groups include psychoeducational, maintenance, activity, and self-help or special problem groups. Psychoeducational and self-help groups are available for families of mentally ill patients.

6. As group leaders, nurses use facilitative communication techniques and role-modeling behaviors.

7. The nurse leader structures the group session by attending to content and process issues.

8. The nurse leader intervenes therapeutically with dominating, uninvolved, hostile, and distracting patients, while continuing to be respectful, guiding patients to improve communication skills.

REFERENCES

Behenck, A., Wesner, A. C., Finkler, D., & Heldt, E. (2017). Contribution of group therapeutic factors to the outcome of Cognitive-Behavioral Therapy for patients with Panic Disorder. *Archives of Psychiatric Nursing, 31*(2), 142–146. https://doi.org/10.1016/j.apnu.2016.09.001.

Van Servellen, G. (1983). *Group and family therapy*. Mosby.

Wright, S., Thompson, N., Yadrich, D., Bruce, A., Bonar, H., Spaulding, R., & Smith, C. (2021). Using Telehealth to assess depression and suicide ideation and provide mental health interventions to groups of chronically ill adolescents and young adults. *Research in Nursing & Health, 44*, 129–137. https://doi.org/10.1002/nur.22089.

Yalom, I., & Leszcz, M. (2020). *The theory and practice of group psychotherapy* (6th ed.). Basic Books.

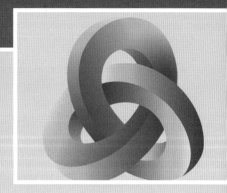

11

Working With the Family

Debbie Steele

 http://evolve.elsevier.com/Keltner

LEARNING OBJECTIVES

- Define the terms *family* and *family* systems.
- Discuss characteristics of healthy families.
- Evaluate the effects of mental disorders on the family system.
- List the factors to be assessed when working with families.

- Describe the skills needed for working therapeutically and collaboratively with families.
- Discuss the issues associated with caring for psychiatric patients within a family context.

Mental illness often changes families' lives and relationships forever. It is a family experience, shared together but suffered separately. *Relational suffering* refers to the suffering experienced by both family members and the individual. Given the influence that symptoms may have on interpersonal relationships, mental illness has a significant impact on family members. Family members face the following challenges: (1) caregiver burden, (2) stigmatization, (3) fear of aggression, (4) potential for mental illness in one family member negatively influencing the mental health of other family members, (5) mourning, (6) shame and guilt, and (7) difficulties in communicating with health care professions. Marshall et al. (2010) reported that it is not always the individual with the illness who suffers the most, but rather it is other family members.

When a family member experiences a mental disorder, the family is likely to be the major source of assistance for the mentally ill individual. Families are the first to observe the changes in behavior accompanying the illness, they will have been confused and concerned by their family member's actions, and they have often tried desperately to obtain the needed care. Nurses who care for individuals with mental disorders need to understand family functioning in order to work collaboratively with families to promote their adjustment to the effects of the mental disorder and improve the chances of recovery.

This chapter explores the characteristics of families, the effects of mental disorders on the family system, and strategies for working therapeutically with families in various settings. The emphasis is on understanding and assessing families as a basis for therapeutic interactions, family conferences, education, support, and referrals rather than focusing on family therapy.

FAMILY AND THE RECOVERY MODEL

Families are important to those with mental health difficulties. All members of the family assume important roles and engage in family interactions that are potentially positive or disempowering amid mental illness. Persons with a mental illness diagnosis perceive that family members both facilitate and hinder their recovery process. While family members are an important source of motivation, morale, and practical support, they may simultaneously be forcing inpatient treatment, displaying a lack of understanding, and acting as a source of stress (Acero et al., 2017). Family roles are largely determined by the developmental period of the family. For example, is the patient a young adult cared for by parents or an elderly adult cared for by adult children? Understanding family dynamics requires the nurse to think interactionally—about the influence of the illness on the family as well as the family influence on the patient (Marshall et al., 2010).

Family caregivers experience significant stressors and moderate to high burdens, which can result in excessive emotional involvement and critical comments. Some patients describe their families as the source of their problems, owing to disruptions in family relationships. In spite of the burden of care, family members are also the main providers of support in the following ways: (1) economically, (2) emotionally, (3) in providing physical assistance, and (4) as a source of knowledge. Individuals with mental illness report the importance of receiving positive support, such as feeling that the family is there for them. Depending on where the patient is in the recovery process, family members will shift from caring for the patient to times when the patient, along with all family members, is able to celebrate greater autonomy and reciprocity. Movement within the cyclical nature of mental illness involves positive risk-taking by both the family members and the individual with a mental disorder (Reupert et al., 2015).

NORM'S NOTES Where would you be without your family? I would not want to consider such a life, and you might not either. When a family member develops mental health problems, other family members are affected. A fundamental role of nurses and other psychiatric professionals is to help families cope with and assist a family member with a mental health disorder and to understand how they may be contributing to the problem or might work toward a resolution. Remember this, because I think it is humbling: When you have done what you know how to do, the family will almost always still be there dealing with the outcomes, whether good or bad.

A NORMAL FAMILY

A normal family is difficult to define, owing to the profound social, economic, and political changes of recent decades, all of which have altered the landscape of family life. Amid the turmoil, families have forged new and varied relationship patterns within and across households as they strive to build long-lasting bonds. One's understanding of a family functioning, from healthy to dysfunctional, must take into account the challenges and changes in family life within a diverse and complex world (Walsh, 2012).

A normal family may be defined as a functional family. Normality is not measured by the lack of symptoms of distress or the severity of problems. Family patterns and roles that are deemed proper or desirable are taught and determined by prevailing societal, ethnic, or religious values. Therefore, a family may be viewed as normal if it fits patterns that are common in ordinary families. Healthy family functioning can be found amid problems; in fact, no families are problem-free. Some stresses and challenges are part of every family's life. However, the ways in which families cope with such issues determine their health. Some family patterns of interaction that would not be considered average would include destructive acts, such as physical or verbal violence. The term *dysfunctional* refers to family patterns that are not working; it is important to not label the family itself as dysfunctional (Walsh, 2012), but rather to focus on such patterns.

FAMILY CHARACTERISTICS

Healthy families can be defined by their effectiveness in building caring and committed relationships with strong bonds. According to Walsh (2012), healthy families can be contrasted with unhealthy families by their ability to adapt to societal changes, as well as the changes that occur naturally within the family cycle.

To define a healthy or functional family, it is necessary to consider the defining characteristics of successful families of all types. Healthy, well-functioning families nurture and support their members and provide stability and cohesion in a rapidly changing world. It is often said in families that "Home is the place you can go and be accepted when the rest of the world rejects you." In today's fast-paced, high-stress society, such nurturing is invaluable. Everyone needs someone to care for them and help them when facing challenges. Knowing that the family will remain together and provide predictability in an unpredictable world can buffer the stresses that individuals face every day.

Successful families also protect their members from dangers by caring for vulnerable members whose age or condition renders them unable to care for themselves independently. For example, infants and children require many years of parental care and supervision. Family members who experience acute or chronic physical and emotional conditions benefit from family care and support. Elderly individuals experiencing physical and mental decline also receive care that is generally provided by family members.

The family of origin provides the platform of truth for children. It is where new members of the family learn what is needed to function in the world, from communication and socialization to values and roles required within the family and in the outside world. Children learn language, communication skills, and religious and secular beliefs, as well as how to be a child, sibling, student, and parent from interactions within the family. In healthy, functional families, communication is open, lines of authority are clear, socialization is encouraged, and respect for self and others is taught, as well as how to relate to each other and others outside the family. Family units serve as a vehicle where members are cared for, valued, and prepared to cope with the society in which they live. The nurturing of individuals as they grow and develop leads to a well-functioning, healthy adult.

These characteristics provide the basis for the family to cope effectively with internal pressures, such as the illness of a member, or external pressures, such as the loss of a job by a parent. During times of stress, a family might experience disruption in one or more of these desirable characteristics; however, the support of caregivers, extended family, and friends can help the family weather the disruption and remain resilient. For example, job loss by the father causes an initial economic and personal crisis. However, if his wife can move to full-time employment and the family can problem solve the crisis together, the father can, for example, return to school to retrain for a better position or find other ways to improve the family's long-term stability.

STAGES OF FAMILY DEVELOPMENT

McGoldrick and Shibusawa (2012) presented the different stages of family life and what is required to accomplish the tasks at each stage. The authors begin with "young adulthood," the stage when the young adult separates from his or her family of origin without cutting off emotionally from the nuclear family. The next stage is referred to as "coupling," the joining of two families, characterized by an overlapping of two family systems to develop a third system. As the couple transitions to becoming a "family with young children," a shift occurs as they move up a generation, becoming caretakers to the younger generation. Once a child is born, the couple maintain an enduring bond as parents to their children, even if they eventually separate. "Families with adolescents" marks a new stage, represented by transitions to adult roles with parents responding to their changing cognitive, emotional, physical, and social needs. "Families at midlife" are busy launching children and moving on to explore new pursuits. This stage necessitates a restructuring of the marital relationship (dealing with the "empty nest"). This phase tends to be the longest in the family life cycle, represented by the greatest number of exits and entries of family members. In the final stage, "families in later life," the couple deals with issues of adjusting to retirement, becoming grandparents, and facing the eventual deaths of their spouse and friends. Declining health and increasing dependence are common as adult children care for their elderly parents.

Families are not static, but knowing the stage of family development a family is dealing with can give the nurse an idea of potential issues and problems. If a family has children of widely varying ages, the family might be dealing with developmental tasks at several levels at the same time. For example, in a blended family, one or both spouses might have adolescents and school-age children from a previous marriage while also dealing with a newborn from their current union. Nurturing an infant and simultaneously guiding an adolescent toward independence requires different parenting techniques and might create stress in the family. Knowledge of appropriate child behavior at each developmental stage of childhood is also an important part of successful parenting that can contribute to the strength of family ties.

CONTEMPORARY FAMILIES

Today, the nuclear family is no longer the predominant family structure. Divorce, remarriage, and same-sex marriages have led to single-parent families, blended families, and families with two parents of the same gender. Some people believe that these changes undermine the integrity of the family, whereas others believe that these new structures demonstrate the flexibility of the family system, allowing the family to remain viable and effective as a vehicle for raising children and maintaining interpersonal support amid the stresses of modern life (Walsh, 2012).

Alterations in family structure parallel other societal changes that have affected how families function. Economic pressures have made two-wage-earner families the norm, necessitating out-of-home care for children and leaving a gap in the supervision of older children and adolescents after school. Statistically, 50% of marriages end in divorce in the United States, which encourages increasingly complex family interactions with parents, stepparents, grandparents, and step-grandparents, not to mention half-siblings and stepsiblings.

Adult children might continue living in their parents' home for an extended time because of divorce, job loss, or financial hardship. Relationships between parents and adult children living in the same household can become strained and, even if cordial, require significant effort to remain harmonious and stable over time as roles and functions shift from what they had been while the children were growing up. Young adults who choose to live independently of their parents often live with a roommate or partner for economic as well as personal reasons (Walsh, 2012).

Society has become more culturally diverse as a result of immigration, intermarriage, and cross-cultural adoption. Issues of assimilation, integration, and maintaining one's cultural identity all affect the structure and function of families. With regard to immigration, cross-cultural marriage, and adoption, the involved parties must balance allegiance to their cultural heritage against the values, norms, and behaviors of the new culture in which they find themselves. Immigrant parents are faced with decisions regarding how much to focus on their own culture and how to free their Americanized children to fit into U.S. culture. The children of immigrants easily adopt the customs of the culture in which they are living, often causing distress and feelings of loss in their immigrant parents and extended family. Assimilation of the younger generation into the new society is necessary for them to fit into the new culture and feel successful, but it might come at a price in terms of their cultural identity (Walsh, 2012).

Discrimination and racism are faced by many immigrants, especially if their cultural norms and appearance are very different from the dominant culture in their new country. Lack of familiarity with the culture, difficulty speaking the language, and lack of job access can cause a ripple effect of low wages and economic hardship that can weaken the family structure.

Alterations in family structure and function, along with societal changes, can create stress in the family. In today's world, communications technology makes everyone constantly aware of world events, which can fuel fear about the future and one's own personal safety and make it more difficult for families to feel secure. In many major cities, random acts of violence, gang wars, and racism result in individuals and their families restricting their daily activities. Such constraints make it more difficult for families to function optimally, although most have shown great resilience in dealing with such threats (Walsh, 2012).

Nurses working with individuals with a diagnosis of a mental disorder must be aware of the needs of modern families. For example, families are more likely to be culturally diverse, requiring the nurse to learn about the values, beliefs, and customs of families from other cultures. Information in this chapter and in Chapter 5 can help nurses to understand and respond to culturally diverse families.

CRITICAL THINKING QUESTION

1. Can a healthy family have a member with a mental disorder?

FAMILY SYSTEMS THEORY

The view of the family as a "system" is an important theoretical framework that is useful for health care professionals, particularly nurses and other professionals who work with mental disorders. The family is conceived as a collective unit made up of individual parts (Nichols, 2013). Every family member plays a critical albeit unique role in the system. It is impossible for change to affect one member of the system without causing a ripple effect of change among the others. The following clinical example may help illustrate the family system concept.

Clinical Example

Gordon is a 14-year-old high school freshman who reports having been depressed for about a year. Recently he has been experiencing suicidal ideation but without a realistic plan. During the assessment, Gordon mentions that he experiences a lot of anxiety at home, especially because his mother screams a lot at him and his siblings. He feels that his mother has high expectations of him and never seems to be satisfied with his efforts. He also explains that his mother and father do not seem to get along and seldom go anywhere together. He also hears his mother frequently yelling at his father. He tends to spend most of his time in his room, isolating himself.

In this clinical example, Gordon would be identified as the patient, and the focus would be on his suicidal ideation. From a family systems' view, the family would be the "identified patient," and changing Gordon's mood would require a change in the family system. If his mother understands how her behavior (screaming, yelling) causes Gordon to feel anxious and depressed, then she can make it a point of learning new ways of communicating with her husband and children. In addition, when Gordon's parents understand the effect their fighting has on the children, they can seek marital counseling. In time, as Gordon's parents change their ways of interacting, Gordon's symptoms are likely to be ameliorated. The changes made by the parents would also have a positive effect on the other children in the home.

The family systems approach provides a solid framework for understanding how families function and how to support their change. Most importantly, the systems view deemphasizes blaming the family's problems on a given family member, particularly a child whose "acting out" behavior may be a natural reaction to a distressing set of circumstances. With accurate identification of the process that sustains painful or stressful conditions in the family, positive changes can lead to

---

BOX 11.1   Family Systems Definitions

Parentification is the process of role reversal whereby a child takes on adult responsibilities within the family. Parentification takes many forms: (1) the child is obliged to act as parent to his or her *own* parent (e.g., helping a drunk mother get into bed), (2) the child or adolescent takes on the role of a confidant or mediator for (or between) the parents (occurs frequently when parents are divorced), and (3) the child is coerced into taking on an adult role (e.g., cases of incest).

Scapegoat refers to a member of the family, usually the identified patient, who is blamed for the conflict in the family. Family members focus on trying to "fix" the identified individual instead of dealing with and resolving the real issues.

Enmeshed refers to a family structure that resists the demands for change. For example, attempts on the part of one member to change, eliciting immediate resistance from other family members. In addition, individual boundaries are not respected (e.g., newly married couple expected to go on family vacation with parents).

Disengaged refers to a family structure where members are distant and disconnected. Family relationships tend to be chaotic, and parental authority is relatively absent. Boundaries tend to be excessively rigid, meaning that the behavior of one family member does not affect other members (i.e., "don't call me if you end up in jail").

Triangulation occurs when there is a conflict between two family members and they attempt to involve a third person who is asked to take a side. For example, conflicted parents may each attempt to garner their child's favor, sympathy, or support.

---

a decrease in the distress experienced by family members. For more information on the family systems framework, see the family systems definitions listed in Box 11.1.

EFFECTS OF MENTAL DISORDERS ON THE FAMILY

Caring for an ill family member is stressful, but the diagnosis of a mental disorder is particularly disturbing for the family. The diagnosis of a mental disorder in a family member can elicit feelings of guilt over possible genetic transmission of the disease to the ill family member by parents, concern over the prognosis and course of the disease, and worry among other family members that they might become mentally ill. The stigma of mental illness leads to shame or embarrassment about how others might view the family. In some cases, parents or spouses are blamed for the onset and continuation of their family member's mental illness. Children of a parent suffering from mental illness may fear becoming "contaminated" by the parent's mental disorder (Van Der Sanders et al., 2015).

Living with someone with a mental disorder has a noticeable influence on social burden and psychological distress among family members. Families must deal with various grief issues, as well as feelings of confusion, anxiety, and bewilderment. There are moments of optimism and hope intermixed with waves of suffering. Overall, the family members will continuously worry about their ill loved one and their situation. There are numerous emotions that overwhelm many families—fear because they do not know what is happening, what will come, or when an episode might repeat itself. Anger, rage, frustration, and sadness are other common emotions. One way in which families may respond to their emotions is keeping the 'secret,' or not talking to anyone about the illness, not even to their own family. This avoidance behavior may reinforce feelings of social isolation due to the fear of rejection by friends, acquaintances, and work relationships (Acero et al., 2017).

In cases of major depression, anxiety, and psychotic disorders, family challenges include monitoring for changes in the patient's health status and needing to protect the patient from serious physical self-harm such as suicidal threats or actions (Miller, 2017). As a result, the family member with a mental illness might exhibit feelings of guilt about the difficulties caused to the family or resignation and hopelessness about the prognosis of the disorder (Gracio et al., 2016; Tsiouri et al., 2015). The family must deal with the ill member's behavior as well as with agencies and institutions available to assist the family member. Law enforcement agencies, courts, social service agencies, schools, hospitals, clinics, and churches are among the many agencies having differing rules and procedures with which the family must negotiate. These agencies might be consulted in the process of obtaining needed care, or contacts might be made as a result of dangerous behavior related to the family member's mental disorder. For example, the family member who is paranoid might believe that a neighbor is planning to harm him or her and consequently might make a threat against the neighbor. This action would bring the family into contact with the local law enforcement agency and the courts. If the family member is committed for treatment, mental health agencies and hospitals might become involved in the person's care. Issues that might surface as a result of a family member's mental disorder could include the following:

- Medication usage—presence and treatment of side effects of medication
- Lack of energy to complete activities of daily living
- Social isolation, avoidance of contact with others
- Acting-out behaviors, particularly threatening or paranoid behavior
- Mood swings
- Denial of disorder, lack of appropriate reasoning or judgment
- Inappropriate or incomprehensible communication
- Persistence of dangerous behavior (e.g., drug or alcohol abuse)
- Manipulation of others to achieve desired goals

When an individual is diagnosed with a mental disorder, there is almost always a change in family functioning. Children who grow up with a seriously mentally ill parent may experience a variety of role changes within the family system. They may take on major responsibilities in order for the family to function, especially if parents are unable to fulfill the children's basic needs. These children may keep silent or seek out support from other adults in their surroundings as their school performance is affected or the parent loses his job. As these children become adults, they may suffer from relational issues or develop a mental illness themselves (Kàllquist & Salzman-Erikson, 2019). Thus, the future of both the individual and the family is potentially jeopardized.

The diagnosis of a mental illness can break a family apart—for example, when a spouse can no longer live with and subject children to an alcoholic or abusive partner—or it can bring family members together. There is a higher probability of divorce in families impacted by serious mental disorders. Divorce has significant negative effects on the mental, social, and economic functioning of all family members, particularly the short- and long-term impact on children (Mojtabai et al., 2017). Kay Redfield Jamison, a professor of psychiatry who also has manic-depressive illness, spoke of her mother in her autobiography (1995) in the following terms: "She could not have known how difficult it would be to deal with madness: had no preparation for what to do with madness—none of us did—but, consistent with her ability to love and her native will, she handled it with empathy and intelligence" (p. 9).

? CRITICAL THINKING QUESTION

2. If the family of a child diagnosed with a mental illness is told that the disorder has a biologic-genetic component, what effect is that statement likely to have on the thoughts and feelings of the child's parents and siblings?

FAMILY REACTIONS TO PSYCHIATRIC TREATMENT AND HOSPITALIZATION

Many family members report feeling little or no support from mental health professionals related to their caregiving burden (Gracio et al., 2016). They feel excluded from the treatment process, due in large part to privacy regulations or medical confidentiality (Van Der Sanders et al., 2015). These concerns are exaggerated when the family member with a diagnosable mental disorder is admitted to a psychiatric facility. The immediate family might not want others to know about the hospitalization, fearing a negative reaction from extended family and friends. The family might be exhausted because of difficulty coping with the patient's bizarre behavior or concern about the safety of all family members.

When the individual must be involuntarily committed to a facility, conflicting emotions can arise on the part of the family. Families are known to initially experience alleviation from stress when the patient is first hospitalized, relieved that the patient is finally in the care of competent professionals. Unfortunately, this emotional reprieve during periods of hospitalization is often only a brief interlude, followed by renewed struggles once the patient is released. Families may experience anxiety and guilt, especially in scenarios where the patient was admitted into the hospital without giving their consent. In cases where the patient refuses admission to an inpatient facility, conflict may emerge in the family system. The seriousness of the patient's mental illness and the acuity of care provided by family members contribute to family burnout. Strained relations between patients and families are a common occurrence as the mental illness negatively alters the relationship between loved ones. For many families, there is the underlying fear in how to relate to the patient without inciting unpredictable or volatile reactions (Miller, 2017).

Admission will be helpful to the entire family if the treatment provided meets the current safety and security needs of the patient and family. Close family members need emotional support due to feeling overwhelmed and exhausted. To help meet their need for support, families need a working relationship with health professionals for the duration of the hospital admission. Families' relationship with staff should consist of genuine concern for their well-being and regular communication with them. In addition, family members' knowledge and presence should be acknowledged and appreciated by all health professionals. Miller (2017) reported that families desire recognition from health professionals for their caregiving role and for having valuable information to share. During hospitalization, family intervention and inclusion is vitally important, involving the collaboration of a range of health care professionals.

Family therapy, in particular, should only be carried out by a professional who has been prepared at the master's or doctoral level because of the complexity of the issues and the skills needed to carry out the treatment. Professionals who are qualified for family therapy are social workers, marriage and family therapists, psychologists, and advanced practice psychiatric nurses. Family therapy is beyond the scope of practice of the baccalaureate-prepared nurse (Maybery et al., 2014).

In the course of family therapy, abuse or assault may be discovered in the family by the health care team. Abused members might experience relief that the *secret* has finally been revealed, but might also experience anger, rejection, or humiliation from exposure of abuse. Fear about the future, fear of retribution, or fear of legal consequences of the abuse might be of concern to family members who have been victimized by another family member. Ensuring the safety of abused family members is necessary for them to confront the pain and suffering caused by the abuse. See Chapter 33 for further information.

NURSE RESPONSE TO PATIENTS AND FAMILIES SEEKING TREATMENT

As frontline mental health professionals, nurses are well positioned to connect with both patients and their families. Nurses have the opportunity to educate, advocate, and emotionally support distraught and overburdened families who are seeking help (Miller, 2017). When a family seeks treatment for any of the problems listed in Box 11.2 or for other problems,

> ### BOX 11.2 Reasons for a Family to Seek Treatment for Mental Health Issues
>
> - Situational crises, such as loss of job or divorce
> - Developmental crises, such as a child diagnosed with autism
> - Relationship problems and conflicts, such as abuse of one or more family members
> - Conflicts between families of origin and current family (family of marriage)
> - Addition of family members through remarriage, adoption, and foster care
> - Family conflicts over treatment
> - Custody conflicts and issues
> - Family exploitation of an ill family member
> - Family confrontation or conflict with caregivers
> - Acute or chronic mental disorder of a family member

the nurse must listen to all parties involved and acknowledge all points of view. The nurse should refrain from perceiving one family member or an entire family as problematic. The nurse and other caregivers must refrain from placing blame either directly or implicitly on an individual family member. The family is not the cause of the mental disorder, and the family member with a mental disorder diagnosis is not the cause of the family's problems (Power et al., 2015).

The family member diagnosed with a mental disorder may not be the sickest member of the family. The term "scapegoating" refers to the family process of identifying one member as the object of displaced conflict or criticism (Nichols, 2013). Often, the individual with the diagnosis is the one who is most sensitive to the disruptions in family life and most desirous of obtaining help to overcome the problem (Walsh, 2012). The nurse can ameliorate some of the scapegoating that might be occurring in a family by consulting directly with the patient and other family members during assessment and treatment. The nurse can offer positive reinforcement about the patient's willingness to engage in the treatment process. Even if the patient is only minimally cooperative with treatment, positive reinforcement can serve to improve the patient's cooperation and boost his or her self-esteem.

ABILITIES NEEDED IN WORKING WITH FAMILIES

The Psychiatric Nurses Association contends that nurses need specific skills and characteristics in order to work effectively with families, among their other roles (Maybery et al., 2014). Self-knowledge, spirituality, assessment skills, and communication skills allow the nurse to collaborate with patients, families, and caregivers and provide appropriate care and possible referrals.

Self-Knowledge

The nurse must recognize and accept his or her own values, beliefs, and biases related to the importance of families and their involvement in the care of their member with a mental disorder diagnosis. The nurse must also avoid allowing personal concerns or crises to interfere with the ability to care appropriately for patients and their families. To do this, the nurse must be aware of and acknowledge his or her own family history and appreciate that all families have strengths and needs (Walsh, 2012). The nurse must model adaptive self-care and stress management techniques, such as regular exercise, healthy eating, and strong support and nurturance from friends and family. Such self-care activities prepare the nurse to assist patients and families in learning similar healthy coping skills to manage their lives.

ASSESSMENT

Interactions among all family members are the raw material for problem solving by the family and nurse. The nurse must become the family's partner in assessment and decision making so that the family can own and be invested in recovery (Maybery et al., 2014). A family assessment guide (Box 11.3) can help the nurse obtain information about family strengths and the issues for which they seek assistance so that the nurse can focus on and address the family's needs. Individual and family strengths are the focus, rather than seeing the problems as deficits. This approach helps family members to see themselves as capable of change rather than suffering at the mercy of their situations and circumstances. Additionally, by better

understanding the importance of symptoms, the family learns valuable skills for managing future issues they might encounter.

Assessments include the following:

- Family characteristics in both the family of origin and the present family
- Developmental stage of the family at the present time
- Family's accomplishment of developmental and daily tasks
- Patient's and family's reasons for seeking treatment and reactions to care
- Effects of mental illness on family members and on the family as a whole
- Family strengths
- Family's understanding of the mental disorder
- Current interaction skills between family members
- Other aspects of the patient, family members, or significant others that might affect care

The nurse's observational skills are important when interacting with members of the family. The nurse should observe the behavior and words of all family members and consider how members relate to each other and to the nurse, rather than focusing on the actions of one individual (the patient) alone. The nurse must consider all available information, its relevance, and its impact before arriving at conclusions about a family. If conclusions are drawn too quickly and with too little information, solutions may be offered that are not likely to be effective; this might discourage the family from seeking help with family stress in the future.

Therapeutic Communication

Therapeutic interactions should be based on the nurse's understanding of the following: families are generally functioning as well as possible, in light of their available resources and abilities; families are capable of managing their problems with the guidance and support of caregivers; all families have strengths that can be utilized amid crises; placing blame does nothing to aid the family and serves only to validate the shame of the family as a whole; and family members act out of frustration or pain when they feel overwhelmed. Nurses should also remember that every interaction with a patient and family represents an opportunity to be therapeutic. Therapeutic interviewing skills include the ability to display respect for all family members and an ability to be nonjudgmental about the family members and the way in which they show their distress.

Specific therapeutic communication techniques used by the nurse vary depending on the stage of the relationship with family members. The most frequently used techniques include active listening, appropriate eye contact, expression of empathy and compassion, sensitivity to verbal and nonverbal cues, validating emotions, clarifying information, summarizing, and supporting the family's efforts. Chapter 8 presents more information concerning therapeutic communication.

Family Psychoeducation

Family psychoeducation refers to the components of treatment that involve educating the family about the nature, course, and treatment of the psychiatric illness (Tsiouri et al., 2015).

BOX 11.3   Family Assessment Guidelines: Possible Questions to Ask

Family Membership and Development
- "Tell me about the members of your immediate (nuclear) family, including ages and gender (male or female)."
- "What other relatives do you have? How are they involved with your immediate family?"

Family Strengths and Needs
- "What do you think is a strength in your family?"
- "What is something you would like to change about your family?"

Family Coping
- "Describe a problem that your family has dealt with successfully."
- "What helped you to deal with this problem successfully?"

Identification of Family Problem
- "What is your perception of the current family problem?"
- "How do you think the current problem should be resolved?"

Family Use of Resources
- "What resources or agencies have you used successfully in the past in dealing with this type of problem?"
- "What does your family do to stay healthy? What does your family do to treat or manage mental, emotional, and physical illness?"
- "What type of help would you like from me (the nurse) in resolving the current problem?"

However, it is not simply family education, per se. It also focuses on the development of problem-solving skills, communication and coping skills, and enhancement of social supports to manage the psychiatric symptoms. Family psychoeducation is considered crucial to the patient's recovery, based on the premise that as family members increase their understanding of the illness, family distress will be reduced and coping skills will be improved, resulting in improved outcomes for the patient. These interventions differ from traditional family therapy in that they do not assume dysfunction in the family.

Family psychoeducation is useful in building a framework around which family members can make sense of mental illness within their family system (Power et al., 2015). Brady, Kangas, and McGill (2017) reported on the importance of educating family members on the negative effects of expressed emotions (EE), which are unsupportive, critical comments. As family interaction is improved through education, caregiver burden is alleviated and patient recovery is promoted (Kolostoumpis et al., 2015).

Successful psychoeducation has also been found to be effective via the Internet. Psychoeducational programs that utilize Internet forums offer users the opportunity to be open and honest about their struggles while attaining important support and education from others. Widemalm and Hjarthag (2015) have reported on the severe feelings of loneliness expressed by children with parents suffering from mental illness. In order to hide the shame related to having a mentally ill parent, these children turned to an Internet forum to seek advice and strategies for dealing with difficult and challenging situations. The anonymity of the Internet allowed these children to express their concerns and lessen their feelings of alienation, loneliness, and social isolation.

Family psychoeducation is similar to the rehabilitation programs that patients and family members go through in medical settings after a family member experiences a stroke or heart attack. Such programs not only speed recovery from acute episodes of the disorder but also enable the patient and family to manage the acute symptoms more effectively, with fewer relapses and rehospitalizations (Brady et al., 2017).

The National Alliance on Mental Illness (NAMI) sponsors the most widely used family psychoeducation intervention, the Family-to-Family (FTF) program. This program consists of a structured curriculum led by trained peers. Family members learn about mental illness, treatment options, self-care, advocacy skills, etc. By attending sessions, family members also have the opportunity to give and receive emotional support and to develop insights into their own experiences around mental illness (Schiffman et al., 2015).

Spirituality

Historically, the physical, psychological, and spiritual have been viewed as interconnected. However, the influence of family members' spiritual and religious beliefs on their illness experience has been one of the areas most neglected by health care professionals. Azman and associates (2017) reported that spiritual and religious approaches are widely used as coping mechanisms to deal with a caregiver's stressful life.

Many family members interpret mental illness as (1) a moral weakness, (2) punishment from a higher being or God, or (3) possession by evil spirits. Caregivers trust in God and pray, believing that God will heal their mentally ill loved one someday. The *Diagnostic and Statistical Manual of Mental Disorders* (DSM-5) recognizes the importance of religious and spiritual assessment and treatment. Specifically, the category of religious or spiritual problems is cited when the focus of clinical attention includes distressing experiences that involve loss or questions of faith and the questioning of spiritual values (American Psychiatric Association [APA], 2013).

Because of their close and frequent contact with patients and families, nurses are in a unique position to create a healing environment for family members to share their stories of illness and suffering, thereby providing a powerful validation of their profound human experience. Nurses create a space within which family members can explore their spirituality through the gift of listening, maintaining curiosity, and inviting reflection on spiritual and religious beliefs. As family members describe their suffering, give meaning to their suffering, wonder about the spiritual nature of their suffering, and share their beliefs about their illness experience, hope and healing become possible. The nurse must be careful to not impose their beliefs and values on the family members. Sensitivity to caregivers' spiritual and religious values, such as mutual love and faith in a higher power, reflects understanding of their burden of care, as well as their attempts to make sense of a painful journey (Damianakis et al., 2018).

The nurse can encourage contact with spiritual resources, such as a minister, priest, or rabbi, when needed or desired by the patient or family. If a family's spiritual beliefs conflict with the prescribed treatment, the nurse should accommodate the beliefs whenever possible. For example, some patients and families are wary of using medication to alter mental function and prefer to rely on prayer as a treatment. However, when a patient is experiencing hallucinations, a reduction in symptoms is more likely to occur with the aid of antipsychotic medication. Nursing care that respects the values and beliefs of the family is more likely to be received and appreciated, in light of the difficult decisions family members face. For example, as the nurse encourages the use of prayer because it is a valued and important component of a family's lifestyle, the family will be more likely to discuss the advantages and disadvantages of medication geared to reduce symptoms.

Collaboration

The nurse must collaborate with patients, families, and colleagues in providing care and helping families reach their goals. Nurses must collaborate with multidisciplinary teams and agencies to advocate for patients and achieve positive family outcomes. Dojeiji, Byszewski, and Wood (2015) have identified three essential dimensions of relationships between involved partners for effective collaboration: (1) shared knowledge, (2) shared goals, and (3) mutual respect for one another's contributions.

Family members have a need for health care professionals to understand how the illness affects the family as a whole.

In addition, family members have a need to share their concerns and stories, providing a unique contribution in their understanding of patient symptoms, behavioral changes, and family challenges. Often, family members express concern that they are not involved in the ways they wish, such as being informed and invited to participate in consultations and meetings with the health care team. Professionals primarily cite privacy laws as the reason why families are not provided with information or invited to be part of discussions related to the patient. Miller (2017) reported that family members experience inconsistencies in how health care professions understand and implement privacy laws, some more forthcoming in releasing information than others. Therefore, nurses should be educated on confidentiality and advocates for the rights of concerned, caring family members.

As much as possible, family members should participate as full collaborators in the planning, delivery, and evaluation of patient care. In addition, to collaborate successfully with all stakeholders in providing comprehensive mental health care, nurses need to recognize their skills, acknowledge the contributions of other team members in problem identification and problem solving, be knowledgeable about resources, and work cooperatively with all involved to attain quality mental health care for the patient and family.

Referrals and Family Support

Referrals are helpful when working with families who have complex needs. The nurse must have the knowledge and skills to support families as they enter the health care system to ensure that they can receive the assistance they require for their specific issues. The nurse should be knowledgeable about the resources to which he or she refers families. The referral is most effective when the patient and family know where to go, whom to meet, the reason for the referral, and what to expect when they get there. If the nurse merely gives the patient and family the name and address of a facility or support person, the probability that the patient and family will follow up is low. The family might not know how to get to the location, might be afraid that the treatment will be harmful or costly, or might fear that the family member will be taken away from them and hospitalized against their wishes. The extra effort made by the nurse to personalize and individualize a referral pays dividends in better continuity of care and better mental health for the entire family.

APPLICATION OF THE NURSING PROCESS TO THE FAMILY

Assessment

The assessment process begins within the context of the nurse-patient-family relationship. Assessment provides the nurse, patient, and family an opportunity to discuss each family member's perspective of how well family members are functioning. Questions might be asked when the patient and the family are together, when only some family members are present without the patient, or when only the patient is

available. Obtaining the viewpoint of as many family members as possible greatly enhances treatment.

Patients who seek treatment might live with their intact family of origin, a parent who has remarried, adoptive parents, foster parents, other relatives, a spouse or significant other, by themselves, or in a residential facility. The nurse must consider living arrangements and the persons supporting the patient who are involved in his or her treatment. Current problems might be an extension of problems that began with the original family or might represent new issues not related to the family of origin.

An assessment should also consider other physical and mental health issues within the family that occur as members cope with a chronic mental disorder. Family members may find themselves losing sleep, not eating healthy meals, and becoming more susceptible to the effects of increased anxiety. Possible symptoms may include headaches, indigestion, ulcers, hypertension, and other stress-related physical problems.

A family assessment guideline can help the nurse think of the family as a system when conducting a family assessment. Examples of questions that the nurse might wish to ask are listed in Box 11.3. These questions are designed as triggers to help the family tell their story, rather than responding to standardized questions that might not reflect the family's issues and concerns. Through nurse-guided discussions, families can be actively engaged in decision making regarding health priorities.

Nursing Diagnosis

Based on the family assessment, the nurse develops priority nursing diagnoses from those approved by the NANDA International or the International Council of Nurses (ICN). Examples of some typical diagnoses are family coping impairment, family process alteration, and risk for caregiver role strain (ICN, 2016). These nursing diagnoses help define the problems that the family is facing, providing a foundation for outcome identification. Although nursing diagnoses are generally stated in terms of deficits, the assessment should include a determination of patient and family strengths that can be used to help overcome deficits or prevent risks for deficits becoming actual patient problems.

Outcome Identification

The nurse works with patients and their families to establish treatment goals based on the family assessment. These goals might be individual goals for a specific family member, goals for the family as a whole, or both. The outcomes or goals identified must be specific, measurable, and achievable within an explicit time frame and under the control of the individual family member. When establishing goals with highly distressed families, the nurse must consider how other agencies should be involved in the treatment process. Agency contact might focus on economic issues, protection for one or more family members, reporting of abuse to a state agency, contacts with police, or actions of a court order.

Planning and Implementation

The skills needed for therapeutic interactions have already been specified earlier in this chapter. Other interventions that the nurse might use when working with patients and their families individually and in groups are listed in the box titled Key Nursing Interventions for Working With Families. Through the process of understanding the patient's and family's perspectives concerning the stresses of living with a

KEY NURSING INTERVENTIONS

For Working With Families

- Provide respect, empathy, support, and acceptance to patients and families.
- Advocate for patients and families in their interactions with other providers, institutions, and organizations.
- Help the family build the patient's self-esteem while being realistic in their expectations of the patient, themselves, and others.
- Facilitate the resolution of normal developmental crises of individuals and families.
- Help families use more adaptive coping skills, facilitating future problem solving.
- Provide referrals to support groups and resources for families who are experiencing normal developmental issues of family life, as well as families dealing with more serious crises.
- Empower families by teaching problem solving, limit setting, and conflict resolution skills.
- Help families validate, clarify, negotiate, and communicate feelings appropriately.
- Assist families in recognizing and coping with abuse issues to maintain safety of all family members.
- Offer feedback to patients and families concerning their progress in dealing with their problems.
- Negotiate role flexibility between patients and their families in response to family needs.
- Be honest with patients and families if abuse must be reported.
- Teach communication and parenting skills.
- Teach families about the causes, manifestations, and treatment of mental disorders.
- Teach families about the desired effects and side effects of medications and symptoms to report to professionals to prevent or minimize relapse.
- Teach and model deescalation techniques.
- Include the patient and family in goal setting and treatment planning.
- Teach and encourage family members to practice self-care.

mental disorder, the nurse can develop interventions that help all parties involved.

Evaluation

Outcomes of working with patients and their families can be measured by determining whether treatment goals have been met and whether patients and families have developed effective solutions. Periodically throughout treatment, the nurse and family must evaluate progress toward the resolution of issues defined by the nurse, patient, and family. When appropriate, the nurse can assist patients and families in reformulating goals and creating posttreatment goals toward which the family can work after the patient's discharge from an inpatient unit or outpatient program. Ongoing nursing evaluation of patient progress and outcome achievement is essential for successful treatment and represents one of the most important phases of the nursing process.

Resources Available to Families

The nurse can assist families in finding helpful resources and arranging for appropriate services. These services might include medical services, social welfare agencies, churches, emergency food services, voluntary agencies, support groups, community health services, and psychiatric home care services. Resources for families include the following:
- Al-Anon/Alateen: http://www.al-anon.org
- Alcoholics Anonymous: http://www.aa.org
- Families Anonymous: http://www.familiesanonymous.org
- Narcotics Anonymous: http://www.na.org
- NAMI and NAMI-CAN (Child/Adolescent Network): http://www.nami.org
- Parents Anonymous: http://www.parentsanonymous.org
- Alzheimer's Association: http://www.alz.org
- Mental Health America: http://www.nmha.org

? CRITICAL THINKING QUESTION

3. What family-oriented approaches would you use with a family that is having difficulty coping with the increasing suicidality of a severely depressed member?

STUDY NOTES

1. Nurses who work with families see many types of contemporary families and should respect their diversity and resilience.
2. Difficulties in accomplishing family tasks and developmental stages reflect the complexities and issues of modern family life.
3. The family of origin influences the communication skills, self-esteem, and coping skills that a person brings to the current family. However, healthy problem-solving and interaction skills can be developed with the assistance of health care professionals and community resources.

4. Having a family member with a mental disorder is stressful and inevitably changes the dynamics within a family.
5. The nursing process with families requires that the nurse possess self-knowledge; assessment, therapeutic, communication, spiritual, and collaboration skills; and skills regarding referrals and family support to help family members cope with the diagnosis of a mental disorder.
6. The nurse must collaborate with the family to assess the function of the family and refer the family to the most appropriate resource for assistance.

REFERENCES

Acero, A., Cano-Proust, A., Castellanos, G., Martin-Lanas, R., & Canga-Armayor, A. (2017). Family identity and severe mental illness: A thematic synthesis of qualitative studies. *European Journal of Social Psychology, 47*, 611–627. https://doi.org/10.1002/ejsp.2240.

American Psychiatric Association. (2013). Diagnostic and Statistical Manual of Mental Disorders: *DSM-5* (5th ed.). Washington: American Psychiatric Association.

Azman, A., Singh, P., & Sulaiman, J. (2017). Caregiver coping with the mentally ill: A qualitative study. *Journal of Mental Health, 26*(2), 98–103. https://doi.org/10.3109/09638237.2015.1124395.

Brady, P., Kangas, M., & McGill, K. (2017). "Family matters": A systematic review of the evidence for family psychoeducation for major depressive disorder. *Journal of Marital and Family Therapy, 43*(2), 245–263. https://doi.org/10.1111/jmft.12204.

Damianakis, T., Wilson, K., & Marziali, E. (2018). Family caregiver support groups: Spiritual reflections' impact on stress management. *Aging & Mental Health, 22*(1), 70–76. https://doi.org/10.1080/13607863.2016.1231169.

Dojeiji, S., Byszewski, S., & Wood, T. (2015). Development and pilot testing the Family Conference Rating Scale: A tool aimed to assess interprofessional patient-centered communication and collaboration competencies. *Journal of Interprofessional Care, 29*(5), 415–420. https://doi.org/10.3109/13561820.2015.1039116.

Gracio, J., Goncalves-Periera, M., & Leff, J. (2016). What do we know about family interventions for psychosis at the process level? A systematic review. *Family Process, 55*(1), 79–90. https://doi.org/10.1111/famp.12155.

International Council of Nurses (ICN). (2016). *CCC-ICNP Equivalency Table for Nursing Diagnoses*. Switzerland: Geneva.

Jamison, K. R. (1995). *An Unquiet Mind*. New York: Vintage.

Kàllquist, A., & Salzman-Erikson, M. (2019). Experiences of having a parent with serious mental disorder: An interpretive meta-synthesis of qualitative literature. *Journal of Child and Family Studies, 28*, 2056–2068. https://doi.org/10.1007/s10826-019-01438-0.

Kolostoumpis, D., et al. (2015). Effectiveness of relatives' psychoeducation on family outcomes in bipolar disorder. *International Journal of Mental Health, 44*, 290–302. https://www.tandfonline.com/doi/full/10.1080/00207411.2015.1076292.

Marshall, A., et al. (2010). Beliefs, suffering, and healing: A clinical practice model for families experiencing mental illness. *Perspectives in Psychiatric Care, 46*(3), 197–208. https://doi.org/10.1111/j.1744-6163.2010.00259.x.

Maybery, D., et al. (2014). Professional differences in family focused practice in the adult mental health system. *Family Process, 53*(4), 608–617. https://doi.org/10.1111/famp.12082.

McGoldrick, M., & Shibusawa, T. (2012). The Family Life Cycle. In F. Walsh (Ed.), *Normal family processes* (3rd ed., pp. 375–398). New York: Guilford.

Miller, D. (2017). Inpatient psychiatric care: Families expectations and perceptions of support received from health professionals. *Perspectives in Psychiatric Care, 53*, 350–356. https://doi.org/10.1111/ppc.12168.

Mojtabai, R., Stuart, E., Hwang, I., Eaton, W., Sampson, N., & Kessler, R. (2017). Long-term effects of mental disorders on marital outcomes in the National Comorbidity Survey ten-year follow-up. *Social Psychiatry and Psychiatric Epidemiology, 52*, 1217–1226. https://doi.org/10.1007/s00127-017-1373-1.

Nichols, M. N. (2013). *Family Therapy: Concepts and Methods* (10th ed.). Boston: Allyn & Bacon.

Power, J., et al. (2015). Working in a family therapy setting with families where a parent has a mental illness: Practice dilemmas and strategies. *Journal of Family Therapy, 37*, 546–562. https://doi.org/10.1111/1467-6427.12052.

Reupert, A., et al. (2015). Place of family in recovery models for those with a mental illness. *International Journal of Mental Health Nursing, 24*, 495–506. https://doi.org/10.1111/inm.12146.

Schiffman, J., et al. (2015). Outcomes of a family peer educational program for families of youth and adults with mental illness. *International Journal of Mental Health, 44*, 303–315. https://doi.org/10.1080/00207411.2015.1076293.

Tsiouri, I., et al. (2015). Does long-term group psychoeducation of parents of individuals with schizophrenia help the family as a system: A quasi-experimental study. *International Journal of Mental Health, 44*, 316–331. https://doi.org/10.1080/00207411.2015.1076294.

Van Der Sanders, R., et al. (2015). Stigma by association among family members of people with a mental illness: A qualitative analysis. *Journal of Community & Applied Social Psychology, 25*, 400–417. https://doi.org/10.1007/s00127-016-1256-x.

Walsh, F. (2012). The New Normal: Diversity and Complexity in 21st-Century Families. In F. Walsh (Ed.), *Normal family processes* (4th ed., pp. 2–27). New York: Guilford.

Widemalm, M., & Hjarthag, F. (2015). The forum as a friend: Parental mental illness and communication on an open forum. *Social Psychiatry and Psychiatric Epidemiology, 50*, 1601–1607. https://doi.org/10.1007/s00127-015-1036-z.

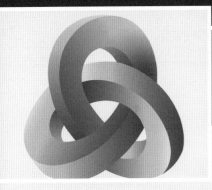

12

Introduction to Psychotropic Drugs

Norman L. Keltner and Peter C. Kowalski

Above all, do no harm.

Hippocrates

http://evolve.elsevier.com/Keltner

LEARNING OBJECTIVES

- Define the role of psychopharmacology in psychotherapeutic management.
- Identify the nurse's responsibilities in administering psychotropic drugs.
- Describe pharmacokinetic and pharmacodynamic processes as they relate to clinical practice.
- Describe the function and inactivation of neurotransmitters.

- Discuss the function of the blood-brain barrier and the significance of lipid solubility.
- State the benefits of teaching patients about psychotropic drugs.
- Describe common reasons why psychiatric patients might not comply with prescribed drug regimens.

PRINCIPLES

Psychopharmacology is the understanding and application of medications to improve and sustain the healthy functioning of the nervous system with the intent to recover, remit, or stabilize mental illness.

From the standpoint of the provider, principles that should guide such treatment include the following:

Treat the person, not the label.

Do your homework.

Know your medications.

Be reasonable.

Solve problems and have an adaptive attitude.

Regarding the first principle, it is essential to understand the person considering treatment via psychopharmacology. One must evaluate that person's request for relief of specific symptoms for specific reasons. What are they asking for? Is a person requesting a medication to relieve depression or anxiety, to improve focus and concentration, to help cope with trauma, to reduce auditory hallucinations, or because someone else wants him to? What is this person's personality like, what temperament does he possess, and what circumstances is he living in that may be causing stress or impairment?

On the second principle, do a thorough pharmacologic history of the person being considered for treatment. Take inventory of past medications used, the amounts prescribed and for how long, the responses, either favorable or <u>adverse</u>, and also the responses of close family members treated for similar conditions.

Regarding the third principle, know your medications. Read the product monograph and literature about the agent. Know the pharmacokinetics and the pharmacodynamics of the psychotropic. Know how it may potentially interact with the body and with other agents that may be co-administered. Listen to pharmaceutical representatives with rational skepticism.

Concerning the fourth principle, establish reasonable expectations for a medication intervention, with tangible goals that can be assessed by the provider and the patient or the patient's family. Articulate a short set of mutually agreed-upon goals or therapeutic targets, to be achieved within a projected period of medication exposure. This involves predictions of likely trajectories of conditions, whether treated or not, based on the natural history of a disorder. Document these therapeutic goals to review in future visits. Ask the patient for their short list of favorable and unfavorable effects to guide medication selection.

Lastly, expect detours and complications, as the work of psychopharmacology necessarily involves limited data and no biomarkers to enhance predictable outcomes. Anticipate with the patient the realities of this kind of work and the need to communicate promptly and effectively should problems arise. Learn from failed medication trials and unintended missteps and adverse effects, for they may point to the right understanding of underlying conditions and solutions in resolving them.

 NORM'S NOTES Take a good look at this chapter. If you read it thoroughly, it will help you to really understand psychotropic drugs. If you don't understand such basics as pharmacokinetics and pharmacodynamics, you will have to memorize each drug. You shouldn't have to do that! You have often heard that nurses need to know the reason for some treatment, some side effect, or some adverse response. The basics found in this chapter form the foundation for understanding the actions of a drug. So take your time—Norm's key to learning important information is *repetition, repetition, repetition.*

NURSING RESPONSIBILITIES

Psychopharmacology is the second component of the psychotherapeutic management model (see Chapter 1 to review this model). Box 12.1 summarizes significant points during the evolution of psychopharmacology. The effectiveness of treatment with antipsychotic, antidepressant, antimanic, and antianxiety drugs has been well established. These drugs have enabled millions of individuals to live increasingly satisfying and productive lives. The least restrictive alternative or environment—a concept that reflects the community mental health effort to allow individuals to live their lives in as unrestrictive an atmosphere as possible—has largely evolved as a result of the impact of these drugs.

The nurse must understand key dimensions of psychotropic drug use. Because nursing provides 24-hour care, the nurse is responsible for assessing drug side effects, evaluating desired effects, and applying preventive care to reduce potential problems. Additionally, the nurse usually makes decisions concerning as-needed (prn) medications.

Unit III provides a discussion of pharmacologic effects (desired effects), pharmacokinetics administration, side effects (undesired effects), and drug interactions. Chapter 34 discusses the use of psychotropic drugs in children and adolescents. Understanding psychopharmacology involves more than memorizing facts. However, it should be noted that *memorization* is not a dirty word. Some basics of pharmacology must be memorized, but the nurse who tries to get by on memorization alone *is a medication error waiting to happen.* Because of our strong belief in the importance of nurses understanding the basics of psychopharmacology, we review the following important concepts:

- Pharmacokinetics
- Pharmacodynamics
- Drug-drug interactions
- Blood-brain barrier
- Neurons and neurotransmitters
- Receptors

This chapter concludes with a few general strategies for helping patients and families understand important

BOX 12.1   Significant Points in the History of Psychotropic Drugs: 1949–2010

1949	Lithium is "discovered" in Australia.
1951	Chlorpromazine, the first antipsychotic, is "discovered" in France.
1952	Monoamine oxidase inhibitors are "discovered" when a tuberculosis drug is found to improve mood.
1958	Tricyclic antidepressants article is published in the *American Journal of Psychiatry.*
1960	Harris publishes the first article on the effectiveness of benzodiazepines in the *Journal of the American Medical Association.*
1980s	A new class of antidepressants, selective serotonin reuptake inhibitors (SSRIs), is developed. The first SSRI marketed is fluoxetine (Prozac).
1990s	Clozapine (Clozaril), the first truly new antipsychotic agent in 40 years, is released in the United States. Risperidone (Risperdal), olanzapine (Zyprexa), quetiapine (Seroquel), ziprasidone (Geodon), and aripiprazole (Abilify) follow over the next decade.
2000s	Drugs used to treat patients with Alzheimer disease are widely available.
2010s	In some years, the top-selling drug of any kind is Abilify (aripiprazole), and a top-10 selling drug is Cymbalta (duloxetine).

considerations in regard to psychotropic drug use. Drug-specific patient teaching content is presented in each chapter.

Most psychoactive drugs are administered orally, which means that they are absorbed either by oral mucosa or by gastrointestinal (GI) mucosa in the small intestine. When absorbed orally, they directly enter the systemic circulation. In the latter case, they enter the trans-hepatic portal system and undergo changes to their chemical structure that makes them easier for the body to excrete, a passage termed "first-pass metabolism." Enteric and liver enzymes convert drugs into metabolites that can be excreted into bile or by the kidneys. A considerable amount of the converted drug will be eliminated by this time. The rest will pass into the systemic circulation and then cross another barrier to reach the central nervous system (CNS), the "blood-brain barrier" or BBB. The BBB is a semipermeable barrier composed of endothelial cells that line the blood vessels vascularizing the CNS. It tightly regulates the transport of molecules and ions between the blood and the brain (Daneman & Prat, 2015). After passing the BBB, a psychoactive drug enters the CNS extracellular fluid and is exposed to receptors on the nerve cell's surface to perform regulation of that receptor. Some psychoactive agents may produce immediate responses, like benzodiazepines inducing antianxiety and sedative effects; others may induce cellular changes and responses over a much longer period, like antidepressants and antipsychotics. Their site of action generally occurs at the gap junction or "synapse" between nerve cells, a space that adjoins two or more neurons in which chemical signals pass from cell to cell via neurotransmitters or chemical messengers.

CRITICAL THINKING QUESTION

1. Some nurses might have little knowledge about some of the drugs they administer. Do you consider this unethical, unprofessional, unsafe, or simply a reality of the nursing profession? Because no one can know every drug, what basic information should a nurse know before giving a medication?

PHARMACOKINETICS: WHAT THE BODY DOES TO THE DRUG

Pharmacokinetics is defined as the effects that the body has on a drug. The four aspects of pharmacokinetics are the following:

- *Absorption*—getting the drug into the bloodstream
- *Distribution*—getting the drug from the bloodstream to the tissues and organs
- *Metabolism*—breaking the drug down into an inactive and typically water-soluble form
- *Excretion*—getting the drug out of the body

Absorption

Drugs taken orally must get out of the GI tract and into the bloodstream to have an effect. For a drug to get out of the GI tract, the drug molecule must pass through the stomach or small intestinal wall into blood vessels. Molecules pass through cell membranes (composed of a phospholipid bilayer) in the following three ways:

1. Small molecules can fit through pores or channels in the membrane.
2. Some drug molecules have special transport systems to ferry them through the membrane.
3. Lipid-soluble drugs (most drugs are lipophilic) can pass through the phospholipid membranes.

Only a certain percentage of an oral drug reaches the systemic circulation, whereas 100% of a drug given intravenously reaches the systemic circulation. The percentage of an oral drug that reaches the systemic circulation is a drug's *bioavailability*. Bioavailability is only a fraction of the dose for many drugs given orally because of incomplete absorption and first-pass metabolism. (First-pass metabolism is the enzymatic breakdown of drugs before they reach systemic circulation.) First-pass metabolism occurs during passage through the gut wall and in a presystemic hepatic exposure. This exposure occurs because the capillaries in the GI tract do not behave as do most capillaries (i.e., dumping into venules), but instead connect with hepatic portal veins, shunting drugs directly from the GI tract to the liver before they reach the general circulation. Some drugs are substantially "used up" in this manner. For example, buspirone (BuSpar), an antianxiety drug, has a bioavailability of 1% to 4%, which means that most of this drug is metabolized before it gets into general circulation. If the first pass through the liver could be eliminated for buspirone by some mechanism, its dose would have to be dramatically reduced.

Drugs with a high first-pass metabolism must be significantly reduced in dose level if given intramuscularly or intravenously.

Distribution

Distribution is the process of the body getting the drug out of the bloodstream and into tissues and organs. If a psychotropic drug cannot leave the bloodstream, it cannot have a therapeutic effect. Lipid-soluble molecules can penetrate capillary membranes as easily as they can penetrate other cell membranes. However, water-soluble (or polar) molecules also leave the circulation because of significant gaps between the cells of the capillary wall. Essentially, because molecules are innately active, water-soluble molecules bounce around inside the capillary until they hit a gap and move into the extracellular fluid. Another distribution issue involves protein binding. Most drugs bind to plasma proteins (mostly albumin) to some degree.

Familiar Psychotropic Drugs	Drug Protein Binding (%)
Sertraline (Zoloft)	99
Diazepam (Valium)	98
Fluoxetine (Prozac)	95
Lorazepam (Ativan)	92
Escitalopram (Lexapro)	55
Venlafaxine (Effexor)	23

Protein binding is important because molecules that are bound to proteins cannot leave the circulation—that is, the protein is simply too large to pass through the gaps in the capillary wall. Protein-bound drugs do not have a pharmacologic effect, cannot be metabolized, and cannot be excreted. Specifically, diazepam (Valium, with 98% protein binding), which has a calming (or anxiolytic) effect, produces its results because of the 2% or so of active drug. Taking diazepam with another drug that can reduce its protein binding to 96% would literally double its effect. Both desired and undesired effects of highly protein-bound drugs result from the activity of the relatively few free drug molecules in circulation. Drug combinations that compete for protein binding sites have the potential of causing significant increases in levels of the free or active drug.

Metabolism

Most drugs must be metabolized to an inactive and water-soluble form to be excreted from the system. Certain conditions (e.g., liver disease, kidney disease) or drug combinations that inhibit metabolism can lead to significant or even deadly results.

Metabolism is the process whereby the body breaks down a drug molecule. Most drugs are metabolized to inactive and water-soluble states in preparation for excretion from the body in the urine. It is important to note that not all drugs are broken down into inactive forms, not all drugs are converted into water-soluble particles, and not all drugs are eliminated via the renal system. More detailed descriptions of metabolism can be found in a general pharmacology text.

Most metabolism occurs in the liver, but it is not the only site; some metabolic activity occurs in the kidneys, lungs, GI tract, and plasma. Enzymes facilitate the metabolic processes and are said to be catalysts because they provoke reactions yet are unaffected by the biochemical reaction. An enzyme is much larger (perhaps 100 times larger) than the drug molecule and is configured in such a way that only molecules matching that specific configuration (i.e., the enzyme's substrates) can be metabolized. A single enzyme performs its metabolic task over and over very rapidly. Acetylcholinesterase (AChE) is the primary enzyme responsible for the hydrolytic metabolism of the neurotransmitter acetylcholine (ACh) into choline and acetate. The enzyme AChE hydrolyzes the neurotransmitter ACh into choline and acetate. That is, it splits a bond and adds hydrogen and the monovalent hydroxide anion = OH− consisting of one atom hydrogen and one of oxygen. ACh molecules that do not bind immediately with a receptor or those released after reacting with a receptor are hydrolyzed almost instantly (in less than 1 m) by AChE (Bittner & Martyn, 2019).

Two enzyme systems are of particular importance to nurses who administer psychotropic drugs: (1) the monoamine oxidase (MAO) system and (2) the cytochrome P-450 (CYP-450) system. The MAO system metabolizes monoamines (e.g., dopamine, norepinephrine, and serotonin) that are already in the body. The other system, CYP-450, breaks down most psychotropic drugs or chemicals brought into the body.

Monoamine Oxidase System

MAO is the enzyme that rapidly inactivates monoamines (e.g., serotonin, dopamine, norepinephrine) by oxidative deanimation and slowly metabolizes noncatecholamines (e.g., ephedrine, phenylephrine). MAO is located in the liver, intestinal wall, and CNS in the terminals and synapses of neurons containing serotonin, norepinephrine, or dopamine (Nestler, Hyman, Holtzman, & Malenka, 2015). In the liver, MAO inactivates tyramine, which is found in many foods, and the biogenic amines found in some drugs. When liver MAO is prevented from metabolizing these amines, serious sympathetic effects can develop. MAO is present in two forms: (1) MAO-A, which inactivates norepinephrine and serotonin, and (2) MAO-B, which inactivates dopamine. Some psychotropic drugs inhibit both MAO-A and MAO-B and are correctly described as *nonselective* MAO inhibitors (these are the agents warned about on many over-the-counter drug containers). A few drugs are selective and inhibit either MAO-A or MAO-B. These agents are described as *selective* MAO inhibitors.

Cytochrome Enzyme System

This complex name (i.e., cytochrome P-450 or CYP-450) can be broken down as follows: cyto stands for microsomal vesicles, P stands for pigmentation (because the enzymes contain red-pigmented heme), and 450 refers to the wavelength

DOPAMINE
Activation (Agonists)
Schizophrenia-like symptoms
Psychosis
Dyskinesias
Hallucinations
Delusions
Nausea
Vomiting
Addictive behaviors
Enhancement of sexual function
Antagonism
Antipsychotic effect
Negative symptoms of schizophrenia
Temperature dysregulation
Antiemetic effect
Parkinsonism and extrapyramidal side effects
Cognitive problems
Sexual dysfunction
Neuroendocrine dysregulation
Depression, anhedonia
Lack of energy, motivation

(in nanometers) at which light absorption occurs (Cozza, Armstrong, & Oesterheld, 2003). This primarily hepatic (with also limited presence in pulmonary, intestinal, renal systems, and plasma and CNS) enzyme system metabolizes most psychotropic drugs, and its purpose is to eliminate xenobiotics, which are chemical compounds foreign to the organism (Box 12.2).

CYP-450 enzymes contain 12 families, with more than 40 individual enzymes found in humans (Burchum & Rosenthal, 2016). Six enzymes account for approximately 90% of CYP-450 enzymes in humans: 1A2, 2B6, 2C9, 2C19, 2D6, and 3 A4.

A family name is denoted by an Arabic number (e.g., CYP-3), the subfamily by a Roman uppercase letter (e.g., CYP-3A), and the individual enzymes by another Arabic number following the letter indicating the subfamily (e.g., CYP-3A4).

BOX 12.2   Psychiatric Medicines with CPIC Dosing Guidelines for the CYP-450 Enzymes

Medication	Gene Enzymes
Amitriptyline	CYP-2C19
	CYP-2D6
Nortriptyline	CYP-2D6
Citalopram and escitalopram	CYP-2C19
Fluvoxamine	CYP-2D6
Paroxetine	CYP-2D6
Sertraline	CYP-2C19
Phenytoin	CYP-2C9

CPIC, Clinical Pharmacogenetics Implementation Consortium. Modified from Gammal, R. S., Gardner, K. N., & Burghardt, K. J. (2016). Where to find guidance on using pharmacogenomics in psychiatric practice. *Current Psychiatry, 15*, 93.

TABLE 12.1　CYP Table

CYP isoform	1A2	2B6	2C9	2C19	2D6	3A4
Summary	Plays minor role, metabolizes ~5% of drugs	Along with CYP2A6, it is involved with metabolizing nicotine	Metabolizes ~20% of all drugs		Metabolizes 25% of drugs	
Inhibitors	Antidepressants Fluvoxamine (potent inhibitor)		Antidepressants Fluoxetine (moderate) Fluvoxamine (moderate) Mood Stabilizers Valproic acid (weak)	Antidepressants Fluvoxamine (potent) Fluoxetine (moderate)	Antidepressants Fluoxetine (potent) Paroxetine (potent) Sertraline Duloxetine (moderate) Bupropion (moderate) Antipsychotics Perphenazine (potent)	Antidepressants Fluoxetine (moderate) Fluvoxamine (moderate)
Inducers	Carbamazepine Cigarettes	Carbamazepine	Carbamazepine	Carbamazepine		Carbamazepine
Substrates	Antidepressants Tricyclics (demethylation) Fluvoxamine Trazodone Duloxetine Mirtazapine Agomelatine Antipsychotics Haloperidol Thioridazine Clozapine Olanzapine Asenapine	Antidepressants Bupropion	Antidepressants Fluoxetine Mood stabilizers Valproic acid Hypnotics Zolpidem Zopiclone	Antidepressants Tricyclics (demethylation) Sertraline Citalopram Escitalopram Moclobemide Anxiolytics Diazepam Clobazam	Antidepressants Tricyclics (hydroxylation) Fluoxetine Fluvoxamine Paroxetine Citalopram, Escitalopram Venlafaxine Mirtazapine Duloxetine Vortioxetine Atomoxetine Antipsychotics Haloperidol Chlorpromazine Fuphenazine Perphenazine Thioridazine Zuclopenthixol Pimozide Clozapine Olanzapine Risperidone Iloperidone Aripiprazole Brexpiprazole	Antidepressants Tricyclics (demethylation) Sertraline Citalopram Escitalopram Venlafaxine Mirtazapine Trazodone Reboxetine Vilazodone Antipsychotics Haloperidol Thioridazine Pimozide Clozapine Quetiapine Risperidone Iloperidone Aripiprazole Brexpiprazole Ziprasidone Lurasidone Cariprazine Anxiolytics Alprazolam Midazolam Tiazolam Mood stabilizers Carbamazepine

Modified from Cytochrome (CYP) P450 Metabolism. (2021). https://www.psychdb.com/meds/cytochrome-p450#substrates-inhibitors-and-inducers.

TABLE 12.2 Psychotropic Drugs That Interact With Tobacco Smoke

Caffeine
Clozapine
Doxepin
Duloxetine
Fluvoxamine
Mirtazapine
Olanzapine
Riluzole (glutamate antagonist)
Thiothixene
Trifluoperazine

Modified from Fankhauser, J. P. (2013). Drug interactions with tobacco smoke: Implications for patient care. *Current Psychiatry, 12*, 12.

A drug that is metabolized by a CYP enzyme is termed a substrate; drugs may inhibit or decrease that enzyme's activity, induce or increase that enzyme's activity, or have no effect on it. Inhibitors increase the plasma concentrations of the drug, or decrease clearance of its substrates. Inducers decrease the plasma concentration of the affected drug, or increase clearance of its substrates.

Although lab testing for CYP-450 enzymes is available, it is expensive, impractical, and should be reserved for limited circumstances. Suspected drug interactions can usually be diagnosed from history and clinical observations (Table 12.1).

Another significant issue when administering psychotropic drugs is the influence that tobacco smoke has on drug pharmacokinetics. Cigarette smoking causes the induction of CYP-450 1A2 (i.e., causes more of this enzyme to be synthesized). Table 12.2 lists the names of psychotropic drugs that are substrates of CYP-450 1A2. Maximal enzyme induction occurs with 7 to 12 cigarettes per day for some agents (e.g., clozapine, olanzapine), which leads to a 40% to 50% reduction in their serum levels (Fankhauser, 2013). The serum level of other drugs may not decline by this much unless the patient is a heavy smoker (≥30 cigarettes per day). Regardless, a patient who smokes half a pack or more of cigarettes per day requires more medication than the patient would have required if he or she did not smoke. Depending on the drug, this could lead to toxic levels developing if the medication is not titrated downward as the patient stops smoking.

These same effects can occur from secondhand smoke as well.

Question: What might happen when a heavy smoker who is taking olanzapine is hospitalized on a nonsmoking unit?
Answer: After a few weeks of nonsmoking, his CYP-450 1A2 level would return to normal, with a subsequent increase in serum levels unless the dose were reduced. With some drugs, this could be dangerous.

Half-Life of Drugs

The half-life of a drug is the amount of time required for 50% of the drug to disappear from the body. If drug X has a half-life of 4 hours, then 50% of the drug will be out of the system in 4 hours. In another 4 hours, only 25% of the original dose will remain. In most cases, it would not matter whether the patient took 100 mg or 300 mg: the amount of drug in the body would decrease by 50% every 4 hours. This action is referred to as *linear kinetics*, and most drugs follow this pattern. This rule has exceptions, most notably in the case of alcohol, in which only a set amount of the drug is metabolized in a given period regardless of the amount ingested (i.e., nonlinear kinetics). If the nurse gives drug X (e.g., 100 mg) at the same time (e.g., three times a day), a steady state is achieved in four half-lives. When discontinuing a drug, four half-lives are required to eliminate 96% of the drug. This period is referred to as the *washout period*.

> ### ? CRITICAL THINKING QUESTION
>
> 2. As stated, most psychotropic drug interactions occur as a result of the effects on the CYP-450 system. If an inhibitor of the CYP-450 3A4 enzyme were given (e.g., grapefruit juice) with psychotropic drugs metabolized by this enzyme (e.g., sertraline, bupropion, diazepam, haloperidol), what would be the effect? (Typically, an entire grapefruit or 8 ounces of juice would be enough to trigger pharmacokinetic changes [Bishop, 2015].)

> ### ? CRITICAL THINKING QUESTION
>
> 3. Prozac has a half-life of approximately 10 days or longer (when norfluoxetine, its active metabolite, is included). How long is the washout period? If a drug known to interact with Prozac is to be given, how long should the interval be between stopping Prozac and beginning the new drug?

Excretion

The kidney excretes most drugs in the urine, but other routes of excretion exist, such as breast milk, bile, feces, saliva, sweat, and the lungs. Factors that can affect excretion include kidney disease, age, and drug competition for active tubular transport.

Clinical relevance: Drugs that are not adequately excreted (e.g., because of kidney disease), particularly drugs excreted unchanged (a few drugs are not metabolized [e.g., lithium, amphetamine]), have a more pronounced effect compared with drugs that are excreted.

PHARMACODYNAMICS: WHAT THE DRUG DOES TO THE BODY

Pharmacodynamics is the effect that a drug has on the body. The two global responses to drugs are the desired, therapeutic effects and the adverse, "side" effects. Drugs that activate receptors are called agonists, and drugs that block receptors are called antagonists. Some psychotropic drugs are agonists, whereas many others are antagonists. Pharmacodynamic effects of particular interest to this discussion are downregulation of receptors and pharmacodynamic tolerance.

Downregulation

Downregulation of receptors is an important concept, primarily because chronic exposure to certain psychotropic drugs causes receptors to change. For example, consistent use of antidepressants causes postsynaptic receptors to decrease in number. Because this downregulation occurs at about the same time that the antidepressant effect develops (approximately 2 to 4 weeks), it is thought by some that reduction in postsynaptic receptors might provide a better explanation for mood elevation than increases in neurotransmitters.

Pharmacodynamic Tolerance

Pharmacodynamic tolerance describes a reduction in receptor sensitivity (or desensitization). A good example is a chronic drinker of alcohol. When the newspaper reports a person driving a car with a blood alcohol level (BAL) of 0.35, the story is likely about a case of pharmacodynamic tolerance. This person's receptors are no longer responding to the ethanol in the way a normal person's receptors would respond. Although at first glance this idea might appear appealing, it really is not. Tolerance to a BAL that could cause deadly respiratory depression does not occur. A person who is functioning at an elevated BAL might drink only a little more alcohol and wind up dead.

Knowledge of downregulatory functions helps the nurse explain the lag time between initiating drug therapy and clinical improvement. Knowledge of pharmacodynamic tolerance aids in teaching patients and families about drug tolerance to some drug effects but little, if any, tolerance to some lethal effects (e.g., respiratory depression) at just slightly higher doses.

Drug-Drug Interactions

There are two types of drug-drug interactions: pharmacokinetic interactions and pharmacodynamic interactions. Pharmacokinetic interactions occur when one of the four pharmacokinetic processes is inhibited or induced. An example of how each pharmacokinetic process might play into a drug interaction follows:

1. *Absorption:* Drug A is taken with another drug that changes stomach pH, affecting absorption of drug A.
2. *Distribution:* Two drugs are both highly protein-bound. Drug A "hogs" most of the binding sites, leaving more of drug B available. Drug B would then have a greater pharmacologic effect.
3. *Metabolism:* Two drugs are metabolized by the CYP-450 enzyme 2D6. One or both drugs could have a higher blood level.
4. *Excretion:* Drug A alters the urinary pH, speeding or hindering the excretion of another drug.

Enzyme induction usually takes several days to weeks to develop, whereas enzyme inhibition develops almost immediately.

Pharmacodynamic interactions are straightforward. On the one hand, two drugs with anticholinergic properties have the potential to have a synergistic or additive effect. On the other hand, two drugs can oppose each other, basically reducing their effectiveness.

THE BLOOD-BRAIN BARRIER

The blood-brain barrier is also an important concept for understanding psychotropic drug activity. The brain, more than other organs of the body, requires a constant internal milieu. Although other parts of the body experience fluctuations in body chemistry, even small changes in the brain produce serious problems. The brain is protected from fluctuations by the blood-brain barrier. This barrier regulates the amount and speed of substances in the blood entering the brain. Water, carbon dioxide, and oxygen readily cross the barrier; other substances are excluded from the brain.

The blood-brain barrier has three dimensions: (1) an anatomic dimension, (2) a physiologic dimension, and (3) a metabolic dimension. The anatomic dimension is the structure of the capillaries that supply blood to the brain and prevent many molecules from slipping through. There are no gaps.

The physiologic dimension is a chemical and transport system that recognizes and allows certain molecules into the brain. Lipid solubility is the most important of the chemical properties that determine whether a molecule can pass through the blood-brain barrier. Highly lipid-soluble substances pass the blood-brain barrier with relative ease. Highly water-soluble substances penetrate this barrier slowly and in insignificant amounts. Nicotine, ethanol, heroin, caffeine, and diazepam (Valium) are examples of highly lipid-soluble substances. This characteristic is clinically important because only drugs that can pass through this barrier in significant amounts are effective in treating a psychiatric or medical disorder of the brain. Certain nonlipid-soluble substances such as glucose, which is the brain's primary energy source, and essential amino acids, which are needed for the synthesis of neurotransmitters, are required for normal brain function. Special transport systems carry these essential substances across the blood-brain barrier.

P-glycoproteins: Another dimension to the physiologic barrier is the *P-glycoprotein efflux transporter system*. This system has various substrates and ferries these molecules back out of the cell about as fast as they enter it. For instance, the P-glycoprotein efflux transporters cause second-generation antihistamines to be nonsedating. These antihistamine drug molecules are transported out of the CNS before they can have a sedating effect (Cozza, Armstrong, & Oesterheld, 2003). Some drugs induce the P-glycoprotein system (e.g., venlafaxine) to produce even greater efflux of certain substrates, causing some drugs to be less effective (Levin, 2012). What is particularly perplexing is that a drug that inhibits P-glycoproteins can cause an increased central effect without causing a change in serum levels. How? When P-glycoproteins are inhibited, more of drug X gets into the brain even though more of the drug has not been taken by the patient. The serum level is unchanged,

TABLE 12.3	Selected Psychotropic Drugs that Affect P-Glycoprotein Efflux Transporters	
Substrates	**Inhibitors**	**Inducers**
Amitriptyline	Amitriptyline	Phenothiazines
Carbamazepine	Carbamazepine	Trazodine
Chlorpromazine	Chlorpromazine	Venlafaxine
Citalopram	Desipramine	—
Nortriptyline	Disulfiram	—
Olanzapine	Fluoxetine	—
Paroxetine	Haloperidol	—
Quetiapine	Imipramine	—
Risperidone	Paroxetine	—
Sertraline	Sertraline	—
Venlafaxine	—	—

Modified from Levin, G. M. (2012). P-glycoproteins: Why this drug transporter may be clinically important. *Current Psychiatry, 11*, 38.

but the effect can be significantly greater. Table 12.3 lists P-glycoprotein substrates, inhibitors, and inducers.

The metabolic barrier prevents molecules from entering the brain by enzymatic action within the endothelial lining of the brain capillaries. For example, levodopa can pass the blood-brain barrier, but much of it is changed to dopamine before it can pass completely through the capillary wall into the brain. The metabolic product, dopamine, does not readily pass this barrier, thus illustrating the third way that the brain protects itself from substances in the peripheral circulation.

Understanding the blood-brain barrier helps the nurse conceptualize, administer, and monitor drug therapy accurately as well as understand addiction to highly lipid-soluble substances such as alcohol and heroin. A comparison of systemic penicillin and dopamine serves as an example for understanding this important principle. If penicillin were the only antibiotic available (which it was at one time), large doses would be needed to treat a CNS infection because this water-soluble drug does not pass through the blood-brain barrier easily. When a large dose of penicillin is given, only a fraction of it enters the brain. Most of the penicillin stays in the peripheral system, which does not cause alarm because

penicillin has relatively few adverse effects. However, dopamine has many adverse effects on the body. The dose needed to penetrate the blood-brain barrier and affect the brain adequately (a central effect) is so large that it would have serious adverse effects on the rest of the body (e.g., cardiac stimulation, a peripheral effect).

NEURONS AND NEUROTRANSMITTERS

The neuronal system is highly complex, with most neurons receiving input from thousands of other neurons. The arborization, or branching, of dendrites continues into late adolescence and early adulthood.

Nerve cells, or neurons, are the basic units of the nervous system. Nerve cells are designed to receive and give information. Dendrites are projections from the neuron; they receive information and transmit it to the cell body. Axons send information from the nerve cell to the dendrites, axons, or cell bodies of other neurons. Axons of one cell are separated from the dendrites, axons, or cell body of another cell by a microscopic space known as a *synapse* (Fig. 12.1). Fig. 12.2 depicts the relationships among neurotransmitters, neurons, and psychotropic drugs.

Information in the form of an electrochemical excitation is communicated between cells in a specific manner. Incoming information from a receptor on the surface of a nerve cell causes the normally stable and mutually balanced electrical charges between the interior and the exterior of the membrane to become destabilized. An action potential is caused by the brief reversal of electrical charges between the inside and the outside of the cell, which is caused by the opening of ion channels in the cell membrane. This causes depolarization of the cell membrane and the subsequent opening of nearby ion channels. This causes the conduction or propagation of nerve signals from the dendrite, through the cell body or nucleus, to the axon of the cell. As the nerve signal passes to the dendrite, vesicles (bubble-like structures with a lipid bilayer containing neurotransmitters) migrate and fuse to the surface of the cell membrane, releasing their contents into the synaptic cleft. This process is repeated in the receiving nerve cell, continuring the cycle of synaptic neurotransmission of information.

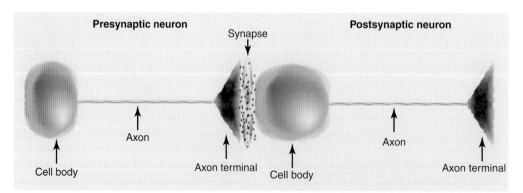

FIG. 12.1 This two-neuron chain shows presynaptic and postsynaptic neurons interconnected by a synapse. The synapse is composed of a synaptic bouton *(triangle)* or presynaptic terminal, the synaptic cleft, and the postsynaptic membrane, which, in this example, is the dendrite or cell body *(circle)* of the postsynaptic neuron.

NEUROTRANSMITTERS

ACETYLCHOLINE (ACh)
DOPAMINE (DA)
GABA
NOREPINEPHRINE (NE)
SEROTONIN (5-HT)

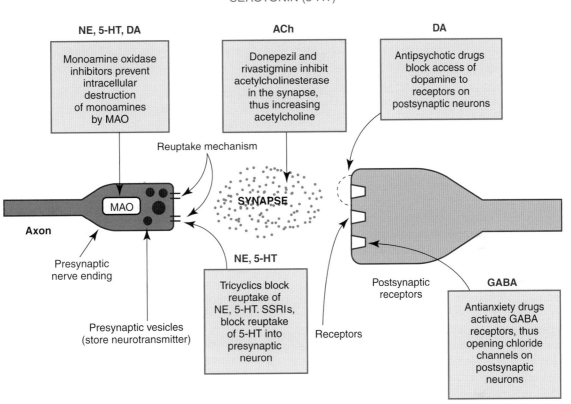

FIG. 12.2 Explanation of the way in which psychotropic drugs affect five major neurotransmitters. *GABA,* γ-aminobutyric acid; *MAO,* monoamine oxidase. (Modified from Stuart, G., & Sundeen, S. [1995]. *Principles and practice of psychiatric nursing* [5th ed.]. Mosby.)

Neurotransmitters are synthesized from natural precursors (e.g., amino acids) in the body (Box 12.3). These precursors are extracted from the bloodstream and synthesized in the cell into neurotransmitters. Neurotransmitters are stored in storage vesicles in the presynaptic terminals of the cell. Neurotransmitters come in many forms, and they combine with specific receptors. For example, the neurotransmitter norepinephrine combines with a norepinephrine receptor. After norepinephrine electrochemically stimulates the norepinephrine receptor, information is transmitted to the cell body, which communicates to the next neuron, and so on. After it is in the synaptic cleft, the neurotransmitter can, until it is inactivated, continue to stimulate the postsynaptic receptor. Neurotransmitters are inactivated by enzymes in the synaptic cleft or by enzymes in the presynaptic terminal, or they are taken up into surrounding glial cells. Knowledge of this inactivation process has facilitated the evolution of psychopharmacology. The most important neurotransmitters for psychiatric nursing students to understand along with related mental disorders are presented in Table 12.4.

RECEPTORS

Receptors are proteins on cell surfaces that respond to endogenous ligands or to drug molecules. A ligand is a transmitter substance or molecule that fits and evokes a response from a receptor. Examples of ligands include drugs, neurotransmitters, hormones, prostaglandins, and leukotrienes. Receptors

---

BOX 12.3 Categories of Neurotransmitters that are Important in Psychiatry[a]

Monoamines
Dopamine
Norepinephrine
Serotonin

Cholinergic
Acetylcholine

Amino Acids
GABA
Glutamate

[a]Peptides not included.
GABA, γ-aminobutyric acid.

TABLE 12.4 Neurotransmitters and Related Mental Disorders[a]

Neurotransmitter-Related State	Mental Disorder
Increase in dopamine	Schizophrenia
Decrease in norepinephrine	Depression
Decrease in serotonin	Depression
Decrease in acetylcholine	Alzheimer disease
Decrease in GABA	Anxiety
Increase in glutamate	Excitotoxicity leading to neuronal death
Decrease in glutamate	Psychotic thinking

[a]Although this explanation is overly simplistic, it nevertheless serves to convey the basic neurotransmitter theories for each related mental disorder and continues to drive drug treatment for those disorders.
GABA, γ-aminobutyric acid.

BOX 12.4 Results of Activating and Antagonizing Serotonin Receptors

Serotonin Activation	Serotonin Antagonism
Antidepressant effect	Depression
Anxiety	Dysthymia
Nausea	Suicidality
Vomiting	Aggressiveness
Other GI disturbances	Obsessive thinking
Sexual dysfunction	Sleep-wake cycle disruption
Reduced appetite and weight loss	Pain
Insomnia	Compulsive behavior
Movement disorders	Anxiety
Temperature dysregulation	Panic
Psychotic thinking	—

GI, Gastrointestinal.

BOX 12.5 Results of Activating and Antagonizing Acetylcholine Receptors

Acetylcholine Activation	Acetylcholine Antagonism
Pupil contraction	Pupil dilation
Decreased heart rate	Increased heart rate
Constriction of bronchi	Dilation of bronchi
Increased respiratory secretions	Decreased respiratory secretions
Increased voiding	Decreased voiding
Salivation	Dry mouth
Increased gastric secretions	Decreased gastric secretions
Increased defecation	Constipation
Sweating	Decreased sweating
Enhancement of cognitive processes	Cognitive slowing

BOX 12.6 Results of Activating and Antagonizing Norepinephrine Receptors

Norepinephrine Activation	Norepinephrine Antagonism
Antidepressant effect	Depressive effect
Vasoconstriction (α_1)	Vasodilation (α_1 antagonism)
Increased heart rate (β_1)	Decreased heart rate (β-blocker)
Bronchial dilation	Sexual dysfunction
Other physical effects	Other physical effects

are configured so that only precisely shaped molecules can fit and subsequently cause or prevent a response. For example, the neurotransmitter serotonin fits serotonin receptors, but ACh molecules do not fit serotonin receptors.

Four primary receptor processes exist (Burchum & Rosenthal, 2016). The two most commonly addressed processes in the literature of psychopharmacology are the ligand-gated ion channel (or first-messenger) process and the G-protein–coupled (or second-messenger) process. When the ligand-gated receptor is activated, an ion channel—such as a sodium, calcium, or chloride channel—opens and the respective ion flows into the cell. Depending on the ion, this action causes cell depolarization (the cell fires) or hyperpolarization (cell firing slows down or the cell does not fire). The process is extremely rapid, usually occurring within milliseconds. ACh (at nicotinic receptors only), γ-aminobutyric acid (GABA), glycine, and glutamate use the first-messenger system. The G-protein–coupled receptor is a more complex process—a biologic cascade of intracellular reactions develop and is slower compared with the first-messenger system. Norepinephrine, serotonin, dopamine, ACh (at muscarinic receptors only), and peptides couple with G-protein or second-messenger receptors. Consequences of selected receptor activation or antagonism are listed in Boxes 12.4–12.6.

Receptors located in the axon terminal and the cell body are called somatodendritic or autoreceptors. Stimulation of these receptors decreases further release of neurotransmitter in negative feedback fashion.

Psychotropic drugs can affect neurotransmitters in several ways:
1. **Block** metabolism (e.g., some antidepressants and drugs for Alzheimer disease)
2. **Block** reuptake (e.g., selective serotonin reuptake inhibitors [SSRIs] and other antidepressants)
3. **Block** receptors (antagonists)
4. **Stimulate** or **block** autoreceptors (see the following discussion on autoreceptors)
5. **Stimulate** receptors (agonists)
6. **Stimulate** receptor affinity (benzodiazepines cause GABA receptors to have a greater attraction for GABA)
7. **Stimulate** the release of a neurotransmitter (e.g., amphetamine stimulates the release of dopamine). The following terms relating to receptors are defined (Box 12.7 for expanded definitions) to facilitate understanding of information presented in the drug chapters (Kowalski, Dowben, & Keltner, 2017).

Receptor antagonism. Receptor antagonism is the process whereby receptor function is compromised related to blocking of that receptor by a psychotropic drug.

BOX 12.7 Expanded Definitions of Agonists, Antagonists, Partial Agonists, and Inverse Agonists

A. Agonists

Agonists are drugs that imitate the endogenous (i.e., a hormone or neurotransmitter) molecule that causes the same neuronal response.

Dopamine agonists—such as ropinirole (Requip) and pramipexole (Mirapex)—are used to treat the motor symptoms of Parkinson disease.

The *exogenous* dopamine agonists have the same effect as the *endogenous* dopamine molecule itself and help to correct the dopamine-starved motor state of the patient with PD. There are agonists for other neurotransmitter systems, too. Perhaps the ones of keenest interest to the psychiatric professional are those that can stimulate the serotonin system. Examples of serotonin agonists include the following:

5-HT1A agonists; for example, buspirone for anxiety

5-HT1B agonists; for example, sumatriptan for migraines

5-HT2A agonists; for example, lysergic acid diethylamide (LSD) for abuse

B. Antagonists

Antagonists attach to a receptor so that an endogenous agonist (e.g., dopamine for dopamine receptors, serotonin for serotonin receptors, etc.) cannot attach. This either blocks a biologic response or reduces the response of the neuron to the endogenous molecule. Many medications fall under this category, including antipsychotics, α-blockers, anticholinergics,

antihistaminergics, β-blockers, calcium channel blockers, and neuromuscular blockers.

C. Partial Agonists

Partial agonists elicit a response that is less robust than the response of an agonist. What is particularly interesting is that a partial agonist can increase endogenous activity in some areas of the brain and slow it down in another area. Aripiprazole (Abilify) increases neuronal activity in the underactive mesocortical dopaminergic tract while decreasing the neuronal activity in the overactive mesolimbic tract. Aripiprazole has a higher affinity for the dopamine receptor than dopamine itself. Dopamine cannot attach to the receptor because its receptor is already occupied.

D. Inverse Agonists

Inverse agonists have an opposite effect to that of an agonist. As Nestler et al. (2009) point out, an inverse agonist is dependent on the receptor having some level of basal activity. That is, many neurons continue to "fire" even in the absence of an agonist—the aforementioned basal (or intrinsic) activity level. When an antagonist is given, basal activity continues in these neurons; thus, neuronal activity is not shut down. An inverse agonist, however, causes an opposite effect to that of an agonist. As these authors note, if an agonist opens an ion channel, the inverse agonist will close the channel. Some inverse agonists that are familiar to many include pimavanserin, naloxone, and naltrexone.

From Kowalski, P. C., Dowben, J. S., & Keltner, N. L. (2017). My dad can beat your dad: Agonists, antagonists, partial agonists, and inverse agonists. *Perspectives in Psychiatric Care, 53*, 76.

Antagonists prevent the endogenous ligand from activating the receptor (Fig. 12.3).

Receptor agonist. A receptor agonist is a drug that fits and activates the receptor in the same manner as the naturally occurring ligand.

Receptor partial agonists. A partial agonist elicits a response that is less robust than that of an agonist.

Receptor inverse agonists. Inverse agonists have an effect opposite to that of agonists.

Autoreceptor. An autoreceptor is the negative feedback mechanism that neurons use to increase or decrease the release of a neurotransmitter; they are typically but not always found on the presynaptic neuron. Autoreceptor *agonists* tell the neuron that enough of the neurotransmitter is present, resulting in a decrease in release of the neurotransmitter. Autoreceptor *antagonists* tell the receptor to release more of the neurotransmitter.

Receptor affinity. Receptor affinity is the attraction or strength of attraction between neurotransmitters and receptors.

Receptor life cycle. Receptors are continually being formed and continually breaking down. The life cycle of the average receptor is short.

Receptor modulation. Some neurotransmitters do not have a direct effect but modify (or modulate) the effect of another neurotransmitter (Fig. 12.4). The following scenario might help to clarify receptor modulation. Picture, if possible, one neuron (#1) synapsing with the synaptic terminal of a

presynaptic neuron (#2), which is synapsing in the traditional way with a third neuron (#3). Neuron #1 influences the release of neurotransmitter from #2, which then affects the amount of neurotransmitter released into the synapse between #2 and #3. Neuron #1 is modulating neuron #2 (see Fig. 12.4).

PATIENT EDUCATION

The importance of patient and family education cannot be overemphasized. Historically, many psychiatric patients and their families have demonstrated little understanding of their medications. Although the emphasis on education has partially remedied this problem, teaching about these potent drugs will always be a nursing priority. Reasons that patients don't take their medications as prescribed include the following (Kalali, Richerson, & Reites, 2016):

1. Lack of knowledge
2. Lack of insight
3. Negative reaction to medication in the past
4. Feeling better, thus thinking that no more medication is needed
5. Side effects
6. Complicated dosing

Nurses have a professional duty to discuss medications and their side effects with patients; they must possess broad knowledge with equal amounts of sensitivity. For example, the nurse might frighten patients with too much

Most response ┈┈┈┈┈ Basal response ┈┈┈┈┈ Inhibited response

Agonist

Partial Agonist

Antagonist

Inverse Agonist

FIG. 12.3 Spectrum of neuronal responses to a ligand. (From Kowalski, P. C., Dowben, J. S., & Keltner, N. L. [2017]. My dad can beat your dad: Agonists, antagonists, partial agonists, and inverse agonists. *Perspectives in Psychiatric Care, 53*, 76.)

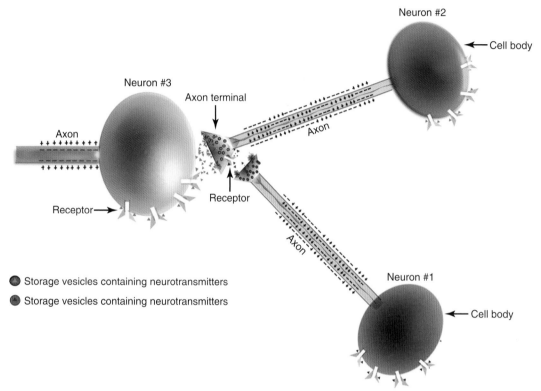

FIG. 12.4 Neuronal modulation.

or inappropriate information. Good professional judgment is important, including teaching patients about what effects are visible, what can be felt, and what the possibilities are of becoming drug-dependent. The nurse should also emphasize the need for regular checkups and tests. Specific areas of education include the following:

1. Discussion of side effects
   - Side effects can directly affect the patient's willingness to adhere to the drug regimen; for example, SSRIs, such as sertraline (Zoloft), are known to reduce libido and sexual functioning. Thus, these drugs indirectly affect spouses as well.
   - Side effects can cause medical problems or even death.
   - Some drugs cause patients to experience emotional flattening, thus dulling responses to the environment, counseling, and family.
   - Some drugs cause cognitive slowing.
   - The nurse should always inquire about the patient's response to a drug—both therapeutic responses and adverse responses.

2. Discussion of safety issues
   - Does the patient take the drug as prescribed?
   - Do the patient and family know which effects should be reported to the nurse or physician?
   - Because some drugs, such as tricyclic antidepressants and lithium, have a narrow therapeutic index, thoughts of self-harm must be discussed.
   - Does the drug have potential for abuse or dependence?
   - Can the drug be discontinued abruptly without effect? Patients should know that many drugs must be tapered gradually.
   - Because many psychotropic drugs cause sedation or drowsiness, discussions concerning the use of hazardous machinery and driving must occur.

3. Attitudes of patient and nurse about medications
   - Because many patients and families believe that the use of medications is a sign of weakness or lack of faith in God, the nurse must discuss these issues.
   - Some nurses do not really "believe" in psychotropic medications. These nurses must examine their own

views and perhaps work in areas of nursing that do not involve psychotropic drugs.
- For patients and families who are resistant to the use of psychotropic agents, the nurse must discuss the potential ramifications of noncompliance.
- Issues of dependence and long-term medication use must be discussed.
- Because many patients and families do not want to become addicted, the nurse must point out the specific addiction potential of any particular drug. Most psychotropic drugs are not addicting.

4. Drug interactions
- Patients and families must be taught to discuss the effects of the addition of over-the-counter drugs, alcohol, and illegal drugs to currently prescribed drugs.
- Patients who see more than one clinician must make potential prescribing professionals aware of all drugs that are currently being taken.

5. Instructions for older adult patients or children of older adult patients
- Because older individuals have a different pharmacokinetic profile than younger adults, special instructions concerning side effects and drug-drug interactions should be tailored for this population.

6. Instructions for pregnant or breast-feeding patients
- Because pregnant or breast-feeding patients have special risks associated with psychotropic drug therapy, special instructions should be tailored for these individuals.

7. Awareness of metabolic differences in diverse races and ethnicities
- Because of genetic differences as well as diet, cultural beliefs and expectations, and lifestyle, patients of different races may achieve the same therapeutic outcome from lower doses of medication than others.
- Gene expression and mutation of certain enzymes (e.g., CYP-450 2D6) have been shown to alter the rate at which medications are metabolized; therefore, some patients are poor metabolizers and others ultrarapid metabolizers. Different doses must be considered to achieve the optimal therapeutic outcome for each individual.

Teaching patients about their medications helps to empower them in their own care and decreases undesirable side effects. Effective teaching can reduce the risks and complications associated with taking psychotropic medications.

? CRITICAL THINKING QUESTION

4. In this chapter, we state that the nurse should use balance when giving information to a patient about a drug. What is the balance between arousing unneeded apprehension in a patient who is vulnerable to suggestion (i.e., giving complete information) and treating that adult patient as a child (i.e., withholding information to protect the patient)? In your role as a student and later as a nurse, you would not want to do either.

■ STUDY NOTES

1. Psychopharmacology is the second component of psychotherapeutic management. Psychotropic drugs have enabled millions of people to live more productive lives in the least restrictive environment.

2. Nurses assess for drug side effects, evaluate desired effects, and make decisions about prn medications.

3. Pharmacokinetic processes include absorption, distribution, metabolism, and excretion of drugs.

4. Absorption is the process whereby drugs leave the GI tract and move into the bloodstream.

5. Bioavailability is the percentage of a drug that reaches the systemic circulation.

6. Distribution refers to the process of drug molecules leaving the bloodstream to reach tissues and organs. Drugs that do not leave the bloodstream cannot have a psychiatric effect.

7. Lipid solubility is a property that affects absorption and distribution. Highly lipid-soluble drugs penetrate the blood-brain barrier easily.

8. Protein binding, the propensity of a drug to bind to serum proteins, also affects drug distribution. Drugs that are bound to serum proteins cannot leave the bloodstream.

9. Metabolism is the process whereby the body breaks down a drug to remove it from the body.

10. The liver is the site of most drug metabolism.

11. The two major enzyme systems associated with psychotropic drugs are the MAO system and the CYP-450 system.

12. An individual enzyme breaks down thousands of drug molecules per second.

13. The CYP-450 system is mentioned often in the current literature on psychotropic drugs.

14. Most drug-drug interactions are related to interference with the CYP-450 system.

15. The half-life of a drug is the length of time required for the body to remove 50% of the original dose. If a *single dose* of a drug is given and the drug has a half-life of 4 hours, 50% of the drug will remain in the body after 4 hours, 25% of the drug will remain after 8 hours, and 12.5% of the drug will remain after 12 hours.

16. Excretion is the removal of drug from the body through the kidneys via the urine.

17. Pharmacodynamics involves the effects of the drug on the body.

18. Drug effects are typically categorized as desired effects or side effects.

19. Downregulation of a receptor refers to a decrease in the number of receptors or to decreased receptor sensitivity.

20. Pharmacodynamic tolerance is a state in which receptors become less sensitive to agonists.

21. Highly lipid-soluble drugs, such as ethanol, heroin, and diazepam (Valium), pass the blood-brain barrier with ease. This characteristic partially accounts for the widespread abuse of these drugs.

22. Only drugs that pass the blood-brain barrier can affect the CNS.

23. Neurotransmitters, which are neurochemical substances in the brain, evoke a neuronal response, are synthesized by cytoplasmic enzymes, and are usually stored in storage vesicles in the presynaptic terminals of the neuron.

24. Both neurotransmitter deficiency and neurotransmitter excess are related to mental disorders; psychotropic drugs are effective because they cause an increase or decrease in the brain's ability to use a specific neurotransmitter.

25. Receptors are proteins on the cell surface that respond to specific ligands.

26. The two receptor processes most important for psychiatric nurses to understand are the first-messenger system and the second-messenger system.

27. The first-messenger system causes a cellular response when a ligand couples with the receptor, which immediately opens an ion channel.

28. The second-messenger system is more complex compared with the first-messenger system. The initial ligand-receptor coupling initiates a series of events that culminate in a neuronal response.

29. The blood-brain barrier protects the brain from the physiologic fluctuations that the body experiences and regulates the amount of substances entering the brain and the speed with which they enter.

30. The P-glycoprotein efflux transporter system ferries molecules out of the cell. Inhibitors of this system allow more of a substrate to stay in the cell, whereas inducers potentiate P-glycoproteins to remove an even greater amount of the substrate.

31. By teaching patients, the nurse can decrease the incidence of side effects and increase effectiveness to the drug regimen. The nurse should use good clinical judgment in deciding what and how to share with patients and their families.

REFERENCES

Bishop, D. L. (2015). Grapefruit juice and psychotropics: How to avoid potential interactions. *Current Psychiatry, 14*(6), 61.

Bittner, E., & Martyn, A. (2019). *Pharmacology and physiology for anesthesia* (2nd ed.). Elsevier.

Burchum, J., & Rosenthal, L. (2016). *Lehne's pharmacology for nursing care.* Elsevier.

Cozza, K. L., Armstrong, S. C., & Oesterheld, J. R. (2003). *Drug interaction principles for medical practice.* American Psychiatric Publishing.

Cytochrome (CYP) P450 Metabolism. (2021). https://www.psychdb.com/meds/cytochrome-p450#substrates-inhibitors-and-inducers.

Daneman, R., & Prat, A. (2015). The blood-brain barrier. *Cold Spring Harbor perspectives in biology, 7*(1), a020412. https://doi.org/10.1101/cshperspect.a020412.

Fankhauser, J. P. (2013). Drug interactions with tobacco smoke: Implications for patient care. *Current Psychiatry, 12*(1), 12.

Gammal, R. S., Gardner, K. N., & Burghardt, K. J. (2016). Where to find guidance on using pharmacogenomics in psychiatric practice. *Current Psychiatry, 15*(9), 93.

Kalali, A., Richerson, S., & Reites, J. (2016). Technology offers tools for ensuring adherence to medical therapy. *Current Psychiatry, 15*(4), 25.

Kowalski, P. C., Dowben, J. S., & Keltner, N. L. (2017). My dad can beat your dad: Agonists, antagonists, partial agonists, and inverse agonists. *Perspectives in Psychiatric Care, 53*(2), 76. https://doi.org/10.1111/ppc.12208.

Levin, G. M. (2012). P-glycoproteins: Why this drug transporter may be clinically important. *Current Psychiatry, 11*(3), 38.

Nestler, E. J., Hyman, S. E., Holtzman, D. M., & Malenka, R. C. (2015). Molecular neuropharmacology (3rd ed.). McGraw-Hill.

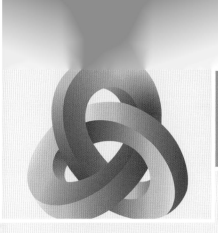

13

Antiparkinsonian Drugs[a]

Joan Grant Keltner

Most people are about as happy as they make up their minds to be.

Abraham Lincoln

(e) http://evolve.elsevier.com/Keltner

LEARNING OBJECTIVES

- Differentiate between Parkinson disease and parkinsonism.
- Discuss the causes and symptoms of parkinsonism.
- Identify the two neurotransmitters primarily associated with Parkinson disease.

- Describe the biochemical relationship between Parkinson disease and extrapyramidal side effects.
- Discuss the side effects of antiparkinsonian drugs.

PARKINSON DISEASE AND EXTRAPYRAMIDAL SIDE EFFECTS

Parkinson disease (PD) is a progressive, chronic, degenerative disease of unknown cause that involves the functional area of the brain called the *extrapyramidal system*. Approximately 0.7% of people aged 65 and older are affected by this disorder, with higher rates in men than in women (Marras et al., 2018). The prevalence of both dementia and depression is about 35% (Hayes, 2019) in individuals with PD (van der Velden et al., 2018). PD is characterized by four cardinal symptoms: (1) tremors, (2) bradykinesia, (3) rigidity, and (4) postural instability. An imbalance of two neurotransmitters—acetylcholine (ACh) and dopamine in the extrapyramidal system associated with these symptoms—is required for normal functioning of the extrapyramidal system. The four primary symptoms and other associated symptoms (e.g., drooling, weight loss, choking, impaired breathing, urinary retention, constipation, difficulty swallowing) occur when these two neurotransmitters are out of balance (Hayes, 2019).

The extrapyramidal system also is associated with the unwanted side effects of various psychotropics, particularly antipsychotics. Historically, it has been assumed that the

newer antipsychotic drugs (atypical or second-/third-generation antipsychotic agents) were less likely to cause extrapyramidal side effects (EPSEs). However, evidence suggests that these differences are more imagined than actual (Hayes, 2019). EPSEs are the result of the biochemical changes similar to those found in PD.

❓ CRITICAL THINKING QUESTION

1. Explain the common symptoms experienced by patients with Parkinson disease and patients on antipsychotics.

Dopamine is synthesized in a couple of areas of the brain, including the midbrain, by pigmented cells in the *substantia nigra* (Latin for "black substance"). Approximately 500,000 of the 100 billion neurons in the brain produce dopamine (Nestler, Hyman, Holtzman, & Malenka, 2015). Cell bodies are located in the substantia nigra, and their axons project to a specific area of the extrapyramidal system called the *basal ganglia* (also known as the *corpus striatum*). The axon terminals of these neurons release dopamine, which activates the dopamine receptors there. This pathway, from the midbrain to the basal ganglia, is known as the *nigrostriatal tract*. In PD, the pigmented neurons of the substantia nigra lose their pigmentation ("blackness"), signifying a decline in dopamine production. Neuronal loss in the substantia nigra that causes

[a]The author would like to acknowledge that the original chapter was written with Norman L. Keltner.

131

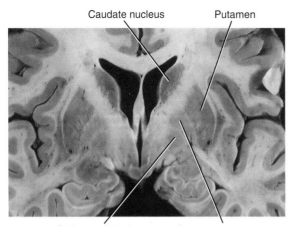

FIG. 13.1 Basal ganglia.

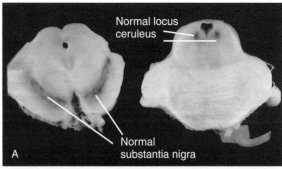

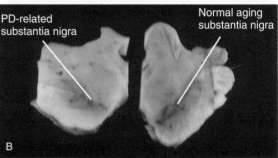

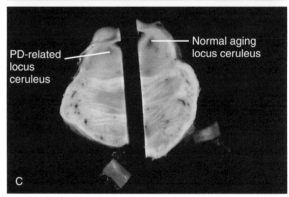

FIG. 13.2 The effects of aging and disease on catecholamine centers in the brainstem. (A) Normal pigment in the substantia nigra *(left)* and locus ceruleus *(right)* of a young man. (B) Mild age-related loss of pigment in the brainstem of a normal individual *(right)* and loss of pigmented neurons in the brainstem of an individual with Parkinson disease *(PD) (left)*. (C) Mild depigmentation of the locus ceruleus (site of norepinephrine synthesis) in an aged individual *(right)* and severe depigmentation in an individual with PD *(left)*. (Courtesy Richard E. Powers, Director, Brain Resource Program, University of Alabama at Birmingham.)

striatal dopamine deficiency and intracellular inclusions containing aggregates of α-synuclein are the hallmarks of PD (Hayes, 2019). A deficiency in dopamine and a subsequent decrease in dopamine transmission to the basal ganglia result in an imbalance with ACh in the basal ganglia. The basal ganglia are shown in Fig. 13.1 in what is referred to as a *coronal* cut of the brain (a slice that runs from top to bottom with the outer edges of this view being close to the ears). Fig. 13.2 illustrates the depigmentation occurring in PD by comparing the substantia nigra and locus ceruleus (where norepinephrine is synthesized) of a young man (see Fig. 13.2A) with those of an older man without PD *(on the right)* and an older man with PD *(on the left)*. This figure clearly shows that normal aging results in a loss of pigmented neurons and that PD dramatically accelerates the process.

NORM'S NOTES As you might have guessed, I love understanding how drugs work and how a certain category of drug helps treat a specific mental disorder. I always start teaching my students about psychotropic drugs by discussing the antiparkinsonian drugs. Studying these drugs and PD itself provides a perfect vehicle for explaining neurotransmitter imbalance (and balance) and neuronal tract degeneration. In some ways, PD could be considered the opposite of schizophrenia, and overtreating schizophrenia can cause PD-type side effects. This is a great place to start.

EPSEs are also caused by an imbalance between ACh and dopamine (Fig. 13.3) but with an important difference: PD is related to neurodegeneration of the substantia nigra at the beginning of the dopamine tracts, whereas EPSEs are caused by the blockade of dopamine receptors in the basal ganglia at the end of the dopamine tracts (Lee & Muzio, 2020).

PD is treated with antiparkinsonian agents that increase dopamine levels (e.g., levodopa/carbidopa [Sinemet], dopamine agonists, or levodopa) and with anticholinergic agents (e.g., benztropine [Cogentin]), or with both (Poewe & Espay, 2020). A potential adjunct to levodopa is catechol-O-methyl transferase (COMT) inhibitors. The enzyme, COMT, converts a portion of the levodopa into a form that is useless to the body. COMT inhibitors work by blocking the COMT enzyme from converting levodopa into a useless form, meaning more levodopa is available to lessen PD symptoms (Hayes, 2019).

EPSEs are treated primarily with anticholinergics because psychosis is thought to be related to an increase in dopamine levels (Table 13.1). To give a dopamine-enhancing drug, such as levodopa, to a patient with schizophrenia would potentially cause psychotic symptoms to increase.

A challenging yet interesting clinical dilemma occurs when an individual suffering from PD develops a PD-psychosis. As

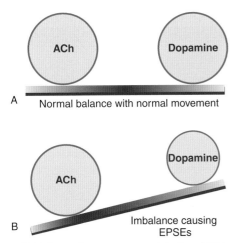

FIG. 13.3 (A) Balance between acetylcholine *(ACh)* and dopamine, resulting in normal movement. (B) Imbalance (too little dopamine) results in extrapyramidal side effects *(EPSEs)*.

BOX 13.1 How Can Parkinson Disease-Related Psychosis Be Treated?

Until very recently, the only truly effective antipsychotic available to treat PD-related psychosis was clozapine. Of course, as you will see in Chapter 14, clozapine has significant side effects. Now, there is a new choice of therapy for psychosis in PD, pimavanserin (Nuplazid). It is a promising new selective serotonin inverse agonist to treat hallucinations and delusions associated with PD-related psychosis. Pimavanserin not only preferentially targets 5-HT2A receptors but also avoids activity at dopamine and other receptors commonly targeted by antipsychotics (Hauser et al., 2020). Like all other antipsychotic drugs, pimavanserin has a black box warning on its package labeling in the United States of the increased prevalence for increasing mortality in elderly patients with dementia-related psychosis. Pimavanserin showed no undesirable effects on motor symptoms in patients with PD who have psychosis (Dashtipour et al., 2021).

PD, Parkinson disease.

noted, almost all antipsychotics will cause the PD to worsen. A newer drug, Pimavanserin, is a nondopaminergic, selective 5-HT2A inverse agonist/antagonist only approved for treatment of hallucinations and delusions associated with Parkinson disease psychoses. Pimavanserin binds mostly to 5-HT2A receptors and to some 5-HT2C receptors but has no binding affinity for dopaminergic, adrenergic, muscarinic, or histaminergic receptors; thus, it does not worsen the motor function in PD and white blood cell count does not need to be monitored (Dashtipour et al., 2021). Box 13.1 provides the latest thinking on this treatment dilemma.

? CRITICAL THINKING QUESTION

2. What is the connection between PD and schizophrenia from a neurotransmitter perspective? (*Hint:* You might need to look at the next chapter.)

Specific Extrapyramidal Side Effects

Although EPSEs are biochemically related to PD, they are not the same as PD. EPSEs are divided into at least seven distinct types. In addition to motor features, PD is also associated with many nonmotor symptoms, which add to overall disability (D'Souza & Hooten, 2020).

Table 13.2 provides further information on these disorders.

- *Akathisia:* Akathisia is a subjective feeling of restlessness that elicits restless legs, jittery feelings, and nervous energy. Akathisia is the most common EPSE and responds poorly to treatment.

- *Akinesia and bradykinesia:* Akinesia refers to an absence of movement, but a slowed movement (i.e., bradykinesia) is more likely. Symptoms include weakness, fatigue, painful muscles, and anergia. Akinesia often responds to anticholinergics.

- *Dystonias:* Dystonias are abnormal postures (i.e., muscle freezing) caused by involuntary muscle spasms. Symptoms manifest as sustained, twisted, and contracted positioning of the limbs, trunk, neck, or mouth. Dystonias tend to appear early in treatment (within about 3 days) and respond to anticholinergic drugs. These agents occasionally must be given parenterally because of the gravity of the situation. Types of dystonias include:
  - Torticollis—contracted positioning of the neck
  - Oculogyric crisis—contracted positioning of the eyes upward
  - Laryngeal—pharyngeal constriction (potentially life-threatening)

- *Drug-induced parkinsonism:* The cardinal symptoms of PD are experienced—tremor, rigidity, bradykinesia, and postural instability (Hayes, 2019).

- *Tardive dyskinesia (TD): Tardive* means "late appearing." This EPSE tends to develop late, after about 6 months of antipsychotic therapy. The dopamine-ACh imbalance does not cause TD, per se; consequently, anticholinergics are not administered for treatment. Anticholinergics generally worsen TD. Long-term use of antipsychotics is

TABLE 13.1 Model for Drug-Induced Parkinsonism

Clinical Manifestation	Theoretical Understanding	Possible Intervention	Effect of Intervention
Positive symptoms of schizophrenia	Increased levels of dopamine given	Dopamine (D$_2$) receptor blockers	Improvement of psychotic symptoms and possible development of EPSEs
EPSEs	Drug-induced imbalance between ACh and dopamine has occurred	Anticholinergic	Continued improvement in psychotic symptoms and amelioration of EPSEs (restored balance between dopamine and ACh)

ACh, Acetylcholine; *EPSEs*, extrapyramidal side effects.

TABLE 13.2 Extrapyramidal Side Effects Caused by Antipsychotic Drugs and Nursing Interventions

EPSE	Nursing Interventions
Akathisia	Be patient and reassure patient who is "jittery" that you understand the need to move and that appropriate drug interventions can help differentiate akathisia and agitation. Because akathisia is a major cause of nonadherence with antipsychotic regimens, switching to a different class of antipsychotic drug might be necessary to achieve adherence
Akinesia/bradykinesia	May or may not respond to anticholinergics. May want to reduce dose or change antipsychotics
Dystonias	If a severe reaction (e.g., oculogyric crisis, torticollis) occurs, give antiparkinsonian drug (e.g., benztropine [Cogentin]) or antihistamine (e.g., diphenhydramine [Benadryl]) immediately, as needed. Offer reassurance. If an order for intramuscular administration has not been written, call the physician at once to obtain the order. When an order for an antiparkinsonian drug is warranted for less severe dystonias, notify the physician
Drug-induced parkinsonism	Assess for major parkinsonism symptoms (tremors, rigidity, and bradykinesia); report to physician. Antiparkinsonian drugs are probably indicated
TD	Assess for signs by using AIMS. Drug holidays might help prevent TD. Anticholinergic agents can worsen TD; question their indiscriminate prophylactic use
Neuroleptic malignant syndrome	Be alert for this potentially fatal side effect. Routinely take temperatures, and encourage adequate water intake for all patients on a regimen of antipsychotic drugs; routinely assess for rigidity, tremor, and similar symptoms
Pisa syndrome	Treat with antiparkinsonian drugs

AIMS, Abnormal inventory movement scale; *EPSEs,* extrapyramidal side effects; *TD,* tardive dyskinesia.

thought to cause dopamine receptors in the basal ganglia to become hypersensitive. Symptoms are bothersome and can be embarrassing. Typical symptoms include tongue writhing, tongue protrusion, teeth grinding, and lip smacking. TD stops with sleep. Although TD movements can be suppressed willfully for a short time, they soon reappear. TD is often irreversible, but if caught in time it can be averted.

- In treating TD, valbenzapine (Ingrezza) is marketed as a vesicular monoamine transport inhibitor, and clinical trials support its efficacy. In a systematic review of 31 randomized controlled trials (RCTs) (i.e., 24 interventions and 1278 participants) to identify the effectiveness of various therapies (e.g., surgical and medical treatments, herbal agents, and electroconvulsive therapy) to treat TD, there was moderate-quality evidence of both valbenazine and extract of Ginkgo biloba, although other studies are needed, especially regarding the latter (Soares-Weiser, et al., 2018). In another systematic review of vesicular monoamine transporter 2 (VMAT-2) inhibitors, valbenazine and deutetrabenazine, empirical data also suggested that these agents are effective in treating TD in both acute and long-term stages, without an increased risk of either depression or suicide (Solmi et al., 2018). Other randomized clinical trials also reported the effectiveness of these two drugs. By comparison, other trials examining treatments for TD are limited methodologically and warrant further investigation (Caroff, 2020).
- *Neuroleptic malignant syndrome:* Neuroleptic malignant syndrome is a potentially lethal side effect of antipsychotic agents. Less than 1% of patients taking antipsychotics develop this problem, with a mortality rate of approximately 6%. Cardinal symptoms include hyperthermia

(temperature typically 101°F to 103°F but can increase to 108°F), rigidity, and autonomic dysfunction. Neuroleptic malignant syndrome can be treated with muscle relaxants and with centrally acting dopaminergics. Benzodiazepines (i.e., lorazepam [Ativan], diazepam [Valium], and clonazepam [Klonopin]) may also be used because of their efficacy in reversing the hypofunctioning GABAergic system that contributes to the neuroleptic malignant syndrome. Other treatment options are bromocriptine plus benzodiazepines for moderate symptoms, while dantrolene, bromocriptine, and benzodiazepines are used for those with significantly more disease severity. Associated complications include rhabdomyolysis and even mortality (Kiyingi et al., 2020). The majority of symptoms resolve within 1 to 2 weeks after withdrawal of antipsychotics; electroconvulsive therapy may be an option for patients with continuing symptoms (Caroff et al., 2021).

- *Pisa syndrome:* Pisa syndrome is a condition marked by the patient leaning to one side. It can be acute or tardive, and older adults are more vulnerable.

Women and elderly adults are more vulnerable to developing EPSEs than others. Box 13.2 lists populations at a higher risk for developing EPSEs from antipsychotics.

BOX 13.2 Populations at Higher Risk for Extrapyramidal Side Effects

1. Women
2. Patients with first episode of schizophrenia
3. Older adults
4. Patients with affective symptoms

From Keltner, N. L., & Folks, D. G. (2005). *Psychotropic drugs* (4th ed.). Mosby.

ANTICHOLINERGICS TO TREAT EXTRAPYRAMIDAL SIDE EFFECTS

Anticholinergic drugs commonly are used to treat EPSEs and work by restoring the imbalance caused by antipsychotic drugs. As noted, both in this chapter and in the next chapter, antipsychotic agents block (or antagonize) dopamine receptors. This dopamine receptor antagonism causes an artificial or iatrogenic parkinsonian-like syndrome, the aforementioned EPSEs. However, restoring the balance with a dopaminergic is inappropriate because, as the chapter on schizophrenia emphasizes, a compelling hypothesis for schizophrenia is the presence of excessive amounts of dopamine. Instead, anticholinergics (drugs that block cholinergic receptors) are used to restore the balance.

The following outline is repetitive but might be helpful:
1. Schizophrenia is linked to excessive dopamine.
2. Antipsychotic drugs block dopamine.
3. Blocked dopamine receptors can cause EPSEs.
4. Antiparkinsonian drugs can fix the problem that antipsychotics create.
5. If dopaminergic antiparkinsonian drugs are given, schizophrenia might worsen.
6. Anticholinergic drugs are given in an attempt to restore ACh-dopamine balance.

Several anticholinergic drugs are available to treat EPSEs. The site of action of these drugs for relieving EPSEs is the central nervous system (CNS). They also have pronounced peripheral effects. The prototype for this class of drugs is atropine, but it is not used to treat EPSEs. Atropine is most commonly used to reduce aspirating during surgery. Benztropine (Cogentin) is the most commonly prescribed anticholinergic for EPSEs, but diphenhydramine (Benadryl) is also effective. The relative anticholinergic potency of selected psychotropic drugs is given in Table 13.3. Table 13.4 lists the adult dosages of anticholinergics.

Chronic use of anticholinergics for EPSEs is not recommended in patients taking antipsychotics, especially those patients receiving second-generation antipsychotics. Negative side effects impact the daily lives of already seriously ill patients, including poor memory, dry mouth, constipation, blurred vision, urinary retention, and tachycardia. Continual monitoring of the effectiveness and necessity of psychiatric medications is essential, using the lowest possible dosage needed, based upon national and international guidelines. If used, anticholinergics should be re-evaluated at least every 3 months for their continuing usage to lessen EPSEs (Caroff, 2020; Lupu et al., 2021; Dur, 2019; Naja & Halaby, 2017).

To illustrate, Lupu et al. (2021) sought to taper or stop the chronic use of anticholinergics in patients with various disorders (i.e., schizophrenia, schizoaffective disorder, or bipolar disorder) who had no EPSEs, yet were taking anticholinergics for at least 6 months. Both education of health providers and clinical pharmacy support were used, and more than 75% of patients were able to either lessen their dosage or stop the use of anticholinergics, with significant improvement in their associated side effects, memory, and quality of life. Of the sample, 10% of patients were restarted on anticholinergics because of a return of EPSEs. These data suggest that some clinically stable patients may benefit from either tapering or stopping the chronic use of anticholinergic medications, with careful monitoring for return of EPSEs. Future clinical trials are needed to further assess the effectiveness of this strategy (Lupu et al., 2021).

Pharmacologic Effects

Antipsychotic drugs block dopamine receptors, frequently causing EPSEs. Many of the symptoms associated with naturally occurring PD—tremors, rigidity, and bradykinesia—are present in drug-induced parkinsonism, along with related symptoms, such as akathisia, dystonia, and dyskinesia. Blockade of dopamine receptors in the basal ganglia (i.e., nigrostriatal tract) produces EPSEs. High-potency antipsychotic agents, such as haloperidol (Haldol), cause EPSEs more often than low-potency or atypical agents. Additionally,

TABLE 13.3 Anticholinergic Effect of Frequently Prescribed Psychotropic Drugs Compared With Benztropine

Drug	Equivalent (mg)	Typical Use
Atropine	0.5	Given before surgery
Benztropine (Cogentin)	1	Antiparkinsonian
Trihexyphenidyl (Artane)	2	Antiparkinsonian
Biperiden (Akineton)	1	Antiparkinsonian
Amitriptyline (Elavil)	10	Antidepressant
Nortriptyline (Pamelor)	60	Antidepressant
Imipramine (Tofranil)	75	Antidepressant
Desipramine (Norpramin)	150	Antidepressant
Clozapine (Clozaril)	15	Antipsychotic
Chlorpromazine (Thorazine)	370	Antipsychotic
Diphenhydramine (Benadryl)	50	Antihistamine

Note: According to this table, 50 mg of Benadryl has the same anticholinergic effect as 1 mg of benztropine.
de Leon, J., Canuso, C., White, A. O., & Simpson, G. M. (1994). A pilot effort to determine benztropine equivalents of anticholinergic medications. *Hospital & Community Psychiatry, 45*(6), 606–607. https://doi.org/10.1176/ps.45.6.606

TABLE 13.4 Anticholinergic Adult Drug Dosages for Extrapyramidal Side Effects

Anticholinergic	Dosage
Benztropine (Cogentin)	EPSEs: 1–4 mg PO or IM once or twice a day For acute dystonic reactions: 1–2 mg IM/IV, then 1–2 mg PO twice a day
Trihexyphenidyl (Artane)	Start with 1 mg daily, then increase Usual dosage range: 5–15 mg/day

EPSEs, Extrapyramidal side effects; *IM*, intramuscularly; *IV*, intravenously; *PO*, orally.

several nonpsychiatric drugs cause EPSEs. These symptoms contribute to the discomfort, anxiety, and frustration of these already troubled patients and are major contributors to nonadherence. Patients taking antipsychotic drugs can experience a gradual or sudden onset of EPSEs.

CRITICAL THINKING QUESTION

3. Although you have not yet read the chapter on antidepressants (Chapter 15), it is known that selective serotonin reuptake inhibitors (SSRIs, such as fluoxetine [Prozac] or paroxetine [Paxil]) can cause EPSEs. Why is this the case?

Side Effects

Although clinicians tend to consider anticholinergic side effects to be less significant than EPSEs, not all patients agree. Anticholinergic drugs produce both CNS and peripheral nervous system (PNS) side effects (Table 13.5). CNS effects include confusion, cognitive impoverishment, agitation, dizziness, drowsiness, and disturbances in behavior. Because the cholinergic system contributes to memory and learning, anticholinergic drugs affect these cognitive functions as well. Ingesting drugs with anticholinergic properties can often explain recent changes in cognition in older adults (EPSEs). Because cognitive decline is a major symptom domain in schizophrenia, giving anticholinergics to patients with schizophrenia has proven to worsen mental abilities (Caroff, 2020; Lupu et al., 2020; Dur, 2019).

CRITICAL THINKING QUESTION

4. Why do older individuals have a more intense response to anticholinergics? (See Box 13.4 for the answer.)

PNS anticholinergic effects, such as dry mouth, blurred vision, nausea, and nervousness, occur in 30% to 50% of patients. Basically, peripheral anticholinergic side effects result from blocking the parasympathetic system (a cholinergic [ACh] system) (Table 13.6). Blurred vision results from pupils that dilate because of the blocking of ACh receptors of the third cranial nerve (CN III; oculomotor nerve). CN III constricts the pupil; when it is blocked, the pupil dilates. Dry mouth results when CN VII and CN IX (facial and glossopharyngeal nerves) are blocked from causing salivation. Decreased tearing is related to blockage of CN VII. Although these problems are annoying, they are not usually major health hazards. However, when the CN X (vagus nerve) is blocked, tachycardia can occur and cause serious problems. Why? See Norm's Notes for the answer.

 NORM'S NOTES The sinoatrial node has a rhythm of 100 to 120 impulses per minute. Hearts do not beat this fast because the parasympathetic system provides a braking action. When anticholinergic drugs are given, part of the brake is removed, which can result in major problems, particularly for older individuals.

Constipation, a problem with patients with parkinsonism secondary to rigidity, can be worsened by anticholinergics as well. Urinary hesitancy and retention and decreased sweating are other PNS effects. Patients who drool or perspire excessively might welcome dry mouth and decreased sweating. However, because of the risk of hyperthermia, reduced sweating may be a significant issue. Box 13.3 lists the more serious risks associated with anticholinergic use.

Nursing Implications for Anticholinergic Drugs
Therapeutic Versus Toxic Dose Levels

Therapeutic dose ranges are listed in Table 13.4. Doses above therapeutic ranges can cause toxic effects. Overdose might result in CNS hyperstimulation (confusion, excitement, hyperpyrexia, agitation, disorientation, delirium, or

---

TABLE 13.5   Peripheral Nervous System Side Effects and Nursing Interventions for Anticholinergics

Side Effects	Nursing Interventions
Dry mouth	Offer sugarless hard candy and chewing gum; encourage frequent rinses; take medication before meals
Nasal congestion	Recommend over-the-counter nasal decongestant, if approved by physician
Urinary hesitation	Introduce running water, privacy, warm water over perineum
Urinary retention	Catheterize for residual fluids; encourage frequent voiding
Blurred vision, photophobia	Provide reassurance (normal vision typically returns in a few weeks); encourage sunglasses; advise caution when driving (tolerance develops). Pilocarpine (a muscarinic agonist that causes pupil constriction) eye drops may be given
Constipation	Give laxatives, as ordered; encourage diet with fiber; recommend 2500–3000 mL of water daily
Mydriasis	If eye pain develops, undiagnosed narrow-angle glaucoma might be the cause; immediate attention is warranted
Decreased sweating	Decreased sweating can lead to fever; take temperature; if fever occurs, reduce body temperature (e.g., sponge baths)
Fever	Advise limited strenuous activity; encourage patient to wear appropriate clothing

Desmarais, J. E., Beauclair, L., & Margolese, H. (2012). Anticholinergics in the era of atypical antipsychotics: Short-term or long- term treatment? *Journal of Psychopharmacology (Oxford, England), 26*(9), 1167–1174. https://doi.org/10.1177/0269881112447988.

TABLE 13.6 Anticholinergic Effects on Cranial Nerves With Parasympathetic Functions

Cranial Nerve	Parasympathetic Function	Anticholinergic Effect
III	Constricts pupils	Mydriasis (dilates pupils), blurred vision
	Alters shape of lens	Impairs accommodation
VII	Salivation	Dry mouth
	Lacrimation	Decreased tearing
	Nasal mucous secretion	Dry nasal passage
IX	Salivation	Dry mouth
	Nasal mucous secretion	Dry nasal passage
X	Slows heart rate	Tachycardia
	Promotes peristalsis	Slows peristalsis; constipation
	Constricts bronchi	Dilates bronchi
	Promotes urination	Urinary hesitancy or retention

hallucinations) or CNS depression (drowsiness, sedation, or coma). The cardiovascular, urinary, and gastrointestinal systems are particularly involved. The eyes are also affected. High fevers are the result of the CNS effects of anticholinergics and their ability to decrease sweating. The goal is to avoid chronic use of anticholinergic drugs, and both nurses and other health providers should work with patients in assessing the effectiveness of their antipsychotic medications and whether these patients potentially can decrease or discontinue the use of anticholinergics without experiencing a return of significant EPSEs.

Use During Pregnancy

Anticholinergics should be used cautiously during pregnancy. Theoretically, these drugs would decrease milk flow during lactation.

Use in Older Adults

As this chapter and other chapters in this text have emphasized, older individuals are particularly sensitive to anticholinergic agents (Box 13.4). Cognitive, cardiovascular, and gastrointestinal side effects are more pronounced in older

BOX 13.3 Risks Associated With Anticholinergic Use

1. Might be lethal in overdose
2. Might induce dependence
3. Might exacerbate tardive dyskinesia
4. Might induce psychosis
5. Might cause erectile dysfunction
6. Might cause paralytic ileus

From Houltram, B., & Scanlan, M. (2004). Extrapyramidal side effects. *Nursing Standard, 18*(43), 39–41. https://doi.org/10.7748/ns2004.07.18.43.39.c3641.

BOX 13.4 Why Older Individuals Have a More Pronounced Reaction to Anticholinergics

Slower metabolism
Slower elimination
Deficits in cholinergic transmission

From Ozbilen, M., & Adams, C. E. (2009). Systematic overview of Cochrane reviews for anticholinergic effects of antipsychotic drugs. *Journal of Clinical Psychopharmacology, 29*(2), 141–146. https://doi.org/ 10.1097/JCP.0b013e31819a91f1.

patients compared with younger patients. Difficulties in older men with prostatic enlargement can be exacerbated with the use of these agents. Cognitive impairment is also associated with anticholinergic drugs (Caroff, 2020; Lupu et al., 2021; Dur, 2019).

Side Effect Interventions

Numerous annoying side effects are associated with anticholinergic drugs (Table 13.5). Several nondrug alternatives to help the patient are listed in Table 13.5.

Interactions With Anticholinergic Drugs

The nurse should alert the patient to the dangers of over-the-counter drugs and other prescription drugs that intensify the atropine-like effects of centrally acting anticholinergics. Other interactions include an intensification of sedative effects when combined with CNS depressants and a decrease in absorption when combined with antacids and antidiarrheal drugs.

Teaching Patients

In addition to teaching appropriate information about side effects, the nurse should emphasize certain points. The patient and family should be advised of the following:

- Avoid discontinuing these drugs abruptly.
- Tapering off over a 1-week period is advised.
- Avoid driving or other hazardous activities until tolerance develops and drowsiness and blurred vision diminish.
- Avoid over-the-counter medications (e.g., cough and cold preparations) that have anticholinergic or antihistamine properties; alcohol, which exacerbates CNS depression; and antacids, which interfere with the absorption of anticholinergics.

Selected Anticholinergic Drugs

Benztropine

Benztropine (Cogentin) is used to treat all parkinsonian-like disorders, including drug-induced EPSEs. Benztropine, which is the most frequently prescribed anticholinergic antiparkinsonian drug, is usually given orally but can be given intramuscularly for nonadherent psychotic patients, and intramuscularly or intravenously for acute dystonic reactions.

Diphenhydramine

Diphenhydramine (Benadryl), the prototype antihistamine, is effective for most parkinsonian-like disorders.

Diphenhydramine can cause considerable sedation in some individuals and little in others; it is considerably less potent than benztropine (see Table 13.3).

Trihexyphenidyl

Trihexyphenidyl (Artane) was the first anticholinergic used extensively for EPSEs. Because trihexyphenidyl is unavailable in parenteral form, its use for acute dystonias is limited.

OTHER TREATMENT OPTIONS FOR EXTRAPYRAMIDAL SIDE EFFECTS

Drugs

Although anticholinergic agents are the mainstay of treatment and prophylaxis of EPSEs, several other agents are available as well, including the following:

- Dopamine agonist—amantadine (Symmetrel)
- Beta blocker—propranolol (Inderal)
- Benzodiazepines—diazepam (Valium), lorazepam (Ativan), clonazepam (Klonopin)

Work with health providers concerning whether reducing the dosage, administering medications only at bedtime, or changing the type of antipsychotic medications (e.g., atypical) contributing to EPSEs would be beneficial (Koola, 2018). Please note that empirical recommendations regarding the best approach to lessen EPSEs in relation to antipsychotic medication is inadequate at this point, with the majority of studies having methodological flaws and being short-term. Hence, conducting longitudinal studies that explore antipsychotic therapy and how to best reduce EPSEs are essential (Bergman et al., 2018).

Vitamins

Both vitamins E and B_6 have some empirical support for their abilities to diminish symptoms associated with TD. Anecdotal evidence also suggests that some patients benefit from vitamin E. Whether this vitamin actually reduces TD symptoms or prevents further deterioration has been debated by many nurses and physicians.

PREVENTION

The best approach to treating EPSEs is prevention. By following a few simple guidelines, both the prescriber and the nurse can reduce EPSE incidence (Hayes, 2019). Enhanced patient care requires the following (in about this order):

1. Establish whether the patient is from a high-risk group (see Box 13.2).
2. Obtain baseline information about EPSEs using a validated tool.
3. Choose an antipsychotic with a lower probability of causing EPSEs (although this is disputed):
   a. High-risk agents—haloperidol (Haldol), fluphenazine (Prolixin), and maybe other traditional antipsychotics.
   b. Lower risk agents—clozapine (Clozaril), quetiapine (Seroquel), and perhaps other atypical antipsychotics.
4. Monitor the patient on a regular basis.
5. If EPSEs develop, consider switching to an atypical drug. If the patient is already taking an atypical drug, lower the dose or change to another atypical drug with a better side effect profile. Add an antiparkinsonian agent but continually monitor its necessity every 3 months.

CASE STUDY

A 25-year-old woman who is taking an antipsychotic drug (haloperidol) starts to experience psychomotor slowing as she walks down the hallway of the hospital. Before she reaches the end of the hall, she requires assistance. Within 2 min of sitting down, her neck becomes rigidly hyperextended, and her eyes roll upward in a fixed stare. Her breathing becomes labored because of the position of her neck, and she is frightened. Because she is also delusional, it is difficult to imagine what this frightening side effect of her medication represents to her. Benztropine, 2 mg, is given intramuscularly and repeated in 15 min because she did not respond as quickly as was hoped. Within another 5 min, she was back to her "normal" self.

STUDY NOTES

1. PD is related to degeneration of the substantia nigra, the dopamine-generating portion of the brain; however, the cause is unknown.
2. EPSEs, a type of parkinsonism (cause known), develop when dopamine receptors in the basal ganglia are blocked by antipsychotic or other drugs.
3. Normal muscle activity requires a balance between dopamine and ACh; consequently, a dopamine deficiency is responsible for symptoms of PD.
4. The four primary symptoms associated with PD are tremors, bradykinesia, rigidity, and postural instability.
5. Drug treatment of PD is based on reestablishing a balance between dopamine and ACh.
6. Drug treatment for EPSEs is based on blocking ACh receptors. Administering a dopaminergic drug could exacerbate psychotic symptoms.
7. The three major anticholinergic antiparkinsonian drugs are benztropine (Cogentin), trihexyphenidyl (Artane), and the classic antihistamine diphenhydramine (Benadryl).
8. Anticholinergic drugs have many side effects. Older individuals are particularly sensitive to these side effects.

REFERENCES

Bergman, H., Rathbone, J., Agarwal, V., Soares-Weiser, K., & Cochrane Schizophrenia Group, (2018). Antipsychotic reduction and/or cessation and antipsychotics as specific treatments for tardive dyskinesia. *Cochrane Database Systematic Reviews, 2018*(2), CD000459. https://doi.org/10.1002/14651858.CD000459.pub3.

Caroff. S. N. (2020). Recent advances in the pharmacology of tardive dyskinesia. *Clinical Psychopharmacology and Neuroscience, 18*(4), 493–506. https://doi.org/10.9758/cpn.2020.18.4.493.

Caroff, S. N., Watson, C. B., & Rosenberg, H. (2021). Drug-induced hyperthermic syndromes in psychiatry. *Clinical Psychopharmacology and Neuroscience, 19*(1), 1–11. https://doi.org/10.9758/cpn.2021.19.1.1.

Dashtipour, K., Gupta, F., Hauser, R. A., Karunapuzha, C. A., & Morgan, J. C. (2021). *Parkinsonson's disease, 2021*, 2603641. https://doi.org/10.1155/2021/2603641.

de Leon, J., Canuso, C., White, A. O., & Simpson, G. M. (1994). A pilot effort to determine benztropine equivalents of anticholinergic medications. *Hospital & Community Psychiatry, 45*(6), 606–607. https://doi.org/10.1176/ps.45.6.606.

Desmarais, J. E., Beauclair, L., & Margolese, H. (2012). Anticholinergics in the era of atypical antipsychotics: Short-term or long-term treatment? *Journal of Psychopharmacology (Oxford, England), 26*(9), 1167–1174. https://doi.org/10.1177/0269881112447988.

D'Souza, R.S., & Hooten, W.M. (2020). Extrapyramidal symptoms. StatPearls [Internet]. StatPearls Publishing. PMID, 30475568. https://www.ncbi.nlm.nih.gov/books/NBK534115/.

Dur, Medi-Cal (2019 September). https://www.hpsj.com/clinical-review-update-concomitant-anticholinergic-and-antipsychotic-use/.

Hauser, R.A. (2020). Parkinson disease treatment & management. http://emedicine.medscape.com/article/1831191-treatment?pa=8YjRX59QoDk7R3fBI8q%2F9okM%2Flm5p3UWbUgQO4%2FUiqCMAa7aoGLqyM94t PnCS7RP5Yi6BJXUtzO3z%2FgRyE PNX%2BejCO3Rk4DWsD37 DrSZWvU%3D.

Hayes. T. M. (2019). Parkinson's disease and parkinsonism. *American Journal of Medicine, 132*(7), 802–807. https://doi.org/10.1016/j.amjmed.2019.03.001.

Houltram, B., & Scanlan, M. (2004). Extrapyramidal side effects. *Nursing Standard, 18*(43), 39–41. https://doi.org/10.7748/ns2004.07.18.43.39.c3641.

Keltner, N. L., & Folks, D. G. (2005). *Psychotropic drugs* (4th ed.). Mosby.

Kiyingi, M., Bongomin, F., Kizito, M., & Kaddumukasa, M. (2020). Neuroleptic malignant syndrome: Early diagnosis saves lives in low-resource settings. *International Medical Case Reports Journal, 13*, 359–362. https://doi.org/10.2147/IMCRJ.S270332.

Koola. M. M. (2018). Anticholinergics to treat antipsychotic-induced extrapyramidal symptoms: Time to avoid this practice. *Asian Journal of Psychiatry, 31*, 100–101. https://doi.org/10.1016/j.ajp.2018.01.009.

Lee, J., & Muzio, M. R. (2020). *Neuroanatomy, extrapyramidal system. In StatPearls [Internet]*. StatPearls Publishing. PMID: 32119429.

Lupu, A. M., MacCamy, K. L., Gannon, J. M., Brar, J. S., & Chengappa, K. R. (2021). Less is more: Deprescribing anticholinergic medications in persons with severe mental illness. *Annals of Clinical Psychiatry, 33*(1), e1–e13. https://doi.org/10.12788/acp.0019.

Marras, C., Beck, J. C., Bower, J. H., et al. (2018). Prevalence of Parkinson's disease across North America. *npj Parkinson's Disease, 4*, 21. https://doi.org/10.1038/s41531-018-0058-0.

Naja, W. J., & Halaby, A. (2017). Anticholinergic use and misuse in psychiatry: A comprehensive and critical review. *Journal of Alcoholism & Drug Dependence, 5*(2), 1000263. https://doi.org/10.4172/2329-6488.1000263.

Nestler, E.J., Hyman, S.E., Holtzman, D.M., & Malenka, R.C. (2015). Molecular neuropharmacology: A foundation for clinical neuroscience (3rd ed.). McGraw-Hill.

Ozbilen, M., & Adams, C. E. (2009). Systematic overview of Cochrane reviews for anticholinergic effects of antipsychotic drugs. *Journal of Clinical Psychopharmacology, 29*(2), 141–146. https://doi.org/10.1097/JCP.0b013e31819a91f1.

Poewe, W., & Espay, A. J. (2020). Long duration response in Parkinson's disease: Levodopa revisited. *Brain, 143*(8), 2332–2335. https://doi.org/10.1093/brain/awaa226.

Solmi, M., Pigato, G., Kane, J. M., & Correll, C. U. (2018). Treatment of tardive dyskinesia with VMAT-2 inhibitors: A systematic review and meta-analysis of randomized controlled trials. *Drug Design Development and Therapy, 2018*, 1215–1238. https://doi.org/10.2147/DDDT.S133205.

Soares-Weiser, K., Rathbone, J., Ogawa, Y., Shinohara, K., Bergman, H., & Cochrane Schizophrenia Group, (2018). Miscellaneous treatments for antipsychotic-induced tardive dyskinesia. *Cochrane Database Systematic Reviews, 2018*(3), CD000208. https://doi.org/10.1002/14651858.pub2.

van der Velden, R. M., Broen, M. P., Kuijf, M. L., & Leentjens, A. F. (2018). Frequency of mood and anxiety fluctuations in Parkinson's disease patients with motor fluctuations: A systematic review. *Movement Disorders, 33*(10), 1521–1527. https://doi.org/10.1002/mds.27465.

14

Antipsychotic Drugs

Marie Smith-East and Norman L. Keltner

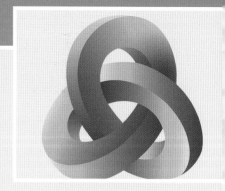

The brain simply does not possess the heart's machine-like, linear functioning. Therefore, targeting individual parts (i.e., receptors) will not equate to fixing the whole organ systematically or predictably.

Willa Xiong, MD (2017)

ⓔ http://evolve.elsevier.com/Keltner

LEARNING OBJECTIVES

- Explain the concept of neurotransmitters, specifically dopamine, in relation to psychosis.
- Identify the clinical uses of first-generation, second-generation (or atypical), and third-generation (also called atypical) antipsychotic drugs.
- Recognize differences between high-potency and low-potency first-generation antipsychotic drugs.
- Identify representative high-potency, low-potency, and atypical antipsychotic drugs, including the specific side effects and interactions of each drug.

- Describe the two theories of atypicality for second-generation antipsychotics.
- Explain the key pharmacodynamic trait that differentiates third-generation antipsychotics.
- Describe signs and symptoms associated with extrapyramidal side effects.
- Describe potential interactions of antipsychotic drugs.
- Discuss implications for teaching patients about antipsychotic drugs.

BLACK BOX WARNING FOR ANTIPSYCHOTICS

Elderly patients with dementia-related psychosis treated with antipsychotic drugs are at increased risk of death.

Antipsychotic drugs are used to treat schizophrenia, schizoaffective disorder, bipolar disorder, and psychotic depressions, as well as various other psychiatric disorders. Additionally, these drugs have numerous off-label uses, such as the treatment of insomnia, tics, delirium, stuttering, and even hiccoughs. Because of their widespread use, spending on antipsychotics in the United States is a multibillion-dollar industry. In fact, recognized as the best-selling prescription (i.e., dollar-sales) in the United States in recent years has been the antipsychotic drug Abilify (the last year of its patent protection).

Antipsychotics were discovered accidentally around 1950. A French scientist was hoping to develop a new antihistamine and, in the process, formulated chlorpromazine, which was initially used to calm presurgery jitters but was soon found to possess antipsychotic properties. Chlorpromazine is considered the first antipsychotic drug.

Before the introduction and acceptance of chlorpromazine and many related drugs, hundreds of thousands of patients with severe psychiatric disturbances were hospitalized, many never to be released. These patients were isolated, physically restrained, and occasionally subjected to psychosurgery (lobotomy). These treatments rarely restored patients to a state that enabled them to function productively or to interact in a reasonably normal way with others.

The role of antipsychotic medications in relapse and recovery of symptoms of schizophrenia and nonaffective psychosis over the past 100 years has been influential, with data suggesting that antipsychotic treatment, particularly during the first 5 years of illness can positively influence the long-term quality of life in these individuals (Begemann et al., 2020; Taylor & Jauhar, 2019). The drugs discussed in this chapter are generally called *antipsychotic agents*, but historically they have also been referred to as *major tranquilizers, ataractics* (drugs that produce calmness or serenity), and *neuroleptics* (Greek for "neuron clasping").

NORM'S NOTES There are two categories of drugs that dominate psychiatric care—antipsychotics and antidepressants. I think that the antipsychotics are the more important category. Many years ago, when I worked in a large state hospital, the antipsychotics had only recently been introduced. Some of the staff had worked there since the 1930s, and I was fascinated with their stories of the pre-Thorazine days when the hospital could only be described as a madhouse—so much pain, so much agony. Although some problems still exist, antipsychotics have made a significant difference in many people's lives.

CLASSIFICATION SYSTEMS: FIRST-GENERATION ANTIPSYCHOTICS, SECOND-GENERATION ANTIPSYCHOTICS, AND THIRD-GENERATION ANTIPSYCHOTICS

Antipsychotic drugs are conceptualized in three ways. The categories are:

1. Traditional or first-generation antipsychotics (FGAs),
2. Atypical or second-generation antipsychotics (SGAs), and
3. Atypical or third-generation antipsychotics (TGAs).

Antipsychotic drugs are listed under these headings in Table 14.1. Antipsychotics have diverse chemical properties, but all effectively reduce various psychiatric symptoms. The type, intensity, and frequency of side effects vary among these drugs because of intrinsic differences.

FGAs, developed between 1950 and 1990, are further divided based on potency.

Subclassification based on potency has support because of its clinical utility. Essentially, the effects of traditional antipsychotics are related to the blockade of a specific type of dopamine receptor (D_2; Box 14.1). Clinical effectiveness occurs when 60% to 70% of these receptors are blocked in a certain area of the brain (which is discussed later in the chapter). Some of the drugs have *high milligrams but low potency*. For example, approximately 100 mg of chlorpromazine (a low-potency traditional drug) is required to achieve the same clinical effect or block the same number of D_2 receptors as 2 mg of haloperidol (a high-potency traditional drug). This classification system is not perfect. A few traditional drugs do not fall comfortably into either a high-potency or a low-potency group (hence a moderate-potency category). Nonetheless, this dichotomy is clinically significant because low-potency drugs tend to cause more intense anticholinergic effects

Drug	Usual Adult Maintenance Range (mg/day)	Rate of EPSEs	Rate of Anticholinergic Effects	Rate of Orthostasis	Rate of Sedation	Rate of Weight Gain
TABLE 14.1 Major Antipsychotic Drugs: Three Generations						
First-Generation Antipsychotics (Traditional)						
High-Potency Drug						
Haloperidol (Haldol)	1–15	High	Low	Low	Low	Low
Moderate-Potency Drug						
Perphenazine	12–64	High	Low	Low	Moderate	Low
Low-Potency Drug						
Chlorpromazine (Thorazine)	200–1000	Moderate	Moderate	High	Moderate	High
Second-Generation Antipsychotics (Atypical)						
Asenapine (Saphris)	10–20	Low	Low	Low	Moderate	Moderate
Clozapine (Clozaril)	75–900	Low	High	High	High	High
Iloperidone (Fanapt)	12–24	Low	Moderate	Moderate	Moderate	Moderate
Lurasidone (Latuda)	40–80	Low	Low	Low	Low	Low
Olanzapine (Zyprexa)	5–20	Low	Moderate	Low	High	High
Paliperidone (Invega)	3–12	Low	Low	Moderate	Moderate	Moderate
Quetiapine (Seroquel)	200–800	Low	Low	Moderate	Moderate	Moderate
Risperidone (Risperdal)	0.5–6.0	Low[a]	Low	Moderate	Moderate	Moderate
Ziprasidone (Geodon)	40–160	Low	Low	Low	Low	Low
Third-Generation Antipsychotics (Atypical)						
Aripiprazole (Abilify)	10–30	Low	Low	Low	Low	Low
Brexpiprazole (Rexulti)	2–4	Low	Low	Low	Low	Low
Cariprazine (Vraylar)	1.5–6	Low	Low	Low	Low	Low

EPSEs, Extrapyramidal side effects.
[a]However, EPSEs develop at high doses.

BOX 14.1 **Effects of Blocking Dopamine D$_2$ Receptors**

60%–70%—optimal clinical effect
~70%—elevated prolactin
~80%—extrapyramidal side effects

From Jindal, R. D., & Keshavan, M. S. (2008). Classifying antipsychotic agents: Need for new terminology. *CNS Drugs, 22*, 1047.

TABLE 14.2 Theoretical Effects of Receptor Blockade

Receptor	Effects
D$_2$	Mesolimbic tract: Antipsychotic effect
	Nigrostriatal tract: EPSEs
	Tuberoinfundibular tract: Prolactin level elevation
	Mesocortical tract: Secondary negative symptoms (caused by antipsychotics)
5-HT$_{2A}$	Improves negative symptoms; decreased EPSEs
M$_1$	Anticholinergic side effects
H$_1$	Sedation, orthostasis, weight gain
Alpha-1	Orthostasis, dizziness, sedation
Alpha-2	Sexual dysfunction
GABA	Lowers seizure threshold; produces anxiety

EPSEs, Extrapyramidal side effects; *GABA*, gamma-aminobutyric acid; *5-HT2A*, 5-hydroxytryptamine 2A; *M1*, cholinergic muscarinic receptors.

(e.g., dry mouth, blurred vision) and antiadrenergic effects (e.g., orthostatic hypotension), whereas high-potency drugs cause more extrapyramidal side effects (EPSEs) and prolactin elevation. Knowing this difference prepares the nurse for the most likely set of side effects. As a general rule, drugs with increased anticholinergic effects, such as chlorpromazine, produce fewer EPSEs (see Table 14.1). Table 14.2 outlines the theoretical effects of a specific receptor blockade.

The SGAs are different. These agents (from 1990 onwards) are often referred to as *atypical* because of the following characteristics:

1. Reduced risk for EPSEs
2. Increased effectiveness in treating negative symptoms (though no antipsychotic has proven to cause a significant improvement in negative symptoms)
3. Minimal risk of tardive dyskinesia (TD)
4. Reduced risk for elevated prolactin

TGAs are different still (i.e., atypical). TGAs cause fewer anticholinergic, prolactin, blood pressure, and cardiac effects. A more complete description of their unique mechanism of action will be provided later.

NEUROCHEMICAL THEORY OF SCHIZOPHRENIA

The neurochemical theory affords the best explanation for the effectiveness of antipsychotic agents. This theory states that increased levels of dopamine in the limbic area of the brain cause schizophrenia and its positive symptoms (e.g., hallucinations, delusions). Because antipsychotic drugs are primarily dopamine blockers, it follows that their effectiveness can be attributed to this dopamine-blocking activity. This theory of schizophrenia is supported by clinical observations and clinical research, both of which demonstrate that high doses of the dopaminergic drugs levodopa and amphetamine can produce schizophrenic symptoms.

However, this explanation does not answer all the questions surrounding the issue, most specifically questions regarding *negative* and cognitive symptoms. Fig. 14.1 provides additional useful information. As shown in Fig. 14.1, the brain has four major dopaminergic tracts. Dopamine is synthesized primarily in the substantia nigra and ventral tegmental area and is delivered to distant sites via dopaminergic tracts. To appreciate the complexity of psychopharmacologic treatment of schizophrenia fully, the student must recognize the existence of dopamine-dependent areas of the brain that communicate with dopamine-synthesizing areas (substantia nigra and ventral tegmental areas in the midbrain) via different neuronal tracts.

Tract 1: The nigrostriatal tract is involved in MOVEMENT. Traditional antipsychotic blockade can *cause EPSEs*.

Tract 2: The tuberoinfundibular tract modulates PITUITARY function. Traditional antipsychotic blockade can lead to *elevation in prolactin levels*.

Tract 3: The mesolimbic tract is involved in EMOTIONAL and SENSORY processes. Traditional antipsychotic blockade normalizes these processes in individuals with schizophrenia, *relieving or eliminating hallucinations and delusions*.

Tract 4: The mesocortical tract is involved in COGNITIVE processes. Traditional antipsychotic blockade can *intensify negative and cognitive problems*.

Traditional antipsychotics can do all of the above, but this is a high price to pay to be free of hallucinations and delusions caused by only one of these tracts (i.e., Tract #3 above).

The ultimate antipsychotic agent might block dopamine receptors in the mesolimbic area (decreasing hallucinations and delusions) and liberate dopamine in the mesocortical area (treating negative and cognitive symptoms), while neither obstructing the function of the nigrostriatal tract (i.e., not causing EPSEs) nor blocking receptors in the tuberoinfundibular tract (i.e., not elevating prolactin levels). SGAs and TGAs were originally said to do this. However, with years of usage and closer analysis, these early pronouncements were somewhat optimistic. It can be said with a large measure of confidence that SGAs and TGAs are significantly less likely to cause EPSEs and hyperprolactinemia.

OVERVIEW

Pharmacologic Effects

Antipsychotic drugs are used primarily to treat psychotic disorders—specifically, schizophrenia, bipolar disorder, and

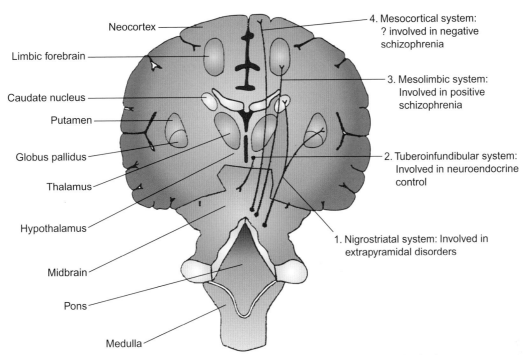

FIG. 14.1 Four dopaminergic tracts are important for understanding the actions of antipsychotic drugs.

Labels (from figure):
- Neocortex
- Limbic forebrain
- Caudate nucleus
- Putamen
- Globus pallidus
- Thalamus
- Hypothalamus
- Midbrain
- Pons
- Medulla
- 4. Mesocortical system: ? involved in negative schizophrenia
- 3. Mesolimbic system: Involved in positive schizophrenia
- 2. Tuberoinfundibular system: Involved in neuroendocrine control
- 1. Nigrostriatal system: Involved in extrapyramidal disorders

other chronic mental illness. Tolerance to their antipsychotic effect is uncommon.

Central nervous system (CNS) effects include emotional quieting and sedation, which explains why these drugs previously were generally referred to as *major tranquilizers*. Emotional quieting enables the patient to take advantage of other forms of therapeutic intervention, for example, the therapeutic nurse-patient relationship and the well-managed milieu.

Sedation decreases insomnia, a frequent complaint of psychotic patients. Whether this is a result of the sedating effect itself or of being free from disturbing thoughts (or a combination of the two) is not fully understood. Not all antipsychotic drugs are significantly sedating and yet are still therapeutic. The conclusion that the effectiveness of antipsychotic agents results from more than their tranquilizing qualities alone is reasonable.

Psychiatric Symptoms Modified by Antipsychotic Drugs

A tranquilizing effect occurs within an hour or so after ingestion. Antipsychotic effects are often observed within the first 2 weeks, with improvement continuing for 6 to 8 weeks (Haddad & Correll, 2018). D_2 blockade develops on the first dose. The lag time required for a clinical response surely indicates that neuronal adaptations must occur before a therapeutic response is seen.

Antipsychotic drugs are most effective in treating the positive symptoms of schizophrenia (Box 14.2). Positive symptoms include hallucinations and delusions. Negative symptoms are less responsive to antipsychotic drugs, including the newer agents. Negative symptoms develop over an extended period and include flattened affect, verbal paucity,

---

BOX 14.2 Positive and Negative Symptoms of Schizophrenia

Positive Symptoms: Caused by Excessive Dopamine in Mesolimbic Tract[a]
Abnormal thoughts
Agitation
Bizarre behavior
Delusions
Excitement
Feelings of persecution
Grandiosity
Hallucinations
Hostility
Illusions
Insomnia
Suspiciousness

Negative Symptoms: Caused by Too Little Dopamine in Mesocortical Tract[a]
Alogia
Anergia
Asocial behavior
Attention deficits
Avolition
Blunted affect
Communication difficulties
Difficulty with abstractions
Passive social withdrawal
Poor grooming and hygiene
Poor rapport
Poverty of speech

[a] This is an oversimplification of what is going on in the frontal and limbic lobes of the brain.

and a lack of drive or goal-directed activity. Referring again to Fig. 14.1, the student can infer that positive symptoms arise from too much dopamine in the limbic area (hyperactive mesolimbic tract) and that negative symptoms arise from too little dopamine in the cortex (hypoactive mesocortical tract). It stands to reason that antipsychotic drugs that are strictly dopamine antagonists are better at decreasing the effect of dopamine in the limbic area than they are at increasing the effect of dopamine in the cerebral cortex. As discussed later in this chapter, atypical agents can increase the dopamine level in one area of the brain while decreasing it in another.

Ultimately, improvement in positive and negative symptoms is the measurement of progress. Psychotic symptoms associated with other mental disorders also improve with these drugs.

Alterations of Perception

As a rule, the more bizarre the behavior of a person experiencing psychotic symptoms (more positive symptoms), the more likely that an antipsychotic drug will be beneficial. Hallucinations and illusions are reduced with these drugs. Even when the symptoms are not fully eradicated, antipsychotic drugs might enable the person to understand that hallucinations and illusions are not real, which is an improvement.

Alterations of Thought

Antipsychotic drugs improve reasoning, decrease ambivalence, and decrease delusions. Because clouded reasoning, ambivalence, and delusional thoughts are frustrating and sometimes frightening, antipsychotic agents can free the patient to think more clearly and communicate better with others.

Alterations of Activity

Individuals with schizophrenia are often hyperactive because of their internal turmoil and, perhaps, their neurochemical state. Antipsychotic drugs slow psychomotor activity.

Alterations in Consciousness

Mental clouding and confusion are anxiety-producing symptoms associated with psychosis. Some mental health professionals believe that these disorders are the most disabling. Antipsychotic drugs are effective in decreasing confusion and clouding.

Alterations in Personal Relationships

Patients with schizophrenia often have histories of social withdrawal and might have few, if any, close personal relationships. If relationships with family members exist, they are often strained. Individuals with schizophrenia may invest little effort in their appearance and may not be particularly careful about their behavior. The combination of introspection, rumination, and self-focused speech produces ineffective communication patterns that reinforce isolation and alienation. In the give-and-take atmosphere of society, individuals with schizophrenia often have little to give and, as a result, are basically socially unattractive to most people. Antipsychotic drugs potentially

can enable patients to become less focused on themselves and more focused on others. The socially damaging, self-absorbed thinking experienced by patients with schizophrenia might be a result of the considerable energy they must expend to maintain some degree of equilibrium in the face of psychological turmoil; this is similar to the way that many people give less attention to their appearance or behavior during an acute illness. Antipsychotic drugs reduce the inner turmoil, freeing psychic energy for normal interpersonal relationships and for the therapeutic nurse–patient relationship.

? CRITICAL THINKING QUESTION

1. If the following are true then…
2. … why is it that patients who receive SGAs do not develop more symptoms of schizophrenia? (Hint: Read my response to the "Very Attentive Student" question later on in this chapter.)
   a. Excessive bioavailability of dopamine causes the positive symptoms of schizophrenia.
   b. SGAs are effective because they increase dopamine (5-HT_{2A} antagonism and all that).

Alterations of Affect

Affective flattening, blunting, inappropriateness, and lability are affective symptoms sometimes associated with schizophrenia that often respond to antipsychotic drugs. However, a flat affect is a cardinal symptom of negative schizophrenia and might respond only to an atypical antipsychotic drug.

Pharmacokinetics

A detailed pharmacokinetic discussion of each antipsychotic agent is beyond the scope of this text. Rather, an overview of significant pharmacokinetic mechanisms is presented.

Absorption of these drugs is variable. Oral drugs are absorbed in 1 to 6 hours, whereas the newer disintegrating tablets are absorbed within 2 minutes. These newer, highly lipid-soluble drugs accumulate in fatty tissue and are released slowly, which might explain why patients who abruptly stop taking their medications continue to experience an antipsychotic effect for some time. This slow release from fatty stores might also account for nonadherence because the patient who stops taking this medication does not experience an immediate return of symptoms. The following clinical example probably represents this phenomenon.

Antipsychotics are highly bound (most between 90% and 99%) to plasma proteins. Physiologic changes that disrupt even slightly this level of protein-binding action might increase the percentage of free drugs and potentially have a more significant effect. As with most highly protein-bound drugs, a greater effect might occur in older adults (who more often experience a decline in serum protein levels).

Antipsychotics are metabolized in the liver by the cytochrome P-450 (CYP-450) enzyme system. The average half-life ranges from 10 to 30 hours, with a few exceptions. Impaired hepatic function extends the half-life and effect of these drugs. As noted in Chapter 24, a much higher percentage

---

Clinical Example: New friends sincere but wrong

Bob, a 58-year-old military veteran with a long history of mental illness, has been taking haloperidol for 30 years. Over that time, the nursing staff at the Veterans' Administration hospital has gotten to know Bob well because he periodically requires hospital-based intervention. One day, Bob calls the nursing office on the psychiatric floor and tells the nurse (i.e., me) that he believes that he can conquer his problems by using "mind over matter." He is going to stop all psychotropic medications. Bob appears to do quite well for a couple of weeks, causing some of the nursing staff (yes, me again) to wonder about the new approach. At the end of 3 weeks, Bob is brought to the hospital in a highly disturbed psychotic state. His medication is reinstituted, and Bob's delusional thoughts subside.

---

of people with schizophrenia smoke compared with the general population. Cigarette smoking (not the nicotine) causes an increase in the CYP-450 1A2 enzyme, which breaks down several antipsychotics, including the following:

SMOKING DECREASES THESE SERUM LEVELS	
Major Substrates of CYP-450 1A2	**Minor Substrates of CYP-450 1A2**
Clozapine	Asenapine
Olanzapine	Chlorpromazine
Thiothixene	Fluphenazine
Trifluoperazine	Haloperidol
	Perphenazine
	Ziprasidone

Formulations.

Oral. Many antipsychotic drugs are available in both oral and parenteral forms. Oral administration is the preferred route for various reasons, including that patients generally prefer this route. However, tablets have consistently created a problem because they are so easy to "cheek." Cheeking occurs when patients place the tablet to one side of the mouth and pretend to swallow it. Nonadherence is thought to be the most important cause of symptom exacerbation and rehospitalization. Psychiatric patients might not want to take their medication for several reasons, including the admission of illness that taking oral medication might imply, paranoid fears of poisoning, or unpleasant reactions or side effects. A few oral versions of these agents dissolve instantly when placed in the mouth.

Long-acting injectables. Parenteral drugs are usually used to treat acutely disturbed patients or patients who represent significant risks. Long-acting injectable forms are also available and require injection only once every 2 to 6 weeks (Jann & Penzak, 2018), although one new long-acting injectable (i.e., Invega Trinza) needs only be administered every 3 months. These long-acting injections prove beneficial for outpatients or acute patients. Specific benefits include increased bioavailability and consistent blood

TABLE 14.3   **Advantages of Long-Acting Injectables**
1. Nonadherence can be distinguished from lack of efficacy
2. The nurse knows when nonadherence began
3. The patient does not need to take the antipsychotic on a daily basis
4. The drug avoids first-pass metabolism, and serum levels are more steady

Derived with permission from Procyshyn, R. M., Bezchlibnyk-Butler, K. Z., & Jeffries, J. J.. (2021). *Clinical handbook of psychotropic drugs* (24th Ed.) ©2021 Hogrefe Publishing www.hogrefe.com. http://doi.org/10.1027/00593-000.

levels. Some long-acting agents and their usual duration of action are:

1. Haloperidol decanoate (Haldol LA) (2 to 4 weeks)
2. Risperidone (Risperdal Consta) (2 weeks)
3. Risperidone (Perseris) (4 weeks)
4. Paliperidone palmitate (Invega Sustenna) (4 weeks)
5. Paliperidone palmitate (Invega Trinza) (3 months)
6. Olanzapine pamoate (Zyprexa Relprevv) (2 to 4 weeks)
7. Aripiprazole (Abilify Maintena) (4 weeks)
8. Aripiprazole lauroxil (Aristada) (4 to 6 weeks)

Table 14.3 lists the advantages of long-acting injectables.

When a patient does not respond to antipsychotic drug therapy, the nurse's assessment of the patient might be quite helpful to the prescriber. Two considerations should be kept in mind when assessing a patient's response:

1. Is the patient actually taking the drug?
2. Has the drug been given a fair trial?

⚇ CRITICAL THINKING QUESTION

2. Refer to the clinical example about Bob. What pharmacokinetic process can explain a rationale for Bob doing fine without medication for a few weeks?

BOX 14.3   Summary of Major Adverse Responses to Antipsychotic Drugs

Anticholinergic Side Effects
Cause: Blockade of cholinergic receptors (muscarinic receptors)
Offending agents: Anticholinergic drugs, such as low-potency antipsychotics and anticholinergic-antiparkinsonian drugs
Signs and symptoms: Constipation, decreased sweating, dilated pupils, dry mouth, slowed bowels, and slowed bladder

Extrapyramidal Side Effects
Cause: Blockade of D_2 receptors
Offending agents: Typically high-potency antipsychotics
Signs and symptoms: Akathisia, akinesia, dystonia, parkinsonism, tardive dyskinesia

Neuroleptic Malignant Syndrome
Cause: Blockade of D_2 receptors
Offending agents: Typically high-potency antipsychotics
Signs and symptoms: High fever and rigidity—can be fatal

Side Effects

Antipsychotic drugs produce numerous side effects because of peripheral nervous system (PNS) and CNS actions (Box 14.3; see Table 14.1).

Anticholinergic Effects: Constipation, Decreased Sweating, Dilated Pupils, Dry Mouth, Slowed Bowel, and Slowed Bladder

PNS anticholinergic effects are a result of the blocking of four cranial nerves (CN) that have parasympathetic components. The exception is decreased sweating, which is a sympathetic system function. The following illustrates these anticholinergic effects:

- CN III: Oculomotor nerve blockade results in mydriasis (dilated pupils) and impaired accommodation. Blurred vision might result.
- CN VII: Facial nerve blockade results in dry mouth, decreased tearing, and dry nasal passages.
- CN IX: Glossopharyngeal nerve blockade results in dry mouth and dry nasal passages.
- CN X: Vagus nerve blockade results in tachycardia, constipation, and urinary hesitation.
  Nursing alert: anticholinergic effects
1. Can increase intraocular pressure, aggravating narrow-angle glaucoma
2. Can intensify prostatic hypertrophy, making urination even more difficult
3. Can trigger arrhythmias and cause death

Antiadrenergic Effects: Decrease in Blood Pressure

Hypotension is the major antiadrenergic effect of antipsychotic drugs. The blocking of alpha-1 receptors is the primary cause of hypotension. Blocking these sympathetic receptors on peripheral blood vessels prevents these vessels from responding (constricting) automatically to changes in position. Hypotension occurs most often in older adults, and when the individual stands or changes positions suddenly (orthostatic hypotension), precautions against falls must be instituted. In a healthy younger person, accommodation usually occurs within a few weeks; however, many patients cannot tolerate orthostatic hypotension for that long. Hypotension also causes a reflex tachycardia that can cause general cardiovascular inefficiency. A reflex tachycardia is, by definition, tachycardia that automatically occurs as an adaptive function to compensate for lower extremity vasodilation. Antipsychotic drugs are prescribed cautiously for individuals with severe hypotension, heart failure, or a history of arrhythmias.

Cardiac Effects: Arrhythmias?

A concern among clinicians who prescribe antipsychotics is that these drugs have a potential for lengthening the QTc interval (a measure of ventricular depolarization and repolarization). Although this concern is not as pronounced as it was previously, prudent practice dictates that attention be paid because lengthening the QTc interval can be associated with a fatal arrhythmia. A normal QTc interval is 330 to 440 ms. Drug-induced lengthening to greater than 450 ms for men and greater than 470 ms for women is considered QTc prolongation. Of the SGAs commonly prescribed, ziprasidone may have the greatest risk of QTc lengthening. Electrocardiographic monitoring is important.

Extrapyramidal Side Effects: Akathisia, Akinesia, Dystonia, Parkinsonism, and Tardive Dyskinesia

The following formula traces the most familiar path leading to rehospitalization:

EPSEs→nonadherence→relapse→rehospitaliztion

Preventing or minimizing EPSEs whenever possible is important. It has been estimated that most patients who receive antipsychotic medications have EPSEs, and EPSEs account for many readmissions. High-potency traditional antipsychotics are most likely, and atypical antipsychotics are least likely to cause EPSEs. Abnormal involuntary movement disorders develop because of drug-induced imbalances between dopamine and acetylcholine in a specific part of the brain. EPSEs can be grouped as follows: akathisia, akinesia, dystonia, TD, drug-induced parkinsonism, Pisa syndrome, and neuroleptic malignant syndrome (NMS). TD, a late-appearing dyskinesia, can be irreversible (Box 14.4).

Akathisia: restlessness. Akathisia is a subjective feeling of restlessness exhibited by restless legs, jittery feelings, and nervous energy. Akathisia, one the most common EPSE, is poorly understood and does not respond as robustly to anticholinergic medications as other pseudoparkinsonism (Patel & Marwaha, 2020). It is a significant reason that patients stop taking medications. Sometimes restless legs syndrome can be mistaken for akathisia and vice versa, but it should be remembered that restless legs syndrome occurs specifically in the lower body.

Akinesia and bradykinesia: slow motion. Akinesia refers to an absence of movement; however, slowed movement, or bradykinesia is more likely. Symptoms include weakness, fatigue, painful muscles, and anergia. Akinesia responds to anticholinergics.

BOX 14.4   Clozapine Treatment Protocol

1. Obtain baseline weight, comprehensive metabolic panel, fasting glucose, fasting lipids, complete blood count.
2. Absolute neutrophil count (ANC) of $\geq 1500/mm^3$ (BEN exception).
3. Weekly ANC for 6 months.
4. Then ANC every 2 weeks for 6 months.
5. Then ANC every 4 weeks after 12 months.

ANC, Absolute neutrophil count; BEN, benign ethnic neutropenia (some ethnic groups normally have lower ANCs).
From Newman, W. J., & Newman, B. M. (2016a). Rediscovering clozapine. *Current Psychiatry, 15*(7), 43.

Dystonia: freezing. Dystonias are abnormal postures caused by involuntary muscle spasms. They elicit a sustained, twisted, and contracted positioning of the limbs, trunk, neck, or mouth. Dystonias tend to appear early in treatment. Types of dystonias include the following:

- Torticollis—contracted positioning of the neck
- Oculogyric crisis—contracted positioning of the eyes upward
- Laryngeal—pharyngeal constriction (potentially life-threatening)

Dystonias respond to anticholinergic drugs, which occasionally must be given parenterally because of the gravity of the situation.

Parkinsonism: bradykinesia, rigidity, tremor. The cardinal symptoms of Parkinson disease, which include tremors, bradykinesia, and rigidity, are present.

Tardive dyskinesia: irreversible? *Tardive* means "late-appearing." TD is an EPSE that tends to develop after approximately 6 months or more of antipsychotic therapy and is not caused by the dopamine-acetylcholine imbalance per se; consequently, anticholinergics are ineffective. Anticholinergics typically worsen the symptoms of TD. Long-term use of antipsychotics is thought to cause dopamine receptors in the basal ganglia to become hypersensitive to dopamine. Symptoms are bothersome and can be embarrassing. Typical symptoms include tongue writhing, tongue protrusion, teeth grinding, and lip-smacking. The symptoms stop with sleep. Although TD movements can be suppressed willfully for a short time, they eventually reappear. Often, TD is irreversible, but it can be reversed if the patient is closely monitored, and the medication is stopped when symptoms first arise. Prevention is the best approach to dealing with TD.

Pisa syndrome. Older individuals are particularly susceptible to this side effect of leaning to one side. Higher doses of antiparkinsonian drugs may be helpful.

Neuroleptic malignant syndrome. NMS is a potentially lethal side effect of antipsychotic agents. The incidence of NMS was formerly much greater than it is today, but with today's careful scrutiny of patients by nurses and physicians, a significant reduction in its incidence and mortality has occurred. NMS occurs most often when high-potency antipsychotic drugs are prescribed (e.g., haloperidol) but not always. NMS is not related to toxic drug levels and might occur after only a few doses. Typically, onset is within a week or so after initiation of an antipsychotic. The cardinal symptoms of NMS are high fever (temperature typically 101°F to 103°F but can increase to 108°F) and rigidity. Related and other symptoms include tremors, impaired ventilation, muteness, altered consciousness, and autonomic hyperactivity. Because an increased temperature is a chief sign of NMS, nurses should monitor temperatures closely. Antipsychotics should not be reinstituted for at least 2 weeks after complete resolution of NMS symptoms.

Endocrine Side Effects

Traditional antipsychotics elevate prolactin levels by blocking D_2 receptors (at about 70% occupancy). Dopamine inhibits prolactin, and when dopamine receptors are blocked,

TABLE 14.4   Consequences of Chronic Prolactin Elevation

Women	Men
Amenorrhea	Impotence
Loss of libido	Loss of libido
Galactorrhea	Gynecomastia
Long-term risk for osteoporosis	Lowered sperm count
Changes in menstrual cycle	Feminization

prolactin levels increase. Many bothersome side effects occur because of chronic elevation of prolactin levels (Table 14.4). FGAs are much more likely to cause hyperprolactinemia.

Metabolic Syndrome

Metabolic syndrome (or insulin resistance syndrome), as a result of antipsychotics, occurs in about one-third of patients and manifests as reduced metabolism of glucose and resistance to insulin by insulin receptors on cells. Type 2 diabetes can result in the associated problems of hyperglycemia, obesity, elevated lipid levels, coagulation abnormalities, and hypertension. SGAs are more likely to cause metabolic syndrome than FGAs or TGAs. The US Food and Drug Administration (FDA) requires drug manufacturers to include a warning about this problem. The following constitute metabolic syndrome (American Heart, 2021; Michael & MacDonald, 2020):

1. Central or abdominal obesity measured by waist circumference (i.e., fat belly)
2. High triglyceride levels or treatment for the same
3. Low HDL cholesterol or treatment for the same
4. Elevated blood pressure or treatment for the same
5. High fasting glucose

Sexual Side Effects

D_2 and alpha-2 blockade, as well as the aforementioned elevated prolactin levels, are thought to be responsible for sexual side effects. Sexual activity can be divided into three phases: desire, arousal, and orgasm. With a little imagination, one could verify that sexual activity pretty much follows that order of events. From a man's perspective, desire is step one. If there is no desire, it is very difficult to go to step two, arousal (i.e., an erection). If step two is accomplished, there is no guarantee that step three, orgasm, will occur.

Desire deficits are most likely caused by dopamine blockade. Because dopamine elevation is linked to schizophrenia, it is difficult to provide dopamine-enhancing agents without exacerbating symptoms. Arousal problems can be treated with sildenafil (Viagra). Invariably, in the authors' experience, the third phase of sexual behavior (orgasm) causes most of the problems. For many men, desire and arousal are not significant issues; however, having an orgasm is significant.

Gastrointestinal Effects

Weight gain can be significant, particularly for patients taking the newer agents. This phenomenon is probably related to the blockade of histamine H_1, 5-hydroxytryptamine 2 C ($5\text{-}HT_{2C}$), and other receptors. Insulin resistance is an outcome and a cause of excessive weight gain. Carbohydrate craving is a common feature.

Clinical Example

Bud, a 23-year-old patient with a diagnosis of schizophrenia, gained 105 pounds in less than 1 year on a particular atypical drug. He was finally switched to another agent and lost about 75 pounds of the extra weight.

Other Side Effects

Other side effects that might occur in patients taking antipsychotic drugs include jaundice, rare but serious blood dyscrasias, susceptibility to hyperthermia, sun-sensitive skin, nasal congestion, wheezing, and memory loss. Because the cholinergic system is implicated in memory and learning, low-potency antipsychotic drugs might play a role in the cognitive symptoms. Clozapine (Clozaril) causes agranulocytosis in a little less than 1% of patients and is potentially fatal. Agranulocytosis is discussed later in this chapter.

Nursing Implications

Therapeutic Versus Toxic Levels

Overdoses of antipsychotic drugs are seldom fatal. An overdose can cause severe CNS depression, hypotension, and EPSEs. Restlessness or agitation, convulsions, hyperthermia, increased anticholinergic symptoms, and arrhythmias are other indicators of an overdose.

Use During Pregnancy

Antipsychotics pose few risks during pregnancy, but human data are limited for some of these drugs. Nonetheless, they should be avoided during the first trimester as the greatest risk for fetal malformations occur then (Procyshyn, Bezchlibnyk-Butler, & Jefferies, 2015). These drugs readily pass the placental barrier, reach significant levels in the fetus, and may cause EPSEs in some newborns. All SGAs are FDA pregnancy category C, which means that in animal studies adverse effects have been demonstrated. Although a number of the antipsychotics have been given during pregnancy without problems arising, all of these drugs potentially worsen or cause glucose intolerance, which can be potentially harmful (Robakis & Williams, 2013).

Use in Older Adults

Because older adults have decreased hepatic metabolism capability, reducing the dose in this age group is prudent. Age-related nigrostriatal and cholinergic degeneration cause pharmacodynamic responses that are more intense than pharmacodynamic responses experienced by younger individuals. Both extrapyramidal and anticholinergic effects can be heightened. Older adults are also at higher risk for TD. A black box warning for atypical agents was issued in 2005, indicating that older adults with dementia-related psychosis

were at increased risk of dying from sudden death or pneumonia when treated with these drugs.

Side Effects

PNS anticholinergic and antiadrenergic effects of antipsychotic drugs are troublesome but not always as serious or as disturbing to the patient as are CNS EPSEs. The nurse can provide several specific interventions to ameliorate side effects or to prevent serious consequences (see the "Peripheral Nervous System Effects and Nursing Interventions" box and the "Extrapyramidal Side Effects and Nursing Interventions" box).

Interactions

Antipsychotic drugs interact with many other drugs. Because these interactions can be serious, the nurse must review offending agents and advise the family and patient accordingly. CNS depressants, such as alcohol, antihistamines, antianxiety drugs, antidepressants, barbiturates, meperidine, and morphine, have additive or pharmacodynamic effects that can cause profound CNS depression. A few of the most common adverse interactions are found in Table 14.5.

? CRITICAL THINKING QUESTION

3. In the "Peripheral Nervous System Effects and Nursing Interventions" box, pilocarpine eye drops are suggested for blurred vision. What category of drug does pilocarpine belong to, and how does it help blurred vision?

Prescription drugs. The nurse should review prescriptions to serve as a safety net for the prescriber who might make an inadvertent error. This safety measure is also important because nurses often act as case managers or advocates for patients who are seeing many caregivers and receiving prescriptions from multiple providers.

TABLE 14.5 Adverse Interactions of Antipsychotics With Selected Drugs

Drug	Effect of Interaction
Amphetamines	Decreased antipsychotic effect
Barbiturates	All cause respiratory depression and increase sedation; all decrease antipsychotic serum levels; hypotension
Benzodiazepines	Increased sedation; respiratory depression is possible
Cigarette smoking	Decreased serum levels of some antipsychotic drugs
Insulin, oral hypoglycemics	Control of diabetes is weakened
Levodopa	Decreased antiparkinsonian effect of levodopa; might exacerbate psychosis
Narcotics	Increased sedation; respiratory depression augmented

PERIPHERAL NERVOUS SYSTEM EFFECTS AND NURSING INTERVENTIONS

PNS Effect	Nursing Interventions
Constipation	Encourage high dietary fiber and increased water intake; give laxatives as ordered.
Decreased sweating	Avoid exposure to extreme heat, if possible.
Dry mouth	Advise patient to take sips of water frequently; provide sugarless hard candies, sugarless gum, and mouth rinses.
Blurred vision	Advise patient to avoid potentially dangerous tasks. Reassure patient that normal vision typically returns in a few weeks, when tolerance to this side effect develops. Pilocarpine eye drops can be used on a short-term basis.
Mydriasis	Advise patient to report eye pain immediately.
Photophobia	Advise patient to wear sunglasses outdoors.
Orthostatic hypotension	Advise patient to get out of bed or chair slowly. If hypotension is a problem, measure blood pressure before each dose is given.
Tachycardia	Tachycardia is usually a reflex response to hypotension. When intervention for hypotension is effective, reflex tachycardia usually decreases.
Urinary retention	Encourage frequent voiding and voiding whenever the urge is present. Older men with benign prostatic hypertrophy are particularly susceptible to urinary retention.
Urinary hesitation	Provide privacy (some individuals struggle to urinate in front of others), run water in the sink, and so on.
Sedation	Help patient get up early and get the day started.
Weight gain	Help patient order an appropriate diet; patient should not take diet pills.

PNS, Peripheral nervous system.

EXTRAPYRAMIDAL SIDE EFFECTS AND NURSING INTERVENTIONS

EPSE	Nursing Interventions
Akathisia	Be patient and reassure the patient who is jittery that you understand the need to move. Because akathisia is a main cause of nonadherence with antipsychotic regimens, a drug change is often necessary.
Dystonias	If a severe reaction occurs, such as oculogyric crisis or torticollis, give benztropine (Cogentin) or diphenhydramine (Benadryl) immediately, as needed, and offer reassurance. For some situations, IM administration of benztropine is required because of the seriousness of the dystonic reaction.
Drug-induced parkinsonism	Antiparkinsonian drugs are probably indicated.
TD	Assess for signs and symptoms by using AIMS. Anticholinergic agents worsen TD.
NMS	Be alert for this potentially fatal side effect. Routinely take temperature and encourage adequate water intake for all patients on a regimen of antipsychotic drugs; routinely assess for rigidity, tremor, and similar symptoms.

AIMS, Abnormal involuntary movement scale; EPSE, extrapyramidal side effect; IM, intramuscular; NMS, neuroleptic malignant syndrome; TD, tardive dyskinesia.

Nonprescription drugs. Many nonprescription drugs have potentially harmful interactive effects with antipsychotic drugs. CNS depressants, such as alcohol, cold and influenza agents, and sleep aids, can have additive effects. Other drugs decrease the effect of antipsychotics. For instance, antacids decrease the absorption of antipsychotic drugs.

Teaching Patients

Teaching patients who are taking antipsychotic drugs is an important dimension of nursing care. The nurse should use discretion in selecting the content of educational sessions because some patients have a tendency to become anxious and paranoid about potential side effects. The nurse should focus on symptoms that can be seen or felt. The patient should be given a simply written description of drug benefits and side effects, with instructions on how to cope with the side effects. Having this information in a written format helps the patient and family be more in control and able to act as collaborators in treatment.

In addition to the education issues already mentioned, the patient and family should be taught the following:

- Avoid immersion in hot water because hypotension might occur, causing falls.
- Use sunscreen to prevent sunburn, and use maximum-strength sunscreen when sunbathing.
- Dress appropriately in hot weather, and drink plenty of water to avoid heatstroke.
- Avoid abrupt withdrawal of medication because EPSEs can occur.
- Take the drug as prescribed. Nonadherence is the leading cause of the return of symptoms and a leading cause of readmission.
- Immediately report signs of a sore throat, malaise, fever, or bleeding. These signs might indicate a blood dyscrasia.

FIRST-GENERATION ANTIPSYCHOTICS (TRADITIONAL): INTRODUCED IN 1950

This section provides additional details about the FGAs. FGAs are inexpensive, so they account for a minuscule amount of the money spent on antipsychotics each year. These drugs are effective, but they have a higher risk for adverse effects. However, some patients do very well on these drugs. They remain viable options because they are effective and much cheaper for patients and payers. Because schizophrenia can be viewed as a lifelong illness, the difference in cost over many years dictates that traditional drugs at least be considered. For example, a 1-month supply of haloperidol costs about $20, whereas a 1-month supply of the new drug cariprazine (Vraylar) costs more than $1000.

Low-Potency First-Generation Antipsychotics: Chlorpromazine

Chlorpromazine (Thorazine) was the first antipsychotic developed. When it became available to state hospitals in the United States, workers viewed it as a godsend. Some patients dramatically improved. Chlorpromazine is a low-potency agent and results in anticholinergic and antiadrenergic effects. It is also sedating and causes significant weight gain. EPSEs are moderately produced.

Moderate-Potency First-Generation Antipsychotics: Perphenazine

Some drugs do not fit into the high-potency versus low-potency conceptual framework. Perphenazine is a moderate-potency drug. Evidence from the landmark Clinical Antipsychotic Trials and Intervention Effectiveness (CATIE) study suggests that perphenazine, when compared with SGAs, was as effective as any of them, with the exception of olanzapine. (Clozapine was not included in this trial.) Because perphenazine is so much less expensive, this can be an attractive alternative to the more expensive atypical agents.

High-Potency First-Generation Antipsychotics: Fluphenazine and Haloperidol

Fluphenazine

Fluphenazine, a high-potency antipsychotic, is commonly prescribed and is considered to be an effective medication. Fluphenazine (Modecate, Prolixin Decanoate), the long-acting form, is beneficial for patients who do not comply with

a daily oral medication regimen. This injection can be given every 2 to 5 weeks.

Haloperidol

Haloperidol (Haldol LA) is a high-potency FGA and the most frequently prescribed one. It tends to cause more EPSEs and fewer anticholinergic side effects than low-potency FGAs. Dr. Henry Nasrallah (2013), a prominent psychiatrist, has questioned whether it should be banned because of the severity of some of its side effects. This injection can be given every 2 to 4 weeks.

SECOND-GENERATION ANTIPSYCHOTICS (ATYPICAL): INTRODUCED IN 1990

Chlorpromazine, the first antipsychotic, was developed around 1950 (SGAs were not marketed until 1990). During this 40-year period, hundreds of antipsychotic formulations were developed. Although the drugs were not significantly different, they were all traditional or FGAs. SGAs are atypical because they work differently (have a different mechanism of action) than the traditional drugs and have a greater effect on negative symptoms. There are two major mechanisms of action that make atypical agents different: (1) they block 5-HT_{2A} receptors (Fig. 14.2); (2) they are faster "on–off" the D_2 receptor.

Serotonin (5-Hydroxytryptamine 2A) Antagonism

Because the 5-HT_{2A} receptor inhibits dopamine release, drugs that are 5-HT_{2A} receptor antagonists liberate dopamine. As previously noted and repeated here, these drugs have the following theoretical features that make them atypical:

1. Reduced risk for EPSEs: 5-HT_{2A} blockade modifies D_2 blockade.
2. Increased effectiveness in treating negative symptoms: dopamine is increased in the frontal lobe.
3. Minimal risk of TD: dopamine receptors do not become hypersensitive.
4. Reduced prolactin level elevation: prolactin-inhibiting factor (i.e., dopamine) is still available.

Each of the four differences is produced by the blockade of 5-HT_{2A} receptors, which putatively liberates dopamine. The reasoning is:

If EPSEs are caused by dopamine D_2 blockade, *SGAs* keep dopamine available and highly competitive for those receptors.

If negative symptoms are caused (at least partially) by decreased dopamine in the cortex, *SGAs* increase dopamine in the cortex.

If prolactin level elevation is caused by a deficiency in dopamine, *SGAs* increase dopamine in this tract.

If TD is caused by irritation of D_2 receptors being continually "grasped" by D_2 antagonists, *SGAs* prevent this from occurring.

In the years after their introduction, SGAs dominated the market. However, they did not live up to their initial promise.

**THE ROLE OF 5-HT$_{2A}$ RECEPTOR ANTAGONISM
IN ANTIPSYCHOTIC EFFECT**

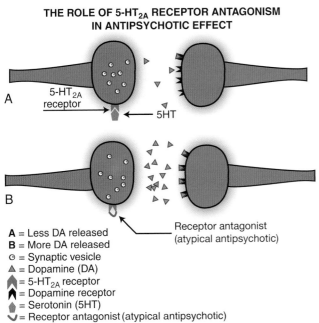

A = Less DA released
B = More DA released
⊙ = Synaptic vesicle
△ = Dopamine (DA)
⋀ = 5-HT$_{2A}$ receptor
⋀ = Dopamine receptor
⬠ = Serotonin (5HT)
⋎ = Receptor antagonist (atypical antipsychotic)

Receptor antagonist
(atypical antipsychotic)

FIG. 14.2 Role of 5-HT$_{2A}$ modulation of dopaminergic neurons and the role of atypical antipsychotics. (A) The 5-HT$_{2A}$ receptor inhibits the presynaptic dopamine neuron. When serotonin fits this receptor, it down-regulates dopamine release and can contribute to extrapyramidal side effects (EPSEs; nigrostriatal tract), hyperprolactinemia (tuberoinfundibular tract), and negative and cognitive symptoms (mesocortical tract). (B) An atypical antipsychotic has blocked the 5-HT$_{2A}$ receptor. This antagonism increases the release of dopamine into the synapse, decreasing EPSEs, stabilizing prolactin, and improving negative and cognitive symptoms. (From Keltner, N. L., & Folks, D. G. [2005]. *Psychotropic drugs* [4th ed.]. Mosby.)

If cognitive symptoms are improved with these drugs, the improvement is not nearly as remarkable as hoped for.

Generally, these agents have a broad affinity for several neurotransmitter systems thought to be implicated in schizophrenia. Additionally, they appear to demonstrate regionally specific activity in the brain. For example, they can modulate mesolimbic function without a significant effect on the nigrostriatal tract. Because of the complexity of these pharmacologic effects, a more refined receptor affinity profile could be developed for each of these drugs. However, this discussion is beyond the scope of this text.

> Very Attentive Nursing Student: "Dr. Keltner, if SGAs increase dopamine and if too much dopamine is the cause of schizophrenia, wouldn't SGAs make schizophrenia worse?"
>
> Keltner: "That is a great question because it shows you are thinking. The answer is there is a paucity of 5-HT$_{2A}$ receptors in the mesolimbic tract, so dopamine is not appreciably increased in that tract, and thus psychotic symptoms are not increased."

Fast-Off Theory

The fast-off theory states that how long a drug is on the D$_2$ receptor is significant. Dopamine antagonists have to "get on"

the receptor to block dopamine from attaching to that same receptor. They eventually have to get off as well. This amount of time can be measured (i.e., how quickly a drug binds to and then dissociates from a receptor or its dissociation constant). The smaller the dissociation constant, the more tightly the drug binds to the receptor. The larger the dissociation constant, the less affinity a drug has for the receptor. In a classic work, Kapur and Seeman (2001) theorized that differences in dissociation from the receptor are what really causes second-generation drugs to be atypical. For example, here are the binding affinities for a few selected antipsychotics and for dopamine itself (Steele, Vance, & Keltner, 2011):

Antipsychotic	Dissociation Constant
Aripiprazole	0.34
Clozapine	126
Dopamine	**1.75**
Haloperidol	0.7
Olanzapine	11
Quetiapine	160
Risperidone	4
Ziprasidone	5

Take note of some important facts in this table: Haloperidol has a significantly stronger binding to D$_2$ than does dopamine itself. So, if dopamine cannot "get back on" the D$_2$ receptor in the nigrostriatal tract, then we would expect significant EPSEs with haloperidol. And, that happens! Also, one sees that risperidone binds more tightly to these receptors than either quetiapine or clozapine and would be predicted to cause a higher level of EPSEs than those two drugs. That is what we see in clinical practice. Risperidone can cause EPSEs, particularly at higher doses.

Potential Negative Effects of Second-Generation Antipsychotics

Although SGAs have numerous significant advantages, they are also known to cause several important adverse effects. These include metabolic dysregulation (see earlier discussion of metabolic syndrome) and its complications—obesity, diabetes, hyperlipidemia, and hypertension. The CATIE study found that 43% of outpatients with schizophrenia met the criteria for metabolic syndrome. Following are the various SGAs.

OLDER SECOND-GENERATION ANTIPSYCHOTICS: 1990 TO 2000

Clozapine

Clozapine (Clozaril), though identified in 1959, was not released to the US retail market until 1990. It was the first truly new antipsychotic agent to be introduced into the United States in 40 years. Clozapine has been referred to as the "gold standard" in the management of treatment-resistant schizophrenia or 20% to 30% of this population. That said, clozapine accounts for only 5% of antipsychotic prescriptions, a phenomenon some refer to as "clozaphobia" (Newman & Newman, 2016a). Although clozapine had been used in Europe and China for some time, it was not approved in the United States because of the seriousness of its major side effects, *neutropenia (white blood cells, [WBC] < 3000 mm³)* and *agranulocytosis (absolute neutrophil count, [ANC] < 500 mm³)*. Because of this side effect, clozapine is indicated only after patients with severe schizophrenia have failed to respond to other antipsychotic drugs. The following summary underscores the severity of this adverse effect.

In Finland, during June and July 1975, 9 of 18 patients who developed clozapine-induced agranulocytosis died (Idänpään-Heikkilä, Alhava, Olkinuora, & Palva, 1975). This alarming event sent shudders through the psychiatric community, and clozapine was not approved in the United States for another 15 years. By the mid-1980s, studies revealed a more optimistic picture of this drug and its effects. However, this picture was still tempered by an excessively high morbidity rate of 1% to 2% for agranulocytosis and a high mortality rate for patients developing this blood dyscrasia. Current investigations have indicated a slightly lower morbidity rate of less than 1%; the mortality rate has also declined significantly. The cause of these drops in WBC and ANC are not known, but Daniel and Gross (2016) speculate that they may be related to clozapine's effects on WBC precursors.

Other side effects of clozapine result from its antagonism of cholinergic, alpha-1, alpha-2, and H₁ receptors. As might be surmised from comparing the receptor-antagonism profile of clozapine with the theoretical effects of receptor blockade shown in Table 14.2, clozapine causes significant side effects, including sedation (> 30%), weight gain (> 30%), tachycardia (17%), constipation (16%), and dizziness (14%) (Newman & Newman, 2016b). Sexual dysfunction and weight gain are particularly troublesome and have social implications.

Clozapine is primarily metabolized by CYP-450 1A2. Most patients with schizophrenia smoke (~70%), and cigarette smoking induces CYP-450 1A2, causing a decreased level of clozapine.

Clinical Example: A bad decision by staff

During a group therapy session in a state public hospital, Bill continually stands up and cannot sit down for long. Bill sits down the moment the group leader instructs him to sit down, but he immediately stands up again. The group leader misinterprets Bill's behavior as defiance. This misinterpretation escalates into a confrontation that culminates when Bill is forcibly restrained and given an as-needed injection of an antipsychotic agent. Had the group leader been more aware of EPSEs, he would have suspected akathisia and would have further recognized that an antipsychotic would make the patient worse.

Clinical Example: Voices gone, but 40 pounds gained!

Joan Smith is a 45-year-old African American, single mother of a teenage boy. Joan is in a program for chronically mentally ill individuals in which staff visit the patients at home (or work) two times per week. Joan is the only person in the program with a full-time job. She works for the federal government answering questions by phone all day. In this organization, people in her position are timed and expected to be talking to "customers" for 6.5 hours per day. Joan has the tremendous handicap of hearing voices constantly. She hears hallucinated voices that compete with the real people she speaks with on the phone most of the day. Joan desperately wants to keep her job because it provides a much better lifestyle than welfare for her and her son (not to mention the self-satisfaction of providing for oneself). At one time, Joan was helped significantly by clozapine, but because her WBC count decreased, she was taken off the medication. While on clozapine, Joan did not hear voices, but she did gain some weight. Joan begged her clinician to place her back on clozapine. After taking 6 months to gain organizational approval, Joan was restarted on clozapine, and she became free of hallucinations. After only a few months, Joan gained about 40 pounds—a terrible trade-off but one that Joan was willing to accept to keep her job.

Agranulocytosis is clinically defined as an absolute neutrophil count less than 500/mm³ and might be caused by bone marrow suppression. Because of its life-threatening potential, this medication must be monitored closely. Box 14.4 outlines the protocols for clozapine therapy.

Clozapine is associated with several other important side effects, including dose-related seizures and excessive salivation. One would think that because clozapine is such a strong anticholinergic, dry mouth and not hypersalivation would be the problem, but that is not the case. Some patients carry paper cups to hold excessive saliva. It seems that although clozapine does block four of the five muscarinic subtypes, it is an agonist at M₄ (Hultfilz, Garris, & Kennedy, 2012). This property accounts for the large amount of "extra" saliva produced in patients taking clozapine.

Risperidone and Paliperidone

Risperidone (Risperdal), approved in 1994, is atypical but different from clozapine. Risperidone has a greater affinity for D₂ receptors and a similar antagonism of 5-HT₂ₐ receptors compared with clozapine; risperidone theoretically has a favorable receptor profile for both positive and negative schizophrenia. The lack of serious side effects associated with risperidone makes it a well-tolerated drug as well. It has little affinity for muscarinic (i.e., cholinergic) receptors, so anticholinergic side effects are minimized (see Table 14.1). In addition, risperidone does not appear to cause agranulocytosis, TD, or NMS, and it appears to be a relatively safe drug. Nonetheless, risperidone significantly blocks alpha-1 and H₁ receptors, resulting in orthostatic hypotension, sedation, and appetite stimulation. At higher doses, patients taking risperidone have experienced EPSEs and hyperprolactinemia (again, note risperidone's dissociation constant). A long-acting intramuscular version is available.

Paliperidone (Invega) is part of the risperidone family and is manufactured by the same company that makes Risperdal. As with many drugs, a metabolite of risperidone has pharmacologic properties similar to the parent drug. In this case, paliperidone is that metabolite: 9-hydroxyrisperidone (risperidone with an additional hydroxyl [OH] group). It has a similar side effect profile as risperidone and presumably achieves its therapeutic effects by antagonism of D_2 and 5-HT_{2A} receptors, as does risperidone. Invega has the advantage of being an extended-release formulation. There is also a long-acting injectable form.

Olanzapine

Olanzapine (Zyprexa), which was released to the market in 1996, is comparable to risperidone in efficacy and side-effect profile and does not cause agranulocytosis. Olanzapine significantly blocks 5-HT_{2A} and D_2 receptors. It also has a high affinity for cholinergic, H_1, and alpha-1 receptors, resulting in anticholinergic effects of sedation, weight gain, and orthostasis. Olanzapine normalizes N-methyl-D-aspartate (NMDA) receptor function in the glutaminergic system, blocking some signs and symptoms associated with schizophrenia. It has a favorable side-effect profile, with few incidents of EPSEs. Olanzapine causes considerable weight gain in some patients. Olanzapine has proven effective in treating acute mania and is an FDA-approved drug for monotherapy for bipolar disorder. A long-acting injectable form is also available. The following clinical example illustrates how olanzapine made a significant difference in one man's life.

Clinical Example: Olanzapine worked!

Charles, a man in his early 30s, was first diagnosed with schizophrenia when he was 19 years old. He experienced a sudden onset and was hospitalized locally five times in 6 months. He was admitted to the state hospital, and clozapine was prescribed within a few weeks. He responded favorably. Charles was discharged from the hospital after 5 months to a day-treatment program and did well in the program while on a regimen of clozapine. As protocols required, he was monitored for blood work on a weekly basis, and after several years experienced a decrease in WBC count. Clozapine therapy was discontinued, and olanzapine therapy was started. Charles did well with olanzapine. His parents described him as being as well or better than he was before he became ill. After years in the day-treatment program and only a few months on olanzapine therapy, he was discharged and now lives on his own.

Quetiapine

Scarecrow, scarecrow, what's that you popping? A powerful pill they call Oxy Contin. But it's so tiny, that it got you dragging. Haven't you heard big things come in small packages. I prefer the oranges with the black O-C. Take two and you cannot move up out ya seat. Some people melt 'em down in a needle and shoot 'em up. But I pop 'em with Seroquel like glue, I am stuck.

Rap song by Lord Infamous

Quetiapine (Seroquel) was made available in 1997. Similar to clozapine, quetiapine has a lower affinity for D_2 receptors than for 5-HT_{2A}. It has little affinity for muscarinic cholinergic receptors; few anticholinergic side effects are expected. However, quetiapine antagonizes alpha-1 receptors, which leads to orthostatic hypotension, and antagonizes H_1 receptors, which leads to sedation and appetite stimulation. Clinically, quetiapine is effective for both positive and negative symptoms, provokes few EPSEs, does not significantly increase serum prolactin levels, and appears to improve elements of cognitive function. As the above-quoted lyrics might suggest, quetiapine is a drug of choice for abuse in jails and prisons. The drug is taken orally, intranasally, and intravenously, and it provides both an anxiolytic and a sedative effect.

Ziprasidone

Ziprasidone (Geodon) is effective for both positive and negative symptoms of schizophrenia. Ziprasidone acts on several neurotransmitter systems, has a high affinity for 5-HT_{2A} receptors, and D_2 receptors moderately block the reuptake of serotonin and norepinephrine and are an agonist for the 5-HT_{1A} receptor. These pharmacologic properties suggest a drug that has the potential to ameliorate depression and anxiety, which are commonly associated with schizophrenia, and causes few EPSEs, few anticholinergic side effects, and mild antihistaminic effects. Ziprasidone appears to cause less weight gain than some other atypical agents. It has been linked to potential cardiac problems related to the lengthening of the QTc interval. Studies have indicated a low potential for drug–drug interactions. Absorption is increased when ziprasidone is given with food.

Effects of 5-HT_{1A} Agonism by Ziprasidone

- Decreased anxiety
- Decreased depressive symptoms
- Improvement in negative symptoms

? CRITICAL THINKING QUESTION

5. Suppose that you are caring for a patient who needs medication but will not take it; for example, a patient with paranoid delusions might truly believe that you are poisoning her with the antipsychotic drug that has been prescribed for her. What are your legal and ethical grounds for nursing care in this situation?

NEWER SECOND-GENERATION ANTIPSYCHOTICS: 2000 TO PRESENT

Asenapine

Asenapine (Saphris) is a newer atypical drug approved in 2009. It is available only as a sublingual tablet, so it is ineffective if swallowed. It is approved for the treatment of both acute schizophrenia and bipolar disorder. It has shown a low tendency to cause EPSEs in preclinical tests, but anecdotal reports suggest that a slightly higher incidence may occur, particularly in the case of akathisia. Beyond giving patients, families, and clinicians another alternative, asenapine is marketed as being more effective in the treatment of cognitive and negative symptoms.

Iloperidone

Iloperidone (Fanapt) is also a newer atypical agent. It is an antagonist of both 5-HT$_{2A}$ and D$_2$ receptors. It blocks histamine and alpha-1 receptors, and weight gain, sedation, and orthostasis are common effects. It is related to risperidone (it is a metabolite of risperidone) and can precipitate EPSEs, prolactin elevation, and hyperprolactinemia.

Lurasidone

The last of the newer atypical agents is lurasidone (Latuda). It, too, blocks 5-HT$_{2A}$ and D$_2$ receptors. It also blocks the 5-HT$_{1A}$ receptor, which is thought to account for antianxiety properties of this drug. Similar to ziprasidone, absorption is improved if taken with food except that Lurasidone does not work without at least 350 calories, whereas with Ziprasidone at least 500 calories are required to reduce variability in patient response to symptoms (Smith-East, 2019). It has a good side-effect profile with few instances of dizziness, orthostatic hypotension, cognitive problems, sedation, or weight gain reported.

THIRD-GENERATION ANTIPSYCHOTICS (ATYPICAL): INTRODUCED IN 2002

The TGAs were introduced with much fanfare in 2002 with the approval of aripiprazole for the treatment of schizophrenia.

It was initially touted as a third-generation drug, then that designation was pulled back by many clinicians because how can you have a third generation if there is just one drug? Well, now there are three drugs that can be designated as TGAs, so they are separated out and rightly so.

A. TGAs are primarily D$_2$ partial agonists, but what does that mean? As Mattingly and Anderson (2016) put it, "...these agents restore homeostatic balance to neurochemical circuit." Well, you might ask, what does that mean? In a nutshell, D$_2$ partial agonists decrease the effects of dopamine in areas of the brain where there is too much dopamine
B. increase the effects of dopamine in areas of the brain where there is too little
C. exert little effect on dopamine where this neurotransmitter activity is normal.

Aripiprazole

Aripiprazole (Abilify) is also referred to as a dopamine system stabilizer. It has also been the #1 best-selling drug in the United States, with about $5.2 billion in sales in 2014 (its last year under patent protection). Dopamine system stabilizers are thought to balance the dopamine systems by increasing dopamine in brain areas in which dopamine is deficient and decreasing dopamine in brain areas in which dopamine is overactive (see immediately above). Fig. 14.3 contrasts the blockade of D$_2$ receptors by traditional drugs (see Fig. 14.3A) with the partial agonism of the same receptors by a drug such as aripiprazole (see Fig. 14.3B). Aripiprazole accomplishes this because it is a partial dopamine agonist, producing activation where lower dopamine tone exists and inhibition at brain sites with high dopaminergic tone. Areas with too much dopamine begin to stabilize because the aripiprazole molecule is less potent than the dopamine molecule; this effect reduces

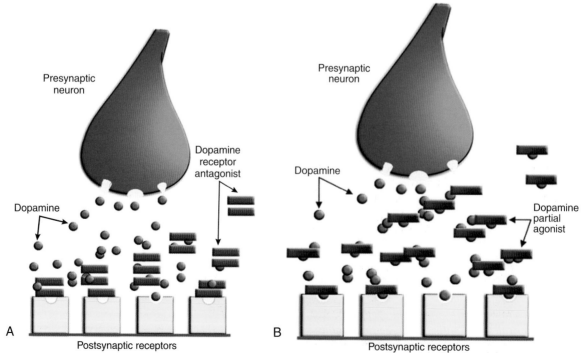

FIG. 14.3 (A) Dopamine receptor antagonism. (B) Dopamine system stabilization. (From Keltner, N. L., & Johnson, V. [2002]. Biological perspectives. Aripiprazole: A third generation of antipsychotics begins? *Perspectives in Psychiatric Care, 38,* 157.)

positive symptoms. Mesocortical areas also begin to stabilize from the opposite direction. Patients begin to feel better, with more energy as negative symptoms subside. Aripiprazole also antagonizes 5-HT$_{2A}$ receptors, as do other atypical drugs, and it is a partial agonist at the 5-HT$_{1A}$ receptor. Clinical studies have suggested a very good side-effect profile.

> **❓ CRITICAL THINKING QUESTION**
>
> 6. In looking at the Dissociation Constant chart, the antipsychotic that stays attached to the D$_2$ receptor the longest is aripiprazole. If staying on the D$_2$ receptor longer correlates to more EPSEs, why doesn't aripiprazole cause more EPSEs than the other drugs listed?

Brexpiprazole

Brexpiprazole (Rexulti) is a TGA. It also provides partial agonist activity at D$_2$ receptors. It was approved in 2015 for the treatment of schizophrenia, and its manufacturer continues to seek FDA approval for other indications. It appears to have a favorable side-effect profile, including reduced incidents of akathisia, restlessness, and insomnia compared to other TGAs.

Cariprazine

Cariprazine (Vraylar) is the newest TGA to be approved (i.e., late 2015). It is said to be an effective partial agonist not only at D$_2$ receptors but also at D$_3$ receptors. All the advantages of D$_3$ partial agonist activity are still not clear, but it is speculated that this might "mediate behavioral abnormalities" caused by glutamate system irregularities (Mattingly & Anderson, 2016). See the following discussion for an overview of the glutamatergic system and schizophrenia.

A NEW THEORY OF SCHIZOPHRENIA

> *… there is consensus that no antipsychotic has emerged as truly efficacious against the enduring cognitive and primary negative symptoms.*
>
> *Diana O. Perkins (2011)*

A new theory of schizophrenia and its treatment has captured a great deal of attention: the glutamate hypothesis. This newest biochemical model of schizophrenia is discussed in more detail in Chapter 24. But first, think about the quotation just given. A lot of ink has already been used explaining how the atypical antipsychotics are better for negative and cognitive symptoms of schizophrenia. They are, but better is not the same as "truly efficacious." This model states that the dopamine hypothesis is inadequate to explain the full range of symptoms we see in patients with schizophrenia. The dopamine hypothesis does a nice job of explaining hallucinations and delusions but a poor job of explaining negative and cognitive symptoms. The argument goes something like this:

1. Dopamine agonists, such as levodopa, do not cause negative and cognitive symptoms.
2. Dopamine antagonists do not "fix" negative and cognitive symptoms.
3. When the dopamine system is stabilized, these symptoms continue.

The glutamate system explains both positive and negative symptoms of schizophrenia. For example, when drug users overdose on phencyclidine (PCP) or ketamine a (K-hole), they demonstrate both positive and negative symptoms of schizophrenia. Because these drugs of abuse are known to block glutamate receptors (i.e., NMDA receptors), drugs that can increase glutamate might have antipsychotic possibilities. However, a fly in the ointment is the fact that glutamate does not pass the blood-brain barrier and that it requires an *obligate co-agonist* (i.e., glycine or a structurally related molecule). At present, the research on co-agonists seems to be going a little better, but this work is still underway. By the time this book is published, most likely, a lot more will be known about these agents.

> **❓ CRITICAL THINKING QUESTION**
>
> 7. Older clinicians (those using FGAs) believed that unless a patient has some level of EPSEs, the patient is not receiving enough medication. What might be the rationale for this view?

▌ STUDY NOTES

1. The dopamine hypothesis of schizophrenia states that an excessive level of dopamine in the brain causes schizophrenia.
2. Antipsychotic drugs block dopamine receptors, reducing the effect of excessive dopamine in the brain, specifically in the mesolimbic tract.
3. Antipsychotic drugs are classified in three ways: traditional or first-generation, atypical second-generation, and atypical third-generation antipsychotics.
4. The traditional agents are divided further into high-potency and low-potency drugs.
5. The desired effects of antipsychotic drugs include sedation, emotional quieting, psychomotor slowing, and alleviation of major symptoms of schizophrenia (e.g., alterations in perceptions, thoughts, consciousness, interpersonal relationships, and affect).
6. Anticholinergic side effects (e.g., dry mouth, blurred vision, constipation) and EPSEs (e.g., akathisia, akinesia, dystonic reactions, drug-induced parkinsonism, Pisa syndrome, and TD) are the major categories of side effects associated with antipsychotic drugs.

7. High-potency antipsychotic drugs, such as haloperidol and fluphenazine, tend to cause more EPSEs. Low-potency antipsychotic drugs, such as chlorpromazine, tend to cause more anticholinergic and antiadrenergic side effects.

8. NMS is a serious adverse effect of antipsychotic drugs (primarily high-potency drugs).

9. Overdoses of antipsychotic drugs are seldom fatal.

10. Antipsychotic drugs interact with other CNS depressants, such as alcohol, meperidine, and morphine, increasing CNS depression.

11. Patient teaching should focus on recognizing side effects and on avoiding CNS depressants.

12. The nurse should routinely assess for NMS by taking the patient's temperature and evaluating for rigidity and tremors.

13. Clozapine, introduced into the United States in 1990, was the first truly new antipsychotic drug in 40 years.

14. Other atypical antipsychotics have a great affinity for D_2 and 5-HT_{2A} receptors, produce few EPSEs, and have had remarkable success in patients resistant to treatment.

15. The atypical antipsychotics go on and off the D_2 receptor much faster than traditional drugs.

16. Clozapine causes agranulocytosis, a potentially fatal illness.

17. Other atypical antipsychotics do not cause life-threatening agranulocytosis.

18. Metabolic syndrome can be a particularly troublesome and serious side effect of atypical agents.

19. Aripiprazole is a TGA; it is also called a dopamine-system-stabilizing antipsychotic. Its mechanism of action is unique: partial agonism of D_2 and 5-HT_{2A} receptors.

REFERENCES

American Heart, Association. (2021). https://www.heart.org/en/health-topics/metabolic-syndrome/symptoms-and-diagnosis-of-metabolic-syndrome.

Begemann, M. J., Thompson, I. A., Veling, W., Gangadin, S. S., Geraets, C. N., van't Hag, E., & Sommer, I. E. (2020). To continue or not to continue? Antipsychotic medication maintenance versus dose-reduction/discontinuation in first episode psychosis: HAMLETT, a pragmatic multicenter single-blind randomized controlled trial. *Trials*, *21*(1), 1–19. https://doi.org/10.1186/s13063-019-3822-5.

Daniel, J. S., & Gross, T. (2016). Managing clozapine-induced neurotropenia and agranulocytosis. *Current Psychiatry*, *15*(12), 51.

Haddad, P. M., & Correll, C. U. (2018). The acute efficacy of antipsychotics in schizophrenia: A review of recent meta-analyses. *Therapeutic Advances in Psychopharmacology*, *8*(11), 303–318. https://doi.org/10.1177/2045125318781475.

Hultfilz, S., Garris, S., & Kennedy, M. L. (2012). Reducing hypersalivation. *Current Psychiatry*, *11*, 6.

Idänpään-Heikkilä, J., Alhava, E., Olkinuora, M., & Palva, I. (1975). Letter: Clozapine and agranulocytosis. *Lancet*, *2*(7935), 611. https://doi.org/10.1016/s0140-6736(75)90206-8.

Jann, M. W., & Penzak, S. R. (2018). Correction to: Long-acting injectable second-generation antipsychotics: An update and comparison between agents. *CNS Drugs*, *32*(3), 603. https://doi.org/10.1007/s40263-018-0531-7.

Jindal, R. D., & Keshavan, M. S. (2008). Classifying antipsychotic agents: Need for new terminology. *CNS Drugs*, *22*, 1047. https://doi.org/10.2165/0023210-200822120-00007.

Kapur, S., & Seeman, P. (2001). Does fast dissociation from the dopamine D2 receptor explain the action of atypical antipsychotics? A new hypothesis. *The American Journal of Psychiatry*, *158*(3), 360–369. https://doi.org/10.1176/appi.ajp.158.3.360.

Keltner, N. L., & Folks, D. G. (2005). *Psychotropic drugs* (4th ed.). Mosby.

Keltner, N. L., & Johnson, V. (2002). Biological perspectives. Aripiprazole: A third generation of antipsychotics begins? *Perspectives in Psychiatric Care*, *38*, 157.

Mattingly, G., & Anderson, R. (2016). Cariprazine for schizophrenia and bipolar I disorder. *Current Psychiatry*, *15*(2), 34.

Michael, S., & MacDonald, K. (2020). Improving rates of metabolic monitoring on an inpatient psychiatric ward. *BMJ Open Quality*, *9*(3), e000748. https://doi.org/10.1136/bmjoq-2019-000748.

Nasrallah. H. A. (2013). Haloperidol clearly is neurotoxic: Should it be banned? *Current Psychiatry*, *12*, 7.

Newman, W. J., & Newman, B. M. (2016a). Rediscovering clozapine: After a turbulent history, current guidance on initiating and monitoring. Current. *Psychiatry*, *15*(7), 42.

Newman, B. M., & Newman, W. J. (2016b). Rediscovering clozapine: Adverse effects develop-what should you do now? *Current Psychiatry*, *15*(8), 40.

Patel J., Marwaha R. Akathisia. [Updated 2020 Nov 29]. In: StatPearls [Internet]. Treasure Island (FL): StatPearls Publishing. https://www.ncbi.nlm.nih.gov/books/NBK519543/.

Perkins. D. O. (2011). Efficacy of available antipsychotics in schizophrenia. *Current Psychiatry*, *10*(Suppl.), S15–S19.

Procyshyn, R. M., Bezchlibnyk-Butler, K. Z., & Jefferies, J. J. (2015). *Clinical handbook of psychotropic drugs* (21st ed.). Hogrefe.

Robakis, T., & Williams, K. E. (2013). Atypical antipsychotics during pregnancy: Make decisions based on available evidence, individualized risk/benefit analysis. *Current Psychiatry*, *12*, 13.

Smith-East, M. (2019). Medication with food: What does it really mean? https://www.myamericannurse.com/medication-with-food-what-does-it-really-mean/.

Steele, D., Vance, D., & Keltner, N. (2011). Antipsychotics and the "fast-off" theory. *Perspectives in Psychiatric Care*, *47*(3), 160. https://doi.org/10.1111/j.1744-6163.2011.00309.x.

Taylor, M., & Jauhar, S. (2019). Are we getting any better at staying better? The long view on relapse and recovery in first episode nonaffective psychosis and schizophrenia. *Therapeutic Advances in Psychopharmacology*, *9*. https://doi.org/10.1177/2045125319870033.

Xiong. W. (2017). The art of psychopharmacology: Avoiding medication changes and slowing down. *Current Psychiatry*, *16*(11), 46.

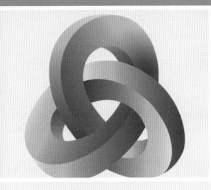

15

Antidepressant Drugs

Norman L. Keltner and Helene Vossos

Most people are about as happy as they make up their minds to be.

Abraham Lincoln

http://evolve.elsevier.com/Keltner

LEARNING OBJECTIVES

- Understand the neurobiologic concepts of depression.
- Describe the differences among the classes of antidepressant drugs.
- Discuss the side effects of antidepressant drugs.
- Identify the symptoms of toxicity for tricyclic antidepressants and monoamine oxidase inhibitors.

- Describe the potential interactions of antidepressant drugs and serotonin syndrome.
- Discuss the implications of teaching patients about antidepressant drugs.
- Identify several nontraditional approaches to treating depression.

BLACK BOX WARNING FOR ANTIDEPRESSANTS

Antidepressants increase the risk of suicidal thoughts and behaviors in patients aged 24 years and younger. Monitor for clinical worsening and emergence of suicidal thoughts and behaviors.

Antidepressants are used in the treatment of depression and other disorders. All antidepressants in this chapter are approved for major depression; however, some have a much more extensive range of effectiveness.

This chapter focuses on the psychopharmacologic classes of drugs used to treat depression (Box 15.1). Depressive disorders are discussed in detail in Chapter 25. The goals of antidepressant medications are as follows:

- Alleviate depressive symptoms
- Restore normal mood
- Prevent recurrence of depression
- Prevent a swing into mania for bipolar patients

BIOCHEMICAL THEORY OF DEPRESSION

Numerous theories exist concerning the cause of depression, but the efficacy of antidepressants is best understood from a neurochemical perspective that had its genesis more than 60 years ago. In the early 1950s, Bein isolated reserpine from *Rauwolfia serpentina*, a naturally occurring medicinal agent used to treat hypertension (Braslow & Marder, 2019). Reserpine was found to have additional value in treating psychosis, but some patients developed profound depression and became suicidal. The researchers related this action of reserpine to norepinephrine (NE) depletion. From this early linking of neurotransmitter depletion to depression, scientists began conceptualizing pharmacologic interventions. The crucial step in the development of antidepressant drugs was the synthesizing of agents that would increase the intrasynaptic availability of certain neurotransmitters, known as "the monoamines," such as NE, serotonin (5-HT), and dopamine (DA) (Fig. 15.1). However, even this staple of common knowledge has its detractors. For example:

IS LOW SEROTONIN REALLY THE CULPRIT?

Not everyone thinks that a serotonin deficiency is a real problem in depression. Dr. Alan Gelenberg from Penn State University makes the unique point, "There's really no evidence that depression is a serotonin-deficiency syndrome. It's like saying that a headache is an aspirin-deficiency syndrome." In other words, just because we can pop an aspirin and gain relief from a headache does not mean we are low on acetylsalicylic acid. It follows then that just because selective serotonin reuptake inhibitors (SSRIs) relieve depression does not mean that we have a serotonin deficiency (Schiele, Zwanzger, & Schwarte, 2021).

BOX 15.1 Classifications of Antidepressants

I Reuptake Inhibiting Antidepressants or Cyclic Antidepressants

- **Selective serotonin reuptake inhibitors (SSRIs):** citalopram, fluoxetine, paroxetine, escitalopram, fluvoxamine, and sertraline.
- **Selective serotonin-norepinephrine reuptake inhibitors (SNRIs):** venlafaxine, desvenlafaxine, duloxetine, and levomilnacipran.
- **Norepinephrine dopamine reuptake inhibitors (NDRIs):** bupropion
- **Novel antidepressants:** To attempt to present this material in the most effective way, a grouping of four more types of cyclic antidepressants will be presented here and following as Novel antidepressants:
  a. Noradrenergic/specific serotonergic agent: mirtazapine
  b. Serotonin-1A agonist/serotonin reuptake inhibitor: vilazodone
  c. Serotonin stimulator/serotonin modulator: vortioxetine
  d. Serotonin-2 antagonists/serotonin reuptake inhibitor (SARI): trazodone and nefazodone.
- **Tricyclic antidepressants (TCAs)** are nonselective, meaning they block the reuptake of both serotonin and norepinephrine: amitriptyline, desipramine, imipramine, maprotiline, nortriptyline.

II Enzyme Inhibiting Agents or Monoamine Oxidase Inhibitors (MAOIs)

- **Nonselective MAOIs** (block both A & B monoamine oxidase): phenelzine and tranylcypromine
- **Selective MAOIs:** MAO-A inhibitor moclobemide and MAO-B Inhibitor selegiline

Beyond the notion of neurotransmitter deficiencies, there are several interrelated biologic hypotheses concerning the etiology of depression, for example, receptor dysregulation, inflammation, methylation, altered genetic output, premature neuronal death, and lack of synaptogenesis (Magid & Reichenberg, 2015).

HOW CAN SO FEW NEURONS MAKE SUCH A BIG DIFFERENCE?

What seems genuinely amazing is that these Big Three neurotransmitters—dopamine, norepinephrine, and serotonin—have so relatively few neurons in the brain that synthesize them. For example, there are about 100,000,000,000 (i.e., 100 hundred billion) neurons in the brain, but only a few synthesize these neurotransmitters that affect our emotions so significantly. For instance:

Neurotransmitter	Number of Synthesizing Neurons[a]	% of All Brain Neurons
Dopamine	500,000	0.0005%
Norepinephrine	100,000	0.0001%
Serotonin	~300,000 ±	~0.0003%

[a]Nestler et al. (2021).

The first complementary view suggests that changes in receptors and genes might be an essential aspect of antidepressant activity. The observation bolsters this suggestion that antidepressants usually require 2 to 4 weeks for a clinical response. Elevations in these neurotransmitter levels occur within hours of treatment initiation, whereas receptor changes take approximately 2 to 4 weeks, and genetic changes take even longer. Interestingly, depression is responsible for 70% of psychiatric hospital admissions and 50% of suicides. According to the National Institute of Mental Health (NIMH), individuals who experience depression do not automatically have a cure with antidepressant medication treatment. Therefore, adjunctive therapy with psychotherapy and addressing lifestyle stressors significantly reduce symptoms (Advokat, Comaty, & Julien, 2019).

NORM'S NOTES These drugs are everywhere and are probably overprescribed. I'd be very surprised if you don't know someone taking an antidepressant (e.g., Cymbalta, Paxil, Zoloft). **One leading authority estimates that six prescriptions are written every second, every hour, of every day in the United States just for the SSRIs.** When really needed, these are great drugs, but just numbing oneself to avoid some pain is not always best. So, even though I think highly of these drugs, I also think that they are overused. Often working through a problem can be the better option. Read this chapter carefully. I guarantee that you will need to be familiar with this information—it could help someone you know.

Antidepressant-mediated genetic modification might be the most crucial current hypothesis describing antidepressant action. This view states that reregulation of the complex workings of the second messenger system is the key to the effectiveness of antidepressants. Fig. 15.2 illustrates the intricacies of the second messenger system. In depression, key genetic products are undersynthesized, and thus depression occurs. Of particular interest is a potential deficiency of brain-derived neurotrophic factor, which, at normal levels, would oppose cellular apoptotic forces (genetically programmed cell death). Left unopposed, apoptosis may be accelerated in some people with depression. Depression might be caused by actual neuronal death, which is caused by dysregulated monoaminergic systems. A related concept is the notion that genetic dysregulation may cause a lack of synaptogenesis (the growth of new synapses) which, in turn, may be the final common pathway leading to depression (Schiele, Zwanzger, & Schwarte, 2021). The efficacy of antidepressants is probably related to regulation of the second messenger system and, by extension, the reregulation of genetic output.

Psychopharmacologic treatment is based on the restoration of normal levels of these neurotransmitters and the consequent neuronal changes (Fig. 15.3). Available antidepressants achieve this goal in several distinct ways. Although the following listing might be complex,

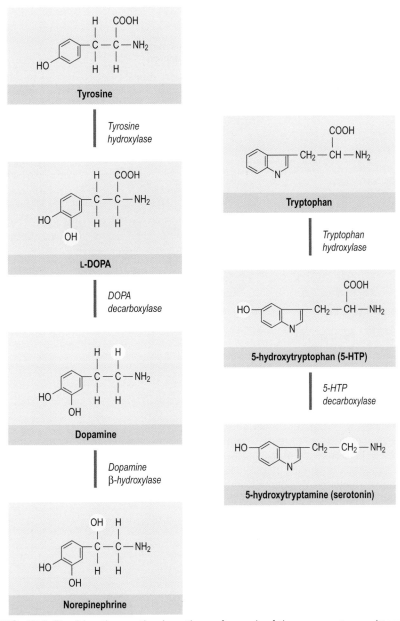

FIG. 15.1 Provides the synthesis pathway for each of these neurotransmitters.

understanding these mechanisms provides a firm understanding of how antidepressants work (also see Box 15.1). Categories of antidepressants are presented in two overarching categories: cyclic antidepressants (or reuptake inhibiting antidepressants) and enzyme inhibiting agents (Advokat, Comaty, & Julien, 2019; Stahl, 2021). Cyclic antidepressants are so named because of their molecular structure (i.e., a ring compound), and many subtypes within this broader category exist. The enzyme inhibiting agents or MAOIs compose a much more homogenous grouping and are prescribed infrequently.

In brief, the pharmacologic treatment of depression is based on the idea that an increase in certain neurotransmitters

produces an antidepressant effect. Thus these two groupings of antidepressant medication increase these neurotransmitters but in two different ways:

Reuptake inhibiting antidepressants increase the "deficient" neurotransmitters by blocking the reuptake of one or more of these neurotransmitters. Hence there are more of these neurotransmitters remaining in the synapse to attach to receiving neurons. As noted, these agents are also called cyclic antidepressants.

Enzyme inhibiting agents or MAOIs increase the "deficient" neurotransmitters by preventing/slowing their metabolic breakdown. Hence there are more of these neurotransmitters to attach to receiving neurons.

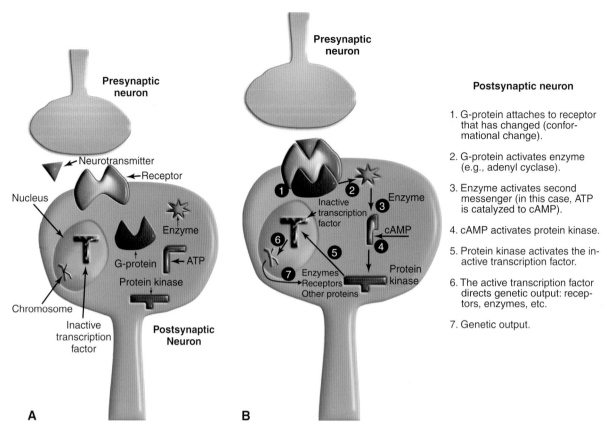

FIG. 15.2 (A) A second messenger system "at rest." Components that are affected by neurotransmitter activation of the second messenger system are labeled. (B) Sequence of events that transpires with second messenger activation. Steps 1 to 7 indicate the sequence, with step 7 providing the genetic output: enzymes, receptors, and other proteins. It is thought that in depression, key genetic products are undersynthesized. Antidepressants "reregulate" the second messenger system. *ATP*, Adenosine triphosphate; *cAMP*, cyclic adenosine monophosphate.

The accompanying numbered list for panel B reads:

Postsynaptic neuron

1. G-protein attaches to receptor that has changed (conformational change).

2. G-protein activates enzyme (e.g., adenyl cyclase).

3. Enzyme activates second messenger (in this case, ATP is catalyzed to cAMP).

4. cAMP activates protein kinase.

5. Protein kinase activates the inactive transcription factor.

6. The active transcription factor directs genetic output: receptors, enzymes, etc.

7. Genetic output.

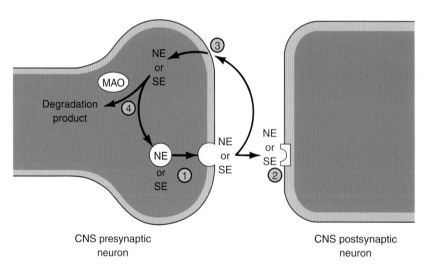

FIG. 15.3 Depression is thought to result from insufficient amines (e.g., norepinephrine, serotonin). In this drawing (1) norepinephrine *(NE)* and serotonin (5-HT) are released into the synapse, (2) they attach to postsynaptic receptors but in depression in insufficient amounts, (3) tricyclic antidepressants nonselectively block the reuptake of NE and 5-HT while selective serotonin reuptake inhibitors selectively block the reuptake of just 5-HT, thus causing larger synaptic concentrations of serotonin, and (4) monoamine oxidase inhibitors *(MAOIs)* prevent the breakdown of NE and 5-HT by MAO, shown here in the presynaptic neuron. The result of the antidepressant actions is an increase in these amines and hopefully relief from depressive symptoms. *CNS*, Central nervous system; *SE*, serotonin.

REUPTAKE INHIBITING ANTIDEPRESSANTS OR CYCLIC ANTIDEPRESSANTS

1. **SSRIs:** citalopram, fluoxetine, paroxetine, escitalopram, fluvoxamine, and sertraline.
2. **Selective serotonin-norepinephrine reuptake inhibitors (SNRIs):** venlafaxine, desvenlafaxine, duloxetine, and levomilnacipran.
3. **Norepinephrine dopamine reuptake inhibitors (NDRIs):** bupropion
4. **Novel antidepressants**: To attempt to present this material in the most effective way, a grouping of four more types of cyclic antidepressants will be presented here and following as novel antidepressants:
   a. Noradrenergic/specific serotonergic agent: mirtazapine
   b. Serotonin-1A agonist/serotonin reuptake inhibitor: vilazodone
   c. Serotonin stimulator/serotonin modulator: vortioxetine
   d. Serotonin-2 antagonists/serotonin reuptake inhibitors (SARIs): trazodone and nefazodone.
5. **Tricyclic antidepressants (TCAs)** are nonselective, meaning they block the reuptake of both serotonin and NE: amitriptyline, desipramine, imipramine, maprotiline, nortriptyline.

BOX 15.2 Innovative Chemical Approaches to Treating Depression

Ketamine: Ketamine is an N-methyl-D-aspartate (NMDA) receptor antagonist. It was approved in 1970 as an anesthetic and then became a "club drug" favorite because of the dissociative state it caused (i.e., a "K-hole"). Recently it has been used for treating depression. It is given intravenously (IV), and relief from depressive symptoms occurs within hours. A major downside is the transient nature of its antidepressant effect.

Botulinum toxin: Botulinum toxin is a very deadly substance. It kills by stopping the release of acetylcholine, that is, paralysis of muscles (e.g., suffocation). It is often used in dermatology to treat wrinkles but is also used to treat migraine, urinary incontinence, excessive sweating, and still other disorders. The explanations for its mechanism of action vary significantly, some being as straightforward as "You feel better when you look better."

Scopolamine: Scopolamine is a potent anticholinergic. It works faster than some antidepressants.

Adjunctive antipsychotics: In combination with antidepressants, some antipsychotics (e.g., aripriprazole, brexipiprazole) have proven effective in major depression.

Anti-inflammatories: This approach is based on the inflammation view of depression.

From Lent, J. L., Arredondo, A., Pugh, M. A., & Austin, P. N. (2019). Ketamine and treatment resistant depression. *American Association of Nurse Anesthetists, 87*(5), 411–419. PMID: 31612847; Franca, K., & Lotti, T. (2017). Botulinum toxin for the treatment of depression. *Dermatology Therapy.* doi:10.1111/dth.12422.

ENZYME INHIBITING AGENTS OR MONOAMINE OXIDASE INHIBITORS

1. **Nonselective MAOIs** (block both A & B monoamine oxidase): phenelzine and tranylcypromine
2. **Selective MAOIs:** MAO-A inhibitor moclobemide and MAO-B inhibitor selegiline.

Antidepressants are not always indicated when individuals report being depressed (e.g., grief); however, when antidepressants are indicated, most patients respond to treatment. Technically, treatment response means that the patient has experienced a 50% reduction in depression severity as measured by a standardized depression scale. Admittedly, depression by its very nature is subjective, and determining whether a symptom has declined by 50% leaves room for error and bias. That said, it is fair to say that these drugs do not cure depression, but long-term use has been successful in reducing symptoms.

Most relapses are associated with patient-initiated tapering off or discontinuance. However, after 2 years, between 10% and 20% of patients who are compliant with these medications experience antidepressant "poop out." It is unknown whether this loss of effectiveness is related to tolerance developing, worsening of the depression, or loss of a placebo effect (Stahl, 2021).

TCAs have been available since the 1950s and are still the first choice of some clinicians. For severe depression, TCAs may be more effective than SSRIs. However, SSRIs and the novel antidepressants are the first-line agents selected by most prescribers for several reasons (which are discussed later in the chapter). MAOIs are usually the last choice because of their serious side effects. Another effective treatment approach, electroconvulsive therapy, is discussed in Chapter 25. Consideration of various forms of psychotherapy and other psychotherapeutic interventions is always indicated. Finally, several new, non-amine approaches are being heralded as changing some basic foundational premises (Lent, Arredondo, Pugh, & Austin, 2019). They are reviewed briefly in Box 15.2. The rationale for this quest lies in the startling statistic that the remission rate for antidepressants is less than 30% (Advokat, Comaty, & Julien, 2019; Stahl, 2021).

REUPTAKE INHIBITING ANTIDEPRESSANTS OR CYCLIC ANTIDEPRESSANTS

Selective Serotonin Reuptake Inhibitors

SSRIs are widely prescribed antidepressants. SSRIs are first-line drugs for treatment of depression because they are effective antidepressants that have fewer side effects than TCAs and are far less dangerous than MAOIs (Table 15.1). SSRIs have fewer anticholinergic, cardiovascular, and sedating side effects. Fluoxetine (Prozac) was the first SSRI marketed in the United States. Stories of near-miraculous recoveries were followed by reports of major problems associated with this drug. Early anecdotal information, coupled

TABLE 15.1   Antidepressants

	DOSAGES AND PHARMACOKINETICS			SPECIFICITY FOR NT REUPTAKE			SIDE EFFECTS					
	Daily Dosage Range (mg)	Half-Life (hours)[a]	Protein Binding (%)	NE	5-HT	DA	Orthostatic Hypotension	Anticholinergic Effects	Insomnia	Sedation	Sexual Dysfunction	GI Effects
Reuptake Inhibiting Antidepressants or Cyclic Antidepressants												
Selective Serotonin Reuptake Inhibitors (SSRIs)							Selective					
Citalopram (Celexa)	10–40	23–45	80	1	4	1	Low	Low	Low	Moderate	High	High
Escitalopram (Lexapro)	10–20	27–32	55	1	4	1	Low	Low	Low	Low	Low	High
Fluoxetine (Prozac)	10–80	48–216	95	1	3	1	Moderate	Low	High	Moderate	High	High
Fluvoxamine (Luvox)	50–300	15–19	80	1	4	1	Low	Low	Moderate	Moderate	High	High
Paroxetine (Paxil)	10–60	3–21	95	1	5	1	Low	Low	Moderate	Moderate	High	High
Sertraline (Zoloft)	25–200	26–98	98	1	4	2	Moderate	Moderate	Moderate	Moderate	High	High
SNRIs, NDRIs, and Novel Antidepressants							Selective					
Bupropion (Wellbutrin)	150–450	8–15	80	1	0/1	2	Low	Low	High	Low	None	Low
Desvenlafaxine (Pristiq)	50	10–11	30	2	4	1	Low	Low	Low	Moderate	Low	Moderate
Duloxetine (Cymbalta)	20–60	8–17	90	3	2	1	Low	Low	Moderate	Low	Low	High
Levomilnacipran (Fetzima)	20–120	12	22	4	3	0	Moderate	Moderate	Low	None	Low	Moderate
Mirtazapine (Remeron)	7.5–45	20–40	85	1	1	0	Moderate	Moderate	None	High	Low	Low
Nefazodone (Serzone)	100–600	2–5	15–23	2	2	2	Moderate	Moderate	Low	High	Low	Moderate
Trazodone (Desyrel)	150–600	4–9	89–95	0	2	1	Moderate	Moderate	Low	High	Low	Moderate
Venlafaxine (Effexor)	75–225	5–11	25	2	4	1	Moderate	Moderate	Moderate	Moderate	Moderate	High
Vilazodone (Viibryd)	10–40	25	96–99	0	4	0	Low	Low	Low	Low	Low	Low

TABLE 15.1 Antidepressants (Continued)

	DOSAGES AND PHARMACOKINETICS			SPECIFICITY FOR NT REUPTAKE			SIDE EFFECTS					
	Daily Dosage Range (mg)	Half-Life (hours)[a]	Protein Binding (%)	NE	5-HT	DA	Orthostatic Hypotension	Anticholinergic Effects	Insomnia	Sedation	Sexual Dysfunction	GI Effects
Vortioxetine (Brintellix)	5–20	57	98	2	4	1	Low	Low	None	Low	Low	Low
Tricyclic Antidepressants (TCAs)							Nonselective					
Amitriptyline (Elavil)	75–300	31–46	97	1	3	1	High	High	Low	Low	Moderate	Low
Clomipramine (Anafranil)	75–300	15–37	97	1	4	1	Moderate	High	Moderate	High	High	Moderate
Desipramine (Norpramin)	75–300	12–24	90–95	5	1	1	Low	Low	Low	Low	Moderate	Low
Imipramine (Tofranil)	75–300	11–25	89–95	2	3	1	Moderate	Moderate	Low	High	High	Moderate
Nortriptyline (Pamelor, Aventyl)	50–150	18–44	92	4	2	1	Low	Moderate	Low	Moderate	Low	Low
Enzyme Inhibiting Antidepressants or Monoamine Oxidase Inhibitors												
Monoamine Oxidase Inhibitors (MAOIs)												
Phenelzine (Nardil)	30–90	2–3	?	—	—	—	Moderate	Moderate	Low	Moderate	High	Moderate
Tranylcypromine (Parnate)	20–60	2–3	?	—	—	—	Moderate	Moderate	High	Low	Moderate	Low

Modified from Procyshyn, R. M., Bezchlibnyk-Butler, K. Z., & Jeffries, J. J. (2015). *Clinical handbook of psychotropic drugs.* Hogrefe; Crutchfield, D. B. (2004). Review of psychotropic drugs. *CNS News Special Edition, 6,* 51.

Scale for receptor antagonism specificity: *1,* Low; *5,* high. *5-HT,* Serotonin; *DA,* dopamine; *GI,* gastrointestinal; *NE,* norepinephrine; *NT,* neurotransmitter.
[a]With active metabolite.

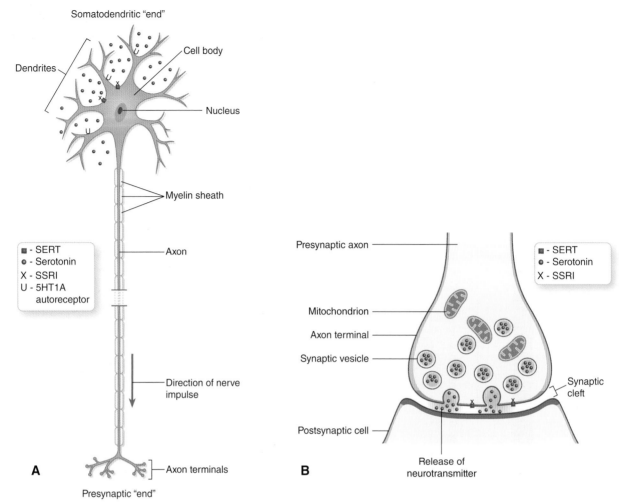

FIG. 15.4 A more complete illustration of how selective serotonin reuptake inhibitors *(SSRIs)* increase serotonin. (A) At the somato-dendritic "end" of the neuron (i.e., cell body [soma] end in the raphe nuclei) four events occur: (1) SSRIs block the reuptake of serotonin via the serotonin transporter *(SERT)*, thus increasing the amount of serotonin available to autoreceptors. (2) Serotonin inundates *5-HT1A* autoreceptors causing them to desensitize. (3) Once 5-HT1A autoreceptors desensitize, they lose their ability to inhibit the synthesis and release of serotonin. (4) Thus causing more serotonin to be released at the presynaptic end of the neuron. (B) At the presynaptic "end" of the neuron: (1) More serotonin is synthesized and released. (2) SSRIs block the reuptake of serotonin back into the neuron. (3) Serotonin accumulates in the synapse. (4) 5-HT postsynaptic receptors desensitize, and a therapeutic result occurs.

with some research findings, associated fluoxetine with sui-cidal and homicidal behaviors. Antidepressants now carry a black box warning cautioning clinicians about the risk of suicidal thinking and behavior when these drugs are pre-scribed to children, adolescents, and young adults. In one recent study, antidepressants were present in 40.2% of sui-cide victims (Petrosky, Ertl, Sheats, et al., 2020). Whether this increase in suicidal ideation is a product of the ener-gizing effects of these drugs (e.g., fluoxetine is an *activating* drug) or is related to more basic mental processes has been debated by clinicians.

Another recognized phenomenon related to SSRIs is a high level of apathy that is apparently induced by these drugs. The antidepressant apathy syndrome manifests as lack of motivation, indifference, disinhibition, and poor atten-tion. Some clinicians have wondered whether some suicides/homicides or marital breakups might be related to antide-pressant-induced indifference and disinhibition. A website, www.ssristories.org, features summaries of violent or adulter-ous behaviors purportedly driven by SSRIs or discontinuance of SSRIs. Some of the contributions are very inflammatory, so good judgment must be used when reading through these listings. Following are some examples:

- February 2017: The suspect in the shooting at the Quebec Mosque was under the influence of alcohol and antidepressants.
- January 2017: "Wealthy philanthropist jumps to her death."

- August 2016: "Attorney for teen accused of encouraging her boyfriend to kill himself raises questions about antidepressants."
- February 2016: Headline, "Citalopram is the Divorce Drug."
- March 2016: "Sarah's Story"—a story of adultery and betrayal she strongly believes was caused by an antidepressant.

It would be difficult to prove a cause-and-effect relationship between these antidepressants and aggressive acts or adultery; nonetheless, some individuals are convinced that a direct connection exists.

Pharmacologic Effect

The antidepressant effect of SSRIs is thought to be linked to their inhibition of serotonin reuptake into neurons. These drugs do not bind significantly to histaminic, cholinergic, dopaminergic, or adrenergic receptors, reducing many of the side effects that people who are taking TCAs experience. Fig. 15.4 illustrates a more complex view of the mechanism of action of SSRIs.

Pharmacokinetics

SSRIs are absorbed in the gastrointestinal (GI) tract. Peak plasma levels are achieved for most of these drugs between 4 and 6 hours. SSRIs are metabolized in the liver and have relatively long serum half-lives. The long half-lives allow once-daily dosing schedules. Both fluoxetine and sertraline have active metabolites that significantly extend their half-lives. Abrupt cessation is associated with the development of specific signs and symptoms (Box 15.3).

Side Effects

As previously noted, SSRIs have few anticholinergic, antihistaminic, or antiadrenergic effects, and they do not cause the same intensity of side effects as those associated with TCAs. Dry mouth, blurred vision, sedation, and cardiovascular symptoms are not as common with these agents as with TCAs; however, these side effects do occur and can be very bothersome for some patients. However, GI symptoms, such as nausea, diarrhea, loose stools, and weight loss or gain, are common. It is believed that activation of 5-hydroxytryptamine 3 (5-HT$_3$) receptors by the elevated levels of serotonin causes these GI symptoms. Hyponatremia has also occurred with these drugs, mostly in older patients. Finally, in slightly more than 20% of patients, excessive sweating occurs (thermoregulation requires a "balance" between DA and serotonin neurons in the hypothalamus [Ramic, Prasko, Gavran, & Spahic, 2020]).

Central nervous system (CNS) effects include headache, dizziness, tremors, anxiety, insomnia, decreased libido, impotence, ejaculatory delay, and decreased orgasm. Of patients prescribed SSRIs, 50% or more may experience sexual dysfunction (Boxes 15.4, 15.5, and 15.6).

BOX 15.4 Sexual Dysfunctions Associated With Selective Serotonin Reuptake Inhibitors

Sexual Sequence	Selective Serotonin Reuptake Inhibitors Can Cause Any or All of the Following:
Desire	Decreased libido
Arousal	Erectile dysfunction or lack of vaginal lubrication
Orgasm	Inability to achieve orgasm (thought to be the most common of these problems)

BOX 15.5 Treatment Strategies for Sexual Dysfunction Related to Selective Serotonin Reuptake Inhibitors

1. Wait and see if improvement in patient occurs naturally.
2. Decrease dosage of selective serotonin reuptake inhibitor (SSRI).
3. Time SSRI dose to maximize probability of sexual satisfaction.
4. Change antidepressants.
5. Augment with other drugs:
   Amantadine: Dopaminergic that inhibits prolactin
   Amphetamines: Increase dopamine
   Bupropion: Increases dopamine
   Sildenafil (Viagra): Enhances erections

BOX 15.3 Is There a Selective Serotonin Reuptake Inhibitor Withdrawal Syndrome?

A question many people have about selective serotonin reuptake inhibitors (SSRIs) is whether a withdrawal syndrome develops on abrupt cessation of these drugs. The answer to this question is yes. Abrupt discontinuation of SSRIs might cause the following symptoms.
Somatic symptoms: Dizziness, lethargy, nausea, vomiting, diarrhea, flu-like symptoms (e.g., headache, fever, sweating, chills, malaise), insomnia, vivid dreams
Psychological symptoms: Anxiety, agitation, irritability, confusion, slowed thinking
Because of its long half-life, fluoxetine is less likely to cause a withdrawal syndrome. Paroxetine is most likely to cause a withdrawal syndrome.

BOX 15.6 Selective Serotonin Reuptake Inhibitors Likely to Cause Sexual Dysfunction

Paroxetine (most likely from anecdotal reports)
Fluoxetine
Citalopram
Sertraline
Escitalopram (least likely)

Concerning the rate of sexual dysfunction, a compounding issue mitigates these percentages. The compounding issue is simply this: patients tend not to report sexual problems if not asked directly, and thus this issue may not be reported at all. Anxiety, insomnia, and sexual dysfunction are thought to be related to serotonin 5-HT$_2$ receptor activation. Anecdotal reports from some practitioners suggest that 70% of patients experience some form of sexual dysfunction. For many individuals, sexual dysfunction is a major factor in decisions about compliance. Nonetheless, because of this overall side effect profile, SSRIs are frequently prescribed. Conversely, the incidence of premature ejaculation seems to be increasing in the general population, and some SSRIs are used to delay orgasm in these men. Although sildenafil (Viagra) has been used for years by men experiencing sexual dysfunction, including SSRI-induced sexual dysfunction, it has been demonstrated that sildenafil is effective in treating anorgasmia in women taking serotonergic antidepressants as well (Burghardt & Gardner, 2013).

Interactions

SSRIs interact with several drugs (Table 15.2), and some of these interactions are related to SSRI inhibition of the cytochrome P-450 enzyme system. Combining SSRIs and MAOIs has proven to be fatal. This phenomenon is called *serotonin syndrome* or *serotonin toxicity* (Box 15.7).

Serotonin Syndrome

One of the most common adverse reactions from SSRIs and/or SNRIs is serotonin syndrome (SS), which may have serious consequences. Although rare, SS is caused by excessive serotonergic action at the 5-HT1A and 5-HT2A receptors in the central and peripheral nervous systems (PNSs). SS may occur within hours to days; patients will present with tremors, hyperthermia, tachycardia, and akathisia (uncontrollable restlessness) (Advokat, Comaty, & Julien, 2019). SSRIs or SNRIs, when taken together or with other "serotonergic" acting medications such as migraine medications known as triptans (i.e., sumatriptan, nartriptan, rizatriptan), have potential

BOX 15.7 Serotonin Syndrome

- Serotonin syndrome can occur if a selective serotonin reuptake inhibitor is combined with the following:
- Drugs that increase serotonin synthesis, such as tryptophan
- Drugs that inhibit serotonin breakdown, such as monoamine oxidase inhibitors
- Drugs that increase the release of serotonin, such as amphetamines, lithium, ecstasy
- Drugs that inhibit serotonin reuptake, such as cocaine, dextromethorphan, some tricyclic antidepressants, venlafaxine
- Drugs that are serotonin agonists, such as buspirone, lysergic acid diethylamide (LSD)
- Signs and symptoms of serotonin syndrome include the following:
  - *Cognitive effects:* Mental confusion, hypomania, hallucinations, agitation, headache, coma
  - *Autonomic effects:* Shivering, sweating, hyperthermia, hypertension, tachycardia, nausea, diarrhea
  - *Somatic effects:* Ataxia, myoclonus (muscle twitching), hyperreflexia, rigidity, tremor

to decrease serotonin metabolism, and an accumulation of serotonin occurs. The signs and symptoms that nurses need to be on the lookout for are altered mental status, diaphoresis, hyperthermia, and tachycardia which may progress to delirium and coma. The nursing intervention is to assess the patient, cool the patient down, hydrate, and notify the practitioner for nursing orders stat. The emergency department would be the best place to send the patient if found in a home healthcare setting with suspicion of SS.

Nursing Implications
Therapeutic Versus Toxic Drug Levels

SSRIs have a low potential for overdose. Even high doses have not resulted in fatalities, though a few have been reported. Toxic symptoms include nausea, vomiting, tremor, myoclonus, and irritability. Treatment is symptomatic and supportive.

Use During Pregnancy

SSRIs or SNRIs in pregnancy and lactation has been changed from classifications of category C drugs (meaning that they should be given only if the benefit justifies the potential risk to the fetus) or category D or X ratings to Pregnancy Categories Prior to New Pregnancy and Lactation Labeling Rule, known now as "PLLR" (Pernia & DeMaagd, 2016; Sujan, Öberg, Quinn, & D'Onofrio, 2019). However, these types of medications should be avoided during the first trimester, specifically as a prudent precaution. The long half-lives of fluoxetine and sertraline might also be significant factors in treating a pregnant patient. The literature, overall, does not find SSRIs to be associated with significant teratogenicity. Hence, these antidepressants are frequently continued during pregnancy. However, neonatal SS has been reported.

TABLE 15.2 Significant Drug Interactions With Selective Serotonin Reuptake Inhibitors

Drug	Effect of Interaction
Irreversible MAOIs	*Avoid*; this combination can be fatal (i.e., serotonin syndrome)
Lithium	Increased lithium levels, increased serotonergic effect
Antipsychotics	Increased EPSEs
Benzodiazepines	Increased benzodiazepine half-life
TCAs	Increased TCA serum levels → toxicity
	Displacement of TCAs from serum proteins → toxicity

EPSEs, Extrapyramidal side effects; *MAOIs*, monoamine oxidase inhibitors; *TCAs*, tricyclic antidepressants.

Neonates who have been exposed to SSRIs in utero and are not breastfed experience a serotonin withdrawal syndrome. This syndrome includes respiratory depression, hypoglycemia, tremor, and lower birth weight. These symptoms seem to have a short duration, and all affected neonates are typically symptom-free within 2 weeks. Nonetheless, pregnant women prescribed SSRIs should be well informed about this possibility. The benefits should outweigh the risks.

Use in Older Adults

SSRIs are safe for use in older adults because of the good side effect profile of these drugs. As with most medications, SSRI dosage levels should be reduced in older adults. However, older adults' potential for weight loss must be monitored. The half-life of paroxetine increases two or three times in older adults, so extra precautions are warranted.

Individual Selective Serotonin Reuptake Inhibitors
Citalopram

Because of its pharmacologic profile (i.e., its weaker inhibition of P-450 enzymes compared with other SSRIs), citalopram (Celexa) has fewer serious drug-drug interactions. Citalopram is composed of stereoisomers that are mirror images of each other. To elaborate, your right hand and left hand are exactly alike but backward—that is, your left hand cannot fit into a right-handed glove. The two reverse-image isomers in citalopram are called *S* and *R*. The belief is that most side effects are caused by the R isomer, and most therapeutic benefits are derived from the S isomer. Fig. 15.5 illustrates this concept.

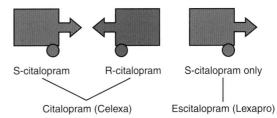

S-citalopram   R-citalopram   S-citalopram only

Citalopram (Celexa)   Escitalopram (Lexapro)

FIG. 15.5 Model demonstrating the mirror-image S and R isomers of citalopram and the S-only isomer of escitalopram.

FIVE IMPORTANT ISSUES RELATED TO ANTIDEPRESSANT USE

1. *Serotonin syndrome:* Drugs that boost intrasynaptic serotonin can cause this syndrome, which comprises hyperthermia, rigidity, cognitive impairments, and autonomic symptoms.
2. *Antidepressant apathy syndrome:* Some people taking these drugs lose interest in life and the events around them.
3. *Antidepressant withdrawal syndrome:* Abrupt discontinuation of these drugs produces withdrawal symptoms.
4. *Antidepressant loss of effectiveness:* Sometimes, these drugs just quit working (also known as drug "poop out").
5. *Antidepressant-induced suicide:* These drugs carry a black box warning about suicide, particularly in 18- to 24-year-old patients early in treatment.

A CLASSIC CASE OF SEROTONIN SYNDROME

Libby Zion was a freshman at Bennington College when she died at age 18 on March 5, 1984. Libby sought care in the emergency department at Cornell Medical Center in New York City. She presented with a temperature of 103.5°F and died 8 hours after being admitted. Other presenting symptoms were agitation, "strange jerking motions" of her body, and a bout of disorientation. Libby had a history of depression and had been prescribed the MAOI phenelzine. The emergency department physicians were unable to diagnose her condition definitively, but they admitted her for hydration and observation. Her death was caused by a combination of meperidine (Demerol) and the MAOI. The physician who prescribed meperidine was an intern. Because of this tragedy, graduate medical education was scrutinized and then criticized for the long hours that intern and resident physicians were expected to work. In defense of these physicians, the concept of serotonin syndrome was very new, with the term not being coined until the early 1980s.

From Brody, J. (2007). A mix of medicines that can be lethal. *New York Times.* http://www.nytimes.com/2007/02/27/health/27brody.html?n=Top/News/Health/Diseases,%20Conditions,%20and%20Health%20Topics/Antidepressants.

Escitalopram

Escitalopram (Lexapro) is related to citalopram; the "es" stands for the S isomer. Theoretically, escitalopram should provide most of the therapeutic benefits of citalopram without all of its side effects. Escitalopram does have a better side effect profile, particularly related to sexual dysfunction, and is prescribed at about half the dosage of citalopram. It has also been approved for treatment of generalized anxiety disorder.

Fluoxetine

Fluoxetine (Prozac) was the first SSRI developed and is frequently prescribed. Other uses include pain management and promoting smoking cessation. Fluoxetine has a long half-life of 10 days or longer (including its active metabolite). This feature makes it an ideal drug for individuals who forget to take their medications on time. A missed dose is not crucial. Drugs that have a high probability for serious interactions (e.g., MAOIs) need to be withheld for 6 weeks or more as fluoxetine is washing out of the system. Prozac is available in a once-weekly formulation for long-term treatment of depression; it is made with a special delayed-release coating. Lastly, fluoxetine is inexpensive compared with other SSRIs.

Fluvoxamine

Fluvoxamine (Luvox) is specifically approved for the treatment of obsessive-compulsive disorder (OCD). Fluvoxamine does not have an active metabolite and has a side effect profile similar to that of other SSRIs. This drug is not often prescribed for depression.

Paroxetine

Paroxetine (Paxil) is a potent serotonin reuptake inhibitor and is approved for the treatment of panic attacks. Because its metabolites are not active, paroxetine has a shorter half-life and poses fewer problems than other SSRIs if it needs to be discontinued. A common side effect is nausea, but this effect rarely leads to dose reduction or drug discontinuation. Paroxetine has also been shown to be effective in the prevention of depressive relapse. Similar to other SSRIs, paroxetine can be given on a once-daily basis and causes sexual side effects. It is approved for treatment of premenstrual dysphoric disorder.

A US Food and Drug Administration (FDA) warning to physicians indicates that paroxetine may be teratogenic. Apparently the risk of birth defects doubles for women taking this drug. The manufacturer has upgraded the pregnancy warning category to D.

Sertraline

Sertraline (Zoloft) is a widely marketed SSRI and was the second drug of this class to be used in the United States. Sertraline can also be given once daily (morning or evening) with or without food. Sertraline causes sexual dysfunction in men and women. Sexual function typically returns to normal 2 to 3 days after drug cessation.

Serotonin Norepinephrine Reuptake Inhibitors
Duloxetine, Venlafaxine, Desvenlafaxine, Levomilnacipran

Duloxetine (Cymbalta), venlafaxine (Effexor), desvenlafaxine (Pristiq), and levomilnacipran (Fetzima) are structurally unrelated to other currently marketed antidepressants. These drugs are classified as SNRIs and can boast the number 1 and the number 2 bestselling antidepressants, Cymbalta and Pristiq. These drugs appear to combine the best qualities of TCAs and SSRIs in that they inhibit the reuptake of both NE and serotonin, similar to TCAs, and, similar to SSRIs, do not bind significantly to muscarinic, histaminergic, or adrenergic receptors. With the exception of levomilnacipran, these drugs also provide a modest increase in intrasynaptic DA by blocking DA reuptake. Theoretically, few anticholinergic, antihistaminic, or antiadrenergic side effects should occur.

Duloxetine (Cymbalta). As noted, this is the best-selling antidepressant. Duloxetine has a good side-effect profile overall. It causes few instances of sedation or insomnia, few headaches, infrequent anticholinergic effects (i.e., dry mouth, blurred vision, constipation), and little dizziness. Cymbalta has been known to cause significant sexual dysfunction, however. It is also approved for the treatment of diabetic neuropathy pain, and both scientific and anecdotal evidence support this indication.

Venlafaxine (Effexor) and desvenlafaxine (Pristiq). Venlafaxine has a side effect profile similar to duloxetine. However, venlafaxine has been documented to increase blood pressure, particularly at higher doses. Venlafaxine has a lower potential for drug interaction than other antidepressants and does not exaggerate the effects of alcohol. Venlafaxine is effective in treating generalized anxiety disorder, social phobias, SSRI-induced sexual dysfunction, OCD, and panic disorders. Desvenlafaxine is an active metabolite of venlafaxine. It appears to have the same good side effect profile, although nausea is a common complaint. One significant exception is that desvenlafaxine has significantly less potential for sexual side effects.

Levomilnacipran (Fetzima). Levomilnacipran (Fetzima), approved in 2013, is one of the newest antidepressants. Levomilnacipran can potently block the reuptake of NE, less so the reuptake of serotonin but not DA. It causes little drowsiness, insomnia, headaches, or anticholinergic effects. It is thought to cause few instances of sexual dysfunction (Advokat, Comaty, & Julien, 2019; Stahl, 2021).

Norepinephrine Dopamine Reuptake Inhibitor
Bupropion

Bupropion (Wellbutrin, Zyban, Aplenzin), an NDRI, is unique in two ways: (1) it is the only antidepressant with DA reuptake inhibition as a major mechanism of action, and (2) it does not affect serotonin systems. Bupropion has a good side effect profile. However, its ability to increase intrasynaptic DA is probably related to its inhibition of NE reuptake. NE reuptake inactivates DA, so by blocking that reuptake, DA impact is greater.

Bupropion should not be given in combination with drugs that increase the DA level. Bupropion has proven to be an effective replacement for, or addition to, SSRIs when these drugs cause sexual dysfunction. Generally, it can be said that DA enhances sexuality and that serotonin inhibits sexual functioning. Because bupropion increases intrasynaptic DA, it offsets SSRI-mediated sexual inhibition and is prescribed in low doses along with SSRIs for this reason. Bupropion has a narrow therapeutic index but is far less lethal than TCAs or MAOIs.

Under the trade name Zyban, bupropion is marketed as a smoking cessation agent. Its effectiveness is probably related to two distinct mechanisms of action:
1. It is a nicotinic antagonist preventing the nicotine from smoking to activate these receptors.
2. It is believed that its DA enhancement effect counters the cravings associated with nicotine withdrawal for smokers who have or who want to quit smoking.

Bupropion is contraindicated for individuals with seizure disorders. However, at typical dosages, it does not seem to be any more epileptogenic than other antidepressants in seizure-free individuals.

Novel Antidepressants

Noradrenergic/Specific Serotonergic Agent (NaSSA)
Serotonin-1A Agonist/Serotonin Reuptake Inhibitor

Serotonin Stimulator/Serotonin Modulator
Serotonin-2 Agonist/Serotonin Reuptake Inhibitors

Mirtazapine—Noradrenergic/Specific Serotonergic Agent

Mirtazapine (Remeron) is an *alpha-2 antagonist with 5-HT$_2$ and 5-HT$_3$ antagonism* that has been approved for major depression. Mirtazapine is thought to have a faster onset of action than the SSRIs. It is also used to reduce SSRI-induced sexual dysfunction. The pharmacologic effect of mirtazapine is different from that of other antidepressants: it selectively blocks alpha-2 autoreceptors, which increases NE and serotonin levels by using the presynaptic feedback system. When this system is blocked, it signals a need for more of these neurotransmitters. Related to its antihistaminic effects, sedation and weight gain are prominent side effects. Paradoxically, sedation decreases at higher dosage levels. An increase in serum cholesterol level occurs in some patients. Mirtazapine's uniqueness is attributable to its antagonism of both 5-HT$_2$ (i.e., reducing sexual dysfunction, anxiety, and insomnia) and 5-HT$_3$ (i.e., reducing GI distress). Remeron is available in an orally dissolvable form that dissolves on the tongue in approximately 30 seconds.

Vilazodone—Serotonin-1A Agonist/Serotonin Reuptake Inhibitor

Vilazodone (Viibryd) can be classified as a serotonin reuptake inhibitor, but it is also a serotonin 1-A agonist. It is a relatively new drug but is already one of the better-selling antidepressants. It has a limited affinity for 5-HT$_{2A}$ receptors and does not cause the level of sexual dysfunction associated with SSRIs. Vilazodone has a greater affinity for 5-HT$_{1A}$ receptors. Presynaptically, these receptors serve as autoreceptors, and when swamped with a serotonin agonist, can no longer regulate serotonin synthesis as before. This causes more serotonin to be made in the neuron and, in turn, released.

Vortioxetine—Serotonin Stimulator/Serotonin Modulator

Vortioxetine (Brintellix) is better thought of as an SRI having minimal effect on NE and DA transporters while significantly increasing the synaptic availability of serotonin. One mechanism causing an increase in serotonin is its affinity for presynaptic 5-HT1A receptors. This affinity causes a rapid desensitization of these receptors, thus freeing up the synthesis of serotonin. This drug also increases acetylcholine levels, perhaps providing a cognitive benefit (i.e., increasing acetylcholine is a primary approach to treating dementia). Vortioxetine has a longer half-life (up to 66 hours) and is highly bound (i.e., 98%) to proteins (Advokat, Comaty, & Julien, 2019; Stahl, 2021).

Trazodone and Nefazodone–Serotonin-2 Agonist/Serotonin Reuptake Inhibitors

Trazodone is now seldom prescribed as an antidepressant but is frequently prescribed for sleep in both depressed and nondepressed individuals. It is not addicting, and it does not produce a high, so it has advantages over benzodiazepines (e.g., diazepam, lorazepam). Nefazodone has been taken off the market in Canada because of hepatoxicity. It is not prescribed often.

TRICYCLIC ANTIDEPRESSANTS

Pharmacologic Effects

Theoretically, the serum level of monoamines (i.e., NE and serotonin) in a depressed person is so low that achieving a normal mood is impossible. TCAs block the reuptake of these released neurotransmitters, increasing the intrasynaptic levels and alleviating the symptoms of depression. In a large meta-analysis, data were included in Advokat, Comaty, & Julien, 2019; and Stahl (2021) that TCAs were significantly more effective than SSRIs for severe depression. Thus it is a fair question to ask why TCAs are not prescribed more often. The short answer may be their side-effect profile—and marketing!

Because reuptake terminates normal neurotransmitter activity, this blocking causes greater neurotransmitter availability and prolongs the stimulating action. Clinical studies have shown that this specific effect occurs quickly, yet there is a lag period of 2 to 4 weeks before an antidepressant effect is experienced.

TCAs can be categorized further as secondary amines or tertiary amines. Drugs that tend to increase the availability of NE more than serotonin are termed *secondary amines*, and drugs that tend to increase serotonin availability more than NE are called *tertiary amines*.

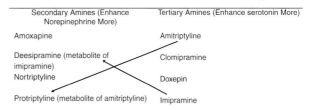

Secondary Amines (Enhance Norepinephrine More)	Tertiary Amines (Enhance serotonin More)
Amoxapine	Amitriptyline
Deesipramine (metabolite of imipramine)	Clomipramine
Nortriptyline	Doxepin
Protriptyline (metabolite of amitriptyline)	Imipramine

Although a strong potentiator of serotonin, clomipramine (Anafranil) is not typically prescribed for depression but is a drug of choice for OCD

Other Therapeutic Effects of Tricyclic Antidepressants

Sedation is a therapeutic effect of some of these drugs because depressed patients commonly experience insomnia and agitation. Tolerance to sedation usually develops.
Lethargy is a common symptom of depression. Some TCAs, described as *activating antidepressants*, might alleviate lethargy.
Improved appetite is another effect of TCAs. Loss of appetite and a consequent loss of weight are symptoms of depression. This effect is probably related to the antihistaminic effect but might be related to improved mood. However, weight gain can be significant and might contribute to a new set of problems.
Anxiety reduction is another positive effect of TCAs.

Urinary hesitancy, although definitely problematic for many patients, can be used therapeutically for childhood enuresis.

Pharmacokinetics and Dosing

TCAs are absorbed well from the GI tract and are usually given orally. TCAs are metabolized in the liver, and some metabolites have antidepressant effects (e.g., desipramine is a metabolite of imipramine; nortriptyline is a metabolite of amitriptyline).

TCAs are highly bound to plasma proteins, so their effects are produced by only a small fraction of free drug; even a small increase in free drug is potentially serious. The relatively long half-lives of these drugs usually allow once-daily dosing schedules. These drugs are initiated at low doses and increased every 3 to 5 days until the patient becomes intolerant of side effects. All TCAs appear to be equally effective.

Side Effects

Patients taking TCAs experience undesirable side effects of both the PNS and the CNS. Tertiary amines (more serotonin-enhancing) have more frequent and more severe side effects than secondary amines (more NE-enhancing).

Peripheral Nervous System Effects

Anticholinergic effects. Anticholinergic effects on the peripheral autonomic nervous system range from annoying to dangerous and include dry mouth, blurred vision, constipation, and urinary hesitancy/retention.

Older adults are most susceptible to these side effects, and older men with benign prostatic hypertrophy are at special risk for bladder problems.

On the other hand, related to this might be the unsettling thought that monoamines may not be the prime suspects in depression after all. Scopolamine is marketed as an anticholinergic, and it works faster than antidepressants. One school of thought suggests that it might be the TCAs' anticholinergic properties that make them the effective antidepressants that they are.

Cardiac effects. Anticholinergic effects on the cardiovascular system are common enough to warrant serious consideration. Essentially, the parasympathetic system serves as a brake for the heart; when this system is blocked by anticholinergics, the brake is released, and the heart speeds up. Although not likely, tachycardias and arrhythmias can lead to myocardial infarction. TCAs can also have a quinidine-like effect that delays conduction. In susceptible patients, this effect can lead to heart block and deadly arrhythmias. These serious outcomes are primarily related to disruption of sodium channels when these agents are taken at very high doses.

Children have shown troublesome cardiovascular responses to TCAs (notably desipramine) that warrant serious consideration. Since these concerns were first noted, several deaths have occurred in children taking these drugs. In each case, sudden death, usually associated with physical activity, was the cause. The serum level might be almost 50% higher in children than in adults at the same dose (Protti, Mandrioli, & Marasca, 2020).

Antiadrenergic effects (orthostasis). These drugs also block alpha-1-adrenergic receptors on peripheral blood vessels and inhibit the body's natural vasoconstricting reaction when a person stands. Blood pooling occurs in the lower extremities, leading to inadequate cerebral perfusion. The heart responds with a reflex tachycardia to help the body adapt.

Central Nervous System Effects

Sedation. Sedation is a common side effect and can be helpful because insomnia is a frequent symptom of depression. Sedation occurs because of histamine H_1 antagonism.

Cognitive or psychiatric effects. CNS effects include confusion, disorientation, delusions, agitation, anxiety, ataxia, insomnia, and nightmares. Blockade of cholinergic receptors accounts for some of these symptoms. TCAs might aggravate existing dementia or mimic dementia.

Suicide

A clear association exists between suicide and depression. Most individuals who commit suicide are found to have demonstrated characteristics of depression. Consequently, considerable evidence exists to support treating depressed individuals who are suicidal with antidepressants. Paradoxically, however, antidepressants can *energize* patients who have been too depressed to act on their suicidal thoughts. Depressed individuals who are suicidal warrant special nursing consideration after antidepressant therapy has been initiated. Further, as discussed later, TCAs are generally highly toxic, which means that the actual drug a patient is taking to treat depression could be used to overdose and die.

Interactions

TCAs are metabolized primarily by P-450 enzymes 2D6, 1A2, and 3A4. Several serious drug interactions occur with TCAs when drugs affecting these same enzymes are used. Other problematic interactions might also occur (Table 15.3).

Central Nervous System Depression

Increased CNS depression might occur when TCAs are taken with CNS depressants (e.g., alcohol, benzodiazepines).

Cardiovascular and Hypertensive Effects

Cardiovascular arrhythmias or hypertension can occur when sympathomimetic drugs are given with TCAs. Because TCAs block the reuptake of NE, sympathomimetic agents cause an increase in NE in the synaptic cleft. Interactants to avoid include NE, DA, ephedrine, and phenylpropanolamine (found in many over-the-counter stimulants). MAOI/TCA combinations are avoided by most clinicians. Severe reactions, including high fever, seizures, and a fatal hypertensive crisis, can occur if MAOIs and TCAs are combined.

Additive Anticholinergic Effects

Additive anticholinergic effects can occur when TCAs are given with other anticholinergic drugs, including antipsychotics, antiparkinsonian drugs, and antihistamines. Older adult patients are especially susceptible.

TABLE 15.3 Significant Drug Interactions With Tricyclic Antidepressants

Drug	Effect of Interaction
MAOIs	Hyperpyrexia, excitability, muscular rigidity, convulsions, fatal hypertensive crisis, mania
Sympathomimetics	Cardiac arrhythmias, hypertension
Warfarin	Increased bleeding
Barbiturates, carbamazepine, phenytoin	Decreased TCA effect
Antipsychotics	Increased EPSEs
Procainamide	Prolongation of cardiac conduction
Anticholinergics	Increased anticholinergic effect
Levodopa	Increased agitation, tremor, and rigidity
Alcohol, anticonvulsants, benzodiazepines	Increased sedation

EPSEs, Extrapyramidal side effects; *MAOIs,* monoamine oxidase inhibitors; *TCA,* tricyclic antidepressant.

Nursing Implications

Therapeutic Versus Toxic Blood Levels

TCAs do not produce euphoria and are not addicting, and the potential for abuse is not great. However, severe toxicity and death can occur. Overdose is an issue and accounts for a high number of intentional suicides. The difference between a therapeutic dose and a lethal dose is small. Outpatients who are at risk for suicide are frequently restricted to a 7-day supply.

Cardiovascular reactions can occur suddenly and cause acute heart failure, even several days after the overdose. Also, cardiovascular reactions can be delayed; that is, they can occur after recovery from overdose. All antidepressant overdoses should be considered serious, and the patient should be admitted to a hospital for monitoring.

The nurse should be aware of several assessment and intervention strategies when a toxic level of TCAs is suspected (see the Key Nursing Interventions for TCA Overdose box).

KEY NURSING INTERVENTIONS

For Tricyclic Antidepressant Overdose

- Monitor blood pressure, heart rate and rhythm, and respirations.
- Maintain patent airway.
- An electrocardiogram is recommended.
- Use cathartics or gastric lavage with activated charcoal to *prevent further drug absorption* (for up to 24 h).
- The antidote for severe TCA poisoning (anticholinergic toxicity) is physostigmine (Antilirium), an acetylcholinesterase inhibitor (inhibits the breakdown of acetylcholine). Physostigmine should be given only to patients with life-threatening symptoms (e.g., coma, convulsions) because of the risk associated with its use.

Use During Pregnancy

TCAs have not been definitively found to cause teratogenic effects but should be avoided in the first trimester. Because depressive symptoms, such as loss of appetite, can interfere with fetal development by preventing adequate fetal weight gain, antidepressants should be prescribed cautiously to pregnant women.

Depressive Symptoms Associated With Serotonin Deficiencies	Depressive Symptoms Associated With Norepinephrine Deficiencies
Anxiety	Fatigue
Panic	Apathy
Phobias	Cognitive disturbances
Posttraumatic stress disorder	Impaired concentration
Obsessions	Focusing attention
Compulsions	Slowed information processing
Eating disorders	Deficiencies in working memory

Although serotonin and norepinephrine deficiencies are both considered causative for depression, Stahl (2021) noted that low levels of these two monoamines produce distinct/different depressive syndromes.

Use in Older Adults

TCAs should be given in reduced doses to older adult patients. The maxim "start low and go slow" is particularly true for these patients. The secondary amines (e.g., desipramine, nortriptyline, protriptyline) are preferred.

Side Effects

Selected side effects and appropriate nursing interventions are listed in the "Side Effects and Nursing Interventions for Antidepressants" box.

Interactions

The nurse should be aware of the drug interactants mentioned in Table 15.3. As a general rule, individuals who are taking TCAs should avoid certain types of drugs, both prescribed and over the counter, including the following:
- Drugs that depress the CNS
- Drugs that have anticholinergic properties
- Drugs that stimulate the CNS
- MAOIs (deaths have occurred)

Teaching Patients

The nurse should discuss the following side effects and important principles with patients and their families:
- A lag period of 2 to 4 weeks occurs before full therapeutic effects are experienced.
- Certain drugs must be avoided, including some over-the-counter preparations.
- Abrupt discontinuation can cause nausea, headache, and malaise.

SIDE EFFECTS AND NURSING INTERVENTIONS FOR ANTIDEPRESSANTS

Side Effects	Interventions
Peripheral Nervous System	
Dry mouth	Advise frequent sips of water, hard candies, and sugarless gum.
Mydriasis	Advise wearing of sunglasses outdoors.
Diminished lacrimation	Suggest artificial tears.
Blurred vision	Caution patient about driving and potential for falls (usually subsides in 1–2 weeks).
Eye pain	Advise patient to report eye pain immediately because it might indicate an acute glaucoma attack.
Urinary hesitancy and retention	Monitor fluid intake. Patients should be told to avoid putting off urinating.
Constipation	Monitor fluid and food intake. Urge patients to heed the urge to defecate. A high-fiber diet and large amounts of water (2500–3000 mL/day) are helpful.
Anhidrosis	Decreased sweating can lead to an increase in body temperature. Adequate fluids, appropriate clothing, and sensible exercise should be stressed.
Cardiovascular effects	Tricyclic antidepressants are contraindicated during the recovery phase of myocardial infarction.
Orthostatic hypotension	Advise patient to rise slowly and dangle the legs before standing.
Central Nervous System	
Sedation	Caution patient about driving.
Delirium or mania	Discontinue the drug and call the physician.
Suicidal patients	Observe patients closely because antidepressants might increase motivation for suicide.

- Eye pain must be reported immediately, particularly in older adults, in which undiagnosed narrow-angle glaucoma can lead to an emergency situation.
- Some side effects lessen after patients adjust to the medication.

Individual Tricyclic Antidepressants

The following brief descriptive statements about TCAs include only the unique features of usage and side effects. This chapter does not discuss the uses and side effects that are common to all the drugs.

Amitriptyline

Amitriptyline is highly anticholinergic and one of the most sedating and cardiotoxic antidepressants.

Desipramine

Desipramine is a secondary amine and a metabolite of imipramine. Desipramine is an *activating antidepressant* and

might be advantageous for patients with apathy, lethargy, and hypersomnia. Because of its aforementioned effects on the cardiovascular system in children, desipramine should be used with care in this age group. It appears to be the most toxic TCA (Advokat, Comaty, & Julien, 2019; Stahl, 2021).

Imipramine

Imipramine is the oldest TCA. None of the newer antidepressants have proven to be more effective. Because of its anticholinergic properties, imipramine has proven to be effective in the treatment of childhood enuresis. Imipramine should be used with care in children because of its cardiovascular effects.

Nortriptyline

Because nortriptyline, a secondary amine TCA, is sedating and has a good side effect profile, it is often prescribed for older adult patients who are depressed, agitated, and experiencing insomnia. It is the least toxic TCA (Zheng, Li, Qi, & Xiao, 2020). Nortriptyline is a metabolite of the tertiary amine, amitriptyline.

ENZYME INHIBITING AGENTS OR MONOAMINE OXIDASE INHIBITORS

MAOIs were the first antidepressants "discovered," but they are usually administered only to hospitalized patients or to individuals who can be closely supervised. Their history is fascinating, and Meyer (2018) does a wonderful job of summarizing it. He notes that after World War II, the government gave large quantities of hydrazine, a chemical used for V2 rocket fuel, to drug companies. From this excess hydrazine, drugs were derived (i.e., isoniazid, iproniazid) that were effective in the treatment of tuberculosis. During the process of treatment, it was further discovered that iproniazid had mood-elevating properties and that it was an MAO inhibitor. From this serendipitous beginning came the first antidepressants.

Their mechanism of action is quite simple: they block enzymatic breakdown of monoamines, thus "leaving" more available for the depressed brain. Many psychiatrists have never prescribed MAOIs because of their toxic potential. Although these drugs are not used much, they warrant mention because they have potentially fatal interactions and can help the student conceptualize significant pharmacokinetic processes.

Two MAOIs that are occasionally used are phenelzine (Nardil) and tranylcypromine (Parnate). They are referred to as *nonselective irreversible inhibitors* because they inhibit both variants of monoamine oxidase: MAO-A and MAO-B (the *nonselective* part) and "stay on" the enzyme until it dies and is replaced (the *irreversible* part). There are also two *selective* MAOIs; one, moclobemide, inhibits only MAO-A, and the other, seligiline, inhibits MAO-B. The former is not available in the United States, and the latter is prescribed for Parkinson disease; thus, neither merit further discussion in this chapter on antidepressants.

Because of the serious adverse reactions to these drugs, especially life-threatening hypertension, the older irreversible MAOIs are almost always prescribed after other antidepressants have failed or for what is called *treatment-resistant depression.* Although some clinicians believe that MAOIs are particularly effective in treating atypical depression (e.g., hypersomnia, somatic anxiety, excessive hunger, extreme sensitivity to rejection), they are still seldom prescribed.

Pharmacologic Effects

MAOIs block monoamine oxidase, a major enzyme involved in the metabolic decomposition and inactivation of NE, serotonin, and DA. This enzyme inhibition lasts for 10 days with the irreversible MAOIs. The inhibition increases the levels of these neurotransmitters in the PNS and CNS. According to the neurochemical theory of depression, depressed individuals have lower than normal levels of these neurotransmitters available. MAOIs help to attain normal levels by slowing the deactivation of these amines. This action is in contrast to TCAs, which help attain normal levels by preventing the reuptake of amines by the neurons. Approximately 2 to 4 weeks is required for the antidepressant effect of MAOIs to occur, although, as is the case with TCAs, the inhibition of monoamine oxidase occurs immediately, thus suggesting that factors other than low levels of specific neurotransmitters are involved in depression.

Absorption, Distribution, and Administration

MAOIs are well absorbed from the GI tract and are given orally. They are metabolized in the liver. Because monoamine oxidase does not decline with age, MAOIs do not present the same age-related risks associated with other drugs.

Side Effects

MAOIs cause CNS, cardiovascular, and anticholinergic side effects. Serious life-threatening reactions can occur when irreversible MAOIs interact with certain drugs or foods (see the following discussion on interactions).

Because MAOIs increase the availability of biogenic amines in the brain, CNS hyperstimulation might occur, causing agitation, acute anxiety attacks, restlessness, insomnia, and euphoria. In individuals thought to have quiescent schizophrenia (an unrecognized, latent form), full schizophrenic episodes have erupted. Hypomania (which is less severe compared with full mania) is a more common effect.

Hypotension is a common cardiovascular effect resulting from a slowdown in the release of NE. In contrast to the effect of TCAs, reflex tachycardia does not occur because other adrenergic nerves also experience the slowed release of NE, and the heart does not speed up reflexively. Hypotension, combined with the absence of a compensatory increased heart rate, can lead to heart failure.

MAOIs can cause anticholinergic effects such as dry mouth, blurred vision, urinary hesitancy, and constipation. Hepatic and hematologic dysfunctions can occur and, although rare, are potentially serious. Blood counts and liver function test results should be obtained before therapy begins.

Interactions

MAOIs have many serious interactions. Potentially lethal interactants include both drugs and foods.

TABLE 15.4 Significant Drug Interactions With Monoamine Oxidase Inhibitors

Drugs	Effect of Interaction
Anticholinergic drugs	Increase anticholinergic response
Anesthetics (general)	Deepen CNS depression
Antihypertensives (diuretics, beta-blockers, hydralazine)	Cause hypotension
CNS depressants	Intensify CNS depression
Sympathomimetics (mixed-acting and indirect-acting): Amphetamines, methylphenidate, dopamine, phenylpropanolamine (in many over-the-counter hay fever, cold, and diet medications)	Precipitate hypertensive crisis, cardiac stimulation, arrhythmias, cerebrovascular hemorrhage
Sympathomimetics (direct-acting): Epinephrine, norepinephrine, isoproterenol; less likely to cause problems	Theoretically should not produce a reaction, but caution is recommended
Serotonergic drugs (e.g., SSRIs)	*Avoid*; this combination can be fatal

Less severe interactions with these drugs also occur with the reversible, selective inhibitors of monoamine oxidase, moclobemide, and seligiline. *CNS*, Central nervous system; *SSRIs*, selective serotonin reuptake inhibitors.

Drug-Drug Interactions

The nurse should be aware of the following types of drug interactions (Table 15.4):

- Drug interactions that cause hypertension
- Drug interactions that cause severe anticholinergic responses
- Drug interactions that cause profound CNS depression

Sympathomimetic drugs are classified as direct-acting drugs, indirect-acting drugs, and mixed-acting drugs (having both direct and indirect properties). Indirect-acting and mixed-acting sympathomimetics cause serious and sometimes fatal hypertension when given with MAOIs. Direct-acting sympathomimetics add new NE to the body, whereas indirect-acting sympathomimetics release existing NE from the neurons. Because MAOIs increase the amount of stored NE in the PNS, a potential exists for indirect-acting and mixed-acting sympathomimetics to induce the release of large amounts of NE. Avoiding these interacting drugs is crucial. Even small amounts can trigger a hypertensive crisis. Typical indirect-acting and mixed-acting sympathomimetics include amphetamines, cocaine, methylphenidate (Ritalin), DA, and ephedrine. Over-the-counter weight-loss and stimulant products contain phenylephrine, phenylpropanolamine, and pseudoephedrine, which are mixed-acting or indirect-acting sympathomimetics. Theoretically, direct-acting sympathomimetics such as NE, epinephrine, and isoproterenol should not trigger the release of existing NE. Finally, MAOIs should not be given in combination with TCAs except in unusually refractory cases and should never be given in combination with SSRIs.

The initial symptoms of hypertensive crisis are palpitation; tightness in the chest; stiff neck; and a throbbing, radiating headache. Extremely high blood pressure with elevation of the heart rate is common. Cardiovascular consequences have included myocardial infarction, cerebral hemorrhage, myocardial ischemia, and arrhythmias. Diaphoresis and pupillary dilation are also prominent signs.

Anticholinergic effects can be severe if other anticholinergic drugs are given with MAOIs. Typical anticholinergic side effects can be reviewed in the discussion of TCA side effects.

Finally, because MAOIs inhibit monoamine oxidase in the liver, some drugs, particularly CNS depressants, are not rapidly metabolized in the liver and result in serum levels high enough to cause serious depression of the CNS.

Meperidine (Demerol) is specifically contraindicated. A marked potentiation of this drug can occur, and deaths have been documented. Hypotensive drugs are also enhanced by MAOIs. The nurse should be aware that MAO inhibition can continue for 10 days after tranylcypromine and phenelzine are discontinued. In other words, the potential for serious interactions continues for some time after MAOIs are discontinued.

Food-Drug Interactions

Food-drug interactions center on the amine tyramine, a decarboxylation product of tyrosine (the precursor to DA, NE, and epinephrine). Tyramine is found in many foods commonly consumed in the North American diet (Box 15.8); however, foods eaten today generally contain less tyramine than foods eaten when these drugs were first prescribed (Meyer, 2018). Only a few foods cause a severe reaction; these include aged cheese, bananas, salami, sauerkraut, soy sauce, all beers on tap, and coffee. However, some clinicians recommend that all high-protein foods that have undergone protein breakdown by aging, fermentation, pickling, or smoking be avoided. Hypertension and hypertensive crisis can develop from this food-drug combination.

Nursing Implications
Therapeutic Versus Toxic Drug Levels

An intensification of the effects already discussed occurs with overdose. A lethal dose of MAOIs is only 6 to 10 times the daily dose (see Table 15.1 for dosages). Careful monitoring when these medications are given is important. "Cheeking" and hoarding of these drugs can be disastrous. If MAOI overdose is indicated, the nurse should know the following:

- Emesis and gastric lavage might be helpful if performed early.
- Monitoring of vital signs is important.
- External cooling is warranted if high fever occurs.
- Hypotension should be treated in the standard manner.

BOX 15.8 Tyramine-Rich Foods to Avoid With Monoamine Oxidase Inhibitors

Alcoholic Beverages
Beer and ale
Chianti and sherry wine
Alcohol-free beer

Dairy Products
All mature cheese: Cheddar, blue, Brie, mozzarella
Sour cream
Yogurt

Fruits and Vegetables
Avocados
Bananas
Fava beans
Canned figs

Meats
Bologna
Chicken liver
Fish, dried
Liver
Meat tenderizer
Pickled herring
Salami
Sausage

Other Foods
Caffeinated coffee, colas, tea (large amounts)
Chocolate
Licorice
Sauerkraut
Soy sauce
Yeast

Use During Pregnancy

MAOIs should be avoided during the first trimester of pregnancy. Later use is justified only when the anticipated benefit outweighs the potential risk to the fetus.

Use in Older Adults

MAOIs might be effective in older patients because monoamine oxidase activity increases with age. However, precautions for orthostatic hypotension should be observed in this age group.

Side Effects

The nurse should be familiar with the common side effects of MAOIs and the appropriate nursing interventions (see the "Side Effects and Nursing Interventions for MAOIs" box).

Interactions and Contraindications

As noted earlier, the nurse must understand that drug-drug and food-drug interactions are serious and potentially fatal.

SIDE EFFECTS AND NURSING INTERVENTIONS FOR MONOAMINE OXIDASE INHIBITORS

Side Effects	Interventions
CNS hyperstimulation	Reassure the patient. Assess for developing psychosis, hypomania, or seizures. If symptoms warrant, withhold the drug and notify the physician.
Hypotension	Monitor blood pressure frequently and intervene to prevent falls and injuries; having patient lie down might help return blood pressure to normal.
Anticholinergic effects	See antidepressant side effects for appropriate nursing interventions.
Hepatic and hematologic dysfunction	Blood counts and liver function tests should be performed. If dysfunction is apparent, monoamine oxidase inhibitor should be discontinued.

CNS, Central nervous system.

MAOIs should not be given in combination with the following drugs:

- Other MAOIs
- TCAs or SSRIs
- Meperidine

Hypertensive crisis is a major concern. If it occurs, the nurse should do the following:

- Discontinue MAOIs and contact the physician.
- Know that therapy to reduce blood pressure is warranted (e.g., an alpha-1 blocker).
- Monitor vital signs.
- Have the patient walk (which decreases blood pressure slightly).

- Manage fever by external cooling.
- Institute supportive nursing care, as indicated.

Teaching Patients

The nurse must be persistent in teaching patients and their families about MAOIs and their side effects. Although most of these drugs are administered in a closely supervised setting, the nurse is nonetheless responsible for educating patients. Because patients taking MAOIs can experience serious reactions to some other drugs and foods, the nurse must clearly convey this information.

NONTRADITIONAL APPROACHES TO DEPRESSION

Supplementation with both vitamin D and L-methylfolate (Deplin) has been demonstrated to be helpful non-psychotropic agents in depression (Advokat, Comaty, & Julien, 2019; Geng, Shaikh, & Han, 2019; Zheng, Li, Qi, & Xiao, 2020). Vitamin D regulates tyrosine hydroxylase, which is needed to convert tyrosine to levodopa and subsequently DA and NE, whereas L-methylfolate modulates the tyrosine hydroxylase (needed for NE and DA synthesis) and tryptophan hydroxylase (needed for serotonin synthesis). Many clinicians supplement antidepressant therapy with these agents.

? CRITICAL THINKING QUESTIONS

1. What is the supposed pharmacologic effect that causes SSRIs to result in sexual dysfunction?
2. Many older, experienced clinicians believe that TCAs are the best drugs for treating depression. Based on your reading about TCAs and the short mention of scopolamine in the text and in Box 15.2, why may that be?

▌ STUDY NOTES

1. According to the neurochemical theory, depression is the result of a decreased availability of the neurotransmitters norepinephrine, serotonin, and possibly dopamine in the brain.
2. Based on this neurochemical theory, there are two overarching approaches to increasing serotonin, norepinephrine, and dopamine:
   Reuptake inhibiting antidepressants
   Enzyme inhibiting antidepressants.
3. Reuptake inhibiting antidepressants are also called cyclic antidepressants because of their molecular structure. They are further divided into selective reuptake inhibitors and nonselective reuptake inhibitors.
4. Among selective reuptake inhibitors, there are several antidepressant classifications:
   SSRIs
   SNRIs
   NDRIs
   Novel antidepressants

5. Among nonselective reuptake inhibitors, there is only one category:
   TCAs
6. Cyclic antidepressants block the reuptake of neurotransmitters back into nerve endings, increasing their availability.
7. Enzyme inhibiting antidepressants include just one classification:
   MAOIs.
8. MAOIs slow the breakdown of these neurotransmitters by inhibiting the enzyme monoamine oxidase, increasing the availability of these neurotransmitters.
9. MAOIs are seldom prescribed because they are dangerous.
10. Newer *novel* antidepressants include mirtazapine, vilazodone, vortioxetine, trazodone, and nefazodone. These agents are also first-line agents in the treatment of depression (although trazodone and nefazodone are less so).

11. Because TCAs have a narrow therapeutic index, amounts even slightly higher than therapeutic doses can be fatal.
12. Patients should be taught about the lag time of 2 to 4 weeks that is required for a full therapeutic effect to be experienced with most antidepressants.
13. Traditional MAOIs interact with certain foods that contain tyramine (e.g., aged cheese, bananas, salami) and with indirect-acting and mixed-acting sympathomimetic drugs (e.g., amphetamines, methylphenidate [Ritalin]) to cause hypertensive crisis.
14. Nontraditional agents such as vitamin D and L-methylfolate have been helpful in the treatment of depression.

REFERENCES

Advokat, C. D., Comaty, J. E., & Julien, R. M. (2019). *Julien's primer of drug action: A comprehensive guide to the actions, uses and side effexors of psychoactive drugs* (14th Ed.). Worth Publishers.

Braslow, J., & Marder, S. R. (2019). History of psychopharmacology. *Annual Review of Clinical Psychology, 15,* 25–50. https://doi.org/10.1146/annurev-clinpsy-050718-095514.

Burghardt, K. J., & Gardner, K. N. (2013). Sildenafil for SSRI-induced sexual dysfunction in women. Current. *Psychiatry, 12,* 29.

Franca, K., & Lotti, T. (2017). Botulinum toxin for the treatment of depression. *Dermatologic Therapy, 30*(2), e12422. https://doi.org/10.1111/dth.12422.

Geng, C., Shaikh, A., Han, W., et al. (2019). Vitamin D and depression: Mechanisms, determination and application. *Asia Pacific Journal of Clinical Nutrition, 28*(4), 689–694. https://doi.org/10.6133/apjcn.201912_28(4).0003.

Lent, J. L., Arredondo, A., Pugh, M. A., & Austin, P. N. (2019). Ketamine and treatment resistant depression. *American Association of Nurse Anesthetists, 87*(5), 411–419. PMID: 31612847.

Magid, M, & Reichenberg, J (2015). Botulinum toxin for depression: An idea that's raising some eyebrows. *Current Psychiatry, 14*(11), 43.

Meyer. J. M. (2018). A concise guide to monoamine oxidase inhibitors: How to avoid drug interactions. *Current Psychiatry, 17*(1), 22–24. 28, 33.

Nestler, E. J., Hyman, S. E., Holtzman, D. M., & Malenka, R. C. (2021). *Molecular neuropharmacology: A foundation for clinical neuroscience.* McGraw Hill.

Pernia, S., & DeMaagd, G. (2016). The new pregnancy and lactation labeling rule. *Pharmacy and Therapeutics, 41*(11), 713–715. https://www.ncbi.nlm.nih.gov/pmc/articles/PMC5083079/.

Petrosky, E., Ertl, A., Sheats, K. J., Wilson, R., Betz, C. J., & Blair, J. M. (2020). Surveillance for violent deaths — National violent death reporting system, 34 states, four California counties, the District of Columbia, and Puerto Rico, 2017. *Surveillance Summaries, 69*(8), 1–37. https://www.cdc.gov/mmwr/volumes/69/ss/ss6908a1.htm.

Protti, M., Mandrioli, R., Marasca, C., et al. (2020). April 13. New-generation, non-SSRI antidepressants: Drug-drug interactions and therapeutic drug monitoring. Part 2: NaSSAs, NRIs, SNDRIs, MASSAs, NDRIs and others. *Medicinal Research Reviews, 40*(5), 1794–1832. https://doi.org/10.1002/med.21671.

Ramic, E., Prasko, S., Gavran, L., & Spahic, E. (2020). Assessment of the antidepressant side effects occurrence in patients treated in primary care. *Materia socio-medica, 32*(2), 131–134. https://doi.org/10.5455/msm.2020.32.131-134.

Schiele, M. A., Zwanzger, P., Schwarte, K., et al. (2021). Serotonin transporter gene promoter hypomethylation as a predictor of antidepressant treatment response in major depression: A replication study. *International Journal of Neuropsychopharmacology, 24*(2), 191–199. https://doi.org/10.1093/ijnp/pyaa081.

Stahl. S. M. (2021). *Stahl's essential psychopharmacology: Prescriber's guide* (7th ed). Cambridge University Press.

Sujan, A. C., Öberg, A. S., Quinn, P. D., & D'Onofrio, B. M. (2019). Annual research review: Maternal antidepressant use during pregnancy and offspring neurodevelopmental problems – A critical review and recommendations for future research. *Journal of Child Psychology and Psychiatry, 60*(4), 356–376. https://doi.org/10.1111/jcpp.13004.

Zheng, W., Li, W., Qi, H., Xiao, L., et al. (2020). Adjunctive folate for major mental disorders: A systematic review. *Journal of Affective Disorders, 267,* 123–130. https:doi.org/10.1016/j.jad/2020.01.096 96, 369.

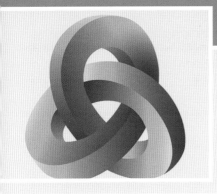

16

Antimanic Drugs

Helene Vossos and Norman L. Keltner

Most people are about as happy as they make up their minds to be.

Abraham Lincoln

ⓔ http://evolve.elsevier.com/Keltner

LEARNING OBJECTIVES

- Explain the mechanism of action of antimanic drugs.
- Discuss the side effects of antimanic drugs.
- Discuss the role of lithium.
- Discuss the role of anticonvulsants.
- Discuss the role of antipsychotics.
- Identify therapeutic versus toxic serum levels of lithium.
- Discuss the implications of teaching patients about antimanic drugs.

Lithium has unique, multiple levels of microscopic to macroscopic mechanisms of action pivotal in psychopharmacology. Lithium is neuroprotective and modulates neurotransmission of dopamine, glutamate, and GABA neurotransmitters. It preceded the introduction of many medications in psychiatry and, in fact, fired the first barrage that initiated the modern era of psychopharmacology.

Flavio Guzman, M.D.
Psychopharmacology Institute.

BLACK BOX WARNING FOR LITHIUM

Lithium toxicity is closely related to serum lithium levels and can occur at doses close to therapeutic levels; start tx only if facility available for prompt accurate serum lithium determinations.

Antimanic drugs or mood stabilizers include lithium and several anticonvulsants. Antipsychotic drugs are also used to treat bipolar spectrum disorder and are very effective (Stahl, 2021). However, no single drug or combination of drugs is always effective. The two poles suggested in the term *bipolar* are dysphoria (or depression) and euphoria (or mania). Although these extremes in emotions are seemingly opposite, they are related. This chapter primarily focuses on the psychopharmacologic classes of drugs used to treat the euphoric end of the bipolar spectrum—the antimanic drugs (Table 16.1). These drug classes include lithium, anticonvulsants, and antipsychotic agents.

There are three overarching issues in treating bipolar disorder:
1. Getting acute mania under control
2. Preventing relapse when remission occurs
3. Returning to the prior level of functioning (i.e., social, occupational, interpersonal)

The focus of treating acute symptoms is on helping the

TREATMENT GOALS FOR BIPOLAR DISORDER

1. Remission
2. Prevention
3. Return to premorbid exacerbation functioning

patient regain control. Box 16.1 lists the typical signs and symptoms associated with acute bipolar disorder (see Chapter 26 for a full discussion of bipolar disorders). *Maintenance therapy* attempts to prevent relapse (about 63% after 2 years [Kishi et al., 2020]), reduce suicide risks, improve functioning, and reduce what are called *subthreshold symptoms* (symptoms not quite reaching a level of clinical diagnostic

TABLE 16.1 Lithium and Anticonvulsants Used for Treatment of Bipolar Disorder

Antimanic Drug	Usual Adult Daily Dosage	Half-Life (hours)	Therapeutic Serum Level	Metabolism	Common Side Effects	Warnings
Lithium	Acute: 900–2400 mg; maintenance: 400–1200 mg	~24	0.6–1.2 mEq/L	95% unchanged	N/V, diarrhea, polyuria, polydipsia, weight gain, tremor, fatigue	Lithium toxicity, teratogenicity
Carbamazepine	800–1000 mg and titrated upward until side effects or serum level reached	12–17; induces own metabolism	4–12 mcg/mL	P-450 enzymes	N/V, dizziness, sedation, rash, HA	Blood dyscrasias, teratogenicity
Divalproex	1000–1500 mg	5–20	50–115 mcg/mL	P-450 enzymes and direct conjugation with glucuronic acid	N/V, sedation, weight gain, hair loss	Hepatotoxicity, teratogenicity, pancreatitis
Lamotrigine	Begin at 25–50 mg and increase by 12.5–25 mg per 2 weeks up to 250 mg bid	~24 with long-term use	4–18 mcg/mL	Attaches to glucuronic acid by conjugation	HA, sedation, cognitive dulling, insomnia, ataxia, N/V, dizziness, diplopia	Serious rash (e.g., Stevens-Johnson), breast-feeding (?)
Oxcarbazepine	600–2400 mg in 2–3 divided doses	7–20 with active metabolites	15–35 mcg/mL	Metabolized to an active metabolite	Fatigue, N/V, dizziness, sedation, diplopia, hyponatremia	Teratogenicity, breast-feeding (?)
Gabapentin	900–4000 mg in 3 divided doses	5–7	NA[a]	Not metabolized	Sedation, fatigue, tremors, nausea, dry mouth, dizziness, diplopia, hyperthermia	Teratogenicity, breast-feeding (?)
Topiramate	Acute: 200–600 mg; maintenance: 50–400 mg	19–23	NA[a]	70% unchanged	Sedation, cognitive blunting, anxiety, tremors, weight loss, dizziness	Breast-feeding, cognitive dulling

[a]Serum concentrations can be measured for these newer antiepileptics, but our understanding of how to utilize this information is limited.
HA, Headache; *NA*, not applicable; *N/V*, nausea and vomiting.
Derived with permission from Procyshyn, R. M., Bezchlibnyk-Butler, K. Z., & Jeffries, J. J. (2021). *Clinical handbook of psychotropic drugs* (24th Ed.) ©2021 Hogrefe Publishing www.hogrefe.com. http://doi.org/10.1027/00593-000.

significance). As noted, relapse is a persistent concern. Box 16.2 illustrates this point through the mnemonic RELAPSE, while Fig. 16.1 points out the clinical difficulties encountered that contribute to relapse.

LITHIUM

Lithium is considered the *gold standard* by many clinicians for the treatment of bipolar spectrum disorder, and a recent large-scale study seems to confirm that conventional wisdom (Rege, 2020). Lithium, a naturally occurring element, is not much different from sodium. However, the differences are significant enough to make lithium useful in treating bipolar disorder. Lithium was discovered in 1817 and named after the Greek word for stone *(lithos)*. It came to be touted as a cure for epilepsy, gout, and other problems. In 1949, an Australian psychiatrist named Dr. Cade reported his research in the *Medical Journal of Australia*, showing lithium to be effective in the treatment of manic depression. Of the manic patients whom he treated, all demonstrated considerable improvement. Lithium's effect was so pronounced that Cade (1949) called the illness a "lithium deficiency disease." Also in 1949, the March 12th issue of the *Journal of the American Medical Association* reported two accounts of fatal lithium

---

BOX 16.1 Signs and Symptoms of Bipolar Disorder—Mania

Elevated mood
Increase in activities
Flight of ideas
Racing thoughts
Inflated self-esteem
Decreased need for sleep
Agitation
More talkative than usual
Pacing, hand wringing
Extreme restlessness
Loses temper often
Significant irresponsible behavior
Increased goal-directed activities (e.g., sexual, social)
Impaired excessive involvement in pleasurable activities, with high potential for painful consequences
Delusions
Hallucinations

BOX 16.2 Mood Disorder RELAPSE

Rhythm disturbances (e.g., shift work, jet lag)
Ending treatment either intentionally or unintentionally
Life change (e.g., divorce, job loss)
Additional drugs (e.g., opiates, steroids, antidepressants [can induce mania])
Physical health changes (e.g., epilepsy, stroke)
Substance use and withdrawal, alcohol, opiates
End of drug response, some patients experience loss of drug response

---

Modified from Rakofsky, J. (2016). RELAPSE: Answers to why a patient is having a new mood episode. *Current Psychiatry, 15*(2), 53.

poisoning in cardiac patients who were given lithium chloride as a salt substitute. These deaths led to a 20-year hibernation for lithium in the United States (Braslow & Marder, 2019). Fears of lithium were compounded by a lack of interest on the part of drug companies. As a natural element, lithium is not patentable; consequently, a drug company might invest research funds only to have another pharmaceutical company legally use the findings. Lithium was not made available in the United States until 1970. Since this time it is now called "The penicillin of psychiatry" (Ruffalo, 2019). Lithium has been prescribed successfully for the past 51 years under prudent assessment and management.

Lithium is a Federal Drug Agency (FDA) approved medication treatment and prophylaxis of the manic phase of manic-depressive illness (Stahl, 2021). About 70% to 80% of individuals who take lithium for long-term prophylaxis and about 50% who are treated for the more acute phase have a therapeutic response to this drug (De Mendiola et al., 2021). Additionally, a growing body of clinical research supports its use as an antidepressant, for augmentation of other antidepressants in refractory depression, and for other disorders. Finally, for reasons not yet understood, lithium seems to have a greater antisuicide effect than the other antimanic drugs (De Mendiola, Hidalgo-Mazzei, Vieta, & Gonzalez-Pinto, 2021; Sarai, Mekala, & Lippmann, 2018).

NORM'S NOTES These drugs are a little more challenging. We have the gold standard (lithium), but antiepileptic drugs are typically first-choice agents, particularly divalproex or valproate (Stahl, 2021). The trick for knowing the reason for antimanic treatment is to find the similarities in action of both antiepileptics and lithium. How do these drugs slow down manic thinking? If you can nail that down, then you are really beginning to learn about psychotropic drugs.

Pharmacologic Effects

Exactly how lithium achieves its normalizing effect on mania is unknown. Its similarity to calcium, sodium, and potassium may be related to its therapeutic effects. For

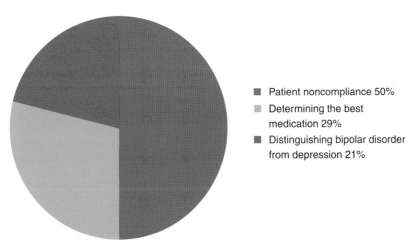

- Patient noncompliance 50%
- Determining the best medication 29%
- Distinguishing bipolar disorder from depression 21%

FIG. 16.1 Difficulties in treating bipolar disorder. As can be seen from this chart, a major difficulty contributing to relapse is the level of patient noncompliance with treatment. (Adapted from Ward, I. [2017]. Pharmacologic options for bipolar disorder. *The Clinical Advisor*, March, 17.)

instance, by substituting for sodium, lithium compromises the ability to release, activate, and respond to neurotransmitters. When taken in therapeutic amounts, lithium inhibits the release of norepinephrine, serotonin, and dopamine, while facilitating their reuptake into presynaptic terminals (Adams, Urban, & Sutter, 2021). The net effect of this action is to decrease the synaptic levels of these neurotransmitters—the very action that one would surmise needs to occur in the hyperactive state of mania. Lithium also normalizes a dysfunctional second messenger system (Nestler, Hyman, Holtzman, & Malenka, 2021). This multistep system eventuates in activation of transcription factors that instruct genes on what proteins to synthesize (e.g., enzymes, receptors, neurotrophic factors). In bipolar disorder, the second messenger system is too active. Lithium and other antimanic agents are thought to reset this system. Lithium specifically prevents the full expression of inositol, a second messenger that increases the release of calcium. Calcium triggers the expulsion of neurotransmitters into the synapse. Lithium reduces neurotransmitter release by modulating the second messenger system.

Using Akkouh et al.'s (2020) neuropsychopharmacologist research model as an explanatory guide, we can expand this information. Lithium can substitute for sodium, normalizing the sodium (Na^+)/potassium (K^+)–activated adenosine triphosphatase (ATPase) pump activity, and it increases the number of sodium pumps. The net effect is a decrease in the intracellular sodium level, which creates a higher threshold for cell depolarization. Apparently, lithium also accelerates calcium removal from the neuronal terminal, normalizing calcium-dependent neurotransmitter release and synthesis, cytoskeletal remodeling, and neuronal excitability. The overall effect is a reduction in neurotransmitter release. Function of γ-aminobutyric acid (GABA)—an inhibitory neurotransmitter system—is also enhanced.

It is unclear exactly how lithium is effective. At least four hypotheses have been advanced (Adams, Urban, & Sutter, 2021; Akkouh et al., 2020; Nestler, Hyman, Holtzman, & Malenka, 2021):

1. Lithium substitutes for sodium and regulates calcium.
2. Lithium inhibits the release and facilitates the reuptake of norepinephrine, serotonin, and dopamine.
3. Lithium regulates the Na^+/K^+-ATPase pump.
4. Lithium stabilizes the second messenger system and regulates intracellular signaling.

Pharmacokinetics

Lithium is well absorbed from the gastrointestinal tract and is given orally in tablets, capsules, or liquid concentrate. Peak blood levels are reached in 1 to 3 hours and 12 hours in the brain. The kidneys excrete more than 95% of the amount ingested unchanged. Lithium is not metabolized. Renal disease lengthens the half-life, necessitating a reduction in dose. Lithium's typical plasma half-life is about 24 hours for these individuals. The absorption and excretion of lithium and sodium are closely linked. Lithium is reabsorbed with sodium in the proximal tubule. Diuretics, particularly diuretics affecting the loop of Henle and the distal tubule (e.g., thiazides), lead to increased retention of lithium, and the dosage may need to be reduced 25% to 50% (Diabetesinsipidus .org, 2017; Stahl, 2021). If dietary sodium intake increases, plasma lithium levels are likely to decrease because lithium is excreted more rapidly. Conversely, if sodium in the diet decreases, or if sodium is lost in ways other than through the kidneys (e.g., sweating, diarrhea), lithium levels increase. These considerations are important; therapeutic serum levels need to be stable because therapeutic levels of lithium are not much lower than toxic levels. Diet and activity levels should not change abruptly.

WHAT GOES WRONG IN BIPOLAR AFFECTIVE DISORDER

What is known about bipolar disorder is that affected individuals have specific signs and symptoms (e.g., elevated mood, grandiosity, irritability, insomnia, anorexia). What is not known is exactly what causes this disorder to happen. The question remains: "What goes wrong in bipolar disorder?" Sadock, Sadock, & Ruiz, 2017 proposed the psychopathology of bipolar affective mood disorder, suggesting that there is a disruption in the monoamine neurotransmitter system (dopamine, norepinephrine, serotonin, histamine, acetylcholine and γ-aminobutyric acid), and ion regulation is the cause. Ion regulation is important for normal mood, also termed euthymia. A key part of ion regulation is the Na^+/K^+-ATPase pump. Bipolar depression and mania are related, and this model proposes a biochemical explanation.

According to this neurotransmitter and ion disturbance, both bipolar depression and mania result from a decrease in Na^+/K^+-ATPase activity. As activity declines, neuronal membranes become irritable, requiring fewer stimuli to provoke cell firing also termed kindling. As sodium accumulates intracellularly because of this faulty pumping action, hyperpolarizing functions of inhibitory neurotransmitters (e.g., GABA) are diminished or an imbalance occurs. Additionally, because neurotransmitter release is calcium-dependent, the presynaptic terminals might release more neurotransmitter because of a related deficiency in sodium-dependent calcium efflux. All these factors contribute to increased neurotransmitter release and firing—or mania.

However, the term *bipolar* means two poles—the pole of mania and the pole of depression. These two poles are related. As the Na^+/K^+-ATPase pump continues to decrease in activity, neuronal irritability reaches a point at which less stimulation triggers depolarization. The neuron fires more easily, but the action potential loses amplitude. This loss of amplitude causes calcium channels to decrease their activity and results in a subsequent reduction in neurotransmitter release. Mania is the first disorder to occur when ion dysregulation occurs, but as the Na^+/K^+-ATPase pump becomes more dysfunctional, the depressive side of bipolar disorder develops. Catatonia might be the ultimate expression of ionic dysregulation (Yoshiteru, Masataka, Hiroaki, Norio, & Kazutaka, 2020). As ions become dysregulated, so does the neurotransmitter system.

Lithium is effective in about 50% of cases; however, 7 to 10 days are often required to achieve a clinical response. Half-life is 18 to 36 hours, although absorption and bioavailability differ on various formulations, such as the immediate-release versus extended-release. Lithium dosage is based on both clinical response and serum lithium levels. The typical dosage for acute mania is 900 to 2400 mg/day, which usually produces a serum level of 0.8 to 1.2 mEq/L. Desirable maintenance blood levels are 0.6 to 1.0 mEq/L, which can be maintained on a dosage of 400 to 1200 mg/day (Procyshyn, Bezchlibnyk-Butler, & Jeffries, 2021). Blood levels greater than 1.5 mEq/L can be toxic, but moderate to severe toxicity typically develops only after blood levels exceed 2 mEq/L. Lithium levels should be checked after 7 days after first initiation, then 7 days after every dose change until the desired level is reached. In older patients, lithium levels should be measured at 7 days, then in 10 to 12 days after first dose initiation to cautiously assess for potential overload of serum lithium levels. This is evidence-based practice to assess potentially renal impaired individuals. Lithium lab sampling should be collected first thing in the morning, 13 hours (12 + 1 hour) after the last evening dose, and before the morning dose if there is twice-a-day dosing (Rege, 2020).

Fig. 16.2 presents an explanation of how lithium works using the biogenic amine theory.

Side Effects

Side effects of lithium are linked to elevated serum blood levels. Blood levels greater than 1.5 mEq/L can be considered toxic although symptoms may present with levels at 1 to 1.2 mEq/L. Common side effects are nausea, dry mouth, diarrhea, and thirst. Moderate side effects include red rash usually on the face. Drowsiness, mild hand tremor, polyuria, weight gain, a bloated feeling, sleeplessness, and lightheadedness are other common side effects. Polyuria and polydipsia occur in about 60% of patients taking lithium (Procyshyn, Bezchlibnyk-Butler, & Jeffries, 2021). Side effects occur at therapeutic levels but usually decrease or cease after 3 to 6 weeks. However, these same side effects increase in severity at toxic serum levels.

Side effects unrelated to serum levels include weight gain, a metallic taste, headache, edema of the hands and ankles, and pruritus. Even at therapeutic levels, lithium can affect thyroid gland function. Approximately 30% of patients develop clinical hypothyroidism, with some needing levothyroxine supplementation (Procyshyn, Bezchlibnyk-Butler, & Jeffries, 2021). Lithium can also impair mental or physical abilities required for driving.

Lithium is generally contraindicated in patients with cardiovascular disease. Lithium might also harm the fetus and is a U.S. Food and Drug Administration (FDA) category Pregnancy and Lactation Labeling Rule (PLLR) (evidence of fetal risk has been established) (Pernia & DeMaagd, 2016; Stahl, 2021). Adverse reactions to toxic blood levels are discussed later in the chapter.

Lithium may negatively affect the kidneys. Lithium therapy is contraindicated for patients with renal disease; if lithium is necessary, close supervision of these patients is recommended. Lithium-induced renal insufficiency (creatinine level consistently >2 mg/100 mL) is apparently uncommon. However, nephrogenic diabetes insipidus (NDI) develops in a significant number of patients taking lithium. NDI is caused by inhibition of the action of antidiuretic hormone (ADH), or vasopressin, on the kidneys, specifically, the distal tubule and collecting duct cells (Diabetesinsipidus.org. (2017). When ADH is blocked, the patient experiences polyuria (defined as urinating >3 L/day). If a patient experiences NDI, lithium is often discontinued, or the dosage is reduced (Advokat et al., 2019).

Mohapatra, Sahoo, and Rath (2016) discussed another major concern with lithium therapy—neuropathy. In their case report, they cited a case study in which an individual developed what appeared to be irreversible neuropathy. This is a very under-recognized condition although healthcare

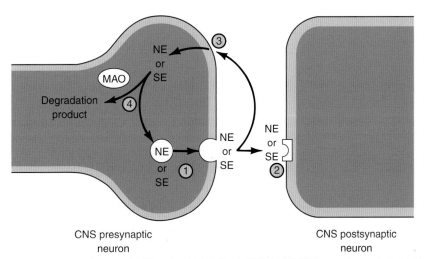

FIG. 16.2 Lithium. *1,* Lithium inhibits release of NE and 5-HT. *2,* Less NE and 5-HT are released. *3,* Lithium enhances reuptake of NE and 5-HT. *4,* MAO prevents degradation of NE and 5-HT. *MAO,* Monoamine oxidase; *NE,* norepinephrine; *SE,* serotonin. (Modified from Clark, J., Queener, S., & Karb, V. [1993]. *Pharmacologic basis of nursing practice* [4th ed.]. St. Louis: Mosby.)

professionals should be aware of this. It is clear from the literature that lithium can cause life-threatening conditions and irreversible neurotoxicity. One case study follows.

CASE EXAMPLE

Billy, a 38-year-old Caucasian man, is now confined to a wheelchair. He was diagnosed with bipolar affective disorder in his early 20s. Billy was arrested and placed in jail. While there, he was given his prescribed amounts of lithium. Billy apparently misled his "outside" prescriber, and that clinician increased the dosage of lithium that Billy was receiving. In essence, Billy said that he was taking his lithium as prescribed, but in reality, he was not. The clinician was aware of therapeutic lithium levels and continued to increase the lithium dosage in an attempt to achieve a therapeutic serum level (0.6 to 1.0 mEq/L). When he was incarcerated, Billy's daily dosage was 2100 mg/day—definitely on the high end. Once he was jailed, the officers made sure that Billy took the correct amount of lithium. In a short while, Billy became sick and then comatose. He was taken to a hospital where he remained for 6 weeks. He came close to dying and a year later still could not walk.

❓ CRITICAL THINKING QUESTION

1. If a person taking lithium experiences serious diarrhea, what will happen to the person's serum level?

Interactions

Familiarity with the drugs that can elevate lithium serum levels is essential. Diuretics (except acetazolamide [Diamox]) decrease lithium excretion and elevate serum lithium levels. Indomethacin and other nonsteroidal antiinflammatory drugs (NSAIDs) reduce renal elimination of lithium by preventing the natural antagonism of ADH by prostaglandin (Diabetesinsupidus.org, 2017), increasing serum lithium levels. Switching to a low-salt diet after treatment commences also elevates serum lithium levels.

Some drugs and other agents decrease serum lithium levels and pose the problem of inadequate treatment and symptom exacerbation. Agents that increase lithium excretion decrease lithium levels. Acetazolamide (Diamox), caffeine, and alcohol are included in this group.

Combining lithium with antipsychotic drugs or benzodiazepines is common. These drugs are ordered with lithium because of lithium's clinical response lag time of 1 to 2 weeks. Antipsychotic agents are prescribed for their antimanic properties and because they produce a tranquilizing effect until lithium produces a clinical response.

Diuretics and NSAIDs increase lithium serum levels, and toxicity can result. A few other drugs and agents decrease lithium levels, and symptom breakthrough can occur. Generally educate patients to avoid nephrotoxic medications concurrently with lithium.

Nursing Implications
Therapeutic Versus Toxic Drug Levels

Therapeutic serum lithium levels are 0.6 to 1.0 mEq/L. The optimal maintenance level is approximately 0.8 mEq/L. Serum levels greater than 1.5 mEq/L can cause adverse reactions. Typically, higher serum levels correspond directly to the severity of the reaction. Mild to moderate toxic reactions occur at 1.5 to 2 mEq/L, and moderate to severe reactions occur at 2 to 3 mEq/L. At serum levels greater than 3 mEq/L, multiple organs and organ systems might be involved, leading to coma and death (Stahl, 2021). Serum levels should be monitored and should not exceed 2 mEq/L.

No antidote is available for lithium poisoning. Discontinuing the drug might be enough when supportive nursing care is available. Gastric lavage has been used successfully. Parenteral normal saline might provide enough volume and sodium to prevent major problems for serum levels less than 2.5 mEq/L. For more severe lithium poisoning, forced diuresis or hemodialysis might be needed.

Use During Pregnancy

Treating bipolar disorder during pregnancy is difficult. Cessation of lithium during pregnancy is suggested because of fetal cardiovascular malformation (i.e., Epstein's anomaly) when lithium is taken in the first trimester in addition to neonatal toxicity if taken thereafter (Rege, 2020; Stahl, 2021). However, whether this toxicity is as common as previously thought is now debated (Rege, 2020). The occurrence of major congenital abnormalities for fetuses of mothers taking lithium is 4% to 12% (Procyshyn, Bezchlibnyk-Butler, & Jeffries, 2021). Postnatal treatment also poses problems because lithium is present in breast milk at 30% to 80% of the mother's serum level.

Therapeutic Serum Levels (0.6–1.0 mEq/L)	Mild to Moderate Toxicity (1.5–2 mEq/L)	Moderate to Severe Toxicity (2–3 mEq/L)	Severe Toxicity (>3 mEq/L)
Hand tremor (fine)	Diarrhea	Previous symptoms *and*	Previous symptoms *and*
Memory problems	Vomiting	Ataxia	Seizures
Goiter	Drowsiness	Giddiness	Organ failure
Hypothyroidism	Dizziness	Tinnitus	Renal failure
Mild diarrhea	Hand tremor (coarse)	Blurred vision	Coma
Anorexia	Muscular weakness	Large output of dilute urine	Death
Nausea	Lack of coordination	Delirium	
Edema	Dry mouth	Nystagmus	
Weight gain			
Polydipsia, polyuria			

HIGHLIGHTING THE EVIDENCE

The pregnancy category of divalproex (Depakote) and other valproates (i.e., valproate sodium [Depacon] and valproic acid [Depakene and Stavzor]) has been changed from X category (risks outweigh any benefit) to Pregnancy and Lactation Labeling Rule (PLLR) for women using these medications while pregnant. This prohibition does not extend to other uses of divalproex such as for epilepsy or bipolar treatment; however, caution and vigilance are warranted (valproates remain a category PLLR drug for these conditions). Children 6 years of age born to women who took divalproex or other valproates throughout their pregnancy had lower IQ scores than children of women treated with other antiepileptics.

From Pernia, S., & DeMaagd, G. (2016). The new pregnancy and lactation labeling rule. *Procyshyn, Bezchlibnyk-Butler, & Jeffries, 2021*(11), 713–715. https://www.ncbi.nlm.nih.gov/pmc/articles/PMC5083079/.

KEY NURSING INTERVENTIONS

For Patients Taking Lithium

- Prepare the patient for expected side effects without instilling anxiety.
- Discuss the side effects that should subside (e.g., nausea, dry mouth, diarrhea, thirst, mild hand tremor, weight gain, bloatedness, insomnia, lightheadedness).
- Identify the side effects that require immediate notification of the physician (e.g., vomiting, severe tremor, sedation, muscle weakness, vertigo).
- Suggest taking lithium with meals to reduce nausea.
- Suggest drinking 10–12 glasses or 2.5 L of water per day to reduce thirst and maintain normal fluid balance.
- Advise the patient to elevate the feet to relieve ankle edema.
- Advise the patient to maintain a consistent dietary sodium intake but to increase sodium if a major increase in perspiration occurs.
- Educate females of child-bearing ages about avoiding unexpected pregnancy.

Use in Older Adults

Older adult patients can benefit from lithium, but because of the severity of side effects and adverse reactions, these patients must be assessed for renal function and dietary history. Lithium-induced reactions are more likely in this age group. Serum levels of 0.4 to 0.8 mEq/L are appropriate for older patients.

Side Effects

Because lithium has a narrow therapeutic index, serum lithium levels should be determined frequently. After the patient is stabilized, monthly or less frequent serum level determinations are usually adequate. Blood levels are usually drawn before the first dose in the morning. However, the nurse should not rely on laboratory tests alone and should continue clinical evaluation of the patient. (See the Key Nursing Interventions for Patients Taking Lithium box.)

Interactions

The nurse should help patients understand the basic mechanisms affecting serum lithium levels. Drug interactions that increase or decrease serum levels should be reviewed. The nurse must impress on all patients, even if they are reluctant to do so, the necessity for alerting all other health care providers that they are receiving lithium treatment.

Teaching Patients

The nurse should teach patients and their families the following precautions:

- Symptoms of minor toxicity, which include vomiting, diarrhea, drowsiness, muscular weakness, and lack of coordination
- Symptoms of major toxicity, which include giddiness, tinnitus, blurred vision, and dilute urine
- Side effects associated with lithium and the proper time to notify the physician
- Avoidance of conception because lithium might harm the fetus
- Avoidance of driving until stabilized on lithium

Box 16.3 provides a complete list of patient guidelines for taking lithium.

BOX 16.3 Patient Guidelines for Taking Lithium

To achieve a therapeutic effect and prevent lithium toxicity, patients taking lithium should be advised of the following:

1. Lithium must be taken on a regular basis, preferably at the same time daily. For example, a patient who is taking lithium on a three-times-daily schedule and forgets a dose should wait until the next scheduled time to take the lithium but should not take twice the amount at that time because lithium toxicity could occur.
2. When lithium treatment is initiated, mild side effects such as a fine hand tremor, increased thirst and urination, nausea, anorexia, and diarrhea or constipation might develop. Most of the mild side effects are transient and do not indicate lithium toxicity. Additionally, in some patients taking lithium, some foods such as celery and butterfat have an unappealing taste.
3. Serious side effects of lithium that necessitate its discontinuance include vomiting, extreme hand tremor, sedation, muscle weakness, and vertigo. The prescribing practitioner should be notified immediately if any of these side effects occur.
4. Lithium and sodium are eliminated from the body through the kidneys. An increase in salt intake increases lithium elimination, and a decrease in salt intake decreases lithium elimination. The patient must maintain a balanced diet and salt intake. The patient should consult with the prescribing practitioner before making any dietary alterations.
5. Various situations can require an adjustment in the amount of lithium administered to a patient; examples are the addition of a new medication to the patient's drug regimen, a new diet, or an illness with fever or excessive sweating.
6. For determination of lithium levels, blood should be drawn in the morning approximately 12 h after the last dose was taken.
7. Kidney function lab tests should be done at least twice per year and thyroid lab tests annually in outpatient stable euthymic patients.

ANTICONVULSANTS

Although lithium is the gold standard for bipolar disorder, many patients do not respond. Most patients with a diagnosis of bipolar disorder have one or more subsequent bouts or exacerbations with the disorder. Because of the seriousness of bipolar disorder, researchers have diligently sought alternatives for patients who do not respond to lithium. An anticonvulsant is often the first drug prescribed. A frequently prescribed drug is divalproex (Depakote), a valproate. Other anticonvulsant alternatives include carbamazepine, gabapentin, lamotrigine, oxcarbazepine, and topiramate. Table 16.2 provides a summary of the evidence for the effectiveness of these drugs for mania, depression, and maintenance therapy. As can be readily identified, not all of these agents are effective for all three dimensions of bipolar spectrum disorder.

Divalproex and Other Valproates

Divalproex (Depakote, a tablet) and other valproates (e.g., valproic acid [Depakene, also as a syrup], valproate sodium [Depacon, an injection]) have been used since the 1960s as antiepileptic agents. In 1995, these drugs were approved for the treatment of mania and have since been considered first-line agents. Valproates appear to be particularly effective for patients with acute mania and for patients with mania secondary to a general medical condition (Guzman, 2019a, b). The effectiveness of the valproates (and all anticonvulsants) might be related to their inhibition of kindling activity in the brain. The concept of kindling can be explained as follows: Just as kindling in the fireplace is the first step in building a fire, some abnormal brain activities might begin as kindling and then spread. A little water can douse the fire when it first starts but is ineffective in the control of a raging fire. The

TABLE 16.2   Evidence Supporting Antiepileptic Drugs for Mood Disorders

Medication	Mania	Depression	Maintenance
Divalproex	XXX	X	XX
Carbamazepine	XXX	X	XX
Lamotrigine	0	0	XXX
Gabapentin	0	0	X
Oxcarbazepine	X	X	X
Topiramate	0	0	X

XXX, Strong evidence; *XX*, moderate evidence; *X*, weak evidence; *0*, no evidence.
Adapted from Gerst, T. M., Smith, T. L., & Patel, N. C. (2010). Antiepileptics for psychiatric illness: find the right match. *Current Psychiatry*, 9, 51.

mechanisms of action listed in the following box normalize and stabilize neuronal activity; this increases the threshold of stimulation needed for cell firing.

HOW VALPROATES WORK

Although the precise nature of the action of valproates is unknown, three mechanisms might be responsible for their antimanic effect:
1. Increase in the inhibitory role of GABA
2. Suppression of sodium influx into the neuron
3. Suppression of calcium influx through specific calcium channels

Advantages of the valproates are that they have a rapid onset, can be used initially without attempting lithium, and are well tolerated with little effect on cognition. Disadvantages include transient hair loss, weight gain, tremors, gastrointestinal upset, and dose-related thrombocytopenia. Polycystic ovary syndrome and general menstrual disturbances in women and reduction in intelligence in children exposed to valproates in utero are major concerns that should be considered (Advokat, Comaty, & Julien, 2019; Stahl, 2021; Guzman, 2019b).

Bioavailability is approximately 80%, with up to 95% protein binding. The drug can be replaced at binding sites by other drugs such as carbamazepine or warfarin, causing toxic effects. Valproates have a half-life of 9 to 16 hours and reach a steady state in 2 to 5 days. Therapeutic serum levels are 50 to 125 mcg/mL or levels slightly higher than for their antiepileptic effects (Stahl, 2021). Valproates are contraindicated for individuals with significant hepatic disease.

Other Anticonvulsants Used to Treat Bipolar Disorder

Carbamazepine

Carbamazepine (Tegretol) is effective for most patients who do not respond to lithium or to the valproates; it also has a faster onset of action compared with lithium. Patients with a rapidly cycling bipolar episode are more likely to be unresponsive to lithium and to respond to carbamazepine. Carbamazepine sometimes might be given in combination with lithium. Carbamazepine's therapeutic antimanic serum levels are 4 to 12 mcg/mL. Although carbamazepine is generally well tolerated, side effects include nausea, anorexia, and occasional vomiting. Sedation and drowsiness are other common side effects. The most serious potential side effect of carbamazepine is agranulocytosis. Complete blood counts should be obtained weekly when this drug treatment is initiated. Drugs that inhibit the cytochrome P-450 3A4 enzyme, such as selective serotonin reuptake inhibitors (i.e., fluoxetine), can cause adverse effects.

Lamotrigine

Lamotrigine (Lamictal) is FDA approved for the treatment of bipolar disorder, including bipolar depression. This drug works by manipulating the GABA system and inhibiting neuronal firing. Other mechanisms of action include blocking of voltage-gated sodium and calcium channels, further inhibiting neuronal conduction. Finally, lamotrigine is believed to inhibit the excitatory neurotransmitter glutamate. Similar to the effects of most drugs, lamotrigine causes numerous side effects; one particular adverse reaction that is especially noteworthy is lamotrigine-induced rash. Lamotrigine can cause moderate skin rashes (about 10% of patients) and potentially fatal Stevens-Johnson syndrome (SJS) (only 1% to 2% of children). Predictors of rash include high initial dose, rapid increase in dosage, missed doses, and young age (Advokat, Comaty, & Julien, 2019; Stahl, 2021).

Oxcarbazepine

Oxcarbazepine (Trileptal) is becoming a commonly prescribed agent for bipolar disorder. Oxcarbazepine is structurally related to carbamazepine and has similar pharmacologic activity. However, it does not cause some of the more serious adverse reactions associated with carbamazepine. Oxcarbazepine also carries the risk of mild to moderate skin rashes and potentially fatal SJS.

Gabapentin

Gabapentin (Neurontin) tends to be used in an adjunctive role and not as monotherapy. As an adjunctive agent, it is believed to be particularly effective if the patient also experiences anxiety. Similar to lamotrigine, gabapentin upregulates the GABA system, blocks sodium and calcium voltage-gated channels, and inhibits glutamate (glutamate increases cell firing).

Topiramate

Topiramate (Topamax) has a mechanism of action similar to that of gabapentin. It increases GABA activity, blocks voltage-gated sodium and calcium channels, and inhibits the excitatory neurotransmitter glutamate. Many patients report weight loss with this drug (the only anticonvulsant known to have this effect). However, whatever positive response this effect has among clinicians and patients is tempered by a cognitive dulling or sedation that some patients have reported.

ANTIPSYCHOTICS

Antipsychotics are discussed in detail in Chapter 14. All atypical antipsychotics except clozapine (although it is effective) have been approved for the treatment of mania. The traditional antipsychotic haloperidol is also effective and may have a more rapid onset of action than either lithium or the atypical agents (Stahl, 2021). These agents have proven to be effective for the treatment of bipolar disorder both as monotherapy and as an adjunct to mood stabilizers. Antipsychotics are particularly beneficial for control of acute mania. A brief description of these drugs is given here.

Aripiprazole: Aripiprazole (Abilify) is a third-generation agent. It has been shown to be effective in the treatment of bipolar disorder.

Asenapine: Asenapine (Saphris) is a second-generation antipsychotic approved for bipolar disorder. It is given sublingually, providing rapid absorption. It is approved by the FDA for treating acute mania, mixed episodes, and as a maintenance medication.

Cariprazine: Cariprazine (Vraylar) is a newer second-generation agent. It is approved by the FDA for treating acute mania, mixed mania (depression and mania), or bipolar depression seen in bipolar 1 disorder.

Clozapine: Clozapine (Clozaril), although not FDA approved, is very effective for the off-label treatment and prophylaxis of acute mania; however, the same concern associated with its more conventional antipsychotic use remains problematic, that is, agranulocytosis. Hematologic close monitoring is required.

Lurasidone: Lurasidone (Latuda) is FDA approved for bipolar depression as monotherapy and as adjunctive therapy for individuals ages 10 and older.

Olanzapine: Olanzapine (Zyprexa) is FDA approved as monotherapy for acute and maintenance treatment of bipolar disorder. Its particular pharmacologic profile might reduce the risk of precipitating a depression after treatment for acute mania. Olanzapine is associated with significant weight gain and hyperglycemia in some patients.

Quetiapine: Quetiapine (Seroquel) is used to treat bipolar disorder. It can control acute mania and rapidly cycling mania and is used prophylactically. Quetiapine is associated with weight gain and hyperglycemia.

Risperidone: Risperidone (Risperdal) has been established as an effective agent for acute bipolar disorder. It does not cause as much weight gain as other mood stabilizers.

Ziprasidone: Ziprasidone (Geodon) has also received approval to be used for treatment of acute bipolar disorder. It causes little or no weight gain and is reported to be well tolerated.

Currently, Abilify Maintena and Risperdal Consta are long-acting injectables (LAIs) approved by the FDA, providing an important option for some patients. Other LAIs include paliperidone, haloperidol, olanzapine, and fluphenazine, which are effectively used off-label (Advokat, Comaty, & Julien, 2019; Stahl, 2021).

OTHER TREATMENTS FOR BIPOLAR DISORDER

Several benzodiazepines (e.g., clonazepam [Klonopin], lorazepam [Ativan]) and calcium channel blockers (e.g., nimodipine, verapamil) have been used with some success in treating bipolar disorder. Agitation, insomnia, and anxiety are probably treatable by the benzodiazepines. Finally, electroconvulsive therapy has proven useful for bipolar disorder and was used effectively before the discovery of lithium and these other drugs. Electroconvulsive therapy is particularly valuable for pregnant patients who have severe symptoms and should avoid medication that is teratogenic (Adams, Urban, & Sutter, 2021; Advokat, Comaty, & Julien, 2019). Note, ECT should be reserved for last resort treatment in pregnant women and updated guidelines are still needed (Leiknes et al., 2015).

WHAT YOU CAN EXPECT TO SEE PRESCRIBED FOR BIPOLAR DISORDER

The first issue is whether the prescriber will attempt to treat bipolar disorder with one medication (monotherapy) or with a combination of antimanic agents. The more common of each follows (Advokat, Comaty, & Julien, 2019; Stahl, 2021):

Monotherapy

First-line approaches	Lithium, a valproate, or medication used for acute stage
Second-line approach	Atypical antipsychotic
Third-line approach	Carbamazepine or lamotrigine or gabapentin or topiramate

Combination Therapy

Atypical approach	Atypical antipsychotic (e.g., olanzapine) *plus* lithium or a valproate
Benzodiazepine approach	Benzodiazepine *plus* lithium or a valproate
Typical approach	Typical antipsychotic (e.g., haloperidol) *plus* lithium or a valproate
Mood stabilizers	*Two or more* mood stabilizers

For Severe Acute Mania

Lithium or a valproate *plus* an atypical antipsychotic

For Bipolar Depression

First-line approaches	Lithium *or* lamotrigine *or* fluoxetine + olanzapine *or* electroconvulsive therapy

STUDY NOTES

1. Antimanic or mood stabilizers are used to treat bipolar disorder (i.e., manic depression).
2. There are two overarching treatment concerns: (a) controlling the symptoms of acute mania and (b) maintenance treatment.
3. Goals of *maintenance treatment* are as follows:
   a. Prevention of relapse
   b. Reduction of suicides
   c. Improvement of functioning
   d. Reduction of subthreshold symptoms
4. Lithium is a naturally occurring element that has been a mainstay of bipolar disorder treatment for more than 50 years in the United States.
5. Other first-line agents used to treat bipolar disorder are anticonvulsants and antipsychotics.
6. Lithium alters intracellular conductance; anticonvulsants act on the GABA system and sodium and calcium voltage-gated channels.
7. Clinically therapeutic serum levels of lithium are 0.6 to 1.0 mEq/L; at higher serum levels, serious or fatal reactions can occur.

8. Common side effects of lithium include nausea, dry mouth, diarrhea, thirst, and mild hand tremor.
9. Lithium has a narrow therapeutic index and a lag time of 7 to 10 days typically.
10. Divalproex and other valproates are effective, have rapid onset of action, and are relatively well tolerated.
11. Carbamazepine has a more rapid onset compared with lithium and is generally well tolerated.
12. Other anticonvulsants, such as lamotrigine, oxcarbazepine, gabapentin, and topiramate, have been proven to be effective in treating bipolar disorder.
13. Use of anticonvulsants, particularly lamotrigine, must be accompanied by close assessment for skin rashes. Some of these rashes, such as Stevens-Johnson syndrome, have proven fatal.
14. Topiramate causes weight loss and is associated with cognitive dulling or sedation.
15. Antipsychotic drugs control the symptoms of acute mania and act as mood stabilizers.

REFERENCES

Adams, M. P., Urban, C. Q., & Sutter, R. E. (2021). *Pharmacology: Connections to nursing practice* (4th ed.). Pearson.

Advokat, C. D., Comaty, J. E., & Julien, R. M. (2019). *Julien's primer of drug action: A comprehensive guide to the actions, uses and side effexors of psychoactive drugs* (14th ed.). Worth Publishers.

Akkouh, I. A., Skrede, S., Holmgren, A., Ersland, K. M., Hansson, L., Bahrami, S., … Hughes, T. (2020). Exploring lithium's transcriptional mechanisms of action in bipolar disorder: A multi-step study. *Neuropsychopharmacology*, 45, 947–955. https://doi.org10.1038/s41386-019-0556-8.

Braslow, J., & Marder, S. R. (2019). History of psychopharmacology. *Annual Review of Clinical Psychology*, 15, 25–50. https://doi.org/10.1146/annurev-clinpsy-050718-095514.

Cade. J. F. (1949). Lithium salts in the treatment of psychotic excitement. *The Medical Journal of Australia*, 36, 349.

De Mendiola, X. P., Hidalgo-Mazzei, D., Vieta, E., & Gonzalez-Pinto, A. (2021). Overview of lithium's use: A nationwide survey. *International Journal of Bipolar Disorders* https://doi.org/10.1186/s40345-020-00215-z. 9/10. https://journalbipolardisorders.springeropen.com/articles/10.1186/s40345-020-00215-z.

Diabetesinsipidus.org. (2017). Lithium induced diabetes insipidus. Author. https://diabetesinsipidus.org/lithium-induced-diabetes-insipidus

Guzman, F. (2019a). Lithium's mechanism of action: an illustrated review. Psychopharmacology Institute. https://psychopharmacologyinstitute.com/publication/lithiums-mechanism-of-action-an-illustrated-review-2212

Guzman, F. (2019b).Valproate in psychiatry: approved indications and off-label uses. Psychopharmacology Institute. https://psychopharmacologyinstitute.com/publication/valproate-in-psychiatry-approved-indications-and-off-label-uses-2188

Kishi, T., Matsuda, Y., Sakuma, K., Okuya, M., Mishima, K., & Iwata, N. (2020). Recurrence rates in stable bipolar disorder patients after drug discontinuation v. drug maintenance: A systematic review and meta-analysis. *Psychological medicine*, 1–9. Advance online publication. https://doi.org/10.1017.

Leiknes, K., Cooke, M., Jarosch-von Schweder, L., Harboe, I., & Hoie, B. (2015). Electroconvulsive therapy during pregnany: A systematic review of case studies. *Archives of Women's Mental Health*, 18, 1–39. https://doi.org/10.1007/s00737-013-0389-0.

Mohapatra, S., Sahoo, M. R., & Rath, N. (2016). Lithium-induced motor neuropathy: An unusual presentation. *Indian Journal of Psychological Medicine*, 38(3), 252–253. https://www.ncbi.nlm.nih.gov/pmc/articles/PMC4904764/.

Nestler, E. J., Hyman, S. E., Holtzman, D. M., & Malenka, R. C. (2021). *Molecular neuropharmacology: A foundation for clinical neuroscience*. McGraw-Hill.

Pernia, S., & DeMaagd, G. (2016). The new pregnancy and lactation labeling rule. *Pharmacy and Therapeutics*, 41(11), 713–715. https://www.ncbi.nlm.nih.gov/pmc/articles/PMC5083079.

Procyshyn, R.M., Bezchlibnyk-Butler, K.Z., & Jeffries, J.J. (2021). *Clinical handbook of psychotropic drugs* (24th Ed.). Hogrefe Publishing. http://www.hogrefe.com.

Rakofsky. J. J. (2016). RELAPSE: Answers to why a patient is having a new mood episode. Current. *Psychiatry*, 15(2), 53.

Rege, S. (2020). Lithium prescribing and monitoring in clinical practice – A practical guide. Psychscenehub.com. https://psychscenehub.com/psychinsights/lithium-prescribing-monitoring-clinical-practice/.

Ruffalo, M.L. (2019). Lithium carbonate: The penicillin of psychiatry. Psychology Today. https://www.psychologytoday.com/us/blog/freud-fluoxetine/201908/lithium-carbonate-the-penicillin-psychiatry

Sadock, B. J., Sadock, V. A., & Ruiz, P. (2017). *Kaplan & Sadock's concise textbook of clinical psychiatry* (4th Ed.). Lippincott Williams & Wilkins.

Sarai, S. K., Mekala, H. M., & Lippmann, S. (2018). Lithium suicide prevention: A brief review and reminder. *Innovations in Clinical Neuroscience*, 15, 30–32. https://www.ncbi.nlm.nih.gov/pmc/articles/PMC6380616/.

Stahl, S. M. (2021). *Essential psychopharmacology* (7th ed.). Cambridge University Press.

Yoshiteru, S., Masataka, S., Hiroaki, O., Norio, Y., & Kazutaka, S. (2020). Successful treatment with lithium in a refractory patient with periodic catatonic features: A case report. *Clinical Neuropharmacology*, 43(3), 84–85. https://doi.org/10.1097/WNF.0000000000390.

17

Antianxiety Drugs

Norman L. Keltner and Helene Vossos

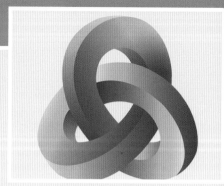

Most people are about as happy as they make up their minds to be.

Abraham Lincoln

 http://evolve.elsevier.com/Keltner

LEARNING OBJECTIVES

- Recognize that the first-line approach to treating anxiety are selective serotonin reuptake inhibitors (SSRIs) and other antidepressants.
- Describe the differences between benzodiazepines and buspirone.
- Identify when benzodiazepines are indicated.
- Discuss the side effects of benzodiazepines.
- Identify benzodiazepines that are appropriate for older adults.
- Identify the specific antidote for benzodiazepine overdose.
- Describe potential drug interactions with benzodiazepines.
- Discuss the implications for teaching patients about antianxiety drugs.

CASE EXAMPLE

Annie dreaded what would happen next—she had been down this road many times before. There she was, minding her own business, just wanting to watch a movie, like any normal person, but then she noticed her breathing was off. Immediately she began to monitor her breathing, and soon it seemed as if she just could not get enough air. She remembered a recent visit to the emergency department when the nurse patiently showed her that her oxygen saturation levels were good. She remembered, but it didn't help. It wasn't that she believed that this time was different, that this time she was going to suffocate. No, that might be a textbook explanation, but it wasn't her explanation. She could not breathe, and knowing that "it was all in her head" did not seem to help. Soon she would be spiraling into symptoms that, like an Old Testament prophet, would beget more apprehension, which would beget more symptoms—palpitations, dizziness, fear of fainting, trembling, feeling that things around her were unreal, fear of going crazy—which would beget more dread. Worst of all, she feared looking foolish. What if she lost control and started gulping big chunks of air down? What if she...? What would they think of her? (Panic Disorder. National Institute of Mental Health, 2016).

People have been seeking relief from anxiety since the beginning of recorded history. Alcohol is the oldest substance used to reduce anxiety, and it has been used by countless millions to self-medicate fears, phobias, and nerves. In more recent times, other drugs have been developed to alleviate anxiety. In the early 1900s, Bromo-Seltzer was advertised as having anxiolytic properties but had to be withdrawn from the market because of its addictive qualities. In the 1930s and 1940s, barbiturates were heralded as having the potential to treat anxiety, but they too were found to have many adverse effects, including seizures, dependence, addiction, and withdrawal.

The first drug that was specific for treating anxiety was meprobamate (Miltown, Equanil), which was developed in 1955 (Braslow & Marder, 2019). This drug, with its ability to calm nerves, blur the reality of stressors, and make people feel better in general, was a national sensation. How it was received probably says far more about the American psyche than about the efficacy of meprobamate. The United States was ready for a drug to buffer the stressors of a busy society. For several years, meprobamate was a widely prescribed medication, but because it was similar to alcohol, Bromo-Seltzer, and barbiturates, problems surfaced. Individuals using meprobamate were subject to abusing it, developed tolerance, and experienced lethal overdoses. Its appeal as an antianxiety agent began to diminish. Fortunately, new agents to calm the trembling hands of a nation besieged with anxiety were waiting in the wings.

Before the end of the 1950s, another class of antianxiety drugs was developed—benzodiazepines. These drugs had advantages over barbiturates in that they were less likely to be abused and were safer when overdoses occurred. Although first synthesized in the 1930s, benzodiazepines were not discovered to have a psychiatric effect until the late 1950s. Eventually, several thousand benzodiazepine derivatives would be synthesized, including familiar drugs such as diazepam (Valium), lorazepam (Ativan), alprazolam (Xanax), chlordiazepoxide (Librium), oxazepam (Serax), and clonazepam (Klonopin). All of these agents manipulate the γ-aminobutyric acid (GABA) system. However, these drugs were also linked to significant problems. Benzodiazepines were abused, induced tolerance, and were implicated in lethal overdoses (although always when combined with other drugs). Many American adults use or have used benzodiazepines.

 NORM'S NOTES Can you spell "addiction"? "Benzos" are great drugs for a short while, but they can be overprescribed and overused. They are very useful when you are really anxious, but almost anyone can get hooked on these drugs in a short time, and long-term use generally does not lead to anything good. Watch out for your patients, your friends, your family, and yourself. It could happen to your mom or dad. And, it can feel like an abyss to come off benzodiazepines.

Clinical researchers and drug manufacturers continue to search for the perfect antianxiety drug—a drug that ameliorates anxiety without significant adverse effects. A nonbenzodiazepine antianxiety agent that has been widely marketed is buspirone (BuSpar). Buspirone does not have the potential for abuse, dependency, and withdrawal associated with benzodiazepines. The SSRIs were developed in the late 1980s. These agents have emerged as a first-line treatment choice for anxiety disorders. Because they are discussed in detail in Chapter 15, this chapter presents only a brief review. Again, this is the primary approach to treating anxiety.

A large group of unrelated drugs appears to have antianxiety properties or at least have been found useful in the treatment of specific anxiety-like syndromes. Examples of drugs with antianxiety properties include some β-blockers (e.g., propranolol [Inderal]), antihistamines, monoamine oxidase inhibitors, tricyclic antidepressants (TCAs), clonidine (Catapres), phenothiazines, hydroxyzine (Vistaril), and opioids. A few of these agents are discussed briefly at the end of the chapter.

MODELS OF ANXIETY

Anxiety and its causes are discussed in Chapter 27. Basically, there are three areas involving causative factors:

BOX 17.1 Autonomic (Adrenergic System) Symptoms of Anxiety

Tachycardia
Dilated pupils
Tremor
Sweating

1. Autonomic nervous system dysregulation
   a. Dysregulation of β-adrenergic receptors
   b. Inhibition of GABA
2. Neuroendocrine overactivity
3. Faulty thinking

The autonomic nervous system overperforms when a person is anxious (Box 17.1, Fig. 17.1). Studies have found that β-agonists, such as isoproterenol, cause anxiety (Table 17.1 for drugs and illnesses that can cause anxiety). Adrenergic autoreceptors (α-2 receptors) also produce anxiety when blocked by drugs. However, α-2 agonists, such as the antihypertensive clonidine, have antianxiety properties. The extension of this thinking suggests that individuals with anxiety are believed to experience α-2 autoreceptor under-functioning, which causes the locus coeruleus, the site of norepinephrine synthesis in the brain, to overproduce norepinephrine. As we discuss later, serotonin-enhancing agents and GABA-modulating drugs play a major role in the treatment of anxiety, which is probably related to the alteration of adrenergic neurons by serotonin.

GABA inhibition might play a role in anxiety because these neurons synapse with adrenergic neurons in the brain. As GABA inhibition is lifted, there is greater inhibition of the adrenergic system. This view is supported by the fact that GABAergic drugs, such as benzodiazepines, decrease anxiety, whereas GABA receptor blockers, such as flumazenil, cause anxiety.

Increased levels of the hormone cortisol, which is secreted by the adrenal cortex in response to increased hypothalamic release of corticotropin-releasing hormone or increased anterior pituitary release of adrenocorticotropic hormone, are related to increased anxiety and insomnia.

People who have anxiety, particularly people who experience panic attacks, tend to engage in negative thinking. These negative thoughts (also known as *what if* or *catastrophic* thinking) can trigger anxiety. Box 17.2 lists the symptoms of a panic attack.

BENZODIAZEPINES

Although benzodiazepines are not considered first-line agents by psychiatric professionals, these drugs are still frequently prescribed by clinicians, so they are extensively discussed in this chapter. Many benzodiazepines are on the market. Table 17.2 presents information on benzodiazepines, including the duration of effect, the usual adult daily dose, the equivalent dose, the elimination half-life, the anxiolytic effect, and the sedative effect. Historically, antianxiety agents

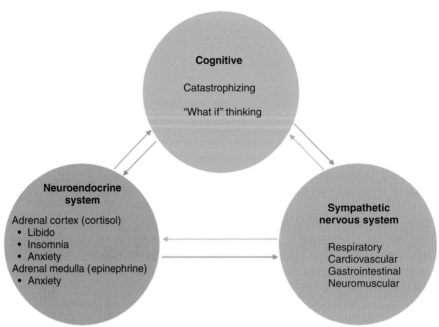

FIG. 17.1 Interacting systems of panic attacks.

TABLE 17.1 Medications and Disorders That Can Cause Anxiety
I. Medications That Can Cause Anxiety
While taking:
Asthma medications (e.g., albuterol)
β-agonists (e.g., isoproterenol)
Herbal drugs (e.g., Ma huang, ginseng)
Corticosteroids (e.g., prednisone)
Antidepressants (e.g., SSRIs, NDRIs, TCAs)
While "withdrawing":
Alcohol
Social drinking (i.e., rebound effect)
Nicotine
Benzodiazepines
Illegal or abused legal drugs:
Methamphetamine
Cocaine
Methylphenidate
Ecstasy
II. Disorders That Can Cause Anxiety
Hypothyroidism
Asthma
Cardiac arrhythmias

NDRIs, Norepinephrine and dopamine reuptake inhibitors; *SSRIs,* selective serotonin reuptake inhibitors; *TCAs,* tricyclic antidepressants.

BOX 17.2 Symptoms Associated With Panic Attacks
Palpitations
Sweating
Trembling or shaking
Shortness of breath
Feeling of choking
Chest pain
Nausea and abdominal distress
Feeling dizzy, unsteady, lightheaded, faint
Derealization
Fear of losing control or going crazy
Fear of dying
Tingling sensations
Chills or hot flashes

have been referred to as *anxiolytics* or *minor tranquilizers.* Benzodiazepines are widely used by both psychiatric and general medicine patients (and might be prescribed more often by nonpsychiatric clinicians). Major indications for benzodiazepines include chronic anxiety, time-limited treatment for crisis, presurgery jitters, acute mania, cannabinoid-induced catatonia, and panic disorder (Adams, Urban, & Sutter, 2021; Beach, Gomez-Bernal, Huffman, & Fricchione, 2017; Tietze, Fuchs, Parsons, O'Connor, & Finlay, 2021).

Anxiety is a subjective experience but can be observed by others (Box 17.3). The anxious person feels excessively alert, is easily startled, is restless, might talk too much, visually scans the environment, has tremors, and might have dilated pupils. Although many people use these drugs as needed, benzodiazepines generally should not be taken for the stressors of everyday life. Benzodiazepines have no therapeutic value in the treatment of psychosis. Box 17.4 outlines mental health and related issues amenable to benzodiazepines.

How Benzodiazepines Work

Benzodiazepines enhance the effects of the inhibitory neurotransmitter GABA. GABA is the major inhibitory

TABLE 17.2 Frequently Prescribed Benzodiazepines and Buspirone

Usual Daily Anxiety Drug Dosage (mg/day)	Equivalent Dose (mg)	Onset of Action	Half-Life (h)	Anxiolytic Effect	Sedative Effect
Benzodiazepine (Shorter Acting)					
Alprazolam (Xanax), 0.75–4[a]	0.50	15–30 min	12–15	XX	X
Lorazepam (Ativan), 2–6[a] (P)	1	15–30 min	10–20	XXX	XX
Oxazepam (Serax), 30–60	30	30–60 min	5–20	XX	X
Temazepam (Restoril), 10–60	30	30–60 min	10–15	X	XXX
Benzodiazepine (Longer Acting)					
Chlordiazepoxide (Librium), 15–100[a] (P)	10	15–30 min	5–30[b]	XX	—
Clonazepam (Klonopin), 0.5–4[a]	0.25–0.5	15–30 min	18–60[b]	XX	X
Diazepam (Valium), 4–40[a] (P)	5	<15 min; IM erratic	20–80[b]	XXX	XX
Nonbenzodiazepine					
Buspirone (BuSpar), 15–0[a]	NA	Slow	2–11[b]	XX	—

[a]Given in divided doses.
[b]With active metabolites.
Modified from Procyshyn, R. M., Bezchlibnyk-Butler, K. Z., Jeffries, J. J. (2021). *Clinical handbook of psychotropic drugs* (24th ed.). Copyright © 2021 by Hogrefe Publishing. http://www.hogrefe.com. http://doi.org/10.1027/00593-000.
N/A, Not applicable; *P*, parenteral form available; *X*, mild effect; *XX*, moderate effect; *XXX*, strong effect.

BOX 17.3 Subjective Symptoms of Anxiety Observable by Others

Patient might be:
- Anxious
- Apprehensive
- Compulsive
- Fearful
- Experiencing feelings of dread
- Irritable
- Intolerant
- Nervous
- Overconcerned
- Panicky
- Phobic
- Preoccupied
- Experiencing repetition in motor activities
- Feeling threatened
- Wound up
- Sensitive to shame
- Worried

BOX 17.4 Conditions Amenable to Benzodiazepine Treatment

Acute agitation
Alcohol withdrawal
Antipsychotic-induced akathisia and tremor
Catatonia
Generalized anxiety disorder
Insomnia
Panic disorder
Social anxiety

neurotransmitter in the brain and is found in roughly 40% of all neurons. GABA attaches to GABA receptors, which trigger the opening of chloride ion channels. Chloride has a hyperpolarizing effect on the neuron, which makes the neuron less responsive to excitatory neurons. Benzodiazepines have the pharmacodynamic property of causing the GABA receptor to respond more robustly to GABA. Specifically, benzodiazepines activate the GABA$_A$ receptor subtype. The overall effect is one of slowing down or halting neuronal firing. Neuronal inhibition is important—as important to brain function as the brake is to the operation of a car. Driving a car

without brakes risks being involved in an accident. A brain without the inhibition of GABA can produce thought acceleration, autonomic dysfunction, excessive anxiety, panic, or even seizure activity—or, to stretch the analogy, a runaway brain. Benzodiazepines help GABA tone down or inhibit the anxiety response to stressors.

GABA is a product of the Krebs cycle. It is synthesized by the decarboxylation of glutamate (i.e., the acid group of the amino acid glutamate is taken off), an amino acid produced from the Krebs cycle.

GABA receptors are located on approximately 40% of all neurons. GABA receptors are composed of five subunits on a particular receptor complex; these subunits can be arranged in any number of configurations. The composition of these subunits determines the functional characteristics of the receptor. Because of these unique configurations, some GABA receptors are selective for specific ligands (molecules that bind to and evoke a response from the receptor). Specific subunit configurations exist for benzodiazepines—a benzodiazepine receptor site. Because the place where benzodiazepines attach to the receptor is different from where GABA attaches, it is said to be an *allosteric* site (Nestler, Hyman, Holtzman, & Malenka, 2021). When attaching to these sites, benzodiazepines enhance the effects of GABA. Because benzodiazepines do not connect directly to the GABA site, the effect created by benzodiazepines is dependent on endogenous GABA. In other words, benzodiazepines would be inactive in the absence of GABA. Other allosteric sites on GABA receptors include sites for barbiturates and alcohol. It is no wonder then that an overdose of any of these three categories of drugs can cause a kind of "drunkenness." Barbiturates are particularly interesting because they both enhance GABA and mimic GABA. They do this by opening chloride channels directly (the GABA site "thinks" the barbiturates are GABA). Barbiturates can cause profound central nervous system (CNS) depression and even death from overdose, whereas the level of CNS depression caused by benzodiazepines is limited (Burchum & Rosenthal, 2021).

Pharmacologic Effects

Benzodiazepines have a generally depressive effect on the CNS, including the limbic system, the thalamus, the hypothalamus, and the reticular activating system (through which incoming sensory information is funneled). Benzodiazepines have the following major therapeutic effects (Adams, Urban, & Sutter, 2021; Advokat, Comaty, & Julien, 2019; Bezchlibnyk-Butler, Jeffries, Procyshyn, & Virani, 2021):

1. They reduce anxiety (at 20% binding to GABA receptors).
2. They promote sleep (at 30% to 50% binding to GABA receptors).
3. They produce hypnosis and amnesia (at 60% binding to GABA receptors).

Because benzodiazepines depress the reticular activating system, incoming stimuli are muted and evoke less reaction. To illustrate the concept of *muting*, two symptoms are highlighted: hyperalertness and environmental scanning. An anxious person uses these defensive reactions to guard against an environment perceived to be threatening. A stressed-out person might overreact to being startled because the body's system is on alert. As the antianxiety agent decreases environmental input, a general relaxing of the anxious posture takes place. The body's reactor is toned down, and the environmental stressors are tuned out.

These drugs can cause several levels of CNS depression, from sedation to anesthesia. Benzodiazepines accomplish this CNS depression by sedating the patient and depressing the inhibitory neurons that affect arousal. The latter effect causes a state of disinhibition, or loosening, of inner impediments to conduct. Disinhibition results in feelings of euphoria and excitement, which can lead to poor judgment. The natural restraint that minimizes social blunders is depressed.

To visualize the potential allure of benzodiazepines, one might imagine a tension continuum, with anxiety at one end and a carefree sense of being at the other. Benzodiazepines have the potential to move an anxious person from the agony of the anxiety end to the relaxed feeling of the carefree end. In therapeutic doses, this degree of shift from anxiety to disinhibition is not gained or sought, but because of the possibility of reaching a carefree zone, benzodiazepines have become drugs of abuse. In addition, many polysubstance abusers use benzodiazepines because of their ability to increase the high of other drugs.

The inhibiting effect of benzodiazepines also accounts for their anticonvulsive activity. Intravenous diazepam and lorazepam are first-line agents for status epilepticus, and clonazepam is regularly prescribed orally as an anticonvulsant.

Paradoxical Reactions to Benzodiazepines

A few people have a paradoxical reaction to benzodiazepines. Symptoms include agitation, emotional lability, talkativeness, and occasionally rage or delirium (Tietze, Fuchs, Parsons, O'Connor, & Finlay, 2021). These reactions suggest the disinhibiting effects on processing in the prefrontal cortex (the area that monitors inhibition and socially acceptable behaviors) are at the root of these untoward responses. Children, older adults, patients with poor impulse control, and individuals with organic brain syndrome are most at risk. Older adults, in particular, are at risk for delirium.

Pharmacokinetics

Benzodiazepines are readily absorbed after oral ingestion; however, intramuscular administration produces slow and inconsistent absorption for most of these drugs (lorazepam is an exception). Benzodiazepines are highly lipid-soluble and readily cross the blood-brain barrier. Benzodiazepines are metabolized by the liver but do not significantly induce their own hepatic metabolism (compared with barbiturates), and they are excreted in the urine. The active metabolites can exert an effect for 10 days. A convenient way of categorizing benzodiazepines is to divide them into drugs with shorter half-lives (≤20 hours) and drugs with longer half-lives (>20 hours). Of the selected benzodiazepines with shorter half-lives listed in Table 17.2, lorazepam, oxazepam, and temazepam (Restoril) are preferable for use in older adults. Chlordiazepoxide (Librium) and diazepam have longer half-lives and have an extended duration of action. These drugs are unsuitable for use in older patients. A benzodiazepine-induced delirium has been associated with the longer-acting drugs in this class (Tidwell, Thomas, Pouliot, Canonico, & Webber, 2018).

Considering only the half-life is misleading. An important factor in half-life determination is the metabolic process that each benzodiazepine undergoes. Most benzodiazepines are oxidized in the liver to active metabolites, but the liver becomes less efficient at metabolizing these drugs over a lifetime because hepatic function and hepatic volume change with age. The half-life of diazepam is approximately 20 hours in a young man but stretches to 80 hours in an 80-year-old man. A few benzodiazepines (e.g., lorazepam, oxazepam, temazepam) rely on conjugation with glucuronic acid to form inactive metabolites. This process is not significantly affected by the aging process. Because the half-lives of these drugs remain stable throughout life, and because these drugs have no active metabolites, they are better suited for use in older adults.

Hepatic metabolism is the primary mechanism for drug disposition. Drugs that interfere with liver metabolism (e.g., alcohol) dangerously compound the effect of benzodiazepines.

Side Effects

CNS side effects such as drowsiness, fatigue, and decreased coordination are commonly exhibited. Some mental impairment and slowing of reflexes also occur. Less frequently, confusion, depression, and headache might be present. Peripheral nervous system effects include occasional constipation, double vision, hypotension, incontinence, and urinary retention. Benzodiazepines can exacerbate narrow-angle glaucoma. Older adults with impaired liver or renal function, and debilitated individuals, experience increased side effects and consequently should receive a decreased amount of these drugs (see Common Side Effects of Benzodiazepines box [Stahl, 2021] and the discussion of pharmacokinetics earlier in the chapter).

COMMON SIDE EFFECTS OF BENZODIAZEPINES

Anterograde amnesia (no new memories)
Ataxia
Confusion
Depression
Drowsiness
Dysarthria
Headache
Impairment of mental functions
Increased reaction time
Lassitude
Lightheadedness
Motor incoordination
Sexual dysfunction
Skin reactions
Weight gain

Data from Charlson, F., Degenhardt, L., McLaren, J., Hall, W., & Lynskey, M. (2009). A systematic review of research examining benzodiazepinerelated mortality. *Pharmacoepidemiology and Drug Safety*, 18, 93.

Dependence, Withdrawal, and Tolerance

In addition to the undesired effects already listed are the triple problems of dependence, withdrawal, and tolerance.

Dependence

Dependence is a state in which the body functions normally when the drug is present and functions abnormally when the drug is absent. Dependence can develop within a few weeks or months of regular use. When a benzodiazepine is withdrawn from a dependent person, symptoms such as agitation, tremor, irritability, insomnia, vomiting, sweating, and convulsions might be experienced. Advokat, Comaty, & Julien, 2019 described three types of benzodiazepine dependence:

1. *Therapeutic dose dependence.* Individuals take the drug as prescribed but develop a need for the drug; they have outgrown the original reason for taking the drug but now need it to get through the day.
2. *Prescribed high-dose dependence.* Individuals are still taking prescribed benzodiazepines but have talked their physician into escalating the dose. Sometimes individuals are receiving prescriptions from more than one clinician.
3. *Recreational benzodiazepine abuse.* Individuals use benzodiazepines outside the traditional medical system. Benzodiazepines are often used to enhance the effects of other abused substances. Typically, the amount of drug used is significantly greater than the amount prescribed for medicinal purposes. For example, a high-end dose of diazepam is 40 mg/day, but recreational abusers often ingest 100 mg daily. Some abusers take benzodiazepines intravenously.

Withdrawal

Abrupt withdrawal from benzodiazepines can cause troublesome to serious effects. Agitation, tremor, irritability, insomnia, vomiting, sweating, convulsions, and psychotic episodes have occurred. Gradual tapering of the dose is imperative. Because GABA is an inhibitory neurotransmitter, releasing its inhibition results in the *"taking off the brake"* phenomenon. Because long-term use of benzodiazepines reduces the number of GABA receptors, abrupt discontinuation of these drugs leaves the brain unable to fulfill inhibitory functions (Advokat, Comaty, & Julien, 2019). The adverse effects previously mentioned occur. The tapering or withdrawal process is highly individual (usually over about 7 weeks) but can take 1 year or longer in some heavily dependent individuals. Table 17.3 provides a more complete list of withdrawal symptoms.

Tolerance

Tolerance to the effects of benzodiazepines occurs, so individuals need an increasing amount of the drug to achieve the same effect. Tolerance to sedation develops quickly (within weeks), whereas tolerance to antianxiety effects occurs slowly (over a few months). Anticonvulsive tolerance also develops slowly, so the use of benzodiazepines for epilepsy is probably ill-advised for most patients. Cognitive and memory effects appear to continue as long as these agents are used (Advokat, Comaty, & Julien, 2019). Tolerance develops to some of the desired effects of benzodiazepines (i.e., hypnotic, anxiolytic, anticonvulsive effects), although tolerance does not appear to develop to the unwanted effects of cognitive and memory deficits. According to several news sources, Michael Jackson was taking 40 Xanax per night. Although the pill strength was not mentioned, this is a large dosage of this benzodiazepine.

Interactions

Benzodiazepines are CNS depressants and interact *additively* with other CNS depressants. Alcohol, TCAs, opioids, antipsychotics, and antihistamines increase the sedative effects of

TABLE 17.3   Symptoms Emerging After Withdrawal From Benzodiazepines

Neurologic	Gastrointestinal	Psychiatric	Other
Convulsions	Nausea	Anxiety	Tachycardia
Insomnia	Vomiting	Irritability	Sweating
Lightheadedness	Diarrhea	Cognitive impairment	—
Involuntary movements	Weight loss	Memory impairment	—
Headache	Decreased appetite	Depression	—
Weakness	—	Confusion	—

benzodiazepines. In addition, grapefruit juice can cause problems because it inhibits the cytochrome P-450 3A4 enzyme, extending the life of several benzodiazepines. Table 17.4 lists major interactants for benzodiazepines.

Nursing Implications

Therapeutic versus toxic drug levels. Benzodiazepines taken alone are relatively safe drugs (Stahl, 2021; Weber & Duchemin, 2018). Overdoses hundreds of times higher than a therapeutic dose have been reported without resulting in death. However, if benzodiazepines are combined with other drugs, such as alcohol or opioids, the effect can be fatal. In fact, benzodiazepines are present in 31% of fatal overdoses (Weber & Duchemin, 2018). Signs and symptoms of overdose include somnolence, confusion, coma, diminished reflexes, and hypotension. Effective treatment begins with emptying the stomach by induced vomiting and gastric lavage, followed by activated charcoal. The nurse should monitor blood pressure, pulse, and respirations and provide supportive care as indicated.

Benzodiazepine receptor antagonist. Flumazenil (Romazicon) blocks the benzodiazepine-binding site on the GABA receptor. It selectively blocks benzodiazepine receptors but does not block adrenergic or cholinergic receptors. Because flumazenil does not stimulate the CNS and does not block other receptors, it usually can be given when benzodiazepine overdose is suspected without fear of unexpected interactions. A response to flumazenil typically occurs within 30 to 60 seconds. Two important considerations when giving flumazenil are that (1) it does not speed up the metabolism or excretion of benzodiazepines, and (2) it has a short duration of action. These considerations present a clinical management problem. If the patient responds to flumazenil, benzodiazepines are present, but because flumazenil does not speed up metabolism and has a short duration of action, the patient might recover only to return to the same state as before flumazenil. This problem requires constant vigilance by the nurse and repeated doses of flumazenil as the body eliminates the benzodiazepine from the system. Flumazenil might not reverse benzodiazepine-induced respiratory depression and can precipitate seizures (Advokat, Comaty, & Julien, 2019; Burchum & Rosenthal, 2021).

Use during pregnancy. The association between benzodiazepine use and fetal abnormalities has not been supported in the first trimester (Weber & Duchemin, 2018). Some concern exists that benzodiazepines might be associated with cleft lip and cleft palate during the entire pregnancy, as there is evidence of a 1% risk of oral cleft malformation (Advokat, Comaty, & Julien, 2019). However, these findings might warrant discontinuance during pregnancy. Additionally, floppy infant syndrome has been associated with benzodiazepine use during labor or in high-dose benzodiazepine use disorder (or benzodiazepine dependence) (Advokat, Comaty, & Julien, 2019). Benzodiazepines are also known to be found in breast milk, so nursing mothers must be cautious and avoid use. If the drug cannot be discontinued without exacerbation of symptoms, tapering to the lowest possible dose is desirable, as is the use of shorter-acting agents, such as alprazolam or lorazepam. Benzodiazepine consumption in breastfeeding is not recommended (Advokat, Comaty, & Julien, 2019; Kimmel and Meltzer-Brody, 2021).

Use in older adults. As mentioned in the discussion on pharmacokinetics, specific benzodiazepines are acceptable for use in older adults, but most are not recommended. This dichotomy is based on metabolic processes. Lorazepam and oxazepam are considered to be the best benzodiazepines for older individuals. Temazepam and occasionally alprazolam are also used in this age group. The other benzodiazepines, including diazepam and chlordiazepoxide, have extended

TABLE 17.4   Major Interactions With Benzodiazepines

Interactant	Interaction
Alcohol and other CNS depressants (e.g., opioids)	Increased sedation, CNS depression
Antacids	Impaired absorption rate of benzodiazepine
Disulfiram (Antabuse) and cimetidine (Tagamet)	Increased plasma level of benzodiazepines that are oxidized (e.g., diazepam)
Phenytoin	Increased anticonvulsant serum level
TCAs	Increased sedation, confusion, impaired motor function
MAOIs	CNS depression
Succinylcholine	Decreased neuromuscular blockage

CNS, Central nervous system; *MAOIs*, monoamine oxidase inhibitors; *TCAs*, tricyclic antidepressants.

half-lives and active metabolites and should not be routinely prescribed for older patients. Benzodiazepines are associated with an increased risk for falls and cognitive problems in senior adults (Weber & Duchemin, 2018).

Side effects. The most common side effects are related to sedation and mental alertness. The patient should be cautioned about driving or operating hazardous machinery. Tolerance to sedation develops quickly. Blood pressure should be monitored routinely. A decrease in systolic blood pressure of 20 mm Hg while the patient is standing warrants withholding the drug and notifying the practitioner.

Interactions. Benzodiazepines interact with many CNS depressants. The nurse should explain this carefully to patients who are taking benzodiazepines. A high percentage of psychiatric patients abuse drugs, so a real potential exists for deadly combinations to be taken. These patients also are likely to develop a cross-tolerance to drugs metabolized in the liver. For example, individuals who develop a tolerance to alcohol have an increased tolerance to diazepam but not when alcohol and diazepam are taken together. Hearing a patient who is experienced in taking diazepam speak with disdain about typical doses is not uncommon—for example, "Ten milligrams of Valium doesn't even touch me!" Although diazepam alone might not touch these patients, diazepam combined with alcohol *will*. The nurse should remind these patients that if they mix diazepam with enough alcohol, they might die.

Teaching patients. Patient education is important because benzodiazepines have tremendous potential for abuse or misuse. Consequently, teaching patients and their families about these drugs is important. The nurse should teach the following precautions:

- Benzodiazepines are not intended for the minor stresses of everyday life.
- Over-the-counter drugs might enhance the actions of benzodiazepines.
- Driving should be avoided until tolerance develops.
- The prescribed dose should not be exceeded.
- Alcohol and other CNS depressants exacerbate the effects of benzodiazepines.
- Hypersensitivity to one benzodiazepine might mean hypersensitivity to another.
- These drugs should not be stopped abruptly.
- A black box warning exists regarding benzodiazepines and opioids or alcohol due to the risk of additive effects that may cause slowed breathing or death.

The Deprescribing of Benzodiazepines

Teaching patients the importance of potential physiological dependence on benzodiazepines is critical in reducing the risk of addiction. Ongoing education with patients is important to discuss the benefits of benzodiazepines short term versus long term, potential risks, rebound anxiety, and a deprescribing plan. For individuals who have taken benzodiazepines over 4 weeks (daily use), tapering over 3 to 6 months is the best practice. This is usually done by a 25% reduction in dose at first, considering 50% less dose in 3 to 6 months while instituting other non-prescription modalities. After

6 months, taper to every other day of no benzodiazepine use until fully deprescribed. Individuals weaning from benzodiazepines should remain in close monitoring with their prescriber (Pottie et al., 2018).

Selected Benzodiazepines

Alprazolam. Alprazolam (Xanax) is particularly useful for generalized anxiety, adjustment disorders, panic disorder, and anxiety associated with depression. It is also prescribed as an anti-tremor agent. Alprazolam has also been used to treat anxiety in acute myocardial infarction. Alprazolam has been criticized for its potential to cause addiction and dependence, and there have been reports of alprazolam-induced violent or aggressive behavior.

Chlordiazepoxide. Chlordiazepoxide (Librium) is prescribed for anxiety disorders, the relief of the symptoms of anxiety, and acute alcohol withdrawal. Chlordiazepoxide is absorbed well orally. Additionally, chlordiazepoxide can be used as an anti-tremor agent. Parenteral chlordiazepoxide is used as an anti-panic agent. Accumulation occurs with this drug as it is hepatically metabolized.

Clonazepam. Clonazepam (Klonopin) is used most often as an anticonvulsant but also has clinical use in the treatment of panic disorder. Clonazepam is weakly lipophilic (i.e., does not sequester readily in adipose tissue), and it has a small volume of distribution. Patients taking clonazepam over the long term should be slowly tapered off this drug because evidence suggests that abrupt withdrawal can precipitate status epilepticus. Clonazepam is also used for benzodiazepine withdrawal.

Diazepam. Diazepam (Valium) is an often prescribed antianxiety agent that has multiple uses related to its CNS depressive effect. In addition to treating anxiety disorders and providing short-term relief from symptoms of anxiety, diazepam is used preoperatively to relieve presurgery jitters, for skeletal muscle spasms (e.g., lower back pain), as a drug of choice (intravenously) for status epilepticus, and as an adjunct for endoscopic procedures. Additionally, diazepam might be useful for symptomatic relief of alcohol withdrawal.

Lorazepam. Lorazepam (Ativan) is used to treat anxiety disorders and can be used as an anti-tremor agent, anti-panic agent, anticonvulsant (parenteral only), and antiemetic for patients with cancer undergoing chemotherapy. Lorazepam 2 mg plus haloperidol 5 mg plus Benadryl 50 mg IM STAT is often used in the emergency department for very agitated or combative patients. The metabolites of lorazepam are inactive, so the effects of this drug do not persist. Patients with impaired liver function can handle this drug better than most other benzodiazepines because lorazepam is metabolized by a conjugative process to inactive metabolites. Lorazepam is recommended for use in older patients when a benzodiazepine is indicated.

Oxazepam. Oxazepam (Serax) is similar to lorazepam in that its metabolite is inactive, and it is metabolized by a conjugative reaction. The drug is effective for a relatively short time (24 hours) and is suitable for patients with liver disorders and for older adults. Oxazepam is used for anxiety associated with depression and for relief from acute alcohol withdrawal.

NONBENZODIAZEPINE: BUSPIRONE

Buspirone (BuSpar), first available in 1986, is a first-line agent for anxiety. It is not a benzodiazepine and does not bind to benzodiazepine recognition sites, but it probably acts as an agonist at the presynaptic serotonin 1 A receptor. Considerable interest exists in buspirone because it differs from benzodiazepines in several important ways. The advantages of buspirone are as follows:

- It is not sedating.
- It does not cause a euphoric high, so it has almost *no abuse potential*.
- It has no cross-tolerance with sedatives or alcohol.
- It does not produce dependence, withdrawal, or tolerance.

Buspirone has one disadvantage:

- It has a delayed onset of antianxiety effect compared with benzodiazepines (1 to 6 weeks).

Buspirone's effects help distinguish anxiety control from the sedative and euphoric actions of older benzodiazepines. Buspirone is particularly effective in reducing symptoms of worry, apprehension, difficulties with concentration and cognition, and irritability. These subjective symptoms are probably more serotonin-based than the more physical symptoms of anxiety (Stahl, 2021). Buspirone does not depress the CNS, and its lack of a sedative effect makes it less attractive for abuse. Because it has no abuse potential, buspirone is not a controlled substance.

Buspirone provides relief from anxiety within 7 to 10 days, but *maximal* therapeutic gain is not achieved until 3 to 6 weeks after treatment is initiated. Buspirone has a relatively short half-life, so it is usually given in divided doses. Buspirone is extensively metabolized after the first pass; 1% to 4% becomes bioavailable. Foods increase its bioavailability by decreasing the first-pass metabolism. Side effects include dizziness, nausea, headache, nervousness, lightheadedness, and excitement. Buspirone is a remarkably safe drug and has few drug interactions.

The benzodiazepine should not be stopped immediately when switching from a benzodiazepine to buspirone. Because of dissimilarities in their pharmacologic properties, benzodiazepines must be tapered (to prevent withdrawal effects) while buspirone is initiated.

SELECTIVE SEROTONIN REUPTAKE INHIBITOR

SSRIs are first-line agents for anxiety spectrum disorders and are discussed in detail in Chapter 15. The fact that these drugs work so well in treating anxiety underscores the overlapping nature of depression and anxiety. They are mentioned only briefly here. Box 17.5 summarizes the typical approach to treating anxiety.

SSRIs are prescribed for generalized anxiety disorder (GAD), obsessive-compulsive disorder (OCD), panic disorder (with panic attacks), posttraumatic stress disorder (PTSD),

---

BOX 17.5 Typical Approach to Treating Anxiety: Staying the Course

People who seek professional help for anxiety are hurting. Although it has been noted in the text that selective serotonin reuptake inhibitors (SSRIs) are the first-line treatment choice, they do not act rapidly. Although it is debated in professional meetings and in scholarly journals, often the anxious individual is prescribed an SSRI and a benzodiazepine. Because the SSRI will take some time to "work," the patient would be too miserable without some extra help. Benzodiazepines provide the immediate help that the patient is seeking. After several weeks or so, the hope is that the patient can be weaned off the benzodiazepine and then rely on the SSRI for relief. As noted in Chapter 15, SSRIs act through the second messenger system. Within weeks, the actual genetic output of the neuron begins to change. In some ways, benzodiazepines are similar to *aspirin*, and SSRIs are similar to *antibiotics*. One medication first treats the symptoms, while the other treats the real problem. It is very important to stay the course with the SSRIs. If there is no improvement in 4 weeks, the dose should be increased every 2–4 weeks until remission of symptoms or until side effects are so troublesome that a dosage increase would be unwise (Advokat, Comaty, & Julien, 2019; Stahl, 2021).

TABLE 17.5 Antidepressants Indicated for Anxiety

Agent	Dosage Class	Dosage Range (mg/day)	Comment (FDA Approval)[a]
Citalopram (Celexa)	SSRI	40–60	OCD
Clomipramine (Anafranil)	SRI/TCA	100–250	OCD
Escitalopram (Lexapro)	SSRI	10–30	GAD, OCD
Fluoxetine (Prozac)	SSRI	20–80	OCD, PD
Fluvoxamine (Luvox)	SSRI	100–300	OCD
Paroxetine (Paxil)	SSRI	40–60	GAD, OCD, PD, SAD
Sertraline (Zoloft)	SSRI	50–200	OCD, PD, PTSD, SAD
Venlafaxine (Effexor XR)	SNRI	75–225	GAD, PD, SAD
Duloxetine (Cymbalta)	SNRI	60–120	GAD

[a]At this writing, this list contains all of the drugs FDA approved for anxiety disorders.

FDA, U.S. Food and Drug Administration; *GAD*, generalized anxiety disorder; *OCD*, obsessive-compulsive disorder; *PD*, panic disorder; *PTSD*, posttraumatic stress disorder; *SAD*, social anxiety disorder; *SNRI*, selective serotonin-norepinephrine reuptake inhibitor; *SRI*, serotonin reuptake inhibitor; *SSRI*, selective serotonin reuptake inhibitor; *TCA*, tricyclic antidepressant.

---

and social phobias. OCD is perhaps the most difficult mental disorder to treat satisfactorily. Several SSRIs are considered first-line approaches to the treatment of OCD (Table 17.5).

TABLE 17.6 Pharmacologic Interventions for Specific Anxiety Disorders

Disorder	Pharmacologic Treatment
Panic Disorder Exhibited as discrete and intense period of anxiety, apprehension, and distress Associated symptoms include palpitations, sweating, trembling, and dyspnea	SSRIs: Perhaps the safest for long-term and prophylactic doses; gradual titration to sertraline 50 mg qd or paroxetine 40 mg qd (minimum effective dosages) Benzodiazepines: Clonazepam (average dosage 1.5 mg/day) and alprazolam (average dosage 3 mg/day) can provide more immediate relief TCAs: Same dosage as that used in treating depressive syndromes, but dose level should be carefully titrated because of risk of a paradoxical effect
Phobic Disorders *Agoraphobia* Fear of being away from home or in situations in which escape is inhibited	Alprazolam at the relatively high dosage of 3–6 mg/day has proven effective TCAs: Dosage typically 150–200 mg/day SSRIs and highly serotonergic TCAs (e.g., clomipramine, amitriptyline, trazodone) are effective for agoraphobia
Social Phobia Persistent fears of situations in which the person is exposed to the scrutiny of others (e.g., stage fright)	β-blockers: Often taken in combination with antidepressants or benzodiazepine; propranolol 10–20 mg tid or qid Benzodiazepines alone or in combination with antidepressants Clonazepam: 0.5 mg bid SSRIs: Low doses initially
Obsessive-Compulsive Disorder Obsessions, compulsions, or both	Clomipramine: 100–200 mg/day Fluvoxamine: 200–300 mg/day Other SSRIs or gabapentin (Neurontin) titrated up to 1800–2400 mg/day
Post-traumatic Stress Disorder[a] Re-experiencing of trauma, avoidance, hyperarousal	SSRIs: Treatment of choice Antipsychotics: Appropriate if psychotic or subsyndromal symptoms occur Mood stabilizers: Appropriate for mood vacillations and irritability

[a]Nestler, E. J., Hyman, S. E., Holtzman, D. M., & Malenka, R. C. (2021). *Molecular neuropharmacology: A foundation for clinical neuroscience.* McGraw-Hill; Weber, S. R., & Duchemin, A. M. (2018). Benzodiazepines: Sensible prescribing in light of the risks. *Current Psychiatry, 17*(2), 22–27.
bid, Twice a day; *qd,* every day; *qid,* four times a day; *SSRIs,* selective serotonin reuptake inhibitors; *TCAs,* tricyclic antidepressants; *tid,* three times a day.

Specifically, citalopram (Celexa), fluoxetine (Prozac), fluvoxamine (Luvox), paroxetine (Paxil), and sertraline (Zoloft) are approved for the treatment of this disorder. SSRIs are probably the most effective as well as the safest agents for prophylaxis and long-term treatment of panic attacks. GABA receptors are thought to be involved in the pathophysiology of panic disorders. It has been theorized that the overwhelming anxiety associated with panic might stem from abnormal serotonin transmission. The effectiveness of SSRIs in panic and other anxiety disorders can be partially explained by serotonin's role in up-regulating GABA transmission in the prefrontal cortex. By up-regulating inhibitory neurons, a more inhibitory effect can be expected. This hypothesis agrees with what we know about symptoms of anxiety.

Venlafaxine and Duloxetine

Venlafaxine (Effexor, Effexor XR) and duloxetine (Cymbalta) are the only selective serotonin-norepinephrine reuptake

inhibitors (SNRIs) approved for GAD. Venlafaxine is also approved for panic disorder and social anxiety disorder. These agents offer a dual approach to treatment because they block the reuptake of both serotonin (at lower doses) and norepinephrine (at medium to higher doses). Doses at the higher ranges are believed to be more effective, possibly because of the increased norepinephrine reuptake inhibition at these ranges. Table 17.6 outlines pharmacologic interventions for specific anxiety disorders.

OTHER DRUGS WITH ANTIANXIETY PROPERTIES

Clomipramine and Other Tricyclic Antidepressants

Clomipramine (Anafranil) is one of two drugs considered most effective for OCD (the other is the SSRI fluvoxamine).

Clomipramine is a serotonin reuptake inhibitor, although it is not as potent as the more traditional SSRIs. The major central side effects of clomipramine include headache, reduced libido, nervousness, myoclonus, and increased appetite. Peripheral effects include dry mouth, constipation, ejaculation failure (42%), erectile dysfunction (20%), and weight gain.

Other TCAs have support for use in patients with anxiety but are not U.S. Food and Drug Administration approved for those conditions: Imipramine (Tofranil) and desipramine (Norpramin), while not officially approved, have proven to be effective for panic-anxiety attacks. Trazodone (Desyrel, Oleptro) has a highly sedative quality and is often prescribed for individuals who are experiencing anxiety (particularly older adults) to facilitate sleep.

Clonidine

Clonidine (Catapres) is an α-2 agonist. Because agonistic stimulation of autoreceptors, such as α-2, causes a decrease in neurotransmitter production, it follows that this drug, which is typically indicated for hypertension, could have antianxiety effects, and it does. Clonidine has also been used successfully in treating nightmares associated with PTSD (Sareen, Stein, & Friedman, 2021).

Gabapentin

Gabapentin (Neurontin) is a commonly used anticonvulsant with antianxiety properties. It has been found to be effective in the treatment of social phobia and moderately effective in the treatment of OCD. It also has been used to augment the antidepressant treatment of PTSD and in chronic pain syndromes (Sareen et al. 2021).

Hydroxyzine

Hydroxyzine (Vistaril, Atarax) also has been used successfully with anxious patients. It is an older agent and was used infrequently for many years but has experienced a "comeback" of sorts. It is an antihistamine (first generation); thus, it blocks histamine and cholinergic receptors. However, it also blocks serotonin receptors, and this mechanism is thought to be responsible for its anxiolytic properties (Entringer, 2020). It has few significant side effects when given in appropriate doses, is inexpensive, is not typically habit-forming, and has many dosage forms.

Antiepileptics: Pregabalin and Levetiracetam

Pregabalin (Lyrica) is molecularly similar to GABA. It is used for the treatment of anxiety spectrum disorders, neuropathic pain, and seizures. It is related to gabapentin in that it inhibits neuronal excitability. It has few drug-drug interactions and does not cause dependence. It is a second-line agent but has been found to be effective. Levetiracetam (Keppra) increases the release of GABA and thus has an antianxiety effect.

Propranolol

Propranolol (Inderal) is a β-blocker that effectively interrupts the physiologic responses of anxiety related to social phobia. As noted earlier, autonomic dysregulation is a factor in anxiety. It makes sense that a drug that blocks these receptors could be effective. Propranolol is less effective than benzodiazepines but is safe and has little abuse potential. Most side effects are transient and mild. However, bradycardia, lightheadedness, and heart block have been reported.

> ### ? CRITICAL THINKING QUESTIONS
>
> 1. Although barbiturates and benzodiazepines both affect GABA receptors, why can an overdose of barbiturates (without coadministration of other drugs) be fatal, whereas an overdose of benzodiazepines (without coadministration of other drugs) is apparently not fatal?
> 2. Flumazenil (Romazicon) is given for benzodiazepine overdose. Why doesn't it serve to reverse the effects of other GABA agonists?

■ STUDY NOTES

1. Antianxiety agents are commonly prescribed psychotropic drugs.
2. SSRIs are first-line agents used to treat anxiety. They are discussed in detail in Chapter 15.
3. The nonbenzodiazepine buspirone is also a first-line agent that is relatively safe and interacts with few other drugs.
4. Benzodiazepines are also commonly used.
5. Diazepam (Valium) is the prototype benzodiazepine; however, other benzodiazepines, particularly alprazolam (Xanax) and lorazepam (Ativan) are used extensively.
6. Benzodiazepines have four basic clinical uses: (a) for chronic anxiety, (b) for time-limited periods in people going through crises, (c) for presurgery nervousness, and (d) for the treatment of panic disorder.
7. The ability to mute incoming stimuli gives benzodiazepines a great potential for abuse.
8. Benzodiazepines can cause physical dependence and produce withdrawal syndrome. Discontinuance should be tapered gradually.
9. Side effects of benzodiazepines include drowsiness, fatigue, ataxia, and other peripheral and central effects; however, tolerance to side effects occurs.
10. Benzodiazepines are safe drugs when taken alone but can be deadly if mixed with other CNS depressants (e.g., alcohol).
11. Benzodiazepines that ultimately rely on conjugation with glucuronic acid to inactive metabolites are more appropriate for older adults (e.g., lorazepam [Ativan], oxazepam [Serax]).

12. Buspirone (BuSpar) is a nonbenzodiazepine and is used extensively for the treatment of anxiety. Buspirone differs from the benzodiazepines in the following ways:
    a. It is not sedating.
    b. It does not cause a euphoric high, so it has almost *no abuse potential*.
    c. It has no cross-tolerance with sedatives or alcohol.
    d. It takes 1 to 6 weeks to be effective.
    e. It does not produce dependence, withdrawal, or tolerance.
    f. It does not cause muscle relaxation.

REFERENCES

Adams, M.P., Urban, C.Q., & Sutter, R.E. (2021). Pharmacology: Connections to nursing practice. (4th ed.) Pearson.

Advokat, C. D., Comaty, J. E., & Julien, R. M. (2019). *Julien's primer of drug action: A comprehensive guide to actions, uses and side effects of psychoactive drugs* (14th Ed.). Worth Publishers.

Beach, S. R., Gomez-Bernal, F., Huffman, J. C., & Fricchione, G. L. (2017). Alternative treatment strategies for catatonia: A systemic review. *General Hospital Psychiatry, 48,* 1–19. https//doi.org./10.1016/j.genhosppsych.2017.06.011.

Bezchlibnyk-Butler, K. Z., Jeffries, J. J., Procyshyn, R. M., & Virani, A. S. (2021). Clinical handbook of psychotropic drugs (20th ed.). Hogrefe Publishing. http://www.hogrefe.com.

Braslow, J., & Marder, S. R. (2019). History of psychopharmacology. *Annual Review of Clinical Psychology, 15,* 25–50. https://doi.org/10.1146/annurev-clinpsy-050718-095514.

Burchum, J., & Rosenthal, L. (2021). *Lehne's pharmacology for nursing care* (10th ed.). Elsevier.

Entringer, S. (2020). Hydroxyzine. https://www.drugs.com/hydroxyzine.html.

Kimmel, M.C. & Meltzer-Brody, S. (2021). Safety of infant exposure to antidepressants and benzodiazepines through breastfeeding. https://www.uptodate.com/contents/safety-of-infant-exposure-to-antidepressants-and-benzodiazepines-through-breastfeeding.

Nestler, E. J., Hyman, S. E., Holtzman, D. M., & Malenka, R. C. (2021). *Molecular neuropharmacology: A foundation for clinical neuroscience.* McGraw-Hill.

Panic disorder: When fear overwhelms. (2016). National Institute of Mental Health (NIMH). https://www.nimh.nih.gov/health/publications/panic-disorder-when-fear-overwhelms/index.shtml.

Pottie, K., Thompson, W., Davies, S., Grenier, J., Sadowski, C. A., Welch, V., … Farrell, B. (2018). Deprescribing benzodiazepine receptor agonists: Evidence-based clinical practice guideline. *The Official Journal of the College of Family Physicians of Canada, 65*(4), 339–351. https://www.cfp.ca/content/64/5/339?mc_cid=f9587cfd0b&mc_eid=c762c3d1ae.

Sareen, J., Stein, M.B. & Friedman, M. (2021). Posttraumatic stress disorder in adults: epidemiology, clinical manifestations, course, assessment and diagnosis. https://www.uptodate.com/contents/posttraumatic-stress-disorder-in-adults-epidemiology-pathophysiology-clinical-manifestations-course-assessment-and-diagnosis?search=psychobiology%20of%20ptsd&topicRef=117909&source=see_link.

Stahl. S. M. (2021). *Essential psychopharmacology* (7th Ed.). Cambridge University Press.

Tidwell, W. P., Thomas, T. L., Pouliot, J., Canonico, A. E., & Webber, A. J. (2018). Treatment of alcohol withdrawal syndrome: Phenobarbital versus CIWA-Ar protocol. *American Journal of Critical Care, 27*(6), 454–460. https://doi.org/10.4037.

Tietze, K.J., Fuchs, B., Parsons, P.E., O'Connor, M.F. & Finlay, G. (2021). Sedative-analgesic medications in critically ill adults: properties, dosage regimens and adverse effects https://www.uptodate.com/contents/sedative-analgesic-medications-in-critically-ill-adults-properties-dosage-regimens-and-adverse-effects?search=Pharmacology%20of%20commonly%20used%20analgesics%20and%20sedatives%20in%20the%20ICU:%20Benzodiazepines,%20propofol,%20and%20opioids&source=search_result&selectedTitle=1~150&usage_type=default&display_rank=1.

Weber, S. R., & Duchemin, A. M. (2018). Benzodiazepines: Sensible prescribing in light of the risks. *Current Psychiatry, 17*(2), 22–27.

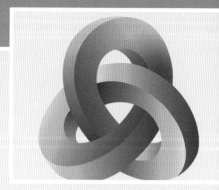

18

Antidementia Drugs

W. Chance Nicholson and Norman L. Keltner

If Afghanistan is the graveyard of empires, then Alzheimer's disease is the graveyard of research dollars.

Allan M. Block, MD (2018)

http://evolve.elsevier.com/Keltner

LEARNING OBJECTIVE

- Identify the drugs used in the treatment of Alzheimer disease and other dementias.

Biological agents used for Alzheimer disease (AD) can be roughly categorized into those for treatment and those for prevention. The use of these agents is not based on evidence that they can slow disease progression, but rather, improve clinical symptomatology or reduce or delay their burden. Neither treatment nor preventive agents provide the definitive approach that patients and families seek. Nevertheless, the available agents provide some relief and alleviate the fear of getting AD. Unfortunately, no new medications have been FDA approved for AD since 2003. There are a few experimental agents that show promise; however, to date, many of these have failed in phase II or III of clinical trials. Although significant limitations exist, current approaches target specific physiologic mechanisms; this hardly resembles the serendipitous approach that dominated drug discovery during the early years of psychopharmacology.

DRUGS USED TO TREAT DEMENTIAS

AD is a degenerative disease that is insidious and devastating. Persons living with AD lose memory-making ability, experience memory loss, cannot find the right words to express themselves, and have generalized cognitive impairment. The neurobiological reasons for this are neuronal death, growth factor dysregulation, and neurotransmitter deficiencies. At this point, the most common approach to treatment attempts to restore neurotransmitter loss. The less common drug approach attempts to, and might, hinder neuronal death. Chapter 28 provides greater detail, but simply, neuronal loss occurs in many places in the brain; however, the hippocampus, where memories are made, is never spared. Neurotransmitter restoration focuses on one primary neurotransmitter, acetylcholine (ACh), recognizing its regulatory relationship with glutamate. While other neurotransmitters degenerate as well, such as the dopamine and the

norepinephrine systems, the focus of this chapter is to introduce ACh as it informs the biological theory, which guided the development of the mainstay pharmacological agents.

AGENTS THAT RESTORE ACETYLCHOLINE

Background

To completely understand the agents used to restore ACh losses, it is important to review related concepts. Cholinergic pathways, enzymes, enzyme inhibition, types of ACh receptors, and types of cholinesterases (ChE) are discussed to facilitate the understanding of how these drugs work.

Cholinergic Pathways

Cholinergic pathways, just one of several neurotransmitter systems affected, are selectively destroyed in AD. Emerging evidence suggests that AD is largely a vascular disorder, with inflammation primarily driving this selective dysfunction. As such, it should be no surprise that the cholinergic pathways regulate cerebral vasodilation and immune cells possess a complete cholinergic system that can synthesize and degrade ACh. Furthermore, the antiinflammatory cholinergic pathway mediates immunoregulation via projections to the cortico-striatal-thalamic and limbic systems and the activation of nicotinic receptors most vulnerable to AD (specifically, $\alpha 7$ and $\alpha 4\beta 2$). ACh transmission is important for memory, learning, attention, and other cognitive functions. Most cholinergic fibers (about 90%) arise from one area, the nucleus basalis of Meynert. As might be suspected, the hippocampus is particularly rich in cholinergic receptors, and the loss of ACh in this area causes the aforementioned memory-making loss. The amygdala, the presumed locus of human emotion, is in front of the hippocampus and plays a role in memorization selection (Ferreira-Vieira et al., 2016). Stated another way, many of our memories are linked to emotional events, so we often remember embarrassing or frightening moments. The amygdala, along with insula and other critical brain areas, coordinates this type of memory-making selection. The amygdala depends heavily on ACh for this function and suffers significantly as ACh pathways decline.

Enzymes

Enzymes are large molecules produced according to specific genetic coding. Enzymes provide the catalytic force that drives production of energy and the material required for the building blocks of life itself.

 NORM'S NOTES There is not a whole lot that our society can do for a patient with AD today, but it is an area of well-funded research, with some promising answers on the horizon. This chapter takes a slightly different approach than the previous drug chapters. Receptors and enzymes are reviewed, because understanding their actions is critical to knowing the "why." If you study this chapter thoroughly, you will have very useful information for patients' families and maybe even for people you know.

Enzyme configuration is such that certain molecules, including neurotransmitters and drugs, fit onto the enzyme and then undergo metabolic change. The enzyme is a catalyst of the metabolic change but is not a participant. Multiple iterations of the enzymatic catalytic activity perpetuate these metabolic cycles. In the case of ChE, a single molecule can metabolize 5000 molecules of ACh every second (Fig. 18.1).

ChE breaks down ACh into the inactive metabolites choline and acetate. Once fragmented, these inactive remnants of ACh can no longer activate cholinergic receptors. Because a loss of ACh is the primary neurotransmitter loss in AD, attempting to prevent the breakdown of ACh has proven to be the most effective means for restoring this neurotransmitter (Hampel et al., 2018).

Enzyme Inhibition

The approach to inhibiting ACh metabolism centers around blocking the enzyme ChE; this is accomplished by introducing molecules into the system that preferentially attach to ChE. When this blocking is accomplished, ACh cannot be metabolized, increasing the availability of this neurotransmitter to postsynaptic cholinergic receptors.

Types of Acetylcholine Receptors

Two types of ACh receptors have been identified in humans: muscarinic receptors and nicotinic receptors. *Muscarinic receptors* are divided into five subtypes; however, for the purpose of this discussion, they are grouped simply as muscarinic receptors. Muscarinic receptors are the primary targets in treating AD. Muscarinic receptors are better known than nicotinic receptors because a blockade of these receptors (i.e., an antimuscarinic or anticholinergic effect) causes many of the side effects frequently encountered by nurses. For instance, dry mouth, dry eyes, blurred vision, urinary hesitancy, and constipation are caused by a blockade of these receptors. An interesting effect of anticholinergic drugs (e.g., diphenhydramine [Benadryl], benztropine mesylate [Cogentin]) that cause these effects is that they can compromise cognition as well. As people age, they become more susceptible to these effects. Stimulating these same receptors improves cognition. That is the therapeutic "bang" that ACh-enhancing agents provide.

The *nicotinic receptor* is best understood as two subtypes: (1) subtypes on the cell bodies of the postganglionic neurons in the autonomic nervous system (N_N); and (2) subtypes on skeletal muscles (N_M). However, there are also central nervous system nicotinic receptors that play a role in cognition and behaviors. When nicotinic receptors are activated, an up-regulation of norepinephrine, glutamate, γ-aminobutyric acid, and dopamine occurs, all of which improve attention, memory, mood, and cognition. Down-regulation of nicotinic receptors is linked to poor attention, sensory gating dysfunction, memory problems, and impaired cognition as is the case in AD, where pronounced loss of nicotinic receptors is observed in the cerebral cortex. As is widely known,

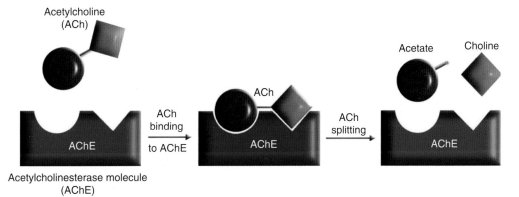

FIG. 18.1 An acetylcholine *(ACh)* molecule and an acetylcholinesterase *(AChE)* molecule *(left panel)*. AChE binds the ACh molecule *(center panel)*. The products of AChE's metabolic activity, acetate and choline *(right panel)*. (Courtesy Vicki Johnson. Modified from Burchum, J., & Rosenthal, L. [2016]. *Lehne's pharmacology for nursing care*. Elsevier.)

nicotinic receptors are stimulated by smoking. However, what is less well known is that smoking and the boosting of brain nicotine is a putatively therapeutic contribution to schizophrenia, attention-deficit hyperactivity disorder, and presumably, cognitive disorders (Keltner & Lillie, 2009). Two very specific nicotinic receptors, α7 and α4β2, have a role in attention and memory. When stimulated by nicotine, these receptors improve those functions. Attention, memory, and learning are cognitive skills enhanced by nicotine stimulation of specific nicotinic receptor subtypes (McLean et al., 2016). A greater appreciation for the potential of nicotinic receptor enhancers and their possible contribution to cognitive improvements has evolved over the last few years. To summarize this section to its most basic bedrock, if one cannot concentrate, one cannot remember; if one cannot remember, one cannot learn.

Types of Cholinesterase

Just as there are two types of monoamine oxidase enzymes, there are two types of ChE that have neuromodulatory properties in the brain and excitatory properties in the periphery. Acetylcholinesterase (AChE) is more common in the brain. The other ChE, butyrylcholinesterase (BChE), is more common in the periphery (Box 18.1). Because a central nervous system effect is required to treat AD, drugs that inhibit both ChEs have greater potential for causing unnecessary and often adverse effects. For example, inhibiting BChE produces nausea and vomiting, diarrhea, facial flushing, sweating, rhinitis, bradycardia, and leg cramps. The ideal drug might selectively inhibit AChE, while not inhibiting BChE.

Cholinesterase Inhibitors

Three drugs known as *cholinesterase inhibitors* target ACh deficiency (Table 18.1). By attaching to and blocking ChE,

BOX 18.1	**Cholinesterases: Primary Site of Action**
Acetylcholinesterase	**Butyrylcholinesterase**
Brain	Periphery
	Plasma
	Skeletal muscles
	Placenta
	Liver

these drugs substantially increase the amount of intrasynaptic ACh available to cholinergic receptors. A fourth drug, tacrine, is mentioned for heuristic and ethical reasons. Tacrine is discussed first.

Tacrine

Tacrine (Cognex) has been discontinued in the United States, but it is still worth reading about because there is a lesson to be learned. Tacrine was the first cholinesterase inhibitor (both AChE and BChE) available for use. It was widely heralded because before tacrine there was little hope for patients with AD. A 1986 article published in the *New England Journal of Medicine* reported that a patient returned to work, while another took up golf after being prescribed tacrine (Keltner, 1994). It was soon revealed that the *research was misrepresented*, and the authors received an unprecedented rebuke by the U.S. Food and Drug Administration (FDA). Tacrine causes significant gastrointestinal disruptions and hepatotoxicity owing to exhaustion of enzymatic resources. This adverse effect led to its withdrawal from the market in 2013.

Donepezil

Donepezil (Aricept) was approved in 1996. It is a reversible inhibitor of ChE with a half-life of approximately 60 to 90 hours and reaches maximum plasma concentrations in 3 to 5 hours. Tacrine inhibits both AChE and BChE, whereas donepezil is much more selective for AChE (1200 to 1 times more selective for AChE), so theoretically, its use should cause fewer peripheral side effects. Other advantages include the absence of hepatotoxicity, once-daily dosing related to a longer half-life, and 100% bioavailability whether taken with or without food. Some peripheral effects have been reported, including gastrointestinal problems and bradycardia, suggesting that selectivity for brain AChE is incomplete (Fig. 18.2). Until more recently, the highest dosage of donepezil was 10 mg/day. However, more recent studies show that donepezil at higher doses has proven helpful to select patients with moderate to severe AD (though side effects and rates of discontinuation are increased) (Haake et al., 2020). What is interesting is the dosage of the new tablet: 23 mg, though studies suggesting benefits of this dose are equivocal. See Box 18.2 for a view of this unusual formulation.

TABLE 18.1	**Antidementia Drugs**				
Drug	**Typical Daily Dosage**	**Half-Life (h)**	**Protein Binding (%)**	**Cytochrome P-450 Enzymes**	**Mechanism of Action**
Donepezil (Aricept)	Oral: 5–10 mg at bedtime	~70	~95	2D6, 3A4	ChE inhibitor
Rivastigmine (Exelon)	Oral: 6–12 mg in two divided doses	~2	~40	Not metabolized	ChE inhibitor
Galantamine (Razadyne)	16–24 mg daily	~7	Insignificant	2D6	ChE inhibitor
Memantine (Namenda)	10 mg in two divided doses or 28 mg once daily (extended-release)	~60–80	~45	Not extensively metabolized	NMDA antagonist

ChE, Cholinesterase; *NMDA*, N-methyl-D-aspartate.
From Stahl, S. M. (2017). *Prescriber's guide: Stahl's essential psychopharmacology.* Cambridge University Press.

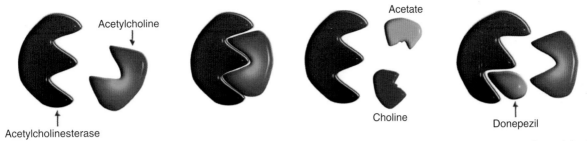

FIG. 18.2 The same process as shown in Fig. 18.1 is illustrated. However, AChE is inhibited from its metabolic activity by the AChE inhibitor donepezil *(last panel)*. ACh survives and builds up in the synapse. *ACh*, Acetylcholine; *AChE*, acetylcholinesterase. (Courtesy Vicki Johnson. Modified from Lehne, R. A. [2003]. *Pharmacology for nursing care*. Saunders.)

BOX 18.2 Exactly 23 Milligrams? Really?

Why would a manufacturer come up with a dosage form of 23 mg? Why not 20 or 25? Is the dosage that precise? Well, maybe, but maybe not. Schwartz and Woloshin (2012) find this a little unconvincing. They suggest that by coming up with a 23 mg tablet and gaining FDA approval, the maker of Aricept can keep its patent going for a few more years. Cynical, you say? Perhaps. But it also has a ring of truth.

Rivastigmine

Rivastigmine (Exelon) was approved for treatment of AD in 2000. It also inhibits ChE, but does so in a slightly different way than the previously described ChE inhibitors. Donepezil is a reversible inhibitor of ChE, whereas rivastigmine is said to be irreversible. Stated another way, donepezil slips off and on ChE continuously, whereas rivastigmine remains attached and forms a covalent bond with the enzyme. Rivastigmine remains effective until the life cycle of the enzyme is complete. Rivastigmine has a relatively short plasma half-life (about 2 hours) but has an inhibition half-life of 10 hours. Essentially, while attached irreversibly to ChE, rivastigmine is not factored into the plasma level.

Rivastigmine is not metabolized by cytochrome P-450 enzymes, so it does not interact with drugs metabolized by this system. With regard to this aspect of drug administration, rivastigmine has an advantage over tacrine and donepezil. Rivastigmine prefers AChE over BChE, but still produces peripheral side effects and, possibly, the highest rate of adverse effects when administered via capsule (Haake et al., 2020).

Galantamine

Galantamine (Razadyne) is the last ChE inhibitor we discuss. It also demonstrates preference for AChE over BChE; however, the ability of galantamine to stimulate presynaptic muscarinic receptors to release more ACh sets it apart. Owing to this latter mechanism, galantamine produces a few more cholinergic side effects, such as gastrointestinal symptoms, but appears to have the lowest mortality of all ACh inhibitors. An added feature with galantamine is its ability to allosterically modulate nicotinic receptors in the brain, particularly in the hippocampus. Galantamine is readily absorbed; it has a bioavailability of about 85% and a half-life of about 6 hours. It has a high volume of distribution and insignificant protein binding. It is metabolized by the cytochrome P-450 enzyme system, so it can interact with drugs catalyzed by this system (Fuenzalida & Arias, 2016).

Summary of Cholinesterase Inhibitors

Elevating ACh levels does not slow the disease process of AD or the other irreversible dementias, though evidence suggests they can delay the need for nursing homes and/or institutionalization. If one of these drugs is discontinued, the patient's cognitive abilities are what they would have been had the drug never been administered. These drugs, all approved for mild to moderate AD, help the patient preserve cognitive performance longer than if he or she had not taken the medication. Eventually, the underlying neurodegeneration becomes so profound that these efforts to bolster ACh no longer mask the devastation of the brain. Emerging evidence suggests that neurotrophic factors (e.g., brain-derived neurotrophic factor [BDNF], nerve growth factor) are instrumental in the maintenance of synaptic plasticity and neurogenesis in the hippocampus of AD via retarding abnormal amyloid production and enhancing repair. Interestingly, while it was initially believed that AChE inhibitors increased and sustained BDNF expression, evidence now suggests that this might not be the case. Longitudinal studies with donepezil and galantamine have challenged this initial belief, thus inviting more research into this area. Along these lines, emerging evidence suggests that rivastigmine could increase nerve growth factor, though this appears to occur independent of ACh inhibition via sigma receptors (most well known in opioids and sertraline literature) (Terada et al., 2018).

AGENTS THAT MAY STYMIE NEURODEGENERATION

AD progressively marches through the brain, leaving dead neurons in its path. Although the analogy of a destroyer marching through the brain does not reflect exactly what occurs, it does come close. Neurons die in several ways.

One such way is *neuronal excitotoxicity*. Excitotoxicity, or very rapid firing of the neuron, is caused by aberrant (i.e., sustained) depolarization (caused by the removal of magnesium channel blockades and the influx of calcium ions into the postsynaptic neuron) of the glutamate–N-methyl-D-aspartate receptor (NMDA) complex. Glutamate is an excitatory neurotransmitter, and NMDA is a glutamate receptor. Importantly, calcium ion permeable NMDA receptors regulate BDNF transcription. Whenever this coupling causes too many neuronal firings, the neuron can die and BDNF transcription is dysregulated; therefore, blocking the NMDA receptor reduces excitotoxicity.

Memantine

Memantine (Namenda) is a noncompetitive NMDA antagonist (Fig. 18.3). Although it is not completely understood, glutamate in a patient with AD becomes overactive via amyloid stimulation (possibly due to increased resting

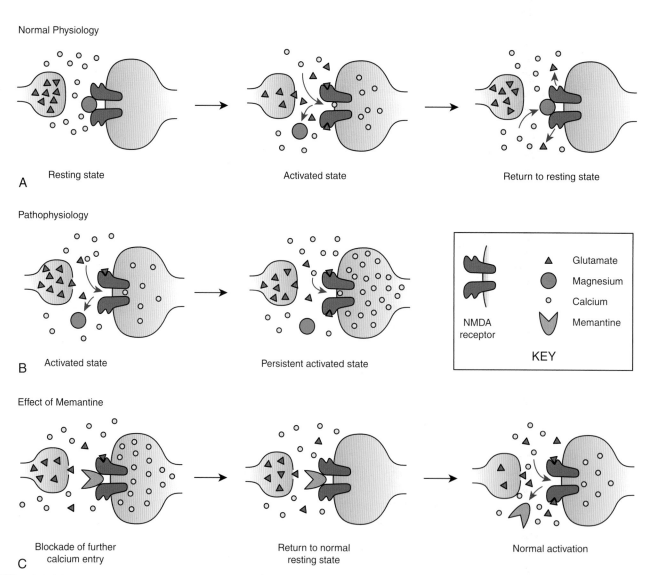

FIG. 18.3 Memantine mechanism of action. (A) Normal physiology. In the resting postsynaptic neuron, magnesium occupies the *N*-methyl-D-aspartate *(NMDA)* receptor channel, blocking calcium entry. Binding of glutamate to the receptor displaces magnesium, allowing calcium to enter. When glutamate dissociates from the receptor, magnesium returns to the channel and blocks further calcium inflow. The brief period of calcium entry constitutes a "signal" in the learning and memory process. (B) Pathophysiology. Slow but steady leakage of glutamate from the presynaptic neuron keeps the NMDA receptor in a constantly activated state, allowing excessive influx of calcium, which can impair memory and learning and eventually cause neuronal death. (C) Effect of memantine. Memantine blocks calcium entry when extracellular glutamate is low and stops further calcium entry, which allows intracellular calcium levels to normalize. When a burst of glutamate is released in response to an action potential, the resulting high level of glutamate is able to displace memantine, causing a brief period of calcium entry. When glutamate diffuses away, memantine reblocks the channel and stops further calcium entry, despite continuing low levels of glutamate in the synapse (not shown). (From Burchum & Rosenthal, 2016. *Lehne's pharmacology for nursing care* [9th ed.]. Elsevier.)

state glutamate concentrations and receptor sensitivity). As a result, glutamate overloads the postsynaptic neurons, thereby generating an insidious excitatory neurodegeneration. By blocking the NMDA receptor, memantine prevents the influx of calcium ions and regulates normal neuronal transmission. Memantine has a moderate affinity to NMDA, which allows it to occupy this receptor during prolonged or abnormal glutamate stimulation. Contrarily, in the presence of transient increases in glutamate (i.e., a normal physiological signal), it will dissociate from the receptor, allowing normal cell activity to resume (BDNF transcription) (Folch et al., 2018).

NMDA receptor antagonists are familiar to nurses in the emergency department because of the use of the drug phencyclidine (PCP). PCP is an NMDA antagonist. Users of the drug exhibit behaviors similar to those of paranoid schizophrenia. They are often violent and then, just as quickly, become nonviolent. The conundrum for the clinician is this: too much NMDA stimulation (i.e., excitotoxicity) can cause neuronal death, whereas too little (i.e., NMDA antagonism) can lead to psychotic behavior. Memantine is formulated so that NMDA stimulation does not occur, and severe behavioral effects do not develop.

Memantine has a long half-life (60 to 80 hours), but it is not metabolized to a great degree. The majority of memantine is excreted unchanged, thus accounting for few, if any, drug interactions. In contrast to the ChE inhibitors, it is approved by the FDA for moderate to severe AD. Memantine is often co-prescribed with donepezil or other ChE inhibitors such as galantamine (Koola, 2020). This combination is effective due to memantine and ChE inhibitors' different intervention points during abnormal AD signaling. When memantine and a ChE inhibitor are combined, reduced NMDA receptor activation occurs, thereby delaying the destruction of cholinergic neurons and normalizing the weakened signals via slowing ACh breakdown in their nerve endings. Of note, there is another NMDA receptor agonist in development called nitromemantine, which has shown promising results in animal trials due to a higher specificity for NMDA receptors and a better side effect profile. Additionally, newer memantine delivery methods are also being studied (such as nanoemulsion) that could increase availability via increased blood-brain barrier penetrability and help sustain its antioxidant properties (Kaur, Nigam, Srivastava, Tyagi, & Dang, 2020).

Secretase Inhibitors

One of the explanations for neurodegeneration in AD is the festering of snipped-off pieces of amyloid precursor proteins, which lead to neuronal death. This cutting is achieved by enzymes known as *secretases*. Secretase inhibition research is an evolving story; however, there is hope associated with these drugs because they get at the core of AD treatment:

preventing neurodestruction (Nie, Vartak, & Li, 2020). At the present time, many serious side effects are associated with these drugs. Chapter 28 provides greater detail about this pathologic process.

DRUGS TO PREVENT ALZHEIMER DISEASE

Drugs used to treat AD are useful and widely prescribed, but they do not stop the destructive onslaught of the disorder. That being the case, it is even more important to find means of preventing AD if possible. Multiple novel strategies are being tested for use that attempt to modify AD progression.

One example of such strategies are dihydropyridine calcium channel blockers. As mentioned previously, AD is grossly informed by vascular dysfunction. With that, it seems reasonable that medications regulating vascular performance might be beneficial as an intervention. Dihydropyridine calcium channel blockers have recently been viewed as a possible new tool in the fight to treat AD. These drugs, including amlodipine (Norvasc), nilvadipine (Escor & others), and nitrendipine (Baypress), are antihypertensives. Hypertension causes small vessel changes, inflammation, and a compromise of the blood-brain barrier. In turn, these conditions may precede cognitive decline. Collectively, dihydropyridines are thought to be able to reduce the influx of calcium ions into amyloid pathways, thereby reducing amyloid aggregation, secretase activity, and amyloid precursor proteins. Evidence suggests that patients taking antihypertensives and statins decrease their probability of developing dementia by 8% to 21% (van Dalen et al., 2021).

Recently, preliminary evidence has suggested that the tyrosine kinase inhibitor nilotinib could penetrate the blood-brain barrier and promote degeneracy of Aβ and tau. The therapeutic effect is decreased hippocampal loss and modulated dopaminergic activity in persons with AD (Turner et al., 2020). Other strategies include antiinflammation, statins, estrogen, antioxidants, vitamins, and antiamyloid immunotherapy. Although no one knows with certainty whether the following drug therapies prevent or forestall AD, evidence has suggested this possibility (Box 18.3). Because most of these drugs are relatively free of severe consequences, they may be worth promoting in the hope that they might be preventive.

❓ CRITICAL THINKING QUESTIONS

1. Why can a large dose of Benadryl cause fuzzy thinking in an older adult?
2. If someone you know has been diagnosed with AD, would it be a good idea for them to start taking a nonsteroidal antiinflammatory drug (NSAID)? (See Box 18.3.)

BOX 18.3   Potential Preventive Strategies for Alzheimer Disease

Strategies	Proposed Mechanism of Action and Evidence
Antiinflammation 1. Prednisone 2. NSAIDs (e.g., ibuprofen, celecoxib)	Pro-inflammatory signaling (e.g., cytokines) promotes persistent deposits of amyloid. 1. Reduces amyloid oligomers, thereby decreasing deposits. Evidence is lacking. 2. Cyclooxygenase (COX) is an enzyme that synthesizes prostaglandins and causes inflammation. Selective COX-2 inhibitors decrease inflammation via regulating secretase. Inconsistent evidence in human trials as a preventative, but effective in animals.
Estrogen	Estrogen to estrogen receptors (ERα) co-localize with neurofibrillary tangles and contribute to tau overexpression (particularly postmenopause), thereby decreasing estrogen levels and neuroprotection. Evidence is mixed. Promising results with conjugated estrogen with medroxy-progesterone improving memory in pre- and postmenopausal women.
Statins	Relationship between high cholesterol levels and amyloid. Reduced cholesterol preserves neuronal function. Act on apolipoprotein E sub-type (ApoE4) to prevent formation of amyloid, thereby reducing tau proteins and neurofibrillary tangles. Evidence supports greater benefit in homozygous ApoE4-genotyped AD (late onset) versus early onset. Benefits as an adjunctive therapy due to its ability to cross blood-brain barrier and improve nervous system function, but insufficient evidence to support them as preventative.
Antioxidants and vitamins 1. B_6, B_{12}, B_9 (folic acid) 2. Vitamin D 3. Vitamin E (α-tocopherol) 4. *Ginko biloba* 5. Polyphenols (e.g., curcumin)	Oxidative stress via lipid, glicidic, protein promote inflammatory or neuritic plaque and neurofibrillary tangles. 1. B vitamins are required for monoamine production, DNA synthesis, and maintenance of phospholipids. Deficiency of these vitamins elevates serum levels of homocysteine (amino acid) and promotes oxidative stress. Evidence is lacking. 2. Insufficient vitamin D promotes oxidative stress and inflammation, thus promoting cognitive dysfunction. Evidence is mixed as preventative. Promising results combining vitamin D and ChE inhibitors for improving cognitive function. 3. Insufficient vitamin E promotes amyloid and tau toxicities via oxidative stress. Strong evidence as a preventative by 2.5- to 4.0-fold. 4. Increases microcirculation blood flow and prevents reduction of synapses, thus increasing neurotrophic factors, which interfere with neuronal apoptosis. Reduces damage caused by amyloid. Strong evidence as a preventative. 5. Block amyloid aggregation pathway, thereby reducing oxidative stress and inflammation. Moderate evidence supports use as preventative.
Antiamyloid immunotherapy	Reduce brain levels of amyloid oligomers by decreasing their deposition via increased circulatory system clearance and redistribution to areas of the brain that promote elimination. Evidence supports their effectiveness in prevention but can have serious toxic side effects.

From Campanari et al. (2014), Cazarim et al. (2016), Geifman et al. (2017), Giraldo et al. (2014), Pasqualetti et al. (2009), Pate et al. (2017), Ramsey and Muskin (2013), and Wang et al. (2016).

■ STUDY NOTES

1. Drugs used to treat dementias can be categorized as (a) drugs for treatment of dementia and (b) drugs for prevention of dementia.

2. The causes of AD can be broadly grouped as (a) neuronal death and (b) neurotransmitter deficiency.

3. The most common drug interventions restore deficient neurotransmitters.

4. The primary neurotransmitter deficiency is ACh.

5. Agents that restore ACh levels do so by blocking the enzyme that metabolizes ACh.

6. ChEs break down ACh. The two types are (a) AChE and (b) BChE.

7. Antidementia drugs attach to ChEs and prevent them from bonding to and subsequently metabolizing ACh.

8. Three drugs are available that are identified as ChE (or AChE or BChE) inhibitors: donepezil, rivastigmine, and galantamine.

9. Memantine is an NMDA receptor inhibitor and has a different mechanism of action.

10. Theoretically, memantine could prevent neuronal death.

11. Other drugs are used to treat dementias.

12. NSAIDs; statins; estrogen; and B, D, and E vitamins are used to prevent AD. However, much research remains to be carried out before such claims can be broadly accepted.

REFERENCES

van Dalen, J. W., Marcum, Z. A., Gray, S. L., Barthold, D., van Charante, E. P. M., van Gool, W. A., ... & Richard, E. (2021). Association of angiotensin II–stimulating antihypertensive use and dementia risk: Post hoc analysis of the preDIVA trial. *Neurology, 96*(1), e67–e80.

Block, A.M. (2018). No improvement in sight for Alzheimer's drug development. https://www.mdedge.com/clinicalneurologynews/article/157645/alzheimers-cognition/no-improvement-sight-alzheimers- drug.

Burchum, J., & Rosenthal, L. (2016). *Lehne's pharmacology for nursing care* (9th Ed.). Elsevier.

Campanari, M. L., García-Ayllón, M. S., Blazquez-Llorca, L., Luk, W. K., Tsim, K., & SÆez-Valero, J. (2014). Acetylcholinesterase protein level is preserved in the Alzheimer's brain. *Journal of Molecular Neuroscience, 53*(3), 446–453. https://doi.org/10.1007/s12031-013-0183-5.

Cazarim, M. D. S., Moriguti, J. C., Ogunjimi, A. T., & Pereira, L. R. L. (2016). Perspectives for treating Alzheimer's disease: A review on promising pharmacological substances. *Sao Paulo Medical Journal, 134*(4), 342–354. https://doi.org/10.1590/1516-3180.2015.01980112.

Ferreira-Vieira, T. H., Guimaraes, I. M., Silva, F. R., & Ribeiro, F. M. (2016). Alzheimer's disease: Targeting the cholinergic system. *Current Neuropharmacology, 14*(1), 101–115. https://doi.org/10.2174/1570159X13666150716165726.

Folch, J., Busquets, O., Ettcheto, M., Sánchez-López, E., Castro-Torres, R. D., Verdaguer, E., ... & Camins, A. (2018). Memantine for the treatment of dementia: a review on its current and future applications. *Journal of Alzheimer's Disease, 62*(3), 1223–1240. https://doi.org/10.3233/JAD-170672.

Fuenzalida, M., & R Arias, H. (2016). Role of nicotinic and muscarinic receptors on synaptic plasticity and neurological diseases. *Current Pharmaceutical Design, 22*(14), 2004–2014. https://doi.org/10.2174/1381612822666160127112021. PMID: 26818867.

Geifman, N., Brinton, R. D., Kennedy, R. E., Schneider, L. S., & Butte, A. J. (2017). Evidence for benefit of statins to modify cognitive decline and risk in Alzheimer's disease. *Alzheimer's Research & Therapy, 9*(1), 10. https://doi.org/10.1186/s13195-017-0237-y.

Giraldo, E., Lloret, A., Fuchsberger, T., & Viæa, J. (2014). Aβ and tau toxicities in Alzheimer's are linked via oxidative stress-induced p38 activation: Protective role of vitamin E. *Redox Biology, 2*, 873–877. https://doi.org/10.1016/j.redox.2014.03.002.

Haake, A., Nguyen, K., Friedman, L., Chakkamparambil, B., & Grossberg, G. T. (2020). An update on the utility and safety of cholinesterase inhibitors for the treatment of Alzheimer's disease. *Expert opinion on drug safety, 19*(2), 147–157. https://doi.org/10.1080/14740338.2020.1721456.

Hampel, H., Mesulam, M. M., Cuello, A. C., Farlow, M. R., Giacobini, E., Grossberg, G. T., ... & Khachaturian, Z. S. (2018). The cholinergic system in the pathophysiology and treatment of Alzheimer's disease. *Brain: A Journal of Neurology, 141*(7), 1917–1933. https://doi.org/10.1093/brain/awy132.

Kaur, A., Nigam, K., Srivastava, S., Tyagi, A., & Dang, S. (2020). Memantine nanoemulsion: A new approach to treat Alzheimer's disease. *Journal of Microencapsulation, 37*(5), 355–365. https://doi.org/10.1080/02652048.2020.1756971.

Keltner, N. L. (1994). Tacrine: A pharmacological approach to Alzheimer's disease. *Journal of Psychosocial and Mental Health Nursing Services, 32*(3), 37.

Keltner, N. L., & Lillie, K. (2009). Nicotinic receptors: Implications for psychiatric care. *Perspectives in Psychiatric Care, 45*, 151.

Koola, M. M. (2020). Galantamine-memantine combination in the treatment of Alzheimer's disease and beyond. *Psychiatry Research, 113409*. https://doi.org/10.1016/j.psychres.2020.113409.

McLean, S. L., Grayson, B., Marsh, S., Zarroug, S. H., Harte, M. K., & Neill, J. C. (2016). Nicotinic α7 and α4β2 agonists enhance the formation and retrieval of recognition memory: Potential mechanisms for cognitive performance enhancement in neurological and psychiatric disorders. *Behavioral Brain Research, 302*, 73–80. http://hdl.handle.net/10454/8460.

Nie, P., Vartak, A., & Li, Y. M. (2020, April). γ-Secretase inhibitors and modulators: Mechanistic insights into the function and regulation of γ-secretase. *Seminars in Cell & Developmental Biology, 105*, 43–53. https://doi.org/10.1016/j.semcdb.2020.03.002.

Pasqualetti, P., Bonomini, C., Dal Forno, G., Paulon, L., Sinforiani, E., Marra, C., ... Rossini, P. M. (2009). A randomized controlled study on effects of ibuprofen on cognitive progression of Alzheimer's disease. *Aging Clinical and Experimental Research, 21*, 102. https://doi.org/10.1007/BF03325217.

Pate, K. M., Rogers, M., Reed, J. W., Munnik, N., Vance, S. Z., & Moss, M. A. (2017). Anthoxanthin polyphenols attenuate Aβ oligomer-induced neuronal responses associated with Alzheimer's disease. *CNS Neuroscience & Therapeutics, 23*(2), 135–144. https://doi.org/10.1111/cns.12659.

Ramsey, D., & Muskin, P. R. (2013). Vitamin deficiencies and mental health: How are they linked? *Current Psychiatry (Edgmont), 12*, 37.

Schwartz, L. M., & Woloshin, S. (2012). How the FDA forgot the evidence. The case of donepezil 23 mg. *BMJ*, Mar 22, 344. doi:10.1136/bmj.e1086. PMID: 22442352.

Turner, R. S., Hebron, M. L., Lawler, A., Mundel, E. E., Yusuf, N., Starr, J. N., ... & Moussa, C. (2020). Nilotinib effects on safety, tolerability, and biomarkers in Alzheimer's disease. *Annals of Neurology, 88*(1), 183–194.

Terada, K., Migita, K., Matsushima, Y., Sugimoto, Y., Kamei, C., Matsumoto, T., ... & Karube, Y. (2018). Cholinesterase inhibitor rivastigmine enhances nerve growth factor-induced neurite outgrowth in PC12 cells via sigma-1 and sigma-2 receptors. *PLoS ONE, 13*(12), e0209250.

Wang, C., et al. (2016). Estrogen receptor-α is localized to neurofibrillary tangles in Alzheimer's disease. *Scientific Reports, 6*, 20352. https://doi.org/10.1038/srep2035.

19

Alternative Preparations and Over-the-Counter Drugs

Marcus Otávio Guimarães Debiasi

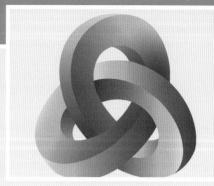

Most people are about as happy as they make up their minds to be.

Abraham Lincoln

(e) http://evolve.elsevier.com/Keltner

LEARNING OBJECTIVES

- Understand the differences between alternative preparations and over-the-counter drugs.
- Define "Integrative Medicine"
- Name common natural products, herbs, and dietary supplements used for psychiatric symptoms, and discuss current research conclusions regarding their efficacy.
- Describe how natural products, herbs, and dietary supplements are regulated.

- Name three dangerous interactions between commonly prescribed psychiatric drugs and over-the-counter drugs or herbal medicines.
- Explain the role of the nurse in assessment and intervention with patients using alternative preparations or over-the-counter drugs.

BACKGROUND

Over-the-Counter Versus Alternative Preparations

Many different products with stated pharmacological properties are available without a prescription in the United States. These can be broadly classified as (1) over-the-counter (OTC) drugs and supplements; or (2) alternative preparations, which primarily include herbal remedies and nutritional supplements. Alternative preparations represent one category of a broader group known as "Complementary Alternative Medicine" (CAM), which includes unconventional diagnostic methods and therapies such as acupuncture, biofeedback, and aromatherapy (to name a few). The main distinction between OTC drugs and alternative preparations is that OTC drugs have gone through the FDA approval process (most OTC drugs at one time could only be obtained with a prescription before approval). In contrast, alternative preparations do not require FDA approval to be marketed to the public. However, for many OTC drugs, sound research and clinical trials have been conducted, while other alternative preparations have been the subject of exploratory research with inconclusive results. Standardization of clinical trials evaluating possible therapeutic benefits of alternative preparations is complicated by variations in the purity and potency of these products. The term "non-prescription products"[a] will be used when addressing both OTC and

alternative preparations; when using the term "conventional therapy," this chapter is referring to all FDA-approved pharmacotherapy (OTC and prescribed).

Focus will be given to commonly used OTC, and alternative preparation products that (1) have significant interactions with commonly prescribed psychotropic drugs; or (2) have intrinsic, psychoactive properties (either as intended responses or as side-effects). Additionally, strategies to elicit information and work with patients using these therapies will be discussed. It is also important to understand that most persons use alternative preparations combined with conventional therapies; the exclusive use of alternative products alone is rare in the United States (National Institute of Health, 2014) (Box 19.1).

NORM'S NOTES CAM is a hot topic and presents a moving target. It is almost impossible to keep up with the various claims on late-night or early morning television advertisements. Some of these agents or remedies work. As for the others, you can hardly tell what works. Maybe they work for some people and not for others. The author of this chapter has done an excellent job selecting the therapies with some support. Nurses should know about them.

---

[a] Although this chapter uses the term "non-prescription products" for both OTC and alternative preparations, the FDA uses the designation of "non-prescription *drug* products" for OTC drugs only.

Government Regulation

The growing popularity of alternative preparations resulted in the creation by the federal government of the Office of Alternative Medicine (OAM) in 1991. After 3 years, the FDA set the requirement that alternative preparations bear the label that "no proof of efficacy, safety, or standards for quality control can be attributed to these products" (Porter, 1995). This agency was last renamed in 2014 as the "National Center for Complementary and Integrative Health" (NCCIH), in part to reflect its focus on CAM in the broader context of their combined use with conventional therapies known as "integrative medicine." The chief mission of NCCIH is to fund research that will evaluate the safety and efficacy of CAM diagnostic methods and therapies available (including alternative preparations). That means that NCCIH taxpayer dollars will be invested in the more realistic context of a trend where most consumers of alternative preparations use them in conjunction with conventional therapies.

OVER-THE-COUNTER DRUGS

There are over 800 different active ingredients marketed as OTC drug products (U.S. Food and Drug Administration, 2015a), each falling within one or more of 80 categories (e.g., analgesics, antihistamines, expectorants), and some have significant interactions with psychotropic medications (Izzo, 2004).

Cold, Cough, Allergy, Bronchodilator, and Antiasthmatic Drugs

Many of these products contain vasoconstrictors, such as phenylephrine and pseudoephedrine, which have sympathomimetic properties. Users should exercise caution when combining these drugs with MAOI antidepressants and stimulants, such as amphetamine derivatives and methylphenidate, both used for attention-deficit hyperactive disorder (ADHD) (Pray, 2006). Some products that treat these conditions also have sedative properties, notably the antihistamines, which carry a warning against "marked drowsiness" and should not be combined with other sedatives, like benzodiazepines or alcohol.

Nicotine and Nicotine Cessation Products

Nicotine increases clearance of many psychotropic medications, including antipsychotics, tricyclic antidepressants, selective serotonin reuptake inhibitors (SSRIs), serotonin-norepinephrine reuptake inhibitors (SNRIs), benzodiazepines, and methadone. Caution is advised when patients stop using nicotine-containing products, as levels of many of these drugs are expected to rise (NSW Health, 2017). Therefore, the nurse is advised to consult a drug guide anytime a patient taking psychotropics ceases to ingest nicotine-containing products.

Caffeine

Caffeine binds to adenosine receptors in the brain to stimulate alertness and even a sense of well-being through secondary, dopaminergic actions in the prefrontal cortex. It also increases levels of circulating catecholamines, triggering a sympathomimetic reaction akin to a "fight-and-flight" response that includes elevated blood pressure and heart rate (hence the colloquialism "coffee nerves" experienced with high doses of caffeine). Natural sources of caffeine include coffee, tea, and chocolate; mild amounts of caffeine have been added to soda-type beverages for nearly a century. More recently, synthetic caffeine has also been added to a variety of food and beverage products to promote arousal, enhance mood, and boost energy—sometimes to amounts as high as 198 mg per serving (a typical serving of coffee averages 80 mg of caffeine). The use of these products as ergogenic, athletic performance enhancers is also common. Although toxic exposure to caffeine is rare, a U.S. National Poison Data System survey found 1480 cases of toxic exposure to caffeinated, non-alcoholic energy drinks in 1 year, including three cases of seizures, two cases of non-ventricular dysrhythmias, and one case of ventricular dysrhythmia. Caffeine tablets often contain 200 mg of caffeine per tablet, and are marketed as weight loss aids, energy boosters, and cognitive enhancers. Although rare, there are a few largely publicized cases of deaths by caffeine intoxication after excessive ingestions of caffeine that, although verging on the excessive, fall well below the considered lethal dose of 5000 mg. In 2011, a 14-year-old Maryland female with a pre-existing cardiac condition died after ingesting two cans of "Monster" energy drink (an estimated 480 mg of caffeine). In 2017, a 16-year-old South Carolina male died of cardiac arrest after ingesting "one 'latte,' a Mountain Dew, and an 'energy drink,'" which amounts to an estimated 472 mg of caffeine. The FDA stipulates 400 mg/day of caffeine as "generally regarded as safe"; with advised intakes by children limited to 2.5 mg/kg/day, whereas reproductive women should limit their intake to no more than 300 mg daily (200 mg if pregnant). Regular caffeine use produces tolerance and physical dependence. Abrupt discontinuation of regular caffeine often induces a withdrawal syndrome, usually characterized by headaches, drowsiness, fatigue, restlessness, and anxiety, lasting 2 to 7 days.

Omeprazole

Omeprazole (Prilosec) is a proton-pump inhibitor (PPI) available as OTC for short- and long-term therapy of gastroesophageal reflux disease (GERD). Omeprazole has been shown to more than double the half-life of diazepam, an anxiolytic (from a mean of 35.9 to 85 hours) (Gugler & Jensen, 1985). Omeprazole also has been shown to raise concentrations of citalopram (Celexa) and sertraline (Zoloft) by more than one-third, whereas escitalopram (Lexapro) serum levels were almost doubled when taken with omeprazole (Gjestad et al., 2015). Lastly, reductions in plasma levels of the antipsychotic clozapine by concomitant use of omeprazole have been demonstrated (Frick et al., 2003).

Esomeprazole

Esomeprazole (Nexium) is also another PPI available as OTC known to raise the concentrations of citalopram (Celexa) by more than one-third and to double serum levels of escitalopram (Lexapro) (Gjestad et al., 2015).

Nonsteroidal Antiinflammatory Drugs

Evidence from epidemiological studies and clinical cases indicate that the concomitant use of SSRIs and NSAIDs increase the risk of gastric bleeding (Helin-Salmivaara, Huttunen, Grönroos, Klaukka, & Huupponen, 2007). The risk of gastrointestinal bleeding is highly increased for patients with bleeding disorders or those on anticoagulant therapy.

ALTERNATIVE PREPARATIONS

Americans spend about twice as much money on natural product supplements as buying eggs (Nahin et al., 2016). This chapter will focus on the 13 most likely alternative preparations that the nurse will encounter in practice.

Herbal Therapies

Naturally derived products are often viewed as valuable alternatives to what has become known as "traditional" or "Western" pharmacotherapy, which is heavily reliant on synthetic drugs developed, manufactured, and marketed by the pharmaceutical industry. Interestingly, a significant portion of synthetic drugs is derived from natural sources (Newman & Cragg, 2016).

For millennia, man has used herbs and natural preparations to promote well-being and prevent, cure, or alleviate suffering and debilitation. Herbal preparations include plant roots, tree barks, berries, leaves, resins, and flowers. Centuries ago, herbal derivatives were sourced and processed by designated individuals who knew the nature and quantities of their ingredients. In contrast, the origins, quality, composition, and levels of impurities of herbal preparations commercially available today through "mainstream" retailers are often questionable. Contamination of alternative preparations by particles ranging from microbes to heavy metals has been widely reported, with outcomes that include lead poisoning, liver failure, encephalopathy, and death.

Some reasons that Americans choose to use natural products, herbs, and dietary supplements include a desire for empowerment, potential enhancement of conventional medical treatments, a desire to try a novel therapy, a belief that conventional medical treatment will not help, accepting the suggestion of a health care professional to try an alternative therapy, and the costs of conventional medical treatments (Barnes, Bloom, & Nahin, 2008). There is also a widespread notion that health supplements and remedies derived from natural sources will always be better tolerated and less harmful than synthetic derivatives. While this is true in some cases, both types of products act at the same basic level: the molecular level (Fig. 19.1). In many instances, bioactive molecules derived from natural sources are extracted through harsh, unnatural chemical procedures, rendering concentrates that often have bioactive substances in quantities that promote toxicity. While the types and quantities of bioactive molecules in synthetic drugs are known, herbal preparations often have several bioactive components, some of which either have not been identified or have unknown properties.

If one considers the basic molecular mechanism of action of natural health supplements, it becomes clear that understanding the intended effects (and side-effects) of these preparations is as important as understanding the same characteristics of synthetic drugs. There are numerous reports in medical and scientific journals of severe reactions to herbs, including liver failure, renal failure, gastrointestinal tract obstruction, cardiac arrhythmias, seizure exacerbation, development of psychiatric symptoms, and fatalities (Clough et al., 2004) (see Fig. 19.1).

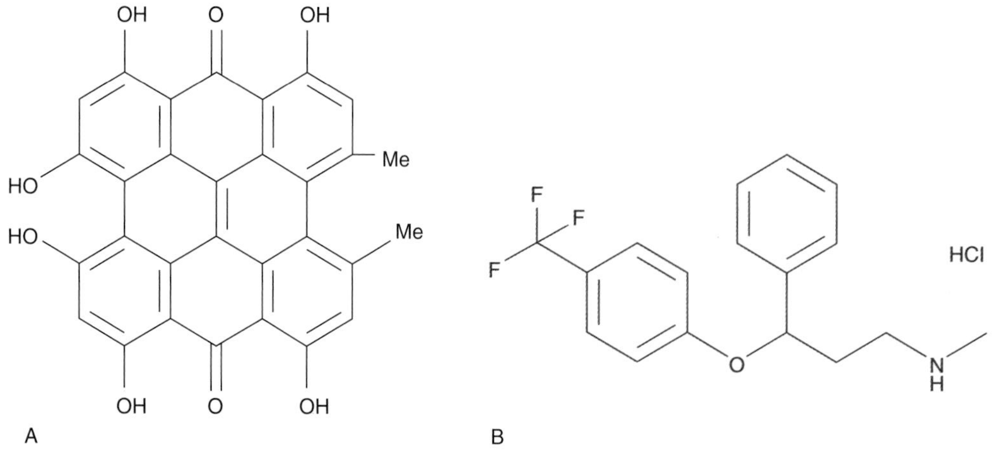

FIG. 19.1 (A) Hypericum, the main bioactive molecule in St. John's wort. (B) Fluoxetine (Prozac).

Understanding drug-drug interactions between natural and synthetic preparations (or even those among different natural preparations) is as important as understanding synthetic drug-drug interactions. Some supplements can decrease or even elevate the effects of certain drugs, potentially causing loss of therapeutic effect or, conversely, producing toxicity just like conventional drug interactions. In this context, most herbal preparations sold are used for mental health–related symptoms, and most people in the United States with self-defined anxiety attacks or severe depression use some form of natural products, herbs, and dietary supplements to treat these conditions. Most users of alternative therapies do not report their use to their health providers; in fact, herbal preparations are often used to augment prescribed psychotropic medications (Parslow & Jorm, 2004).

HERBAL PREPARATIONS TO TREAT ANXIETY AND DEPRESSION

Herbal preparations are among the most frequently tried alternative therapies for depression (Lee & Bae, 2017). Table 19.1 summarizes herbals used for psychiatric symptoms. The use of herbal preparations for mental health–related symptoms is so common that it has been called part of the "hidden mental health network" (Simon et al., 2004).

Interestingly, one study examining preferences for treatment of mental health–related symptoms in the general public did *not* identify treatment with psychotropic medication or even visiting a psychiatrist as the first treatment choice (except in the case of schizophrenia). Instead, alternative therapies or psychotherapy was more likely to be utilized (Riedel-Heller, Matschinger, & Angermeyer, 2005).

St. John's Wort

Primarily used as a treatment for mild-to-moderate depression, St. John's wort *(Hypericum perforatum)* preparations are available as capsules, tea leaves, or tinctures, and are among the top-selling botanical products in the United States. Two recent meta-analyses investigating the effectiveness of St. John's wort for depression found that it might be as efficacious as and better tolerated than conventional antidepressants for mild depression (Haller, Anheyer, Cramer, & Dobos, 2019; Ng, Venkatanarayanan, & Ho, 2017). St. John's wort is also commonly used to treat seasonal affective disorder, sleep disorders, anxiety disorders, and even ADHD. However, evidence of the efficacy of St. John's wort for these conditions is still lacking (Sarris, 2013). The precise mechanism of action of St. John's wort is still a matter of scrutiny and debate; however, most accept that a broad range of different, biologically active components present in the plant act synergistically on different brain neurotransmitter systems to produce its antidepressant effects (Schmidt & Butterweck, 2015). However, there have been case reports of St. John's wort exacerbating mania and increasing the risk for serotonin syndrome; thus, it should not be taken with other antidepressants, particularly SSRIs.

TABLE 19.1   Herbals Used for Psychiatric Symptoms

Herbal Product	Contraindications	Adverse Side Effects	Drug Interactions
Angelica	Diabetes Peptic ulcer disease Bleeding disorders Pregnancy Breast-feeding	CV: Decreased BP GI: Anorexia, flatulence, spasms, dyspepsia Integumentary: Photosensitivity, phototoxicity, dermatitis	Increased PTT with anticoagulants
Chamomile	Known abortifacient Cross-sensitivity to sunflowers, ragweed, and members of aster family *(Echinacea)*	Hypersensitivity—allergic reactions Burning of face, mouth, eyes, and mucous membranes	Anticoagulants Increases effects of CNS drugs
Ginkgo biloba	Pregnancy Breast-feeding Peptic ulcer disease and other bleeding problems	Headache, anxiety, restlessness	Trazodone
Kava *(Piper methysticum)*	Hepatotoxicity (?) Liver failure (?)	Scaling, yellowing of skin Overdose	Antiparkinsonian agents Benzodiazepines CNS depressants More data needed
Melatonin			
St. John's wort *(Hypericum perforatum)*	Pregnancy Breast-feeding	Dizziness, insomnia, restlessness, constipation, abdominal cramps, photosensitivity	Protease inhibitors Olanzapine (Zyprexa) Oral contraceptives
Valerian *(Valeriana officinalis)*	Pregnancy Breast-feeding	Dependence	MAOIs, Warfarin, Phenytoin

BP, Blood pressure; *CNS*, central nervous system; *CV*, cardiovascular; *GI*, gastrointestinal; *MAOIs*, monoamine oxidase inhibitors; *PTT*, prothrombin time.
From Keltner, N., & Folks, D. (2005). *Drugs used in alternative and complementary medicine.* Mosby.

S-Adenosyl-L-methionine

Introduced in the United States as a dietary supplement in 1999, *S*-Adenosyl-*L*-methionine (SAM-e) is widely used in Europe and Canada; in fact, it is available as a prescription drug in Germany. SAM-e is an endogenous molecule essential for the functioning of over 100 metabolic reactions within cells (Cheng & Blumenthal, 1999), including the synthesis of folate, which in turn is a metabolic component for the synthesis of the neurotransmitters norepinephrine, serotonin, and dopamine. Numerous clinical trials investigated the alleged antidepressant properties of Sam-e starting in the early 1970s; however, results have been complicated by inadequate sample size, methodological disparities, and bias. Best results were achieved with parenteral formulations, and although the effectiveness of SAM-e as an oral antidepressant is still unclear, it shows promise as monotherapy or adjuvant to antidepressant treatment (Cuomo et al., 2020). SAM-e is considered safe, with no evidence of hepatotoxicity and serious side effects. Most importantly, a double-blind, randomized clinical trial demonstrated SAM-e to be safe when used with SSRIs (Papakostas, Mischoulon, Shyu, Alpert, & Fava, 2010); however, caution is advised when SAM-e is used in combination with MAOIs due to the risk of serotonin syndrome.

Kava

Kava is a root derivative from a subspecies of the pepper plant *(Piper methysticum)*; it is ubiquitous to many Pacific Islands and prized for its purported "ability to soothe the worried mind." It is widely incorporated into traditional religious and social ceremonies of those cultures. Although 15 different bioactive pyrone molecules have been identified in the kava plant (Sarris, Panossian, Schweitzer, Stough, & Scholey, 2011), their precise mechanism of action is not entirely understood. There is, however, an indication that kava, like benzodiazepines, acts upon GABA receptors to enhance their intrinsic activity. Evidence suggestive of the efficacy of kava in treating anxiety has been broadly documented; for example, a meta-analysis of randomized clinical trials found kava to have anxiolytic properties that were significantly higher than placebo in 10 out of 11 studies reviewed (Pittler & Ernst, 2003). Comparable results were found in another meta-analysis looking at six randomized clinical trials that evaluated the anxiolytic properties of kava in non-psychotic anxiety disorders (Witte et al., 2005). Finally, a more recent systematic review concluded that, although promising, current evidence is insufficient to determine the efficacy of kava in the treatment of anxiety disorders (Ooi, Henderson, & Pak, 2018).

However, there have been reports of severe hepatotoxicity caused by concentrated kava extracts manufactured in Germany and Switzerland (Rakel, 2017) and from traditional beverages prepared at Pacific Island locations, with some patients needing liver transplantations and even dying. These unfortunate events ultimately caused the retraction of kava-containing products from the market by regulatory authorities in Germany, Canada, Switzerland, and France (kava preparations are still available in the United States). Although those often represent extreme cases resulting from excessive consumption, prior history of liver failure, concomitant use of hepatotoxic drugs, or contamination of preparations (Christl et al., 2009), kava should be used with caution. Liver tests should be performed on those using it daily, and it should not be used daily for more than 4 months (Rakel, 2017). Individuals with liver problems, those who use medications extensively metabolized by the liver, and persons who consume alcohol daily should not use kava preparations (Blumenthal, Brinckmann, & Wollschlaeger, 2003). Patients using kava should also be warned about signs and symptoms of hepatotoxicity, such as jaundice, malaise, and nausea.

Clinical Example

Sherry S., a 26-year-old African American woman, was admitted to the psychiatric unit for depression with psychotic features. Sherry received a 1-mg injection of lorazepam (Ativan) in the emergency department. On admission to the unit, Sherry was noted to have slurred speech, poor coordination, and slow responses. Sherry has not been on any scheduled or prescribed medications, but the nurse found a bottle of kava among Sherry's belongings. Sherry's excessive reaction to the lorazepam was most likely due to her concomitant use of the herbal preparation kava.

Valerian

More than 250 different species of valerian are native to Europe and Asia. The variety used for anxiety comes from the plant *Valeriana officinalis*. Considerable difference exists in the potency of valerian, depending on the manufacturing process. Most studies evaluating the therapeutic properties of valerian have focused on the treatment of sleep disturbances; it is effective in decreasing sleep latency, nocturnal awakening, and promoting a subjective sense of "good sleep" (Beaubrun & Gray, 2000). Another study compared the sedative properties of valerian, triazolam, temazepam, and diphenhydramine, with valerian providing sedation equivalent to that of the other drugs studied, with a slightly better side effect profile (Glass et al., 2003). Fewer studies exist that evaluate the use of valerian to treat anxiety disorders, with mixed results reported. In fact, a rigorous, systematic review of available studies found just one well-designed randomized clinical trial, with no evidence supporting anxiolytic properties of valerian (Miyasaka et al., 2006). One study where valerian was used in combination with St. John's wort found the combination superior to placebo and comparable to diazepam (Panijel, 1985) for treating anxiety. Like kava, valerian appears to exert sedative effects via modulation of GABA receptor activity (a property shared with benzodiazepines). Valerian is not effective for short-term treatment of anxiety and insomnia, as it may take several weeks for it to become effective (Rakel, 2017).

Chamomile

Several therapeutic properties have been attributed to chamomile, including sedation and anxiolysis. Although there is no firmly established scientific evidence supporting these claims, one randomized clinical trial found chamomile to significantly reduce moderate-to-severe symptoms of generalized anxiety disorder (GAD) (Mao et al., 2016). Another open-label, randomized control trial using chamomile extracts for treatment of GAD found anxiolytic responses significantly greater than placebo treatment lasting for up to 8 weeks (Keefe et al., 2016). Interestingly, isolated bioactive components of chamomile have been found to produce arterial vasodilation, which may explain the sedative properties commonly attributed to chamomile (Roberts et al., 2013).

Angelica

Several studies have attributed neuroprotective properties to angelica derivatives via antiapoptotic, antioxidative, and anti-inflammatory mechanisms (Sowndhararajan & Kim, 2017), indicating a promising role of angelica preparations in the treatment of neurodegenerative disorders. Angelica has also been shown to cause significant muscle relaxation without changes in the level of consciousness. Studies on the use of angelica for anxiety disorders remain insufficient, but it remains a promising anxiolytic herb for treating anxiety because of its potential to facilitate relaxation without impairing cognition and motor behavior. In laboratory testing, angelica essential oils decreased aggressive behavior and increased social interaction in mice (Min et al., 2005). There is insufficient evidence of efficacy and safety for the use of angelica at present.

Cannabidiol

With the enacting of the latest Farm Bill by the U.S. Congress in 2018, the production and sale of cannabidiol (CBD) from industrial hemp were legalized at the federal level. The legislation has resulted in a true explosion of sales of CBD products, fueled by marketing claims touting near-miraculous effects on conditions ranging from chronic pain, anxiety, sleep, and stress relief (to name a few). Also, public interest and research effort evaluating the properties, safety, and potential uses of CBD have increased significantly.

The human endocannabinoid system plays an important, regulatory role at virtually all organs and systems, mediating processes such as immunity, inflammation, response to anxiety and stress, digestion, and overall homeostasis (VanDolah, Bauer, & Mauck, 2019).

CBD is a non-psychoactive derivative of the *cannabis* plant with modulatory human endocannabinoid system components. It is now widely available for sale in many states (primarily as oil preparations meant to be ingested sublingually, but also as edibles and even inhalants). CBD is the most abundant cannabinoid found in the *cannabis* plant (there are over one hundred other cannabinoids also present), and in its pure form, it lacks the psychoactive properties of the *marijuana* plant. Although CBD oil (marketed under the tradename of Epidolex) has been granted FDA approval for use as adjunct treatment of a rare, severe form of epilepsy, this will not be the focus of this chapter, as most consumers use CBD to treat anxiety, stress, and sleep problems (Moltke & Hindocha, 2021).

Human laboratory studies and clinical trials have been conducted for conditions that include epilepsy, anxiety, pain and inflammation, schizophrenia, substance use disorders, posttraumatic stress disorder (among others). Evidence of efficacy for any conditions other than epilepsy has not yet been demonstrated (Sholler et al., 2020).

With respect to safety, clinical trials have reported adverse effects that include diarrhea, somnolence, decreased appetite, and vomiting (Huestis et al., 2019). Moreover, CBD caused the elevation of certain liver enzymes in a significant portion of participants in CBD clinical trials, suggesting potential for hepatotoxicity (Lattanzi et al., 2020). Caution is advised to persons using CBD with pre-existing hepatic conditions or using drugs and substances known to increase the risk of hepatotoxicity.

Finally, CBD alters the function of several CYP-450 liver metabolizing enzymes and is a substrate of the CYP2C9 and CYP3A4 subsets. Data from *in vivo* studies demonstrated that CBD increases plasma concentrations of CYP2C substrates (e.g., diazepam), including a threefold increase in levels of the anticonvulsant clobazam and increased hepatotoxicity with decreased clearance of valproic acid (Vázquez, García-Carnelli, Maldonado, & Fagiolino, 2021).

As of the writing of this chapter, a significant portion of the aspects of CBD production and commerce regulation remain at the state level (case in point: there are still four states where the sale and use of CBD are banned, despite broader legalization at the federal level). Caution is also advised as reports of patients taking CBD and testing positive for THC (the psychoactive ingredient of *marijuana*) have occurred (Bonn-Miller et al., 2017). As with any alternative preparations mentioned, there is wide variation in potency, purity, and levels of contaminants among CBD-based products available. Lastly, prices of CBD products stand among the highest among all alternative preparations—an expense hardly justifiable considering its unproven effectiveness as an alternative therapy and potential for adverse reactions.

HERBAL PREPARATIONS FOR MEMORY AND DEMENTIA

Ginkgo

Ginkgo biloba is another top-selling herbal preparation in the United States. It has been the subject of at least 18 clinical trials evaluating the effects of EGb-761 (its bioactive derivative product) in cognition and memory (Nash & Shah, 2015). Many of these studies focused on potential therapeutic uses in Alzheimer's disease. Evidence gathered indicates that a daily regimen of 240 mg of EGb-761 may be efficacious in stabilizing or slowing cognitive decline in persons with dementia (Gavrilova et al., 2014). In 2018, nine countries, including China, Germany, and Singapore, published guidelines for treating dementia and mild cognitive impairment using EGb-761 (Kandiah, Ong, Ng, Mamun, & Reshma, 2019). Concerns about the safety of ginkgo were raised when it induced tumors in animal models (National Toxicology Program, 2013; Rider et al., 2014) and when a higher incidence of colon and breast cancer among trial participants receiving ginkgo derivatives (Biggs et al., 2010) was demonstrated.

Additionally, a study involving a large Veterans Administration population found an increased risk of adverse bleeding events when warfarin is taken in conjunction with ginkgo (Stoddard et al., 2015). Due to ginkgo's anticoagulant properties (Chung et al., 1987), caution should be advised when taking ginkgo with other drugs sharing anticoagulant properties (Mahady, 2002). Increased levels of omeprazole clearance were observed when taken with ginkgo derivatives (Yin, Tomlinson, Waye, Chow, & Chow, 2004). Ginkgo has antihypertensive properties, and caution should be exerted when combining ginkgo with antihypertensive drugs. Finally, increased clearance of insulin and oral hypoglycemics by ginkgo has been demonstrated (Kudolo, 2001), potentially raising blood sugar levels, particularly among diabetics taking insulin or oral hypoglycemics.

VITAMIN, MINERAL, AND NUTRITIONAL SUPPLEMENT THERAPIES

Melatonin

Lack of synchronicity between the circadian clock and the external environment increases the risk of metabolic disturbances, cardiac disease, cancer, psychiatric disorders (Baron & Reid, 2014), and "circadian rhythm sleep-wake disorders" (Williams, McLin, Dressman, & Neubauer, 2016). For example, epidemiological studies have shown increased breast cancer rates among night-shift nurses (Davis & Mirick, 2006). Melatonin is an endogenous biomolecule that has been implicated in regulating the circadian rhythm of sleep (Gandhi et al., 2015); it is also a potent antioxidant (Tan, Manchester, Esteban-Zubero, Zhou, & Reiter, 2015). As an exogenous supplement, melatonin has been postulated to promote sleep by re-synchronizing the circadian clock (Arendt, 2003), with evidence suggesting that melatonin reduces sleep onset latency, duration, and quality, and the number of nocturnal awakenings. Melatonin supplements have also been demonstrated to be safe, well-tolerated, and non-habit forming (Geoffroy, Etain, Franchi, Bellivier, & Ritter, 2015).

Vitamins C and E

Evidence suggests that supplementation of combined vitamins C and E is associated with reduced risks of cognitive decline (Basambombo et al., 2017) and might even benefit patients at risk of Alzheimer's-type dementia development (Zandi et al., 2004).

Vitamin D

Vitamin D deficiency has been associated with depression. Clinical studies have demonstrated reduced risks of depression in persons with high vitamin D levels (Callegari et al., 2016). Evidence suggests that vitamin D supplementation alleviates symptoms of depression (Murphy & Wagner, 2008).

Folate

Folate deficiency has been correlated with the risk of the development of depressive disorders. Studies have shown that augmentation with a folate supplement increases medication response in both treatment-naïve and treatment-resistant depressed patients regardless of whether they have folate deficiency (Owen, 2013).

Niacin (Vitamin B$_3$)

Niacin (vitamin B$_3$, also known as nicotinic acid) is present in meat, poultry, fish, enriched and whole-grain bread, and fortified cereals. Niacin deficiency is rare, primarily found in persons with severe dietary deficiencies, malabsorption syndromes, those receiving dialysis and high intake of corn-derived products, and human immunodeficiency virus (HIV) (Murray et al., 2001). Neurologic manifestations of niacin deficiency include headache, insomnia, depression, loss of memory, psychosis, and coma (Polavarapu & Hasbani, 2017).

Pyridoxine (Vitamin B$_6$)

Pyridoxine (vitamin B$_6$) is found in fortified cereals, beans, poultry, meat, fish, and some fruits and vegetables, with deficiencies usually restricted to malnourished elderly and alcoholics (Pray, 2006). Pyridoxine is essential for the proper function of the nervous system, and deficiencies have been linked to neuropathies (Ghavanini & Kimpinski, 2014) and the onset of seizures (Lee et al., 2015). Supplementation must be done carefully, as excessive levels may cause sensory neuropathy and ataxia (Ghavanini & Kimpinski, 2014).

Cyanocobalamin (Vitamin B$_{12}$)

Cyanocobalamin is found in animal-derived foods, putting vegetarians and their breast-fed infants at risk for deficiencies; persons with specific malabsorption syndromes are also at risk. Neurologic manifestations of vitamin B$_{12}$ deficiency include paresthesias, loss of balance, depression, confusion, and psychosis (Healthon, Savage, Brust, Garrett, & Lindebaum, 1991; Lindebaum et al., 1988). Both parenteral cyanocobalamin treatment and high-dose oral vitamin B$_{12}$ treatment (1000 to 2000 µg daily) are effective therapies (Stabler, 2013).

Omega-3 Fatty Acids

Omega-3 fatty acids belong to the highly unsaturated fatty acids (HUFAs), abundantly found in neuronal membrane phospholipids; these are not synthesized by humans and must come from dietary sources or supplementation, such as fish oil and flaxseed oil (Bozzatello, Brignolo, De Grandi, & Bellino, 2016). Omega-3 fatty acid supplementation has been shown to alter the composition and biochemical properties of neuronal membranes and synapses (Garland & Hallahan, 2006; Ross, Seguin, & Sieswerda, 2007). These phenomena provided a biochemical, theoretical foundation for clinical trials involving omega-3 fatty-acid supplementation for psychiatric disorders, including schizophrenia, depression, bipolar disorder, obsessive-compulsive disorder, ADHD, autism spectrum disorders, borderline personality disorder, aggression, and substance use disorders. A meta-analysis of these trials found modest, positive results for depression, schizophrenia, ADHD, autism, and substance use disorders (Bozzatello, Brignolo, De Grandi, & Bellino, 2016); however, these were inconclusive and often contradictory when compared to their counterpart trial results, with the best and most consistent evidence pointing to the utility of omega-3 fatty acid in bipolar disorder of the predominantly depressed type. Omega-3 fatty acids are considered safe and well tolerated.

Obtaining and Delivering Information

One study revealed that 16% of prescription medication users also took at least one herb or supplement (Kaufman et al., 2002), with older adults as the largest consumers of non-prescription products (Qato et al., 2008). The rate of alternative preparations used by patients is significantly underestimated by healthcare providers, with one study showing less than 3 out of 10 patients disclosing their use of alternative preparations to their providers (Robinson & McGrail, 2004). Sometimes a dose adjustment of a prescribed medication needs to be made based on concomitant use of a non-prescribed product; alternatively, a non-prescription product may need to be discontinued for prescribed medication to be fully effective. Although it is not within the nurse's scope of practice to adjust prescribed medication dosages and schedules, they must safeguard patients against harm by promptly informing the primary provider of possible pharmacological interactions between conventional and alternative agents.

From the perspective of patients, the main reasons for nondisclosures are usually centered on a perception that the practitioner is disinterested or the expectation of a negative response from the provider, with disinterest or even hostility, should patients disclose their use of alternative treatments. Patients may also have preconceived notions that alternative therapies do not interfere with conventional treatments.

From the provider side, it appears that an antagonistic attitude towards alternative therapies, poor awareness of their use by their patients, and minimal proactivity towards collecting that information are the main contributors to nondisclosure.

Given these realities, the nurse must be proactive in eliciting that information; they must do so with a sense of respect, openness, and interest. The nurse need not be a content expert; however, more awareness of the different modalities of alternative treatments usually translates into less nondisclosure.

GENERAL CONCERNS REGARDING HERBS AND SUPPLEMENTS

Safety and Efficacy of Alternative Preparations

Among manufacturers, there is significant variability between sourcing of raw materials, extraction, processing, and formulation of herbal derivatives, causing substantial differences in potency and levels of impurities of these products (sometimes even within the same brand marketed). The American Herbal Products Association and the American Botanical Council are serious, reputable institutions focusing on promoting the responsible use of herbal medicine, and they have attempted to regulate these products. Unfortunately, these organizations simply do not have the resources and authority necessary to regulate this industry adequately. For example, every month, the FDA issues an average of six warning letters to manufacturers of alternative products for violations ranging from adulterated products, false claims, manufacturing irregularities, and improper labeling (in February of 2021 alone, a total of ten such communications were issued). Moreover, a statement released in 2019 by the FDA commissioner announced steps towards ensuring that (a) products are safe and adequately labeled, (b) the public is promptly informed of infractions by manufacturers, sellers, and marketers of alternative preparations, and (c) enforcement of rules on bad actors is expedited and rigorously enforced. Also, some non-profit, private entities were created to ensure the purity, potency, and identity of alternative preparations. For example, the United States Pharmacopeia (USP) supports a program whereby companies submit their products for testing and, if the product meets their standards, a "USP" seal of approval is allowed on the product's label. A list of over 100 products can be found at their website http://www.quality-supplements.org/). NSF International, a company renowned for protecting consumers via rigorous testing of various manufactured products, has a division that tests dietary supplements (http://www.nsf.org/services/by-industry/dietary-supplements/) to assure consumers of the safety and quality of these products. ConsumerLab.com is another reputable private company whose mission is "to identify the best quality health and nutritional products through independent testing," where members can access a database of over 1000 tested products (http://www.consumerlab.com/). It is important to remember that quality assurance does not equate to safety, as some alternative products may cause harm or produce untoward reactions with other drugs solely by virtue of their natural, inherent properties (Box 19.2).

BOX 19.2 General Precautions for Consumers and Health Care Professionals Regarding Herbals

- Avoid products with multiple herbs. Check the active and inactive ingredients for possible combinations and additives.
- Avoid imported herbs because of differences in dose effects.
- Buy only from reputable, established companies and with the *United States Pharmacopeia* (USP) or the NSF seal of approval.
- Always inform the health care provider of any use of herbal products, including topicals and any complementary health practices used.
- Health care providers need a full picture of what is done to manage health; communication can be facilitated by using the NCCIH, Time to Talk campaign tips (available at https://nccih.nih.gov/news/multimedia/gallery/asktell.htm).
- Discontinue if any unusual side effects occur and report negative side effects or adverse reactions to the FDA at www.fda.gov/medwatch, or call 1-800-332-1088.
- Avoid herbals during pregnancy, when attempting to get pregnant and during breastfeeding.
- Avoid self-medicating with herbals before a medical illness has been ruled out.

❓ CRITICAL THINKING QUESTION

1. What are the implications for patients who self-medicate with over-the-counter drugs? Are there any dangers? What are the possible benefits?

FUTURE DIRECTIONS OF INTEGRATIVE HEALTH CARE

The creation of the National Center for Complementary and Integrative Health by the U.S. National Institutes of Health in 2014 sends a clear signal that alternative therapies have become a significant component of the American healthcare model and that removing that alternative from over 50 million consumers in the United States is simply not feasible. Although much remains to be accomplished to ensure the safety of alternative preparations, significant progress has been made, with both the government and private enterprises providing valuable resources for regulation, education, research, and quality assurance of these products; however, improvements have been modest at best. Continued improvement will likely only come through drastic changes and investment in regulation, standardization, and funding for research and education concerning alternative preparations. Moreover, the pooling of resources into collaborative partnerships based on equivalent representation and mutual respect between the fields of botanical and conventional medicine needs to be established. Also, partnerships between educational institutions and the reputable segments of the private sector already doing a valuable job with researching, testing, and endorsing alternative products should maximize efficiency in achieving these integrative goals. These efforts take considerable time and resources; some matters, though, are of extreme urgency. Since over 50 million people regularly consume unregulated therapeutic products offered by what many consider to be a "runaway industry," the FDA will have to extend its arm for a firmer grasp on the alternative preparation industry to fulfill its mission to protect public health by assuring safety, helping speed innovations to get science-based information to use these medicines. Lastly, greater emphasis and a broader introduction of integrative medicine as part of the curricula of the schools of health professions should promote a more realistic view of the variables that inform medical care, thus generating more efficient and cost-effective treatment plans.

NORM'S NOTES The use of alternative and complementary therapies is widespread and still growing. Traditional medicine has been unable to meet the needs of a public that believes good health is a right. The statistical table of the prevalence of mental disorders in Chapter 2 and all psychopathology chapters reflects data that have not changed much for about 30 years. However, during that time, many new, supposedly wonderful medications were discovered. The conventional psychotropic drug industry is a multibillion-dollar concern, but the actual number of people with a drug-treatable disorder has increased. Consequently, many Americans now look outside the traditional psychiatric drug manufacturing complex to see whether they can "fix" themselves. The alternative and complementary approach to mental health care derives, in part, from this disillusionment and disappointment.

REFERENCES

Arendt, J. (2003). Importance and relevance of melatonin to human biological rhythms. *Journal of Neuroendocrinology, 15*(4), 427–431. https://doi.org/10.1046/j.1365-2826.2003.00987.x.

Barnes, P. M., Bloom, B., & Nahin, R. L. (2008). Complementary and alternative medicine use among adults and children: United States, 2007. *National Health Statistics Reports, (12)*, 1–23.

Baron, K. G., & Reid, K. J. (2014). Circadian misalignment and health. *International Review of psychiatry (Abingdon, England), 26*(2), 139–154. https://doi.org/10.3109/09540261.2014.911149.

Basambombo, L. L., Carmichael, P. H., Côté, S., & Laurin, D. (2017). Use of Vitamin E and C supplements for the prevention of cognitive decline. *The Annals of Pharmacotherapy, 51*(2), 118–124. https://doi.org/10.1177/1060028016673072.

Beaubrun, G., & Gray, E. (2000). A review of herbal medicines for psychiatric disorders. *Psychiatric Services, 51*(9), 1130–1134.

Biggs, M. L., Sorkin, B. C., Nahin, R. L., Kuller, L. H., & Fitzpatrick, A. L. (2010). Ginkgo biloba and risk of cancer: Secondary analysis of the Ginkgo Evaluation of Memory (GEM) Study. *Pharmacoepidemiology and Drug Safety, 19*(7), 694–698. https://doi.org/10.1002/pds.1979.

Blumenthal, M., Brinckmann, J., & Wollschlaeger, B. (2003). *The ABC clinical guide to herbs.* American Botanical Council.

Bonn-Miller, M.O., Loflin, M.J.E., Thomas, B.F., Marcu, J.P., Hyke, T., & Vandrey, R. (2017). Labeling accuracy of cannabidiol extracts sold online. *The Journal of the American Medical Association, 318*(17), 1708–1709. https://www.ncbi.nlm.nih.gov/pmc/articles/PMC5818782/.

Bozzatello, P., Brignolo, E., De Grandi, E., & Bellino, S. (2016). Supplementation with omega-3 fatty acids in psychiatric disorders: A review of literature data. *Journal of Clinical Medicine, 5*(8), 67. https://doi.org/10.3390/jcm5080067.

Callegari, E. T., Reavley, N., Gorelik, A., Garland, S. M., Wark, J. D., & Safe-D study team (2017). Serum 25-hydroxyvitamin D and mental health in young Australian women: Results from the Safe-D study. *Journal of Affective Disorders, 224*, 48–55. https://doi.org/10.1016/j.jad.2016.10.002.

Cheng, X., & Blumenthal, R. (1999). *S-Adenosylmethionine-Dependent Methyltransferases.* https://doi.org/10.1142/4098.

Christl, S. U., Seifert, A., & Seeler, D. (2009). Toxic hepatitis after consumption of traditional kava preparation. *Journal of Travel Medicine, 16*(1), 55–56. https://doi.org/10.1111/j.1708-8305.2008.00259.x.

Chung, K. F., Dent, G., McCusker, M., Guinot, P., Page, C. P., & Barnes, P. J. (1987). Effect of a ginkgolide mixture (BN 52063) in antagonising skin and platelet responses to platelet activating factor in man. *Lancet, 1*(8527), 248–251. https://doi.org/10.1016/s0140-6736(87)90066-3.

Clough, A. R., Rowley, K., & O'Dea, K. (2004). Kava use, dyslipidaemia and biomarkers of dietary quality in Aboriginal people in Arnhem Land in the Northern Territory (NT), Australia. *European Journal of Clinical Nutrition*, 58(7), 1090–1093. https://doi.org/10.1038/sj.ejcn.1601921.

Cuomo, A., Crescenzi, B., Bolognesi, S., Goracci, A., Koukouna, D., Rossi, R., & Fagiolini, A. (2020). S-Adenosylmethionine (SAMe) in major depressive disorder (MDD): A clinician-oriented systematic review. *Annals of General Psychiatry*, 19, 50. https://www.ncbi.nlm.nih.gov/pmc/articles/PMC7487540/.

Davis, S., & Mirick, D. K. (2006). Circadian disruption, shift work and the risk of cancer: A summary of the evidence and studies in Seattle. *Cancer Causes & Control: CCC*, 17(4), 539–545. https://doi.org/10.1007/s10552-005-9010-9.

Frick, A., Kopitz, J., & Bergemann, N. (2003). Omeprazole reduces clozapine plasma concentrations. A case report. *Pharmacopsychiatry*, 36(3), 121–123. https://doi.org/10.1055/s-2003-39980.

Gandhi, A. V., Mosser, E. A., Oikonomou, G., & Prober, D. A. (2015). Melatonin is required for the circadian regulation of sleep. *Neuron*, 85(6), 1193–1199. https://doi.org/10.1016/j.neuron.2015.02.016.

Garland, M. R., & Hallahan, B. (2006). Essential fatty acids and their role in conditions characterised by impulsivity. *International Review of Psychiatry*, 18(2), 99–105. https://doi.org/10.1080/09540260600582009.

Gavrilova, S. I., Preuss, U. W., Wong, J. W., Hoerr, R., Kaschel, R., Bachinskaya, N., & GIMCIPlus Study Group (2014). Efficacy and safety of Ginkgo biloba extract EGb 761 in mild cognitive impairment with neuropsychiatric symptoms: A randomized, placebo-controlled, double-blind, multi-center trial. *International Journal of Geriatric Psychiatry*, 29(10), 1087–1095. https://doi.org/10.1002/gps.4103.

Geoffroy, P. A., Etain, B., Franchi, J. A., Bellivier, F., & Ritter, P. (2015). Melatonin and melatonin agonists as adjunctive treatments in bipolar disorders. *Current Pharmaceutical Design*, 21(23), 3352–3358. https://doi.org/10.2174/1381612821666150619093448.

Ghavanini, A. A., & Kimpinski, K. (2014). Revisiting the evidence for neuropathy caused by pyridoxine deficiency and excess. *Journal of Clinical Neuromuscular Disease*, 16(1), 25–31. https://doi.org/10.1097/CND.0000000000000049.

Gjestad, C., Westin, A. A., Skogvoll, E., & Spigset, O. (2015). Effect of proton pump inhibitors on the serum concentrations of the selective serotonin reuptake inhibitors citalopram, escitalopram, and sertraline. *Therapeutic Drug Monitoring*, 37(1), 90–97. https://doi.org/10.1097/FTD.0000000000000101.

Glass, J. R., Sproule, B. A., Herrmann, N., Streiner, D., & Busto, U. E. (2003). Acute pharmacological effects of temazepam, diphenhydramine, and valerian in healthy elderly subjects. *Journal of Clinical Psychopharmacology*, 23(3), 260–268. https://doi.org/10.1097/01.jcp.0000084033.22282.b6.

Gugler, R., & Jensen, J. C. (1985). Omeprazole inhibits oxidative drug metabolism. Studies with diazepam and phenytoin in vivo and 7-ethoxycoumarin in vitro. *Gastroenterology*, 89(6), 1235–1241.

Haller, H., Anheyer, D., Cramer, H., & Dobos, G. (2019). Complementary therapies for clinical depression: An overview of systematic reviews. *British Medical Journal*, 9(8), e028527. https://doi.org/10.1136/bmjopen-2018-028527.

Helin-Salmivaara, A., Huttunen, T., Grönroos, J. M., Klaukka, T., & Huupponen, R. (2007). Risk of serious upper gastrointestinal events with concurrent use of NSAIDs and SSRIs: A case-control study in the general population. *European Journal of Clinical Pharmacology*, 63(4), 403–408. https://doi.org/10.1007/s00228-007-0263-y.

Huestis, M., Solimini, R., Pichini, S., Pacifici, R., Carlier, J., & Busardò, F. (2019). Cannabidiol adverse effects and toxicity. *Current Neuropharmacology*, 17(10), 974–989. https://www.ncbi.nlm.nih.gov/pmc/articles/PMC7052834/.

Izzo, A. A. (2004). Drug interactions with St. John's Wort (Hypericum perforatum): A review of the clinical evidence. *International Journal of Clinical Pharmacology and Therapeutics*, 42(3), 139–148. https://doi.org/10.5414/cpp42139.

Kandiah, N., Ong, P., Ng, L., Mamun, K., & Reshma, A. (2019). Treatment of dementia and mild cognitive impairment with or without cerebrovascular disease: Expert consensus on the use of *Ginkgo biloba* extract, EGb-761. *CNS Neuroscience & Therapeutics*, 25(2), 288–298. https://www.ncbi.nlm.nih.gov/pmc/articles/PMC6488894/.

Kaufman, D. W., Kelly, J. P., Rosenberg, L., Anderson, T. E., & Mitchell, A. A. (2002). Recent patterns of medication use in the ambulatory adult population of the United States: The Slone survey. *The Journal of the American Medical Association*, 287(3), 337–344. https://doi.org/10.1001/jama.287.3.337.

Keefe, J. R., Mao, J. J., Soeller, I., Li, Q. S., & Amsterdam, J. D. (2016). Short-term open-label chamomile (Matricaria chamomilla L.) therapy of moderate to severe generalized anxiety disorder. *Phytomedicine: International Journal of Phytotherapy and Phytopharmacology*, 23(14), 1699–1705. https://doi.org/10.1016/j.phymed.2016.10.013.

Kudolo, G. B. (2001). The effect of 3-month ingestion of Ginkgo biloba extract (EGb 761) on pancreatic beta-cell function in response to glucose loading in individuals with non-insulin-dependent diabetes mellitus. *Journal of Clinical Pharmacology*, 41(6), 600–611. https://doi.org/10.1177/00912700122010483.

Lattanzi, S., Brigo, F., Trinka, E., Zaccara, G., Striano, P., Del Giovane, C., & Silvestrini, M. (2020). Adjunctive cannabidiol in patients with Dravet Syndrome: A systematic review and meta-analysis of efficacy and safety. *CNS Drugs*, 34(3), 229–241. https://doi.org/10.1007/s40263-020-00708-6.

Lee, G., & Bae, H. (2017). Therapeutic effects of phytochemicals and medicinal herbs on depression. *BioMed Research International*, April, 6596241. https://doi.org/10.1155/2017/6596241.

Mahady. G. B. (2002). Ginkgo biloba for the prevention and treatment of cardiovascular disease: A review of the literature. *The Journal of Cardiovascular Nursing*, 16(4), 21–32. https://doi.org/10.1097/00005082-200207000-00004.

Mao, J. J., Xie, S. X., Keefe, J. R., Soeller, I., Li, Q. S., & Amsterdam, J. D. (2016). Long-term chamomile (Matricaria chamomilla L.) treatment for generalized anxiety disorder: A randomized clinical trial. *Phytomedicine: International Journal of Phytotherapy and Phytopharmacology*, 23(14), 1735–1742. https://doi.org/10.1016/j.phymed.2016.10.012.

Min, L., Chen, S. W., Li, W. J., Wang, R., Li, Y. L., Wang, W. J., & Mi, X. J. (2005). The effects of angelica essential oil in social interaction and hole-board tests. *Pharmacology, Biochemistry, and Behavior*, 81(4), 838–842. https://doi.org/10.1016/j.pbb.2005.05.015.

Miyasaka, L. S., Atallah, A. N., & Soares, B. G. (2006). Valerian for anxiety disorders. *The Cochrane Database of Systematic Reviews*, 4, CD004515. https://doi.org/10.1002/14651858.CD004515.pub2.

Moltke, J., & Hindocha, C. (2021). Reasons for cannabidiol use: A cross-sectional study of CBD users, focusing on self-perceived stress, anxiety, and sleep problems. *Journal of Cannabis Research, 3*(1), 5. https://doi.org/10.1186/s42238-021-00061-5.

Murphy, P. K., & Wagner, C. L. (2008). Vitamin D and mood disorders among women: An integrative review. *Journal of Midwifery & Women's Health, 53*(5), 440–446. https://doi.org/10.1016/j.jmwh.2008.04.014.

Murray, M. F., Langan, M., & MacGregor, R. R. (2001). Increased plasma tryptophan in HIV-infected patients treated with pharmacologic doses of nicotinamide. *Nutrition, 17*(7-8), 654–656. https://doi.org/10.1016/s0899-9007(01)00568-8.

Nahin, R. L., Barnes, P. M., & Stussman, B. J. (2016). Expenditures on complementary health approaches: United States, 2012. *National Health Statistics Reports, 95*, 1–11. https://www.cdc.gov/nchs/data/nhsr/nhsr095.pdf.

Nash, K. M., & Shah, Z. A. (2015). Current perspectives on the beneficial role of ginkgo biloba in neurological and cerebrovascular disorders. *Integrative Medicine Insights, 10*, 1–9. https://doi.org/10.4137/IMI.S25054.

National Institute of Health. (2014). "NIH complementary and integrative health agency gets new name.": *NCCIH. December* 17 https://nccih.nih.gov/news/press/12172014.

National Toxicology Program. (2013). Toxicology and carcinogenesis studies of Ginkgo biloba extract (CAS No. 90045-36-6) in F344/N rats and B6C3F1/N mice (Gavage studies). *National Toxicology Program Technical Report Series, 578*, 1–183.

Newman, D., & Cragg, G. (2016). Natural products as sources of new drugs from 1981 to 2014. *Journal of Natural Products, 79*(3), 629–661. https://pubs.acs.org/doi/10.1021/acs.jnatprod.5b01055.

Ng, Q. X., Venkatanarayanan, N., & Ho, C. Y. (2017). Clinical use of Hypericum perforatum (St John's wort) in depression: A meta-analysis. *Journal of Affective Disorders, 210*, 211–221. https://doi.org/10.1016/j.jad.2016.12.048.

NSW Health. (2017). "Medication Interactions with Smoking and Smoking Cessation." *NSW Government Health.* http://www.health.nsw.gov.au/tobacco/Publications/tool-14-medication-intera.pdf.

Ooi, S. L., Henderson, P., & Pak, S. C. (2018). Kava for generalized anxiety disorder: A review of current evidence. *Journal of Alternative and Complementary Medicine, 24*(8), 770–780. https://doi.org/10.1089/acm.2018.0001.

Owen, R. T. (2013). Folate augmentation of antidepressant response. *Drugs of Today, 49*(12), 791–798. https://doi.org/10.1358/dot.2013.49.12.2086138.

Panijel, M. (1985). The treatment of moderate states of anxiety: Randomized double-blind study comparing the clinical effectiveness of a phytomedicine with diazepam. *Therapiwoche, 41*, 4659–4668.

Papakostas, G. I., Mischoulon, D., Shyu, I., Alpert, J. E., & Fava, M. (2010). S-adenosyl methionine (SAMe) augmentation of serotonin reuptake inhibitors for antidepressant nonresponders with major depressive disorder: A double-blind, randomized clinical trial. *The American Journal of Psychiatry, 167*(8), 942–948. https://doi.org/10.1176/appi.ajp.2009.09081198.

Parslow, R. A., & Jorm, A. F. (2004). Use of prescription medications and complementary and alternative medicines to treat depressive and anxiety symptoms: Results from a community sample. *Journal of Affective Disorders, 82*(1), 77–84. https://doi.org/10.1016/j.jad.2003.09.013.

Pittler, M., & Edzard Ernst, E. (2003). Kava extract versus placebo for treating anxiety. *Cochrane Database of Systematic Reviews.* https://doi.org/10.1002/14651858.CD003383.

Polavarapu, A., & Hasbani, D. (2017). Neurological complications of nutritional deficiencies. *Seminars in Pediatric Neurology.* https://doi.org/10.1016/j.spen.2016.12.002.

Porter, D. (1995). Dietary Supplement Health and Education Act of 1994. *Nutrition Today, 30*(2), 89.

Pray, W. S. (2006). *Nonprescription product therapeutics.* Lippincott Williams & Wilkins.

Qato, D., Alexander, G., Conti, R., Johnson, M., Schumm, P., & Tessler Lindau, S. (2008). Use of prescription and over-the-counter medications and dietary supplements among older adults in the United States. *The Journal of the American Medical Association, 300*(24), 2867–2878. https://www.ncbi.nlm.nih.gov/pmc/articles/PMC2702513/.

Rakel, D. (2017). Integrative medicine: *Elsevier Health Sciences.*

Rider, C., Nyska, A., Michelle, C., Kissling, G., Cynthia Smith, C., et al. (2014). Toxicity and carcinogenicity studies of Ginkgo biloba extract in rat and mouse: Liver, thyroid, and nose are targets. *Toxicologic Pathology, 42*(5), 830–843. https://www.ncbi.nlm.nih.gov/pmc/articles/PMC3929544/.

Riedel-Heller, S. G., Matschinger, H., & Angermeyer, M. C. (2005). Mental disorders—Who and what might help? Help-seeking and treatment preferences of the lay public. *Social Psychiatry and Psychiatric Epidemiology, 40*(2), 167–174. https://doi.org/10.1007/s00127-005-0863-8.

Roberts, R. E., Allen, S., Chang, A. P., Henderson, H., Hobson, G. C., Karania, B., … Alexander, S. P. (2013). Distinct mechanisms of relaxation to bioactive components from chamomile species in porcine isolated blood vessels. *Toxicology and Applied Pharmacology, 272*(3), 797–805. https://doi.org/10.1016/j.taap.2013.06.021.

Robinson, A., & McGrail, M. R. (2004). Disclosure of CAM use to medical practitioners: A review of qualitative and quantitative studies. *Complementary Therapies in Medicine, 12*(2-3), 90–98. https://doi.org/10.1016/j.ctim.2004.09.006.

Ross, B. M., Seguin, J., & Sieswerda, L. E. (2007). Omega-3 fatty acids as treatments for mental illness: Which disorder and which fatty acid? *Lipids in Health and Disease, 6*, 21. https://doi.org/10.1186/1476-511X-6-21.

Sarris, J. (2013). St. John's wort for the treatment of psychiatric disorders. *The Psychiatric Clinics of North America, 36*(1), 65–72. https://doi.org/10.1016/j.psc.2013.01.004.

Sarris, J., Panossian, A., Schweitzer, I., Stough, C., & Scholey, A. (2011). Herbal medicine for depression, anxiety and insomnia: A review of psychopharmacology and clinical evidence. *European Neuropsychopharmacology: The Journal of the European College of Neuropsychopharmacology, 21*(12), 841–860. https://doi.org/10.1016/j.euroneuro.2011.04.002.

Schmidt, M., & Butterweck, V. (2015). The mechanisms of action of St. John's wort: An update. *Wiener Medizinische Wochenschrift (1946), 165*(11-12), 229–235. https://doi.org/10.1007/s10354-015-0372-7.

Sholler, D., Schoene, L., & Spindle, T. (2020). Therapeutic efficacy of cannabidiol (CBD): A review of the evidence from clinical trials and human laboratory studies. *Current Addiction Reports, 7*, 405–412.

Simon, G. E., Cherkin, D. C., Sherman, K. J., Eisenberg, D. M., Deyo, R. A., & Davis, R. B. (2004). Mental health visits to complementary and alternative medicine providers. *General*

Hospital Psychiatry, 26(3), 171–177. https://doi.org/10.1016/j.genhosppsych.2004.01.002.

Skidmore-Roth, L (2009). Mosbys nursing drug reference. Mosby.

Sowndhararajan, K., & Kim, S. (2017). Neuroprotective and cognitive enhancement potentials of Angelica Gigas Nakai Root: A Review. *Scientia Pharmaceutica, 85*(2), 21. https://doi.org/10.3390/scipharm85020021.

Stabler, S. P. (2013). Clinical practice. Vitamin B12 deficiency. *The New England Journal of Medicine, 368*(2), 149–160. https://doi.org/10.1056/NEJMcp1113996.

Stoddard, G. J., Archer, M., Shane-McWhorter, L., Bray, B. E., Redd, D. F., Proulx, J., & Zeng-Treitler, Q. (2015). Ginkgo and warfarin interaction in a large Veterans Administration population. *AMIA. Annual Symposium Proceedings. AMIA Symposium, 2015*, 1174–1183.

Tan, D. X., Manchester, L. C., Esteban-Zubero, E., Zhou, Z., & Reiter, R. J. (2015). Melatonin as a potent and inducible endogenous antioxidant: Synthesis and metabolism. *Molecules, 20*(10), 18886–18906. https://doi.org/10.3390/molecules201018886.

U.S. Food and Drug Administration. (2015a). "Drug Applications for Over-the-Counter (OTC) Drugs. Center for Drug Evaluation and Research. https://www.fda.gov/Drugs/Development ApprovalProcess/HowDrugsareDevelopedandApproved/ ApprovalApplications/Over-the-CounterDrugs/default.htm.

VanDolah, H. J., Bauer, B. A., & Mauck, K. F. (2019). Clinicians' guide to cannabidiol and hemp oils. *Mayo Clinic Proceedings, 94*(9), 1840–1851. https://doi.org/10.1016/j.mayocp.2019.01.003.

Williams, W. P., 3rd, McLin,, D. E., 3rd, Dressman, M. A., & Neubauer, D. N. (2016). Comparative review of approved melatonin agonists for the treatment of circadian rhythm sleep-wake disorders. *Pharmacotherapy, 36*(9), 1028–1041. https://doi.org/10.1002/phar.1822.

Witte, S., Loew, D., & Gaus, W. (2005). Meta-analysis of the efficacy of the acetonic kava-kava extract WS1490 in patients with non-psychotic anxiety disorders. *Phytotherapy Research, 19*(3), 183–188. https://doi.org/10.1002/ptr.1609.

Yin, O. Q., Tomlinson, B., Waye, M. M., Chow, A. H., & Chow, M. S. (2004). Pharmacogenetics and herb-drug interactions: Experience with Ginkgo biloba and omeprazole. *Pharmacogenetics, 14*(12), 841–850. https://doi.org/10.1097/00008571-200412000-00007.

Zandi, P. P., Anthony, J. C., Khachaturian, A. S., Stone, S. V., Gustafson, D., Tschanz, J. T., … Cache County Study Group, (2004). Reduced risk of Alzheimer disease in users of antioxidant vitamin supplements: The Cache County Study. *Archives of Neurology, 61*(1), 82–88. https://doi.org/10.1001/archneur.61.1.82.

20

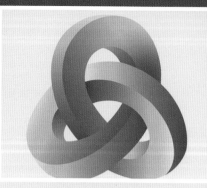

Introduction to Milieu Management

Debbie Steele

Most people are about as happy as they make up their minds to be.

Abraham Lincoln

ⓔ http://evolve.elsevier.com/Keltner

LEARNING OBJECTIVES

- Define the terms therapeutic milieu, therapeutic environment, and therapeutic community.
- Describe the goal of managing the therapeutic environment in the care of psychiatric patients.

- Identify the elements of the therapeutic environment.
- Discuss several ways in which nurses can influence the therapeutic environment.

Note to Students: *Political, social, economic, and other forces have resulted in a health care system that changes quickly. These forces dictate the setting in which care takes place. For example, managed care insurance plans favor the use of less expensive forms of treatment than the inpatient unit. Although hospitals used to employ most psychiatric nurses, a great number of psychiatric nurses currently practice in community settings. Despite the rapidly changing mental health system, treatment principles remain the same when the nurse is guided by the professional definition of nursing—that is, facilitation of healing and alleviation of suffering through the treatment of human responses in the care of individuals and families (American Nurses Association, n.d.). The treatment environment is affected by many variables, but it is the nurse's involvement in creating a therapeutic environment that ultimately determines the overall atmosphere of the treatment setting. This role is true in any specialty area, but it is the focus of psychiatric nursing and therefore the purpose for including these chapters.*

There is an international initiative to integrate recovery-oriented practices into the delivery of all mental health services. For example, the President's New Freedom Commission on Mental Health reported that recovery is the most important goal for the mental health system (Substance Abuse and Mental Health Services Administration [SAMHSA], 2006). For years, nurses have been posed to facilitate and nurture

recovery from mental illnesses and substance abuse (Chang et al., 2018).

Within the therapeutic nurse/patient relationship, nurses are being challenged to integrate recovery into all of their practices (McLoughlin et al., 2013). A therapeutic environment is a vital ingredient in facilitating the journey of recovery for patients within all health care settings. Attention to the therapeutic environment ensures protection of patients from potentially harmful effects and maximizes opportunities for patients to learn something about themselves and their difficulties in everyday living.

The terms *therapeutic environment* and *therapeutic milieu* are sometimes used interchangeably to describe the atmosphere of a psychiatric setting. Strictly speaking, a therapeutic milieu refers to a formalized treatment modality called *milieu therapy*. Regardless of the term used, all treatment environments have an impact on patient outcomes. This is also true in nonpsychiatric patient care environments (e.g., medical surgical, intensive care, postpartum units), even when the environment is not avowed the primacy given in a psychiatric setting. A significant responsibility of psychiatric nurses is the management of the environment, one of the three tools of the psychotherapeutic management model described in Chapter 1.

Patients cannot be in an inpatient setting without being affected by the environment. When you really understand this, it will change your understanding of nursing. Here's the question: How can you shape an environment to make it more therapeutic? This chapter presents a history of the concept of milieu therapy, followed by a discussion of components that are essential for creating a therapeutic environment.

HISTORICAL OVERVIEW

The discussion in this section focuses on *milieu therapy* as it applies to hospital inpatient settings. It is assumed that similar principles could be applied in most treatment settings.

For many years, custodial care was the norm in inpatient settings. Custodial care referred to a *mindset* in which patient care focused exclusively on the patient's activities of daily living, such as hygiene, nutrition, elimination, and safety needs. Custodial care was a paternalistic system in which the staff knew what was best for the patient. Few attempts were made to allow the patient to participate in his or her own treatment, and beyond basic needs, there were no efforts to provide structured treatment activities. After World War II, some professionals were concerned that many opportunities to enhance treatment were being missed. Schwartz & Stanton, 1954 noted the discrepancy between "what could be and what was" in the hospital. They believed that a better result from hospitalization might be realized if *all* dimensions of care were focused on their potential for therapeutic benefit.

The most notable figure of this time was Maxwell Jones. In 1953, Jones wrote his landmark book, *The Therapeutic Community*, in which he described the benefits of an environment that was therapeutic in and of itself. Jones (1953) proposed patient involvement in decision making through daily group meetings, termed *therapeutic community meetings*. In these daily meetings, patients participated in planning ward activities. Patient self-responsibility was an important concept in the therapeutic community, whereby patients were expected to take an active role in their treatment. Increasingly, the importance of the patients' contribution to their own treatment was recognized, and this approach replaced the paternalistic system of the professional treatment team knowing best. Milieu therapy and therapeutic community came to reflect the idea of comprehensive use of the environment as a tool to facilitate the recovery of patients experiencing psychiatric and mental health problems.

The environment of the acute inpatient psychiatric facility of today is significantly different from that of the 1960s and 1970s. In particular, the number of units or beds is much fewer. The patients' average length of stay is greatly reduced. The acuity of psychotic and detained patients is higher, as is the increased risk of violence. Contemporary psychiatric units have become short-term intensive care settings to contain and resolve crises. At times, coercive methods are necessary to prevent violence, particularly with highly psychotic and manic patients. Coercive treatments include involuntary holds, seclusion, and physical and chemical restraints. A high level of care is needed to balance the competing needs embedded in crisis control and recovery approaches to acute inpatient hospitalization (Hornik-Lurie et al., 2018).

Staff members are presented with the challenge of applying therapeutic milieu principles in an environment in which the primary directive is rapid stabilization of symptoms and return of the patient to a less expensive community-based treatment program. All of these factors pose a great challenge to staff members who are expected, and who themselves expect, to create a therapeutic as well as a safe environment for the patients in their charge. The constant change and demands associated with a rapid turnover of patients require nurses to reevaluate the environment continuously in tandem and in coordination with the entire multidisciplinary team.

THE JOINT COMMISSION: ENVIRONMENT OF CARE ISSUES

The Joint Commission requires that institutions routinely evaluate the environment for its ongoing effectiveness to provide care. Additionally, the facility must establish a social environment supporting its basic philosophy. Box 20.1 lists The Joint Commission environment of care standards for inpatient psychiatric units. These standards also apply to outpatient clinics and counseling centers.

BOX 20.1 The Joint Commission Environment of Care Standards

Environmental safety is attained through:
- Ongoing assessment and maintenance of all equipment
- Hazard surveillance
- Reporting and investigation of safety issues
- Monitoring of safety management techniques and procedures
- Orientation programs that address safety issues

A health care facility ensures the security of all people through:
- Mechanisms for addressing security issues
- Provision of appropriate identification for all staff, patients, and visitors
- Security orientation programs
- Mechanisms for handling emergencies
- Mechanisms for interacting with the media

The social environment must provide:
- Space for storage of grooming and hygiene articles
- Closet and drawer space for personal property
- Clothing that is suitable for clinical conditions

The physical setting must provide:
- Adequate privacy to ensure respect for patients
- Door locks consistent with program goals
- Availability of telephones that allow for private conversations
- Sleeping rooms with doors for privacy unless clinically contraindicated
- Furnishings suitable to the population served
- Access to the outdoors unless contraindicated for therapeutic reasons

From The Joint Commission. (2021). *Comprehensive accreditation manual.* https://store.jcrinc.com/2021-comprehensive-accreditation-manuals/.

A day treatment program for patients with chronic mental illness is housed in a large rustic building in a rural county in a southeastern state in the United States. Within easy walking distance of the day treatment program are two group homes. Many of the residents from the group home are also patients at the day treatment center. The therapeutic environment for the day treatment program includes a range of structured treatment activities, such as educational classes; group and individual therapy; and basic living skills such as making a budget, reading food labels for nutrition, planning meals, and job skills. For the patients living in the group home, many of these activities are enhanced and reinforced by trained staff members who structure the days and evenings at the group home. Both treatment settings manage the environment to make it therapeutic for patients.

NURSING AND THE THERAPEUTIC ENVIRONMENT

Florence Nightingale recognized the importance of the environment on the patient's recovery. The aim of the therapeutic environment is to create a relationship of trust—a cooperation between the nurse and patient in which the patient is able to organize his life, while both the patient and nurse are aware of the patient's vulnerabilities. The nurse and patient both work purposely and effectively toward the attainment of patient recovery (Voogt et al., 2015).

Nurses draw on their therapeutic relationship with patients to create connecting learning experiences in the treatment environment. Interactions with patients are opportunities to help them learn and adapt to their problems in daily living. Distortions, conflicts, and inappropriate behavior are dealt with in the here and now of each interaction and relate back to the patient's treatment plan.

Psychiatric nurses must take an active role to ensure that the environment is therapeutic. Paying attention to one's personal values, reactions, and preconceptions is one aspect of keeping the environment therapeutic. Other important elements involve altering the environment through a careful, active, and coordinated process of providing structured therapeutic activities and interactions. For example, inpatient education groups have been found to have a positive effect on patients' well-being and ability to cope with their illness (Bersani et al., 2017). Ensuring that patients have information related to their disease process and participation in decision making concerning their own care is facilitated by effective communication skills of the nurse and positive nurse-patient interactions. Stewart, 2015 found that patients expressed a desire for more and better quality connection with nursing staff, either formally through therapeutic interventions or through informal conversations and communication. It was important and meaningful to patients when nurses took the time to sit with them; patients also felt listened to when nurses took action to follow through on their requests. Nurses with high emotional intelligence and the ability to manage relationships using their social skills have a positive effect on patients. Basogul and associates (2019) found that psychiatric nurses' interpersonal styles, attitudes, awareness of their emotions, and experience are significant determinants of the rate of their exposure to violence in the workplace.

HIGHLIGHTING THE EVIDENCE

Evidence-Based Practice

Voogt et al. (2015) studied how patients experience the acute inpatient psychiatric structure. They found the following nursing factors important to them:

- The nurse knows and understands the patient's situation
- The nurse remains connected with the patient
- The nurse helps and teaches the patient to handle unit rules, times, and habits
- The nurse explains the treatment plan
- The nurse helps moderate the patient's thinking

In addition, the researchers reported what the patient expects from nursing interventions:

- wants to be taken seriously
- wants to know what to do
- wants to maintain autonomy

Elements of the Treatment Environment

The environment provides a context in which patients can move forward toward their goal of optimal health. The following interrelated elements provide the foundation necessary for the nurse to manage the environment effectively:

- Safety
- Structure
- Norms
- Limit setting
- Balance

Safety

Safety is primary to all other aspects of the environment. Safety involves both physical and psychological protection. In acute mental health units, safety is always the priority. Nurses working with severely depressed patients in inpatient settings have 24-hour responsibility for caring for people at risk for suicide. The nurse and patient work cooperatively toward the goal of attaining internal and external safety for the patient. Nurses and other team members endeavor to provide patients with a safe hospital environment to prevent harm. Environmental interventions include removing harmful items (e.g., belts, shoelaces, keys) and placing them in a locked container. Patients are placed on 24-hour-a-day observations on a one-to-one basis. To minimize the distress caused by the process, the patient should be informed of the plan of care, including the level of observations. Additionally, nurses should strive to form a human-to-human connection with the patient. The provision of a therapeutic relationship helps patients address their suicidal feelings and allows the nurse to convey to the patient that his or her life has value. The nurse creates and provides an environment where the patient can begin to explore and discuss painful emotions.

The nurse understands the importance of demonstrating unconditional acceptance, tolerance, and understanding as an integral part of a safe and caring environment. The role of the nurse is primarily to address the patient's need for emotional and physical security.

Management of the unit environment also includes protection from physical harm as a result of patients' verbal and physical aggression. Aggression implies an attitude of hostility or intent to do harm. Nurses should create and adhere closely to the nursing policies and procedures developed for prevention of aggression. These policies usually involve intervening before an aggressive event occurs by such actions as sending a patient to his or her room, talking one to one with a patient, assisting with problem solving in conflicts between patients, administering as-needed (prn) medications, and using seclusion or restraints to control behavior as a last resort. Intervening before situations escalate requires that the nurse be aware of the unit environment at all times, either by direct observation or through the reports of psychiatric technicians and aides. The relationship between the nurse and psychiatric technicians or other unlicensed assistive personnel needs to involve an active, team-oriented approach for mutual understanding of goals for the patient. Most psychiatric units require the documentation of safety observations (often termed *rounds*) on patients, at a frequency ranging from hourly checks to constant observation. The routine and prescribed safety observations on a psychiatric unit are done with the safety of both staff and patients in mind and are essential for maintaining the safety of the environment.

Environmental care is focused on protecting patients from all threatening events. To this end, it might be necessary to restrict visitors known to upset patients. Intrusive behaviors such as getting in other people's private space or bullying others about personal characteristics need to be dealt with by staff to protect patients from this destructive behavior in the treatment environment. Safety cannot be fully accomplished unless the nurses are regularly out among the patients in the environment.

Psychiatric patients are a vulnerable population because of the ease with which their illness can be blamed for any allegations they might make; it is essential to be attentive to complaints of abuse made by patients. Patients with paranoia, delusions, or personality disorders might perceive events as abusive; however, all allegations require the attention of the treatment team. Incident reports, follow-up by management, and notification of patient representatives or advocates might be necessary when allegations of abuse are made. Complaints against staff members are especially difficult for staff committed to the care of their patients, but it is important to be attentive to patterns suggestive of patients being exploited by staff members and to take action when suspicious or confirmed patterns are discovered. Patients need to know that staff members will not harm them and will not permit anyone else to do so. Posting patient rights, including telephone numbers to access assistance for violations of these rights, creates feelings of safety by empowering patients in an environment that can leave them feeling vulnerable.

Providing emotional safety is an essential element of the therapeutic milieu. Hawamdeh and Fakhry (2014) reported on interventions that nurses found important within the nurse-patient relationship. These elements included accessibility, reassurance, comfort, genuineness, openness, trust, security, and provision of physical care. Accessibility involves giving time and priority to patients, which results in building and strengthening the nurse-patient bond. "Being there" for patients allows them to better tolerate their struggles, the pain, and the associated sorrow of living with a mental disorder. Providing reassurance and comfort to patients when they are experiencing distress, fear, or suspicion will put them at ease as their questions and concerns are addressed. Expressing understanding about a patient's difficult experience helps establish trust and provides a sense of not being alone and abandoned. An emphasis on patients' physical care is also critical to the nurse-patient relationship. All of these interventions relay to patients that nurses are there for them to meet their emotional and physical needs, establishing themselves as someone the patients can rely on.

Clinical Example

John is angry with another patient and is threatening him with bodily harm. The nurse intervenes by directing John that she will escort him to his room. The nurse stays with John and encourages him to talk about what he is feeling. "I understand that you are upset, can you share with me what is going on for you?"

Structure

Structure refers to the physical environment, daily schedules of treatment activities, and informal rules of interacting between patients and staff. Structure is an essential component of a therapeutic milieu. Nurses lead activities such as patient education and unit community groups. Teaching about medications, side effects, and aftercare support for both patients and families is an important function of the psychiatric nurse in inpatient settings.

Psychosocial groups led by social workers or trained therapists are incorporated into the daily schedule of patient events. Patients also may be offered individual or family therapy, depending on available resources.

Recreation and art are important aspects of the structured treatment environment. Occupational or recreational therapists ideally fulfill this function. Recreation and art therapy provide an opportunity for patients to socialize and interact with others. They also serve as a welcome distraction from painful feelings and distressing perceptions. The goal of recreation therapy is to use leisure, recreation, and sport activities to treat, improve, or maintain the physical, mental, and emotional well-being of patients served. Interventions include structured activities that enhance specific functional skills, organized sports, and fitness activities. A few examples of recreational activities include bingo, basketball, Ping-Pong, cards, and games. Group exercise programs delivered by trained personnel have been found to be well received by individuals in acute psychiatric hospitals (Stanton et al., 2016).

Art therapy is a form of psychotherapy that uses some form of art as its primary mode of expression and communication and includes dance or movement, drama, and music. Art psychotherapy enhances an individual's creativity, emotional expression, communication, insight, and ability to relate to themselves and others. Art therapy has also been used to enhance the patients' cognitive understanding of their disorder, their sense of self, interpersonal contact, self-esteem, and social competency (Qui et al., 2017). Art therapy is an established approach, recommended for the treatment of psychosis, especially in relation to negative symptoms (Stickley et al., 2018). Through art therapy, patients are able to understand and make sense of themselves and others. As patients are provided a means of relating to their experiences in new and different ways, they feel a sense of validation and normalcy.

Nurses and the various therapists work together as a team in determining which scheduled activities are in accord with the current level of functioning and within the ability of each patient on the unit. For example, a depressed inpatient may be at a higher level of functioning than a patient experiencing perceptual disturbances associated with psychosis.

The physical design of the unit is also an aspect of structure. Adequate space, areas for socializing and receiving visitors, telephones, and areas for privacy all are required elements of a therapeutic environment. Additionally, patients need a central location to interact with each other; often, this is the day room. Research has shown that participating in art therapy produces outcomes which support recovery, specifically enhancing connectedness and improving hope (Stickley et al., 2018).

Norms

Norms are specific expectations of behavior that permeate the treatment environment; they are intended to promote safety and trust in the environment through the sanctioning of socially acceptable behaviors and consistency about what to expect. Norms create an environment that is predictable and applicable to all patients. Individuals experiencing psychosis may not understand why they are in the hospital, how long they will be there, what will be provided, and what is required of them. The communication of expectations related to norms enables respect and protection of the patients' integrity. Many of the behavioral norms are related to activities of daily living. For example, patients are expected to bathe, brush their hair and teeth, and dress appropriately to the environment. Other types of norms are focused on personal responsibility, such as the expectations that (1) patients will not harm themselves or others, (2) patients will attend and participate in group meetings and other unit activities, and (3) patients will focus on their personal treatment plan. How norms are communicated is of particular importance in an inpatient setting where some of the patients may be there involuntarily. Whenever possible, patients should be offered a sense of control, and staff should avert power struggles with patients whose tolerance and

resilience are tenuous. Norms related to unit rules and activities were clearly articulated by a patient as follows, "You might not like some of the things you have to do and you might not agree with the rules, but you can kinda see how it's best in the long run cause you have so many different people and problems to deal with; I guess it keeps it smooth."

Clinical Example

The nurse and the patient together develop mutual relational interventions via open dialogue, negotiation, and collaboration. For example, instead of the nurse passively ignoring an unkempt patient who is disoriented and easily agitated, the nurse can say, "I am wondering what would happen if you took a shower?" or "When would you like to take a shower?"

Limit Setting

Limit setting refers to how nurses establish boundaries and clarify expectations about appropriate behavior within the mental health milieu. Applying limit setting therapeutically is important to ensure safety and promote a structured therapeutic environment. Specific means of sharing limits involves an attitude of making unit rules and expectations clear, as well as encouraging patients to take responsibility for self. Key concepts that support this strategy involve patients being advised of unit rules on admission and at frequent intervals, depending on their capacity to comprehend and attend to these rules. Written copies of unit rules should be provided to each patient and posted on the unit in a highly visible location. Although limits are a natural part of daily living, patients who are new to a unit cannot be expected to understand all the rules. Unit expectations should be communicated impartially and with a nonjudgmental attitude.

At times, limit setting is employed to prevent or limit inappropriate, aggressive, or unsafe behavior of patients. In these cases, de-escalation is employed by the nurse in a nonconfrontational manner to prevent a further disturbance of behavior. It is also sometimes necessary to set limits or address behaviors such as excessive requests, overt and covert sexual advances, and refusal to participate in treatment activities.

HIGHLIGHTING THE EVIDENCE

Current Research

El-Azzab and associates (2019) explored patients' and nurses' perspectives of limit setting in a psychiatric hospital. The findings of the study indicated that limit setting reduced the patient's violent and aggressive behavior, clarified what was the appropriate and expected behavior of the patients, and that limit setting helped patients to feel physically and emotionally secure. However, some patients had negative experiences with limit settings that contributed to the enforcement of misconceptions and negative opinions about nurses' behavior. Furthermore, patients reported the need for more explanations about the use of limit-setting strategies. The researchers concluded that limits set by nurses that felt like rejection was related to patient hostility toward the nurse.

CRITICAL THINKING QUESTION

1. How can limit setting be viewed as coercive by patients in acute psychiatric units?

Balance

Balance, perhaps more than any other element of managing the therapeutic environment, represents the value of developing expertise in nursing. Balance involves the process of gradually allowing independent behaviors in a dependent situation. It might be necessary to make specific judgments about a patient's readiness to assume certain responsibilities for his or her care versus providing assistance when the patient might be unable to act on his or her own behalf. Making this decision requires the nurse to weigh the multiple and competing needs of the patient involved, as well as the needs of other patients and staff on the unit. How aggressive incidents are perceived and managed by nurses illustrates the importance of a balanced approach. For example, although de-escalation is the expected method for dealing with patients' aggression, Hallett and Dickens (2015) emphasized the importance of timing in terms of nursing interventions. Being deliberate in spending time with patients and seeking their perspective can prove beneficial in preventing misunderstandings and subsequent violence. However, exploration of the patients' perspective is essential not just in relation to aggressive incidents. Patients who are depressed and anxious can also benefit from

the development of this practice. Instead of focusing on the behavior of a patient, nurses are encouraged to seek to understand the nature of the patient's problem within the context of the unit. An overall proactive stance can be accomplished as nurses approach patient deficits and needs based on an accurate, comprehensive evaluation. Consistency in responding to patients' behaviors and requests is essential in providing a safe, therapeutic environment.

 CRITICAL THINKING QUESTION

2. How can consistency and follow-through by nurses contribute to a therapeutic environment?

THE NURSE AS MANAGER OF THE TREATMENT ENVIRONMENT

Environmental modification is an important intervention of the psychiatric nurse and entails using the elements of safety, structure, norms, limit setting, and balance to achieve patients' treatment goals. Through environmental modification, the nurse can enhance the therapeutic environment for the patient. Physical arrangements, safety issues, and other features can create an atmosphere in which patients can learn new behaviors or become aware of their personal strengths. Responsiveness to the needs of patients necessitates that nursing staff continually review environmental norms, rules, and

---

◎ CARE PLAN

Assessment	**Problems:** A 23-year-old man has been unable to manage the auditory hallucinations (voices) telling him to cut (self-mutilate).
	1. Patient states that he thinks God wants him to cut, admitting to auditory hallucinations.
	2. Patient's mood is anxious with constricted affect.
	3. Patient tends to isolate in his room.
	4. Patient expresses negative symptoms such as avolition.
	5. Patient has gained 40 lb in the past year (on antipsychotics).
	6. Patient is religiously preoccupied.
Diagnosis	Risk for self-mutilation related to command hallucinations telling him to cut.
Outcomes	**Short-term goals**
Date met: _____	Patient will explore thoughts related to anxious feelings with staff.
Date met: _____	Patient will report a decrease in anxiety based on a scale of 1–10.
Date met: _____	Patient will participate in groups and recreation and art therapy every day.
Date met: _____	Patient will verbally contract for safety with nurse every shift.
	Long-term goals
Date met: _____	Patient will report confidence in ability to manage command hallucinations.
Date met: _____	Patient will participate in follow-up individual and family psychotherapy.
Planning and Interventions	**Nurse-patient relationship:** Assist patient to identify and explore feelings of anxiety related to thoughts of self-mutilation; encourage patient to participate in all psychoeducational and therapy groups; encourage patient to participate in recreational and art programs to divert thoughts away from command hallucinations; assess for presence and content of auditory hallucinations; and verbally contract for safety every shift.
	Psychopharmacology: Aripiprazole (Abilify) 10 mg PO every day; discuss role of medications and related side effects.
	Milieu management: Support patient's efforts to decrease anxiety. Encourage patient to spend time in the day room interacting with other patients. Monitor progress in using the diversion techniques and their effectiveness. Cooperate with patient in ongoing treatment plan.

regulations as an important aspect of managing and modifying the environment. Flexibility in maintaining a therapeutic environment is accomplished by this ongoing evaluation of effectiveness. The care plan illustrates how environmental modification is used as a tool for meeting the patients' treatment goals. One of the most challenging and rewarding aspects of psychiatric nursing is the ability to affect the experience of patients in the hospital in a positive, therapeutic, and creative way.

From the patient's perspective, being forced into treatment activities by nursing staff may interfere with the development of a therapeutic nurse-patient relationship. Occasionally, disagreement over rules is the precipitating factor leading to patient aggression. Rules on a psychiatric unit are intended for safety, but they can turn into a battle for control (El-Azzab et al., 2019). A high level of skill is required of nurses as they manage rules and norms in the treatment environment. A delicate balance exists between enhancement of the nurse-patient relationship and expectations related to unit rules.

Excessive focus on rules and efficiency may become the tendency of some nursing staff members, whereas the priority of maintaining the therapeutic relationship is paramount for others. An experienced nurse instinctively relates to the uniqueness of each patient, based on his or her training and skills. Awareness of the patient's perspective, coupled with consistency and creativity among the nursing staff, can go a long way in creating a therapeutic, yet safe milieu.

> ### ? CRITICAL THINKING QUESTION
>
> 3. A 23-year-old man with a diagnosis of schizophrenia, undifferentiated type, has been admitted to a psychiatric hospital because of recent thoughts related to self-mutilation. The patient lives with his mother, who does not feel comfortable in her ability to keep her son from harming himself. How might the use of a therapeutic environment assist this patient and family?

▮ STUDY NOTES

1. Environmental modification is the purposeful use of all interpersonal and environmental forces to enhance the mental health of psychiatric patients through the development of a therapeutic environment.
2. Because nurses use environmental modification as a tool for assisting patients, nurses have a significant part of the responsibility for shaping the therapeutic environment.
3. The Joint Commission has very clear standards regarding the effects of the environment of care on inpatient psychiatric settings. Safety and a functional environment conducive to patient care are major priorities of the environment of care.
4. Historically, nurses provided only custodial care, but after World War II, Jones (1953) and others conceptualized an environment in which all aspects of the psychiatric

patient's day would be used to promote mental health; this was termed *milieu therapy*.
5. The use of inpatient psychiatric settings has diminished as biologically-based treatments have gained prominence and community care has become the preferred setting for treatment. In all settings, safety is a priority goal.
6. Principles of milieu therapy can also be applied to community settings.
7. All treatment environments can be therapeutic or nontherapeutic.
8. Psychiatric nurses manage the treatment environment by modification of five elements: safety, structure, norms, limit setting, and balance.
9. Creating and managing a therapeutic environment requires the psychiatric nurse to be compassionate, caring, committed, consistent, and collaborative.

REFERENCES

American Nurses Association (n.d.). What is Nursing? https://www.nursingworld.org/practice-policy/workforce/what-is-nursing/.

Bersani, F., Biondi, M., Coviello, M., & Fagiolini, A. (2017). Psychoeducational interventions focused on healthy living improves psychopathological severity and lifestyle quality in psychiatric patients: Preliminary findings from a controlled study. *Journal of Mental Health, 26*(3), 271–275. https://doi.org/10.1080/09638237.2017.1294741.

Basogul, C., Arabaci, L., Buyukbayram, A., Aktas, Y., & Uzunoglu, G. (2019). Emotional intelligence and personality characteristics of psychiatric nurses and their situations of exposure to violence. *Perspectives of Psychiatric Care, 55*, 255–261. https://doi.org/10.1111/ppc.12358.

El-Azzab, S., Mohamed, S., & El-Nady, M. (2019). Using of limit setting strategies at psychiatric hospital: Patients and nurses

perspectives. *International Journal of Nursing, 6*(1), 117–126. https://doi.org/DOI:10.15640/ijn.v6n1a13.

Hallett, N., & Dickens, G. (2015). De-escalation: A survey of clinical staff in a secure mental health inpatient service. *International Journal of Mental Health Nursing, 24*, 324–333. https://doi.org/10.1111/inm.12136.

Hawamdeh, S., & Fakhry, R. (2014). Therapeutic relationships from the psychiatric nurses' perspectives: An interpretative phenomenological study. *Perspectives in Psychiatric Care, 50*, 178–185. https://doi.org/10.1111/ppc.12039.

Hornik-Lurie, T., Shalev, A., Haknazar, L., & Epstein, P. (2018). Implementing recovery-oriented interventions with staff in a psychiatric hospital: A mixed-methods study. *Journal of Psychiatric Mental Health Nursing, 25*(9-10), 569–581. https://doi.org/10.1111/jpm.12502.

Jones, M. (1953). *The therapeutic community*. Basic Books.

McLoughlin, K. A., et al. (2013). Recovery-oriented practices of psychiatric-mental health nursing staff in an acute hospital setting. *Journal of the American Psychiatric Nurses Association, 19*, 1. https://doi.org/10.1177/1078390313490025.

Qui, H., Ye, Z., Liang, M., & Huang, Y. (2017). Effect of an art brut therapy program called go beyond the schizophrenia (GBTS) on prison inmates with schizophrenia in mainland China – A randomized, longitudinal, and controlled trial. *Clinical Psychology & Psychotherapy, 24*, 1069–1078. https://doi.org/10.1002/cpp.2069.

Schwartz, A., & Stanton, M. (1954). *The mental hospital.* Basic Books.

Stanton, R., et al. (2016). Participation in and satisfaction with an exercise program for inpatient mental health consumers. *Perspectives in Psychiatric Care, 52*, 62–67. https://doi.org/10.1111/ppc.12108.

Stewart, D., et al. (2015). Thematic analysis of psychiatric patients' perception of nursing staff. *International Journal of Mental Health Nursing, 24*, 82–90. https://doi.org/10.1111/inm.12107.

Stickley, T., Wright, N., & Slade, M. (2018). The art of recovery: Outcomes from participatory arts activities for people using mental health services. *Journal of Mental Health, 27*(4), 367–373. https://doi.org/10.1080/09638237.2018.1437609.

Substance Abuse and Mental Health Services Administration [SAMHSA]. (2006). National consensus statement on mental health recovery. http://www.samhsa.gov/samhsa_news/volumexiv_2/article4.htm.

The Joint Commission. (2021). Comprehensive accreditation manual. https://store.jcrinc.com/2021-comprehensive-accreditation-manuals/.

Voogt, L. A., et al. (2015). The patient's perspective on "providing structure" in psychiatric inpatient care: An interview study. *Perspectives in Psychiatric Care, 51*, 136–147. https://doi.org/10.1111/ppc.12076.

21

Variables Affecting the Therapeutic Environment: Violence and Suicide

Debbie Steele

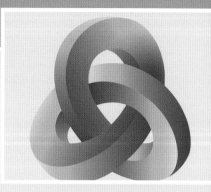

http://evolve.elsevier.com/Keltner

LEARNING OBJECTIVES

- Discuss the impact of recovery-oriented care on the inpatient psychiatric milieu.
- Describe the five stages of the assault cycle.
- Explain the nursing interventions appropriate to the escalation and crisis phases of the assault cycle.
- Describe the nursing care of patients in seclusion and restraints.

- Differentiate between suicidal ideation, threats, gestures, attempts, and completion.
- Discuss nursing interventions related to suicidality.
- Describe the impact that aggressive and suicidal patients have on nursing staff.

In Chapter 20, management of the treatment environment was presented as a process whereby the nurse modifies elements of the treatment environment, including safety, structure, norms, limit setting, and balance. The psychiatric nurse must be aware of each of these essential elements while making decisions about how to modify various aspects of the environment to meet the treatment needs of patients. In this chapter, the focus is on the issues of violence and suicidality, particularly in the inpatient setting.

CURRENT TRENDS

Psychiatric inpatient and outpatient settings have changed significantly over the past 30 years. In 1990, the average inpatient psychiatric stay was 1 month, whereas the average stay today is between 3 and 10 days, with many admissions lasting only 3 or 4 days—even for patients with active psychosis. These short hospital admissions are referred to as micro-hospitalizations.

As a result of insurance and managed care restrictions, patients must meet stringent criteria to be admitted for a psychiatric hospitalization (i.e., imminent danger to self or others or grave disability). The cost-efficient managed care approach forces inpatient units to rapidly return the patient to the community for less expensive treatment options. This trend has resulted in high turnover and even higher patient acuity rates.

Patients admitted to psychiatric hospitals are among the sickest, with sometimes limited resources, frequent readmissions, few placement alternatives, and bouts of distressing emotions, thoughts, and behavior. While the goal of patients' admission is to promote psychological wellbeing and safety, the environment of the psychiatric unit can become physically and emotionally dangerous for all. When patients are experiencing emotional instability due to feeling ignored or controlled, aggression and violence may occur. In many cases, the very methods and structures of the inpatient unit can (re)create and perpetuate experiences of trauma and violence against patients and health care providers (Campbell et al., 2019). Despite the competing risks and needs, the Substance Abuse and Mental Health Services Administration, American Psychiatric Association, American Psychiatric Nurses Association, and the United Nations Convention on the Rights of Persons with Disabilities have pushed to eliminate the use of seclusion and restraint in psychiatric treatment. As part of this mandate, nurses are required to use less restrictive measures before using the more restrictive interventions of seclusion and restraints. The professional discourse regarding the use of seclusion and restraints is ongoing and revolves around whether these restrictive measures constitute a therapeutic intervention, an emergency measure, or a tool for control and submission. Currently, the use of seclusion and restraints remains a constant in acute psychiatric facilities (Jacob et al., 2016).

NORM'S NOTES If there is one aspect of psychiatric nursing that most students (and many practicing nurses) fear, it is confrontation with an angry, aggressive, or violent mentally ill person. I don't blame you for feeling that way—in some ways, this fear is reasonable because it can motivate you to learn the material in this chapter. Aggressive outbursts, both verbal and physical, do happen, but the good news is that they do not occur nearly as often as you might imagine. This chapter provides important concepts on how to de-escalate aggressiveness when it occurs.

AGGRESSION AND VIOLENCE

The potential for aggression in hospital psychiatric units is a well-known environmental hazard. In addition to the emotional and physical danger that disruptive inpatients present to themselves, peers, and hospital staff, their actions are frightening and disturb the therapeutic environment. At its worst, violent behavior can result in serious injury or death.

Violence in an inpatient psychiatric unit cannot always be predicted. It is important to be able to intervene when early warning signs are evident as nurses spend time providing direct contact with patients. Nurses cannot know what is occurring on the unit unless they interact with their patients at frequent, regular intervals. Expert nurses use their assessment skills and previous experiences to interpret inappropriate behavior within the context and knowledge of a patient's pathology. Understanding the patient's experience is considered a crucial factor in anticipating aggressive behavior. The nurse's presence and ability to be with the patient as a unique person in a stressful situation is essential to dealing with potentially violent patients. The necessity of staff-patient interaction cannot be overemphasized.

Although there are no guarantees against the occurrence of violence on psychiatric units, one variable affecting the risk of aggression is staff training. Aggressiveness is known to result from the complex interactions among patients, nursing personnel, and the culture of the specific unit (Jacob et al., 2016). Issues that contribute to a patient's becoming violent include not feeling heard or understood, unmet expectations, substance withdrawal, feeling out of control, being retraumatized, and receiving upsetting information (Parrish, 2019). Strategies for decreasing the potential for violence focus on enhancing the nurse-patient relationship by improving communication skills, advocating for clients, being available, using continual clinical assessment skills, providing patient education in an open dialog, and collaborating with patients in treatment planning.

Social learning theory provides a helpful explanation of the dynamics underlying aggressiveness and violence. In short, patients' aggression serves a vital role in communicating their emotional distress. Fear and insecurity are general feelings on inpatient units. Patients do not know each other; they may be afraid of authoritarian nursing styles.

Staff-patient interaction has been found to account for 39% of aggressive and violent incidents (i.e., limiting patient's freedom, denying a patient request). How patients react when confronted or ignored is predetermined based on their childhood learning and conditioning. Patients who experienced adverse childhood experiences (abuse and neglect) are more likely to be easily triggered when faced with conflict on the unit. Patients' hypersensitivity is believed to stem from growing up in an environment where their negative emotions were often rejected, punished, or ignored by caregivers (Liu et al., 2015). Nurses' beliefs about the causes of aggression and violence determine the strategies they will implement when faced with emotionally charged situations (Dickens, Piccirillo, & Alderman, 2013).

One of the main reasons for aggression is the patient's inability to express their emotional distress and needs effectively. Therefore, noncoercive de-escalation is the intervention of choice in managing acute agitation and frustration (Roppolo et al., 2020). The following steps are known to be helpful:

- Respect the patient's personal space. Use connecting language (i.e., soft voice, slow movements, eye contact)
- Be calm and supportive
- Establish rapport and maintain an alliance
- Be concise; do not provoke
- Identify the patient's feelings, wants, and needs
- Validate and normalize the patient's emotional distress
- Listen closely to what the patient is saying
- Offer choices and optimism
- Set clear limits and clearly explain what will happen

Working with psychiatric patients who may become irritable and aggressive requires nurses to be aware of their own emotional vulnerabilities, how they respond when triggered, and their methods to achieve and maintain a safe work environment. Nurses cannot defuse patients' anger or aggression when they are in a similar state. Responding to aggression with aggression sets up a vicious cycle that will predictably result in escalation and the need for force and, ultimately, restraints.

When patients become aggressive, nurses might experience fear, a feeling of professional inadequacy, or a sense of failure. They might become overly coercive and engage in power struggles with patients. A nurse's participation in physically controlling violent patients can damage the chances of developing or continuing a therapeutic relationship. However, when nurses view patients' aggressive behaviors as a form of communication and focus on assisting patients in processing their emotional distress, the therapeutic relationship is strengthened. How nursing staff speak to patients demonstrates that they are listening to and understanding their concerns. Caring dialogue is known to have a soothing and threat-regulating effect on patients (Veale et al., 2015).

? CRITICAL THINKING QUESTION

1. A visitor to the unit begins to hit a patient. How would you handle this situation?

MANAGEMENT OF INPATIENT AGGRESSION

In acute psychiatric settings, using coercive measures to care for aggression is still common despite the considerable efforts made to reduce its usage. De-escalation, medication, physical restraint, and seclusion are the therapeutic measures used by nursing staff to care for aggression and violence in the acute psychiatric setting. Spinzy and associates (2018) researched patients' perspectives of restraints and found that they verbalized an ambivalent attitude. On the one hand, they viewed physical restraint as sometimes justified. On the other, they viewed them as an experience that evoked many negative emotions, which could be ameliorated by nursing contact (Spinzy et al., 2018). A high skill level is required of psychiatric nurses who regularly find themselves in this clinically complex situation.

Consequently, most of the in-service staff training conducted in acute psychiatric hospitals revolves around teaching nurses and other personnel how to de-escalate agitated patients and how to perform coercive measures safely when patients become aggressive and dangerous to themselves and others. Psychiatric nurses are conflicted in their professional roles and personal ethics. For example, the nurse's role to maintain unit safety by utilizing coercive measures contradicts the ethical principles of patient autonomy and human rights consistent with the recovery movement (Al-Maraira et al., 2019). Current research is focused on identifying evidence-based interventions to reduce mechanical restraint, such as cognitive milieu therapy (CMT), patient/staff education, patient participation, cultural changes, and patient-centered care. CMT is enhanced training in psychosocial approaches that promote open dialogue and collaborative problem solving between nursing staff and patients. Other measures include the provision of extra monitoring and/or support for those patients assessed to be at risk for aggression; assessing for a history of trauma to determine vulnerabilities and triggers; assessing what has worked in the past to care for patient aggression; measures emphasizing preventative interventions with at-risk patients (Lykke et al., 2020).

NURSING INTERVENTIONS BASED ON THE ASSAULT CYCLE

The assault cycle can be used as a framework for nursing interventions that aim to prevent aggression and violence. On the most basic level, the goal of all interventions is to avoid physical and emotional harm to patients and staff. Smith's stress model (1981) describes the assault cycle with five stages of a predictable pattern or chain of aggressive responses to emotional or physical stress. Patients who are repeatedly assaultive exhibit behavior patterns that are ritualistic, stereotypical, and automatic. As the acuity of the aggressive response increases, a comparable decrease occurs in patients' problem-solving abilities, creativity, spontaneity, and behavioral options. The five-phase assault cycle includes the following:

1. *Triggering phase.* The stress-producing event occurs, initiating the stress responses (associated with overwhelming emotions of fear).

2. *Escalation phase.* Responses represent escalating behaviors that indicate a movement toward the loss of control (characterized by illogical and irrational thoughts).
3. *Crisis phase.* During this period of emotional and physical crisis, loss of control occurs (anger and rage are expressed to defend oneself).
4. *Recovery phase.* In this period of cooling down, the person slows down and returns to normal responses (fear of danger wanes).
5. *Postcrisis depression phase.* In this period, the person attempts reconciliation with others (despair over disconnection occurs).

An overview of the assault cycle follows, interspersed with nursing interventions based on de-escalation techniques. De-escalation is defined as specific connecting and disarming skills utilized by skilled helpers to prevent aggressive behaviors and reduce the use of seclusion and restraints. Nurses help patients who become triggered to feel less threatened through verbal and physical expression of empathy, alliance, and nonconfrontational limit setting based on mutual respect. Simply put, de-escalation is defusing or "talking down" the agitated patient into a calmer state with the goal of preventing aggressive or violent behavior. De-escalation comprises a specific set of learned skills, as explained next (Table 21.1).

Triggering Phase

The triggering phase is characterized by the automatic, negative emotional response that patients have to stressful events that may occur while they are on the unit. Initially, as patients' negative emotions are aroused, their responses are nonviolent and present no danger to others. The behavior reflects patients' usual coping and defense mechanisms. The nurse must assess how patients have coped with negative emotions in the past so that when they are triggered, the nurse becomes proactive and assists patients in coping appropriately with their emotions. For example, suppose a patient's stressor is another individual in the immediate environment. In that case, the two patients can be separated, and nurses can talk with each patient individually to promote safe ventilation of emotions.

Agitation, commonly, although not always, precedes aggression. Thus, specific strategies to prevent aggression often try to intercede at the onset of a triggering event, reflected in behaviors such as pacing, restlessness, intrusive behavior, annoyance, and confusion. At this point, the nurse focuses on redirecting the patient by being supportive and using empathic and understanding statements. The nurse speaks softly in calm, clear, simple statements, avoiding any challenge to the patient. Aggressive, confrontational, or threatening approaches at this time usually result in escalation. Although ventilation is encouraged, other techniques found to be useful include relaxation techniques, such as deep breathing. Patients' display of agitation is socially embarrassing for them and counterproductive, leaving them with feelings of vulnerability and loss of autonomy. To protect the dignity of patients and the rights and safety of others, patients can be asked to take a "time out" in their rooms or at least move to a quieter area; other patients might be asked to leave

TABLE 21.1   Interventions Based on Assault Cycle

Phase	Behaviors	Nursing Interventions
Triggering phase: +1 to +2 level of anxiety	Muscle tension, changes in voice quality, tapping of fingers, pacing, repeated verbalizations, restlessness, irritability, anxiety, suspiciousness, perspiration, tremors, glaring, changes in breathing	Convey empathic support. Encourage ventilation. Use clear, calm, simple statements. Normalize the patient's feelings. Collaborate with patient by discussing alternative solutions. If needed, go with the patient to a quiet area. Offer safe tension reduction measures. If needed, offer oral medications (prn).
Escalation phase: +2 to +3 level of anxiety	Pale or flushed face, screaming, anger, swearing, agitation, hypersensitivity, threats, demands, readiness to retaliate, tautness, loss of reasoning ability, provocative behaviors, clenched fists	Take charge with calm, firm directions. Accompany patient to a quiet room for "time out." Offer oral medications (prn) if ordered. Ask the staff to be on standby at a distance. Prepare for a "show of concern."
Crisis phase: +3 to +4 level of anxiety	Loss of self-control, fighting, hitting, rage, kicking, scratching, throwing things	Use seclusion, restraints, or IM/po medications (prn), as ordered. Initiate intensive nursing care.
Recovery phase: +3 to +2 level of anxiety	Accusations, recriminations, lowering of voice, decreased body tension, change in conversational content, more normal responses, relaxation	Continue intensive nursing care. Process the incident with staff and other patients. Assess patient and staff injuries. Evaluate patient's progress toward de-escalation
Postcrisis depression phase: +2 to +1 level of anxiety	Crying, apologies, reconciliatory interactions, repression of assaultive feelings (which might later appear as hostility, passive aggression)	Process incident with patient. Validate the patient's situation and feelings. Progressively reduce the degree of restraint and seclusion. Facilitate reentry to unit.

IM, Intramuscular; *prn*, as needed.

the scene. It is important for nurses to compliment patients for their use of positive solutions.

Additional nursing interventions include helping patients identify productive coping skills that have worked in the past. Common suggestions may include journaling, exercising, working with clay, or walking up and down the hall. Oral antianxiety or antipsychotic medications can also be offered. A focus on the patients' strengths and past successes needs to be integrated into the approach of nursing staff to patients through this process.

Clinical Example

John Henderson has been a patient on the unit for 3 days. While talking to his wife on the telephone, he becomes upset and raises his voice at her. The nurse calmly suggests that he tell his wife that he will continue their conversation later. He hangs up the telephone and starts pacing in the hallway. The nurse says, "Tell me what you are upset about." For 15 minutes, he describes the telephone conversation in detail, expresses anger toward his wife, and says he is afraid that she will divorce him. As the nurse listens attentively, validating and normalizing his emotional distress, John begins to softly cry, wiping his tears with the back of his hand.

Escalation Phase

The escalation phase is characterized by an escalation of dangerous behaviors such as swearing, screaming, and

threatening. De-escalation techniques in this phase include allowing the patient whatever time is necessary to reduce their anxiety, fear, or anger. Telling aggressive patients that nurses are there to "support" them helps to reframe the situation from a confrontational to a collaborative encounter (Goetz & Taylor-Trujillo, 2012). For example, at a safe distance, the nurse calls the patient by name and states in a calm, confident manner that the nurse is there to assist the patient in working through their feelings. The nurse avoids sudden movements and loud tones so as not to appear attacking.

Medications may help acute agitation if less restrictive measures are not successful. Medications are intended to relieve the symptoms without oversedating the patient, so the lowest possible dose is recommended. The patient needs to be involved in deciding the type and route of medication administered. Oral medications are usually as effective as intramuscular medications and are more readily received by patients. However, IM administration may be necessary as a last resort. The medications most commonly used are antipsychotics and benzodiazepines. The etiology of the patient's agitation influences medication choice (Roppolo et al., 2020). Among the oral antianxiety medications, lorazepam (Ativan) and alprazolam (Xanax) are often the drugs of choice because they take effect rapidly and have relatively few side effects. Lorazepam might be given via the IM route. Among the antipsychotics, the medications that can be given orally (quetiapine [Seroquel]) or orally or intramuscularly (haloperidol [Haldol] and ziprasidone [Geodon]) have lower sedating effects but help decrease agitation.

Given the principle of the least restrictive environment, the nurse first offers a time out in a quiet room in a kind but firm manner. If this measure is ineffective, more restrictive measures might be instituted when the patient's behavior compromises the culture of safety. Other staff members might be called to be on standby, but they should initially try to remain out of the patient's view. When patients are potentially violent, their physical proximity to others is perceived as much closer than it is, and they might feel threatened.

If the patient cannot use their coping skills effectively and safety is threatened, the nurse asks for staff assistance for a stronger "show of concern" (Goetz & Taylor-Trujillo, 2012). This action involves having four to six staff members within sight of the patient but at a greater distance from the patient than the primary nurse so that they do not appear ready to attack the patient. Frequently, when the patient becomes aware of the other staff members and is informed that the staff will help the patient control their behavior, the patient can gain reasonable composure, cooperate with the nurse's request, take the medications, and go to a quieter room with a staff escort. If these interventions do not work, the patient is usually close to entering the crisis phase.

Crisis Phase

The crisis phase is reached when the patient is approaching an attack on the environment, self, other patients, or staff. Verbal limits are ineffective, and external control by the staff is essential. In these emergencies or crises, immediate seclusion, restraint, or the administration of stat. medications becomes necessary. The patient has the right to refuse medication, but staff might give it in the presence of an *immediate* physical threat to others. These actions should be supported by emergency protocols that the physicians and hospital have approved, and any actions taken should be carefully and thoroughly documented in the patient's records.

The staff must deal with psychiatric emergencies in coordinated and organized ways as practiced during staff in-service trainings on de-escalation and self-defense. All staff members should master self-protection techniques against behaviors such as kicking, hitting, and biting. Facilities must provide de-escalation programs for all staff members on a yearly basis. Staff members who are well trained in de-escalation techniques are less likely to be victims of patient assaults.

Seclusion

Seclusion is the involuntary confinement of placing a patient alone in a specially designed, lockable room equipped with a security window or a camera for observation. There are many ethical and humanitarian concerns about the use of seclusion. Patients report on the negative impact, feelings of fear, anger, and being abandoned. Secluding a patient also has detrimental effects on nursing staff, who experience emotional distress and powerlessness (Mann-Poll et al., 2018).

Nurses decide to initiate and terminate the seclusion of patients according to established protocols and are involved in the care of patients during seclusion. The principle of seclusion is *containment*: restricting patients so that they do not hurt themselves or others, decreasing stimulation, and increasing intensive nursing care. Disruptive or inappropriate sexual behaviors are other reasons for seclusion. Seclusion is viewed as a preventive strategy to *avoid* aggressive assaults as well as a responsive action. Time out, closer supervision, quiet interactions, and medication are therapeutically effective when used appropriately for brief periods.

The degree of seclusion depends on the patient's current status. The patient who can choose time out voluntarily might be willing to stay in their room and talk about the distressing situation. Others may be escorted by two staff members without bodily contact to a seclusion room containing only a bed (bolted to the floor) and a mattress or just a mattress on the floor. This type of room decreases stimuli, protects the patient from injury, prevents destruction of property, and provides for the patient's privacy. The door, lockable from the outside, keeps the patient from leaving the room if needed. Dangerous articles (e.g., belts, sharp objects such as pens and keys, shoes, eyeglasses) are taken away from the patient.

Restraint

Restraint is a coercive measure used to prevent or restrict a patient's movement through human power or mechanical means when harm is imminent (Geoffrion et al., 2018). The staff must take immediate action when they assess that aggression is escalating. Six to eight staff members (including hospital security officers if insufficient unit staff members are available) are needed to control a patient *safely* and ensure that no injuries occur to the staff, patient, or other patients on the unit. The number of staff required should not be underestimated because of the patient's size, age, or gender. Some agencies include information about patients' previous athletic interests and accomplishments (e.g., weightlifting or a black belt in karate) on the admission form.

Details of restraint procedures, including therapeutic holds for children, are not described here, but a general outline is presented. To prepare for managing an aggressive patient, staff members remove their own glasses, rings, earrings, pins, watches, keys, and anything else that might cause injury to the patient or staff. Furniture and objects that can be used as weapons are removed from the area. One staff member becomes the team leader in organizing and directing the planned, coordinated approach, while the original staff member continues talking with the patient. At least one staff member takes the other patients to a safe place and stays with them.

The team approaches the patient calmly, in a "show of concern." The patient is told that the team is there to help, will not hurt the patient, and will not allow the patient to hurt anyone else. The nurse should inform the patient that although physical contact is employed as a last resort, the minimum amount of force will be used to ensure that everyone is safe. During physical contact, the team should continue to interact with the aggressive patient in such a manner as to cease physical contact at the first available opportunity. As two team members approach from each side and take control of the patient's arms, three other staff members quickly take control of the patient's legs and head so that the patient can be carried to the room or held on the floor until a bed is brought to the patient. Physical contact is protective and defensive, not aggressive. One staff member brings the restraint cuffs, opens doors, and moves obstacles. A nurse prepares the IM medication if needed.

In the seclusion room, the patient is usually placed on the bed on their back. Patients are placed in four-point restraint or two-point restraint as deemed necessary. As the name implies, four-point restraint is used to secure the wrists and ankles of a patient to a bed or stretcher, and just the wrists are secured in a two-point restraint (Jegede et al., 2017). The patients' privacy and dignity need to be maintained during restraint application. Four or more trained staff apply the physical restraints with one person at each extremity and one person at the head of the bed, being careful to avoid using excessive force or compromising the patient's ability to breathe (Roppolo et al., 2020). Wrist and ankle restraints are applied to extremities and secured to the frame of the bed. The restraints are tight enough to inhibit slipping out of them but not tight enough to interfere with circulation. The patient should be free of all belongings that might be used to cause harm to self or others. Medications might be administered at this time. A waist restraint or a restraint blanket (or any combination of these) is applied *only* if the patient is at risk of injury because of fighting the restraints. Before staff members leave, they check the patient for injuries and observe the patient for the ability to move safely in the restraints. Within 1 hour, an order to restrain the patient must be obtained, and a physician must perform a face-to-face evaluation of the patient. Federal, state, and hospital regulations or policies govern the extent to which the nurse and physician must evaluate the patient for the need to continue the restraints by the physician in a face-to-face examination and in the progress notes by the nurse and physician (Jegede et al., 2017).

Care of Patients in Seclusion or Restraints

When a patient is placed in seclusion or restraints, intensive nursing care is instituted. The patient is continuously observed directly or by a video monitor. Other patients are not allowed to be near a restrained patient. The patient's mental status, response to and side effects of medications, hydration, nutrition, elimination, range of motion, vital signs, and hygiene are monitored. Immediate attention to any injuries resulting from the incident or the restraints is critical and requires documentation. Every 2 hours, with two staff members present, the restraints are removed one at a time, for 10 minutes each, to allow range-of-motion activities. Change of position and skincare are also important. Restricting visitors, telephone calls, and diversional materials, such as radios and magazines, reduces stimuli; however, regular staff contact decreases the patient's sense of isolation and loneliness.

Recovery and Postcrisis Depression Phase

In this phase, patients are assured that they are not being punished while in seclusion and will be allowed back in the milieu as soon as possible. Patients must be assisted in relaxing, sleeping, and benefiting from this phase of cooling down and reconciliation. The time that patients are in restraints or seclusion should be a supportive, restorative time. Otherwise, patients remain afraid, frustrated, and angry, possibly leading to future aggression. After patients are calm, they are encouraged to discuss the circumstances of what happened to them from their perspective. They need to feel heard and understood without judgment or condescension. Plans are discussed about how the patient and nurse can handle similar situations differently in the future.

Patients are ready to be released from restraints when they can verbalize feeling less anxious and agitated and have an increased attention span, reality orientation, and sound judgment. Patients might be kept in the seclusion room briefly to assess their reaction to release from the restraints. Patients need assistance to reenter the unit with as little fear and embarrassment as possible. The nurse's role is to help other patients accept these patients back into the unit.

Immediately after a patient has been secluded and restrained, a code event review is initiated to ensure that no staff injuries have occurred, evaluate how the situation was handled, and give mutual support and feedback. This debriefing by staff involves focusing on the specifics of the event and the success of techniques used or not used. Data are collected, such as the patient's aggression level, response effectiveness, safety issues, and future recommendations. This review of events reinforces safety education and identifies areas for improvement (Goetz & Taylor-Trujillo, 2012). In addition, careful documentation must be recorded in the patient's chart to include the patient's behaviors before, during, and after the incident and a rationale for using physical control interventions, seclusion, and restraint. Staff perceptions are compared for accuracy. Documentation is descriptive, sequential, organized, and specific about what was seen, heard, and felt; what was said and by whom; who was notified; and what actions were taken and will be taken. The request for and granting of a physician's order for seclusion or restraint are also recorded.

Other patients' reactions to restraint and seclusion situations should be discussed openly and explored in a unit meeting with staff. The reasons for and the purpose of seclusion and restraint need to be discussed in a forthright and honest manner. Patients must have the opportunity to share their concerns, reactions, and fears and be reminded to approach staff if they begin feeling upset and angry. It is important for patients on the unit to know that the safety of all patients is the primary concern, not punishment or mere control of a patient's behavior. Although restraints and seclusion are sometimes necessary, they remain a method of last resort.

? CRITICAL THINKING QUESTION

2. Why is it important for other patients to share their opinions and reactions about the seclusion and restraint of a patient on the unit?

In light of these new philosophical changes, nurses often express concern and strong opinions when the topic of restraint reduction arises. Dahan and associates (2018) conducted a study to explore staff members' attitudes after they participated in the physical act of restraining a patient. Staff members who took part in restraining a patient were more focused on security and care and less focused on the patient's experience of feeling humiliated and offended. These findings reflect the conflicting feelings and attitudes of staff members about the use and need of restraints. Because staff and patient safety are perceived to be at risk, the idea of staff being discouraged from placing the patient in restraints may lead to nursing staff having a decreased sense of security in their environment. The barriers to restraint reduction are real and complex, requiring additional research and broad-based system change.

Making a change in the culture of safety on inpatient psychiatric units has been the subject of much research for years. There are two types of restraints—physical and chemical. Even though restraints are efficacious in the face of aggression and violence, their use has adverse psychological effects on both patients and staff. These two diametrically opposed dynamics represent the state of the current research on restraints (Jacob et al., 2016).

Blair and associates (2017) reported on a pilot study for reducing aggression and violence. The study consisted of multiple interventions: (1) frequent use of the Brøset Violence Checklist (BVC), (2) mandated staff education in crisis intervention and trauma-informed care, (3) increased frequency of physician re-assessment of the need for seclusion and restraint, (4) formal administrative review of all seclusion and restraint events, and (5) environmental enhancements, such as the use of comfort rooms. Staff education included a standardized 8-hour crisis intervention course that emphasized de-escalation techniques and a 2-day training program focused on a trauma-informed model of care to reduce nursing behaviors that can exacerbate "trauma reactions" in patients. The frequency of physician review was increased to every 2 hours. The Medical Director and the Director of Nursing examine all seclusion and restraint events. They conduct all reviews, the format for which included assessment of the patient (e.g., checklist scores, history of violence, medications prescribed), and the specific de-escalation interventions used during the event. The results of this study indicated a decrease in seclusion but did not significantly reduce the use of restraints.

McLoughlin and associates (2013) noted the need for more formal education in integrating de-escalation and the recovery model for nurses and patients. As expected, seasoned nurses are reluctant to incorporate recovery-oriented practices such as self-management and personal responsibility into acute psychiatric settings because of safety concerns. It may be more challenging to integrate recovery principles with children and adults who are displaying psychosis. Modification becomes necessary based on the individual's needs and circumstances. With patients who cannot make sound decisions related to their safety and well-being, it becomes the nurses' responsibility to do more for these individuals when they can do less and do less for the individuals when they can do more for themselves. Nurses must assess the situation continually and seek to empower individuals in their decision making as they move toward enhanced self-direction.

Although this chapter has focused on nursing interventions related to aggression and violence in acute psychiatric hospitals, aggressive behavior may occur in any setting, including medical and surgical units, nursing homes, community health settings, clinics, and especially emergency departments (Fernández-Costa et al., 2020).

The emergency department (ED) is one of the most vulnerable hospital environments for patient violence due to the high volume of acutely agitated patients who have the potential to escalate and exhibit verbal or physical assaults. Acute agitation is a symptom, like pain, with many potential etiologies that need to be investigated. The potential causes for acute agitation, particularly in the ED, may include physical disease (i.e., pain, withdrawal, hyperglycemia), panic, trauma, mania, psychosis, sensory or cognitive disturbances, and difficulty communicating needs. Even if a patient has a known history of psychiatric disorders, comorbid physical disease and other acute triggers should be ruled out (Gerson et al., 2019; Roppolo et al., 2020).

SUICIDE

Suicide occurs when individuals direct violence at themselves with the intent to end their lives, dying as a result of their actions. The issue of suicidality can be viewed on a continuum ranging from suicidal ideation to completed suicide. *Suicidal ideation* involves a person's thoughts and wishes related to wanting to die. Suicidal ideas may vary from relatively nonspecific thoughts that life is not worth living to specific thoughts of death, including intent and a plan. Threats, gestures, and attempts may accompany suicidal ideation. *Suicidal threats* involve an individual's declaration of intent to end their life. *Suicidal gestures* are coping strategies used by suicidal individuals; these nonlethal self-injury acts include cutting or burning the skin and ingesting small amounts of drugs. *Suicide attempts* are the actual implementation of a self-injurious act with the express purpose of ending one's life. Suicide attempts are considered self-destructive behavior severe enough to warrant medical contact. *Completed suicide* is the term used exclusively when individuals have successfully ended their lives. According to the CDC, in 2020, suicide was the 10th leading cause of death for all ages in the United States, the second leading cause of death for ages 10 to 34, and the fourth leading cause for ages 35 to 54 (Hedegaard et al., 2020).

All human beings periodically experience psychological burdens, pain, and stress during their lifetime, and having transient thoughts of wanting to die may be a natural response to emotional pain. Most people develop non-suicidal strategies for coping with the inevitable suffering in life; for some people, suicide becomes a solution to these overwhelming feelings. Intolerable psychological pain is an important predictor of suicidal thoughts and behavior. Amid the intolerable psychological pain, suicide can become a gripping and viable means of escape (Lear et al., 2018).

Suicidal behavior can be considered a problem-solving behavior reflecting a person's way of relating to the world. For example, an individual with HIV may consider suicidal behavior to enhance a sense of control over life. Fantasizing about the time, place, and method of one's death allows a person to feel a sense of escape from the suffering. Imagining the possibility of an escape may make it easier for the individual to carry on and endure emotional pain. Contemplation of suicide and suicidal gestures or attempts, once relinquished, often are met with a sense of relief. Suicide may serve several functions: (1) an escape, (2) a means of ensuring control, (3) a solution, and (4) a cry for help.

Shneidman, a suicidologist, coined the term *psychache* to describe the agony associated with suicidality. "Psychache is the hurt, anguish, or ache that takes hold in the mind. It is intrinsically psychological—the pain of excessively felt shame, guilt, fear, anxiety, loneliness, angst, dread of growing old or of dying badly… Suicide happens when the psychache is deemed unbearable, and death is actively sought to stop the unceasing flow of painful consciousness" (Shneidman, 1996). When suicidal individuals can no longer bear their pain and suffering, crisis intervention becomes necessary. For some individuals, hospitalization becomes the best choice for providing safety from harm.

Risk Factors

Chronic mental disorders most closely associated with risk for suicide include major depressive disorder, bipolar disorder, borderline personality disorder, posttraumatic stress disorder (PTSD), schizophrenia, and substance abuse. Medical illnesses, especially conditions associated with chronic pain, also increase suicide risk. A mental disorder diagnosis is considered to be the most reliable risk factor for committed suicides. More than 90% of individuals who attempt or commit suicide have a diagnosable psychiatric illness (Sher, 2019).

Suicide is one of the leading causes of premature death among individuals with schizophrenia and other psychotic disorders, occurring at a significantly greater rate than in the general population. Studies have reported that up to 50% of those suffering from schizophrenia experienced suicidal ideation and/or suicidal attempts at some time during their lives. Suicide risk factors in schizophrenia include depressive symptoms, frequent psychiatric admissions, male sex,

substance abuse, and onset at first psychotic break (Sher & Kahn, 2019). The negative contents of command hallucinations telling an individual to self-harm are significant risk factors for attempted suicide. Therefore, assessing for the presence of auditory hallucinations should be included when assessing these patients for suicide risk (Singh et al., 2016).

Veterans have typically had higher rates of suicide than the general population, and these rates have been increasing at an alarming rate since the early 2000s. It is estimated that in the United States, approximately 22 veterans die by suicide every day. Combat exposure increases the risk for suicide, as many soldiers experience emotional, physical, and medical health problems after deployment and discharge from service (Wood, Wood, Watson, Sheffield, & Hauter, 2020). Jobes (2013) suggested that one of the major obstacles to treatment of active soldiers is related to the Army culture; seeing a "shrink" is widely perceived as a "career ender." In addition, soldiers have access to lethal means, guns, and other weapons (Chu et al., 2016; Jobes, 2013) (see Box 21.1 for risk factors associated with suicide).

Suicide is the leading cause of death in psychiatric hospitals and is reportedly the most distressing event on an inpatient unit. Suicidality is one of the most common reasons for acute psychiatric hospital admissions and one of the most challenging clinical conditions facing mental health nurses. Ensuring patient safety is one of the primary purposes of psychiatric inpatient settings. Therefore, all patients in these settings should be assessed for suicide risk (Fosse et al., 2017; DeSantis et al., 2015). Environmental factors known to influence the occurrence of inpatient suicide include inadequate patient intake assessments, inadequate staffing levels, insufficient staff orientation and training, infrequent patient observations, inadequate communication, and patient assignment to inappropriate units. Hanging, suffocation, and jumping are the most frequent methods of suicide in inpatient settings. Exposed pipes, fire safety sprinkler heads, and curtain rods are all high-risk environmental hazards. Patient items such as belts, shoelaces, and drawstring pants are also potentially dangerous. Additional precautions to be employed on inpatient units to decrease the possibility of suicidal attempts are provided by The Joint Commission (Box 21.2).

BOX 21.1 Risk Factors Associated With Suicide

- History of trauma or abuse as a child
- History of prior suicide attempts
- Alcohol and drug abuse
- Family history of suicide
- Economic loss
- Bereavement
- Serious illness; physical or chronic pain
- Social isolation
- Access to lethal means
- Recent release from inpatient psychiatric hospitalization

BOX 21.2 The Joint Commission Tips for Preventing Inpatient Suicides

Environmental factors that mitigate inpatient suicides include the following:

- Breakaway bars, rods, showerheads
- Low-flushing toilets, weight-tested for safety
- Adequate visualization of high-risk areas
- Use of monitoring equipment
- Suicide risk assessments with psychometric properties
- Checking for contraband on admission
- Observation at frequency prescribed by risk
- Engagement of family and friends
- Identification of high-risk populations
- Prescribed observation checklist
- Consideration of staff assignment, including consideration of circadian rhythms, workloads, and time pressures
- Staff performance reviews and quality improvement protocols
- Provisions for shift change
- Using medications to treat conditions that contribute to risk

From Joint Commission on Accreditation of Healthcare Organizations. (2019). *Comprehensive accreditation manual for hospitals.* JCAHO.

HIGHLIGHTING THE EVIDENCE

In a phenomenological study, Shamsaei and associates (2020) offered insight into the suffering experienced by suicide attempt survivors. The authors found three prominent themes: mental pain, social challenges, and a need for love and belonging. A brief description of each theme follows:

Mental pain: Living with sadness and emptiness; feeling embarrassed and ashamed of the suicide attempt; feeling that the world (family) is better off without them

Social challenges: Lacking social connections, experiencing financial difficulties, and seeking out social support services

Need for love and belonging: Needing to feel understood, needing to experience empathy from others

Nursing Practice Implications: Patients may be admitted to an ED or acute psychiatric hospital following a suicide attempt. Recognizing the dynamics of what these patients are experiencing is helpful as nurses interact and seek to provide emotional care and support.

From Shamsaei, F., Yaghmaei, S., & Hghighi, M. (2020). Exploring the lived experiences of the suicide attempt survivors: A phenomenological approach. *International Journal of Qualitative Studies on Health and Well-being, 15*(1), 175478.

Assessment of Suicidal Patients

Patients being evaluated or treated for mental health conditions often experience suicidal ideation. The Joint Commission (2019) recommends that all patients treated for behavioral health conditions be evaluated with a validated suicide screening tool. Screening tools should be age-appropriate for the population to the extent possible. Examples of validated screening tools include the ED Safe Secondary Screener, the PHQ-9, the Patient Safety Screener, the TASR Adolescent Screener, the ASQ Suicide Risk Screening Tool, and the Columbia-Suicide Severity Rating Scale. Individuals identified as at risk for suicide require further assessment and steps to protect them from attempting suicide. Suicide assessments should be performed on admission and discharge and at frequent intervals as warranted (i.e., change in mental status, medication, or treatment protocol). A suicide risk assessment addresses suicidal thoughts, intent, plan, and lethality of a suicide plan.

A suicidal patient is fraught with conflicting thoughts and feelings, particularly ambiguity about the future. The more depressed and hopeless the patient, the more detailed the plan, the more lethal and accessible the method, the greater the likelihood that a suicidal attempt will be successful. In some cases, the impulsive behaviors of suicidal individuals experiencing ambiguous feelings about taking their own life can prove to be fatal. Intended and unintended death is more likely to occur when a more lethal method is utilized.

Suicide Interventions

The following general guidelines are useful for nurses who work with suicidal patients:

1. Developing the nurse-patient relationship built on trust and understanding is the most important component of positive patient outcomes. As trust is developed, the patient is more apt to reveal information vital to determining the likelihood of an imminent crisis related to suicidal ideation.
2. The first step in the assessment of potential suicidality is asking the patient about suicidal thoughts. Nurses ask directly about thoughts of suicide as part of the screening. Sample screening questions include: Have you had any thoughts about wanting to harm yourself? Have you felt like you don't want to live anymore? Identification of suicidal ideation allows nurses to focus on ensuring patient safety in light of the presence of self-harming cognitions.
3. If a patient endorses suicidal ideation, the nurse should ask about the plan (i.e., how the patient intends to accomplish the suicide). Patients who share a well-developed plan with intent and means are considered at increased risk for suicide attempts and suicide completion.
   a. Ask the patient directly if they intend to commit suicide and the means they would use to end their life.
   b. Lethality associated with suicidality is related to accessibility—the means to commit suicide.
   c. If a patient mentions using a gun, family members should be notified either to remove any firearms from home entirely or to lock guns and ammunition securely in two separate locations.
   d. If the patient mentions overdosing on drugs, the same recommendations are applied to restricting access to

potentially lethal prescriptions, over-the-counter medications, and alcohol.

4. When asking a patient about a suicidal plan, it is important for the nurse to understand the following:

   a. Talking to patients about their suicidal intentions does not drive them to suicide. Asking patients direct questions elicits useful information and may provide patients with a sense of relief (e.g., "Finally, someone hears me").

   b. Many people who have died due to suicide did not mean to die; they tragically miscalculated. Many people who die as a result of suicide do so accidentally.

5. Previous attempts are known to be a risk factor associated with suicide. It is essential to ask the patient about previous suicide attempts.

   a. The nurse should ask about the method of the previous attempt.

   b. The nurse should ask how the patient was rescued.

   c. The nurse should ask about the patient's response to treatment and follow-up care.

6. Patients should be evaluated for major depressive symptoms, recent losses, alcohol or drug abuse, and command hallucinations, all of which place individuals at an increased risk for suicide.

7. The nurse should communicate openness and acceptance of the suicidal patient's feelings and life situation. The nurse should encourage exploration and open expression of suicidal feelings, allowing patients to understand their problems better within an emotionally safe nurse-patient relationship.

8. Close observation, also called *one-to-one observation*, is the standard of care for patients experiencing suicidal thoughts, severe anxiety, and agitation. Suicidal patients on inpatient psychiatric units are regularly assessed using one of two levels of suicide prevention:

   a. Frequent observation (sometimes referred to as *level 1*) is used for patients who are not considered at immediate risk of attempting suicide. The nursing staff provides periodic observation (every 15 minutes) and monitors drug-taking, eating utensils, shaving gear, and other potentially dangerous devices in the environment. The staff communicates concern and control with this close observation of patients and their environment. Patients are asked to seek out a staff member should they begin to contemplate self-injurious behavior. Although still utilized, having patients sign a no-suicide contract has not been found to deter harmful behavior. Suicidal patients who are admitted to an inpatient unit commonly start to feel better almost immediately. As a result of the safe environment provided, patients may deny having suicidal thoughts shortly after admission. Simply having a structured, safe environment can diminish feelings of

---

◎ CARE PLAN

A 23-year-old man diagnosed with schizophrenia, paranoid type, has been admitted to a psychiatric hospital because of command hallucinations telling him to kill himself. The patient lives with his mother, who does not feel confident in her ability to keep her son from harming himself. How might nursing care assist this patient and family?

Assessment

Problems:

1. Patient admits to auditory hallucinations commanding him to kill himself.
2. Patient is easily agitated and increasingly paranoid.
3. Patient tends to isolate in his room.
4. Patient is religiously preoccupied.
5. Patient is logical, linear, organized, and coherent.
6. Patient can contract for suicide while hospitalized but not after discharge.
7. Patient denies substance abuse and dependence.

Diagnosis   Risk for suicide related to command hallucinations commanding him to kill himself.

Outcomes   **Short-term goals**

Date met: _____   Patient will explore suicidal thoughts with staff.

Date met: _____   Patient will contract for safety with nurse every shift.

Date met: _____   Patient will connect suicidal thoughts to current stressors.

Long-term goals:

Date met: _____   Patient will report ability to manage suicidal thoughts.

Date met: _____   Patient will participate in follow-up individual and family psychotherapy.

Planning and   **Nurse-patient relationship:** Assess for presence of suicidal ideation. Assess severity of suicidality,
Interventions   asking patient about intent and plan related to suicidal thoughts. Contract for safety every shift. Allow patient to share feelings such as hopelessness, helplessness, shame, and despair. Assist patient in connecting suicidal thoughts to current stressors.

Psychopharmacology: Paliperidone (Invega) 12 mg PO every morning; discuss role of medications and related side effects.

Milieu management: Continuous observation with restrictions, such as confinement on the unit. Keep environment free of harmful objects. Encourage patient to spend time in day room interacting with other patients. Collaborate with patient in ongoing treatment plan.

helplessness and hopelessness. As patients are removed from their stressful situations and have the opportunity to interact with caring mental health professionals, they have the opportunity to think more clearly and feel some relief. However, the nurse must understand that maintaining a safe environment is the primary cause of the patient's more positive feelings and thinking. Frequent observation and other safety measures should be continued even when a patient no longer endorses suicidal ideation while hospitalized.

  b. Continuous observation (sometimes referred to as *level 2*) is used for patients who present an immediate and serious threat of suicidal behavior. In level 2, uninterrupted observation is typically required. This approach is an expensive use of human resources but provides the needed environmental, emotional, and behavioral support. Patients at serious risk are usually confined to the unit, have restrictions on visitors, take meals, and have bathroom supervision.

Research studies provide evidence that a patient's risk for suicide is high after discharge from acute psychiatric inpatient or emergency department settings (Forte et al. 2019). It is important to develop a safety plan with the patient and provide the number of crisis call centers before discharge. Continuity of care is best provided through careful and thoughtful patient and family discharge planning:

- Explain the uneven recovery path from their illness, especially depression (e.g., "There are likely to be times when you feel worse and times when you will feel better. Contact our health care clinician if you start having difficulty dealing with your depressive thoughts").
- Teach the patient and family about the signs of increased suicide risk, especially sleep disturbance, anxiety, agitation, and suicidal expressions and behaviors.
- Document if the patient does not wish to permit contact with family.
- Provide information for a follow-up appointment, which may include contacting the current provider or scheduling an appointment.
- If the presence of firearms has been identified, document safety instructions given to patient and significant others.
- Provide prescriptions that allow for a reasonable supply of medication to last until the first follow-up appointment (when indicated).
- Provide information about local mental health resources with contact information.

Evidence-based therapies for suicidal patients include dialectical behavior therapy (DPT) and cognitive therapy for suicide prevention (CBT-SP). The goal of individual therapy is to instill a new set of targets that focus on (1) radical acceptance of one's past, present, and realistic limitations on the future; and (2) skills to tolerate distress without impulsivity or destructively reducing it (Linehan & Wilks, 2015). Most importantly, infusing a sense of hopefulness is essential for those facing suicidality. Hope is the crucial ingredient needed to replace suicidal tendencies with an active pursuit of life with purpose and meaning (Jobes, 2013).

? CRITICAL THINKING QUESTION

3. What positive and negative effects can an inpatient hospitalization have on a patient's emotional recovery?

BURNOUT AND SECONDARY TRAUMATIZATION

Burnout is highly prevalent among mental healthcare clinicians, the highest among medical specialties. Burnout has been associated with physical and psychological problems in nurses (Eliacin et al., 2018). The daily stress of dealing with patients with emotional and behavioral problems can be taxing for nursing staff caring for patients in acute psychiatric hospitals. Psychiatric nurses must manage violent and suicidal patients, yet they are charged with keeping the environment safe for all patients and staff. This negative workplace experience results in negative feelings, such as fear and anxiety. Stressors such as these take their toll on the nurse in the form of burnout (also known as *emotional exhaustion*), secondary traumatization, and PTSD.

Burnout is a psychological experience caused by long-term involvement in emotionally demanding situations. Although a subjective phenomenon, burnout has a clear relationship with the organizational setting in which it occurs. It is a process that involves intense emotional labor leading to symptoms such as emotional exhaustion (i.e., a sense of feeling overwhelmed by workplace demands), depersonalization (i.e., developing cynical attitudes toward job and clients served), and reduced personal achievement (i.e., feeling like their job doesn't make a difference) (Eliacin et al., 2018). Once burnout begins, it will have an impact on job performance, perhaps leading to low morale, disinterest, avoidance, complaining, and adverse reactions to others. The human tendency toward burnout is juxtaposed with the high level of professionalism expected of psychiatric nurses. This tendency leads to a spiraling process of decreased effectiveness in nurse-patient interactions at all levels so that assistance may be required (Box 21.3).

In recent decades, increased attention has been given to the effects of trauma on individuals. The professional literature related to working with trauma revealed the phenomenon of vicarious traumatization, also called *secondary traumatization, helper stress,* or *compassion fatigue.* Secondary traumatization consists of cognitive and behavioral symptoms in

---

BOX 21.3   Resources for Burnout

It is important that nurses seek out assistance for preventing and recovering from burnout. Examples of professional resources include Dr. Vidette Todaro-Franceschi's book, *Compassion Fatigue and Burnout in Nursing: Enhancing Professional Quality of Life* (Springer Publishing Company, 2019) and the American Nurses Association (http://www.nursingworld.org). Involvement in one's professional association can be an excellent resource for new and experienced nurses.

the nurse due to exposure to patients' suffering. The nurse's vulnerability to the client's traumatic experience evokes an emotional response within the nurse. Exposure to the clients' experience of suffering is a direct result of the nurse's empathic presence. The development of secondary traumatization impacts how the nurse experiences self, others, and the world. Secondary traumatization is the "cost of caring" for those in emotional pain. (Hubbard et al., 2017).

Being injured by a patient is similar emotionally to being a victim of crime and can lead to PTSD. Experiencing physical and emotional harm at the workplace can destroy the staff member's sense of trust in others and sense of control of their life. The staff member often expresses guilt, vulnerability, irritability, depression, anxiety, nightmares, grief, and fear of the patient who caused the injury. The assault might be minimized, and feelings might be denied if emotional support and debriefing are not provided after the medical examination and treatment have been completed. If the injured staff member is away from work for a while, the rest of the staff might be unaware that their emotions have subsided much more than the emotions of their injured colleague. To ensure that the staff victim achieves an emotional resolution of the incident, supportive interventions should be available (Hubbard et al., 2017). Peer support programs that understand the dynamics of assault and the typical responses of victims are important. The needs of the victim determine the type of support and counseling initiated and maintained. In addition, victims are encouraged to share their feelings with family or significant others. This process aims to facilitate emotional resolution, help the person remain productive, and decrease the chance of resignation and development of PTSD. More research is needed that focuses on the cumulative effects of vicarious traumatization, coupled with direct trauma and violence, on inpatient psychiatric nursing staff.

CLINICAL SUPERVISION FOR PSYCHIATRIC NURSES

Clinical supervision is one intervention known to assist psychiatric nurses who experience high-stress levels associated with the overwhelming responsibility of caring for patients and families with complex and difficult mental health care needs. This stress management strategy helps nurses to avoid burnout and job-related stress. Clinical supervision provides a structured mechanism of allowing nurses to reflect on their day-to-day practices and validate their complex and challenging clinical decisions. As psychiatric nurses are provided an opportunity to examine their attitudes, reactions, and conflicts with patients, they find new ways of approaching patient problems. Activities such as clinical supervision also help nurses develop sensitivity to the patient.

Clinical supervision is recognized as a vital component of modern, effective psychiatric care. Traditionally, mental health care professions have an established culture of clinical supervision. For example, clinical social workers consider supervision to be essential for sustaining reflective practice. Clinical supervision is defined as a formal relationship-based education and training that is work-focused. Supervisors aim to manage, support, develop, and evaluate the work of supervisees through corrective feedback. Supervision differs from related activities such as mentoring and coaching. Although psychiatric nursing employs a form of clinical supervision, the manner practiced by other mental health professions remains more of an aspiration than a reality. Clinical supervision within the nursing arena is most frequently seen as part of management, rather than properly regarded as nonhierarchical, nonjudgmental, and focused on the nurse (supervisee) rather than the organization. The benefits of supervision serve to clarify values, promote self-awareness, provide a role model, evaluate best practices in health care, and protect against burnout. Good supervision contributes to general well-being, knowledge, confidence, morale, understanding, and job satisfaction.

Clinical supervision is used not only to address the emotional impact of patient encounters but also to examine issues within the team and the broader workplace setting. Two approaches to supervision are equally effective: one-to-one sessions and group meetings. Clinical supervision, done properly, provides a checks-and-balances system built to promote professional development that ultimately benefits the nurse, the patients, and the rest of the nursing staff. Research shows that this type of organizational support to nurses translates into improved patient outcomes.

EFFECTIVE FUNCTIONING IN THE ACUTE PSYCHIATRIC SETTING

At the close of this chapter, discussing the new era of psychiatric care is in order.

In light of the high patient acuity seen in psychiatric hospitals, current practices continue to rely on medications, seclusion and restraints, rapid turnover, and a revolving door. As previously mentioned, recovery-oriented care is a patient-led and family-led initiative that emphasizes collaboration between patients and providers to ensure that treatment respects patients' preferences and perspectives. This influential movement is expected to continue to play a pivotal role in restructuring mental health services in the future. Because nurses are educated to provide holistic patient-centered care, they may find themselves trapped between the medical model and recovery principles. Psychiatric nurses are weighed down by administrative, technical, and crisis tasks that take them away from collaborating with and empowering patients. This conflict can lead to burnout for nurses and other hospital staff. More recently, efforts have taken place to reconcile the divergent approaches of mental health care personnel and consumers (individuals diagnosed with mental disorders). Organizational changes are needed, such as inviting consumers to serve on boards of mental health care facilities to be a part of the review process for state-funded agencies.

STUDY NOTES

1. An increase in patient acuity and a more rapid turnover in admissions and discharges in psychiatric hospitals creates stress for staff members and patients.
2. The assault cycle describes the predictable phases of aggression: triggering, escalation, crisis, recovery, and depression.
3. Verbal and physical aggression requires safe, immediate interventions based on the principle of the least restrictive alternative.
4. Tension reduction, medications, physical control, seclusion, and restraints are to be used judiciously in the escalation and crisis phases of the assault cycle.
5. Patients in seclusion and restraints require intensive physical and emotional nursing care.
6. Suicide is a complex issue—a spectrum ranging from ideation to completed suicide.
7. Identifying patients at imminent risk for suicide in the inpatient setting is a critical clinical challenge.
8. The nurse needs to communicate openness and acceptance of the suicidal patient's feelings and life situation.
9. Open expression of suicidal feelings allows patients to understand their problems better within an emotionally safe nurse-patient relationship.
10. Hopelessness, meaninglessness, and feeling out of control are common emotions associated with suicidal ideation.
11. Caring for aggressive and suicidal patients continuously can lead to burnout and secondary traumatization.
12. Clinical supervision for nursing staff can be a tool to facilitate emotional support for nurses, improve morale, and increase the nurse's ability to maintain therapeutic relationships with patients.
13. Recovery-oriented care has influenced treatment settings by providing feedback to staff about the patient's perspective of the treatment environment.

REFERENCES

Al-Maraira, O., Hayajneh, F., & Shehadeh, J. (2019). Psychiatric staff attitudes toward coercive measures: An experimental design. *Perspective in Psychiatric Care, 55*(4), 734–742. https://doi.org/10.1111/ppc.12422.

American Nurses Association. http://www.nursingworld.org.

Blair, E., Woolley, S., Szarek, B., & Mucha, T. (2017). Reduction of seclusion and restraint in inpatient psychiatric setting: A pilot study. *Psychiatric Quarterly, 88*(1), 1–7. https://doi.org/10.1007/s11126-016-9428-0.

Campbell, V., Foley, H., Vianna, K., & Brunger, F. (2019). Folie du système? Preventing violence against nurses in in-patient psychiatry. *Psychiatric Quarterly, 90*, 413–420. https://doi.org/10.1007/s11126-019-09636-1.

Chu. C., et al. (2016). The interactive effects of the capability for suicide and major depressive episodes on suicidal behavior in a military sample. *Cognitive Therapy and Research, 40*, 22–30. https://doi.org/10.1007/s10608-015-9727-z.

Dahan, S., Levi, G., Behrbalk, P., & Bronstein, I. (2018). The impact of 'being there': Psychiatric staff attitudes on the use of restraint. *Psychiatric Quarterly, 89*, 191–199. https://doi.org/10.1007/s11126-017-9524-9.

DeSantis, M., Myrick, H., Lamis, D., & Pelic, C. (2015). Suicide-specific safety in the inpatient psychiatric unit. *Issues in Mental Health Nursing, 36*(3), 190–199. https://doi.org/10.3109/01612840.2014.961625.

Dickens. G., Piccirillo. M., & Alderman., N. (2013). Causes and management of aggression and violence in a forensic mental health service: Perspectives of nurses and patients. *International Journal of Mental Health Nursing, 22*(6), 532–544. https://doi.org/10.1111/j.1447-0349.2012.00888.x.

Eliacin, J., Flanagan, M., Monroe-DeVita, M., & Wasmuth, S. (2018). Social capital and burnout among mental healthcare providers. *Journal of Mental Health, 27*(5), 388–394. https://doi.org/10.1080/09638237.2017.1417570.

Fernández-Costa, D., Gómez-Salgado, J., Fagundo-Rivera, J., Martín-Pereira, J., Prieto-Callejero, B., & García-Iglesias, J. J. (2020). Alternatives to the use of mechanical restraints in the management of agitation or aggressions of psychiatric patients: A scoping review. *Journal of Clinical Medicine, 9*(9), 2791. https://doi.org/10.3390/jcm9092791.

Forte, A., Buscajoni, A., & Fiorillo, A. (2019). Suicide risk following hospital discharge: A review. *Harvard Review of Psychiatry, 27*(4), 209–216. https://doi.org/10.1097/HRP.0000000000000222.

Fosse, R., Ryberg, W., Carlsson, M., & Hammer, J. (2017). Predictors of suicide in the patient population admitted to a locked-door psychiatric acute ward. *PLoS ONE, 12*(3), 1–13. https://doi.org/10.1371/journal.pone.0173958.

Geoffrion, S., Concalves, J., Giguerre, C., & Guay, S. (2018). Impact of a program for the management of aggressive behaviors on seclusion and restraint use in two high-risk units of a mental health institute. *Psychiatric Quarterly, 89*, 95–102. https://doi.org/10.1007/s11126-017-9519-6.

Gerson, R., Malas, N., Feuer, V., Silver, G. H., Prasad, R., & Mroczkowski, M. M. (2019). Best practices for evaluation and treatment of agitated children and adolescents (BETA) in the emergency department: Consensus statement of the American Association for Emergency Psychiatry. *The Western Journal of Emergency Medicine, 20*(2), 409–418. https://doi.org/10.5811/westjem.2019.1.41344.

Goetz, S. B., & Taylor-Trujillo, A. (2012). A change in culture: Violence prevention in an acute behavioral health setting. *Journal of the American Psychiatric Nurses Association, 18*, 96. https://doi.org/10.1177/1078390312439469.

Hedegaard, H., Curtin, S., & Warner, M. (2020). Increase in suicide mortality in the United States, 1999-2018. *NCHS Data Brief, 362*, 1–7. https://www.cdc.gov/nchs/data/databriefs/db362-h.pdf.

Jacob. T., et al. (2016). Patterns of restraint utilization in a community hospital's psychiatric inpatient units. *Psychiatric Quarterly, 87*, 31–48. https://doi.org/10.1007/s11126-015-9353-7.

Jegede, O., Ahmed, S., Olupona, T., & Akerele, E. (2017). Restraints utilization in a psychiatric emergency room. *International Journal of Mental Health*, 46(2), 125–132. https://doi.org/10.1080/00207411.2017.1295781.

Jobes. D. A. (2013). Reflections on suicide among soldiers. *Psychiatry: Interpersonal and Biological Processes*, 76(2), 126–131. https://doi.org/10.1521/psyc.2013.76.2.126.

The Joint Commission. (2019). *R3 Report Issue 18: National patient safety goals for suicide prevention.* https://www.jointcommission.org/standards/r3-report/r3-report-issue-18-national-patient-safety-goal-for-suicide-prevention/.

Lear, M., Stacy, S., & Pepper, C. (2018). Interpersonal needs and psychological pain: The role of brooding and rejection sensitivity. *Death Studies*, 42(8), 521–528. https://doi.org/10.1080/07481187.2017.1393029.

Linehan, M., & Wilks, C. (2015). The course and evolution of dialectical behavior therapy. *American Journal of Psychotherapy*, 69(2), 97–110. https://doi.org/10.1176/appi.psychotherapy.2015.69.2.97.

Liu. S., et al. (2015). Cumulative contribution of child maltreatment to emotional experiences and regulatory intent in intimate adult interactions. *Journal of Aggression, Maltreatment & Trauma*, 24(6), 636–655. https://doi.org/10.1080/10926771.2015.1049768.

Lykke, J., Hjorthoj, C., Thomsen, C., & Austin, S. (2020). Prevalence, predictors, and patterns of mechanical restraint use for inpatients with dual diagnosis. *Perspectives in Psychiatric Care*, 56(1), 20–27. https://doi.org/10.1111/ppc.12367.

Mann-Poll, P., Smit, A., Noorthoorn, E., & Janssen, W. (2018). Long-term impact of a tailored seclusion reduction program: Evidence for change? *Psychiatric Quarterly*, 89, 733–746. https://doi.org/10.1007/s11126-018-9571-x.

McLoughlin. K. A., et al. (2013). Recovery-oriented practices of psychiatric-mental health nursing staff in an acute hospital setting. *Journal of the American Psychiatric Nurses Association*, 19, 1. https://doi.org/10.1177/1078390313490025.

Parrish. E. (2019). Violence against nurses: Increased awareness. *Perspectives in Psychiatric Care*, 55(2), 139. https://doi.org/10.1111/ppc.12378.

Roppolo, L.P., Morris, D.W., Khan, F., Downs, R., Metzger, J., Carder, T., Wilson, M.P. (2020). Improving the management of acutely agitated patients in the emergency department through implementation of Project BETA (Best Practices in the Evaluation and Treatment of Agitation). *Journal of the American College of Emergency Physicians Open*, 1(5), 898–907. https://doi.org/10.1002/emp2.12138.

Shamsaei, F., Yaghmaei, S., & Hghighi, M. (2020). Exploring the lived experiences of the suicide attempt survivors: A phenomenological approach. *International Journal of Qualitative Studies in Health and Well-being*, 15(1), 1745478. https://doi.org/10.1080/17482631.2020.1745478.

Sher. L. (2019). Resilience as a focus of suicide research and prevention. *Acta Psychiatrica Scandinavica*, 140(2), 169–180. https://doi.org/10.1111/acps.13059.

Sher, L., & Kahn, R. (2019). Family interventions and prevention of suicide in first episode schizophrenia. *Acta Psychiatrica Scandinavica*, 139(5), 484. https://doi.org/10.1111/acps.13018.

Shneidman. E. (1996). *The suicidal mind.* Oxford University Press.

Singh, H., Chandra, P., & Reddi, V. (2016). Clinical correlates of suicide in suicidal patients with schizophrenia spectrum disorders and affective disorders. *Indian Journal of Psychological Medicine*, 38(6), 517–523. https://doi.org/10.4103/0253-7176.194910.

Smith. P. (1981). Empirically based models for viewing the dynamics of violence. In K. Babich (Ed.), *Assessing patient violence in the health care setting.* Western Interstate Commission for Higher Education.

Spinzy, Y., Marei, S., Segev, A., & Cohen-Rappaport, G. (2018). Listening to the patient's perspective: Psychiatric inpatients attitudes toward physical restraint. *Psychiatric Quarterly*, 89, 691–696. https://doi.org/10.1007/s11126-018-9565-8.

Todaro-Franceschi. V. (2019). *Compassion fatigue and burnout in nursing: Enhancing professional quality of life.* Springer Publishing Company.

Veale. D., et al. (2015). A new therapeutic community: Development of a compassion-focused and contextual behavioral environment. *Clinical Psychology & Psychology*, 22(4), 285–303. https://doi.org/10.1002/cpp.1897.

Wood, D., Wood, B., Watson, A., Sheffield, D., & Hauter, H. (2020). Veteran suicide risk factors: A national sample of nonveterans and veteran men who died by suicide. *Health & Social Work*, 45(1), 23–30. https://doi.org/10.1093/hsw/hlz037.

22

Therapeutic Environment in Various Treatment Settings

Debbie Steele

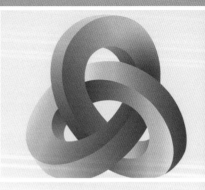

http://evolve.elsevier.com/Keltner

LEARNING OBJECTIVES

- Describe the various treatment activities used in the following inpatient psychiatric settings:
  Intensive care or acute psychiatric units (locked units)
  Child-adolescent psychiatric units
  Acute substance abuse units
  Co-occurring disorders units
  Medical-psychiatric units
  Geropsychiatric units

  State psychiatric hospitals
  State forensic hospitals
- Describe the treatment environment of community psychiatric settings, including:
  Group homes
  Partial hospitalization
  Day treatment centers

Inpatient and outpatient psychiatric treatment centers provide a multitude of unique needs for patients with mental disorders. The therapeutic environment is enhanced through the use of various structured activities arranged by a multidisciplinary team. In this chapter, key activities are described, along with an explanation of the various inpatient and outpatient treatment settings.

INPATIENT SETTINGS

Treatment Activities

The following types of therapeutic activities are offered in psychiatric settings in both inpatient and outpatient environments: (1) occupational therapy, (2) recreational therapy, (3) psychoeducation, (4) group therapy, (5) spirituality groups,

NORM'S NOTES I have mentioned the importance of the environment, but as I noted in Chapter 1, one size does not fit all. How can you apply these concepts to different types of settings? Does it even matter? Both answers are "yes." You can't get away from your environment, and the people under your care can't get away from their environment. This chapter provides some ideas about how the concept of environmental manipulation can foster a therapeutic atmosphere in many diverse settings. What might be therapeutic in one setting might not be therapeutic in another.

and (6) community meetings. Many different disciplines are involved in enhancing the effectiveness of the therapeutic modalities offered to patients in the recovery process.

Occupational Therapy

Occupational therapists are trained professionals concerned with the functional abilities of patients, as these abilities affect their capacity to work and perform tasks of daily living (Noyes, Sokolow, & Arbesman, 2018). In general, occupational therapists work with mental health patients to build functional life skills, develop job skills, improve social participation, and pursue leisure activities. Occupational therapists practice in acute psychiatric hospitals, state hospitals, forensic hospitals, partial hospital programs, and as community case managers. In acute psychiatric hospitals, the emphasis is on assessment and assisting patients with problem-solving skills. Arts and crafts, games, sports, and gym activities may be supervised by occupational therapists. In partial hospital programs, occupational and educational issues may be the target of intervention. Occupational therapists who work in community settings provide life skills, coping mechanisms, and training to improve patients' performance and participation in employment and educational endeavors (Stoffel, Reed, & Brown, 2019). Specific therapy approaches and classes are selected by occupational therapists and patients based on a functional assessment of patients' strengths and challenges (Lannigan et al., 2019).

Recreational Therapy

Leisure time is important for all individuals and is useful in promoting mental health. For the psychiatric patient, recreational activities are an important intervention in meeting treatment outcomes. Recreational therapists and occupational therapists assist patients in finding activities that help them learn to balance work and play. Individualized plans of care may involve exercise groups, such as aerobics or strength training. The level and type of exercise are determined by the abilities of the patient. The benefits of exercise in modulating depression and anxiety have been well documented. Exercise therapy is also a therapeutic outlet for agitation and aggression.

HIGHLIGHTING THE EVIDENCE

The Wellness Recovery Action Plan (WRAP) is an evidence-based approach to group therapy that is consistent with recovery-oriented care. WRAP can be used in various mental health settings by certified peer specialists or other staff. The WRAP approach is designed to help patients create their own plan of care for staying well through a process of (1) decreasing and preventing intrusive or troubling behaviors and thoughts, (2) increasing personal empowerment, (3) improving quality of life, and (4) assisting individuals in achieving their own life goals and dreams (Copeland, n.d.). Pratt, MacGregor, Reid, & Given, 2013 conducted a study on the WRAP approach in Scotland. The authors found that WRAP groups offered participants information about the concept of recovery that most had not heard before, leading some participants to develop a useful, powerful new perspective of their experience. Participants described feeling that they were capable of taking ownership of their own well-being for the first time. As stated by one participant, "WRAP offers a reminder of what you are like when you are well, and that offered hope and uncovered strategies for overcoming challenges when encountering an episode of illness" (p. 7).

Psychoeducation

Psychoeducation is a combination of education, cognitive-behavior therapy, and group therapy. The intent is to provide the patient and family information about the mental illness, including its treatment. The goal is fourfold: (1) enhance patient competence, (2) provide insight into the mental disorder, (3) promote relapse prevention, and (4) prevent suicide and other crises (Sarkhel et al., 2020). Psychoeducation involves interaction and clarification on a number of issues, including interpersonal, social, biological, and pharmacological perspectives. The goal of psychoeducation is to provide social support and assist patients in their adaptation to living with a chronic illness. Empirical evidence has shown that understanding mental illness helps patients and their families cope more positively with the illness. Numerous studies have demonstrated the value of psychoeducation groups in reducing relapse and rehospitalization rates, promoting medication use, improving quality of life and social functioning, and altering negative family reactions

(Economou, 2015). Passley-Clarke (2019) reported on the benefits of nurses teaching patients about illness management and the recovery model in acute psychiatric hospitals; findings indicated that patients reported insight into how to improve their mental health as well as decreased readmissions on the inpatient unit.

Based on the target population and setting, psychoeducation can be individual, family, group, or community based. Because families often assume much of the care burden for patients with chronic mental illness, the inclusion of family members in psychoeducational groups is essential (Lucksted et al., 2013; Onwumere, Grice, & Kuipers, 2016; Tsiouri, 2015). Box 22.1 lists examples of topics appropriate for psychoeducational groups (Sarkhel et al., 2020). Theoretically, any member of the treatment team could offer psychoeducational groups, and in many cases, the psychiatric nurse uses this format for patient and family teaching, particularly in preparation for discharge.

Group Therapy

Group therapy is a beneficial and effective treatment option employed in many psychiatric settings. Groups are a cost-effective method of promoting social interaction and access to psychotherapeutic interventions. The many benefits associated with group therapy include: (1) an opportunity to address issues with input from others (gain new insight, knowledge, and perspective), (2) feeling of acceptance and a sense of belonging, and (3) being accountable to a group of people with similar struggles (Radcliffe & Bird, 2016). Group therapy is a type of therapeutic environment of its own because it uses many of the important principles known to benefit patients with psychiatric disorders, such as openness, giving and receiving feedback, respect, privacy, acceptance, interdependence, and individual responsibility. Group therapy is an important part of hospitalized patients' therapeutic experiences, even during short stays. Group therapy may be more effective when members are in a community group over a long period of time, allowing some of the unique curative factors of group work to develop.

BOX 22.1 Examples of Topics for Psychoeducational Groups

- Recognizing signs of relapse
- Need for individual and family psychotherapy
- Need for social support
- Coping with stress
- Understanding triggers and emotions
- Symptoms of specific mental illnesses
- Managing medications and side effects
- Suicide prevention
- Knowing when to seek help
- Getting along with family members
- Returning to work
- Anger management
- Interpersonal skills
- Living skills

Groups can be formatted in many ways: open or closed, process-oriented or psychoeducational, time-limited or ongoing. The type of group therapy depends on the purpose intended. For example, process-oriented groups may address such issues as isolation and anxiety. Box 22.2 lists the various types of group therapy practiced in psychiatric settings. Group therapy is applicable to the full spectrum of mental disorders, including child, adult, and elderly populations.

Support Groups

The National Alliance of Mental Illness (NAMI) has peer-led support groups for any adult who is in recovery of a mental health disorder, as well as family support groups for the loved ones of those experiencing mental health issues. Members of the group gain insight from the challenges and successes of others facing similar experiences (NAMI National Alliance of Mental Illness, n.d.).

HIGHLIGHTING THE EVIDENCE

Current Research

In a study by Florensa, Keliat, Wardani, and Suliotiowati (2019), cognitive behavioral group therapy (CBGT) and family psychoeducation (FPE) were utilized in the treatment of adolescents experiencing depression and anxiety. The result indicated that peer support through CBGT, as well as teaching caregivers about mental illness, were effective in increasing self-esteem and reducing anxiety and prodromal early psychosis symptoms in adolescents.

Spirituality Groups

Spirituality, religion, and faith can help patients and family members find meaning and cope with mental health disorders. Some turn to spirituality in times of crisis or to help them manage their recovery process (NAMI National Alliance of Mental Illness, n.d.). Although spirituality groups are not typically offered in psychiatric treatment settings, The Joint Commission has standards requiring the assessment and interdisciplinary planning for the spiritual concerns and needs of patients. A chaplain or other mental health professional conducts these groups; the focus of these groups is usually on topics such as forgiveness, grieving, and finding meaning in life. During the group meetings, the group leader encourages the patients to be present with one another and share stories, beliefs, spiritual journeys, suffering, and acceptance. An important overall goal of the spirituality group is to help patients in their personal quest for spiritual, emotional, and relational growth and healing. As patients grow spiritually, they find increased strength and power to help them cope with and overcome the problems and challenges in their lives. Patients vary in their response to these groups, but they seem to respond well to a non-directive approach that involves unconditional positive regard, empathy, and congruence.

Community Meetings

Community meetings provide a forum for addressing the daily needs associated with community living and may take place in an inpatient or community setting. For example, a halfway house may have daily morning meetings to welcome new residents, review program rules, and make general announcements about the day's activities. Community meetings allow patients to initiate discussions of community or individual concern and receive feedback from staff and other patients. Patient-patient and patient-staff conflicts may occur, requiring a skilled group leader to assist the involved individuals in handling the situation in a positive fashion. Common patient-patient concerns involve control of the television, the radio being played too loudly, and personal hygiene (e.g., someone is not bathing regularly). Community meetings are not forums for discussing the individual treatment needs and issues of patients; rather, they serve to address daily aspects of being in the treatment environment.

Inpatient Psychiatric Environments

This section provides an overview of the various inpatient treatment environments available to patients with mental health disorders. Each of these therapeutic settings focus on a particular population with unique needs. The various activities described earlier in the chapter play an integral role in the structure of these therapeutic environments.

Intensive Care or Acute Psychiatric Units (Locked Units)

Acute psychiatric units provide 24-hour structured inpatient treatment within a locked setting. Treatment emphasis is on short-term, intense therapeutic interventions designed to provide the patient with rapid evaluation and stabilization of symptoms. Criteria for admission to an acute psychiatric unit includes danger to self, danger to others, and gravely disabled. Patients may be admitted on either a voluntary or an involuntary basis. The severity of patients' illnesses tends to be quite high, requiring close supervision and intervention by nursing staff. The presenting problems include acute and severe or persistent mental illnesses, organic brain syndrome, detoxification from alcohol or drugs, acute situational or emotional distress, suicide threats or attempts, and medication adjustments. Staff includes psychiatrists, social workers, registered nurses, certified psych techs, psychologists, marriage and family therapists, and occupational or recreational therapists.

Child-Adolescent Inpatient Units

Child-adolescent inpatient units offer comprehensive psychiatric assessment, stabilization, and short-stay intensive treatment to children and adolescents aged 3 to 17 years old who have complex psychiatric conditions. Common conditions that are treated on these units include mood disorders, conduct disorder, autism, ADHD, personality disorders, schizophrenia and other psychotic disorders, substance abuse, and eating disorders. Staff consists of an extensive interdisciplinary team (Box 22.3).

The child-adolescent unit must meet specific age-appropriate criteria in terms of the physical environment and the treatment activities offered. Patients' schedules include time for individual, group, and family therapy; psychopharmacology consultation; and schoolwork. Time is also included for patients to play with their peers. Cognitive-behavioral therapy is the most common approach utilized with this population. Time-out, level or step programs, skills training groups, and seclusion all are approaches used to protect patients from harming themselves or others. Medication use to control disordered children and youth are highly utilized yet very controversial. Huefner and associates (2014) studied the effects of significantly reducing psychotropic medication rates in an intensive residential setting. The researchers found that the reduced use of psychotropics did not result in increased rates of problem behavior or the use of seclusion or personal restraints. See Chapter 34 for further discussion of the child and adolescent population.

Child and family-centered care is an essential element in the care of children admitted to psychiatric inpatient units. Interventions include individual and group parent education sessions as well as family evaluations and treatment (Lamers et al., 2015). Treatment focus is on the patient and family working together to address the issues that led to the hospitalization. Attachment-based family therapy (ABFT) is an evidence-based model that focuses on the developmental needs of adolescents. Devacht, Bosmans, Dewulf, Levy, and Diamond (2019) reported on a 3-year implementation of ABFT on an inpatient young adult psychiatric unit; results indicated that the young adults experienced an increased motivation to participate in treatment, were more connected in the parent–child relationship, and had a significant decrease in aggressive behavior. This study reinforces that parental participation is critical to all aspects of care, and vital to the successful return of children to their home, school, and community. Essential elements of the child and family-centered care approach need to be modified to take into account the special circumstances associated with adolescents and children who have grown up entirely in foster care or group home settings.

Acute Substance Abuse Treatment Centers

Substance abuse treatment centers provide detoxification and acute inpatient medical and psychiatric stabilization and treatment to individuals who are seeking help with an identified drug or alcohol problem. Admission criteria are based on the need for an inpatient level of care that may include detoxification from alcohol or opioids (including prescription narcotics) and detoxification and stabilization for patients in pain management programs. Therapeutic activities on substance abuse units include rigorous patient education, mindfulness, breathing techniques to manage acute negative affect and cravings, and cognitive restructuring techniques targeting the interactions of cognitions, emotions, and behaviors (McGovern et al., 2015). See Chapter 31 for further discussion of patients with substance-related problems.

Clinical Example

Mary is a 37-year-old white woman who has experienced episodes of depression since her early twenties. Mary takes Paxil CR, 25 mg daily, for depression. A recent series of stressors involving her work and marriage precipitated an inpatient admission. Mary is married to a man with an alcohol problem and a pattern of irresponsibility related to family finances. Mary's husband recently informed her that he has a girlfriend and wants a divorce. Yesterday, she took an overdose of Paxil and called her husband in despair. Her husband called the police who brought her to a local emergency department. Mary was treated and later that day was admitted to an acute psychiatric unit. During group therapy, Mary is encouraged to journal, writing down her feelings. In recreation therapy, Mary uses a stationary bicycle to help elevate her mood. The occupational therapist assists Mary in creating a ceramic cup. While participating in individual therapy with the social worker, Mary becomes aware of the effect of her actions on her children. The nurse interacts with Mary to acknowledge and validate her emotional distress as she shares her story in their one-to-one therapeutic interactions.

Clinical Example

Sara is a 42-year-old white woman who has been drinking alcohol excessively and taking alprazolam (Xanax) for the past 3 years. Sara's withdrawal symptoms were managed on the inpatient substance abuse unit. Sara attends educational sessions about addiction, alcoholism, and attachment traumas (Fletcher, Nutton, & Brend, 2015). She also attends group therapy, where she talks about many underlying unaddressed feelings of grief about her late mother's death. As Sara progresses through treatment, she will participate in numerous therapy groups aimed at helping her avoid relapse after discharge.

Co-Occurring Disorders Inpatient Units

Inpatient units for patients with co-occurring disorders focus on the treatment of substance abuse and mental illness in a psychiatric hospital setting. The goals of treatment involve simultaneous resolution of the medical and psychological crises. In addition to alleviating the symptoms and distress of withdrawal, an important goal is to introduce the patient to the long-term goal of initiating and maintaining sobriety and recovery (Salloum & Brown, 2017). Treatment plans address the patients' substance abuse or dependence, psychiatric illness, and the relationship between the co-occurring disorders. Helpful nursing interventions include sharing knowledge and information on various drugs and their effects on patient's behavior, mood, and daily functioning, as well as on the pharmacological interactions that occur when taking prescribed medications while consuming alcohol and/or illicit drugs (Brahim, Hanganu, & Gros, 2020). During hospitalization, patients begin to build the skills, knowledge, and motivation to abstain from substance misuse and maintain gains achieved toward positive outcomes. These patients are at increased risk of suicide, violence, and discharge against medical advice. After patients are stabilized medically and psychologically, they are referred to co-occurring disorder programs in the community setting.

HIGHLIGHTING THE EVIDENCE

Co-Occurring Disorders
Ulibarri, Ulloa, and Salazar (2015) conducted research to determine the role of trauma among Latino women diagnosed with co-occurring disorders. The researchers reported significant relationships between childhood sexual abuse, depressive symptoms, posttraumatic stress disorder (PTSD) symptoms, and alcohol/drug abuse. Findings suggest that mental health and substance use services should incorporate treatment for trauma, which may be at the root of comorbid mental health and substance abuse issues.

MEDICAL-PSYCHIATRIC HOSPITAL UNITS

Medical-psychiatric units are specially designed for mentally ill patients with coexisting medical problems who are in need of hospitalization. These specialized units are equipped to address the comorbid conditions simultaneously, improving outcomes. Nurses working on these units must have knowledge of psychological disorders, psychotropic drugs, medical diseases, and medications. The focus of therapeutic activities depends on the nature of the psychological and medical infirmity. Some geriatric psychiatric units have been reclassified as medical-psychiatric units because of the large number of medical problems in this population. Integrating mental health services within medical inpatient settings has been found to improve health outcomes for patients with comorbid medical and mental health illnesses (Pudalov, Swogger, & Wittink, 2018).

Clinical Example
Marvin is a single 74-year-old African American man with a history of mild Alzheimer disease, diabetes, and congestive heart failure. He was brought to the emergency department with a blood sugar level of 643 mg/dL and severe dehydration. Marvin stopped taking his medications recently because he was forgetting about them most days. He has been walking the streets and preaching to people in fast-food restaurants. Last night, the McDonald's store manager found Marvin babbling and acting "drunk." The manager called the police, who then escorted Marvin to the local emergency department. Typically, Marvin's diabetes is difficult to control. After Marvin was rehydrated and his blood sugar level restabilized, he was admitted to the integrated medical-psychiatric unit for close observation of his medical status and cognitive deficits. Marvin's daughter participated in psychoeducation on cognitive disorders, diabetes, and congestive heart failure. The social worker met with Marvin and his family to discuss home care after discharge.

Geropsychiatric Units

Population demographics reflect an increasingly aging population with medically complex conditions. Patients on geropsychiatric units have a psychiatric disorder, one or more acute or chronic health conditions, and an array of normal age-related physical changes. The most commonly occurring mental disorders include cognitive disorders (Alzheimer disease) and depression (Varghese & Dahale, 2018). Additionally, older patients are at increased risk for medical complications related to hypertension, kidney disease, Parkinson disease, heart disease, and numerous other chronic physical problems.

Specific considerations related to the treatment environment are dictated by the unique needs of this medically compromised older adult population with psychiatric problems. The physical structure of geropsychiatric units must be designed with the frail, elderly, cognitively impaired patient in mind. For example, the unit should be free of unnecessary noise to counter the vulnerability of older patients to sensory overstimulation. Due to their high level of acuity, a smaller unit with fewer patients is beneficial to enhance interactions between patients and staff, to increase safety, and to foster a therapeutic environment.

Older patients with dementia may experience confusion and disorientation leading to difficulty navigating the hospital environment. Interventions such as environmental cues have been found to be helpful in geropsychiatric settings. Environmental cues may include (1) large orientation boards on which the date, time, and location of daily events are posted; (2) clearly marked names or graphic images (e.g., bathrooms, bedrooms with patients' names on the doors); and (3) color coding of different locations.

Falls are of great concern on the geropsychiatric unit. The older adult population in this setting takes multiple prescribed drugs, increasing their susceptibility to drug interactions and falls. Because elderly patients are likely to have impairment in mobility, balance, and vision, increased lighting and simple, uncluttered rooms facilitate comfort and safety.

The importance of the environment for patients in a geropsychiatric unit is evident by the increasing number of studies on facility design and planning. These studies have shown an association between the environmental design of the unit and patients' level of improvement in regard to variables such as self-care, agitation, and mood. Group therapy, for patients able to participate, might involve issues such as grief and loss. For less cognitively functional patients, group therapy might involve reminiscence activities such as sharing real-life stories. See Chapters 28 and 35 for discussion of the unique care needs of the geriatric patient.

State Psychiatric Hospitals

Traditionally, state psychiatric hospitals provided long-term treatment to individuals with intellectual and developmental disabilities, chronic psychiatric disorders, and forensic cases. In 1999, there was an aggressive movement toward deinstitutionalization as a result of the Olmstead decision, making "unjustified isolation" of individuals with cognitive disabilities in institutions a violation of the Americans with Disabilities Act. More patients are now being treated in the community, are homeless, or are incarcerated. These huge shifts have resulted in state psychiatric hospitals housing patients with more serious mental health issues and/or patients who are perceived to be a danger to the community. Specifically, an increased number of forensic patients have been admitted to state psychiatric hospitals for pretrial evaluations or to receive treatment services. These individuals tend to remain at the state psychiatric hospitals for long periods of time. The occurrence of violence/aggression in state psychiatric hospitals is a major concern that influences the dynamic of the units/wards and requires intensive and predetermined measures (Wik, 2018). The environment at state psychiatric hospitals is highly restrictive. In some facilities, *treatment malls* are built and used to provide programs focused on rehabilitation and recovery. The rehabilitative focused approach employs (1) skills-based relapse prevention programs to decrease recidivism rates; (2) cognitive-behavioral programs to decrease symptom severity; and (3) psychoeducation to improve patients' knowledge of their illness. Daily and weekly activities, such as community meetings, anger management, gardening, and computer skills groups, are geared toward the goal of community reintegration.

State Forensic Hospitals

Patients confined to state forensic facilities have a diagnosable mental illness and have been convicted by a court of a criminal offense. These patients have committed crimes carried out under the influence of a severe mental illness and are deemed too dangerous to reside in the community (Hörberg, 2015). State forensic hospitals are the most restrictive of all treatment environments; they are a secure environment with strict rules and regulations to ensure safety for the general population. The buildings are designed with maximum security to prevent patients from escaping. Guard-controlled doors, metal detectors, and strategically placed checkpoints throughout the facility are common features of state forensic facilities.

Notorious individuals who exemplify the types of patients cared for by forensic psychiatric nurses include Andrea Yates, the Texas woman who drowned her five children, and Lee Malvo, the teenager who participated in the Washington, DC, sniper shootings with his father figure, John Muhammad.

The involuntary nature of being committed to a forensic hospital for treatment equates to patients losing basic human rights. However, treatment in forensic settings is justified by reasons of public safety; a patient's right for autonomy is subjugated to public safety. Compulsory treatments may be used, such as compelling patients into taking medication intended to manage symptoms or reduce their risk of behaving violently (Lau, Brackman, Mokros, & Habermeyer, 2020). A major risk factor for interpersonal violence is the use of illicit substances, which is known to be common among forensic psychiatry patients (MacCall, 2017). Coercive measures may become necessary (i.e., seclusion, restraints) in the management of dangerous behavior against self or others.

Psychiatric nurses in forensic settings must possess a unique set of skills and competencies. The primary role of the nurse is to provide a therapeutic relationship with patients, while at the same time monitoring and responding to risks of violence toward themselves and others (Vincze, Fredriksson, & Wiklund Gustin, 2015). The anxiety of working around potentially dangerous patients results in nurses sometimes distancing themselves from patients. Therefore, nurses working in forensic psychiatric settings must develop self-awareness to manage their feelings, oftentimes experienced as fear. Nurses are expected to demonstrate respect for the humanity of the patient regardless of the crime committed. Nurses must interact with these offenders in an ethical manner, cognizant of the fact that they are mentally ill. Providing care to this population is very complex, and requires a high degree of training and education.

COMMUNITY TREATMENT SETTINGS

As the focus of psychiatric care has shifted away from inpatient and state psychiatric hospitals, community treatment programs have increased. At the present time, much psychiatric care takes place in group homes and day programs, or through support offered to patients and their family members via home health visits. Psychiatric patients in these community settings are more acutely ill than ever before. This section focuses on the unique aspects of community psychiatric treatment.

HIGHLIGHTING THE EVIDENCE

Evidence-Based Practice

Patients in forensic settings are a vulnerable group due to their suffering from a severe mental illness, having committed a crime, and residing in an institutional environment with a high level of security. Hörberg (2018) discusses a caring science perspective that can be utilized by nurses in their interactions with this population.

Seeking to understand patients' perspectives enables their self-reflection and serves as a foundation for caring.

Expressing a desire to know how patients understand their situation confirms them as experts of themselves.

Group supervision can assist nurses in developing the art of understanding, while enhancing a reflective attitude towards one's own and others' actions.

A caring science perspective can contribute to a comprehensive view, assisted by the perspectives from other team members.

? CRITICAL THINKING QUESTION

1. How has the trend for hospitalized psychiatric patients to be more acutely ill now than they were in the past affected the nursing profession?

? CRITICAL THINKING QUESTION

2. Should society be investing resources into the treatment of patients who have committed heinous crimes? How would it be determined that a patient was rehabilitated?

Group Homes

A group home is a moderately sized, approximately 6- to 12-bed program located in a neighborhood setting that is staffed with nonclinical paraprofessionals who provide specialized services offered within the context of a "24/7" homelike milieu. It is a structured service program that creates a physically, emotionally, and psychologically safe environment for children, adolescents, or adults with moderate psychological needs who are either too young or lack the skills necessary to function in an independent living situation. A group home is designed to serve as an alternative living arrangement to the family home. Staff members are expected to support the residents in life skills development. Residents are expected to abide by the house rules, which are clearly communicated during community group meetings. Therapeutic activities, such as psychoeducation, individual and group therapy, and medication management, may be offered in-house or accessed through community providers as needed. Nursing staff are not always employed in these settings, but rather serve as consultants.

Group homes, or residential treatment centers, are oftentimes utilized to house large numbers of children in foster care or children experiencing behavioral issues. Group homes for children or adolescents require a 24-hour structured supportive and educational milieu. Children may be having moderate to severe functional problems in school or community settings (e.g., school suspension, involvement with the law) due to their inability to accept age-appropriate direction or supervision from the parent or guardian. Typically, the poor impulse control experienced by the child or adolescent is expressed through periodic verbal aggression directed toward self and others, interfering with the development of successful interpersonal relationships. For some older children and adolescents convicted of sexually aggressive behavior, a specialized group home setting may be an option over a locked juvenile detention facility.

The majority of residential treatment centers for adults are focused on helping men and women free themselves from addiction, while encouraging them to take recovery ownership. Other types of residential centers treat eating disorders, autism spectrum disorder, co-occurring disorders, as well as chronic mental disorders, such as PTSD, depression, anxiety, schizophrenia, and borderline personality disorder. Services offered may include one-on-one therapy sessions, cognitive-behavioral and dialectical therapy, trauma awareness, medically supported detox, as well as gardening, yoga, dance/movement, and art therapy.

Partial Hospitalization

Partial hospitalization is a short-term treatment program for patients transitioning from an acute psychiatric inpatient facility. As a result of brief inpatient hospital stays, psychiatric patients with severe and enduring symptoms are often poorly stabilized before their hospital discharge, and so require ongoing intensive treatment. Patients admitted to partial hospitalization programs spend 4 to 6 hours a day, 5 days a week in the care of doctors, nurses, and therapists. There is a significant benefit for patients as they experience a therapeutic milieu with a high degree of structure, personalized treatment, and socialization.

The goal of the partial hospitalization approach is to reduce the likelihood of rehospitalization and to facilitate successful integration into a less restrictive setting. The partial hospitalization facility is usually connected with a hospital. The program provides specialized psychiatric rehabilitation services, including psychoeducation, psychiatric medication evaluation and monitoring, case management services, and individual psychotherapy. Regulatory agencies and third-party payers require a registered nurse in these facilities to, at the minimum, attend to urgent care matters that might arise and assist with medication administration and management. Treatment is structured similarly to the inpatient environment, but patients are considered safe enough to be able to return to their residence in the evening. After completing a partial hospitalization program, patients are stepped down to a community mental health center for day treatment or outpatient care.

Day Treatment

Day treatment programs focus on patient stabilization, rehabilitation, and recovery in a community outpatient setting. The programs are designed to assist participants in (1) learning new skills to enhance current levels of functioning and independence, (2) achieving life goals and maintaining community living, and (3) developing self-awareness through the exploration and development of intrapersonal strengths and interpersonal relationships. Day treatment is similar to the partial hospitalization program in that patients attend the scheduled activities for a prescribed number of hours and specified frequency. Day treatment programs represent a midpoint between hospitalization and outpatient clinic visits.

Pec and associates (2018) tested whether a psychodynamically based group program might improve symptoms, social functions, or quality of life in patients with schizophrenia spectrum disorders. Eighty-one patients diagnosed with schizophrenia spectrum disorders participated in a 9-month psychodynamically based psychotherapeutic day program. The results showed that the higher functioning patients improved in their clinical status and quality of life.

Clinical Example

Peter is a 25-year-old single, white man with schizophrenia who lives with his mother. He has a history of multiple hospitalizations. Typical symptoms include paranoid delusions, acute agitation, impulsiveness, and verbally threatening behavior. The staff at the day treatment center is collaborating with Peter to plan an individualized treatment program. His counselor has daily interactions with Peter to teach and promote more socially appropriate behavior through modeling and mentoring. Peter's mother attends parenting classes offered through the day treatment center, which has enhanced her relationship with Peter tremendously.

Day Treatment Center for Patients With Co-Occurring Disorders

The term *co-occurring disorders* refers to the comorbidity of a mental disorder and a substance addiction disorder. Researchers have found that about half of those who experience a mental illness during their lives will also experience a substance use disorder and vice versa. The onset of mental illness and substance use disorders often occurs during adolescence, and those who develop problems earlier typically have a greater risk for severe symptoms as adults (NIDA, 2020). Patients with co-occurring disorders are more difficult to treat successfully than patients with either substance abuse diagnosis or a mental disorder. Rather than parallel treatment for mental health and addictions, patients receive intensive, coordinated community-based mental health and substance abuse treatment provided by a team of professionals.

Interventions found to be successful at day treatment centers are extensive and comprehensive. Group sessions are useful in motivating patients with co-occurring disorders to set goals. (See Box 22.4 for examples of co-occurring disorder groups.) Day treatment centers offer an integrated approach that focuses on patients developing coping skills to manage the anxiety, frustration, and problems of daily living. Lectures, videos, and discussions on relapse prevention are crucial aspects of the program and assist patients in identifying their high-risk situations and in practicing alternative coping strategies. These patients are encouraged to attend Alcoholics Anonymous or Narcotics Anonymous groups and to secure a sponsor.

BOX 22.4 Co-Occurring Disorder Groups

- Medication management
- Community meetings
- Wellness classes
- Vocational classes
- Family psychoeducation

SUMMARY

This chapter has provided an overview of the various psychotherapeutic environments in inpatient and outpatient settings. There is a continuum of care ranging from intensive care psychiatric inpatient hospitalization to day treatment centers for patients with psychiatric disorders. Nurses fill a wide variety of health care roles depending on the treatment setting; in most settings, they are responsible for providing psychoeducation related to mental disorders and medication regimens. Additionally, nurses are responsible for managing the therapeutic milieu and coordinating the various interdisciplinary activities. In settings where paraprofessionals are responsible for the various activities, such as group homes, nurses may serve as consultants. Regardless of the setting, the goal of treatment is the stabilization, rehabilitation, and recovery of patients with psychiatric disorders.

STUDY NOTES

1. A variety of health care professionals are involved in the treatment milieu of a psychiatric facility, including physicians, nurses, psychologists, social workers, chaplains, and occupational and recreational therapists.

2. Members of the treatment team as well as patients attend therapeutic community meetings to welcome new patients, review milieu rules, and make general announcements about the day's activities. (*Note:* Not all units have therapeutic community meetings.)

3. Various treatment activities are employed within psychiatric settings, such as group therapy, recreational therapy, exercise therapy, spirituality groups, and psychoeducation.

4. Patients in intensive care or acute, locked psychiatric units are sometimes admitted involuntarily and usually need close supervision and intervention by nursing staff.

5. A special focus of the child-adolescent psychiatric unit is the inclusion of parents in the treatment program.

6. Medical-psychiatric units are specialty psychiatric environments that address the needs of patients with a chronic medical illness and coexisting psychiatric problems.

7. The abuse of substances may be an attempt to cope with the distressing emotions associated with past trauma.

8. Patients with both a substance abuse problem and a psychiatric diagnosis can be treated on co-occurring disorder units, which provide a therapeutic, supportive approach.

9. Geropsychiatric units address specialized needs of older adults, including environmental modifications necessary due to sensory losses and other safety factors.

10. A forensic hospital is the most restrictive of all treatment environments.

11. Significant levels of psychiatric care are provided in group homes, partial hospitalization programs, and other community settings.

12. Preparing patients to live in the community requires an emphasis on social skills, independent living skills, and prevention of relapse and rehospitalization.

REFERENCES

Brahim, L., Hanganu, C., & Gros, C. (2020). Understanding helpful nursing care from the perspective of mental health inpatients with a dual diagnosis: A qualitative descriptive study. *Journal of the American Psychiatric Nursing Association, 26*(3), 250–261. https://doi.org/10.1177/1078390319878773.

Copeland, M. (n.d.). The Wellness Recovery Action Plan (WRAP). https://copelandcenter.com/wellness-recovery-action-plan-wrap.

Devacht, I., Bosmans, G., Dewulf, S., Levy, S., & Diamond, G. (2019). Attachment-based family therapy in a psychiatric inpatient unit for young adults. *Australian and New Zealand Journal of Family Therapy, 40*(3), 330–343. https://doi.org/10.1002/anzf.1383.

Economou, M. (2015). Psychoeducation: A multifaceted intervention. *International Journal of Mental Health, 44*(4), 259–262. https://doi.org/10.1080/00207411.2015.1076288.

Fletcher, K., Nutton, J., & Brend, D. (2015). Attachment, a matter of substance: The potential of attachment theory in the treatment of addictions. *Clinical Social Work Journal, 43*, 109–117. https://doi.org/10.1007/s10615-014-0502-5.

Florensa, M., Keliat, B., Wardani, I., & Suliotiowati, N. (2019). Promoting the mental health of adolescents through cognitive behavioral group therapy and family psychoeducation. *Comprehensive Child and Adolescent Nursing, 42*(1), 267–276. https://doi.org/10.1080/24694193.2019.1594459.

Hörberg. U. (2015). Caring science and the development of forensic psychiatric care. *Perspectives in Psychiatric Care, 51*(4), 277–284. https://doi.org/10.1111/ppc.12092.

Hörberg. U. (2018). 'The art of understanding in forensic psychiatric care' — From a caring science perspective based on a lifeworld approach. *Journal of Mental Health Nursing, 39*(9), 802–809. https://doi.org/10.1080/01612840.2018.1496499.

Huefner. J., et al. (2014). Reducing psychotropic medications in an intensive residential treatment center. *Journal of Child & Family Studies, 23*, 675–685. https://doi.org/10.1007/s10826-012-9628-7.

Lamers. A., et al. (2015). A measure of the parent-team alliance in youth residential psychiatry: The Revised Short-Term Working Alliance Inventory. *Child Youth Care Forum, 44*, 801–817. https://doi.org/10.1007/s10566-015-9306-1.

Lannigan, E. G., & Noyes, S. (2019). Occupational therapy interventions for adults living with serious mental illness. *American Journal of Occupational Therapy, 73*(5), 1–5. https://doi.org/10.5014/ajot.2019.735001.

Lau, S., Brackman, N., Mokros, A., & Habermeyer, E. (2020). Aims to reduce coercive measures in forensic inpatient treatment: A 9-year observational study. *Frontiers in Psychiatry, 11*, 1–8. https://doi.org/10.3389/fpsyt.2020.00465.

Lucksted, A., Medoff, D., Burland, J., Stewart, B., Fang, L. J., Brown, C., … Dixon, L. B. (2013). Sustained outcomes of a peer-taught family education program on mental illness. *Acta psychiatrica Scandinavica, 127*(4), 279–286. https://doi.org/10.1111/j.1600-0447.2012.01901.x.

MacCall. C. (2017). Drug testing in forensic mental health settings. *Addiction, 112*(4), 729–730. https://doi.org/10.1111/add.13727.

McGovern. M., et al. (2015). A randomized controlled trial of treatments for co-occurring substance use disorders and post-traumatic stress disorder. *Addiction, 110*(7), 1194–1204.

NAMI National Alliance of Mental Illness (n.d.). NAMI Family Support Group. Support & Education. https://www.nami.org/Support-Education/Support-Groups/NAMI-Family-Support-Group.

NIDA. (2020). Part 1: Common Comorbidities with Substance Use Disorders Research Report Part 1: The Connection Between Substance Use Disorders and Mental Illness https://www.drugabuse.gov/publications/research-reports/common-comorbidities-substance-use-disorders/part-1-connection-between-substance-use-disorders-mental-illness.

Noyes, S., Sokolow, H., & Arbesman, M. (2018). Evidence for occupational therapy intervention with employment and education for adults with serious mental illness: A systematic review. *The American Occupational Therapy Association, 72*(5), 1–10. https://doi.org/10.5014/ajot.2018.033068.

Onwumere, J., Grice, S., & Kuipers, E. (2016). Delivering cognitive-behavioral family interventions for schizophrenia. *Australian Psychologist, 51*(1), 52–61. https://doi.org/10.1111/ap.12179.

Passley-Clarke. J. (2019). Implementation of recovery education on an inpatient psychiatric unit. *Journal of the American Psychiatric Nursing Association, 25*(6), 501–507. https://doi.org/10.1177/1078390318810413.

Pec, O., Bob, P., Pec, J., & Hrubcova, A. (2018). Psychodynamic day treatment programme for patients with schizophrenia spectrum disorders: Dynamics and predictors of therapeutic change. *Psychology and Psychotherapy: Theory, Research, and Practice, 91*(2), 157–168. https://doi.org/10.1111/papt.12153.

Pratt, R., MacGregor, A., Reid, S., & Given. L. (2013). Experience of wellness recovery action planning in self-help and mutual support groups for people with lived experience of mental health difficulties. *The Scientific World Journal,* 180587. https://doi.org/10.1155/2013/180587.

Pudalov, L., Swogger, M., & Wittink, M. (2018). Towards integrated medical and mental healthcare in the inpatient setting: What is the role of psychology? *International Review of Psychiatry, 30*(6), 210–223. https://doi.org/10.1080/09540261.2018.1552125.

Radcliffe, J., & Bird, L. (2016). Talking therapy groups on acute psychiatric wards: Patients' experience of two structured group formats. *BJPsych bulletin, 40*(4), 187–191. https://doi.org/10.1192/pb.bp.114.047274.

Salloum, I. M., & Brown, E. S. (2017). Management of comorbid bipolar disorder and substance use disorders. *The American Journal of Drug and Alcohol Abuse, 43*(4), 366–376. https://doi.org/10.1080/00952990.2017.1292279.

Stoffel, V., Reed, K., & Brown, C. (2019). The unfolding history of occupational therapy in mental health. In C. Brown, V. Stoffel, & J. Munoz (Eds.), Occupational therapy in mental health: A vision for participation (2nd ed., pp. 11–28). F.A. Davis.

Tsiouri, I., et al. (2015). Does long-term group psychoeducation of parents of individuals with schizophrenia help the family as a system? A quasi-experimental study. *International Journal of Mental Health, 44*(4), 316–331. https://doi.org/10.1080/00207411.2015.1076294.

Ulibarri, M., Ulloa, E., & Salazar, M. (2015). Association between mental health, substance use, and sexual abuse experiences among Latinas. *Journal of Child Sexual Abuse, 24*(1), 35–54. https://doi.org/10.1080/10538712.2015.976303.

Varghese, M., & Dahale, A. B. (2018). The geropsychiatric interview—Assessment and diagnosis. *Indian Journal of Psychiatry, 60*(3), 301–311. https://doi.org/10.4103/0019-5545.224471.

Vincze, M., Fredriksson, L., & Wiklund Gustin, L. (2015). To do good might hurt bad: Exploring nurses' understanding and approach to suffering in forensic psychiatric settings. *International Journal of Mental Health Nursing, 24*(2), 149–157. https://doi.org/10.1111/inm.12116.

Wik, A. (2018). Elevating patient/staff safety in state psychiatric hospitals. National Association of State Mental Health Program Directors Research Institute (NRI). https://www.nri-inc.org/media/1465/2018-elevatingpatient_endnotesfinal.pdf.

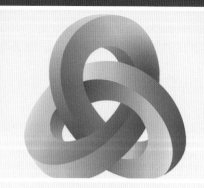

23

Introduction to Psychopathology

W. Chance Nicholson and Norman L. Keltner

Old paradigm: Caring teachers urged caring students to be more caring.
New paradigm: Caring is not enough. Psychiatric nurses must
understand psychobiology and psychopharmacology.

http://evolve.elsevier.com/Keltner

LEARNING OBJECTIVES

- Describe the extent of mental illness in the United States.
- Identify the most common mental disorders in the United States.

- List the three requirements for understanding psychopathology.
- Describe several guidelines applicable to all aspects of psychotherapeutic management.

According to the National Institute of Mental Health (2021), approximately 20% of the US adult population is affected by mental disorders during a given year. As noted in Table 23.1, anxiety disorders are the most prevalent, followed by mood, substance use, and posttraumatic stress disorders. This table, which is also found in Chapter 2 and in most chapters in this unit, lists prevalence rates for a 12-month period. Among specific disorders, major depression (one type of mood disorder) and phobias are most common. Table 23.2 provides the data for lifetime prevalence rates for the most common mental and substance use disorders. Many individuals have a comorbid status; for example, an individual may be depressed and anxious and abuse a substance or have some other combination of disorders. Many of these individuals do not seek professional help, suggesting a great reservoir of unmet mental health needs in the United States.

The incidence of psychopathology is high, and the nurse's understanding of psychopathology is basic for effective psychotherapeutic management of mental disorders. Understanding psychopathology requires the following standards:

1. Knowledge should be organized.
2. Operational definitions should be formed.
3. Criteria for diagnosis should be developed.

Several diagnostic systems have been developed, but this text relies on criteria from the *Diagnostic and Statistical Manual of Mental Disorders (DSM)*, which is published by the American Psychiatric Association and is the official diagnostic manual in use in the United States. The current version, *DSM-5* (American Psychiatric Association, 2013), is the seventh version since the *DSM* was first published in 1952 (*DSM-I, DSM-II, DSM-III, DSM-III-R, DSM-IV,* and *DSM-IV-TR*). Because diagnostic consistency among clinicians is so important, psychiatric experts are constantly evaluating and updating criteria for this manual. All chapters in this unit are developed around *DSM* criteria. *DSM-IV-TR* and previous editions used a multiaxial system to capture more than the criteria describing patient symptoms. These axes looked at contributing factors, such as medical conditions, childhood trauma, and environmental problems. *DSM-5* does not use this approach; instead, a chapter is dedicated to "other conditions that may be a focus of concern."

Interestingly, some psychiatrists are beginning to doubt that there is nearly as much diagnostic distinction as such a lengthy tome (about 1000 pages) would suggest. Goodkind and colleagues (2015) point out that when looking at the six major forms of serious mental illness (i.e., schizophrenia, bipolar disorder, major depression, obsessive-compulsive disorder, anxiety, and addiction), they all show brain shrinkage in the same three brain areas. Further, serious mental disorders tend to share the same genes. Without meaning to do so, these genetic and structural similarities (Nasrallah, 2015)

TABLE 23.1 Twelve-Month Prevalence Rate of Mental Disorders in the United States[a]

Disorders	Approximate Percentage >17 Years Old (%)[a] (Unless Noted for Children)	Gender Overrepresentation
Anxiety disorders	19.1 overall	
Agoraphobia	1.7	Female
Panic disorder	2.4	Female
Panic attacks	11.2	Female
Social anxiety	7	Female
Specific phobia	7–9	Female
Separation anxiety	1.2	Equal
Generalized anxiety disorder	2	Female
Posttraumatic stress disorder	3.6	Female
Obsessive-compulsive disorder	1.2	Equal
Major depression	7.8	Female
Bipolar disorder I and II	2.8	BD I: ~ Equal
Attention-deficit/ hyperactivity disorder	5 in children; 2.5 in adults	Males
Substance use disorders	8.9 overall	
Alcohol use disorder	8.5 in adults; 2.5 in 12- to 17-year-olds	Males
Drug use disorders	1.4	Males
Schizophrenia	1	~ Equal

[a]Not one source has all of this information. This information has been derived from the following sources: Kessler, R. C., Petukhova, M., Sampson, N. A., Zaslavsky, A. M., & Wittchen, H. U. (2012). Twelve-month and lifetime prevalence and lifetime morbid risk of anxiety and mood disorders in the United States. *International Journal of Methods of Psychiatric Research, 21*, 169; SAMHSA. (2009). *Results from the 2008 national survey on drug use and health: National findings*; American Psychiatric Association. (2013). *Diagnostic and statistical manual of mental disorders* (5th ed.). APA.

TABLE 23.2 Lifetime Prevalence Rates for Mental Disorders in the United States

Disorders	Lifetime Prevalence Rate (%)
Anxiety disorders (all)	28.8
Panic disorder	6.8
Agoraphobia disorder	3.7
Social phobia	13
Separation anxiety	8.7
Specific phobia	18.4
Generalized anxiety disorder	9
Posttraumatic stress disorder	10.1
Obsessive-compulsive disorder	2.7
Mood disorders (all)	20.8
Major depressive disorder	29.9
Bipolar disorders I and II	4.1
Dysthymia	2.5
Cyclothymia	0.4–1
Schizophrenia	0.3–0.7
Schizoaffective	0.34
Substance abuse disorder (all)	14.6
Alcohol use disorder	13.2
Drug use disorder	7.9
Attention-deficit/hyperactivity disorder	8.1
Any mental or chemical abuse disorder	46.4

Not one source has all of this information. This information has been derived from the following sources: Kessler, R. C., Berglund, P., Demler, O., Jin, R., Merikangas, K. R., & Walters, E. E. (2005). Lifetime prevalence and age-of-onset distributions of DSM-IV disorders in the national comorbidity survey replication. *Archives of General Psychiatry, 62*, 593; Kessler, R. C., Petukhova, M., Sampson, N. A., Zaslavsky, A. M., & Wittchen, H. U. (2012). Twelve-month and lifetime prevalence and lifetime morbid risk of anxiety and mood disorders in the United States. *International Journal of Methods of Psychiatric Research, 21*, 169; SAMHSA. (2009). *Results from the 2008 national survey on drug use and health: National findings*; American Psychiatric Association. (2013). *Diagnostic and statistical manual of mental disorders*. (5th ed.). APA.

NORM'S NOTES This chapter provides an overview of some statistics about mental illness and a rationale for the nurse's need to know psychopathologic concepts. A disturbing point that you cannot detect from seeing Table 23.1 is that things are not getting better. I can see it because I've been around a long time and know the older stats. Even though billions of dollars have been spent, in reality, more people have mental disorders today than they did 35 years ago. I must admit I'm a little discouraged.

seem to support Dr. Henrich Neumann's (1859) observation when he encouraged professionals "…to throw overboard the whole business of classification. There is but one type of mental disturbance, and we call it insanity" (cited by Lehman, 1980).

BEHAVIOR

Patients' behaviors are described to help the student identify behavioral phenomena. Some behaviors can be observed directly (objective assessment or signs), whereas the patient must report other behaviors (subjective assessment or symptoms). Knowledge of these signs and symptoms helps the nurse anticipate and plan appropriate interventions.

ETIOLOGY

For many years, psychiatric clinicians have typically fallen into one of two camps with regard to what causes mental disorders: those who subscribe to the nature argument and believe that mental disorders arise from *nature* (e.g., organic, biologic, genetic) and those who subscribe to the nurture argument and believe that mental disorders arise from *nurture* (e.g., psychodynamic, functional, environmental stressors, early life experiences). In recent years, most clinicians have come to recognize that both views provide valuable insights into the complexities of the human mind. Research has suggested that some life experiences (i.e., nurture) change biology (i.e., nature), underscoring a more holistic view of mental illness. Threads of the "nature versus nurture" argument (or the "biologic versus psychodynamic" argument) are presented in discussions of etiologies; however, the overriding theme of this unit is the recognition of the unifying symptoms that point to the contributions of each etiologic factor.

PSYCHOTHERAPEUTIC MANAGEMENT

Sections on psychotherapeutic management in each chapter draw on the general intervention strategies presented in Units II to IV to develop appropriate interventions for each disorder. In addition, a case study and a related nursing care plan are presented for each disorder. A sample nursing care plan is found at the end of this chapter. The following rules provide relevant guidelines for all aspects of psychotherapeutic management:

- Provide support for patients
- Provide empathetic care and concern
- Strengthen patients' self-efficacy
- Treat patients as experts in their lives
- Prevent failure or embarrassment
- Treat patients as individuals
- Provide reality testing
- Handle hostility therapeutically
- Be calm and matter-of-fact about norms and limits

NURSES NEED TO UNDERSTAND PSYCHOPATHOLOGY

Nurses cannot gain a true understanding of patients with mental disorders until they understand mental disorders. Psychiatric nursing is more than warm, caring feelings about patients. Although being affirming and kind are important attributes, more is required of an effective psychiatric nurse. This "more" is based on an understanding of psychopathology.

A psychiatric nurse can no more effectively plan and provide psychiatric care without an understanding of psychopathology than a medical-surgical nurse can plan and provide care without an understanding of pathophysiology. In this unit, the authors provide a discussion of psychopathology for each disorder. We have included chapters on the following mental disorders: schizophrenia, depression, bipolar disorders, anxiety-related disorders, cognitive disorders, personality disorders, sexual disorders, substance-related disorders, and eating disorders.

A crucial element of assessment is the usage of rating scales that can be used in the clinical setting. The following are five

---

◎ CARE PLAN

Name: _____   **Admission Date:** _____

DSM-5 Diagnosis: _____

Assessment   **Areas of strength:** _____
                               Problems: _____
Diagnoses   _____
                               _____
                               _____

Outcomes   **Short-term goals**
Date met: _____
Date met: _____
Date met: _____

Date met: _____   **Long-term goals**
Date met: _____
Planning and Interventions **Nurse-patient relationship:** _____
                               _____
                               _____
                               _____
                               Psychopharmacology: _____
                               Milieu management: _____
                               _____
Evaluation   _____
Referrals   _____

assessment tools that can be used in both the inpatient and outpatient environment (Gupta & Wood, 2017).

1. Patient Health Questionnaire (PHQ)

   The PHQ-S is a nine-question, self-reporting tool that helps in the detection of depression.

2. Mood Disorder Questionnaire (MDQ)

   The MDQ is a brief, three-item scale to help recognize bipolar disorder.

3. Generalized Anxiety Disorder (GAD)

   The GAD is a seven-point scale that is also self-administered. The GAD, as expected, facilitates the assessment of anxiety.

4. CAGE

   The CAGE questionnaire is a familiar four-item scale that helps identify substance abuse.

5. Columbia Suicide Severity Rating Scale (C-SSRS)

The C-SSRS measures the severity of suicidal ideation. It can be completed by the patient or the nurse. However, specific training in the use of the C-SSRS is recommended. The advantage of utilizing these scales is that they have undergone scientific scrutiny and have proven to be objective, reliable, valid, norm-based, and practical (Gupta & Wood, 2017).

? CRITICAL THINKING QUESTION

1. The biologic versus psychodynamic argument has gone on for a long time. Why is it important to be open to both points of view? Although you might not have used the same words, you probably had a bias one way or the other before you started nursing school. What was your bias?

STUDY NOTES

1. According to the NIMH, about 20% or more of Americans have some type of mental or addictive disorder in any given 12-month period.

2. Anxiety disorders are the most common category of mental disorders, followed by mood disorders, impulse-control disorders, and substance use disorders.

3. Understanding psychopathology is fundamental for effective psychotherapeutic management; it requires organizing knowledge, defining terms operationally, and developing criteria for diagnosis.

4. *DSM-5* is the official diagnostic system for psychiatry used in the United States.

5. Etiologic explanations of mental disorders can be broadly placed in one of two categories: biologic (natural or organic causes) and psychological (nurturing, psychodynamic, or functional causes).

6. Guidelines appropriate for all aspects of psychiatric care include empathetic and supportive care, strengthening self-efficacy, preventing failure or embarrassment, person-centered care, reinforcing reality, and handling patients' hostility calmly and matter-of-factly.

7. Practical and reliable assessment scales are available for the nurse to use in both the inpatient and outpatient settings.

REFERENCES

American Psychiatric Association. (2013). *Diagnostic and statistical manual of mental disorders* (5th ed.). APA.

Goodkind, M., Eickhoff, S. B., Oathes, D. J., Jiang, Y., Chang, A., Jones-Hagata, L. B., … Etkin, A. (2015). Identification of a common neurobiological substrate for mental illness. *JAMA Psychiatry, 72*(4), 305–315. https://doi.org/10.1001/jamapsychiatry.2014.2206.

Gupta, S., & Wood, J. M. (2017). Using rating scales in a clinical setting: A guide for psychiatrists. *Current Psychiatry, 16*(2), 21–25. https://www.mdedge.com/psychiatry/article/130311/practice-management/using-rating-scales-clinical-setting-guide.

Kessler, R. C., Berglund, P., Demler, O., Jin, R., Merikangas, K. R., & Walters, E. E. (2005). Lifetime prevalence and age-of-onset distributions of DSM-IV disorders in the National Comorbidity Survey Replication. *Archives of General Psychiatry, 62*(6), 593–602. https://doi.org/10.1001/archpsyc.62.6.593.

Kessler, R. C., Petukhova, M., et al. (2012). Twelve-month and lifetime prevalence and lifetime morbid risk of anxiety and mood disorders in the United States. *International Journal of Methods of Psychiatric Research, 21*, 169. https://www.ncbi.nlm.nih.gov/pmc/articles/PMC4005415/.

Lehman. H. E. (1980). Schizophrenia: History. In H. I. Kaplan (Ed.), *Comprehensive textbook of psychiatry*. Williams & Wilkins.

Nasrallah. H. A. (2015). Is there only 1 neurobiological psychiatric disorder with different clinical expressions? *Current Psychiatry, 14*, 10. http://www.moodclinic.ca/wp-content/uploads/2019/09/010_0715CP_FromTheEditor_FINAL.pdf.

Reeves, W. C., Strine, T., Pratt, L., et al. (2013). Mental illness surveillance among adults in the United States. *Supplement, CDC, 60*(3), 1–32. http://www.cdc.gov/mmwr.

SAMHSA. (2009). Results from the 2008 national survey on drug use and health: National findings. http://www.samhsa.gov/data/nsduh/2k8nsduh/2k8Results.htm.

24

Schizophrenia Spectrum and Other Psychotic Disorders

Norman L. Keltner and Marie Smith-East

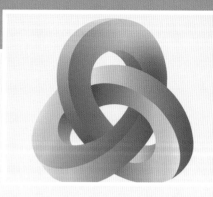

…when a man with a gun walks into an FBI office hearing voices and complaining that the CIA is pushing him to become a member of al-Qaeda, he is asking to be treated for his psychosis. Instead, he was given some anti-anxiety medication, released after three days, and given his gun back, which he then took to Ft. Lauderdale.

Dr. E. Fuller Torrey and John D. Snook, commenting on the state of psychiatric care in America. (Feb 14, 2017, "A Ray of Hope for Mental Health," National Review Online)

ⓔ http://evolve.elsevier.com/Keltner

LEARNING OBJECTIVES

- Define the term *schizophrenia*.
- Describe the major historical figures, events, and theories that have contributed to the current understanding of schizophrenia.
- Identify Bleuler's "four A's."
- Recognize the *DSM-5* criteria and terminology for schizophrenia.
- Differentiate and describe type I (positive) and type II (negative) subtypes.
- Recognize and describe objective and subjective symptoms of schizophrenia.
- Identify biologic explanations for schizophrenia.
- Describe two psychodynamic explanations for schizophrenia.
- Develop a nursing care plan for patients with schizophrenia.
- Identify the major drugs used in the treatment of schizophrenia, their mechanisms of action, their target symptoms, and their major side effects.
- Evaluate the effectiveness of nursing interventions for patients with schizophrenia.

There are three inescapable "facts" about schizophrenia:
1. *Age at onset: Onset is almost always during late adolescence or early adulthood.*
2. *Role of stress: Onset and relapse are almost always related to stress.*
3. *Efficacy of dopamine antagonists: Drugs that block dopamine receptors are therapeutic.*

Dr. Daniel Weinberger (1987) wrote these words over 30 years ago, and they remain accurate today. Psychosis, described as losing touch with reality (National Institute of Mental Health NIMH, 2021), affects one's highest mental functions. Drastic shifts in thoughts, language, and emotions are noted. Common symptoms of psychosis include hallucinations, delusions, and difficulty with thought organization. Psychosis can be present in schizophrenia, acute mania, depression, drug intoxication, dementia, and delirium and can be caused by brain trauma. Schizophrenia is one of the most common causes of psychosis and is the focus of this chapter.

SCHIZOPHRENIA

A changing personality does not characterize schizophrenia as some think. The popular notion of a dramatic personality change comes far short of capturing the devastating effect that schizophrenia has on the life of a person and the person's family. Globally, schizophrenia is associated with considerable disability, and its presentation could affect the individual's educational and occupational performance. Simply stated, schizophrenia is one of the most complex illnesses that the nurse may encounter and is often connected with societal stigma despite being treatable (World Health Organization WHO, 2019).

NORM'S NOTES This might be the most important chapter in this book. Although schizophrenia affects only about 1% of the adult population (Table 24.1), it is a devastating disorder because it has ripple effects that disproportionately impact society. These are the people whom you might walk by (or around) in our cities, not wanting to interact with them at all. They might scare you at times or offend in other ways. After you read this chapter and have a good clinical experience, I think that your attitude about these individuals will change.

Schizophrenia is a diagnostic term used to describe a major psychotic disorder characterized by disturbances in the following areas:

- Perception (e.g., hallucinations)
- Thought processes (e.g., flight of ideas, derailment)
- Reality testing (e.g., delusions)
- Feeling (e.g., flat or inappropriate affect)
- Behavior (e.g., social withdrawal)
- Attention (e.g., inability to concentrate)
- Motivation (e.g., cannot initiate or persist in goal-directed activities)

Contributing to overall deterioration is a decline in psychosocial functioning. It affects men and women almost equally; however, gender differences do exist. Box 24.1 highlights some of the gender differences in the expression of this disorder.

Studies have shown that approximately 1% of the population experiences schizophrenia during their lifetime. Although its prevalence rate and symptom presentation are fairly constant worldwide, inner-city residents, people from lower socioeconomic classes, and individuals who experience early childhood trauma are more likely to be affected; (American Psychiatric Association [APA], 2013). Economic costs are in the tens of billions of dollars each year. The cost of human suffering is incalculable.

Historical Perspective

Benedict Morel was the first to name the psychiatric symptoms of schizophrenia (see Box 24.2 for a historical summary). In 1860, while treating an adolescent boy, Morel used *dementia praecox* (precocious senility) to describe the group of symptoms he observed. Kahlbaum (in 1871) and Hecker (in 1874) added to the diagnostic nomenclature with their categories *catatonia* and *hebephrenia*. In 1878, Kraepelin added the term *paranoia* and engaged in a rigorous study of what is now called *schizophrenia*. Kraepelin found commonalities among the three mental disorders (catatonia, hebephrenia, and paranoia) and grouped them in 1899 under the diagnostic term that Morel had coined 40 years before—*dementia praecox*. Kraepelin believed that schizophrenia resulted from neuropathologic factors; he envisioned a progressively deteriorating course, resulting in disabling mental impairment with little hope of recovery.

TABLE 24.1 Twelve-Month Prevalence Rate of Mental Disorders in the United States[a]

Disorders	Approximate Percentage >17 Years Old (%)[a] (Unless Noted for Children)	Gender Over-Representation
Anxiety disorders	18.1 overall	
Agoraphobia	1.7	Female
Panic disorder	2.4	Female
Panic attacks	11.2	Female
Social anxiety	7	Female
Specific phobia	7–9	Female
Separation anxiety	1.2	Equal
Generalized anxiety disorder	2	Female
Posttraumatic stress disorder	3.4	Female
Obsessive-compulsive disorder	1.2	Equal
Major depression	8.6	Female
Bipolar disorder I and II	1.8	BD I: ~ Equal BD II: Female
Autism spectrum disorders	1 in children	Male
Disruptive, impulse control, and conduct disorders	8.9 overall	
Conduct disorders[a]	4 in children	Male
Attention-deficit/ hyperactivity disorder[a]	5 in children; 2.5 in adults	Male
Substance use disorders	8.9 overall	
Alcohol use disorder	8.5 in adults; 2.5 in 12- to 17-year-olds	Male
Other substances	1.4	Male
Schizophrenia	1.1	~ Equal

[a]These statistics apply to individuals over 17 years of age unless specifically noted for children.
Modified from Kessler, R. C., Petukhova, M., Sampson, N. A., Zaslavsky, A. M., & Wittchen, H.-U. (2012). Twelve-month and lifetime prevalence and lifetime morbid risk of anxiety and mood disorders in the United States. *International Journal of Methods of Psychiatric Research, 21*, 169; American Psychiatric Association. (2013). *Diagnostic and statistical manual of mental disorders* (5th ed.). APA.

BOX 24.1 Typical Gender-Based Differences in Schizophrenia

- Age of onset is typically 4–6 years earlier in men.
- Men have a more severe course.
- Women have more positive symptoms (e.g., hallucinations).
- Estrogen modulates dopamine function and presumably plays a protective role for women.
- Women are more compliant with medications.
- Women tend to have lower blood levels and longer half-lives of medications.

BOX 24.2   Evolution of Schizophrenia Subtyping

1860	Morel coins the term *dementia praecox*.
1871	Kahlbaum uses the term *catatonia* to describe patients immobilized by psychological factors.
1874	Hecker uses the term *hebephrenia* to describe patients with silly, bizarre, and regressed behaviors.
1878	Kraepelin adds the term *paranoia* to describe highly suspicious patients.
1899	Kraepelin groups all three patient categories under the heading *dementia praecox*.
The 1900s	Bleuler introduces the term *schizophrenia* to describe these mental disorders.
1952	*DSM-I:* Includes 9 subtypes for schizophrenia.
1968	*DSM-II:* Includes 11 subtypes.
1980	*DSM-III:* Reduced to 5 subtypes: disorganized, catatonic, paranoid, undifferentiated, and residual.
1982	Schizophrenia is categorized based on symptoms: positive (type I) and negative (type II).
1994	*DSM-IV:* Includes same subtypes as *DSM-III*.
1997	American Psychiatric Association recognizes the addition of the subtype "disorganized" to the positive and negative subtyping concept.
2000	*DSM-IV-TR:* Includes same subtypes.
2013	*DSM-5:* Removes subtypes.

It was left to Bleuler in the early 1900s to coin the term *schizophrenia* in a book subtitled *The Group of Schizophrenias.* Bleuler believed that schizophrenia does not always follow a course of deterioration (making the term *dementia* inappropriate). It does not always occur early in life (making the term *praecox* also inappropriate). Bleuler broadened Kraepelin's concept by focusing on symptoms and identified four primary symptoms that he believed were present in all individuals with schizophrenia. All four of these classic symptoms begin with the letter "A" (Bleuler's "four A's"), which facilitates memorization: *a*ffect disturbance, *a*utism, *a*ssociative looseness, and *a*mbivalence.

Kraepelin and Bleuler, two historical giants of psychiatry, founded two divergent views of schizophrenia. In using the diagnostic category of dementia praecox, Kraepelin revealed a conceptual alignment between schizophrenia and disorders such as Alzheimer disease, which have a less optimistic prognosis. Bleuler developed a school of thought that was much broader and more optimistic than that of Kraepelin. Based on Bleuler's wider grouping, pessimism eased, and some clinicians began to see improvements in their patients. Although Kraepelin based his views on biology, Bleuler, influenced by the master analyst Freud and other psychodynamic theorists, sought psychological explanations for schizophrenia. For most of the 20th century, Freud's psychoanalytic explanations and, by extension, Bleuler's thinking dominated the understanding of schizophrenia. However, as the limitations of "talking" cures became more evident, mental health professionals became less interested in the psychodynamic approach. In the past

40 years or so, a resurgence of interest in biologic research has resulted in a renewed respect for Kraepelin's work.

? CRITICAL THINKING QUESTION

1. When clinicians think that their patients could get better, the patients seem to improve. What do you make of this?

Course of Illness

Schizophrenia typically first occurs in adolescence or early adulthood, during which brain maturation is almost complete. There are three overlapping phases of the disorder:

- *Acute phase:* The patient experiences severe psychotic symptoms.
- *Stabilizing phase:* The patient is getting better.
- *Stable phase:* The patient might still experience hallucinations and delusions in this phase, but they are not as severe or disabling as they were during the acute phase.

Most patients alternate between acute and stable phases.

Clinical Example: Hallucinating but stable

Billy is a 39-year-old man living in a psychiatric residential facility who attends a day treatment program Monday through Friday. Although Billy experiences hallucinations frequently, most often visual hallucinations, he is stabilized. All staff members agree that Billy is not a danger to himself or others and that the day treatment program is more appropriate for him than a state hospital.

? CRITICAL THINKING QUESTION

2. Why do you think Kraepelin was so pessimistic about the patients whom he saw with dementia praecox?

DSM-5 Terminology and Criteria

Schizophrenia spectrum and other psychotic disorders include schizophrenia, schizoaffective disorder, schizophreniform disorder, delusional disorder, brief psychotic disorder, and schizotypal personality disorder. Key features that define this spectrum of disorders include the presence of one or more of the following: delusions, hallucinations, disordered thinking and/or speech, abnormal behavior such as catatonia, and negative symptoms (DSM-5, 2013).

Positive and Negative Symptoms of Schizophrenia

Schizophrenia is known to have positive and negative symptoms (Box 24.3). Positive symptoms are an embellishment or exaggeration of normal cognition and perception. The symptoms are additional. Positive symptoms are believed to result from elevated dopamine levels affecting the limbic areas of the brain.

DSM-5 CRITERIA

Schizophrenia

Diagnostic Criteria

A. Two (or more) of the following, each present for a significant portion of time during a 1-month period (or less if successfully treated). At least one of these must be (1), (2), or (3):
  1. Delusions.
  2. Hallucinations.
  3. Disorganized speech (e.g., frequent derailment or incoherence).
  4. Grossly disorganized or catatonic behavior.
  5. Negative symptoms (i.e., diminished emotional expression or avolition).

B. For a significant portion of the time since the onset of the disturbance, the level of functioning in one or more major areas, such as work, interpersonal relations, or self-care, is markedly below the level achieved before the onset (or when the onset is in childhood or adolescence, there is failure to achieve expected level of interpersonal, academic, or occupational functioning).

C. Continuous signs of the disturbance persist for at least 6 months. This 6-month period must include at least 1 month of symptoms (or less if successfully treated) that meet criterion A (i.e., active-phase symptoms) and may include periods of prodromal or residual symptoms. During these prodromal or residual periods, the signs of the disturbance may be manifested by only negative symptoms or by two or more symptoms listed in criterion A present in an attenuated form (e.g., odd beliefs, unusual perceptual experiences).

D. Schizoaffective disorder and depressive or bipolar disorder with psychotic features have been ruled out because either (1) no major depressive or manic episodes have occurred concurrently with the active-phase symptoms; or (2) if mood episodes have occurred during active-phase symptoms, they have been present for a minority of the total duration of the active and residual periods of the illness.

E. The disturbance is not attributable to the physiological effects of a substance (e.g., a drug of abuse, a medication) or another medical condition.

F. If there is a history of autism spectrum disorder or a communication disorder of childhood onset, the additional diagnosis of schizophrenia is made only if prominent delusions or hallucinations, in addition to the other required symptoms of schizophrenia, are also present for at least 1 month (or less if successfully treated).

Specify if

The following course specifiers are only to be used after a 1-year duration of the disorder and if they are not in contradiction to the diagnostic course criteria.

First episode, currently in acute episode: First manifestation of the disorder meeting the defining diagnostic symptom and time criteria. An acute episode is a time period in which the symptom criteria are fulfilled.

First episode, currently in partial remission: Partial remission is when an improvement after a previous episode is maintained. The defining criteria of the disorder are only partially fulfilled.

First episode, currently in full remission: Full remission is a period of time after a previous episode during which no disorder-specific symptoms are present.

Multiple episodes, currently in acute episode: Multiple episodes may be determined after a minimum of two episodes (i.e., after a first episode, remission, and a minimum of one relapse).

Multiple episodes, currently in partial remission

Multiple episodes, currently in full remission

Continuous: Symptoms fulfilling the diagnostic symptom criteria of the disorder remain for the majority of the illness course, with subthreshold symptom periods being very brief relative to the overall course.

Unspecified

Specify if

With catatonia (refer to the criteria for catatonia associated with another mental disorder, pp. 119–120, for definition).

Coding note: Use additional code 293.89 (F06.1) catatonia associated with schizophrenia to indicate the presence of comorbid catatonia.

Specify Current Severity

Severity is rated by a quantitative assessment of the primary symptoms of psychosis, including delusions, hallucinations, disorganized speech, abnormal psychomotor behavior, and negative symptoms. Each of these symptoms may be rated for its current severity (most severe in the last 7 days) on a 5-point scale ranging from 0 (not present) to 4 (present and severe). (See Clinical-Rated Dimensions of Psychosis Symptom Severity in the chapter "Assessment Measure.")

Note: Diagnosis of schizophrenia can be made without using this severity specifier.

From the American Psychiatric Association. (2013). *Diagnostic and statistical manual of mental disorders* (5th ed.). APA.

Clinical Example: Positive symptoms

John is sitting in the day room on the psychiatric unit when his eyes begin to dart back and forth, and he becomes increasingly anxious. You ask, "John, are you hearing something that I cannot hear?" "Can't you hear them?" he replies. "They are going to get me." John's auditory hallucination is a positive symptom because it exaggerates a normal perception ("hearing" without an auditory stimulus).

The negative symptoms of schizophrenia are experienced as an absence or diminution of normal cognition and perception (e.g., lack of affect, lack of energy). Unfortunately, many negative symptoms linger for years in some patients (Khan et al., 2017). Negative symptoms are related, at least in part, to a hypodopaminergic process. These symptoms are also associated with structural changes in the brain. Pathoanatomy consistently mentioned in the literature includes decreased cerebral blood flow and increased ventricular brain ratios (i.e., enlarged

BOX 24.3   Positive and Negative Symptoms of Schizophrenia[a]

Positive Symptoms: Caused by Excessive Dopamine in Mesolimbic Tract[a]

Abnormal thoughts
Agitation
Bizarre behavior
Delusions
Excitement
Feelings of persecution
Grandiosity
Hallucinations
Hostility
Illusions
Insomnia
Suspiciousness

Negative Symptoms: Caused by Too Little Dopamine in Mesocortical Tract[a]

Alogia
Anergia
Asocial behavior
Attention deficits
Avolition
Blunted affect
Communication difficulties
Difficulty with abstractions
Passive social withdrawal
Poor grooming and hygiene
Poor rapport
Poverty of speech

[a]This is an oversimplification of what occurs in the limbic and frontal lobes of the brain.

ventricles). Decreased frontal blood flow is most pronounced in the dorsolateral prefrontal cortex. Ventricular enlargement can be detected with the naked eye on computed tomography (CT) and magnetic resonance imaging (MRI). Other patho-anatomic features that might contribute to negative symptoms include a modest reduction in brain weight (and much less so than in Alzheimer disease) and cerebral atrophy.

Clinical Example: Negative symptoms

Philip Wilson has a long history of mental problems. Mr. Wilson is a patient in the state hospital system. The summary note written by the nursing team leader includes the following observation: "Mr. Wilson is isolative and, for the most part, expressionless. He spends long hours sitting and staring out of the window. Attempts to engage Mr. Wilson in unit activities have not been successful."

Negative symptoms are associated with increased morbidity among schizophrenic patients due to the following risk factors that enhance their expression:

- Antipsychotic medications
- Hospitalizations
- Loss of social supports
- Socioeconomic decline

Therefore, early assessment and treatment of these patients are needed to arrest chronic, gradual decompensation.

Clinical Example: Lack of connectedness

Merritt is a homeless man with a long history of mental illness. He has not seen his family in many years. Although his family was supportive, they became overwhelmed as he continuously became worse with shorter periods of remission. At this point, even modest improvements in his mental health are compromised by his lack of social support.

According to biologic theory, typical antipsychotic drugs (drugs that antagonize dopamine D2 receptors primarily) are likely to benefit positive symptoms due to a hyperdopaminergic process. In contrast, negative symptoms are thought to be more structurally related and a partially hypodopaminergic process. Traditional antipsychotics have relatively little effect and might cause negative symptoms to worsen. The more excessive the positive symptoms, the greater is the likelihood of a favorable response to antipsychotics. As noted in Chapter 14, atypical antipsychotic drugs may benefit negative symptoms because they affect dopamine receptors and antagonize serotonin 5-hydroxytryptamine 2A receptors, which liberate dopamine in cortical areas, that is, correcting the hypodopaminergic state. Most of these newer drugs are expensive as long as they are patent-protected.

Behavior

People who are treated for mental problems come to the attention of mental health professionals in one of two ways. The first is when people seek help. They do so because they have experienced such troubling subjective symptoms that they want professional intervention. However, professional help often is not sought until people have exhausted self-help aids, friends, and family. The second way in which people come to the attention of the mental health system is that they draw attention to themselves through behaviors that *bother*, *concern*, or *frighten* other people. These indicators of a mental disorder are apparent to others and are called *objective signs*. As discussed in Chapter 3, the patient sometimes resists help, and they must be treated on an involuntary basis.

Subjective and objective categories are not as discrete as they might appear at first. For example, hallucinations are subjective phenomena but might easily cause objective signs that get the attention of others (e.g., a person who talks back to an auditory hallucination). Nonetheless, dividing the expressions of schizophrenia into subjective symptoms and objective signs is a rational and convenient approach for understanding this mental disorder. Several rating scales for the severity of schizophrenia have been developed, and psychiatric nurses must be familiar with them. Six significant alterations occur in schizophrenia and can be grouped into objective signs or subjective symptoms (Box 24.4). Alterations in personal relationships and alterations of activity are highly visible to others (objective signs), whereas altered perceptions, thought, consciousness, and affect are more subjective in nature.

Two Objective Signs

Alterations in personal relationships. Patients with schizophrenia have troubled interpersonal relationships. Often, these problems develop over a long period, well before schizophrenia is diagnosed, and become more pronounced as the illness progresses. It is common to hear that a person was asocial, a loner, or a social misfit before being diagnosed.

Frequently, patients become less concerned with their appearance and might not bathe without persistent prodding. Table manners and other social skills might diminish to the point at which patients are offensive to others. Patients are focused on internal processes to the extent that their external social world collapses. Schizophrenia can cause a diminished energy level (anergia), which also complicates social interactions.

Interpersonal communication becomes inadequate and might be inappropriate. Again, internal processes are at work. Hostility, a common theme, also distances these individuals from others. Finally, people with schizophrenia withdraw, further compromising their ability to engage in meaningful social interactions.

BOX 24.4 Objective and Subjective Behavioral Disorders in Schizophrenia

Objective Signs

Alterations in Personal Relationships
- Decreased attention to appearance and social relationships
- Inadequate or inappropriate communication
- Hostility
- Withdrawal

Alterations of Activity
- Psychomotor agitation
- Catatonic rigidity
- Echopraxia (repetitive movements)
- Stereotypy (repetitive acts or words)

Subjective Symptoms

Altered Perception
- Hallucinations
- Illusions
- Paranoid thinking

Alterations of Thought
- Loose associations
- Retardation
- Blocking
- Autism
- Ambivalence
- Delusions
- Poverty of speech
- Ideas of reference
- Mutism

Altered Consciousness
- Confusion
- Incoherent speech
- Clouding
- Sense of "going crazy"

Alterations of Affect
- Inappropriate, blunted, flattened, or labile affect
- Apathy
- Ambivalence
- Overreaction
- Anhedonia

Clinical Example: Loneliness and schizophrenia

William is a white man in his early 40s with schizophrenia. He can be seen walking near the university. He nearly always wears the same clothes. He arrives early at Starbucks almost every morning. He never buys anything, but the young woman working there gives him a glass of water. He doesn't talk. He sits and sips. He is obese and typically smelly. He has nowhere to go, no one to see, and no friends.

Alterations of activity. Patients with schizophrenia also display alterations of activity. Patients might be too active (psychomotor agitation)—they are unable to sit still and continually pace—or they might be inactive or catatonic. These symptoms respond to antipsychotic drugs but can also be caused by them. The following clinical example illustrates this point.

Clinical Example: Symptoms or side effects?

The nurse must be careful in assessing alterations in activity level. *Restlessness* might be caused by akathisia (an extrapyramidal side effect [EPSE]) or might be a manifestation of schizophrenia. *Rigidity* might be a sign of drug-related parkinsonism (also an EPSE), not catatonia. Accurate assessment of EPSEs of antipsychotic drugs is critical. Although it is appropriate to administer an as-needed (prn) dose of haloperidol for psychomotor agitation or catatonia, this same drug would intensify akathisia and other EPSEs.

Four Subjective Symptoms

Subjective symptoms, by definition, are experienced by patients in a personal way. Patients might hide these symptoms from others. For example, if a patient experiences the delusion that he is a famous person, he might be able to keep it to himself. Some clinicians advise patients who resist psychiatric care to "keep your symptoms to yourself, and no one will ever know." Presumably, some individuals in society are not reporting their subjective symptoms to anyone and are avoiding psychiatric intervention. For the most part, however, subjective symptoms of schizophrenia spill over into behavior in public view. Subjective symptoms can be grouped into four categories.

Altered perception. Altered perception includes hallucinations, illusions, and paranoid thinking. Hallucinations are false sensory perceptions and can be auditory, visual, olfactory, tactile, gustatory, or somatic (strange body sensations). Auditory hallucinations are the most common in schizophrenia and often take the form of accusations ("You slut," "You're worthless") or commands ("Get away from these people"); however, many "normal" people (~10% to 15%) also report auditory hallucinations (Crowner, 2014). Visual hallucinations are not as common in schizophrenia. (The nurse might suspect a toxic process such as drugs or fever if visual hallucinations are present.) A hyperdopaminergic state probably causes hallucinations.

Illusions are misinterpretations of real external stimuli. For example, a tree might be mistaken for a threatening person. Illusions are often associated with physical illness as well as schizophrenia.

Clinical Example: Delirium versus schizophrenia

Delirium: While lying in a hospital bed with a low-grade fever, Gladys, a 68-year-old woman, asks, "Are those cobwebs on the wall?" Her son responds, "No, Mama, those are just shadows from your bedside lamp." Gladys laughs and says, "I guess my mind is going."

Schizophrenia: Tim, a patient in a day treatment program, mistakes a tennis shoe on the porch for a rat.

Paranoid thinking is characterized by a persistent interpretation of the actions of others as threatening or demeaning. Paranoid themes can color delusions and hallucinations as well as the ordinary behavior of others. The student needs to differentiate paranoid thinking associated with a paranoid personality disorder from paranoid delusions in schizophrenia (Wilcox & Duffy, 2016). Paranoid thinking is less severe than paranoid delusions. Paranoid thinking might be corrected with facts, whereas paranoid delusions cannot be dispelled.

Clinical Example: Schizophrenia versus delusional disorders

Paranoid personality disorder: Bill, a patient at the mental health clinic, has sought help because of trouble on the job and at home. His ability to get along with people has deteriorated to the point that he has no friends. Bill's wife has started divorce proceedings, and he has sought treatment, hoping that she will change her mind. Over the last few years, Bill has been obsessed with the thought that his wife is cheating on him. He follows her when she leaves the house, sometimes listens to her telephone calls, and has confronted her with accusations

of infidelity. Whenever he finds that he is mistaken, he is relieved for a while and apologizes for not trusting her, but soon he begins to have the same paranoid thoughts. His paranoid thinking has caused alterations in his personal relationships.

Delusional disorder, persecutory type: Chuck is rational in almost every social situation and can hold a job, though some of his workmates find him odd at times. However, Chuck firmly believes that he is being followed by foreign agents even though his work does not entail anything related to the government.

Paranoid schizophrenia: Fred is a 28-year-old unemployed laborer. The police recently brought Fred to the emergency department. Fred had been at the downtown bus station preaching loudly to all who passed by. He spoke of a conspiracy of African Americans and Jews who plan to take over America. Fred tells the emergency department nurse that he feared for his life. He adds that he has proof that the FBI was behind President Kennedy's assassination.

Alterations of thought. Alterations of thought are common in schizophrenia and are sometimes disturbing and frightening. Antipsychotic drugs are often beneficial. Common thought disorders include thought blocking, ambivalence, loose associations, delusions, poverty of speech, and concrete thinking.

Thought blocking is a slowing of mental activity. A patient might state, "I just can't think." Blocking is the interruption of a thought and the inability to recall it. This symptom is very disturbing to patients and sometimes frightening. Blocking might be caused by the intrusion of hallucinations, delusions, or emotional factors. The following is a common example of blocking that could happen to anyone.

Clinical Example: Blocking, but no meds needed

Joe, a 55-year-old teacher, is in the middle of a lecture when he loses his "train of thought." He cannot remember what point he is developing or where to go next. He stalls for time, realizing that he is in a potentially embarrassing situation. Finally, he finds his notes and proceeds, a little shaken and distracted but able to continue.

Ambivalence is a state in which two opposite, strong feelings exist simultaneously. Patients might be both attracted to and repelled by a person, object, or goal. Ambivalence (e.g., love/hate) toward a domineering parent is common. Another common example is the simultaneous need for and fear of people, resulting in immobilization. Their ambivalence might immobilize patients with schizophrenia regarding a simple matter, such as deciding whether to drink orange juice or milk for breakfast. In these cases, it is therapeutic for the nurse to make patient decisions if patients allow this. The following clinical example illustrates ambivalence that occurs in some families, and it is not meant to depict schizophrenia ambivalence.

Loose association is a pattern of speech in which a person's ideas slip off one track onto another that is completely unrelated or only slightly related. An occasional change of topic without obvious connection, known as tangentiality, does not indicate loose associations. A more severe form of loose association is known as word salad. The single words spoken do not seem to be related to one another.

EXAMPLES OF LOOSE ASSOCIATIONS AND WORD SALAD

The following example of loose associations is based on a conversation with Bill, a 46-year-old patient attending day treatment. Because of the severity of his disorder, he was admitted to a state hospital shortly after this interaction.

Nurse: "How are you doing today, Bill?"

Bill: "Do it. Get it on with monster woman. Do it. Sure Bill, sure. Do it. Prevented. There goes the doctor. Kills a woman to have a baby. Fish woman. Purple bologna. That was good. Was that a 38, 25, or 44–45 magnum? White hair. A pig. Ham social security. USDA. USGI grocery store. Paycheck. Money. Funny. Money. Meat. Charles Atlas. Arnold. Hercules. Destroyed Bill. Destroyed Charles Atlas. Charley. Charles Manson. Manchild Part I of Bill. Charley Manson Bill. Helter Skelter. White people. Bride of Frankenstein blood drinkers."

As is readily apparent, Bill's communication pattern at this time is incoherent. With effort, one can see some of the underlying connections of these disconnected words and phrases, but overall, Bill's dialogue cannot be followed.

Delusions are fixed, false beliefs and can take many forms. They are described as fixed beliefs because they cannot be changed by logical persuasion. They are described as false because they are not based on reality. Delusional content often relates to life experiences and can include erotomanic, somatic, grandiose, religious, nihilistic, referential, and paranoid content. An example of each type follows:

- *Erotomanic*: A patient believes that Sandra Bullock is in love with him.
- *Somatic:* After medical tests confirm otherwise, a patient still insists, "I have cancer in my stomach."
- *Grandiose delusions:* A patient states, "I am the president."
- *Religious delusions:* A woman attempts to kill her children because she believes the devil wants her to do so.
- *Nihilistic delusions:* A patient believes he is dead.
- *Delusions of reference:* "The TV is talking about me. The guests on *Oprah* are making fun of me."
- *Delusions of influence:* "I can control her with my thoughts."
- *Persecutory:* "They all think that I am a homosexual."
- *Jealous:* A patient believes her husband or lover is unfaithful.

Related phenomena sometimes encountered are the bizarre delusions that thoughts can be inserted or withdrawn by others: "Other people can read my mind"; "My thoughts are being broadcast so that everyone can hear." Finally, three very interesting delusions, all identified in France, have been reviewed by Riggs et al. (2017):

Cotard Delusion: persistent feelings of non-existence.

Folie a Deux: the sharing of a delusional belief among two or more people.

Capgras Delusion: someone/someplace/something is an imposter.

Poverty of speech is manifested by the inability to formulate and articulate thoughts that are relevant to the discussion at hand. Vocabulary is markedly limited in individuals who experience poverty of speech.

Concrete thinking is the inability to conceptualize the meanings of words and phrases. For example, a concrete response to the proverb "People who live in glass houses should not throw stones" might be "The glass would break." These individuals are likely to misinterpret jokes or similes. For example, the meaning of "a diamond in the rough" or "cool as a cucumber" might be lost on a person exhibiting concrete thinking.

Altered consciousness. Altered consciousness is perhaps the most troubling symptom to patients; however, it is also often responsive to antipsychotic drugs. Manifestations of altered consciousness include confusion, incoherent speech, clouding, and a sense of going crazy. The last manifestation of altered consciousness—going crazy—deserves special mention. Many students are surprised when they enter a psychiatric facility to find that patients are not "crazy." Although psychiatric patients by definition are struggling with mental disorders, psychiatric units are not wild, bizarre environments. Patients can readily differentiate between the normal struggle of dealing with a mental disorder and the feeling of going crazy (loss of control). The student will observe that patients on the psychiatric unit define a fellow patient who has become wild or who is loudly talking to himself or herself as "crazy." In other words, this behavior is unusual—even in a psychiatric unit. Referring to the discussion of incompetence in Chapter 3, the student can appreciate why the designation of incompetence is reserved for only a select few individuals.

Alterations of affect. Alterations of affect vary and include inappropriate, flattened, blunted, or labile affects; apathy; ambivalence; and overreaction. For example, responding to bad news with laughter is an affective response that is inappropriate and does not match the circumstances. If a patient cannot generate much affect, and the response to the bad news is understated, the affect is *blunted* or *dull*. The inability to generate any affective response is referred to as a *flattened affect*. Labile affect is a condition in which emotional tone changes quickly. A patient might be telling a happy story, suddenly begin to cry, and quickly become violent.

Apathy, defined as a lack of concern or interest, is the inability to generate a normal response to people, situations, or the environment.

Another alteration of affect is the tendency to overreact to events. A trauma-informed framework helps understand emotional reactivity. Patients with schizophrenia may overreact when triggered due to past childhood trauma. The emotional outbursts, especially when frequent, tend to offend the sensitivities of people nearby.

Etiology

Many authorities suggest that multiple factors must cause schizophrenia because no single theory satisfactorily explains the disorder. Explanations can be categorized broadly into biologic or psychological (psychodynamic) causes. These two categories parallel the nature versus nurture debate discussed in Chapter 23. Biologic and psychodynamic theories are discussed here, followed by a vulnerability-stress model. This eclectic approach seems to describe the major forces at work in the genesis and outcomes of schizophrenia.

Biologic Theories: Biochemical, Neurostructural, Genetic, and Perinatal Factors

People don't cause schizophrenia; they merely blame each other for doing so.

Dr. E. Fuller Torrey

Biologic theorists posit that anatomic or physiologic abnormalities cause schizophrenia. Biologic explanations include biochemical, neurostructural, genetic, and perinatal risk factors, and other theories. Biologic explanations have driven the development of biologic interventions, such as psychotropic drugs.

Some clinicians have been reluctant to endorse biologic theories because the exclusive use of biologic approaches, such as psychotropic drugs, excludes interpersonal factors. However, the psychotherapeutic management model recognizes the importance of both biologic and interpersonal interventions.

A positive result of biologic theories has been the minimization of the blaming that is inherent in other explanations. Just as viewing alcoholism as an illness has helped clinicians, families, and patients to get beyond blaming and on to treatment, biologic theories have facilitated the treatment of schizophrenia. To illustrate, just as diabetic patients must learn to cope with their illness (e.g., a lifestyle change), psychiatric patients must learn to cope with the limitations of their illness. Over 100 biological factors or biomarkers

have been identified (Ma, Rolls, Liu, Liu, Jiao, Wang, & Wan, 2019). Significant biological issues are discussed here.

Biochemical theories. Biochemical theory can be traced to 1952 when Delay and Deniker reported the antipsychotic effects of the dopamine receptor antagonist, chlorpromazine. The prevailing biochemical explanation is referred to as the *dopamine hypothesis*. According to this hypothesis, excessive dopaminergic activity in limbic areas causes acute positive symptoms of schizophrenia (hallucinations, delusions, and thought disorders). Excessive dopamine might result from increased dopamine synthesis, increased dopamine release, or an increase in the number and activity of dopamine receptors. It is also known that drugs that increase dopamine, such as levodopa and amphetamines, can cause a psychotic state. This hypothesis is attractive because it is easy to grasp and because drugs that block dopamine seem to be extremely effective in the treatment of schizophrenia. However, it takes days, weeks, or months to establish the clinical effectiveness of these drugs, whereas the central nervous system dopamine receptors are blocked within a few minutes. Therefore, it seems that the dopamine hypothesis is too simplistic and that other factors are involved in explaining the effectiveness of antipsychotic drugs.

The following are the apparent positive effects of smoking on schizophrenia (see the box entitled "Cigarette Smoking and Schizophrenia") caused by stimulation of nicotinic receptors in the brain:

1. Improved cognition
2. Improved negative symptoms
3. Protective effects against EPSEs
4. Improved auditory gating
5. Improved memory and attention

The dopamine hypothesis, although limited in explanatory power, continues to have great educational value for the following reasons:

1. Drugs that increase dopamine (i.e., dopaminergics, such as levodopa and amphetamine) can cause psychotic symptoms.
2. Drugs that block dopamine (i.e., antipsychotics) alleviate psychotic symptoms.

Other proposed neurotransmitter contributors to schizophrenia include serotonin and glutamate. Serotonin inhibits dopamine synthesis and release; serotonin antagonists potentially increase dopamine levels. This characteristic is one of the neurophysiologic properties presumed to cause atypical antipsychotics to be effective. These agents are referred to as *serotonin-dopamine antagonists* by some clinicians and manufacturers.

Glutamate, a product of the Krebs cycle, also has been proposed as a factor in schizophrenia. Glutamate contributes to the regulation of N-methyl-D-aspartate (NMDA) receptors, which are necessary for cognitive processes. Too little glutamate can lead to hallucinations. For example, the street drug phencyclidine (PCP) antagonizes NMDA receptors and can cause a psychotic state. Excessive levels of glutamate lead to overstimulation of the NMDA receptors, increasing intracellular calcium levels and causing increased neuronal

CIGARETTE SMOKING AND SCHIZOPHRENIA

People with schizophrenia tend to smoke a lot. One out of two cigarettes sold in the United States is smoked by a person with mental health or substance use disorders (Anthenelli, 2016). Although approximately 21% of the general public smokes, studies have indicated that 74% of individuals with schizophrenia smoke (El-Mallakh et al., 2016). The difference in cigarette use between this population and the general population is significant, but there are noticeably fewer attempts at smoking cessation (Cieslak & Freudenreich, 2018). Some researchers have argued that depriving the person with schizophrenia of the joys of smoking would be unduly cruel—smoking presumably is one of the few pleasures they have. Others have decried these weak attempts at smoking cessation programs for individuals with serious mental illness and see them as nothing less than discriminatory.

Why do people with schizophrenia smoke so much? The answer to this question probably lies in the biochemical changes produced by nicotine. All drugs of abuse cause changes in brain dopamine levels. Dopamine axons from the ventral tegmental area are afferents through the reward pathway, including the putative pleasure nucleus, the nucleus accumbens. Nicotine increases the release of dopamine in the nucleus accumbens. This occurs because nicotinic receptors synapse on dopamine afferents in the reward pathway—that is, nicotine modulates dopamine release. Nicotine also modulates dopamine afferents to the prefrontal cortex (mesocortical tract). When coupled with the supposition that negative symptoms are related to a hypodopaminergic process, nicotinic stimulation of dopamine in prefrontal areas might produce a therapeutic effect. In other words, the answer to the question, "Why do patients with schizophrenia smoke so much?" is simply this: It makes them feel better. Despite recognizing the significant health risks of smoking among individuals with schizophrenia, predictors for smoking aside from nicotine dependence also include education, motivation to quit, and relief (Kowalczyk et al., 2017). A study by Miller et al. (2017) reported on smokers described as "ever-users" who reported that they felt regular cigarettes significantly helped reduce symptoms of depression and anxiety, impaired concentration, and paranoia compared with e-cigarettes.

firing. This cellular excess is referred to as *excitotoxicity* and can cause neuronal death. Cell death plays a role in schizophrenia. Treatment with glutamate has not been particularly promising at this point.

Neurostructural theories. Neurostructural theorists have proposed that schizophrenia, particularly negative symptoms, is significantly the result of pathoanatomy. The three specific neurostructural changes mentioned most often are:

1. Enlarged ventricles (often referred to as increased ventricular brain ratios)
2. Brain atrophy
3. Decreased cerebral blood flow

Ventricular brain ratios. The finding that a significant subgroup of individuals with schizophrenia has enlarged ventricles was first reported by Johnstone and colleagues in the 1970s. Individuals with enlarged ventricles have a poor prognosis and exhibit negative symptoms.

Although ventricular enlargement is not peculiar to schizophrenia, anatomic findings are substantially different from findings for neurodegenerative disorders, such as Alzheimer disease. Ventricular enlargement in schizophrenia is not associated with a neurodegenerative process; that is, one would not expect to find a gradual increase in ventricular volume over time in a patient with schizophrenia. However, in a patient with Alzheimer disease, ventricles continue to increase in volume as brain cells die. Not all patients with schizophrenia have abnormally enlarged ventricles. About 50% of these patients fall within the range of control or normal subjects. This overlapping effect has led researchers to study monozygotic twins when one twin has schizophrenia. In documented cases in which the affected twin had ventricles falling within the normal range, enlarged ventricles can be demonstrated only when contrasted with the ventricles of the unaffected (i.e., non-schizophrenia) twin.

Brain atrophy. More than 100 years ago, Alzheimer described brain cell loss in schizophrenia. Brain imaging has suggested anatomic pathology in cortical and subcortical areas and confirmed by postmortem examinations of individuals with schizophrenia. Limbic, hippocampal, and thalamic structures; temporal lobes; the amygdala; and the substantia nigra are specific lobes and nuclei found to have undergone neuropathologic changes.

Neuroimaging and cerebral blood flow studies have revealed structural, functional, and neurochemical modifications that are more prominent in the cortex and subcortical regions of the brain (Keshavan et al., 2020). Individuals with atrophic changes also have decreased cortical blood flow, particularly in the prefrontal cortex, with decreases noted in metabolic activity (Kindler et al., 2018). Thus, cognitive demands, such as organizing, planning, learning from experience, problem solving, introspection, and critical judgment, are compromised.

Genetic theories. The relatives of patients with schizophrenia have a greater incidence of the disorder than chance alone would allow. Although a huge amount of resources have been directed at finding the genetic cause of schizophrenia, the results are not specific. There are thousands of fixed positions located on a chromosome (also referred to as loci) that have been linked to schizophrenia (Ma et al., 2019) and behavioral traits (personality, psychological, lifestyle, and nutritional) that are associated with elevated genetic risk for schizophrenia (Socrates et al., 2021).

The genetic risk for schizophrenia is shown in Box 24.5. Of particular interest to clinicians is the risk associated with having a parent with schizophrenia. This high incidence (15%) alone does not adequately address the debate of nature (genetics) versus nurture (upbringing). For instance, a parent

BOX 24.5 Commonly Reported Heritable Risks for Schizophrenia	
Identical twin affected	50%
Fraternal twin affected	15%
Brother or sister affected	10%
One parent affected	15%
Aunt/uncle/cousin affected	2%
General population/no affected relative	1%

with a mental disorder might rear children inadequately to the extent that the children are predisposed to schizophrenia based on parenting skills, not genetics.

Researchers have studied monozygotic (identical) and dizygotic (fraternal) twins to control the nurture variable. Monozygotic twins have consistently shown a higher concordancy rate (meaning both twins do or do not have symptoms of schizophrenia). Concordancy rates are 50% for monozygotic twins. This rate is 50 times higher than the risk for the general population, and it is 3 times higher than the risk for dizygotic or fraternal twins.

These findings seem to establish the genetic or natural basis of schizophrenia; however, extraneous variables cannot be explained. For example, many monozygotic twins are dressed alike and often are misidentified; their upbringing might be identical, too. Some experts argue that it is no wonder that monozygotic twins have a high concordancy rate. Unless researchers can control the environmental variable, the relative impact of nature and nurture cannot be reported with confidence.

To control for the variable of environment, studies have been conducted of monozygotic twins who were separated at birth and reared apart. Monozygotic concordancy rates remained significantly higher in these studies.

❓ CRITICAL THINKING QUESTION

3. What would be a balanced approach to understanding the risk factors associated with schizophrenia?

Perinatal risk factors. Multiple nongenetic factors influence the development of schizophrenia. Some researchers believe that schizophrenia can be linked to prenatal exposure to influenza; birth during the winter; prenatal exposure to lead; minor malformations developing during early gestation; exposure to viruses from house cats; and pregnancy complications, particularly during labor and delivery. The research about the influenza epidemic is inconclusive, but there is evidence that individuals with schizophrenia are more likely to have been born in the winter months (APA, 2013). Research of cohorts conceived during devastating influenza epidemics has revealed a meaningfully higher incidence of schizophrenia in products of conception (i.e., children) during this time.

Psychodynamic Theories and Childhood Trauma

Psychodynamic theories of schizophrenia, which at one time held much sway in psychiatric circles, describe schizophrenia as being linked to an earlier Freudian stage called primary narcissism where the id is not separated from the ego (the rational part of the mind), leading to the individual losing touch with reality (Rupani & DeSousa, 2017). There is research linking childhood trauma to more vulnerability in developing schizophrenia. Additive effects of childhood trauma have been associated with increased positive symptoms, depressive symptoms, and poorer cognitive function in patients with schizophrenia (Popovic et al., 2019). The common theme of these explanations is the internal reaction to life stressors or conflicts. These explanations include developmental and family theories.

Developmental theories of schizophrenia. During the early part of the 20th century, Meyer and Freud emphasized the significance of developmental psychiatry. They believed that the seeds of mental health and illness are sown in childhood. An extension of their arguments is that events in early life can cause severe problems such as schizophrenia. The work of two developmental theorists, Erik Erikson (1902–1994) and Harry Stack Sullivan (1892–1949), increases understanding of schizophrenia. Erikson, who theorized an eight-stage model of human development, saw the first step, trust or mistrust, as crucial to later interpersonal relationships. A child who is deprived of a nurturing, loving environment or who is neglected or rejected is vulnerable to mental disturbances. Inadequate passage through this stage predisposes the person to mistrust, isolative behaviors, and other asocial behaviors—the very behaviors found in schizophrenia. Therapeutic intervention focuses on the reestablishment of trust through consistent, safe, and secure relationships.

Sullivan, using different terms, expressed essentially the same ideas. The absence of warm, nurturing attention during the early years blocks the expression of these same affective responses in later years. Without this capacity, a person exhibits disordered social interactions and other disturbances. These individuals learn to avoid interpersonal interactions because these interactions are painful and even dangerous.

Family theories of schizophrenia. Family theories of schizophrenia are linked naturally to developmental theories. If early life experiences are crucial in development, the argument is made that the family—the environment in which most people grow—is significant to developing mental health or illness. Lack of a loving and nurturing primary caregiver, inconsistent family behaviors, and faulty communication patterns are thought to be responsible for mental problems in later life.

Outdated and harmful theories specifically tailored to the families of individuals with schizophrenia were the schizophrenogenic mother theory and the double-bind theory. The word *schizophrenogenic* literally means "to cause schizophrenia." Perhaps this definition has been the greatest disservice of psychodynamic theories. Essentially, this notion states that the blame for schizophrenia can be placed on the mother. The double-bind theory described family practices in which the child was damned if he did and damned if he didn't. An example often used was the child who was expected to do well in school but was criticized for taking time away from the family to study. Acocella (2000) captured some of the ideology behind these assertions:

> Psychoanalysis took a while to conquer the United States, but once it did, after the Second World War, its dominance was unquestioned, and its arrogance breathtaking. Schizophrenia, autism, and numerous other disorders were blamed on the mother, with no evidence, just utter certainty. (p. 11)

Some clinicians refer to family theories as "blame theories." Families have been viewed as causative agents, saboteurs of treatment, toxic influences, and patients themselves. Sometimes families have been treated with hostility and distrust. Because families bear the brunt of preprofessional and postprofessional care of these patients, it is important to work with families without alienating them.

Although most professionals have abandoned these harmful notions, some laypeople still labor under these misconceptions. Hence, they are mentioned in this textbook.

Clinical Example: Unbelievable but true—I

Many of us think back to our childhood and remember birthday parties and games, such as hide-and-seek and baseball games. Al thinks back to his past and remembers molestation, cruelty, and punishment. Al has been diagnosed with schizophrenia since the age of 20. But as one brother said, "Al ain't never been right."

Al is the next-to-youngest of eight children. According to Al, more than half of his siblings have a major mental illness. Al states, "My mama had schizophrenia for 10 years, then God saved her." When asked about his relationship with his mother now, Al states that she left the rest of the family after "Daddy" died. When questioned about his father, Al speaks of how his father used to beat his mother and the children. Al recalls seeing his father beat one brother so severely that he thought the boy might die. Al further described a beating he received from his father that left him bleeding. When asked why he thought his father beat him, Al responded, "He got mad a lot. I forgot to get firewood like he told me."

In discussing his illness, Al is asked to describe when he first started hearing voices. He replies, "When I was little after those boys did that to me. I was out fixing my bicycle, and I heard the devil talk to me over and over." Al reports numerous incidents of abuse during his life. During the interview, Al states his belief that his schizophrenia is God's punishment for his actions.

Al's first documented psychiatric episode occurred many years ago. In the psychological evaluation emanating from this experience, the psychiatrist noted hallucinations and delusions; Al described spaceships and command hallucinations, and he stated that he had killed Christ. His

---

condition deteriorated further, and he was committed to a public hospital. During his hospitalization, Al was given a diagnosis of schizophrenia.

Today, Al lives in a residential group home and attends day treatment. He continues to experience both auditory and visual hallucinations. Although he is prescribed two atypical antipsychotic drugs, symptom control varies from day to day.

Vulnerability-Stress Model of Schizophrenia

Most clinicians and researchers generally believe that schizophrenia has multifactorial causes, with many susceptibility genes interacting with numerous environmental factors to yield what is called schizophrenia. Dr. Insel (2004), Director of the National Institute of Mental Health, referred to schizophrenia as a "perfect storm" of events.

As previously stated, no single theory adequately answers the questions about the genesis of schizophrenia. The vulnerability-stress model addresses the various forces that cause schizophrenia in some cases and in other cases cause the broader schizophrenia spectrum problems of schizoaffective disorders and schizophrenia-related personality disorders. This model recognizes that both biologic (including genetic) and psychodynamic predispositions to schizophrenia, when coupled with stressful life events, can precipitate a process of schizophrenia. According to this model, people with a predisposition to schizophrenia might (but not always) avoid serious psychiatric disease if they are protected from the stresses of life. Individuals with a similar vulnerability might develop schizophrenia if exposed to stressors. This point illustrates that a wealthy person might be spared the brunt of some stressors because of wealth, whereas a poor person, struggling to meet basic needs, confronts stressors on a daily basis. According to this model, the poor person is more likely to display symptoms of schizophrenia.

As noted earlier, schizophrenia is over-represented among poor people. Individuals with schizophrenia tend to drift downward socioeconomically. This unenviable status enhances their vulnerability by exposing them to constant stressors.

Student Example: The straw that broke the...

This situation is easily applied to you and your peers. Students who need to deal only with the stress of nursing school have it hard enough. Students who must deal with the stress of nursing school plus significant financial and family responsibilities have a heavier load to manage. When a family crisis or change in work status comes along, the student who already has multiple stressors often has a more difficult time adjusting to life demands.

SPECIAL ISSUES RELATED TO SCHIZOPHRENIA

Many special issues need to be clarified to help the student focus on the breadth of concerns involved in the psychiatric nursing care of patients with schizophrenia. Box 24.6 lists key objectives when working with patients and families.

BOX 24.6   Key Objectives for Treating Patients With Schizophrenia

- Work with the family.
- Treat depression.
- Minimize stressful interactions.
- Treat substance abuse.
- Avoid lengthy, intense verbal interactions.

Comorbid Medical Illnesses

There are many special issues related to schizophrenia, but the issue of most concern is the high concordancy rate of other medical problems superimposed on schizophrenia. This is referred to as *comorbidity*. The majority of patients with schizophrenia have a comorbid condition. Specifically, there is a higher incidence of hypertension, diabetes, cardiovascular disease, metabolic syndrome, and accelerated aging in patients with schizophrenia (Table 24.2). Further, studies conclude that as measured by body mass index, 86% of women and 70% of men with schizophrenia are overweight or obese (Koch & Thomas, 2016). An overall life expectancy decrease of about 25 to 30 years has been consistently found in mortality studies among this diagnostic group and appears not to have lessened over time (Hjorthoj, Stürup, McGrath, & Nordentoft, 2017; Nasrallah, 2016). This situation (i.e., poor health, premature death) is confounded. It can be perpetuated by some psychotropic medications used to treat schizophrenia, lack of exercise, inadequate nutrition, and comorbid substance use disorders. Metabolic syndrome (see Chapter 14) is a very serious issue among patients taking antipsychotic drugs.

Families of Individuals With Schizophrenia

Families have often been blamed for the problems of individuals with schizophrenia. It is no wonder that some families are suspicious of professionals who might view the family as the villain. It is also not surprising that many of these families have little desire to be studied.

TABLE 24.2   Accelerated Aging of Relatively Young People in Schizophrenia

Central nervous system	Reduced brain volume and gray matter volume
Musculoskeletal	Altered nerve conduction; reduced bone density
Skin	Aging skin
Eyes	More cataracts
Endocrine	Low estrogen, low androgen, thyroid dysfunction
Cardiovascular	Systolic hypertension; increased pulse pressure
Telomeres[a]	Significantly higher rates of telomere loss.

[a]Telomeres are located at the end of chromosomes and govern cell replication.
Modified from Nasrallah, H. A. (2016). Accelerated aging in schizophrenia: Shorted telomeres, mitochondrial dysfunction, inflammation, and oxidative stress. *Current Psychiatry, 15*(11), 21.

Although research has substantiated the state of turmoil in these families, many clinicians argue that dysfunctional families are not the cause of schizophrenia but rather the result of having a family member with this illness. Nevertheless, when a family becomes destabilized, there is a high probability that the dysfunctional family will destabilize the member with schizophrenia.

Individuals with schizophrenia can be a disruptive influence on the family, particularly when they are not responding to prescribed medications or when they use mind-altering drugs. Although there is a consensus that negative features (e.g., emotionally overinvolved, hostile, and critical attitudes) are present in many families of patients with schizophrenia, these families are studied after schizophrenia has been identified—years after the illness might have disrupted the family. This observation leads to the "chicken or egg" question raised previously: Do disruptive families cause individuals to have schizophrenia, or do individuals with schizophrenia cause families to become disruptive, or both?

Although blame might be warranted in some family situations, in most cases, it is not. Blaming the family leads to a sense of alienation between the family and the treatment team. Nurses should remember that families bear the brunt of care outside the hospital. Most discharged psychiatric patients are sent home to live with their families; the family's stake in the patient's care is obvious. As time goes on, these families tend to become increasingly isolated and feel more frustrated, helpless, and hopeless, even though they care very much about the patient.

Clinical Example: A burned-out family

Pete is 24 years old. At age 19, he began having symptoms that eventually led to a diagnosis of schizophrenia. Through several hospitalizations and outpatient treatment programs, he continued to live at home with his parents. Pete started having delusions that people were watching him. His paranoid thinking reached such levels that his presence in the home completely disrupted family life. Pete would barricade himself in his room, believed that his parents were part of a conspiracy to spy on him, and occasionally became physically violent. After a fourth hospitalization 2 years earlier, Pete's parents informed the treatment team that he was no longer welcome in their home. They verbalized their fear of Pete and worried about how he was affecting his younger siblings in the home. Although his parents live within 50 miles of Pete, they seldom visit.

Depression and Suicide in Schizophrenia

Depressive symptoms are frequently a part of the psychopathology of schizophrenia, with some studies suggesting that approximately 25% of patients with schizophrenia experience depression (Siris, 2012). These symptoms can occur at any time during the illness, including years after the acute phase, but they do respond to antidepressants. A related phenomenon is the high incidence of suicide attempts (20%) and deaths (5% to 10%) among patients with schizophrenia

(APA, 2013). Suicide is the leading cause of premature death in patients with schizophrenia. There are several risk factors associated with the high prevalence of suicide (APA, 2013):

1. Depression related to schizophrenia
2. Hopelessness related to schizophrenia
3. Being unemployed
4. Comorbid substance use

Cognitive Dysfunction

It is well established that patients with schizophrenia have cognitive impairment. For example, memory, attention, and executive function are affected. Research has shown that cognitive deficits are a better predictor of declining abilities to engage in basic activities of daily living than positive or negative symptoms. Because cognitive ability directly influences so many aspects of successful living, it is important to discuss this aspect of schizophrenia with patients and family members.

Relapse

Stopping prescribed medications and exposure to significant stressors are the most common causes of relapse, occurring in 80% of patients within 5 years (Gardner & Nasrallah, 2015). Psychoeducation aimed at these issues is important.

Stress

Earl is a 36-year-old African American man who lives in a board and care home in a suburb of Birmingham, Alabama. He receives a monthly check for $700 that goes to his board and care home operator; $655 is deducted for his room and board. He theoretically has $45 per month to spend on sodas, cigarettes, clothes, snacks, or for a trip to McDonald's. However, he does not get to "hold" his money, and, according to Earl, he does not always get the full amount. This level of poverty is a stressor for Earl, as it would be to anyone.

One of the three inescapable facts noted at the beginning of this chapter is the role of stress at onset and in relapse. According to the vulnerability-stress model, people with schizophrenia are vulnerable to stress. Common stressors can be categorized as follows:

1. Biologic (e.g., medical illness)
2. Psychosocial (e.g., loss of a relationship)
3. Sociocultural (e.g., homelessness)
4. Emotional (e.g., persistent criticism)

The therapeutic mandate is to minimize the impact of stress on vulnerable individuals. The following two basic strategies are used:

1. Reducing stress and stressor accumulation
2. Developing healthy relationship skills

Because of their economic and social status, many individuals with schizophrenia routinely face significant stressors. Stated another way, some individuals most vulnerable to stress have more stress to handle. Helping patients learn to identify and avoid stressful events is an important task for the psychiatric nurse.

Substance Use Disorders in People With Schizophrenia

Substance use disorders are the most common comorbid psychiatric condition associated with schizophrenia, and substance use seems to be increasing. A high percentage of people with schizophrenia abuse alcohol, drugs, or both. Alcohol, marijuana, and cocaine account for most of the drugs of choice. Several studies (Hahn, 2018; Wainberg, Jacobs, di Forti, & Tripathy, 2021; National Institute on Drug Abuse NIDA, 2020) found that younger individuals may be especially vulnerable to psychosis, including the earlier and more frequent onset of psychosis, resulting from using cannabis. Substance use disorders have a negative effect on the treatment of patients with schizophrenia and are associated with poor outcomes. When substance use disorders begin, the individual is less likely to take prescribed medications and accept treatments and is more likely to become hostile, violent, and suicidal. Substance use disorders probably account for the overrepresentation of individuals with schizophrenia who are jailed. For example, alcohol causes disinhibition, aggressiveness, and poor judgment. These symptoms are already present in patients with severe mental illness. These same symptoms and related lack of social skills hinder patients with schizophrenia from fully benefiting from treatment programs, such as Alcoholics Anonymous and Narcotics Anonymous.

 CRITICAL THINKING QUESTION

4. Why do you think the rate of substance abuse is so high among individuals with schizophrenia?

Work

The lack of work, the inability to work, and the lack of a desire to work are all features of schizophrenia. Because work, or what one does for a living, is a major defining characteristic in society, the fact that many people with schizophrenia do not work adds to their inability to fit in. The major problem confronting these individuals is not so much a lack of skill but an inability to cope on the job socially. Routine behaviors such as joking, inviting someone out, or having insight into how one affects others are the major obstacles to a productive work life for people with schizophrenia.

Psychosis-Induced Polydipsia

Psychosis-induced polydipsia, or compulsive water drinking (4 to 10 L/day), is seen in a significant number of patients with psychosis (Kowalski et al., 2014). The desire to drink probably occurs because of thirst and osmotic dysregulation; it is characterized by a compulsive approach to water ingestion. The main concern associated with polydipsia is hyponatremia. Hyponatremia causes lightheadedness, weakness, lethargy, muscle cramps, nausea and vomiting, confusion, convulsions, and coma. Treatment includes frequent weighings, restricted fluid intake, sodium replacement, and positive reinforcement.

CONTINUUM OF CARE FOR PEOPLE WITH SCHIZOPHRENIA

Rather than starting to release patients in a few locales and measuring the outcome, officials implemented the policy in cities and counties across the United States virtually simultaneously, based on widespread hope that the new drugs would cure people and the widespread belief in state legislatures that the policy would save taxpayers money.

Dr. E. Fuller Torrey

By "policy," Torrey (1997) means deinstitutionalization, and driven by this policy, an array of services, or a continuum of care, has developed. Most clinicians agree that a community setting is good for some patients, and an institutional setting is better for others. The continuum of care for patients with schizophrenia includes the following:

- Acute symptoms—short-term hospitalization
- Treatment-resistant—long-term hospitalization
- Stable but chronic—day treatment
- Some level of supervision is needed—if the family is unable, supportive housing, including foster care, a board and care home, or a nursing home

PSYCHOTHERAPEUTIC MANAGEMENT

Most patients with schizophrenia go on for years struggling alone without anyone to help them become stronger than their symptoms.

P.J. Ruocchio

Think about Ruocchio's statement, specifically "...struggling alone without anyone to help them become stronger than their symptoms." What an utterly profound insight. Remember it whenever you care for a patient with schizophrenia. Psychotherapeutic management is aimed at helping patients become stronger than their symptoms. The nursing interventions used in the treatment of patients with schizophrenia are derived from the appropriate development of the nursing care plan.

Psychotherapeutic Nurse-Patient Relationship

Pharmacotherapy can improve some of the symptoms of schizophrenia but has a limited effect on social impairments that characterize the disorder and limit functioning and quality of life

Huxley, Rendall & Sederer Huxley and Rendall (2000, p. 187)

Huxley is still right. Drugs can do a lot, but there is more to it than the old "diagnose and adios" mentality in some agencies. The objective of the psychotherapeutic nurse–patient relationship is to build a therapeutic alliance with patients. A long-term relationship in which trust has developed is probably more significant and therapeutic than a particular theory of care. Insight therapy has limited usefulness with this population. In contrast, less invasive modalities, such as supportive therapy, problem solving, and relationship skills training that focus on emotions and behavior, are more helpful. Long-term, trusting relationships yield better outcomes with psychological resources.

The objective of this section is to provide basic concepts for working with patients with schizophrenia. General principles for developing a therapeutic nurse–patient relationship are presented. In addition, the "Key Nursing Interventions for Developing the Therapeutic Nurse–Patient Relationship" box lists some of these specific principles and some patient comments that the student might encounter. Examples of therapeutic responses by the nurse are also given.

General principles for developing a therapeutic nurse–patient relationship include the following:

- Be calm when talking to patients. *Rationale:* Anxiety is contagious.
- Accept patients as they are, but do not accept all behaviors. *Rationale:* Everyone wants to be accepted.
- Keep promises. *Rationale:* Dependability builds trust.
- Be consistent. *Rationale:* Consistency increases trust.
- Be honest. *Rationale:* Honesty strengthens trust.
- Do not deny hallucinations or delusions. *Rationale:* The nurse can validate the patient's experience and also simply state his or her perception of reality.
- Orient patients to time, person, and place, if indicated. *Rationale:* Orientation reinforces reality. However, use good judgment. To be continually reminded that you are disoriented takes an emotional toll.
- Do not touch patients without warning them. *Rationale:* Suspicious patients might perceive a touch as a threat and retaliate.
- Avoid whispering or laughing when patients are unable to hear all of a conversation. *Rationale:* Have you ever wondered whether you were the subject of discussion when you were around people who whispered or giggled? Suspicious patients interpret these actions as a personal affront.
- Reinforce positive behaviors. *Rationale:* Appropriate reinforcement can increase positive behaviors.
- Avoid competitive activities with some patients. *Rationale:* Competition is threatening and can lead to decreased self-esteem. (Remember junior high?)
- Do not embarrass patients. *Rationale:* Patients with schizophrenia often avoid social contact because they fear embarrassment.
- For withdrawn patients, start with one-to-one interactions. *Rationale:* Even in group situations, it is probably most therapeutic for interactions to be a series of nurse-patient interactions rather than patient-patient interactions. Nurse–patient interactions are less threatening to patients and can evolve into a wider circle of social interaction.
- Encourage and validate verbalization of feelings. *Rationale:* Patients will feel understood and accepted when their experiences are acknowledged.

PATIENT AND FAMILY EDUCATION

Schizophrenia

Illness

Schizophrenia is a brain disease that disrupts perceptions, thinking, feelings, and behaviors. It can cause distortions of reality; delusions; hallucinations; and changes in speech patterns, moods, and behaviors. It disrupts the person's ability to function, socialize, and work.

Medications

1. Some medications for schizophrenia might cause uncomfortable but typically temporary side effects. Some of these side effects can be lessened with other medications, nondrug interventions, or both.

2. Due to these side effects, the patient might not want to take the prescribed medications. The physician needs to know this immediately.
3. The patient must continue taking the medications, even after feeling better or the symptoms of illness are no longer evident.

Other Issues

Discuss early symptoms with the patient, which might indicate the beginning of a relapse. Agree with the patient about the actions that family, friends, or both will take to get appropriate help.

KEY NURSING INTERVENTIONS

For Developing the Therapeutic Nurse-Patient Relationship

The following are specific interventions and examples for developing a therapeutic nurse–patient relationship, including examples of appropriate responses. These examples are meant to illustrate some of the common situations described in the text. Each patient is unique, and that uniqueness might necessitate a variation of the suggested response.

Intervention	Rationale
Do not argue with patients about delusions. Delusions are often frightening, and the patient's experience can be validated.	Escalation of emotions is counterproductive to the nurse–patient relationship. Reflect reality, and attempt to distract patients in a matter-of-fact manner. *Patient:* The FBI and the Mafia are both after me. *Nurse:* That sounds really frightening. I want you to know that you are safe here. Let's go into the day room and talk. Proceed to talk about occupational therapy efforts (or a similar topic) focusing on the patient's real world.
Do not deny hallucinations.	*Patient:* The voices are calling me terrible names. *Nurse:* That must be really hard for you. The patient looks around the room, eyes darting to the corners of the room. *Nurse:* It looks like you might be listening to something. Are you hearing voices? This effort might lead to identifying and avoiding triggering events. *Patient:* I started hearing the voices last night right after I went to bed. *Nurse:* Tell me about your evening last night. There might be a link between something that happened and your hearing voices again.
Focus on real people and real events.	This helps patients stay in touch with reality. *Patient:* I keep hearing the voices. *Nurse:* I understand, is there anything else going on in your life that is difficult for you right now? Let's go to the day room and talk. Talking about what is going on in the patient's daily life may relieve some of their stress.
Be diligent in attempting to understand patients.	It is therapeutic to help patients communicate what they want to say; however, use good judgment. Pushing too hard to understand can be frustrating for the patient. *Patient:* I could have been bitten. It was never a dog's day. *Nurse:* I am not sure what you are saying, but I want to understand. Are you talking about almost being hurt?
Attempt to balance siding with inappropriate behavior and crushing a fragile ego.	Time and effort help the nurse learn to negotiate artfully between these potentially negative outcomes. *Patient:* I am going to hit that bastard if he says another word to me. *Nurse:* I know you are upset with him. Let's talk about other ways you can deal with this situation. If a patient is acting odd, and the nurse suspects they are hallucinating, the patient should be asked about it. Help patients to identify the stressors that might precipitate hallucinations or delusions.

BOX 24.7   Nursing Interventions to Increase Drug Adherence

- Observe patients for side effects and intervene accordingly. Akathisia is a troubling side effect that patients cannot tolerate.
- When giving tablets or pills, make sure that patients do not "cheek" the medications (hide the medication in cheeks or mouth) to spit them out or hoard them for later.
- At discharge, teach patients and their families about drugs, including side effects, potential interactions, and dosage schedules.
- Long-acting injectable drugs are effective for patients.

Psychopharmacology

Lieberman (1997) compared the discovery of antipsychotic drugs to the discovery of insulin. The development of this class of medications revolutionized mental health treatment. The student is encouraged to review Chapter 14, which provides a complete discussion of antipsychotic drugs.

Although antipsychotic medications are the basis for treatment for patients with schizophrenia, many do not adhere to taking their medications as prescribed (Smith-East, Powers, & Vossos, 2018). Box 24.7 lists some strategies to promote adherence to drug therapy. Box 24.8 reviews major side effects. As many experienced clinicians have thought, more recent findings imply that how a patient responds to an antipsychotic initially (first 2 to 4 weeks) is a good predictor of how well a patient will respond to that particular medication in the long run.

Milieu Management

Milieu management is an important dimension of the psychiatric nursing care of patients with schizophrenia because it is clear that drugs alone are not enough. A therapeutic treatment approach is best developed with all three components of psychotherapeutic management in place.

Therapeutic manipulation of the environment can occur at both the inpatient and outpatient levels and helps patients function better. As a rule of thumb, low-intensity, calm environments benefit patients with schizophrenia. General principles that specifically address the environment of patients with schizophrenia follow.

For disruptive patients:
- Set limits on disruptive behavior.
- Decrease environmental stimuli. For example, many nurses find that soft or classical music calms an environment, whereas hard rock or loud music creates agitation.
- Observe escalating patients frequently to intervene. Intervention (e.g., medication) before acting out protects patients and others physically and prevents embarrassment for escalating patients.
- Modify the environment to minimize objects that can be used as weapons. Some units use furniture so heavy that most people cannot lift it. "Unit safety is an outcome based on nursing interventions" (Ray, Perkins, Roberts, & Fuller, 2017, p. 26).
- Be careful in stating what the staff will do if a patient acts out; however, follow through once a violation occurs (e.g., "You will have to leave the day room now so you can settle down").

BOX 24.8   Review of Major Side Effects of Antipsychotic Drugs

Dopamine D$_2$ blockade in the nigrostriatal tract, causing *EPSEs*
  Parkinsonism
  Akathisia
  Dystonias
  Neuroleptic malignant syndrome
  Pisa syndrome
Muscarinic blockade in parasympathetic systems, causing *anticholinergic effects*
  Dry mouth
  Blurred vision
  Constipation
  Urinary hesitation
  Tachycardia
Hypersensitivity to dopamine in the nigrostriatal tract, causing *tardive dyskinesia*
  Elevated prolactin related to dopamine blockade in the tuberoinfundibular tract, causing *amenorrhea, galactorrhea, impotence,* and *decreased libido*
Histamine blockade, causing *sedation*
  Alpha-1 blockade, causing *orthostatic hypotension*

EPSEs, Extrapyramidal side effects.

- When isolating patients, provide safety by evaluating the patient's hydration, nutrition, elimination, and circulation.

For withdrawn patients:
- Arrange nonthreatening activities involving patients doing something (e.g., walking around the yard outside, painting).
- Arrange furniture in a semicircle or around a table, which forces patients to sit with someone. Interactions are permitted in this situation but should not be demanded. Sit in silence with patients who are not ready to respond. Some may move the chair away despite the nurse's efforts.
- Help patients to participate in decision making as appropriate.
- Reinforce appropriate grooming and hygiene.
- Provide psychosocial rehabilitation—training in community living, social skills, and health care skills.

For suspicious patients:
- Be matter-of-fact when interacting with these patients.
- Staff members should not laugh or whisper around patients unless the patients can hear what is being said. The nurse should clarify any misperceptions that patients have.
- Do not touch suspicious patients without warning. Avoid close physical contact.
- Be consistent in activities (time, staff, approach).
- Maintain eye contact.

For patients with impaired communication:
- Be patient and do not pressure patients to make sense.
- Do not place patients in group activities that would frustrate them, damage their self-esteem, or overtax their abilities.
- Provide opportunities for purposeful psychomotor activity.

For patients with hallucinations:
- Attempt to provide distracting activities.
- Be patient with patients when they are experiencing disordered perceptions.
- Monitor television selections. Some programs seem to cause more perceptual problems than others (e.g., horror movies).

- Monitor for command hallucinations that might increase the potential for patients to become dangerous.
- Have staff members available in the day room so that patients can talk to real people about real people or real events.
  For disorganized patients:
- Move patients to a less stimulating environment.
- Provide a calm environment; the staff should appear calm.
- Provide safe and relatively simple activities for these patients.

Clinical Example: Unbelievable but true—II

When I was in nursing school, a hospital where we trained, placed a woman in a four-point restraint but did not lock the door or stay with her. Another patient raped her.

CASE STUDY

The police bring Bill Wilson, a 25-year-old man, to the hospital. He was in a downtown bus station preaching loudly. He states in the emergency department that he had spoken to God and that God had told him to save San Francisco. He admits to hearing both God and Satan arguing and is terrified at times. In talking with his family, staff members discover that Bill was a solid student until about a year ago. He began to struggle in school but continued to pass his coursework. He dropped out of school 3 months ago. His family believes that his problem started when his girlfriend of 4 years broke off their engagement.

According to his family, Bill began hearing voices a couple of weeks ago, but the family lost contact with him until they were notified of this hospitalization. Bill's family is committed to helping him. Bill is oriented to time, place, and person on admission to the unit but states, "God has chosen me to be his special angel. I must save the sinners of San Francisco." Bill then stands up and turns his head rapidly from side to side. When asked why he is turning his head, he says, "God and Satan are arguing about what I should do."

OTHER SCHIZOPHRENIA SPECTRUM DISORDERS

In addition to schizophrenia, several other psychotic disorders are described in *DSM-5* with which the student should be familiar. Interventions for these disorders are directed at prominent symptoms and are the same as the interventions used for the symptoms of patients with schizophrenia.

CASE STUDY

Emma Rice, a 40-year-old woman with a history of multiple admissions, is admitted to the psychiatric unit. She was found wandering downtown incoherent and disheveled. During the assessment interview, Emma is noted to have a flat affect and is withdrawn. She reports not seeing her family for 5 years and cannot remember when she last held a job. There is no history of hallucinatory or delusional thought content in this recent occurrence. The staff knows Emma and knows that, during past admissions, she has responded to the less expensive haloperidol. After admission, Emma says, "Let me go. Go on, onward, backward. (pause) Emma hide, died." When asked where she lives, Emma slowly responds, "Over there, somewhere, anywhere, nowhere." Emma's board and care operator knows her well and has indicated that a bed is being held for Emma.

Clinical Example: A life gone to hell

Patty is a 42-year-old white woman referred to the county mental health department by her sister after attempting suicide by combining a large number of benzodiazepines with a six-pack of beer. Patty states that most of her "mental" problems began when she became pregnant at age 18. At the time, she was unmarried and alienated from her parents. Patty raised her daughter, Billie, alone until she eventually married at 23. At age 25, Patty became pregnant again and gave birth to a son. Her husband, an alcoholic, had abused Patty to some extent, but the abusive behavior became more frequent and more severe as Patty entered her early thirties. There had been suspicion that he had sexually abused Billie, but nothing conclusive was documented. Patty and her husband divorced when the boy was 7 years old. The court awarded the child to the husband. Today, Patty has little contact with her daughter, son, ex-husband, or parents. She frequently has auditory hallucinations telling her to kill herself and has nightmares about killing her son and ex-husband. She attends a day treatment program 5 days a week and lives in a one-bedroom apartment alone. Patty is very sad and always looks at the floor. She is consumed with guilt. She does not initiate conversation with others at the day treatment program. She states that she continues to hear voices and thinks about suicide all the time.

Delusional Disorder

People with delusional disorder display symptoms similar to those seen in schizophrenia. However, substantial differences exist and necessitate a diagnostic differentiation. The following symptoms differentiate delusional disorders from schizophrenia (APA, 2013):

- Delusion persists for at least 1 month.
- The patients have never met the criteria for schizophrenia.
- The behavior of these patients is relatively normal except for their delusions.
- If mood episodes have occurred concurrently with delusions, their total duration has been relatively brief.
- The symptoms are *not* the direct result of a substance-induced or medical condition.
- If hallucinations are present, they are not prominent.

Brief Psychotic Disorder

A brief psychotic disorder is the same as schizophrenia, only shorter in duration. It lasts less than 1 month and is not related to a mood disorder, a general medical condition, or a substance-induced disorder (APA, 2013). At least one of the following psychotic disturbances must be present: delusions, hallucinations, disorganized speech, or grossly disorganized or catatonic behavior. *DSM-5* cautions against applying these standards to people from a culture in which they are exhibiting acceptable behavior.

Schizophreniform Disorder

Patients with schizophreniform disorder display typical symptoms of schizophrenia and last at least 1 month but no longer than 6 months. This cautious approach spares an individual the lifelong diagnosis of schizophrenia until professionals are sure of the diagnosis.

Schizoaffective Disorder

Schizoaffective disorder is a psychosis characterized by both affective (mood disorder) and schizophrenia (thought disorder) symptoms, with substantial loss of occupational and social functioning. It is about one-third as common as schizophrenia (APA, 2013). Because this disorder is a hybrid of two disorders believed to have different biochemical origins, schizoaffective disorder is a puzzle to many clinicians. Affective disorders cause people to be extremely depressed or elated, and schizophrenia is expressed as positive, negative, or disorganized symptoms. The fact that patients with affective disorders can experience positive and negative symptoms and that patients with schizophrenia experience mood changes partially explains the difficulty in diagnosis.

In this disorder, schizophrenia symptoms are dominant but are accompanied by major depressive or manic symptoms. Patients with schizoaffective disorder will have experienced delusions or hallucinations in the absence of a prominent mood disturbance. Still, mood disorder symptoms are present for most of the total disorder's duration (APA, 2013). The prognosis for schizoaffective disorder is better than the prognosis for schizophrenia but is significantly less optimistic than the prognosis for mood disorders.

❓ CRITICAL THINKING QUESTION

5. If a first-degree relative of yours had schizophrenia, what behavior might cause you to refuse to live with that person?

FUTURE DIRECTIONS

An evolving area of research focuses on early identification and intervention in schizophrenia. The National Institute of Mental Health, the primary source of funding for neuroscientific mental illness studies, has made this area of research a funding priority. It has long been known that early treatment of schizophrenia symptoms results in better outcomes. Similarly, there is some indication that identifying the prodromal manifestations of schizophrenia might alter the course of the illness. The ability to offer screening tests, such as blood tests, brain imaging, and checking for simple but often overlooked signs, such as impaired smell and eye-tracking, offers the hope of reducing the disabling effects of schizophrenia. Box 24.9 lists some behavioral early warning signs of schizophrenia. If several of these signs are present in a young person, it behooves the nurse to suggest professional evaluation even if the person is just a neighbor. As stated, the earlier, the better.

BOX 24.9   Early Warning Signs of Schizophrenia

- Deterioration of personal hygiene
- Suspiciousness, paranoia, or uneasiness with others
- Social withdrawal, isolation, and reclusiveness
- Unusual, intense new ideas, strange feelings, or not having feelings at all
- Trouble thinking clearly or concentrating
- Dropping out of activities or out of life
- Decline in academic or athletic interests
- Difficulty telling reality from fantasy
- Confused speech or trouble communicating

From National Institute of Mental Health NIMH, 2016. Fact sheet: Early warning signs of psychosis. https://www.nimh.nih.gov/health/topics/schizophrenia/raise/fact-sheet-early-warning-signs-of-psychosis.

PRINCIPLES OF PSYCHOTHERAPEUTIC MANAGEMENT

Nurse-Patient Relationship Principles
Focus on behavior, not "deeper" meaning
A long-term relationship is most therapeutic
Accept the patient but not all behaviors
Be consistent
Do not deny hallucinations and delusions
Avoid whispering or laughing if the patient cannot hear all of the conversation

Psychotropic Drugs
Traditional Antipsychotics
Haloperidol (Haldol)
Fluphenazine (Prolixin)
Chlorpromazine (Thorazine)

Atypical Antipsychotics (Second and Third Generation)
Aripiprazole (Abilify)
Brexpiprazole (Rexulti)

Cariprazine (Vraylar)
Asenapine (Saphris)
Clozapine (Clozaril)
Iloperidone (Fanapt)
Lurasidone (Latuda)
Olanzapine (Zyprexa)
Paliperidone (Invega)
Quetiapine (Seroquel)
Risperidone (Risperdal)
Ziprasidone (Geodon)

Milieu Management Principles
Modify the environment to decrease stimulation and increase safety
Staff consistency is crucial
Arrange the environment to reduce withdrawn behavior
Monitor television watching
Protect the patient's self-esteem

◎ CARE PLAN

Name: Bill Wilson   Admission Date: _____

DSM-5 Diagnosis: Schizophrenia

Assessment	**Areas of strength:** Past accomplishments; past good heterosexual interpersonal relationships; alert, oriented to time, place, person; acute symptoms respond to medications; family support.
	Problems: Religious hallucinations, religious delusions, thought disorder; broken engagement; dropped out of school.
Diagnoses	Disturbed sensory perception (auditory) related to thought disturbance, as evidenced by hallucinations.
	Anxiety related to disturbed perceptions, as evidenced by fear and extraneous movements.
Outcomes	**Short-term goals**
Date met: _____	The patient will voice relief from hallucinations.
Date met: _____	The patient will report decreased fear of others.
Date met: _____	The patient will discuss feelings about the loss of a girlfriend.
	Long-term goals
Date met: _____	The patient will verbalize the need for medication and counseling.
Date met: _____	The patient will make an appointment for an outpatient program assessment in mid-July.
Date met: _____	The patient will return to school in September.
Planning and Interventions	**Nurse-patient relationship:** Do not deny hallucinations and delusions; encourage being in the here and now; encourage identification of strengths and accomplishments; encourage expressing feelings about broken engagement; discuss plans for immediate future.
	Psychopharmacology: Olanzapine (Zyprexa) 10 mg qd.
	Milieu management: Provide distracting activities; monitor television, particularly religious programming and movies with satanic themes; encourage participation in self-esteem and anger management groups.
Evaluation	Patient responding to Zyprexa.
Referrals	Will see Ms. White, RN, MSN, once a week as an outpatient. Appointment in 3 weeks with R. Jones for education counseling.

◎ CARE PLAN

Name: Bill Wilson   Admission Date: _____

DSM-5 Diagnosis: Schizophrenia

Assessment	**Areas of strength:** Board and care operator knows Emma well and wants her back. The staff knows and understands Emma.
	Problems: Affective flattening, loose associations, withdrawn, chronic course of illness, no family support.
Diagnoses	Impaired verbal communication related to thought disturbance, as evidenced by impaired articulation and loose association of ideas.
	Bathing and hygiene self-care deficit related to thought disturbance, as evidenced by the inability to maintain appearance at a satisfactory level.
	Social isolation related to a lack of trust, as evidenced by the absence of supportive significant other.
Outcomes	**Short-term goals**
Date met: _____	The patient will talk coherently.
Date met: _____	The patient will carry out activities of daily living.
Date met: _____	The patient will participate in nonthreatening activities.
	Long-term goals
Date met: _____	Patient will maintain outpatient program.
Date met: _____	The patient will return to board and care.
Date met: _____	The patient will comply with the medication regimen.
Planning and Interventions	**Nurse-patient relationship:** Be patient; treat as an adult; encourage hygiene and appropriate dress; reinforce positive social behaviors; start with one-to-one interactions with the nurse and then encourage independent social behaviors.
	Psychopharmacology: Haloperidol (Haldol) 5 mg bid PO (concentrate). A long-acting form may be needed on discharge.
	Milieu management: Start patient in occupational therapy by the end of the week; invite patient to sit with staff and other patients; encourage her to make decisions about meals or other simple tasks; provide resocialization group experience and community living education.
Evaluation	The patient stabilized on medications.
Referrals	Will see Ms. Brown, RN, MSN, once a week and will attend outpatient resocialization group five times a week. The board and care operator will monitor drugs and arrange transportation.

NEXT-GENERATION NCLEX EXAMINATION-STYLE CASE STUDY

Managing the Client Newly Diagnosed With Schizophrenia

Scenario: A 17-year-old male presented at the community hospital's emergency department (ED) accompanied by both parents. The client appeared disheveled and exhibited poor attention to personal hygiene while pacing about the examining room. The parents reported that their son has become increasingly agitated and verbally aggressive over the last 6 months stating, "He has given up attending high school. He spends most of his time watching one television channel while participating in chat rooms that focus on political movements." The parents add, "He's up all night; then he sleeps about 3–4 hours during the day." The client states, "A voice in my head keeps telling me that I have to make bad people stop ruining our country." The parents added, "He's different from most teenagers, but we got really concerned when he became so fixated on politics that he stopped going to class."

The teen was admitted for a psychiatric evaluation based on the suspicion he was a risk for injury to himself or others. He was diagnosed with schizophrenia, first episode (currently in the first episode) by the health care provider. Inpatient treatment was begun immediately. After a 10-day hospitalization in the hospital's mental health unit, the client's condition was stabilized, and he was discharged to his parents' home. Discharge planning included a prescription for oral risperidone 1 mg bid.

The client and his parents received education regarding the medication prescribed and recognizing and managing signs of relapse. The client is to return for a follow-up visit with the health care provider in 6 weeks.

At the follow-up visit, the client is appropriately dressed and displaying appropriate personal hygiene. He sits quietly in the examination room while the assessment and visit are conducted. During the history, the client confirms feeling dizzy upon standing. The physical assessment is unremarkable except for a noted weight gain of 6 pounds. He denies hearing voices and reports that "This guy on television is talking to me specifically, so I have to listen to the news every day." His parents add that he has yet to resume his schoolwork while he is spending much less time on his computer. The client states, "I'm just not interested in much of anything anymore." They add that he always appears very tired and sleeps 13–14 h a day. The client confirms he takes his medication and has begun smoking a pack of cigarettes daily, and often drinks beer when it is in the refrigerator.

Item Type: Matrix

Use an X to indicate which assessment finding is associated with each of the listed client's health conditions. All assessment findings should be used once.

Assessment Finding	Mental Health Diagnosis	Side Effects of Treatment	Comorbid Condition
Referential Thinking (regarding thinking the television announcer is talking specifically to the client)			
Beginning smoking			
Drinking alcohol			
Dizziness upon standing			
Weight gain of 6 pounds			
Somnolence (sleeping 13–14 h daily)			
Apathy ("I'm just not interested in much of anything anymore.")			

Answer(s):

Assessment Finding	Mental Health Diagnosis	Side Effects of Treatment	Comorbid Condition
Referential Thinking (regarding thinking the television announcer is talking specifically to the client)	X		
Beginning smoking			X
Drinking alcohol			X
Dizziness upon standing		X	
Weight gain of 6 pounds		X	
Somnolence (sleeping 13–14 h daily)		X	
Apathy ("I'm just not interested in much of anything anymore.")	X		

Rationales: The client has been diagnosed with schizophrenia, first episode (currently in the first episode) based on positive and negative symptoms. Positive symptoms include alterations in perception (the senses), disorganized thinking, and odd behaviors. For this client, positive symptoms are exhibited in hearing voices that are not present, referential thinking, and odd behaviors such as fixating on one television network and the topic of politics.

Negative symptoms include apathy—a general disinterest in pleasurable activities or activities of daily living (ADLs), emotional flatness, and impaired function. For this client, negative symptoms

are exhibited in the form of apathy that includes stating he is not interested in anything and neglecting personal hygiene.

Side effects of risperidone (and other second-generation antipsychotic drugs) include hypotension and orthostatic hypotension, sedation, somnolence, and (eventually) metabolic syndrome (which includes weight gain). Metabolic syndrome, which a health care provider must diagnose, is characterized by three of five risk factors: a large waistline, high triglycerides, low HDL levels, high blood pressure, and high fasting blood sugar. Type II diabetes can also develop due to weight gain and the adverse effect on insulin sensitivity and secretion. With this understanding at this time, dizziness upon standing (orthostatic hypotension), weight gain (of 6 pounds in 6 weeks), and somnolence (sleeping 13–14 h daily) are identified as side effects of risperidone.

Many patients diagnosed with schizophrenia have a comorbid condition. A high percentage of people with schizophrenia misuse alcohol, drugs including nicotine, or both. Misuse of alcohol and tobacco is believed to be common coping mechanisms that contribute to the general poor health of patients with mental health conditions, particularly schizophrenia.

Cognitive Skill: Analyze Cues

Reference

Keltner, N. L., & Steele, D. (2021). Chapter 14: Antipsychotic drugs and Chapter 24: Schizophrenia spectrum and other psychotic disorders. *Psychiatric nursing* (9th ed.). : Elsevier.

STUDY NOTES

1. The concept of schizophrenia has evolved over the last 150 years.
2. *DSM-5* is the major source for diagnostic criteria for schizophrenia.
3. Bleuler identified what he thought to be the four primary symptoms of schizophrenia (also known as Bleuler's "four A's"): (1) *a*ffective disturbances, (2) loose *a*ssociations, (3) *a*mbivalence, and (4) *a*utism.
4. Some clinicians conceptualize schizophrenia as having only two subtypes: positive symptoms and negative symptoms.
5. Objective signs of schizophrenia include alterations in personal relationships and activity.
6. Subjective symptoms of schizophrenia include alterations in perception, thought, consciousness, and affect.
7. Causative theories for schizophrenia are numerous and include both biologic theories (dopamine hypothesis, pathoanatomy, and genetic theories) and psychodynamic theories (developmental and family theories).
8. The dopamine hypothesis—that schizophrenia is a result of the increased bioavailability of dopamine in the brain—is a widely held theory of schizophrenia.
9. Antipsychotic drugs block dopamine receptors and relieve acute symptoms of schizophrenia.
10. Nursing interventions include developing a therapeutic nurse-patient relationship. Several general principles underlie the nurse's interactions with patients who have schizophrenia, including being calm, accepting, dependable, consistent, and honest.
11. In addition to these basic principles, several basic interventions are therapeutic for most patients with schizophrenia:

   Basic Don'ts for the Nurse: Do not deny hallucinations and delusions, do not touch patients without warning, do not whisper or laugh when patients cannot hear the conversation, do not compete with patients, and do not embarrass patients.

   Basics Do's for the Nurse: Do provide reality testing, do assist with orientation when appropriate, do reinforce positive behaviors, and do encourage verbalization of feelings.
12. Psychopharmacology is an important part of the nurse's role in caring for patients with schizophrenia. Understanding the importance of adherence to the medication regimen is critical.
13. Nurses are typically responsible for the environment. Strategies for working with disruptive, withdrawn, suspicious, and disorganized patients are crucial for developing a therapeutic environment.
14. Other psychoses listed in *DSM-5* include schizoaffective disorder, delusional disorder, brief psychotic disorder, and schizophreniform disorder.

REFERENCES

Acocella, J. (2000). The empty couch. *The New Yorker, 8*(11), 200.

American Psychiatric Association. (2013). *Diagnostic and statistical manual of mental disorders* (5th ed.). APA.

Anthenelli, R. M. (2016). Forget the myths and help your psychiatric patients quit smoking. *Current Psychiatry, 15*(10), 23.

Cieslak, K., & Freudenreich, O. (2018). 4 ways to help your patients with schizophrenia quit smoking. *Current Psychiatry, 17*(2), 28–33.

Crowner, M. (2014). Hearing voices, time traveling, and being hit with a high-heeled shoe. *Current Psychiatry, 13*, 57.

El-Mallakh, P., McPeak, D., Khara, M., & Okoli, C. T. (2016). Smoking behaviors and medical co-morbidities in patients with mental illnesses. *Archives of Psychiatric Nursing, 30*(2016), 740.

Gardner, K. N., & Nasrallah, H. A. (2015). Managing first episode psychosis: An early stage of schizophrenia with distinct treatment needs. *Current Psychiatry, 14*(5), 32.

Hahn, B. (2018). The potential of cannabidiol treatment for cannabis users with recent-onset psychosis. *Schizophrenia Bulletin, 44*(1), 46–53. https://doi.org/10.1093/schbul/sbx105.

Hjorthoj, C., Stürup, A. E., McGrath, J. J., & Nordentoft, M. (2017). Years of potential life lost and life expectancy in schizophrenia: A systematic review and meta-analysis. *The Lancet Psychiatry, 4*(4), 295–301. https://doi.org/10.1016/S2215-0366(17)30078-0.

Huxley, N. A., Rendall, M., & Sederer, L. (2000). Psychosocial treatments in schizophrenia: A review of the past 20 years. *The Journal of Nervous and Mental Disease, 199*, 187.

Keshavan, M. S., Collin, G., Guimond, S., Kelly, S., Prasad, K. M., & Lizano, P. (2020). Neuroimaging in schizophrenia. *Neuroimaging Clinics, 30*(1), 73–83. https://doi.org/10.1016/j.nic.2019.09.007.

Kessler, R. C., Petukhova, M., Sampson, N. A., Zaslavsky, A. M., & Wittchen, H.-U. (2012). Twelve-month and lifetime prevalence and lifetime morbid risk of anxiety and mood disorders in the

United States. *International Journal of Methods of Psychiatric Research, 21,* 169.

Khan, A. Y., Kalia, R., Ide, G. D., & Ghavami, M. (2017). Residual symptoms of schizophrenia: What are realistic treatment goals? *Current Psychiatry, 16*(3), 35.

Kindler, J., Schultze-Lutter, F., Hauf, M., Dierks, T., Federspiel, A., Walther, S.,... & Hubl, D. (2018). Increased striatal and reduced prefrontal cerebral blood flow in clinical high risk for psychosis. *Schizophrenia Bulletin, 44*(1), 182–192. https://doi.org/10.1093/schbul/sbx070.

Koch, J., & Thomas, C. J. (2016). Using lipid guidelines to manage metabolic syndrome for patients taking an antipsychotic. *Current Psychiatry, 15*(7), 59.

Kowalczyk, W. J., Wehring, H. J., Burton, G., Raley, H., Feldman, S., Heishman, S. J., & Kelly, D. L. (2017). Predictors of the perception of smoking health risks in smokers with or without schizophrenia. *Journal of Dual Diagnosis, 13*(1), 29–35. https://doi.org/10.1080/15504263.2016.1260190.

Kowalski, P. C., Dowben, J. S., & Keltner, N. L. (2014). Hyponatremia: A side effect of psychosis. *Perspectives in Psychiatric Care, 50*(2014), 221.

Lieberman, J. A. (1997). Atypical antipsychotic drugs: The next generation of therapy. *Decade of the Brain, 8,* 1.

Ma, L., Rolls, E. T., Liu, X., Liu, Y., Jiao, Z., Wang, Y.,... & Wan, L. (2019). Multi-scale analysis of schizophrenia risk genes, brain structure, and clinical symptoms reveals integrative clues for subtyping schizophrenia patients. *Journal of Molecular Cell Biology, 11*(8), 678–687. https://doi.org/10.1093/jmcb/mjy071.

Malhotra, A. K., Marder, S. R., & Weiden, P. J. (2014). Cognitive impairment and poor functional outcomes in schizophrenia. *Supplement to Current Psychiatry,* 1–8.

Miller, B. J., Wang, A., Wong, J., Paletta, N., & Buckley, P. F. (2017). Electronic cigarette use in patients with schizophrenia: Prevalence and attitudes. *Annals of Clinical Psychiatry: Official Journal of the American Academy of Clinical Psychiatrists, 29*(1), 4–10.

Nasrallah, H. A. (2016). Accelerated aging in schizophrenia: Shortened telomeres, mitochondrial dysfunction, inflammation, and oxidative stress. *Current Psychiatry, 15*(11), 21.

National Institute of Mental Health (NIMH). (2021). Schizophrenia. Retrieved from https://www.nimh.nih.gov/health/publications/schizophrenia/.

National Institute of Mental Health (NIMH). (2016). https://www.nimh.nih.gov/health/topics/schizophrenia/raise/fact-sheet-early-warning-signs-of-psychosis.

National Institute on Drug Abuse (NIDA). (2020). Is there a link between marijuana use and psychiatric disorders? Retrieved from https://www.drugabuse.gov/publications/research-reports/marijuana/there-link-between-marijuana-use-psychiatric-disorders.

Popovic, D., Schmitt, A., Kaurani, L., Senner, F., Papiol, S., Malchow, B.,... & Falkai, P. (2019). Childhood trauma in schizophrenia: Current findings and research perspectives. *Frontiers in Neuroscience, 13,* 274. https://doi.org/10.3389/fnins.2019.00274.

Ray, R., Perkins, E., Roberts, P., & Fuller, L. (2017). The impact of nursing protocols on continuous special observation. *Journal of the American Psychiatric Nurses Association, 23*(1), 19.

Riggs, S., Perry, T., Dowben, J., & Burson, R. (2017). Vive la France: Three delusional disorders originally reported in the French medical literature. *Perspectives in Psychiatric Care, 53,* 5.

Rupani, K., & De Sousa, A. (2017). Psychodynamic theories of Schizophrenia–revisited. *Indian Journal of Mental Health, 4*(1).

Siris, S. G. (2012). Treating 'depression' in patients with schizophrenia. *Current Psychiatry, 11,* 35.

Smith-East, M., Powers, L., & Vossos, H. (2018). Management of schizophrenia spectrum disorders in the outpatient setting: A quality improvement project. *Journal of Doctoral Nursing Practice, 11*(1), 72–78. https://doi.org/10.1891/2380-9418.11.1.72.

Socrates, A., Maxwell, J., Glanville, K. P., Di Forti, M., Murray, R. M., Vassos, E., & O'Reilly, P. F. (2021). Investigating the effects of genetic risk of schizophrenia on behavioural traits. *NPJ Schizophrenia, 7*(1), 1–9. https://doi.org/10.1038/s41537-020-00131-2.

Torrey, E. F. (1997). The release of the mentally ill from institutions: A well-intentioned disaster. *The Chronicle of Higher Education, 43,* B4.

Wainberg, M., Jacobs, G. R., di Forti, M., & Tripathy, S. J. (2021). Cannabis, schizophrenia genetic risk, and psychotic experiences: A cross-sectional study of 109,308 participants from the UK Biobank. *Translational Psychiatry, 11*(1), 1–9. https://doi.org/10.1038/s41398-021-01330-w.

Weinberger. D. R. (1987). Implications of normal brain development for the pathogenesis of schizophrenia. *Archives of General Psychiatry, 44,* 660.

Wilcox, J. A., & Duffy, P. R. (2016). They're out to get me!: Evaluating rational fears and bizarre delusions in paranoia. *Current Psychiatry, 15*(10), 29.

World Health Organization (WHO). (2019). https://www.who.int/news-room/fact-sheets/detail/schizophrenia.

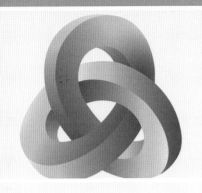

25

Depressive Disorders

Debbie Steele

Most people are about as happy as they make up their minds to be.

Abraham Lincoln

ⓔ http://evolve.elsevier.com/Keltner

LEARNING OBJECTIVES

- Recognize the *DSM-5* criteria for depressive disorders.
- Compare and contrast the following depressive disorders: major depressive disorder, disruptive mood dysregulation disorder, persistent depressive disorder (dysthymia), and premenstrual dysphoric disorder.
- Describe the biologic and psychodynamic explanations for depressive disorders.
- Describe effective nursing interventions for depressed patients.

- Identify the major indications for electroconvulsive therapy (ECT).
- Describe the nurse's role in caring for patients before and after ECT.
- Recognize warning signs of suicide.
- Describe interventions to prevent suicide.
- Describe family issues related to depressive disorder.

Depression is a devastating and pervasive disorder that leaves hundreds of millions of people in need of treatment throughout their lifetimes. The existence of depression has been documented since biblical times. Historically, many important individuals have experienced the devastating effects of depression, including King Saul, Job, Elijah, Jeremiah, Mary, and Abraham Lincoln, Ernest Hemingway, Eugene O'Neill, and Winston Churchill. Contemporary superstars like rapper Scarface, as well as actors Brooke Shields, Ashley Judd, and Drew Carey, are known to have this disorder. Normal feelings of sadness are appropriate in many situations; it would be abnormal not to feel sad on occasion, as when a loved one dies, or other losses occur. However, these feelings are usually short-lived and do not persist or alter the person's ability to function. When an individual's mood causes clinically significant distress or impairment in social or occupational functioning, a diagnosis of depressive disorder is warranted. Because there is a notable connection between major depressive disorder (MDD) and suicide, early diagnosis and intervention may increase the chances of a favorable outcome. A discussion of suicide and depression is presented at the end of the chapter. Demographic factors and prevalence rates of depressive disorders are shown in Table 25.1A and B.

DEPRESSIVE DISORDERS

The American Psychiatric Association recognizes eight major types of depressive disorders (American Psychiatric Association, 2013): MDD, disruptive mood dysregulation disorder, persistent depressive disorder (dysthymia), premenstrual dysphoric disorder, substance-induced or medication-induced depressive disorder, depressive disorder secondary to a medical condition or treatment of a medical condition, other known depressive disorders, and depressive disorder of unknown etiology. All of the depressive disorders share the common features of sadness, feeling empty, irritable mood, and somatic and cognitive changes that significantly affect the person's ability to function. This chapter focuses on the four most common types of depressive disorders.

MAJOR DEPRESSIVE DISORDER

MDD is characterized by one or more major depressive episodes, which are defined by at least 2 weeks of depressed mood or loss of interest accompanied by at least four additional symptoms. Individuals may describe their mood as depressed, sad, hopeless, discouraged, or "down in the dumps." Loss of interest or pleasure may be portrayed as

279

feeling "blah," having no feelings, not caring anymore, and social withdrawal. Individuals may present with physical complaints such as insomnia and fatigue. The presentation of psychomotor agitation (inability to sit still, pacing, handwringing, and rubbing the skin) or retardation (slowed speech, thinking, and body movements) is associated with greater severity of the disorder, as is the presence of excessive or inappropriate guilt. Weight gain and suicidality are more evident when recurrent depressive episodes occur. In children and adolescents, an irritable or cranky mood may be the prevalent symptom. Major depression is a disorder of *severity* and is treatable through therapy and medication management. *DSM-5* criteria for MDD are presented in the box labeled *DSM-5* Criteria (American Psychiatric Association, 2013).

NORM'S NOTES The discussion of depressive disorders in *DSM-5*, although written by physicians and psychologists, is used by psychiatric nurses. Advance practice nurses use the language of *DSM-5* in their practice as they diagnose, plan care for, and treat individuals with depression. *DSM-5* provides the common language necessary for an interdisciplinary team approach to patient care. Nursing rhetoric regarding depressive disorders can be difficult for individuals outside the nursing profession to understand. However, particular nursing terms have been accepted as standard medical terms. For example, *activities of daily living* is a common term used in the evaluation of depressed patients and their ability to function. As psychiatric nurses continue to develop theories and research useful in understanding the responses of depressed patients, they incorporate language found in *DSM-5* as well as nursing rhetoric.

DISRUPTIVE MOOD DYSREGULATION DISORDER

The diagnostic term *disruptive mood dysregulation disorder* is typically applied to children and adolescents 6 to 18 years old. This term, which was new to the *DSM-5* in 2013, was created in an effort to differentiate between children with severe irritability as opposed to children who present with classic, episodic bipolar disorder (American Psychiatric Association, 2013). The prominent feature is severe, chronic irritability interspersed with an angry mood. The severe irritability is

DSM-5 CRITERIA

Major Depressive Disorder

Diagnostic Criteria

A. Five (or more) of the following symptoms have been present during the same 2-week period and represent a change from previous functioning; at least one of the symptoms is either (1) depressed mood or (2) loss of interest or pleasure. Note: Do not include symptoms that are clearly attributable to another medical condition.

1. Depressed mood most of the day, nearly every day, as indicated by either subjective report (e.g., feels sad, empty, hopeless) or observation made by others (e.g., appears tearful). (Note: In children and adolescents, can be irritable mood)
2. Markedly diminished interest or pleasure in all, or almost all, activities most of the day, nearly every day (as indicated by either subjective account or observation).
3. Significant weight loss when not dieting or weight gain (e.g., a change of more than 5% of body weight in a month) or decrease or increase in appetite nearly every day. (Note: In children, consider failure to make expected weight gain.)
4. Insomnia or hypersomnia nearly every day.
5. Psychomotor agitation or retardation nearly every day (observable by others, not merely subjective feelings of restlessness or being slowed down).
6. Fatigue or loss of energy nearly every day.
7. Feelings of worthlessness or excessive or inappropriate guilt (which may be delusional) nearly every day (not merely self-reproach or guilt about being sick).
8. Diminished ability to think or concentrate or indecisiveness nearly every day (either by subjective account or as observed by others).

9. Recurrent thoughts of death (not just fear of dying), recurrent suicidal ideation without a specific plan, or a suicide attempt or a specific plan for committing suicide.

B. The symptoms cause clinically significant distress or impairment in social, occupational, or other important areas of functioning.

C. The episode is not attributable to the physiological effects of a substance or to another medical condition.

D. Note: Criteria A to C represent a major depressive episode.

E. Note: Responses to a significant loss (e.g., bereavement, financial ruin, losses from a natural disaster, a serious medical illness or disability) may include feelings of intense sadness, rumination about the loss, insomnia, poor appetite, and weight loss noted by criterion A, which may resemble a depressive episode. Although such symptoms may be understandable or considered appropriate to the loss, the presence of a major depressive episode in addition to the normal response to a significant loss should also be carefully considered. This decision inevitably requires the exercise of clinical judgment based on the individual's history and the cultural norms for the expression of distress in the context of loss.

F. The occurrence of the major depressive episode is not better explained by schizoaffective disorder, schizophrenia, schizophreniform disorder, delusional disorder, or other specific and unspecified schizophrenia spectrum and other psychotic disorders.

G. There has never been a manic episode or a hypomanic episode.

H. Note: This exclusion does not apply if all the manic-like or hypomanic-like episodes are substance-induced or are attributable to the physiological effects of another medical condition.

From the American Psychiatric Association. (2013). *Diagnostic and statistical manual of mental disorders* (5th ed.). APA.

TABLE 25.1 12-Month Prevalence Rates of Mental Disorders and Depressive Disorders in the United States

A. 12-Month Prevalence Rate of Mental Disorders in the United States[a]

Disorders	Approximate Percentage Above 17 Years Old (%)[a] (Unless Noted for Children)	Gender Overrepresentation
Anxiety disorders	18.1 overall	
Agoraphobia	1.7	Female
Panic disorder	2.4	Female
Panic attacks	11.2	Female
Social anxiety	7	Female
Specific phobia	7–9	Female
Separation anxiety	1.2	Equal
Generalized anxiety disorder	2	Female
Posttraumatic stress disorder	3.4	Female
Obsessive-compulsive disorder	1.2	Equal
Major depression	8.6	Female
Bipolar disorder I and II	1.8	BD I: About equal BD II: Female
Autism spectrum disorders	1 in children	Male
Disruptive, impulse control, and conduct disorders	8.9 overall	
Conduct disorders[a]	4 in children	Male
Attention-deficit/hyperactivity disorder[a]	5 in children; 2.5 in adults	Male
Substance use disorders	8.9 overall	
Alcohol use disorder	8.5 in adults; 2.5 in 12- to 17-year-olds	Male
Drug use disorders	1.4	Male
Schizophrenia	1.1	About equal

B. 12-Month Prevalence Rate of Depressive Disorders in the United States[b]

Disorders	Approximate Percentage Above 17 Years (%)	Gender Overrepresentation
Major depressive disorder	7	Female
Disruptive mood dysregulation disorder	2–5[c]	Male
Persistent depressive disorder	0.5–1.5	Unknown
Premenstrual dysphoric disorder	1.8	Female only

[a]No one source has all of this information. This information has been derived from the following sources: Kessler, R. C., Petukhova, M., Sampson, N. A., Zaslavsky, A. M., & Wittchen. H. (2012). Twelve-month and lifetime prevalence and lifetime morbid risk of anxiety and mood disorders in the United States. *International Journal of Methods of Psychiatric Research, 21*, 169; NIMH. (2017). NIMH-Funded National Comorbidity Study Replication (NCS-R) Study: Mental Illness Exacts Heavy Toll, Beginning in Youth.
[b]From American Psychiatric Association. (2013). *Diagnostic and statistical manual of mental disorders* (5th ed.). APA.
[c]Ages 6–18.

manifested as frequent temper outbursts in response to frustration at least three times a week. These outbursts appear in the form of verbal rages or physical aggression or both toward people or property. The onset of disruptive mood dysregulation disorder must occur before 10 years of age. Because of their severe irritability and low frustration tolerance, affected children generally experience marked disruption in family and peer relationships as well as school performance. Family therapy is vital in the treatment process of children diagnosed with this disorder (Stebbins & Corcoran, 2016). Behavioral management strategies are often utilized for the treatment of frequent outbursts. Pharmacologic management includes stimulants, selective serotonin reuptake inhibitors, mood stabilizers, and antipsychotic medications (Miller et al., 2018).

PERSISTENT DEPRESSIVE DISORDER

Persistent depressive disorder is a highly prevalent form of unipolar depression that has a chronic course. Persistent depressive disorder is diagnosed when a person has a depressed mood that occurs for most of the day and has lasted for at least 2 years (at least 1 year for children and adolescents). There are three subtypes: (1) chronic depression with mild severity, known as *dysthymia*; (2) major depressive episodes that occur continuously or intermittently with incomplete recovery between episodes; and (3) major depressive episodes superimposed on dysthymia, known as *double depression*. The criteria for dysthymia are almost identical to the criteria for MDD; however, the symptoms may be more subtle and unremitting. Individuals describe their moods as sad or "down in the dumps." Because of the chronicity of the disorder, the depressive symptoms become a part of the individual's day-to-day experience (i.e., "I've always been this way"). In addition, the individual may complain of sleeping and eating disturbances, fatigue, low self-esteem, difficulty making decisions, and feelings of hopelessness.

PREMENSTRUAL DYSPHORIC DISORDER

Premenstrual dysphoric disorder is characterized by the presence of mood swings, sudden tearfulness, irritability or anger, depressed mood, and/or anxiety that occur before and during menstruation. Other symptoms include lethargy, fatigue, sleep disturbances, difficulty concentrating, changes in appetite, and a sense of being overwhelmed or out of control. Physical symptoms such as breast tenderness or swelling, pain, and a sensation of bloating or weight gain may be present. Typically, symptoms occur during the late luteal phase of the menstrual cycle, about 1 week before the onset of menses. The intensity and expression of symptoms vary based on social and cultural background, family perspective, and religious beliefs. Treatment includes simple dietary changes such as high fiber and calcium supplements. Low doses of antidepressants can be taken continuously throughout the menstrual cycle or just during the luteal phase (Danis et al., 2020).

Depressive Disorder Specifiers

Each of the depressive disorders described previously can be categorized further into subtypes, also called *specifiers*. These provide more clarity to the presentation of the depressive disorders. Examples include *atypical features, anxious features, mixed features, melancholic features, catatonic features, peripartum onset, psychotic features*, and *seasonal pattern*. Overarching symptoms are the same across these subgroups, but variances in expression occur.

Atypical depression is characterized by symptoms that typically do not appear in MDD. For example, the individual's mood may brighten considerably in response to actual or potential positive events. Other symptoms include increased appetite or weight gain, hypersomnia, leaden paralysis (a heavy feeling in the arms and legs), and extreme sensitivity to interpersonal rejection.

Anxious depression is characterized by anxious distress during a depressive episode. Prominent symptoms include feeling keyed up, tense, or unusually restless, and fearing loss of control, difficulty concentrating, or that something awful may happen. Higher levels of anxiety are associated with higher suicide risk.

Mixed depression is characterized by manic or hypomanic symptoms occurring within a major depressive episode. Manic or hypomanic symptoms appear as an elevated, expansive mood; inflated self-esteem; grandiosity; being more talkative than normal; experiencing a flight of ideas; having racing thoughts; or displaying increased energy or goal-directed behavior. This type of MDD is associated with increased or excessive involvement in activities that have a high potential for painful consequences (e.g., buying sprees, sexual indiscretions, foolish business investments). During these periods, the individual has a decreased need for sleep and feeling rested despite sleeping less than usual.

Melancholic depression is characterized by anhedonia (loss of pleasure in activities) and an inability to be cheered up. At least three of the following depressive symptoms are found in melancholic patients: profound despondency, despair, or moroseness; depression worse in the morning; early-morning awakening; marked psychomotor retardation or agitation; significant anorexia or weight loss; and excessive or inappropriate guilt. This diagnosis is oftentimes associated with dexamethasone non-suppression and elevated cortisol levels.

Catatonic features are marked by significant psychomotor alterations, including immobility, or excessive motor activity, mutism, echolalia (parrot-like repetition of words), and inappropriate posturing. Although this symptom is more often associated with schizophrenia, more cases actually occur in patients with mood disorders.

Peripartum depression or "baby blues," which occurs during pregnancy or in the first 30 days postpartum, is the most frequent psychiatric affliction related to childbearing (Kleinman & Reizer, 2018). Common symptoms include mood swings, difficulty sleeping, fatigue, and anxiety, as well as irritability, pervasive depressed mood, and panic (Sahin & Seven, 2019). Peripartum depression is associated with a host of factors: unplanned pregnancy, history of previous depression, history of physical or sexual abuse, perinatal or delivery complications, relationship problems, lack of social support, and adverse neonatal outcomes (Mukherjee, Fennie, Coxe, Madhivanan, & Trepka, 2018). Postpartum depression is associated with difficulty parenting and subsequent child behavioral problems. In worst-case scenarios, the mother may be at risk of harming herself or her baby (Kleinman & Reizer, 2018).

In *psychotic depression*, a person has delusions and hallucinations in conjunction with mood disturbances. These perceptual problems can be differentiated between mood-congruent and mood-incongruent psychosis. With mood-congruent psychosis, the content of the delusions and hallucinations is consistent with the depressive themes of personal inadequacy, guilt, disease, or death. With mood-incongruent psychosis, the delusions or hallucinations involve bizarre content. Psychotic depression is associated with a poorer prognosis compared with other forms of depression. Antidepressant and antipsychotic use for psychotic depression are associated with a poorer response than nondelusional major depression (Østergaard et al., 2015).

Seasonal depression occurs in conjunction with a seasonal change, most often beginning in fall or winter and remitting in spring (in the Northern Hemisphere). Less commonly, there may be depressive episodes in the summer. As might be expected, the higher the latitude, the more likely it is that this type of depression will occur. Prominent symptoms include depressed mood, decreased energy, hypersomnia, overeating, weight gain, and a craving for carbohydrates.

Occurrence in Specific Populations

Adults

Depression (all types) is one of the most prevalent mental health problems in the United States. It results in severe impairments that interfere with an individual's ability to carry out major life activities (NIMH, Depression, n.d.). The lifetime risk for depression in women is 10% to 20%; in men, the lifetime risk is about 5% to 10% (American Psychiatric Association, 2013). By later life, the risk becomes about 50:50 (Patten et al., 2016). According to the National Institute of Mental Health, 17 million adults in the United States have experienced at least one major depressive episode; this number represents 7 % of all U.S. adults. The prevalence of major depression is higher among adult females (8.7%) compared to males (5.3%).

Although depression can occur at any age, the average age of adult onset is between 18 and 25 years. Some individuals have a single episode of major depression, recover, and never experience another depressive episode. However, about 80% of individuals who experience a single episode eventually have recurrent episodes. The prevalence rates appear to be unrelated to ethnicity; however, low-income groups and individuals with a positive family history of depression are at increased risk (up to three times greater risk).

Children and Adolescents

The occurrence of depression in children and adolescents can be more devastating than in adults. Children with depressed parents are at greater risk of developing the disorder than children with parents who are not clinically depressed, and the onset of childhood depression predicts continued depression as an adult. Nurses need to be able to assess children and their families for possible symptoms of depression and to develop appropriate interventions for them. Certain events might predispose children and adolescents to develop MDD, including the following:

1. Traumatic loss of parents through divorce, separation, or death
2. Bereavement related to the death of other individuals or pets close to the child
3. Impaired caregiving
4. Witnessing domestic violence
5. Emotional abuse and/or neglect
6. Physical and/or sexual abuse
7. Significant physical illness or injury

Culture, Age, and Gender

Individuals from certain ethnic, racial, or cultural groups might express depressive symptoms differently than European Americans. For example, people from Hispanic, Latino, and Mediterranean groups might describe their sadness or guilt somatically, feeling nervous or having headaches or stomachaches. Individuals from Asian cultures might describe themselves as being out of balance or feeling weak and nervous. Native American and Asian American groups withdraw for meditation and personal growth as part of their culture to cope with symptoms of depression. Chapter 5 presents more specific information on the expression of emotional states in different ethnic, racial, and cultural groups.

Nurses and other health care providers can misinterpret symptoms of depression in children, adolescents, men, and older adults. For example, depressive symptoms in children and adolescents are known to be expressed as irritability and outbursts. Men may have difficulty identifying their depression and often exhibit atypical symptoms such as anger (Athanasiadis et al., 2018). This may reflect why women are diagnosed with depression twice as often as men. Finally, recognizing symptoms of depression in older adults is particularly challenging because many symptoms of depression are similar to symptoms of dementia, diabetes, and cardiac conditions. In older adults living with depression, the depression may not appear as sadness; instead, they may demonstrate loss of interest, frailty, cognitive impairment, suicidal ideation, unexplained somatic complaints, and loneliness (Melrose, 2018).

FACTS ABOUT DEPRESSION

1. The prevalence of MDD is higher among adult females (8.7%) compared to males (5.3%).
2. The prevalence of MDD is highest among adults reporting two or more races.
3. An estimated 17.3 million adults in the United States had at least one major depressive episode in the past year. This number represented 7.1% of all U.S. adults.
4. The first onset of major depression typically occurs between the ages of 18 and 25 years.
5. Most individuals with one episode of major depression have another episode (the average is five or six episodes over a lifetime).
6. Stress plays a role in the onset and exacerbation of depression.

NIMH. (n.d.). *Major depression.* https://www.nimh.nih.gov/health/statistics/major-depression.html.

❓ CRITICAL THINKING QUESTION

1. What factors do you think contribute to the high levels of depression in the United States? _____

BEHAVIORAL SYMPTOMS OF DEPRESSION

Depression results in both objective and subjective behaviors. Objective signs, such as agitation, can be observed by the nurse. Painful subjective symptoms, such as hopelessness and isolation, might be hidden by depressed individuals. Objective and subjective symptoms in depression are difficult to differentiate. The nurse is encouraged to observe for visible signs of depression and to be aware of, assess for, and expect subjective symptoms such as irritability and anger.

Clinical Example

Mrs. Lewis is a 50-year-old woman who presents with anhedonia, tearfulness, suicidal ideation, loss of energy and sexual interest, and insomnia. Although she feels hopeless about the future and worries that she will never get better, she denies that she is really depressed. Mrs. Lewis is an extremely devout woman and believes that someone truly walking with the Lord would not find himself or herself in depression. Mrs. Lewis believes that she is a burden to her family; she also has fears related to her physical health. Mrs. Lewis feels guilty for not being able to handle her situation. Her husband, also a religious person, has been dutifully patient throughout all this turmoil but is growing tired of her pessimism, crying, and lack of interest in sex. The nurse suspects that a breakup of this 25-year marriage might occur if Mrs. Lewis does not respond to treatment.

Objective Signs

Depressed patients often demonstrate behavior that is noticeable to others, but they might not want to talk to anyone and might seek to be alone. If someone intrudes into the negative thinking of such a person's inner world, he or she might become irritable and strike out at the intruder. Two general areas of objective signs are alterations of activity and altered social interactions.

Alterations of Activity

Depressed patients may exhibit psychomotor agitation or retardation. Psychomotor agitation appears as pacing, hand-wringing, and the inability to sit still. These patients may pull or rub their hair, skin, clothing, or other objects. Tying and retying shoelaces and buttoning and unbuttoning a shirt or blouse are common behaviors. Psychomotor retardation is marked by a slowing of speech, increased pauses before answering, soft or monotonous speech, decreased frequency of speech (poverty of speech), and muteness. In addition, a general slowing of body movements occurs. These patients may say that they are "tired all the time," even when they are not physically active. For example, a patient might have difficulty getting up from a chair to turn off the television. Even the smallest task might seem unbearable.

The involvement in daily living activities declines as well. Depressed individuals often neglect attending to their basic personal hygiene, such as bathing, shaving, putting on clean clothes, or wiping their mouths after eating. However, these objective signs are probably a result of more than a lack of energy. Apathy—a lack of feeling, absence of emotion, or an inability to be motivated—plays an important role in these behaviors as well. An extreme extension of these anergic symptoms is seen when a depressed person lies in bed and becomes incontinent or constipated because he or she cannot muster the energy (both physical and psychological) to walk to the bathroom.

Depressed people usually experience a change in eating behaviors that result in either the gain or loss of weight. Sleeping patterns change as well. Depressed individuals may experience insomnia (difficulty falling asleep), middle insomnia (difficulty remaining asleep), or terminal insomnia (early morning awakening). Hypersomnia (increased or prolonged sleeping or both) is an atypical symptom of depression. Depressed people may deny that they are depressed yet spend hours alone. In this case, the nurse should not confuse a request to "go to my room and lie down" with hypersomnia. Many depressed people want to lie down but do not sleep. There, in the solitude of an empty room, these individuals may descend into uninterrupted, self-defeating contemplations.

Clinical Example

Jan Treback is a 60-year-old white woman who has been successful in business for many years. She recently became very upset at work when her boss confronted her. Jan had not been happy when the company's CEO assigned her to a new boss 6 months earlier. The new boss was overbearing, and Jan felt that she was not trusted, even though she had worked for this same business for 25 years.

Jan had left work because she felt too upset to stay and basically was told by the Human Resources Department to take some time off. She decided to see a psychiatrist and a therapist. The psychiatrist started Jan on citalopram. The therapist diagnosed persistent depressive disorder based on Jan's reported symptoms of feeling blue most days for most of her adult life. She had a tendency to overeat, felt fatigued most days, never felt that she got enough sleep, and sometimes isolated herself. She denies a history of suicidal ideation. She lived with her daughter and granddaughter and had been divorced for more than 30 years.

Altered Social Interactions

Depressed individuals often have poor social skills that are linked directly to other symptoms of depression. Underachievement causes a lack of productivity on the job and at home. The overwhelming negative thought of these individuals reduces their ability to focus on other people, their ideas, and their problems. Depression causes problems with concentration, the development of ideas, and problem solving. In addition, they find conversations difficult to maintain, and only with great effort can a depressed person sustain a facial expression of interest and concern. Depressed individuals tend to withdraw from social interaction with others. Hobbies and vocations that they once actively pursued become unimportant and may be abandoned or engaged in halfheartedly. Finally, the body language of depression (e.g., saddened facial expression, drooping posture) tends to be a social barrier.

Subjective Symptoms
Alterations of Affect

Alterations of affect are the symptoms primarily associated with depression, which is reasonable because these disturbances dominate the inner world of a depressed person. The term *affect* describes the emotional range that outwardly reflects one's feelings, mood, and emotional tone. Some of the terms used to describe affect include *flat*, *blunted*, and *labile.* Congruency of affect and mood is demonstrated when there is consistency between the two (flat affect being congruent with depressed mood). For depressed individuals, affect and mood may also be incongruent, observed as labile affect incongruent with depressed mood.

Anxiety, doom and gloom, fear, self-destructive thoughts, and panic are all products of the depressed mind. Because of this anguish, depressed individuals vacillate between sadness and apathy. When the pain becomes too great, they shut down and become numb. Although most laypeople consider sadness to be the universal symptom of distress, apathy actually comes closer to being continually present in depressed individuals.

Inappropriate guilt is often associated with depression. Guilt may manifest as an overreaction to some current failing or might be associated with an indiscretion in the distant past that cannot be forgiven. Guilt can also take the form of accepting responsibility for occurrences in which the person had little impact or take the form of obsessional preoccupation with such thoughts as "What if I had only …?" The person becomes immobilized with "should haves" and "could haves." An even more morbid extension of guilt is the psychotic delusion of guilt for calamities that happened far away, even on the other side of the world.

Anxiety is a companion of depression. Depressed individuals are filled with anxiousness and dread, fearing that something awful may happen. For example, a ringing telephone holds the potential for catastrophic news. The anxiety may manifest as feeling unusually restless, tense, and keyed up. In addition, the depressed individual may fear losing control.

Worthlessness can range from a feeling of inadequacy to total devaluation. Depressed individuals might scan the environment for clues to their inadequacy. As one person remarked, "I knew I wasn't any good; it just took a while to figure out why." Some individuals have a hypersensitivity to how they are perceived by others, always assuming the worst.

Alterations of Cognition

Alterations of cognition include ambivalence and indecision, inability to concentrate, confusion, loss of interest and motivation, memory problems, pessimism, self-blame, self-deprecation, self-destructive thoughts, thoughts of death and dying, and fear. The inability of depressed individuals to make a decision is particularly difficult for others to understand. They express much vacillation when faced with even a simple decision. Once a decision is made, depressed individuals might be obsessed with "what if" questions. Major decisions can be immobilizing.

Alterations of a Physical Nature

Alterations of a physical nature are common in depressed individuals. Almost all parts of the body can be affected. Common physiologic symptoms include abdominal pain, anorexia, chest pain, constipation, dizziness, fatigue, headache, indigestion, insomnia, menstrual changes, nausea and vomiting, and sexual dysfunction. Additionally, as mentioned in the previous discussion of cultural aspects, cultural practices of some ethnic and racial groups might mimic depressive symptoms, or depression might be expressed somatically.

These subjective symptoms come to the attention of the nurse because of the numerous somatic complaints that depressed individuals often express. Some people become preoccupied with their bodies to the extent that every twinge and body change is greeted with great alarm and dread. One recovering depressed patient joked, "I have had a hundred heart attacks." The monitoring of body functions is common in the general population; however, overinvestment in self-assessment by depressed individuals can be overwhelming.

Alterations of Perception

Some depressed individuals have altered perceptions or psychotic features. Delusions and hallucinations are typically congruent with the depressed themes of personal inadequacy, guilt, disease, death, or deserved punishment. Somatic delusions (e.g., "My body is full of cancer") and nihilistic delusions (e.g., "My brain is dying") are common forms of psychotic delusions in depressed individuals.

ETIOLOGY OF DEPRESSION

Biologic Theories of Depression

The etiology of depression has been biologically attributed to alterations in neurochemical, genetic, endocrine, and circadian rhythm functions and changes in brain anatomy. These alterations produce physical and psychological changes expressed as depression.

Neurochemical Theories

Research findings suggest that neurochemical depression results when levels of certain neurotransmitters are altered. The biogenic amines norepinephrine and serotonin are most often mentioned, but dopamine, another biogenic amine, is involved as well. Fig. 25.1 illustrates the proposed roles of the three key monoamines. Dysregulation of acetylcholine and gamma-aminobutyric acid (GABA) might contribute to the development of biochemical depression as well. More specifically, when the levels of these neurotransmitters are altered at receptor sites or when receptor sensitivity changes, a neurochemical depression might result.

It might be appealing to conceptualize depression as a decreased level of serotonin and norepinephrine or to suggest that depression can be successfully treated by increasing the bioavailability of these amines. However, doing so oversimplifies both the problem and the solution. A more informed way of looking at depression is to think of it as a monoaminergic dysregulation. It is not so much that monoamines are lacking but that the cells they activate have lost the capacity to respond in a healthy manner; intracellular processes no longer effectively produce the transcription factors necessary for neuronal development. When the receptor is occupied with serotonin (or norepinephrine), a cascade of intracellular events is initiated (i.e., the second-messenger system). This

Proposed Roles for the Three Key Monoamine Systems

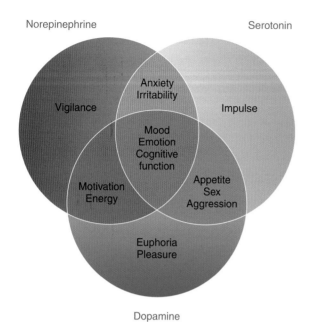

FIG. 25.1 Proposed roles for the three key monoamine systems. From Healy, D., & McMonagle, T. (1997). The enhancement of social functioning as a therapeutic principle in the management of depression. *Journal of Psychopharmacology, 11* (Suppl.), S25.

cascade results in the production of proteins such as enzymes, receptors, and neuroprotective proteins. When some part of this process is dysfunctional, the end products needed for cell sustenance are compromised. Antidepressants may stabilize this intraneuronal environment.

Other hypotheses include the sensitivity of both presynaptic and postsynaptic receptors and the modulating effects of acetylcholine and GABA on aminergic systems (Keltner et al., 2001a). For example, it is believed that beta autoreceptors, which normally inhibit the release of norepinephrine, are downregulated by antidepressants, disinhibiting norepinephrine release (i.e., increasing synaptic norepinephrine). Too many norepinephrine or serotonin receptors might be thought of as a positive situation. However, excessive receptors or their upregulation indicates insufficient levels of these neurotransmitters. This action is an example of the body compensating for decreased monoamine availability. However, all the upregulation and downregulation of receptors can also result from the intracellular response to antidepressants, as mentioned earlier. Finally, peptides, dietary practices, and nutritional status are being examined for their biochemical roles in the development of depression because food intake affects the development of the precursor amino acids required for neurotransmitter synthesis. There is still much to learn about the biochemistry of depression.

Genetic Theories

Other researchers have contended that depression might be genetically based and that heredity might predispose individuals to develop depression. Several studies have examined the incidence of depression in twins. A meta-analysis of twin studies estimated that MDD heritability is about 35%, indicating the importance of non-genetic factors. Epidemiological studies have suggested that stressful life events are associated with a high risk for MDD. The current working hypothesis is that highly complex genetic and environmental factors work together to determine susceptibility to MDD (Uchida et al., 2018). An example of environmental factors: mothers who are depressed tend to rear children who are more susceptible to depression. Researchers are still trying to determine the genetic, inherited, and psychosocial causes of depression.

Endocrine Theories

Endocrine changes related to depression have also been investigated. Normally, the hypothalamic-pituitary-adrenal (HPA) axis is a system that mediates the stress response. However, in some depressed people, this system malfunctions and creates cortisol, thyroid, and hormonal abnormalities. Dysregulation of the HPA axis results in hypercortisolemia (in about 40% to 60% of depressed patients), non-suppression by dexamethasone, and elevated levels of corticotropin-releasing factor (CRF) (Keltner et al., 2001b; Michelson, 2009). The hypersecretion of cortisol is the result of overexpression of the CRF gene (leading to increased CRF synthesis) and an increase in CRF-producing neurons in the hypothalamus. This action leads to an increased pituitary release of adrenocorticotropic hormone (ACTH) and subsequent hypersecretion of cortisol by the adrenal glands. Nemeroff (1998) noted that early life exposure to overwhelming trauma literally changes the expression of CRF neurons in the hypothalamus. The diathesis-stress model suggests that early childhood trauma makes some individuals more vulnerable to environmental stressors. Negative experiences, such as inadequate parenting and childhood sexual and physical abuse, are most likely to negatively impact the development of individuals who carry vulnerability factors. The assumption is that a stressor can activate the diathesis, or vulnerability factor, and may transform it into psychopathology, such as depression (Stoltz et al., 2017). Essentially, trauma brought about by childhood stressors causes a long-term or even permanent hyperactivity of central corticotropin-releasing hormones, leaving the adult highly vulnerable to stress.

Circadian Rhythm Theories

There is robust evidence of sleep disturbances in depression, which has led to several hypotheses to explain this association. However, it is unclear if disrupted circadian rhythms cause depression or if depression causes disturbed sleep/wake cycles (Zaki et al., 2018). Sleep disturbances are reported in 60% to 90% of individuals with MDDs, depending on the severity of depression (Wichniak et al., 2013). Changes in sleep patterns, insomnia, and hypersomnia are included in the diagnostic criteria for major depressive episodes in the *DSM-5*. Individuals who are experiencing stressful events are prone to disruption to the circadian system, as well as destabilization of mood. The onset of depression is associated with shift work, jet lag, and other stressful situations that disrupt the circadian system (Malhi & Kuiper, 2013).

Changes in Brain Anatomy

Evidence exists indicating that depression might result from or cause atrophy of specific brain locations. Researchers utilizing brain-imaging methods, have identified brain atrophy in cortical and limbic regions of depressed individuals, particularly decreased volumes in the prefrontal cortex (PFC) and hippocampus (Uchida et al., 2018). One of the leading neurobiologic hypotheses on chronic depression has been associated with a pronounced reduction in serum brain-derived neurotrophic factors over time. Brain-derived neurotrophic factor is a member of the neurotrophic family of growth factors involved in the plasticity of neurons in several regions of the brain (Bus et al., 2015). Chronic stress and major depressive episodes may reduce the expression of neurotrophic factors, which leads to premature neuronal death and atrophy in specific brain regions. Long-term treatment with typical antidepressants leads to an increase in neurotrophic factors and improves neuronal and synaptic plasticity (Uchida et al., 2018).

Psychological Theories of Depression

The psychological explanations for depression flow from psychoanalytic, cognitive, interpersonal, and behavioral perspectives. In addition, related psychosocial-psychodynamic views explain depression from three general themes, individually or combined, as follows: (1) adverse early life experiences, (2) intrapsychic conflicts, and (3) reactions to life events (i.e., stressors).

Psychoanalytic theorists have contended that depression occurs as a result of an important loss in early life (Freud, 1957). Freud's model of psychoanalysis conceptualized the unconscious wishes of an individual, triggered by the loss of a loved person or object (object loss) in childhood. This loss predisposes the adult to depression when adult losses trigger the memory of the childhood loss. Psychoanalysis investigates a wide array of unconscious contents, including traumatic memories, defense mechanisms, and intrapsychic and interpersonal strategies. This therapy seeks to make sense of emotional suffering and the individual's need to understand the roots of their pain (Azzone, 2018).

Cognitive theorists believe that cognition affects emotion and behavior, and altering cognitions lead to corresponding changes in emotions and behaviors (Beck, 2021). Depressed individuals see themselves, others, and daily events in a negative light. These negative beliefs are grounded in early childhood losses (e.g., often the loss of a parent through death, separation, or divorce) and serves as the basis for how the depressed person makes decisions and sees himself or herself in relation to other persons and occurrences. Cognitive therapy aims at symptom removal by identifying and correcting distorted, negative, moment-by-moment maladaptive thinking and seeks to prevent recurrence by correcting dysfunctional assumptions, attitudes, and core

beliefs. Cognitive approaches are often used in conjunction with antidepressants.

Interpersonal theorists believe that individuals are social beings who seek out and thrive in their interactions with others. Yet, relationship difficulties can also be a huge source of distress, leading to the onset and maintenance of depression. Three main categories of interpersonal functioning are affected: reduced satisfaction in one's relationships, low levels of perceived social support, and interpersonal skill deficits. Individuals with depression display higher levels of interpersonal distress, experience social isolation, and can become hostile or withdrawn in their relationships (D'Iuso et al., 2018).

Behavioral theorists propose that a person develops depression due to feelings of helplessness and unworthiness related to dysfunctional expectations about the future. Behavioral experiments are designed and utilized to increase engagement in adaptive activities and decrease engagement in activities that maintain the depression (Kubi et al., 2017),

Debilitating Early Life Experiences

Adult depression and suicidality have been established as common outcomes of adverse childhood experiences (ACEs). Adverse childhood experiences are defined as those experiences that occur before the age of 18, including abuse and household dysfunction, and cause extreme distress. Developmental theorists view the early years of life as the foundation for lifelong mental health, focusing on the importance of a solid, nurturing early life environment. Children who grow up in a home where there are significant caregiver issues such as violence, incarceration, addiction, poverty, abusive and/or neglectful parenting are predisposed to depression and other mood disorders. Interventions include teaching clients about emotional regulation and practicing trauma-informed care that provides clients insights into the impact of ACEs on their lives (Zyromski et al., 2018).

Intrapsychic Conflict

Intrapsychic conflict refers to the conflicts that people experience when they have mixed emotions about a behavior, event, or situation. For instance, an individual who has been brought up to refrain from sexual activity but who also has strong urges to experience sex has a conflict. Refraining from sexual activity increases sexual frustration, and engaging in sexual activity might cause anxiety, guilt, and fear. People are faced with intrapsychic conflicts all the time. Persistent and unsuccessful resolution of these conflicts can lead to depression.

Reactions to Life Events (Stress)

Extensive literature documents the role of life stress in the development, severity, and course of depression. Common stressors include loss of a loved one and job, academic failure, peer difficulties, family and financial difficulties (Shapero et al., 2019). Reacting to these stressors with grief and sadness is normal; when normal becomes abnormal is still unclear.

Clinical Example

Elle is a 45-year-old, well-educated, intelligent white woman who has been in and out of therapy over the course of 15 to 20 years. Elle grew up in northern Mississippi with two brothers and a very physically and emotionally abusive father. Elle reports that when she was quite young, her mother left home and did not return for several years. Elle left home at age 17, was married twice, and divorced shortly after each marriage. She has a history of depression and attempted suicide 20 years earlier. After many turbulent years, she started going to bars in hopes "that I might get killed." She refers to this period as her "death hunt days." After a recent emotional and financial collapse, Elle returned to her father's home, where he continues to control her life in every way. She has commented that her life is so futile that she would rather be dead.

ASSESSMENT OF DEPRESSION

Assessment of depression may be accomplished through both nonbiologic and biologic assessment methods. For an accurate assessment of depression, the following should be addressed:

1. History and onset of symptoms
2. Presence of comorbid substance, alcohol, and medication use
3. Physical examination to rule out the presence of medical conditions (Box 25.1)
4. Presence of comorbid psychiatric disorders
5. Patient resources and social support systems
6. Interpersonal and coping abilities
7. Level of stressors
8. Presence of suicidal ideation

Nurses can be instrumental in collecting all this information because they are often the health care professionals who initially assess patients and develop the database for use in the general diagnostic and nursing process.

Cultural Issues and Assessing Depression

The selection of an assessment instrument is based on the nurse's clinical knowledge and experience as well as on the age and mental capacity of the person being assessed. Only limited measures have been developed and normed for use in different ethnic, racial, and cultural groups. The lack of measurement specificity for these populations can lead to misdiagnosis or underdiagnosis. Because some researchers have contended that culturally competent measures predict relevant criteria more accurately than non-culturally competent measures, this assessment deficiency should be viewed as clinically significant. Routine review of cultural competence issues facilitates accurate and valid assessment for all patients.

Assessment of Depression
Depression in Older Adults

Depression in older adults is a major health concern. Depressive symptoms in the elderly are common, but because of the overlapping symptoms of physical illness and the depressive side effects of many medications, diagnosis is complex. Depression-causing illnesses that share symptoms with depression are listed in Box 25.1.

If depression is related to a medical illness, treatment of the illness often returns the depressed mood to normal. However, MDD and medical illnesses can coexist, and appropriate treatment for all disorders is necessary. The nurse

GRIEF

If you live long enough, you will experience grief—an intense but normal response to loss—typically the loss of someone very close to you. Often, we think of grief as a reaction to death, but it can also be a reaction to divorce, relocation to another part of the country, terminal illness (e.g., anticipatory grief), or natural disaster. As noted, grief is normal. To lose someone close—for example, a mother, father, brother, sister, wife, husband, or child—and not experience grief is abnormal.

Grief can be distinguished from a major depressive episode; in grief, the predominant affect is a feeling of emptiness and loss, whereas a major depressive episode consists of a persistently depressed mood and the inability to anticipate happiness or pleasure. The sadness in grief tends to decrease in intensity over days to weeks and occurs in waves, the "pangs of grief." These waves are associated with thoughts or reminders of the deceased. The pain of grief may even be accompanied by positive emotions and humor in thinking about the deceased loved ones. If a bereaved individual thinks about death and dying, these thoughts are possibly about joining the deceased, whereas, in a major depressive episode, thoughts are focused on stopping the pain associated with feelings of worthlessness and hopelessness (American Psychiatric Association, 2013).

The grief response typically lasts about 6 months. People experiencing grief report a choking sensation, emptiness, shortness of breath, weakness, and sighing. They also use the term *waves* to verbalize how these feelings roll over them. After about 6 months, the grieving person begins to return to normal, but pangs of grief can continue to occur for some time.

We have all been acquainted with individuals who have lost family members. It is not unusual for old photographs to be displayed on pianos or on the wall of the home. On occasion, when looking at the photos even 20 years later, loved ones will experience a wave of grief from time to time.

Differentiating grief and depression is not always simple, but the following guidelines can be useful:

Grief	Depression
Follows a known loss	Cumulative response to losses in life
Time-limited and improves	Persistent and recurrent
Responsive to social contacts	May avoid social contacts
Rarely suicidal	Suicidal ideations common
Typically does not need antidepressants	Responsive to antidepressants and therapy

BOX 25.1 Medical Conditions Commonly Associated With Depression

Central Nervous System Disorders
Alzheimer disease
Amyotrophic lateral sclerosis
Brain tumor
Cerebrovascular accident (stroke)
Chronic subdural hematoma
Multiple sclerosis
Normal-pressure hydrocephalus
Parkinson disease
Subarachnoid hemorrhage

Collagen Vascular Diseases
Polymyalgia rheumatica
Rheumatoid arthritis
Systemic lupus erythematosus
Temporal arteritis

Toxic-Metabolic Disturbances and Endocrinopathies
Addison disease
Cushing disease
Diabetes mellitus
Electrolyte disorders
Hypercortisolemia
Hypoglycemia
Hypothyroidism

Metal intoxication
Parathyroid disorders
Uremia

Infections
AIDS
Encephalitis
Hepatitis
Infectious mononucleosis
Influenza
Syphilis
Tuberculosis
Viral pneumonia

Neoplastic Disorders
Carcinoma of head of pancreas
Chronic myelogenous leukemia
Lymphoma
Other malignant disease
Small cell carcinoma of lung

Other
Chronic fatigue syndrome
Chronic obstructive pulmonary disease
Decreased bone density

Modified from Ford, C. V., & Folks, D. G. (1985). Psychiatric disorders in geriatric medical/surgical patients: II. Review of clinical experience in consultation. *Southern Medical Journal, 78*, 397; Michelson, D. (2009). Depression: Body and brain. *Biological Psychiatry, 66*, 405.

should also be aware that some people who are given a diagnosis of dementia may actually be depressed (referred to as *pseudodementia*). It is important to differentiate between depression and dementia. Depression and dementia can also occur together, in which case both disorders must be treated. Comorbid MDD and dementia tend to occur early in the course of Alzheimer's disease.

Depression manifesting in later life may be related to grief issues confronted by older adults, including the loss of a spouse, family members, children, jobs, housing, income, mobility, and health. As a result of these inevitable losses, older adults are at increased risk of suicide. Men have an increased risk over women. Older white men have the highest risk of suicide in the elderly population. Suicide is discussed at the end of this chapter.

Nonbiologic Assessment Measures

Nonbiologic assessments comprise standardized verbal and written measurement scales. Obtained data from the assessments can be used in conjunction with *DSM-5* criteria to provide a more accurate diagnosis regarding MDDs. Various instruments can be used for assessment purposes. The Beck Depression Inventory, the Hamilton Depression Scale, and the Geriatric Depression Scale are important examples of these assessment tools.

Biologic Assessment Measures

Polysomnographic measurements. Polysomnographic findings (i.e., examination of sleep patterns) and hypnograms

are used to assess depression in adults. Disturbances in rapid eye movement (REM) sleep are believed to be associated with depression. REM sleep usually begins within 70 to 100 minutes of a person falling asleep and increases in length throughout the night. Important biomarkers of depression include increased REM density (frequency of REM) and altered distribution of delta (slow-wave) sleep throughout the sleep period (Wichniak et al., 2013). Antidepressants or sleep aids are utilized to restore the normal pattern of REM sleep.

PUTTING IT ALL TOGETHER

PSYCHOTHERAPEUTIC MANAGEMENT

The nurse uses the nursing process to develop appropriate nursing interventions and strategies, expected outcomes, and evaluation of the outcomes in depressed patients. The intervention strategy described in this book, psychotherapeutic management, emphasizes the nurse-patient relationship, psychopharmacology, and milieu management. The case study and care plan presented in this section are geared toward nursing management of the depressed patient who is being treated in any health care environment. Within the current managed care environment, most depressed patients are rarely hospitalized; if they are hospitalized, it is for short periods of time (3 to 5 days). Consequently, the nursing management of depressed individuals primarily occurs in medical settings or outpatient clinics. At any rate, it is imperative that nurses in any setting be familiar with the *DSM-5* criteria of MDDs and with the information regarding mood disorders presented in this chapter.

Nurse-Patient Relationship

The objective of this section is to provide specific principles of therapeutic communication for nurses who work with depressed patients.

1. Depressed individuals have a fragile view of self. The most effective approach to bolster such self-views is to accept patients as they are (negative attitude and all), help them focus on their strengths (accomplishments), provide successful experiences with positive feedback, keep self-help strategies simple, and help patients avoid embarrassing social blunders (e.g., smelly clothes, unkempt appearance).

2. Development of a meaningful relationship in which depressed individuals are valued as human beings is important to their sense of personal worth. It is important for the nurse to be honest and to work on developing trust. Doing specific things that are in the best interest of each patient develops a trusting relationship. For example, a patient might wish to tell the nurse something of clinical significance but does not want the nurse to share the information with other staff members. The nurse builds trust by telling the patient that significant information will be shared only with staff members who have a need to know. In this way, the patient learns to trust the nurse as a professional whose primary concern is to help the patient.

3. The nurse who works effectively with depressed patients must have a sincere concern for patients and be empathic. The nurse acknowledges and validates the emotional pain and suffering conveyed by patients in a kind and gentle manner. Normalizing their emotional experiences provides patients with a sense of being understood. Empathy is important in the healing of emotional pain, especially the sense of feeling alone in the world.

4. It is usually ineffective to outline logically why a patient is a worthwhile human being. However, the nurse can point out small visible accomplishments and strengths—for example, "Your hair looks nice today." The nurse can look for ways to provide appropriate compliments as they are noticed.

5. Depressed individuals can become dependent on the mental health system. The nurse should recognize the importance of modeling a relationship that is interdependent. The nurse should interact in a way that promotes patient feedback to promote change.

6. The nurse should not attempt to manipulate patients out of being depressed. For example, pointing out less fortunate people in the hope that such an action might bring depressed individuals to their senses provides, at best, short-lived relief based on the misfortune of others.

7. The nurse should never argue with a patient over hallucinations, delusions, or negative beliefs. The nurse may describe his or her perception of reality and move on to

discuss what the patient is feeling in regard to such perceptions. Talking about the patient's fears and sadness is therapeutic and helps the patient to feel safe in the nurse-patient relationship.

8. Depressed individuals will tend to get angry when triggered (Fig. 25.2). Sometimes, they even surprise themselves with the outbursts they experience. It is important for the nurse to learn to handle hostility therapeutically by recognizing the emotional pain, not taking it personally, and not retaliating in word, deed, or some passive-aggressive form. Encouraging verbal expressions of powerful emotions helps release patients' tension.

9. The nurse can help withdrawn patients manage their social isolation by spending time with them (even without speaking), providing nonthreatening one-to-one time with them, being sensitive to their emotional states, and being accepting of them.

10. Depressed individuals can have difficulty making simple decisions. It is not therapeutic to badger patients into making a decision, but it is therapeutic to provide decision-making opportunities that patients are able to manage. Initially, the nurse might have to make decisions for patients—for example, "It's time for your bath" or "Here's your apple juice." When possible, the nurse can help guide patients to appropriate decisions by using problem-solving techniques—that is, identifying options, the advantages and disadvantages of each, and the potential consequences of each decision. (See box titled "Key Nursing Interventions for Depressed Patients.")

PSYCHOPHARMACOLOGY

To understand the range of information required for effective psychopharmacologic intervention, the student is encouraged to review Chapter 15, which provides a complete discussion

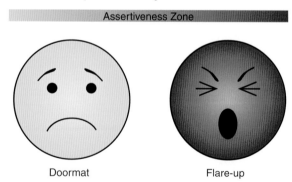

Interpersonal Style Continuum

Assertiveness Zone

Doormat   Flare-up

FIG. 25.2 Depressed individuals often adopt an interpersonal style that causes them to be "doormats"; that is, they allow people to walk all over them. Sometimes the individual who pretends to not care explodes when he or she has had too much. These outbursts are typically followed by recrimination and regret. The nurse can help patients learn to avoid these extremes of interpersonal behavior by teaching them to use clearer communication techniques.

KEY NURSING INTERVENTIONS

For Depressed Patients

The psychiatric nurse should consider the following intervention principles in working with depressed patients.

Intervention	Rationale
Accept patients where they are and focus on their strengths.	Depressed persons have a negative view of self, and this is the best approach to recapturing some sense of value.
Present situations to these patients that do not require decision-making (e.g., "It's time to go for a walk").	Depressed patients struggle to make simple decisions. By reinforcing patients' efforts to make simple decisions, the nurse helps them to move toward health.
Respond to anger therapeutically. Deescalation techniques include being calm, using a soft voice, reassuring the patient that you understand.	When triggered, depressed persons can lash out in anger. By understanding that anger is a reflection of their immense emotional pain, the nurse can focus on the moment and help patients move toward feeling less threatened.
Spend time with withdrawn patients.	Withdrawn patients are aware of their surroundings. By spending time (frequent but brief contact) with these patients, the nurse communicates the patients' worth. Tell patients that you will be available when they feel more comfortable talking.
Involve patients in activities through which they can experience success.	People can feel good about themselves in several ways. One way to develop self-worth is through accomplishment.

of antidepressant drugs. A brief review of critical parameters of antidepressant drug administration is given in Box 25.2 and in the box headed Side Effects of Antidepressant Drugs.

Milieu Management

Milieu management is an important dimension of the psychiatric nursing care of depressed patients. The student is referred to Unit IV for a discussion of milieu management. General principles that specifically address the environment of depressed patients are presented here.

For Patients With a Negative View of Self

- Encourage depressed patients to participate in activities, including groups, where they can experience success and receive positive feedback. Most people develop a sense of self-worth through mastery or accomplishment. Simply telling patients that they are okay is not convincing. Provide for successful experiences, however small.

BOX 25.2 Important Points for Administering Antidepressant Drugs

- Most antidepressants have a lag time of 2–4 weeks before a full clinical effect occurs.
- Many reports suggest that these drugs might provoke suicidal ideation and behavior.
- Suicidal patients may "cheek" these drugs to build up a supply for an overdose. Tricyclic antidepressants (TCAs) have a narrow therapeutic index.
- Monitor vital signs of patients who take TCAs and mono-amine oxidase inhibitors (MAOIs):
  1. TCAs can cause orthostatic hypotension, reflex tachycardia, and arrhythmias.
  2. MAOIs have the potential for triggering a hypertensive crisis.
- Monitor sexual side effects of selective serotonin reuptake inhibitors (SSRIs) because they occur frequently, and patients may stop taking them.
- Be aware of the drug-drug and food-drug interactions associated with MAOIs.
- Observe for early signs of toxicity:
  1. TCAs: Drowsiness, tachycardia, mydriasis, hypotension, agitation, vomiting, confusion, fever, restlessness, sweating
  2. MAOIs: Dizziness, vertigo, fatigue
  3. SSRIs: Have a low probability of causing toxicity

SIDE EFFECTS OF ANTIDEPRESSANT DRUGS

Antidepressants (TCAs, SSRIs)
Sexual dysfunction (depressed libido, arousal, or orgasm)
Dry mouth
Nasal congestion
Urinary hesitancy
Urinary retention
Blurred vision
Constipation
Sedation, ataxia
Confusion
Orthostatic hypotension
Arrhythmias, tachycardia, palpitations
Decreased sweating

MAOIs
Overstimulation (e.g., agitation, hypomania)
Blurred vision, hypotension, dry mouth, constipation
Hypertensive crisis related to food-drug or drug-drug interactions

MAOIs, Monoamine oxidase inhibitors; *SSRIs,* selective serotonin reuptake inhibitors; *TCAs,* tricyclic antidepressants.

- Provide assertiveness training. Many depressed individuals feel alone in the world because of their interactional problems; their communication history is typically a lifetime of feeling misunderstood, punctuated by periodic outbursts of anger when they get triggered. Assertiveness training helps these patients learn to express their feelings and needs along the way; thus, the extremes of "withdrawal" and "flare-up" are avoided.

- Help patients avoid embarrassing themselves through socially unacceptable appearance or behavior. Many appearance problems are related directly to depressed individuals' preoccupation, apathy, and decreased energy level. For example, food stains on clothes, food in a beard, an unattended runny nose, uncombed hair, urine on trousers, and an unzipped fly may be seen in depressed individuals who cannot pay attention to these hygienic concerns. Help patients to shower and dress appropriately. Remind patients to go to the bathroom. In some cases, it is better to encourage patients to walk with the nurse (e.g., to the bathroom area or to the shower).

For Withdrawn Patients

- Keep contacts with withdrawn patients brief but frequent. Depressed patients often do not want anyone around or, at least, they may not wish to be spoken to or addressed. Their wishes are not a good indicator of what should be done. Spending time with patients is constructive; allowing patients to isolate themselves is not constructive. Patients need to know they are accepted right where they are before they feel comfortable verbalizing their inner world.
- Many patients are insistent about going to their rooms to lie down. They might stay there all day if the nurse did not intervene. Locking a patient's room for periods throughout the day might be required to keep a withdrawn or isolated patient from disappearing for hours at a time. Sitting in silence during an activity is better than ruminating in isolation.

For Anorectic Patients

- The nursing staff must take responsibility for ensuring that depressed patients eat. It is irresponsible to set a tray down in front of a depressed person, particularly in his or her room, and then leave. The nurse must encourage patients to eat and might even spoon-feed them if required.
- Allow patients to participate in selecting preferred foods from the menu.
- Promote a proper diet, adequate fluids, and exercise. Provide small frequent meals. Record intake.
- Constipation is a side effect not only of antidepressants but also of depression. A diet with adequate fiber content and sufficient fluids is important. Monitoring and recording bowel elimination is also important.
- If patients will eat food brought from home, permit them to do so.

For Patients With Sleep Disturbances

- Depressed individuals want to sleep, but many have insomnia. Tremendous fatigue is experienced by these patients because the sleep they manage to get is usually not restful. Patients often wake up looking and feeling exhausted. The nursing staff should record the amount and quality of patients' actual sleep. Patients who lie down during the day might be isolating themselves and not sleeping. An

accurate understanding of how much the patient has slept helps the nurse formulate an intervention strategy.

- People with insomnia often engage in self-defeating behaviors, such as daytime napping and drinking stimulants (e.g., coffee, colas). Eliminating these behaviors increases the likelihood of nighttime sleep.

CRITICAL THINKING QUESTION

2. Should adults in their right minds be allowed to commit suicide?

SOMATIC THERAPIES

Somatic therapies are treatment approaches that use physiologic or physical interventions to effect behavioral change. The most common form of somatic therapy is electroconvulsive therapy (ECT), which is discussed here in detail. Box 25.3 outlines early efforts in somatic therapy, summarizing the history of insulin-coma therapy and initial convulsive therapies. Other somatic therapies used to treat depression include transcranial magnetic stimulation (TMS), bright light therapy (BLT), and vagus nerve stimulation (VNS).

ECT and psychosurgery emerged as treatment forms in the 1930s. The roots of ECT lie in the misconception of early-20th-century psychiatrists that epilepsy and schizophrenia were incompatible (Abrams, 1997). Advocates of ECT and psychosurgery envisioned and promised dramatic relief from the curse of mental illness. Over time, inappropriate use and

BOX 25.3 Early Somatic Therapies

Insulin-Shock Therapy: 1933
Insulin-shock therapy was introduced in 1933 by Manfred Sakel, a Viennese physician, after he accidentally discovered that giving too much insulin to a psychotic diabetic patient produced a reduction in the patient's symptoms. Insulin-shock therapy gained a wide following for some time in hopes of alleviating the debilitating symptoms of psychosis (Colaizzi, 1996; Dorman, 1995).

First Convulsive Therapies: 1934
Meduna, a Hungarian, was the originator of convulsive therapy. In 1934, Meduna introduced camphor oil-induced and then metrazol-induced convulsion therapy based on his pathologic observation that the glial cells of patients with schizophrenia were different from the glial cells of patients with epilepsy. Meduna erroneously concluded that schizophrenia and epilepsy were mutually exclusive disorders (Abrams, 1997). Fink (1999) chronicled one of Meduna's first patients, a 33-year-old man who had been psychotic, mute, and withdrawn for 4 years:

Two days after the fifth (camphor oil) injection, on February 10 in the morning, for the first time in four years, he got out of his bed, began to talk, requested breakfast, dressed himself without help, was interested in everything around him, and asked about his disease and how long he has been in the hospital. When the patient was told he has been in the hospital for 4 years, he did not believe it! (p. 88) disappointing results, coupled with the development of psychotropic drugs and a growing general distrust of psychiatric hospitals, created climate of hostility toward these therapies and their practitioners. In the 1960s and early 1970s, the use of both therapies came to a virtual standstill. However, in the last 30 years, ECT has emerged again as a useful treatment alternative when more traditional approaches have failed. With rigid treatment criteria and careful pretreatment evaluation, many psychiatric patients respond to these somatic therapies.

 NORM'S NOTES Somatic therapies, especially electroconvulsive therapy (ECT), are terribly misunderstood. If antidepressants are not working for someone with severe depression, ECT can usually help. If you know someone who just cannot seem to improve with the various antidepressant medications available, particularly if that person has entertained thoughts of suicide, please talk to someone in his or her family about this option. The kind of procedure you see in older movies has not been used in most hospitals (in industrialized countries) since the 1960s. Modern ECT is safe and effective, and it saves lives.

ELECTROCONVULSIVE THERAPY

Cerletti and Bini (Cerletti's assistant), two Italian psychiatrists, introduced ECT in 1938. The first patient had schizophrenia and, after 11 treatments, experienced a full recovery. The first ECT treatment in the United States was in 1940. ECT was previously commonly referred to as *electroshock therapy* (EST) or simply *shock therapy*. Both terms are considered pejorative today.

During ECT, an electric current is passed through the brain, causing a seizure. Historically, this seizure resulted in a full grand mal convulsion accompanied by the various complications of these convulsions—muscle soreness, fractures, dislocations, sprains, and tongue lacerations. These seizures and the resulting grotesque facial grimaces have been dramatically captured on film and graphically detailed in the literature. In films and novels, ECT has been portrayed as a devious tool used by psychiatrists and psychiatric nurses who are themselves demented. The novel *One Flew Over the Cuckoo's Nest*, by Ken Kesey, and the 1975 movie of the same name created a firestorm of hostility against the use of ECT. In his book, Kesey portrayed ECT as an agent used to maintain control over sane but highly individualistic patients. This public attack on ECT, linked with reports of inappropriate use, virtually stopped the use of ECT in the United States. Inappropriate use of ECT included administering it for almost all conditions and, from the accounts of former patients, using it as punishment for noncompliant behavior.

However, despite the negative perceptions, ECT remains a viable treatment approach because many mental health professionals know it to be an effective treatment. In the process

of waiting to evaluate the efficacy of other treatments, many patients have suffered needlessly. Many clinicians now argue that ECT should be considered earlier in the treatment process because it is the most effective antidepressant. About 100,000 patients receive ECT treatments annually in the United States (Smith, 2001).

Modern Electroconvulsive Therapy

Although no one knows for sure how it works, ECT has been found to be a highly effective treatment option for severe mood disorders and acute and chronic psychoses (Obbels et al., 2018; Tørring et al., 2017). During ECT, an electric current is passed through the brain for seconds at a time to induce seizures. The seizures resulting from ECT should last from 30 to 90 seconds to be considered therapeutic. The patient is monitored by an electroencephalogram to monitor seizure activity and is also monitored with an oximeter to ensure optimal oxygenation.

ECT is typically administered 2 to 3 times a week until remission or up to 12 treatments (Obbels et al., 2018; Popiolek et al., 2019). There are two basic medications always used for ECT. These medications are anesthetics (to induce a hypnotic state) and muscle relaxants (to prevent seizure-related injuries). See Box 25.4 for a list of medications and their uses for ECT. Any medications that the patient is on to treat their psychiatric disorder can be continued during ECT except those that impede the induction of a seizure (e.g., anticonvulsants and benzodiazepines). Cardiac medications, antihypertensives, and antigastric medications can typically be continued (Zolezz, 2016).

Nursing Responsibilities After Electroconvulsive Therapy

1. The nurse or anesthesiologist mechanically ventilates the patient with 100% oxygen until the patient can breathe unassisted.
2. Blood pressure, oxygen saturation, and heart rate are monitored.
3. The nurse monitors for respiratory problems.
4. ECT causes confusion and disorientation; it is important to help with reorientation (time, place, person) as the patient emerges from this groggy state.
5. The nurse may have to administer a benzodiazepine as needed for agitation.
6. Observation is necessary until the patient is oriented and steady, particularly when he or she first attempts to stand.
7. All aspects of the treatment should be carefully documented in the patient's record.

❓ CRITICAL THINKING QUESTION

3. ECT is more effective than antidepressants in the treatment of severe depression. Nonetheless, there is a reluctance to use ECT. If you or a member of your family were severely depressed, which of these two treatment forms would you want? Carefully consider the stigma of ECT as well as the effects of anesthesia and transient memory loss.

Indications for Electroconvulsive Therapy: Major Depression

Although ECT was originally developed for schizophrenia, its primary indication soon shifted to patients who were severely depressed, particularly patients manifesting acute psychotic episodes and catatonia (Omori et al., 2019). Severely depressed patients account for about 85% to 90% of all patients receiving ECT. ECT should be started with patients that are not responding to antipsychotic medications such as antidepressants and benzodiazepines, particularly those who are suicidal and catatonic (Leroy et al., 2018).

Clinical Example

Penny Jones is a 48-year-old woman who worked for the postal service until 3 weeks earlier. She was admitted to an acute psychiatric facility accompanied by her daughter, who indicated that her mother had lost 30 lb during the preceding 4 months. The daughter further described her mother as having a poor appetite, being isolative, awakening early in the morning with the inability to fall back to sleep, and verbalizing thoughts with suicidal ideation. The daughter stated that her mother's actions scare her. Ms. Jones states that life is intolerable, and she does not want to live anymore without Jerry, her husband, who died 5 months ago.

Ms. Jones sought psychiatric help immediately and was prescribed sertraline 25 mg/day for 1 week and then 50 mg/day. She improved slightly but then relapsed into a deeper depression and continued to verbalize suicidal thoughts. Based on her poor response to antidepressants and her risk for suicide, a course of six ECT treatments was prescribed. Ms. Jones tolerated the procedures well. Her suicidal ideations ceased, she began interacting with others spontaneously, and she regained her appetite. She was discharged during the third week of her hospitalization.

Disorders, depressive symptoms, and conditions that respond to ECT are listed in Table 25.2 (Swartz, 1993).

Contraindications to Electroconvulsive Therapy

Although ECT is a potentially lifesaving procedure, there are a few contraindications to its use. Before initiating ECT, clinicians should consider the risks and benefits of using ECT if any of the conditions listed in Box 25.4 are present.

Disadvantages of Electroconvulsive Therapy

ECT has been found to be more effective than antidepressants for certain groups of patients with severe mental illness. However, ECT does not offer a permanent cure. While it does provide temporary relief, and many patients are able to remain free of depression for long periods, others might never need treatment again. For others, another series of treatments might be warranted within a few months. Some psychiatrists order maintenance or a continuation of ECT, once weekly to once every 4 weeks, aimed at preventing

TABLE 25.2 Disorders, Depressive Symptoms, and Conditions That Respond to Electroconvulsive Therapy

Disorders	Depressive Symptoms	Conditions
Severe depression	Anhedonia	Tardive dystonia
Refractory depression	Anorexia	Tardive dyskinesia
Catatonia	Delusions	Akathisia
Mania	Insomnia	Parkinsonian symptoms
Some types of schizophrenia	Muteness	Neuroleptic malignant syndrome
	Psychomotor retardation	
	Suicidal ideations	

BOX 25.4 Contraindications to Electroconvulsive Therapy

Delusional disorders
Patients with a substance abuse problem
Personality disorders
Patients with preexisting neurological disorders, such as Parkinson's disease or dementia
Patients who have a history of not responding to an acute course of ECT
Patients with cardiovascular disease
Patients with recent cerebral hemorrhage or stroke
Patients with an intracranial lesion with elevated intracranial pressure
Patients with bleeding or unstable vascular aneurysm
Patients with severe pulmonary disease

Omori, W et al., (2019). Shared preventive factors associated with relapse after a response to electroconvulsive therapy in four major psychiatric disorders. *Psychiatry and Clinical Neurosciences, 73*, 495. Zolezz, M. (2016). Medication management during electroconvulsive therapy. *Neuropsychiatric Disease and Treatment, 12*, 932.

relapse or recurrence (Nordenskjöld et al., 2011; Omori et al., 2019).

Immediate side effects of ECT include nausea, headache, jaw pain or muscle ache, and cognitive deficits (Su et al., 2019). Takagi and associates (2018) evaluated the short- and long-term cognitive effects of ECT and reported the presence of transient cognitive decline without permanent changes. Historically, researchers have concluded that autobiographical memory loss or retrograde amnesia are long-term side effects of ECT. In elderly patients, ECT was found to be safe and effective; however, long-term cognitive side-effects were present in a small minority of patients (Obbels et al., 2018).

ECT produces cardiovascular stress in patients. During ECT, there is a brief parasympathetic effect followed by sympathetic stimulation while inducing the seizure. Heart rate and blood pressure may decrease or increase during the

BOX 25.5 Medications used during the ECT procedure

Anesthetic induction agents-
Rapidly induce hypnotic state

Methohexital
Thiopental
Propofol
Etomidate
Ketamine

Neuromuscular blocking agents-
Decrease bone and soft tissue injury

Succinylcholine (suxamethonium)
Rocuronium
Atracurium
Mivacurium

Antihypertensives as needed-
Reduce tachycardia and hypertension

β-Blockers (atenolol, esmolol, and labetalol)
Calcium channel blockers (nifedipine and nicardipine)

Anticholinergics as needed-
Treat bradycardia and hypotension

Glycopyrrolate
Atropine

Narcotics as needed

Fentanyl
Remifentanil
Alfentanil

Modified from Zolezz, M. (2016). Medication management during electroconvulsive therapy. *Neuropsychiatric Disease and Treatment*, *12*, 933. Originally published by and adapted with permission from Dove Medical Press Ltd.

procedure, putting patients at risk for an acute coronary or cerebrovascular event. Several medications are used to prevent or to attenuate the hemodynamic response to ECT (e.g., nitroglycerine, fentanyl, labetalol, esmolol, clonidine, and dexmedetomidine (Parikh et al., 2017) (Box 25.5).

ECT remains underutilized because of fears of cognitive and medical risks, including the risk of death. Torring and associates (2017) assessed the mortality rate of ECT by means of a systematic review and found that death caused by ECT is an extremely rare event. ECT has a lower mortality rate than general anesthesia: 2.1 deaths per 100,000 patients versus 3.4 deaths per 100,000 patients.

OTHER SOMATIC THERAPIES

Vagus Nerve Stimulation

VNS is used for treatment-resistant or refractory depression. VNS involves the implantation of an electrode on the left cervical vagus nerve. The electrode is connected to a pulse generator, situated subcutaneously in the left thoracic region. The pulse generator transmits intermittent electrical stimulation to the vagus nerve. Because of the invasive nature of this treatment, patients only meet the criteria for implantation after a duration of depression of 2 years without remission, as well as lack of response after at least four full trials of antidepressants (Giuseppe et al., 2014).

Bright Light Therapy

BLT, formerly called *phototherapy*, exposes patients to intense light (5000 lux-hours) each day. The rationale for this treatment comes from several studies plus anecdotal reports indicating that environmental factors play a role in mood disorders. Seasonal affective disorder results from decreased exposure to sunlight and usually occurs in and around the winter season. BLT, used for individuals with seasonal affective disorder, relieves symptoms of depression. Apparently, morning administration is most beneficial.

BLT works in just a few days. The precise mechanism of action of how exposure to intense light produces an antidepressant effect is unclear; however, it is believed that its therapeutic effect is mediated by the eyes, not the skin. Other conditions thought to respond to BLT include bulimia, sleep maintenance insomnia, and nonseasonal depression. Because phototherapy produces few if any significant adverse effects (e.g., nausea, eye irritation), the risk-to-benefit ratio favors its use. Contraindications include glaucoma, cataracts, and the use of photosensitizing medications.

? CRITICAL THINKING QUESTION

4. Does it make sense that bright light could improve a person's mental health? Does a sunny day help your mood?

Repetitive Transcranial Magnetic Stimulation

Repetitive TMS is a non-invasive brain stimulation tool that produces a magnetic field over the brain, influencing brain activity. TMS is indicated for those with nonrefractory or treatment-resistant depression. This treatment apparently increases the release of neurotransmitters or downregulates beta-adrenergic receptors (or both), ameliorating depressive symptoms and possibly other mood disorders. Because TMS does not require anesthesia, it would be an attractive alternative to ECT if conclusive evidence of its efficacy could be demonstrated. Recent studies suggest that only minimal improvement is observed in patients treated with repetitive TMS (Lepping et al., 2014). Adverse effects include seizures in previously seizure-free individuals, headache, and transient hearing loss. Patients with metal implanted in their bodies (e.g., plates), pacemakers, heart disease, or increased intracranial pressure should be carefully evaluated before receiving TMS.

SUICIDE AND DEPRESSION

Most people who commit suicide die accidentally.
Anonymous

The death by suicide of psychiatric patients is of particular importance to the nurse because of opportunities for assessment and intervention. Suicide is a complex phenomenon influenced by a person's cultural beliefs, values, and norms. Suicide can occur in children, adolescents, and adults. Because suicide is such an important topic, it is addressed separately in Chapter 21. Nurses should be aware that suicide is not exclusively committed by people with the diagnosis of major depression. The psychiatric nurse must continually assess for suicide potential among all patients, especially patients with schizophrenia and substance abuse. However, even when individuals with a "nondepression" background kill themselves, they are typically experiencing a period of despair. Specifically, a significant number of people (approximately 10%) with the diagnosis of schizophrenia commit suicide, and the number is even greater for people with alcoholism. Alcoholics typically kill themselves in response to loss (e.g., divorce, separation, being fired) and when they have been drinking. The following topics are worth reiterating in case the reader has not had time to review Chapter 21: the nomenclature of suicide, suicide risk assessment, and the most likely victims of suicide.

Suicide Nomenclature

Following is a brief description of suicide nomenclature:
Suicidal ideation level: Suicidal ideation includes a person's thoughts regarding suicide as well as suicidal gestures and threats.
Suicidal gestures: Suicidal gestures are a person's nonlethal self-injury acts, including cutting or burning of skin areas or ingesting small amounts of drugs. Others often see these gestures as attention-getting measures and do not consider them to be serious problems that might lead to a suicide attempt or completion.
Suicidal threats: Suicidal threats are a person's verbal statements that might declare their intent to commit suicide. Threats often precede an actual suicide attempt.
Suicide attempts: Suicide attempts involve the actual implementation of a self-injurious act with the express purpose of ending one's life.

Suicide Risk Assessment

It is important for the nurse to assess the suicidal potential of psychiatric patients because these patients are at an increased risk of self-harm. Most facilities provide the nurse with a format for evaluating suicidal lethality. The crucial variables are the plan, the method, and the provision for rescue.

Plan

A more developed plan is associated with a higher risk of suicide. People who have carefully developed a suicide plan are more serious about suicide and present a higher risk compared with people who have no plan. Although impulsive suicide attempts can result in death, generally, they are often less lethal because the lack of planning sometimes foils the effort.

Method

Some methods of attempting suicide are more lethal than others. Accessibility of the means to commit suicide is important as well. Having a gun on hand is more lethal than having three bottles of pills on hand. A crucial factor in determining the lethality of a particular method is the amount of time between initiation of the suicide method and delivery of the lethal impact of that method. For instance, a person using a gun has no opportunity to avoid the bullet once the trigger is pulled. However, sitting in the garage with the motor running affords some time to choose an alternative to self-destruction, as does taking an overdose of certain drugs. Lethal methods of suicide include the use of guns, jumping from a high place, hanging, poisoning from carbon monoxide or other gases, and overdosing with certain drugs (e.g., barbiturates, alcohol, and other central nervous system depressants). Methods that are less likely to be lethal include wrist cutting and overdosing on aspirin or diazepam (Valium).

Rescue

The person who deliberately attempts to deceive would-be rescuers has an increased lethality potential. For instance, a woman who says she is going to the ocean for the weekend and then drives to the mountains makes it difficult for family and friends to intervene. A person who leaves a note or makes a telephone call before making an attempt is more likely to be rescued.

Summary

The more detailed the plan, the more lethal and accessible the method, and the more effort exerted to block rescue, the greater the likelihood the effort to commit suicide will be successful. However, impulsive efforts of suicidal individuals with rescuers in sight have proved fatal, particularly when a lethal method (e.g., a gun) has been selected.

Suicide Victims

(A). In the past 20 years, the suicide rate in the United States has increased 35%. Suicide is the second leading traumatic cause of death and the tenth leading cause of death in the United States. Males are four times more likely to commit suicide than females. Among males, the suicide rate is highest for those aged 75 and older; among females, the suicide rate is highest for those aged 45 to 64. The rates of suicide are highest for American Indians, then Non-Hispanic males and females, followed by White males and females (NIMH, Suicide, n.d.).

It is well known in suicidology that mental disorders play a significant role in almost all suicides. This is often referred to as the 90% statistic. Depression is the mental disorder with the strongest relationship to suicide. Although men are known to commit suicide more frequently than women, the rate of depression is higher in women than in men. Hjelmeland and Knizek (2017) propose that suicidality can only be understood from a contextual perspective that includes a sociocultural lens; what it means to those who live it. Box 25.6 lists risk factors that have been related empirically to completed suicide.

BOX 25.6 Risk Factors for Completed Suicide

Male
Native American or Non-Hispanic
Older age
Relationship difficulties
Hopelessness
Medical illness
Severe anhedonia
Living alone
Prior suicide attempts
Unemployment or financial problems
Sexual identity and HIV/AIDS

CRITICAL THINKING QUESTION

5. How would you differentiate between a suicidal gesture and a suicidal threat in assessing a depressed patient?

CASE STUDY

Will S. is a 35-year-old African American man who has been in and out of mental health facilities for several years. Before his formal entrance into the mental health system, he had had several brushes with the law, primarily related to driving under the influence (DUI) of alcohol. It is thought that Will was self-medicating with alcohol and other substances long before he was able to admit that he had a problem. Will developed hepatitis B through sexual activity 1 year after being diagnosed with major depression. Following this diagnosis, Will attempted to kill himself on at least five occasions. During a brief period of his depression, he developed auditory hallucinations accusing him of being gay. Although this was a relatively brief episode and did not recur, Will is very troubled by it, believing that these hallucinations make him "certifiably crazy." Will now lives with his widowed father, who seems to be very pleased to have Will "back home again." Will continues to attend an outpatient program 3 days a week. He verbalizes wanting to go back to work but cannot seem to get moving. A long-standing fear of crowds and people remains. As Will says, "I'm not out of the woods, but I am a lot better than I was."

CARE PLAN

Name: Will S.   **Admission Date:** _____
DSM-5 Diagnosis: Major depression

Assessment	**Areas of strength:** Will understands his disease, has a good relationship with his father, is willing to acknowledge his problems and work on them and is motivated to go back to work.
	Problems: Will verbalizes motivation but seems "stuck"; he enjoys living with his father, but is he too dependent for a 35-year-old man; he continues to be intimidated by crowds and people and has a suicidal history.
Diagnoses	Risk for self-injury related to depression as evidenced by a history of suicide attempts.
	Social isolation related to anxiety, as evidenced by withdrawal from people and uncommunicative behavior.
Outcomes	**Short-term goals**
Date met: _____	Learn and develop relationship skills for dealing with other patients at a mental health treatment center.
Date met: _____	Participate in class activities at the mental health treatment center.
Date met: _____	Develop socialization skills.
Date met: _____	Talk about his feelings with others at the treatment center.
	Long-term goals
Date met: _____	Seek out information about jobs at his skill level.
Date met: _____	Practice relationship skills learned at the mental health treatment center in public areas.
Date met: _____	Take steps to continue psychotherapy after discharge.
Planning and Interventions	**Nurse-patient relationship:** Develop a trusting relationship based on honesty and genuine concern for the patient. Spend time with him, and reinforce his strengths and accomplishments. Help patient develop relationship skills, addressing his fears and sadness.
	Psychopharmacology: Risperidone 3 mg qd; sertraline 50 mg qd; alprazolam 1 mg prn.
	Milieu management: Minimize patient's tendency to isolate himself by encouraging social interaction. As tolerated, draw patient into group situations. Keep patient's environment safe to prevent self-injury.
Evaluation	Patient is doing better but still tends to avoid large groups of people. He is consistently taking his medications, and no psychotic behavior has been observed or reported.
Referrals	Refer patient to a therapist for individual therapy.
	National Alliance of Mental Illness (NAMI) meetings

👥 PATIENT AND FAMILY EDUCATION

Depression

Illness

Depression is a life-altering process or state. Depression can be precipitated by overwhelming life stresses, including loss (e.g., death, divorce, job), medications, medical illnesses, and specific chemical variances in the brain. These precipitating factors are not mutually exclusive and might interact to produce depression. For example, chronic exposure to intense childhood and adult stress and trauma alters brain chemistry. Support for the chemical variance view has increased over the last 3 decades as medications known to relieve depressive states focus on correcting the chemical imbalances previously noted. Nine cardinal symptoms define depression: (1) depressed mood, (2) apathy, (3) changes in weight, (4) sleep disturbances, (5) movement disturbances, (6) lack of energy, (7) sense of worthlessness, (8) inability to concentrate, and (9) thoughts of death. An individual with five of these symptoms (depressed mood or apathy must always be present) meets the criteria for a diagnosis of depression.

Medications

1. The most popular antidepressants are selective serotonin reuptake inhibitors (SSRIs). Well-known drugs in this category include fluoxetine (Prozac), sertraline (Zoloft), paroxetine (Paxil), escitalopram (Lexapro), and citalopram (Celexa). These drugs are effective and have few side effects. However, sexual dysfunction, defined as a loss of interest in sex or the inability to perform sexually, is common and disturbing to many patients. This side effect motivates some patients to stop taking their SSRI. Other medications can be added that might restore sexual vitality (e.g., bupropion [Wellbutrin], sildenafil [Viagra]).
2. An older group of medications, referred to as tricyclic antidepressants (TCAs), are still commonly prescribed (e.g., amitriptyline [Elavil], nortriptyline [Pamelor], desipramine [Norpramin]). Although they have a higher rate of side effects than SSRIs, TCAs are equally effective and are considerably less expensive. The most common side effects are a decrease in blood pressure when standing, dry mouth, constipation, and a racing heart (at times).
3. Numerous other agents are also available (e.g., Wellbutrin, venlafaxine [Effexor], mirtazapine [Remeron], desvenlafaxine [Pristiq], vilazodone [Viibryd], vortioxetine [Brintellix]). All these drugs seem to be tolerated by most people.

Other Issues

It is easy to be dismayed with a depressed person—to wonder why that person simply cannot snap out of it. If a family member feels this way, it might help to compare the situation with that of someone with diabetes. Individuals with diabetes have a reduced level of insulin; they cannot just snap out of it. The same is true of a depressed person. However, just as the person with diabetes is not powerless, the person who is depressed also is not powerless. For example, individuals with diabetes who do not adhere to a diabetic diet or take medications as prescribed can make their condition become worse. Likewise, an individual with depression might have to avoid certain substances, associations, and situations.

▌ STUDY NOTES

1. Major depressive disorder, disruptive mood dysregulation disorder, persistent depressive disorder, and premenstrual dysphoric disorder are significant depressive disorders.
2. *DSM-5* defines major depression as an episode of depression without a history of manic episodes.
3. Disruptive mood dysregulation disorder is diagnosed primarily in children and adolescents who experience frequent outbursts of rage and physical aggression.
4. Persistent depressive disorder is characterized by its chronicity.
5. Reacting to a disappointment or loss with sadness, guilt, or depression is normal; however, if any of these reactions persist too long, a diagnosable depression may be warranted.
6. There is a high correlation between depression and suicide.
7. There are several subtypes of depression, including atypical depression, melancholic depression, catatonic depression, peripartum depression, psychotic depression, and seasonal depression.
8. Depression is common in the United States. Women have a lifetime risk of 10% to 20%, and men have a lifetime risk of about 5% to 10%.
9. Many early-life traumas are associated with depression in children and adults.
10. People from different ethnic and cultural groups might experience depression differently.
11. Objective signs of depression include alterations in activity and social interactions.
12. Subjective symptoms of depression include alterations in affect, cognition, physical and somatic concerns, and perception.
13. Biologic explanations for depression include neurotransmitter, genetic, endocrine, and circadian rhythm dysfunctions. Psychological explanations include debilitating, early-life experiences, intrapsychic conflicts, and reactions to stressful and traumatic life events.
14. Assessment of depression includes consideration of cultural influences, age (older adults are particularly vulnerable), nonbiologic standardized tests, and biologic indices.

15. Psychotherapeutic management includes developing a therapeutic nurse-patient relationship, administering antidepressant drugs when appropriate, and providing a well-managed milieu with a particular emphasis on safety.

16. Somatic therapies are treatment approaches that use physiologic or physical interventions to effect behavioral change.

17. The most common form of somatic therapy is ECT, which involves an electrical current passing through the brain, causing a grand mal seizure.

18. The psychiatric nurse should assess for suicidal ideation in depressed patients.

19. Greater than 70% of all suicides are committed by men. Elderly men are at particularly high risk.

20. In assessing the lethality of suicide, the psychiatric nurse should consider the plan, the method, and the prevention of rescue.

REFERENCES

Abrams, R. (1997). *Electroconvulsive therapy*. Oxford University Press.

American Psychiatric Association. (2013). *Diagnostic and statistical manual of mental disorders* (5th ed.). APA.

Athanasiadis, C., Gough, B., & Robertson, S. (2018). What do counsellors need to know about male depression? *British Journal of Guidance & Counselling, 46*(5), 596–604. https://doi.org/10.1080/03069885.2017.1346232.

Azzone, P. (2018). Understanding the crisis: Five core issues in contemporary psychoanalysis. *International Forum of Psychoanalysis, 27*(4), 255–265. https://doi.org/10.1080/0803706X.2016.1221134.

Beck, J. (2021). *Cognitive behavioral therapy: Basics and beyond* (3rd ed.). The Guilford Press.

Bus, B. A., Molendijk, M., Tendolkar, I., et al. (2015). Chronic depression is associated with a pronounced decrease in serum brain-derived neurotrophic factor over time. *Molecular Psychiatry, 20*(5), 602–608. https://doi.org/10.1038/mp.2014.83.

Colaizzi, J. (1996). Transorbital lobotomy at Eastern State Hospital (1951–1954). *Journal of Psychosocial Nursing and Mental Health Services, 34*(12), 16.

Danis, P., Drew, A., Lingow, S., & Kurz, S. (2020). Evidence-based tools for premenstrual disorders. *Journal of Family Practice, 69*(1), E9–E17. https://cdn.mdedge.com/files/s3fs-public/JFP06901e9.PDF.

D'luso, D., Dobson, K., Watkins-Martin, K., Beaulieu, L., & Drapeau, M. (2018). Bridging the gap between cognitive and interpersonal variables in depression. *Counselling and Psychotherapy Research, 18*(3), 274–285. https://doi.org/10.1002/capr.12167.

Dorman, J. (1995). The history of psychosurgery. *Texas Medicine, 91*, 54.

Freud, S. (1957). *Mourning and melancholia: Vol. 14*. Hogarth Press.

Giuseppe, T., Franzini, A., Messina, G., Savino, M., & Gambini, O. (2014). Vagus nerve stimulation therapy in treatment-resistant depression: A series report. *Psychiatry and Clinical Neurosciences, 68*(8), 606–611. https://doi.org/10.1111/pcn.12166.

Healy, D., & McMonagle, T. (1997). The enhancement of social functioning as a therapeutic principle in the management of depression. *Journal of Psychopharmacology, 11*(Suppl), S25.

Hjelmeland, H., & Knizek, B. (2017). Suicide and mental disorders: A discourse of politics, power, and vested interests. *Death Studies, 41*(8), 481–492. https://doi.org/10.1080/07481187.2017.1332905.

Keltner, N. L., Hogan, B., & Guy, D. M. (2001a). Dopaminergic and serotonergic receptor function in the CNS. *Perspectives in Psychiatric Care, 37*, 65.

Keltner, N. L., Hogan, B., Knight, T., & Royals, A. (2001b). Adrenergic, cholinergic, GABAergic, and glutaminergic receptor function in the CNS. *Perspectives in Psychiatric Care, 37*, 140. http://scholars.uab.edu/display/pub1728212.

Kleinman, C., & Reizer, A. (2018). Negative caregiving representations and postpartum depression: The mediating roles of parenting efficacy and relationship satisfaction. *Health Care for Women International, 39*(1), 79–94. https://doi.org/10.1080/07399332.2017.1369080.

Kubi, T., D'Astolfo, L., Glombiewski, J., Doering, B., & Rief, W. (2017). Focusing on situation-specific expectations in major depression as basis for behavioural experiments - Development of the Depressive Expectations Scale. *Psychology and Psychotherapy: Theory, Research and Practice, 90*(3), 336–352. https://doi.org/10.1111/papt.12114.

Lepping, P., Schönfeldt-Lecuona, C., Sambhi, R. S., Lanka, S. V., Lane, S., Whittington, R., Leucht, S., & Poole, R. (2014). A systematic review of the clinical relevance of repetitive transcranial magnetic stimulation. *Acta Psychiatrica Scandinavica, 130*(5), 326–341. https://doi.org/10.1111/acps.12276.

Leroy, A, Naudet, F, & Vaiva, G, et al. (2018). Is electroconvulsive therapy an evidence-based treatment for catatonia? A systematic review and meta-analysis. *European Archives of Psychiatry and Clinical Neuroscience, 268*(7), 675–687. https://doi.org/10.1007/s00406-017-0819-5.

Malhi, G. S., & Kuiper, S. (2013). Chronobiology of mood disorders. *Acta Psychiatrica Scandinavica, 128*, 2–15. https://doi.org/10.1111/acps.12173.

Melrose, S. (2018). Late life depression: Nursing actions that can help. *Perspectives in Psychiatric Care, 55*(3), 453–458. https://doi.org/10.1111/ppc.12341.

Michelson, D. (2009). Depression: Body and brain. *Biological Psychiatry, 66*(5), 405. https://doi.org/10.1016/j.biopsych.2009.06.002.

Miller, L., Hlastala, S., Mufson, L., & Leibenluft, E. (2018). Interpersonal psychotherapy for mood and behavior regulation: A pilot randomized trial. *Depression and Anxiety, 35*(6), 574–582. https://doi.org/10.1002/da.22761.

Mukherjee, S., Fennie, K., Coxe, S., Madhivanan, P., & Trepka, M. (2018). Racial and ethnic differences in the relationship between antenatal stressful life events and postpartum depression among women in the United States: Does provider communication on perinatal depression minimize the risk? *Ethnicity & Health*, 23(5), 542–565. https://doi.org/10.1080/13557858.2017.1280137.

Nemeroff, C. B. (1998). The neurobiology of depression. *Scientific American*, 278, 42.

NIMH, (n.d.). Major Depression. https://www.nimh.nih.gov/health/statistics/major-depression.shtml#part_155029.

NIMH, (n.d.). Suicide. https://www.nimh.nih.gov/health/statistics/suicide.shtml.

Nordenskjöld, A., von Knorring, L., & Engström, I. (2011). Rehospitalization rate after continued electroconvulsive therapy—A retrospective chart review of patients with severe depression. *Nordic Journal of Psychiatry*, 65(1), 26–31. https://doi.org/10.3109/08039488.2010.485327.

Obbels, J., Verwijk, E., Vansteelandt, K., Dols, A., & Bouchaert, F. (2018). Long-term neurocognitive functioning after electroconvulsive therapy in patients with late-life depression. *Acta Psychiatrica Scandinavica*, 138(3), 223–231. https://doi.org/10.1111/acps.12942.

Omori, W., Itagaki, K., Kajitani, N., Abe, H., Okada-Tsuchioka, M., & Okamoto, Y. (2019). Shared preventive factors associated with relapse after a response to electroconvulsive therapy in four major psychiatric disorders. *Psychiatry and Clinical Neurosciences*, 73(8), 494–500. https://doi.org/10.1111/pcn.12859.

Østergaard, S. D., Rothschild, A., Flint, A., et al. (2015). Rating scales measuring the severity of psychotic depression. *Acta Psychiatrica Scandinavica*, 132(5), 335–344. https://doi.org/10.1111/acps.12449.

Parikh, D., Garg, S., Dalvi, N., Surana, P., Sannakki, D., & Tendolkar, B. (2017). Outcome of four pretreatment regimes on hemodynamics during electroconvulsive therapy: A double-blind randomized controlled crossover trial. *Annals of Cardiac Anaesthesia*, 20(1), 93–99. https://doi.org/10.4103/0971-9784.197844.

Patten, S. B., Williams, J., Lavorato, D., Wang, J., Bulloch, A., & Sajobi, T. (2016). The association between major depression prevalence and sex becomes weaker with age. *Social Psychiatry and Psychiatric Epidemiology*, 51, 201–210. https://doi.org/10.1007/s00127-015-1166-3.

Popiolek, K., Bejerot, S., Brus, O., Hammar, A., Landen, M., & Lundberg, J. (2019). Electroconvulsive therapy in bipolar depression - Effectiveness and prognostic factors. *Acta Psychiatrica Scandinavica*, 140(3), 196–204. https://pubmed.ncbi.nlm.nih.gov/31334829/.

Sahin, E., & Seven, M. (2019). Depressive symptoms during pregnancy and postpartum: A prospective cohort study. *Perspectives in Psychiatric Care*, 55(3), 430–437. https://doi.org/10.1111/ppc.12334.

Shapero, B., Curley, E., Black, C., & Alloy, L. (2019). The interactive association of proximal life stress and cumulative HPA axis functioning with depressive symptoms. *Depression and Anxiety*, 36(11), 1089–1101. https://doi.org/10.1002/da.22957.

Smith, D. (2001). Shock and disbelief. *Atlantic Monthly*, 287, 79.

Stebbins, M., & Corcoran, J. (2016). Pediatric bipolar disorder: The child psychiatrist perspective. *Child and Adolescent Social Work Journal*, 33(2), 115–122. https://doi.org/10.1007/s10560-015-0411-7.

Stoltz, S., Beijers, R., Smeekers, S., & Deković, M. (2017). Diathesis stress or differential susceptibility? Testing longitudinal associations between parenting, temperament, and children's problem behavior. *Social Development*, 26(4), 783–796. https://doi.org/10.1111/sode.12237.

Su, L., Jia, Y., Liang, S., Shi, S., Mellor, D., & Xu, Y. (2019). Multicenter randomized control trial of bifrontal, bitemporal, and right unilateral electroconvulsive therapy in major depression. *Psychiatry and Clinical Neurosciences*, 73(10), 636–641. https://doi.org/10.1111/pcn.12907.

Takagi, S., Takeuchi, T., Yamamoto, N., Fujita, M., Furuta, K., & Ishikawa, H. (2018). Short- and long-term evaluation of cognitive functions after electroconvulsive therapy in Japanese population. *Psychiatry and Clinical Neurosciences*, 72(2), 95–102. https://doi.org/10.1111/pcn.12614.

Tørring, N., Sanghani, S., Petrides, G., Kellner, C., & Østergaard, S. (2017). The mortality rate of electroconvulsive therapy: A systematic review and pooled analysis. *Acta Psychiatrica Scandinavica*, 135(5), 388–397. https://doi.org/10.1111/acps.12721.

Uchida, S., Yamagata, H., Seki, T., & Watanabe, Y. (2018). Epigenetic mechanisms of major depression: Targeting neuronal plasticity. *Psychiatry and Clinical Neurosciences*, 72(4), 212–227. https://doi.org/10.1111/pcn.12621.

Wichniak, A., Wierzbicka, A., & Jernajczyk, W. (2013). Sleep as a biomarker for depression. *International Review of Psychiatry*, 25(5), 632–645. https://doi.org/10.3109/09540261.2013.812067.

Zaki, N., Spence, D. W., BaHammam, A. S., Pandi-Perumal, S. R., Cardinali, D. P., & Brown, G. M. (2018). Chronobiological theories of mood disorder. *European Archives of Psychiatry and Clinical Neuroscience*, 268(2), 107–118. https://doi.org/10.1007/s00406-017-0835-5.

Zolezz, M. (2016). Medication management during electroconvulsive therapy. *Neuropsychiatric Disease and Treatment*, 12, 931–939. https://doi.org/10.2147/NDT.S100908.

Zyromski, B., Dollarhide, C., Aras, Y., Geiger, X., Oehrtman, J., & Clarke, H. (2018). Beyond complex trauma: An existential view of adverse childhood experiences. *Journal of Humanistic Counseling*, 57(3), 156–171. https://doi.org/10.1002/johc.12080. Clinics of North America, 77, 443.

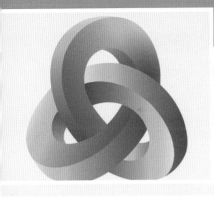

26

Bipolar Disorders

Helene Vossos and Norman L. Keltner

http://evolve.elsevier.com/Keltner

LEARNING OBJECTIVES

- Recognize the *DSM-5* criteria and terminology for bipolar disorder.
- Describe the objective and subjective symptoms of bipolar disorder.
- Explain the biologic and psychosocial hypotheses for bipolar disorder.

- Describe the psychotherapeutic management issues related to bipolar disorder.
- Formulate a nursing care plan for bipolar disorder using the psychotherapeutic management model.

Nothing is more addictive than the high of a manic euphoria. Once you have tasted that soaring, exhilarating, invincible, phantasmagorical feeling of "It's great to be me! I can do anything!" once you've experienced the rush of your mind in overdrive, the creativity pouring through it, the connectivity of burgeoning lateral thinking, the ridiculous ease of witty repartee, the unutterable knowledge of your own immensity, your own infinity, then life without another mania is a dreary prospect indeed.

M. Orum

GENERAL DESCRIPTION OF BIPOLAR DISORDER

Bipolar affective disorder is a spectrum of mood disorders in which individuals experience the extremes of mood polarity and fluctuations. Individuals might feel euphoric or very depressed. A depressive episode is not required for this diagnosis, but a manic episode is required. Bipolar disorder has been deemed the most expensive mental health disorder (CDC, 2020).

Box 26.1 lists the symptoms likely to occur in either a manic episode or a depressive episode. Bipolar disorder can be traced from earliest recorded history to the present day. Thousands of years ago, the Greeks recognized the vacillation between extremes of elation and depression. Other people have also observed and recorded wide mood swings for the historical record. Although the term *bipolar disorder (BD)* is the accepted diagnostic terminology, historically, the terms *manic-depressive* or *bipolar affective disorder* were used and

still might be heard. These terms are used interchangeably at times in this chapter.

Epidemiologic research has indicated that about 6 million women and men in the United States (about 2% of the adult population) experience bipolar disorders yearly (BD I, BD II, and cyclothymic disorder, all to be described later) (American Psychiatric Association [APA], 2013). The median age of onset is 20, with up to 20% of these individuals experiencing mood symptoms starting as early as late adolescence. Men have an earlier age onset, with 90% of both genders diagnosed before 50 and 10% diagnosed after 50 (CDC, 2020; Carlino et al., 2013). Slightly close to 1% of the US population has the more debilitating BD I symptoms secondary to co-occurring substance use disorders (dual diagnosis), anxiety disorder, posttraumatic stress disorder, or medical comorbidity (APA, 2013; Boland, Verduin, & Ruiz, 2021; NAMI, 2017a, 2017b). Approximately 4.1% of the US population have major bipolar disorders at some point during their lifetime (APA, 2013). Another 2% have what has been referred to as *subthreshold bipolar disorder*, or a bipolar spectrum disorder; this simply means that many people do not meet the criteria for a diagnosis but experience distressing depressive symptoms (Advokat et al., 2019). A full 25% of patients with bipolar disorder are elderly (aged 60 years or older) (APA, 2013; Sajatovic et al., 2017). Because statistics can be mind-numbing, they are repeated for clarity as follows (APA, 2013; CDC, 2020):

1. 0.6% have BD I over the course of 1 year.
2. 1.8% have BD I or BD II over the course of 1 year.
3. 1% may experience cyclothymic disorder over their lifetime.
4. 4.1% develop BD I or BD II in their lifetime.
5. Median age of onset is 20.

BOX 26.1   Symptoms Occurring During Manic and Depressive Episodes

Manic Episode
Elevated mood
Grandiosity, inflated self-esteem
Irritability
Anger
Insomnia
Low appetite
Flamboyant gestures
Flight of ideas, racing thoughts
Distractibility
Hyperactivity
Involvement in pleasurable activities
Loud, rapid speech; talkative
High energy
Increased interest in sex
High rate of suicide
Excessive makeup

Other Symptoms
Labile mood
Delusions

Hallucinations
Depressed mood
Low self-esteem

Depressive Episode
Withdrawal
Passivity
Insomnia, daytime sleepiness
Anorexia
Sluggish thinking
Difficulty concentrating, distractibility
Anergia
Diminished interest in activities, inappropriate or excessive guilt
Decrease in speech
Fatigue
Decreased interest in sex
High rate of suicide

Other Symptoms
Memory loss
Abnormal thoughts about death
Weight loss

BOX 26.2   Facts About Bipolar Disorder

1. Average age of onset is early 20s for both men and women.
2. BD I occurs about equally in men and women.
3. Up to 50% of patients with bipolar disorders are nonadherent with medications.
4. In a given year, BD I affects >0.6% of the adult population.
5. Each year, all bipolar disorders affect more than 1.8% of the adult population.
6. People with bipolar disorders account for almost one-fourth (20%) of all completed suicides.
7. About 37% of patients with bipolar disorders relapse in the first year, and only 24% regain a "normal" life.
8. Untreated, a person with a bipolar disorder might experience 10 or more episodes over a lifetime.
9. Bipolar disorder runs in families.
10. Chronic interpersonal and occupational difficulties are experienced by 60% of people with bipolar disorders.

BD I, Bipolar I disorder.
From American Psychiatric Association. (2013). *Diagnostic and statistical manual of mental disorders* (5th ed.). APA; and Anonymous. (2008). Improving outcomes in bipolar disorder. Psychosocial therapies augment medication, but challenges remain. *Harvard Mental Health Letter, 24*(12), 1–3.

6. 10% are over the age of 50.
7. 25% are over the age of 60 or older.

Similar to schizophrenia, onset tends to be in late adolescence to early 20s, and symptoms are recurrent for 90% of affected individuals (Box 26.2). The few individuals who have a later onset typically experience a less severe course. However, they have been in previous treatment for major depressive disorder (unipolar depression) for at least 10 years (Advokat et al. 2019). BD I appears to be almost equally common among men and women, but with evidence of a difference in order of expression. If the first episode is a manic episode, it

more likely occurred in a man, but for both women and men, depression is more likely to be experienced first (APA, 2013). There is also some support for the belief that pregnancy often causes exacerbations in women with a history of bipolar disorder. There are reports of differential incidence based on ethnicity as a lower incidence of bipolar spectrum disorders in Afro-Caribbean individuals. Some individuals are often misdiagnosed with schizophrenia secondary to psychotic symptoms in the severe manic phase, although a diagnosis of bipolar 1 disorder would be more appropriate. This misdiagnosis is understandable because these two disorders share common characteristics as 75% of individuals with bipolar mania have psychotic symptoms (Advokat et al. 2019). Table 26.1 compares the 12-month prevalence rate of bipolar disorders with other mental disorders. Table 26.2 outlines the similarities between BD I and schizophrenia.

 NORM'S NOTES This is a fascinating subject. Note Ms. Orum's quote at the beginning of the chapter. She is honest—she was addicted to the euphoric highs (manic phase) of manic depression. When you meet people with this condition, you might be intimidated because they are moving so fast mentally. Their thoughts can fly so quickly that you cannot keep up, but you are there to be therapeutic. This is where your instructor really needs to guide you. Talking to a person in a manic state is one of the most challenging situations in psychiatric nursing.

DSM-5 TERMINOLOGY AND CRITERIA

DSM-5 defines several variations under the category of bipolar disorders, as previously noted. To understand *DSM-5*

TABLE 26.1 12-Month Prevalence Rate of Mental Disorders in the United States

Disorders	Approximate Percentage > 18 Years Old (%)[a] (Unless Noted for Children)	Gender Representation
Anxiety disorders	19.1 overall	Female = Male
Agoraphobia	1.3	Female
Panic disorder	2.7	Female
Panic attacks	11.2	Female
Social anxiety	7.1	Female
Specific phobia	9	Female
Separation anxiety	1.2	Female = Male
Generalized anxiety disorder	2.7	Female
Posttraumatic stress disorder	3.6	Female
Obsessive-compulsive disorder	1.2	Female > Male
Major depressive disorder	8.7	Female > Male
Bipolar disorder I and II	2.9	BD I: Female = Male BD II: Female
Autism spectrum disorders	1.9 in children	Male > Female
Disruptive, impulse control, and conduct disorders	8.9 overall	
Conduct disorders[a]	4 in children	Male
Attention-deficit/hyperactivity disorder[a]	8.7 in children; 4.4 in adults	Male > Female
Substance use disorders	8.9 overall	
Alcohol use disorder	8.5 in adults; 2.5 in 12- to 17-year-olds	Male
Drug use disorders	1.4	Male
Schizophrenia	1.1	Female = Male

[a]No one source has all this information.
This information has been derived from the following sources: *NIMH. (2017). NIMH-Funded National Comorbidity Study Replication (NCS-R) study: Mental illness exacts heavy toll, beginning in youth*; American Psychiatric Association. (2013). *Diagnostic and statistical manual of mental disorders* (5th ed.). APA.

diagnostic categories, the student must be able to distinguish the basic syndromes presented, such as the manic episode and the hypomanic episode.

FOR INSTRUCTORS' EYES ONLY

I can still remember something from my psychiatric rotation 50+ years ago. I was talking with a group of patients. "My" patient, a young woman, was in the later stages of the acute manic phase of BD, which had led to her hospitalization. She was older than I was, more intelligent than I was, college-educated, and knew a lot more about life in general. She used a word I did not know, *façade*. Part of me wanted to go with the flow as if I knew the word, but I am glad I didn't. I told her I did not know what the word meant. My instructor, who overheard the conversation, later praised me for being honest, noting that all therapeutic relationships are built on honesty. As they say, she caught me doing something right, and as simple as that moment was, it meant a lot to a 19-year-old fellow and still does. You can work with more intelligent and better-educated patients if you know some basic psychiatric nursing principles and are honest. (Students, I told you not to read this!)

❓ CRITICAL THINKING QUESTIONS

1. Can a person fall within the bipolar spectrum but not meet the *DSM-5* criteria for bipolar disorder?
2. Does the patient with bipolar disorder spend more time in a manic mood or a depressed mood?

TABLE 26.2 Similarities Between Bipolar I Disorder and Schizophrenia

	Bipolar I	Schizophrenia
Gender affected	Equal	Equal
Mean age of onset	20s	20s
Genetic factors	Yes	Yes
One affected parent	30% risk	15% risk
Two affected parents	75% risk	35% risk
Identical twin	70%	50%
Course	Chronic	Chronic
Suicide	20%	4.9%
Cigarette smoking	Increased	Increased
Substance abuse	Increased	Increased
Ventricular enlargement	Yes	Yes
Hippocampal volume	Reduced	Reduced
Very sensitive to stress	Yes	Yes

Dome, P., Rihmer, Z., & Gonda, X. (2019). Suicide risk in bipolar disorder: A brief review. *Medicina, 55*(8), 403; NIMH. (2018). Schizophrenia.

Manic Episodes

Manic episodes are characterized by an elevated, expansive, or irritable mood and are fundamental to the diagnosis of BD I. To meet diagnostic criteria, the symptoms must persist for at least 1 week (or less time if hospitalization is required). Symptoms are listed in Box 26.1. Manic episodes usually begin suddenly, escalate rapidly, and last a few days to several months. Judgment is impaired, social blunders occur, and involvement with alcohol and drugs is common. Onset is usually in the early 20 s. Individuals experiencing a manic episode have an inflated view of their importance, sometimes reaching grandiosity (e.g., "I'm so important that the president needs my advice on international affairs").

The impairment is sufficiently serious that functioning deteriorates at home, work, school, or social contexts. Other symptoms include a decreased need for sleep, talkativeness, racing thoughts, and distractibility. The mind seems to go faster and faster. Individuals experiencing a manic episode might engage in risky behavior, such as sexual relationships that are not in keeping with their everyday conduct. People might speculate on a risky business venture because they understand the big picture of business. People have lost everything in these periods of manic thinking. Excess is common: spending sprees, sexual indiscretions, loud clothing, and excessive makeup are often seen in individuals in a manic state. Hospitalization is frequently required to prevent harm to the person or others. Manic episodes can also be part of other mental disorders or a general medical condition (Box 26.3), or they might be substance-induced (Box 26.4).

Relapse is a fact of life with mania. Research suggests that 24% of patients relapse in six months, 37% of patients relapse in 1 year, 61% relapse within 4 years, and 73% relapse within 5 years (Advokat et al. 2019; Baldessarini et al., 2019). Box 26.5 illustrates the suspected causes of the high rate of relapse. Fig. 26.1 illustrates some of the difficulties encountered when treating people with bipolar disorder.

Many famous people have had bipolar disorder. Although many historical figures could be mentioned, perhaps more

BOX 26.3   Medical Conditions That Cause Mania

Anoxia
Hyperthyroidism
Hemodialysis
Lyme disease
Hypercalcemia
AIDS
Stroke
Brain tumor
Multiple sclerosis
Normal-pressure hydrocephalus
Other neurologic disorders

BOX 26.4   Drugs That Can Cause Mania

Antidepressants
Steroids
Anticholinergics
Stimulants
Levodopa

DSM-5 CRITERIA

Bipolar I Disorder

Diagnostic Criteria
To diagnose bipolar I disorder, it is necessary to meet the following criteria for a manic episode. The manic episode may have been preceded by and may be followed by hypomanic or major depressive episodes.

Manic Episode
A. A distinct period of abnormally and persistently elevated, expansive, or irritable mood and abnormally and persistently increased goal-directed activity or energy, lasting at least 1 week and present most of the day, nearly every day (or any duration if hospitalization is necessary).
B. During the period of mood disturbance and increased energy or activity, three (or more) of the following symptoms (four if the mood is only irritable) are present to a significant degree and represent a noticeable change from usual behavior:
  1. Inflated self-esteem or grandiosity
  2. Decreased need for sleep (e.g., feels rested after only 3 h of sleep)
  3. More talkative than usual or pressure to keep talking
  4. Flight of ideas or subjective experience that thoughts are racing
  5. Distractibility (i.e., attention too easily drawn to unimportant or irrelevant external stimuli), as reported or observed
  6. Increase in goal-directed activity (either socially, at work or school, or sexually) or psychomotor agitation (i.e., purposeless non–goal-directed activity)
  7. Excessive involvement in activities that have a high potential for painful consequences (e.g., engaging in unrestrained buying sprees, sexual indiscretions, or foolish business investments)
C. The mood disturbance is sufficiently severe to cause marked impairment in social or occupational functioning or to necessitate hospitalization to prevent harm to self or others, or there are psychotic features.
D. The episode is not attributable to the physiological effects of a substance (e.g., a drug of abuse, a medication, other treatment) or another medical condition.
Note: A full manic episode that emerges during antidepressant treatment (e.g., medication, electroconvulsive therapy) but persists at a fully syndromal level beyond the physiological effect of that treatment is sufficient evidence for a manic episode and, therefore, a bipolar I diagnosis.
Note: Criteria A–D constitute a manic episode. At least one lifetime manic episode is required for the diagnosis of bipolar I disorder.

From American Psychiatric Association. (2013). *Diagnostic and statistical manual of mental disorders* (5th ed.). APA.

BOX 26.5 Mood Disorder Relapse

Rhythm disturbances—e.g., shift work, jet lag

Ending treatment—either intentional or unintentional

Life change—e.g., divorce, job loss

Additional drugs—e.g., opiates, steroids, antidepressants (can induce mania)

Physical health changes—e.g., epilepsy, stroke

Substance use and withdrawal—alcohol, opiates

End of drug response—some patients experience loss of drug response

Modified from Rakofsky, J., & Rapaport, M. (2018). Mood disorders. *Continuum (Minneapolis Minn), 24*(3), 804–827.

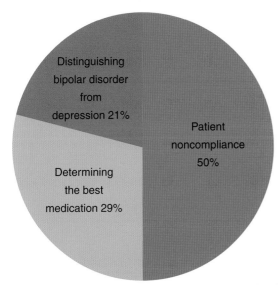

FIG. 26.1 The most difficult aspect of treating bipolar disorder patients. (Adapted from Bezchlibnyk-Butler, K. Z., Jeffries, J. J., Procyshyn, R. M., & Virani, A. S. (2021). *Clinical handbook of psychotropic drugs* [20th ed.]. Hogrefe Publishing; Advokat, C. D., Comaty, J. E., & Julien, R. M. [2019]. *Julien's primer of drug action: A comprehensive guide to actions, uses and side effects of psychoactive drugs* [14th ed.]. Worth Publishers; Stahl, S. M. [2021]. *Essential psychopharmacology* [7th ed.]. Cambridge University Press.)

meaningful to nursing students would be contemporary figures from American culture (http://famousbipolarpeople.com/index.html (2021):

Tim Burton (Author/director)

Robert Downey Jr. (Actor)

Carrie Fisher (Actress, deceased)

Demi Lovato (Actress/singer)

Wolfgang Armadeus Mozart (Musician, deceased)

Sinead O'Connor (Singer)

Jane Pauley (TV personality)

Jean-Claude Van Damme (Actor)

Catherine Zeta-Jones (Actress)

The following clinical example outlines the success and then the failure of a successful businessman.

Clinical Example

Bill is a 50-year-old former chief executive officer of a computer software company. Bill built the company from scratch into a multimillion-dollar-a-year endeavor. It was his second time developing a profitable business from the ground up. While in his early 30s, Bill left a nationally recognized computer company and went into business on his own. Within 3 years, his company was remarkably profitable, with what seemed an unlimited potential. However, 4 years later, the business was bankrupt. He started a second business about 10 years later and experienced even more success with it. Eventually, the new business became insolvent as well. The reason that both businesses failed is directly linked to Bill's bipolar disorder. Although he credits the energy and goal-directed drive associated with the illness for helping him achieve great success, grandiose (e.g., unwarranted expansion, excessive spending) and unrealistic (e.g., he believed the government could not function without his computer applications) thinking eventually drove his business into the ground. As he puts it, "I also lost two businesses, two wives, and three children because of this illness." Both episodes of bipolar disorder required hospitalization.

Bill has never really recovered from the financial and personal setbacks of his last nervous breakdown. He now lives in a county-operated apartment complex with other people who have a persistent mental disorder. Bill has a limited income and, although significantly improved, continues to display mood lability and other residual symptoms. He volunteers at a community mental health center and acknowledges that he most likely will never be a wheeler-dealer again. He can laugh about the good old days when he would drive into a Cadillac dealership and buy two cars—one for himself and one for his girlfriend of the moment.

Hypomanic Episodes

Manias, at least in the early and mild phases, are described as intoxicating states that give rise to great personal pleasure, with a streaming flow of thoughts, and unbounding energy that allows translation of new ideas into creativity, papers and projects.

Adapted from: Dr. Kay Redfield Jamison (2017)

The hypomanic episode is similar to the manic episode but denotes a less severe level of impairment. Because patients feel good about themselves and their lives, hypomania is perceived as normal. Both BD II and cyclothymia diagnoses require evidence of a hypomanic episode. Because the severity level is subjective, *DSM-5* attempts to differentiate hypomanic from manic episodes with more objective criteria. For a hypomanic episode to be diagnosed, the episode's length must be at least 4 days in duration but not severe enough to warrant hospitalization. In addition, the episode is not severe enough to cause "marked impairment" at home, work, school, or in the social milieu but is observable by others and is distinct from the person's typical behavior. The episode is characterized by an abnormal period of persistent elevated, expansive, or irritable mood. Also, the individual must experience at least three of the following symptoms:

- Increased self-esteem or grandiosity
- Decreased need for sleep
- Increased talkativeness
- Subjective sense that thoughts are racing
- Distractibility
- Increase in goal-directed activity (usually social, occupational, educational, or sexual) or motor agitation
- Excessive involvement in pleasurable activities that have a high potential for painful consequences

Depressive Episodes

Bipolar depression causes more suffering and is more disabling than manic or hypomanic symptoms (NAMI, 2017a, 2017b). Depression is the first symptom in more than 50% of patients with bipolar disorder and lasts a lot longer (NAMI, 2017a, 2017b). These patients are in a state of depression about 70% of the time. Bipolar depression differs significantly from unipolar ("regular" major depression) and tends to be more debilitating. Bipolar depression typically develops at a younger age than unipolar depression, and the patient is more likely to express paranoid thoughts, be irritable, and experience hallucinations.

BIPOLAR DISORDERS

DSM-5 bipolar affective diagnoses are based on understanding the spectrum of manic episodes, hypomanic episodes, and major depressive episodes. As noted, *DSM-5* divides bipolar diagnoses into BD I, BD II, cyclothymic disorders, and substance- or medication-induced bipolar disorder.

Bipolar Diagnoses
Bipolar I Disorder

BD I is the most significant of the bipolar disorders. In BD I, the patient experiences swings between manic episodes (defined earlier) and major depression (defined in Chapter 25). Fig. 26.2 illustrates the subtle differences in the bipolar disorders. *DSM-5* provides numerous *specifiers*—for example:

With rapid cycling—at least for mood episodes in the previous year (women more likely)

With melancholic features—loss of pleasure in all, or almost all activities

With psychotic features—delusions or hallucinations present

With anxious distress—feeling keyed up, difficulty concentrating

Bipolar II Disorder

BD II is similar to BD I, with the main exception being that the person has never experienced a manic episode but only a hypomanic episode. In this disorder, the person has experienced significant depression (lasting at least 2 weeks) but has experienced a hypomanic episode (lasting at least 4 days) rather than a full manic episode. There seems to be a higher incidence of this disorder among women. Over the course of a few years, 5% to 15% of individuals with BD II go on to develop a full manic episode (APA, 2013).

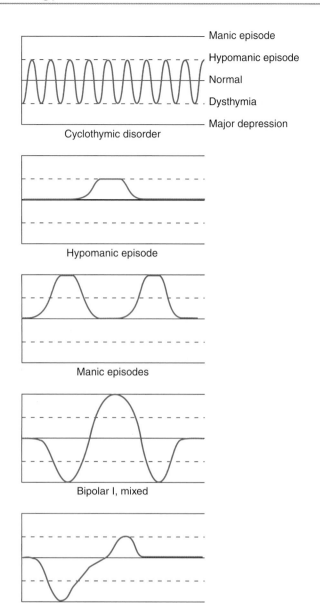

FIG. 26.2 Differences in the bipolar disorders on the mood continuum. By understanding this figure, the student can conceptualize the differences among these bipolar disorders.

❓ CRITICAL THINKING QUESTION

3. What do you think of the following statement? "There are many people in American society who could be diagnosed as hypomanic. Many high-level, workaholic executives are hypomanic and just don't know it."

Cyclothymic Disorder

Cyclothymic disorder is defined as a swing between a hypomanic and depressive episode involving numerous (cycling) periods of hypomania to depressive episodes that are distinct from each other. The swings in either direction are not severe enough to warrant the ultimate diagnosis of a manic episode or a major depressive episode. Using a pendulum as a metaphor, the person experiencing cyclothymic disorder swings from one side to the other but never reaches the extremes of the arc. The person is elated and expansive but does not meet the criteria for a manic episode. Cyclothymic disorder is characterized by symptoms for at least 2 years, without symptom remission for more than 2 months. The person experiences numerous hypomanic episodes and numerous dysthymic-level episodes. Cyclothymic disorder is equally distributed between men and women, with a lifetime risk of 0.4% to 1%. About 15% to 50% of these individuals develop full-blown bipolar disorder (APA, 2013).

Behavior

Objective Behavior

The person experiencing a manic episode appears enthusiastic, energetic, and euphoric. Other people around the person recognize these behaviors as excessive from baseline. Objective behaviors include speech disturbances, the individual's social, interpersonal, and occupational relationships, and activity and appearance. Violent behavior, divorce, spousal and child abuse, job loss, and academic failure are common features of this illness.

Clinical Example

Sue is a 45-year-old Jewish woman who was admitted for bipolar disorder. Police were called to the Greyhound bus station, where they found Sue annoying customers. She claimed to be a Messianic Jew and was preaching to anyone who would politely listen. She resisted the officers and repeatedly stated that she was the "woman at the well" and had married Christ. On arriving on the unit, Sue had excessive bright-red lipstick on, dramatically enhanced eyebrows, and turquoise eye shadow. The rest of her clothing appeared unattended, and she was dirty and smelly. She is known to the hospital staff and was prescribed and received lithium after her initial physical assessment. This drug had been quite effective in the past.

Disturbed speech patterns. The following are examples of disturbed speech patterns of manic individuals:

- Rapid speech
- Pressured speech
- Loud speech
- Easily distracted

Manic patients might speak loudly in a rapid-fire fashion; they monopolize the dialogue and deflect attempts by others to contribute to the dialogue. Conversations are filled with jokes and puns. Sarcastic and biting remarks are common. Even though mental health professionals are aware of this tendency, the ability of manic patients to find a weak spot often frustrates, embarrasses, and angers mental health professionals. The tendency to complain often and loudly is also present. Manic patients can engage staff members in debate and place them on the defensive. Speech is often dramatic, and it is common for manic individuals to burst into song.

Speech is often pressured (i.e., they have a compulsion or strong need to talk).

These patients also are easily distracted. For example, while in the middle of a meaningful discussion, a patient might be distracted by a bird flying outside the window and change the topic of the conversation to flying. This phenomenon, in which patients jump from topic to topic, is referred to as a *flight of ideas*.

Altered social, interpersonal, and occupational relationships. Manic individuals often have changes in their relationship patterns, such as the following:

- Failed relationships
- Job loss and job failure
- Overbearing behavior
- Increased sex drive
- Alienation of family

Clinical Example

Demographics: A young man (Bob, age 30) and a young woman (Mary, age 26) are engaged, with a wedding date planned for the near future.

Background: Both are college-educated, with up-and-coming careers.

The setting: Mary flies into a rage and breaks off the engagement when Bob asks her if she will let the pets out. Mary leaves for 3 weeks and then returns the day before a relative's funeral. Bob attends with her, and she introduces him as her fiancé.

The crisis: After the funeral, she tells Bob, "I got married to my old boyfriend while I was gone. It was a mistake. I went to see my doctor. He thinks I have bipolar disorder."

As this clinical example suggests (Advokat, Comaty, & Julien, 2019; Boland, Verduin, & Ruiz, 2021), a manic episode can cause chaos in an individual's life and for the people close to that individual.

Manic patients irritate others with their impulsive behaviors, fault-finding, anger, and blaming. This disorder destroys relationships. In a classic article, Janowsky et al., (1970) list five tendencies that cause social, interpersonal, and occupational problems for bipolar patients:

1. *Manipulation of the self-esteem of others.* Patients use coercive techniques to increase or decrease another's self-esteem. It is easy to fall prey to the manipulation of praise (e.g., "No one here really understands me but you"). It is just as easy to feel the ego-deflating wrath when plans are thwarted. Some insightful nurses have remarked about feeling like "having been played like a yo-yo."

2. *Ability to find vulnerability in others.* Manic patients can exploit weakness in others or create conflicts among staff members.

3. *Ability to shift responsibility.* Patients shift personal responsibility (e.g., being late) to someone else through the technique mentioned earlier. Nurses are particularly vulnerable in this area because they are trained to take responsibility for their patients' concerns.

4. *Limit testing.* Manic patients keep pushing the limits established by the treatment setting. If a limit is relaxed, these patients push it even more.
5. *Alienation of family.* Manic patients can drive away their families with their behavior. The cyclic nature of the disorder at first inspires hope in the family. After numerous cycles, families often sink into a demoralized state. Divorce related to child and spousal abuse is common during severe manic episodes.

 NORM'S NOTES Each semester, many students question why a patient's family is distant or even out of the picture altogether. In other words, some students suspect that the family has abandoned the patient. My advice is something you have heard all your life: There are two sides to every story. Some families give up too easily, and others have exhausted all avenues to make things work—and they didn't work. Right or wrong, many tired and demoralized families have flown a white flag and retreated.

The same behaviors that drive away family also drive away friends, lovers, bosses, coworkers, ministers, and nonpsychiatric health care providers.

Several trends have been noted among individuals with bipolar disorder:
1. Failed relationships are common for individuals who do not receive adequate treatment.
2. Most individuals report difficulties maintaining long-term friendships.
3. Job loss and job change are common.
4. A need to engage people, even strangers, in conversation characterizes bipolar disorder. Although at first behavior such as this attracts others, soon the overbearing and intrusive nature of the conversation alienates and even frightens people.
5. Mood lability can cause these individuals to fall in and out of love rapidly, with all the associated problems for themselves and others.

The effects of bipolar illness permeate all types of relationships. The expansive mood overflows into excesses as well. The otherwise faithful spouse might become sexually promiscuous, the otherwise thrifty homemaker might go on a shopping or spending spree, and the conservative investor might make a dangerously speculative investment. Divorce rates are two to three times higher than for comparable couples (APA, 2013).

Alterations in activity and appearance. Manic patients are often hyperactive and agitated. Overt manifestations, such as pacing, flamboyant gestures, colorful dress, singing, and excessive use of makeup, are common. Patients also might dress sloppily and omit personal grooming; they might not need sleep or perhaps need only a few hours per night. Some patients have gone for days without sleep, and reports of manic patients dropping from exhaustion, particularly before the modern era of psychopharmacology, were common. Many manic patients have poor nutrition because they stop eating; they simply do not have the patience, the ability to sit still long enough, or the desire to eat.

Subjective Behavior

Alterations of affect. Manic patients experience euphoria and high regard for themselves. The inflated self-image can reach levels of grandiosity. Subjectively, the person going through a manic episode experiences an elevated mood, a feeling of joy, and a sense of greatness. A certain sense of invincibility leads to the social, interpersonal, and occupational problems already discussed.

Another significant symptom is a labile or quickly changing affect. Rapid mood swings are exhibited as changing from elation to irritability or from happiness to anger. For example, a 69-year-old woman was laughing and talking about her acquaintance with former president Bush. "You know, my husband's name was George." She abruptly began to cry. "He is dead, you know." She quickly returned to the topic of her importance, becoming very excited, with an elevated mood.

Alterations of perception. Delusions and hallucinations occur, and their content is typically consistent with mood. For example, if a patient is grandiose about their importance to the government, a mood-congruent delusion might include paranoid thinking about being pursued by enemy forces.

Etiology

Psychosocial theories. At one time, most psychiatric professionals believed that psychological difficulties caused bipolar illness or manic-depressive illness. Developmental theorists have hypothesized that faulty family dynamics during early life are responsible for manic behaviors in later life. According to this view, the mother (or primary caregiver) enjoys being the giver of life and resents autonomy. As the child grows more independent, the mother becomes unhappy, so to please the mother, the child becomes more dependent—that is, to gain affection, the child at an early age learns to deny their own natural tendencies. According to this view, the unnatural tension between dependence and independence and the inherent ambivalence in this family environment can be a causative factor in bipolar illness. Others have suggested that the polar events (e.g., approval or disapproval) of childhood are so significant for some people that an adult emotional counterpart to the emotional roller coaster results—for example, receiving approval (elation) and disapproval (depression). Although some psychosocial explanations seem more credible than others, many professionals believe that family dynamics play an important role in the genesis of manic-depressive illness.

Another psychosocial hypothesis explains manic episodes as a defense against or massive denial of depression. According to this view, manic-depressive individuals go through life appearing to be independent and excessive to others (e.g., too pushy, too talkative, and too manipulative), only to be eventually blocked by someone who no longer tolerates being pushed, talked to, or manipulated. When this happens, the manic individual (who is overdependent) can become psychotic.

Neurotransmitter and Structural Hypotheses

Although some professionals still believe in the importance of psychological influences, most are aware of the role of biology. Just as depression seems to be caused by neurotransmitter deficiency, manic episodes also seem to be related to excessive levels of norepinephrine and dopamine, an imbalance between cholinergic and noradrenergic systems, or a serotonin deficiency. Rakofsky and Rapaport (2018) proposed that bipolar disorder, including manic and depressive symptoms, arises from ion dysregulation, mainly altered serotonin metabolites (Boland, Verduin, & Ruiz, 2021). Box 26.6 summarizes this interesting hypothesis. *If* the ion view is correct, *then* differences between "normal" depression (or unipolar depression) and the depression associated with bipolar disorder can be more clearly appreciated. A common diagnostic mistake is making an incorrect diagnosis of significant depression in someone experiencing the depressive aspect of bipolar disorder. Prescribing an antidepressant would be appropriate for unipolar depression, but such a treatment strategy is controversial when a patient has bipolar depression. Giving an antidepressant to a patient with bipolar depression often pushes the individual into a manic state (APA, 2013). Nonetheless, treating bipolar depression with antidepressants is common but usually is tried only after several other options have failed.

A more compelling view of altered neurobiochemistry in bipolar disorder has been reported by Boland, Verduin, & Ruiz, 2021 and Rakofsky and Rapaport (2018). In the study of molecular psychiatry, Baldessarini et al. (2019) outlined the evidence for a breakdown in the complicated second messenger systems of neurons. In the multistep second messenger system, intracellular processes are triggered when a neurotransmitter binds to a receptor. First, a protein (called a *G-protein*) attaches to the underbelly of the receptor complex, which activates the attachment of an enzyme. This enzyme stimulates another intracellular entity (often either cyclic adenosine monophosphate or inositol), which causes the activation of protein kinases that turn on transcription factors in the nucleus. At this point, the transcription factors can instruct genes to synthesize factors such as enzymes, receptors, or reuptake proteins (i.e., the proteins that cause the neuron to function). Baldessarini et al. (2019) showed that in bipolar disorder, there is greater activity than normal with G-proteins and protein kinases and other steps in the second messenger system. (See Fig. 15.2 for a summary of the second messenger system.)

Biologic findings also suggest that brain lesions, white matter changes, and loss of periventricular gray matter are more common in people with bipolar disorder. Knowing what to make of these structural findings is difficult, but the neurotransmitter hypotheses are consistent with explanations of the putative mechanisms of some antimanic drugs.

Genetic Considerations

It seems clear that genetics has a role in bipolar disorder (APA, 2013). Monozygotic (identical) twins have a very high concordance rate (up to 80%), whereas dizygotic (fraternal) twins have a slightly higher rate than normal siblings and other close relatives. Siblings and close relatives have a higher incidence of manic-depressive illness than the general population, and cyclothymic characteristics are shared among family members of bipolar patients. The following risks have been established for developing bipolar disorder (Soares et al., 2018):

1. First-degree relative—15% to 30%
2. Increases with two affected first-degree relatives—up to 75%
3. Identical twin with bipolar disorder—70%

Significant issues arise surrounding family planning counseling for women with bipolar illness, including the heritability of the disease, the stress of parenthood, and an ill parent's effect

---

BOX 26.6 What Goes Wrong in Bipolar Disorder

Individuals with bipolar disorder have specific signs and symptoms (e.g., elevated mood, grandiosity, irritability, insomnia, anorexia). What is not known is exactly what causes this disorder to happen. The question remains: "What goes wrong in bipolar disorder?" Nestler, Hyman, Holtzman, & Malenka, 2021 indicate a convincing model for the pathology of bipolar disorder, suggesting that a disruption in ion regulation is the cause. Ion regulation is important for normal mood. A key part of ion regulation is the sodium (Na^+) and potassium (K^+)–activated adenosine triphosphatase (ATPase) pump. As this chapter explores, bipolar depression and mania are related, and this model proposes a biochemical explanation (Boland, Verduin & Ruiz, 2021).

According to this model, both bipolar depression and mania result from a decrease in Na^+,K^+-ATPase activity. As activity declines, neuronal membranes become irritable, requiring fewer stimuli to provoke cell firing. As Na^+ accumulates intracellularly because of this faulty pumping action, hyperpolarizing functions of inhibitory neurotransmitters (e.g.,

gamma-aminobutyric acid) are diminished. In addition, because neurotransmitter release is calcium-dependent, the presynaptic terminals might release more neurotransmitter because of a related deficiency in Na^+-dependent calcium efflux. All these factors contribute to increased neurotransmitter release and firing—or mania.

However, the term *bipolar* means "two poles"—the pole of mania and the pole of depression. These two poles are related. As the Na^+, K^+-ATPase pump continues to decrease in activity, neuronal irritability reaches a point whereby less stimulation triggers depolarization. The neuron fires more easily, but the action potential loses amplitude. This loss of amplitude causes calcium channels to decrease their activity and results in a subsequent reduction in neurotransmitter release. Mania is the first disorder to occur when ion dysregulation occurs, but as the Na^+, K^+-ATPase pump becomes more dysfunctional, the depressive side of bipolar disorder develops. Catatonia might be the ultimate expression of ionic dysregulation.

on a child. The teratogenicity of lithium, carbamazepine, and valproic acid is a concern when treating a pregnant woman with bipolar disorder. Consequently, pregnant women with bipolar disorder should be prescribed these drugs only when the risk of not doing so is greater than the risk of fetal insult. Because of these teratogenic effects, atypical antipsychotic medications are more likely to be prescribed to pregnant women.

Comorbidity

About 87% of individuals with a manic-hypomanic disorder have a comorbid mental health disorder (Merikangas et al., 2007). Comorbid mental disorders that occur in up to 75% of patients with bipolar disorders include borderline personality disorder, attention-deficit/hyperactivity disorder, generalized anxiety disorder, panic disorder, social phobias, obsessive-compulsive disorder, substance use disorder, and posttraumatic stress disorder (American Psychiatric Association, 2013; Boland, Verduin, & Ruiz, 2021).

A. Abuse of alcohol and other substances is more common among individuals with bipolar disorder than individuals with any other *DSM-5* diagnosis. More than 50% of individuals diagnosed with bipolar disorder abuse alcohol (APA, 2013). In addition, individuals known to abuse drugs are much more likely to have bipolar disorder than the general public. Patients with bipolar disorder who abuse drugs have higher hospitalization rates and poorer chances of recovery than their peers who do not use drugs. For instance, recent studies have shown that methamphetamine abuse may mimic the manic state of bipolar disorder, and the accompanying psychotic symptoms may persist long after abstinence from this substance (Chiang et al., 2019). When alcohol use is superimposed on co-occurring bipolar disorder and substance abuse, early depression is a frequent outcome. Some clinicians believe that most first-time diagnoses of bipolar disorder are made in the emergency department, related to the consequences of alcohol or other substance abuse. SAMHSA (2016) researchers have reported a high rate of substance abuse in patients with bipolar disorder, including substance abuse as a SYMPTOM or common co-occurrence of bipolar disorder.

B. Substance abuse is an attempt to SELF-MEDICATE bipolar disorder symptoms.

C. Substance abuse CAUSES bipolar disorders.

The use and abuse of alcohol and other substances cause several problems for the patient with bipolar disorder:

1. Relapse rates increase with more hospitalizations,
2. Response to lithium decreases,
3. Remission is delayed,
4. Poor treatment compliance occurs,
5. Poor treatment outcomes are common with more suicide attempts.

Individuals with bipolar disorder often have numerous comorbid medical conditions. As deadly as suicide, 15% of individuals with bipolar disorder, compared to the general population, have a metabolic syndrome and its progeny cardiovascular diseases with a higher mortality rate (American Psychiatric Association, 2013; Boland, Verduin, & Ruiz, 2021).

▌PUTTING IT ALL TOGETHER

PSYCHOTHERAPEUTIC MANAGEMENT

There are three treatment goals when working with patients with bipolar disorder:

1. Getting acute mania under control
2. Preventing relapse when remission occurs
3. Returning to the prior level of functioning (i.e., social, occupational, interpersonal)

Nurse-Patient Relationship

The "Key Nursing Interventions for a Manic Episode" box lists specific interventions for patients who experience manic episodes.

- *Matter-of-fact tone.* A matter-of-fact tone minimizes the need for the patient to respond defensively and avoids power struggles. The nurse conveys both control of the situation and empathy by providing emotional support and responding to patients in a matter-of-fact manner.

- *Clear, concise directions and comments.* Working with hyperactive patients who are highly talkative, easily distracted, experience flight of ideas, and have poor judgment and a labile affect is difficult. When the nurse is confronted with talkative patients, it is not unusual for the nurse to use familiar skills. For example, most people learn not to interrupt another person until a pause. The pause might never come with manic patients. To be effective, the nurse might need to raise their hand and say, "Wait just a minute. I do not want to be rude, but I would like to say something." As a patient starts improving, the nurse might work out a nonverbal signal to indicate when the patient needs to stop and let someone else speak. Although manic patients are talkative, there is a tendency for the talk to be superficial. When talking to hyperactive patients, the nurse should keep remarks brief and straightforward. Many patients literally cannot tolerate a lengthy discussion of any subject.

- *Limit setting.* When the nurse is leading a group, a talkative patient can be disruptive because of the following tendencies:
  - Manipulation of the self-esteem of others
  - Ability to find vulnerability of others
  - Ability to shift responsibility to others
  - Limit testing

These patients have the ability to damage the self-esteem of other patients, ridicule the nurse, blame others, pick fights, create problems between patients, and manipulate others. The nurse needs to protect vulnerable patients and keep them from being drawn into manic patients' anger. When the nurse can remain calm instead of becoming angry, it helps manic patients and the other patients in the group. This calmness should be based on an understanding of psychopathology; otherwise, the nurse might simply be an unhealthy defense (e.g., "You cannot bother me; you are not important enough"). The nurse does not want to convey that they are engaged in an adult version of the childish behavior of plugging the ears and saying, "I can't hear you." It is also important to avoid arguing with patients about unit rules and limits. Do not debate these issues with patients. Simply state the unit policy and move on. Debating and arguing reinforce the tendencies mentioned earlier.

Psychopharmacology

Medication adherence in BD is a priority because of the potential neurodegeneration in BD and the neuroprotective effects of mood stabilizers and some atypical antipsychotics (Pakpour et al., 2017). However, nonadherence is a significant consideration. Box 26.7 provides a nursing strategy for enhancing adherence.

The efficacy of lithium and other mood stabilizers in treating bipolar disorder has been recognized for years. Checking the blood levels of lithium is crucial because this drug has a narrow therapeutic index. Maintenance blood levels between 0.6 and 1.0 mEq/L are standard and can usually be maintained on a dosage of 400 to 1200 mg/day. There are several alternatives to lithium. Anticonvulsants and atypical medications are typically prescribed as adjunctive therapy.

KEY NURSING INTERVENTIONS

For a Manic Episode

Patients Too Busy to Eat
The nurse should use the following interventions to maintain the patient's body weight:
1. Provide patients with foods that can be eaten on the run (sometimes called *finger foods*) because some patients cannot sit long enough to eat.
2. Provide high-protein, high-calorie snacks for patients. A vitamin supplement might be indicated.
3. Weigh patients regularly (sometimes weighing daily is needed).

Patients Who Cannot Sleep
Manic patients experience insomnia. The nurse can help patients maximize the opportunity for sleep by doing the following:
1. Provide a quiet place to sleep.
2. Structure patients' days so that there are fewer stimulating activities toward bedtime.

3. Do not allow caffeinated drinks before bedtime.
4. Assess the amount of rest that patients are receiving. Manic patients cannot judge the need for rest, and exhaustion and death have resulted from lack of rest.

Other Nursing Interventions
- Reinforce reality. Manic patients also experience disturbances in perception. The intervention strategies outlined for other patients with disturbing perceptions are recommended for manic patients as well.
- Respond to legitimate complaints. Although many frivolous complaints arise, the nurse must respond to legitimate complaints to defuse irritability and develop trust.
- Redirect patients into more healthy activity. The bipolar patient's distractibility serves as an intervention tool when the patient engages in nonproductive behavior.

PATIENT AND FAMILY EDUCATION

Bipolar Disorder

Illness
Bipolar disorder is a brain disorder that disrupts mood. The patient might experience extreme moods—bouncing from depression to euphoria (or mania)—or might primarily exhibit symptoms of mania. About 0.6% of the adult population has BD I. Manic episodes are characterized by an elevated mood, irritability, inflated self-esteem, decreased need for sleep, talkativeness, distractibility, and excessive involvement in pleasurable activities. The disorder is typically diagnosed first in the early 20s and occurs about equally in men and women. Because of the pursuit of pleasurable activities, many patients with bipolar disorder overspend, become sexually involved in situations that they would normally avoid, and invest in unwise business dealings. Both dress and language can become loud and excessive. Involvement with drugs and alcohol is common.

Medications
Lithium has been the mainstay of treatment for patients with bipolar disorders; however, it is not prescribed as much as it previously was. It has some troubling side effects, so the physician or nurse practitioner may prescribe divalproex sodium (Depakote) or a second-generation antipsychotic instead. Although lithium is adequate for most patients, it can cause problems because the difference is slight between a therapeutic dose and a harmful dose (or toxic dose). Because of this concern, patients diagnosed with bipolar disorder must have their blood frequently tested for lithium content. After long-term and stable use of lithium, blood draws become less frequent.

Antiepileptic drugs such as divalproex sodium are also used to treat bipolar disorder. Divalproex sodium is an excellent drug and the most often prescribed drug for bipolar disorder. It has fewer side effects than lithium and is safer all around. Although safer than lithium, divalproex sodium and other antiepileptic drugs also produce some significant serious side effects.

Atypical antipsychotic agents have been approved to treat bipolar disorder as well. These drugs are effective but have been known to cause substantial weight gain.

Other Issues
Patients with bipolar disorder can be challenging to live with. Their self-importance, nonstop behavior, talkativeness, style of dress, and irritability can overwhelm a family member. However, these individuals can be remarkably creative and productive. When living or dealing with individuals with this diagnosis, it is vital to be matter-of-fact, clear, and concise in communication; to set limits; and redirect critical negativism into healthier activities. Although difficult at times, the psychiatric nurse needs to avoid personalizing the negative, sarcastic, and rude comments that these individuals might direct toward the nurse. Solid research supports family therapy over individual therapy. Working within the context of the family has been found to reduce relapse dramatically.

BOX 26.7 Nursing Strategies to Improve Adherence

A. Expressing empathy so that patients feel understood and accepted
B. Encouraging patients to recognize a personally meaningful discrepancy between their goals and their current state to motivate change
C. Supporting patients' confidence in their ability to change (self-efficacy)

Adapted from Pakpour, A. H., Modabbernia, A., Lin, C.-Y., Saffari, M., Ahmadzad Asl, M., & Webb, T. L. (2017). Promoting medication adherence among patients with bipolar disorder: A multicenter randomized controlled trial of a multifaceted intervention. *Psychological Medicine, 47*(14), 2528–2539. doi:10.1017/S003329171700109X. PMID: 28446253.

Antipsychotics are very valuable drugs. The most beneficial anticonvulsants are the valproates, particularly divalproex sodium (Depakote). It is a frequently prescribed drug for bipolar disorder now with at least twice the prescriptions of lithium. Other effective anticonvulsants include carbamazepine (Tegretol) and lamotrigine (Lamictal). Lamotrigine has a unique niche because it is particularly effective in treating the depressive phase of bipolar disorder. Newer anticonvulsants such as gabapentin (Neurontin), oxcarbazepine (Trileptal), and topiramate (Topamax) are also used occasionally. Atypical antipsychotics are also approved for the treatment of acute manic episodes. The best options for treating an acute manic episode are the antipsychotics aripiprazole, cariprazine, haloperidol, risperidone, and olanzapine (Baldessarini et al. 2019; Stahl, 2021).

The use of antidepressants to treat bipolar depression is debatable because these drugs can trigger mania. Further, there is very little data to support the effectiveness of antidepressants in these patients (NAMI, 2017a, 2017b). Sanchez, Shoaib, and Aggarwal (2015) developed a mnemonic: "No SAD Me." The basics of this sound advice include:

1. **No**n-antidepressant therapy should be considered (e.g., lithium, quetiapine).
2. **S**afe-to-use adjunctive antidepressants can be considered if relapse occurs.
3. **A**void antidepressant monotherapy.
4. **D**o not use tricyclic antidepressants (TCAs) or venlafaxine. Both carry a high risk of "inducing pathologically elevated states of mood and behavior."
5. **M**onitor closely.

Combining the antidepressant fluoxetine with the antipsychotic olanzapine and/or quetiapine has proven effective (Baldessarini et al. 2019). Recent reports suggest that the dopamine agonist ropinirole, used for Parkinson's disease, may be very beneficial (Capote et al., 2018). These drugs are discussed in detail in Chapters 14 and 15.

Finally, for severe acute mania, unresponsive to the drugs listed previously, electroconvulsive therapy or benzodiazepines may be beneficial. Dr. Stephen Stahl (2021) indicates that different antipsychotics and mood stabilizers failed whereas benzodiazepines such as lorazepam may be utilized as adjunctive pharmacotherapy for individuals with acute mania so severe. Benzodiazepines may prevent a further decline, especially in an acute setting.

Milieu Management

Milieu management is an essential dimension of the nursing care of manic patients. These patients test the unit or day treatment program perhaps more than any other group of patients.

1. *Safety.* The nurse must prevent manic patients from hurting themselves or others. Manic patients can become angry when things do not go their way. This pathologic irritability leads to arguments, fights, self-injury (e.g., hitting the wall, not paying attention to the environment), and hurting others. It is reassuring to patients to realize that the staff will not let them harm themselves or others.

2. *Consistency among staff.* Because manic patients tend to create conflict, pick on vulnerable individuals (patients and staff), blame others, test limits, and shift responsibility to others, the nurse must carefully develop a care plan. Nursing and other staff members should often meet to defuse conflict and clarify communication. All staff members should be aware of intervention strategies and agree to abide consistently by team decisions. Inexperienced staff members must guard against falling prey to esteem-building statements that tend to split the staff (e.g., "You're the only one who understands.").

3. *Reduction of environmental stimuli.* Because manic patients are hyperactive, talkative, irritable, and angry, it is important to decrease environmental stimuli. Patients are distractible and respond to all sorts of environmental cues; it is important to modify the environment as much as possible. Helpful environmental modifications include limited activities with others, gross motor activities (e.g., walking, sweeping, aerobics) to discharge some of the need to be active, and a public room with no television or compact disc player.

4. *Dealing with patients who are escalating.* Manic patients can become hostile and aggressive. The staff needs to deal with this aggressiveness in a calm, confident manner. For patients who are escalating, an antipsychotic drug can be administered to prevent physical aggressiveness, and potential weapons (e.g., chairs, pool cues) can be removed. Limits and the consequences of violating these limits should be reviewed. Do not include limits that are not significant. It is countertherapeutic to defend a poor policy, and it is also countertherapeutic to allow patients to debate a unit issue. It is therapeutic to follow through with appropriate action should a patient violate a unit norm or lead to sexual misconduct on the unit.

5. *Reinforcement of appropriate hygiene and dress.* Patients with bipolar disorder often forget hygiene behaviors, appearing disheveled and unclean at times. Simple reminders to shower, brush teeth, and wear clean clothes can correct some problems. The nurse should also monitor for flamboyant and suggestive dress that might ultimately embarrass the patient.

6. *Nutrition and sleep issues.* Both inadequate nutrition and inadequate sleep patterns plague patients with bipolar disorder.

7. *Routines.* One of the most important contributions the nurse can make is the establishment of routines. A routine bedtime, mealtime, and wake-up time can be immensely therapeutic to patients with bipolar disorder.

CASE STUDY

Mr. Casey Bates, a 50-year-old attorney, was admitted to the unit with the diagnosis of bipolar I disorder, manic type. The police arrested him after he started a fight with three Hispanic men in a bar. He had been drinking heavily. He was hyperactive, distractible, irritable, talkative, and demanding on admission. He demonstrated flight of ideas and was verbally hostile concerning a Hispanic coworker, whom he accused of sleeping with his wife. Mr. Bates has vowed to get even. He made several comments about Hispanics in general while looking at Mr. Lopez, a Hispanic nurse.

This is Mr. Bates's third hospitalization. The first occurred 12 years ago when he contracted a *Candida* infection after having sexual intercourse with his wife. The second hospitalization occurred recently. No precipitating event was recorded, and Mr.

Bates does not recollect anything unusual about the second admission.

Mr. Bates has responded well to lithium in the past; he was also given olanzapine during his last hospitalization because of his agitation. Between hospitalizations, Mr. Bates has functioned well and is considered a good attorney. His partners appreciate his perfectionist tendencies. Mrs. Bates states that Mr. Bates has not slept in 3 days and has not stopped to eat for some time (the actual length of time is unclear). She reports a good marriage until Mr. Bates stopped taking his lithium, which he says he will no longer take. She wants him to "get better and come home." The head nurse decides to streamline the admission process because of Mr. Bates's agitated state. He is taken to a quiet area and given peanut butter crackers and milk.

BOX 26.8 Mood Disorder Questionnaire

Instructions: Check the answer that best applies to you. Please answer each question as best as you can.

	Yes	No
1. Has there ever been a period of time when you were not your usual self and …		
…you felt so good or so hyper that other people thought you were not your normal self, or you were so hyper that you got into trouble?	O	O
…you were so irritable that you shouted at people or started fights or arguments?	O	O
… you got much more self-confident than usual?	O	O
…you got much less sleep than usual and found you didn't really miss it?	O	O
…you were much more talkative or spoke faster than usual?	O	O
…thoughts raced through your head, or you couldn't slow your mind down?	O	O
…you were so easily distracted by things around you that you had trouble concentrating or staying on track?	O	O
…you had much more energy than usual?	O	O
…you were much more active or did many more things than usual?	O	O
…you were much more social or outgoing than usual; for example, you telephoned friends in the middle of the night?	O	O
…you were much more interested in sex than usual?	O	O
…you did things that were unusual for you or that other people might have thought were excessive, foolish, or risky?	O	O
2. If you checked YES to more than 1 of the above, have several of these ever happened during the same period of time? *Please check one response only.*	O	O
3. How much of a problem did any of these cause you—like being able to work; having family, money, or legal troubles; getting into arguments or fights?	O	O

Please check one response only.

O No problem O Minor Problem O Moderate Problem O Serious Problem

	Yes	No
4. Have any of your blood relatives (i.e., children, siblings, parents, grandparents, aunts, uncles) had manic-depressive illness or bipolar disorder?	O	O
5. Has a health professional ever told you that you have manic-depressive illness or bipolar disorder?	O	O

How to score: Further medical assessment for bipolar disorder is warranted if a patient:
Answers: Yes to 7 or more of the events in #1
AND
Answers: Yes to question #2
AND
Answers: Moderate problem or serious problem to question #3
From the Hirschfeld, et al. (2000): University of Texas Medical Branch. *Mood disorder questionnaire.* https://sadag.org/images/pdf/mdq.pdf.

Mood Disorder Rating Scales

The Young Mania Rating Scale (YMRS) and Mood Disorder Questionnaire (MDQ) are two popular rating scales. While both are good scales, the MDQ is newer and slightly handier in the clinical area to uncover a history of mania and thus will be highlighted here (Box 26.8). The MDQ is a five-question scale, with question 1 asking about 13 common signs or symptoms of mania/hypomania. If 7 of the 13 signs/symptoms in question 1 are acknowledged, a "yes" is given to question 2, and a "moderate" or "severe" is provided for question 3, then the MDQ is considered positive (Thomas, 2021; Rakofsky & Rapaport, 2018). The MDQ has a specificity of 97%, which means that nonmanic people are rarely identified as bipolar (Thomas, 2021).

◎ CARE PLAN

Name: Casey Bates   *Admission Date:* _____
DSM-5 Diagnosis: Bipolar I disorder

Assessment	**Areas of strength:** Patient's marriage is solid between hospitalizations. Patient's partners like him and are eager for him to return to work. Patient has good adjustment between hospitalizations. He has responded well to lithium in the past.
	Problems: Patient is threatening and irritating others. Patient has legal problems from bar fight. Patient is threatening to get even with his wife's alleged lover. Patient has not complied with medication regimen recently and states that he will not take lithium.
Diagnoses	Risk for other directed violence related to mania, delusions, irritability, and verbal hostility.
	Nutrition, altered: less than body requirements related to anorexia and hyperactivity, as evidenced by lack of interest in food.

Outcomes   **Short-term goals**
Date met: _____   Patient will not hurt anyone while in hospital.
Date met: _____   Patient will comply with medication regimen.
Date met: _____   Patient will comply with unit norms and limits.

Long-term goals
Date met: _____   Patient will remain free of manic episodes.
Date met: _____   Patient will continue to take lithium on outpatient basis.
Date met: _____   Patient will resolve legal problems.

Planning and Interventions	**Nurse-patient relationship:** Talk to patient in a matter-of-fact tone and clearly indicate that aggressive behaviors are unacceptable. Set firm, clear limits. Do not engage in debates over unit policy or limits. Keep comments brief and straightforward. Do not respond to sarcastic remarks with anger. Reinforce good behavior and confront (carefully) unacceptable behavior.
	Psychopharmacology: Lithium carbonate 600 mg tid PO (concentrate); olanzapine 15 mg HS.
	Milieu management: Provide quiet room and decrease stimuli. Do not include in group activities for a few days. Provide opportunities for rest, and monitor sleep. Provide finger foods and weigh daily. Set limits.
Evaluation	Mr. Bates is less agitated and is taking lithium on schedule. He is beginning to talk less about his wife's alleged infidelity. He has not lost weight. He continues to test limits.
Referrals	Schedule outpatient appointment and give patient and wife a telephone number for a manic-depressive support group.

NEXT-GENERATION NCLEX® EXAMINATION-STYLE CASE STUDY

Scenario: Prioritizing care for a client experiencing mania related bipolar disorder I

A 35-year-old named Gwen presents at the local emergency department reporting, "I need to talk to whoever is in charge; I have the cure for Covid. Hurry! I can make it all go away right now! Don't you try to stop me; get out of my way." The woman appears agitated and is becoming increasingly more verbally and physically aggressive, demanding, "I need to see the boss, and I'm going to hurt you if you get in my way." Security intervenes, and Gwen is admitted to the emergency department due to being a risk to self or others.

Gwen volunteers that she was once diagnosed with bipolar I but has not been medication-adherent because, "Medication hurts my creative energy. I don't take that stuff, and a few beers help calm me when I get too nervous." Vital signs include BP 130/70, P 90, R 18.

Item Type: Cloze
Complete the following sentences by choosing from the list of options. Only one choice should be used per column.
The nurse would first expect _____1_____
to _____2_____ for the purpose of _____3_____.

Option for 1	Option for 2	Option for 3
Substance abuse assessment	Minimize risk of harm to self and other	Introduction of coping skills mood
Initiation of outpatient treatment	Minimize mood disturbance	Stabilization of symptoms
Inpatient hospitalization	Evaluate use of alcohol	Eliminate substance abuse

▌ STUDY NOTES

1. Bipolar affective disorders (e.g., BD I and BD II) occur in about 1.8% of the adult population in any given 12-month period. About 4.1% of Americans are affected by these disorders in their lifetime.

2. Manic episodes are characterized by a distinct period (1 week at least or shorter if hospitalized) during which there is an abnormal and persistent elevated, expansive, or irritable mood. These symptoms tend to occur suddenly and escalate rapidly, lasting a few days to several months. At least three other symptoms are required (see Box 26.1).

3. Hypomanic episodes are characterized by the set of symptoms that occur in manic episodes, except that the symptoms are not as severe; occur over 4 days; do not

4. BD I is described as a swing in mood from a manic episode to major depression.

5. BD II is described as a swing in mood from a hypomanic episode to major depression.

6. Cyclothymic disorder is described as a swing in mood from a hypomanic episode to dysthymia (depressive episode not as severe as episodes with major depression).

7. Objective signs of bipolar illness include altered speech patterns; altered social, interpersonal, and occupational relationships; and altered activity and appearance.

8. Subjective symptoms of bipolar illness include alterations in affect and perception.

9. Psychosocial theories of bipolar illness include theories about family dynamics and psychoanalytic explanations.

10. Biologic explanations of bipolar disorder include excessive levels of neurotransmitters (norepinephrine and dopamine) and genetics (up to 70% concordance rates among identical twins in some studies).

11. Lithium is still the gold standard treatment for bipolar disorders; however, the valproates (e.g., valproic acid [Depakene], divalproex sodium [Depakote]) and second-generation antipsychotics are prescribed more often.

REFERENCES

Advokat, C. D., Comaty, J. E., & Julien, R. M. (2019). *Julien's primer of drug action: A comprehensive guide to actions, uses and side effects of psychoactive drugs* (14th ed.). Worth Publishers.

American Psychiatric Association. (2013). *Diagnostic and statistical manual of mental disorders* (5th ed.). APA.

Baldessarini, R. J., Tondo, L., & Vazquez, G. H. (2019). Pharmacological treatment of adult bipolar disorder. *Molecular Psychiatry*, (2), 198–217. https://doi.org/10.1038/s41380-018-0044-2.

Bezchlibnyk-Butler, K. Z., Jeffries, J. J., Procyshyn, R. M., & Virani, A. S. (2021). *Clinical handbook of psychotropic drugs* (20th ed). Hogrefe Publishing.

Boland, R., Verduin, M. L., & Ruiz, P. (2021). *Kaplan & Sadock's synopsis of psychiatry* (12th ed.). Wolters Kluwer.

Capote, H. A., Rainka, M., Westphal, E. S., Beecher, J., & Gengo, F. M. (2018). Ropinirole in bipolar disorder: Rate of manic switching and change in disease severity. *Perspectives in Psychiatric Care*, 54(2), 100–106. https://doi.org/10.1111/ppc.12205.

Carlino, A., Stinnett, J., & Kim, D. (2013). New onset of bipolar disorder in late life. *Psychosomatics. Jan-Feb.*, 54(1), 94–97. https://doi.org/10.1016/j.psm.2012.01.006. https://www.ncbi.nlm.nih.gov/pmc/articles/PMC3914401/.

CDC. (2020). Mental Health. https://www.cdc.gov/mentalhealth/

Chiang, M., Lombadi, D., Du, J., Makrum, U., Sitthichai, R., Harrington, A., … Fan, X. (2019). Methamphetamine-associated psychosis: Clinical presentation, biological basis, and treatment options. *Human Psychopharmacology*, 34(5). https://doi.org/10.1002/hup.2710.

Dome, P., Rihmer, Z., & Gonda, X. (2019). Suicide risk in bipolar disorder: A brief review. *Medicina*, 55(8), 403. https://doi.org/10.3390/medicina55080403.

Jamison, K. R. (2017). *Setting the river on fire: A study of genius, mania and character*. Knopf.

Janowsky, D. S., Leff, M., & Epstein, R. S. (1970). Playing the manic game. *Archives of General Psychiatry*, 22, 252–261. https://doi.org/10.1001/archpsyc.1970.01740270060008.

Merikangas, K. R., Akiskal, H. S., Angst, J., Greenberg, P. E., Hirschfeld, R., Petukova, M., & Kessler, R. C. (2007). Prevalence, severity, and comorbidity of 12-month DSM-IV disorders in the National Comorbidity Survey Replication. *Archives of General Psychiatry*, 64, 543–552. https://doi.org/10.1001/archpsyc.64.5.534.

NAMI. (2017a). Bipolar disorder. https://www.nami.org/Learn-More/Mental-Health-Conditions/Bipolar-Disorder.

NIMH. (2017b). NIMH-Funded National Comorbidity Study Replication (NCS-R) Study: Mental Illness Exacts Heavy Toll, Beginning in Youth. https://www.nimh.nih.gov/health/topics/ncsr-study/nimh-funded-national-comorbidity-survey-replication-ncs-r-study-mental-illness-exacts-heavy-toll-beginning-in-youth.

NIMH. (2018). Schizophrenia. https://www.nimh.nih.gov/health/statistics/schizophrenia.shtml.

Nestler, E. J., Hyman, S. E., Holtzman, D. M., & Malenka, R. C. (2021). *Molecular neuropharmacology: A foundation for clinical neuroscience*. McGraw-Hill.

Orum, M. (1996). *Fairytales in reality*. Seraline.

Pakpour, A. H., Modabbernia, A., Lin, C. Y., Saffari, M., Asl, M., & Webb, T. L. (2017). Promoting medication adherence among patients with bipolar disorder: A multicenter randomized controlled trial of a multifacted intervention. *Psychological Medicine*, 47(14), 2528–2539. https://doi.org/10.1017/S003329171700109X. PMID: 28446253.

Rakofsky, J., & Rapaport, M. (2018). Mood disorders. *Behavioral Neurology and Psychiatry*, 24(3), 804–827. https://doi.org/10.1212/CON.0000000000000604.

Sanchez, S., Shoaib, H., & Aggarwal, R. (2015). 'No SAD Me': A memory device for treating bipolar depression with an antidepressant. *Current Psychiatry*, 14(2), 52.

Sajatovic, M., Kales, H. C., & Mulsant, B. H. (2017). Prescribing antipsychotics in geriatric patients: Focus on schizophrenia and bipolar disorder. *Current Psychiatry*, 16(10), 20.

Soares, J. C., Walss-Bass, C., & Brambilla, P. (2018). *Bipolar disorder vulnerability: Perspectives from pediatric and high-risk populations*. Elsevier.

Stahl, S. M. (2021). *Essential psychopharmacology* (7th ed.). Cambridge University Press.

SAMHSA. (2016). An introduction to bipolar disorder and co-occurring substance use disorders. https://store.samhsa.gov/sites/default/files/d7/priv/sma16–4960.pdf

Thomas, S. (2021). Psychiatric rating scales for bipolar disorder. https://www.neurotransmitter.net/bipolarscales.html

27

Anxiety-Related, Obsessive-Compulsive, Trauma- and Stressor-Related, Somatic, and Dissociative Disorders

Debbie Steele

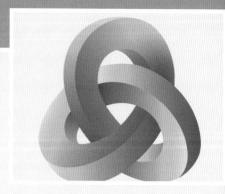

http://evolve.elsevier.com/Keltner

LEARNING OBJECTIVES

- Explain the relationships between stressors and the neurochemical, emotional, and physiologic responses to anxiety.
- Recognize the special terms related to anxiety-related disorders, obsessive-compulsive disorders, trauma- and stressor-related disorders, somatic disorders, and dissociative disorders.
- Describe the *Diagnostic and Statistical Manual of Mental Disorders*, 5th edition (*DSM-5*), criteria for these disorders.

- Describe objective and subjective symptoms of these disorders.
- Develop nursing care plans for individuals with these disorders.
- Evaluate the effectiveness of nursing interventions for individuals with these disorders.
- Recognize unique issues related to the care of individuals and their families with these disorders.

The disorders discussed in this chapter are classified in *DSM-5* as anxiety-related disorders, obsessive-compulsive and related disorders, trauma- and stressor-related disorders, somatic symptom and related disorders, and dissociative disorders. All of these disorders are rooted in stress, anxiety, or fear; it is important to understand their dynamics and how they affect individuals and manifest as mental disorders. When the dynamics of these disorders are understood, appropriate nursing interventions can be instituted.

STRESS

Stress in a person's life is normal, unavoidable, and imminent. Stress is the physiological reaction to a threat or pressure, manifested as physical symptoms of exhaustion or energy loss and psychological symptoms, such as tension or anxiety. The stress response plays an important adaptive role in restoring an individual back to homeostasis. Adaptation to stressors involves a specific repertoire of cognitive, behavioral, and physiologic responses. However, these responses, though essential for survival, can become dysregulated and result in acute and chronic diseases (Gold, 2015). Although stress is typically equated with distress, it is not wholly negative or

something that we should avoid in life. For example, stress can facilitate performance and promote active coping, such as when people are pursuing goals that are important to them. Commonly, people believe that efforts to cope with stress should focus on eliminating stress rather than seeking to optimize stress responses. That is, stress is a problem to be solved rather than an opportunity that needs a response (Jamieson et al., 2018).

Stress models provide nurses with a framework for understanding how stress affects individuals and their responses. Stress models developed by Selye (1956) and Lazarus (1966, 2006) provide essential concepts that are important for nurses to know as they care for vulnerable patients, especially patients who have experienced acute or chronic trauma. The ability to acclimate to stressors leads to conflict resolution, whereas the inability to adapt effectively might result in physical or mental disorders or even death (Fig. 27.1).

Selye Stress Adaptation Model

Hans Selye is known for the general adaptation syndrome, which describes the stereotypical responses or reactions to a stressor. Selye viewed stressors as positive or negative occurrences that produced an emotion requiring a

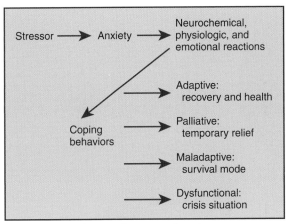

FIG. 27.1 Process of anxiety.

TABLE 27.1	**Stress Adaptation Syndrome**	
Stage I: Alarm Stage	**Stage II: Resistance Stage**	**Stage III: Exhaustion Stage**
Mobilization of the body's defensive forces and activation of the potential for "fight or flight"; increase in alertness to mobilize defenses to alleviate stressor (+1 – +2 anxiety).	The body attempts to adapt to the ongoing stress and tries to return to normal, within the person's capabilities (+2 – +3 anxiety).	Loss of ability to resist stress because of depletion of body resources; decreased resistance to disease (+3 – +4 anxiety).

response. Interactions with the environment and others inevitably produce stress; how a person responds to the stressor is unique and depends on individualized perceptions of the stressor. Generalized adaptation syndrome or stress adaptation syndrome is a three-stage process that the body goes through when it is exposed to stress: (1) alarm, (2) resistance, and (3) exhaustion. The three stages are summarized in Table 27.1.

Alarm

The first stage is the alarm reaction ("fight or flight" response) to a stressor. The body is activated in response to the stressor in order to maintain homeostasis. Allostasis is the term used to describe the biological response to stressors to regain stability. Primary mediators of allostasis involve the hypothalamic-pituitary-adrenal (HPA) axis. A cascade of hormones is released, particularly adrenaline and cortisol (a stress hormone). The adrenaline gives a person a boost of energy, increasing the heart rate, blood pressure, and glucose levels. These physiological changes are governed by the autonomic nervous system (ANS), particularly the sympathetic branch.

The levels of anxiety experienced in this stage are mild (+1) to moderate (+2). When the stressor continues and is not adaptively or effectively resolved, individuals experience the next stage.

Resistance

Restoration of allostasis leads to the second stage of resistance. Here the body tries to counteract the physiological changes that happened during the alarm stage. The resistance stage is governed by the parasympathetic branch of the ANS, which tries to return the body to normal by reducing the amount of cortisol produced. The heart rate and blood pressure begin to return to normal.

If the stressful situation diminishes, the body will begin to return to normal. However, if the stressor remains, the body will stay in a state of alert as stress hormones continue to be produced. In this stage, a person may struggle to concentrate and become irritable. The levels of anxiety experienced are moderate (+2) to severe (+3). As stressors are prolonged and not alleviated, individuals may experience the next stage.

Exhaustion

In stage three, the body's capacity to withstand prolonged stressors is experienced as exhaustion and depleted resources. When the acute response to stress persists and becomes chronic, vulnerability to physical disease and psychopathology occurs. The levels of anxiety experienced are severe (+3) to panic (+4).

Lazarus Interactional Model of Stress and Coping

Lazarus & Folkman, 1984 transactional model of stress and coping emphasizes the bidirectional and reciprocal relationship between individuals and their environment. According to Lazarus and Folkman, stress occurs when an individual perceives the environmental demand as greater than one's ability to deal with it. In other words, stress is experienced when the individual appraises the environmental demand as taxing or exceeding his capability and endangering his well-being. Anxiety is a normal response to a threat (Lazarus, 1966). The significance of the threat or what it means to the individual is of primary importance. For one person, a particular event might be viewed as a challenge; for another, the same event might be viewed as a severe threat or problem.

Cognitive appraisal occurs at multiple points during the stress experience. Primary appraisal is immediate as the individual is triggered and whether the situation has the potential to harm the individual (i.e., a perceived threat) or is benign. Secondary appraisal occurs next as the individual determines if he has the capacity required to cope with the threat. Possible strategies or solutions, as well as resources and supports, are examined. *Reappraisal* occurs as new or additional information has been received, allowing the individual to reconsider or reframe a stressful situation in a way that changes its meaning (Raymond et al., 2019).

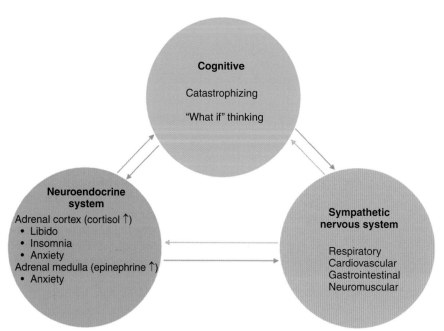

FIG. 27.2 Interacting systems of panic attacks. (From Keltner, N. L., Perry, B. A., & Williams, A. R. [2003]. Panic disorder: A tightening vortex of misery. *Perspectives in Psychiatric Care, 39*, 41.)

Personal and environmental factors influence appraisal—commitments, beliefs, values, feelings, emotions, and views of what is important. A seemingly appropriate solution might not be useful because it conflicts with individual values and beliefs. For example, a passive wife might be unable to be assertive with her husband because she was taught and believes that women should be quiet and submissive.

Stress contributes to a myriad of mental health concerns and is oftentimes the primary presenting concern for patients seeking mental health treatment. Stressful events often create demands which overwhelm the individual. Occasionally, personal resources or social supports are inadequate. Theories and models for stress and coping are helpful tools for understanding the stress process and developing interventions to combat stress-related illnesses (Butts & Gutierrez, 2018). Nurses help patients become aware of the consequences of their behavior and compassionately challenge unworkable actions. (See Fig. 27.2 for prevalence rates of anxiety and other disorders.)

Patients' appraisal of stressors or problems includes their perception of the stressors, the resources or supports they have to help them cope, and the way in which their beliefs and values influence that coping. For example, an individual who is independent, has sufficient income and savings and a supportive family, and believes that divorce is acceptable is likely to cope differently with a partner's affair than an individual who is dependent, unemployed, without close family, and who believes that divorce is not an option. Nurses aim to work alongside patients as they confront unworkable agendas, helping them acknowledge that previous problem-solving methods may not be working or may be a part of the problem. The Chinese finger trap is a popular metaphor that illustrates the process of maintaining unworkable action. As

an individual inserts his fingers into the Chinese finger trap toy and tries to forcefully pull their fingers out on each side, one becomes more and more emotionally distressed. The more the individual struggles and fights, the less likely they are to escape, illustrating that their current approach is not working. Nurses help clients explore the workability of their actions and reassess their appraisal of the stressful experience. The nurse helps explore the workability of the patient's stress-related appraisals, helps the client to clarify his values, and supports the client in committing to action in accordance with his values (Butts & Gutierrez, 2018). Patients may also benefit from classes on stress management, relaxation training, mindfulness, and biofeedback.

ANXIETY

The cardinal manifestation of the stress response is anxiety (Gold, 2015). Anxiety has been described as follows:

- Subjective experience that can be detected only by objective behaviors that result from it
- Emotional pain
- Apprehension, fearfulness, or a sense of powerlessness resulting from a threat that is less visible or definable than fear that has a visible object or trigger
- Warning sign of a perceived danger or threat
- Emotional response that triggers behaviors (automatic relief behaviors) aimed at eliminating the anxiety
- Alerting an individual to prepare for self-defense
- Occurring in degrees
- Contagious; communicated from one person to another
- Part of a process, not an isolated phenomenon

Facing a stressful situation results in predictable emotional and physiological changes. Research on anxiety has identified its biological cascade. Stress responses involve the activation of the sympathetic-adrenal-medullary (SAM) and the HPA axes. The SAM axis rapidly releases catecholamines, whereas the HPA axis, through a hormonal cascade, leads to the release of epinephrine and cortisol by the adrenal glands. The activation of both axes represents the reactivity phase of the acute stress response (Raymond et al., 2019). Additionally, insulin resistance, mild inflammation, and a prothrombotic state emerge to prepare for injuries during fight-or-flight experiences. To conserve calories during the stress response, the growth hormone, gonadal, and thyroid axes are disinhibited. Intracellular changes include neurogenesis, enhanced neural plasticity, and an effectual endoplasmic reticulum response to stress (Gold, 2015). The information in this section is meant to convey the significance of the effects of stressful events on the body. For readers particularly interested in psychobiology, the material presented here can be related to the information in Chapter 4.

Major neurochemical changes identified as affected by stressful episodes include the following (Gold, 2015; Raymond et al., 2019):

- Increased regional epinephrine and norepinephrine turnover in the locus ceruleus and cortex
- Increased corticotropin-releasing hormone
- Moderate reduction of dopamine release in the nucleus accumbens
- Increased cortisol levels
- Activation of the sympathetic nervous system
- Decrease in serotonin neurotransmission
- Activation of the glutamate system
- Rise in plasma glucose
- Release of cytokines and 20 other compounds with proinflammatory and prothrombotic effects

Anxiety-related responses are essential for survival. Naturally, a person's attention is going to be focused on any threatening stressor. The dorsolateral prefrontal cortex exerts cognitive control over fear-related thoughts and behaviors. During stress, it is downregulated, and cognition shifts automatically to stored memories so that access to previous experiences is accessible. Emotional memories become particularly accessible during stressful events, which are stored in the amygdala and hippocampus. They can emerge in the context of exposure to a stressful situation that activated the stress system in years past. The secretion of cortisol and norepinephrine during stress promotes the retrieval of these emotional memories. The accumulation of multiple emotional memories acquired over a lifetime predisposes individuals to stress-related disorders (Gold, 2015).

A stress cycle may begin with physical and psychological symptoms that cause additional stress, negative thinking, and fears. These reactions lead to reactivation of the

TABLE 27.2 Twelve-Month Prevalence Rate of Mental Disorders in the United States

Disorders	Approximate Percentage > 17 Years Old (%)[a] (Unless Noted for Children)	Gender Overrepresentation
Anxiety disorders	18.1 overall	
Agoraphobia	1.7	Female
Panic disorder	2.4	Female
Panic attacks	11.2	Female
Social anxiety	7	Female
Specific phobia	7–9	Female
Separation anxiety	1.2	Equal
Generalized anxiety disorder	2	Female
Posttraumatic stress disorder	3.4	Female
Obsessive-compulsive disorder	1.2	Equal
Major depression	8.6	Female
Bipolar disorder I and II	1.8	BD I: ~ Equal BD II: Female
Autism spectrum disorders	1 in children	Male
Disruptive, impulse control, and conduct disorders	8.9 overall	
Conduct disorders[a]	4 in children	Male
Attention-deficit/hyperactivity disorder[a]	5 in children; 2.5 in adults	Male
Substance use disorders	8.9 overall	
Alcohol use disorder	8.5 in adults; 2.5 in 12- to 17-year-olds	Male
Drug use disorders	1.4	Male
Schizophrenia	1.1	~ Equal

[a]No one source has all of this information.
This information has been derived from the following sources: Kessler, R. C., Petukhova, M., Sampson, N. A., Zaslavsky, A. M., & Wittchen, H.-U. (2012). Twelve-month and lifetime prevalence and lifetime morbid risk of anxiety and mood disorders in the United States. *International Journal of Methods of Psychiatric Research, 21,* 169; Substance Abuse and Mental Health Services Administration. (n.d.). *Results from the 2010 national survey on drug use and health: Summary of national findings.* American Psychiatric Association. (2013). *Diagnostic and statistical manual of mental disorders* (5th ed.). APA.

stress response, resulting in increasingly severe symptoms, increasingly frequent symptoms, or both. Eventually, other symptoms might develop, such as memory loss, mood disturbances, insomnia, gastrointestinal disturbances, hypertension, palpitations, insulin resistance, decreased immune function, and cardiovascular disease (Yaribeygi et al., 2017). In contrast, if the original stress is resolved, the body can return to normal (a relaxation response) through activation of the parasympathetic nervous system and decreased activity in the hypothalamus and pituitary gland.

ANXIETY-RELATED DISORDERS

Anxiety-related disorders involve the subset of disorders discussed here: (1) anxiety disorders, (2) obsessive-compulsive and related disorders, (3) trauma- and stressor-related disorders, (4) dissociative disorders, and (5) somatic symptom and related disorders (see box titled "*DSM-5* Diagnoses for Anxiety-Related Disorders"). Anxiety disorders share features of excessive anxiety, fear, and related behavioral disturbances. Anxiety disorders include (1) generalized anxiety disorder (GAD), (2) social anxiety disorder (social phobia), (3) specific phobias, (4) panic disorder, and (5) agoraphobia (Table 27.2).

GENERALIZED ANXIETY DISORDER

An individual with GAD experiences *excessive or unreasonable worry or apprehension.* The intensity of the worry is out of proportion to the actual likelihood of the anticipated event. The anxiety or worry is chronic, excessive, or unreasonable and may concern everyday events, such as job responsibilities, health, and finances. These individuals have great difficulty in controlling the anxiety, and "worry" becomes a habitual way of coping to prevent a negative occurrence or something bad from happening. Decreased concentration and memory problems often exist. Physical symptoms of anxiety—such as difficulty sleeping, fatigue, and muscle tension—are also part of the disorder. The anxiety causes significant distress and impairment of interpersonal, social, or occupational functioning (see box titled "*DSM-5* Criteria for Generalized Anxiety Disorder").

Etiology and Course

The etiology of GAD is not entirely known. Noradrenergic, serotonergic, and other neurotransmitter systems appear to play a role in the body's response to stress, beginning in childhood. Many believe that low serotonin system activity and elevated noradrenergic system activity are responsible for the development of GAD. The stress and anxiety associated with childhood and adult trauma have been found to contribute to pathological worry. GAD has been linked to high rates of comorbidity, particularly major depressive disorder and substance abuse. Those who suffer from GAD may experience a high rate of health care utilization (Ebberwein, Hopper, Vedala, & Macaluso, 2020; Munir & Takov, 2020).

Further research is needed to clarify the neurobiological mechanisms involved in GAD.

***DSM-5* DIAGNOSES**

For Anxiety-Related Disorders

Anxiety Disorders
Generalized anxiety disorder (GAD)
Panic disorder
Agoraphobia
Specific phobias
Social anxiety disorder (social phobia)

Obsessive-Compulsive and Related Disorders
Obsessive-compulsive disorder (OCD)
Body dysmorphic disorder
Hoarding disorder
Trichotillomania (hair-pulling disorder)
Excoriation (skin-picking disorder)

Trauma- and Stressor-Related Disorders
Posttraumatic stress disorder (PTSD)
Acute stress disorder (ASD)
Adjustment disorder

Somatic Symptom and Related Disorders
Somatic symptom disorder
Illness anxiety disorder
Conversion disorder
Factitious disorder

Dissociative Disorders
Dissociative identity disorder (DID)
Dissociative amnesia
Depersonalization/derealization disorder

From the American Psychiatric Association. (2013). *Diagnostic and statistical manual of mental disorders* (5th ed.). APA.

NORM'S NOTES Anxiety is the most common mental disorder. There are all types of stressors that just get to us, day in and day out. Some people refer to this phenomenon as *life.* On top of that, some of us just don't handle life as well as others. Among your classmates, you have already identified some people who handle things better than others. Why? There are many reasons, and this chapter will help you understand them better. It will also look at some types of anxiety that probably go well beyond anything you have experienced. Just as the chapter on depression can hit a little close to home, so can this chapter.

Psychosocial and environmental factors have been found to play a role in the development of GAD. Prominent theories of GAD suggest that worrying serves to regulate painful emotional experiences (Vasey et al., 2017). For example, worrying is a verbal-linguistic activity that allows individuals to avoid more vivid and threatening mental images and emotions.

Similar theories propose that worrying is a result of emotional dysregulation, particularly related to feelings of shame. Shame is a distressing emotion that is experienced when individuals perceive themselves to be inadequate, worthless, or inferior. Worrying motivates them to withdraw and hide in order to conceal their flaws and avoid social isolation (Shahar, Bar-Kalifa, & Hen-Weissberg, 2015). The median age of onset for GAD is 30 years, and women are more likely to develop the disorder than men. Many affected individuals report that they have felt anxious and nervous all their lives (American Psychiatric Association, 2013).

DSM-5 CRITERIA
For Generalized Anxiety Disorder

1. Excessive anxiety and worry (apprehensive expectation) occurring more days than not for at least 6 months about a number of events or activities (such as work or school performance).
2. The individual finds it difficult to control the worry.
3. The anxiety and worry are associated with three or more of the following six symptoms, with at least some symptoms having been present for more days than not for the past 6 months (note: only one item is required in children):
   - Restlessness or feeling keyed up or on edge
   - Being easily fatigued
   - Difficulty concentrating or mind going blank
   - Irritability
   - Muscle tension
   - Sleep disturbance (difficulty falling or staying asleep, or restless, unsatisfying sleep)
4. The anxiety, worry, or physical symptoms cause clinically significant distress or impairment in social, occupational, or other important areas of functioning.
5. The disturbance is not attributable to the physiologic effects of a substance (e.g., a drug of abuse, a medication) or another medical condition (e.g., hyperthyroidism).
6. The disturbance is not better explained by another mental disorder (e.g., anxiety or worry about having panic attacks in panic disorder, negative evaluation in social anxiety disorder [social phobia], contamination or other obsessions in obsessive-compulsive disorder, separation from attachment figures in separation anxiety disorder, reminders of traumatic events in posttraumatic stress disorder, gaining weight in anorexia nervosa, physical complaints in somatic symptom disorder, perceived appearance flaws in body dysmorphic disorder, having a serious illness in illness anxiety disorder, or the content of delusional beliefs in schizophrenia or delusional disorder).

From the *American Psychiatric Association. (2013). Diagnostic and statistical manual of mental disorders* (5th ed.). APA.

PUTTING IT ALL TOGETHER
PSYCHOTHERAPEUTIC MANAGEMENT
Nurse-Patient Relationship

The first step in the nurse-patient relationship is for the nurse to assess patients' level of anxiety and its associated symptoms.

Most importantly, patients need support and reassurance from the nurse. The nurse promotes trust through acceptance of patients' positive and negative feelings and acknowledgment of their discomfort. Conveying empathy tells patients that the nurse is concerned and understanding and does not minimize the level of distress. For example, the nurse might say, "This must be uncomfortable and painful for you." To help patients manage and reduce their level of anxiety, the nurse should use the interventions found in the box titled "Key Nursing Interventions for Reducing Anxiety."

After the anxiety level has been reduced to a more manageable and comfortable level, the nurse should begin to assist patients in examining their coping behaviors. Through the use of problem-solving methods, adaptive coping skills can increase. The nurse helps the individual to replace ineffective, maladaptive worrying with effective coping methods for dealing with anxiety (see box titled "Key Nursing Interventions for Problem Solving").

The process of helping individuals learn to use adaptive coping behaviors requires patience and the awareness that individuals learn and change at their own pace. The nurse must also be aware of his or her own verbal and nonverbal behavior in working with these patients because anxiety is contagious. The nurse should manage his or her own stress and anxiety so that the work between the nurse and the patient is not compromised. The nurse's role is to educate the patient about the illness, including the effects of anxiety on the patient's life and on family members.

Psychopharmacology

Antidepressants, such as selective serotonin reuptake inhibitors (SSRIs) and selective serotonin-norepinephrine reuptake inhibitors (SNRIs), are the first-line agents for treating GAD and comorbid disorders such as depression (Munir & Takov, 2020). Because GAD is a chronic disorder, antidepressants are better than benzodiazepines owing to the possibility of dependency and tolerance with the latter's long-term use. Benzodiazepines are sometimes used on a short-term basis when a quick-acting medication is needed until the antidepressant takes effect. The benzodiazepine is then slowly tapered, if necessary, and discontinued. Tricyclic antidepressants (TCAs) are seldom used because they have more serious side effects than SSRIs.

Buspirone, a nonaddicting nonbenzodiazepine, is useful for cognitive symptoms of worry, irritability, and apprehension. Typically, it is used as a second-line agent behind SSRIs and SNRIs when a patient does not respond to or cannot tolerate their side effects (Wilson & Tripp, 2020).

Milieu Management

Patients with GAD can benefit from a variety of activities. Cognitive-behavioral therapy (CBT) is effective for patients with GAD; it is known to be the gold standard for anxiety disorders. CBT employs strategies that enable better management of the psychological and physiologic symptoms of anxiety. Behavioral techniques such as meditation, yoga, and mindfulness have been researched in the treatment of GAD (Khalsa et al., 2015). In

KEY NURSING INTERVENTIONS

For Reducing Anxiety

1. Provide a calm, quiet environment. *Rationale:* To identify and reduce stimulation, which includes exposure to situations and interactions with other patients that might provoke anxiety.
2. Ask patients to identify what and how they feel. *Rationale:* To help patients increase their recognition of what is happening to them.
3. Encourage patients to describe and discuss their feelings with you. *Rationale:* To help patients increase their awareness of the connection between feelings and behaviors.
4. Help patients identify possible causes of their feelings. *Rationale:* To help patients connect their feelings with earlier experiences.

5. Listen carefully for patients' expressions of helplessness and hopelessness. *Rationale:* To assess for self-harm; patients might be suicidal because they want to escape their pain and do not think that they will ever feel better. A comorbid major depression may also be present.
6. Ask patients whether they feel suicidal or have a plan to hurt themselves. *Rationale:* To assess for self-harm, same as above, and to initiate suicide precautions if necessary.
7. Plan and involve patients in activities such as going for walks or playing recreational games. *Rationale:* To help patients release nervous energy and discourage preoccupation with the self.

KEY NURSING INTERVENTIONS

For Problem Solving

1. Discuss with patients their successful present and previous coping mechanisms. *Rationale:* To reinforce effective adaptive behaviors.
2. Explore with patients the meaning of their problems and conflicts. *Rationale:* To help patients appraise stressors, explore their personal values, and define the scope and seriousness of their problems.
3. Use supportive exploration and teaching. *Rationale:* To increase patients' insight into the negative effects of their maladaptive and dysfunctional coping behaviors.

4. Help patients to explore alternative solutions and behaviors. *Rationale:* To increase adaptive coping mechanisms.
5. Encourage patients to test new adaptive coping behaviors through role-playing or implementation. *Rationale:* To provide an opportunity for patients to practice new behaviors.
6. Teach patients relaxation exercises. *Rationale:* To reduce the level of anxiety. These techniques help patients to manage or control anxiety on their own.
7. Promote the use of hobbies and recreational activities. *Rationale:* To help patients deal with routine feelings of stress and anxiety.

addition, the use of relaxation exercises, tapes, and biofeedback helps decrease tension and promote relaxation and comfort.

Groups that focus on stress management, problem solving, self-esteem, assertiveness, and goal setting are helpful for coping with stress. Depending on the issues and concerns of each patient, various groups can be helpful.

PANIC DISORDER

Patients with panic disorder experience recurrent panic attacks and are worried about having more attacks. A panic attack is an abrupt surge of intense fear or discomfort that peaks within 10 minutes. In addition to somatic symptoms, patients who experience panic attacks fear that they are losing control over themselves, "going crazy," having a heart attack, or dying from a life-threatening illness.

According to the *DSM-5*, panic attacks are (1) unexpected, occurring out of the blue, such as when an individual is emerging from sleep, or (2) situationally bound, meaning that they occur in anticipation of or on exposure to a trigger situation. These patients avoid places where a panic attack has occurred or could occur. The frequency of panic attacks varies widely, from weekly to yearly. Women are more prone to have panic attacks than men (2:1). Panic attacks are among the most frequently occurring symptoms in psychiatric populations (Liu et al., 2015).

Research Article: Facing Adversity: Authentic Stories of Living and Working with Panic Attacks

Perrone et al., (2013) conducted a phenomenologic study on the effects of panic attacks. Those who experienced panic attacks shared the devastation of how their lives were instantly disrupted at home and work. The first couple of years were particularly traumatic as their lives shifted abruptly from wellness to chronic illness—lives fractured by fear, shame, and stigma. In particular, many individuals experienced fear of sharing their condition with employers, afraid that their sudden, frequent, unpredictable absences would not be understood and that they would not qualify for sick leave. This lack of empathy can result in isolation as such individuals resort to wearing a mask of normalcy.

Etiology

Multiple theories exist as to the possible etiology of panic disorder. The potential role of a chemical imbalance has been researched, including abnormalities in gamma-aminobutyric acid, cortisol, and serotonin. Neural circuitry may play a role in panic disorder whereby certain areas of the brain are hyperexcitable in some individuals making

CASE STUDY

Sandra Johnson, 41 years old, was admitted to the emergency department of a local hospital. Her symptoms were shortness of breath, hyperventilation, palpitations, chest pain, choking sensation, and fear of dying. She stated that these symptoms had occurred unexpectedly while she was cooking dinner. She thought she was having a heart attack.

These attacks had happened three times before. The first attack occurred 2 months earlier. This prompted her to visit her family physician, who performed an electrocardiogram and a stress test and conducted a complete physical examination. All results were negative for any physiologic cause of the symptoms. After the second attack, Mrs. Johnson stated that she took 2 weeks off from work because she was worried about having another attack. She had been employed for 5 years as a secretary for a small insurance agency. Just before she was about to return to work, she experienced another attack. After this third attack, she decided not to return to work and to quit her job. She was unable to leave the house to go grocery shopping, drive the children to activities, or go out socially with friends. Her husband, 42 years old, stated that he and their three daughters, aged 15, 12, and 9 years, were very concerned about her and had been helping her with daily tasks.

After her husband left the emergency department, Mrs. Johnson began to cry, stating that she is letting her family down. She cannot work or even leave the house because she is so afraid of being unable to control another attack. She does not understand what is happening to her and wants medication to help her feel better.

them more prone to developing the disorder. Genetic factors may play a role in the development of panic disorder; first-degree relatives have a 40% increased risk of developing the disorder.

Adverse childhood events have been reported to be a precursor to panic disorder (Cackovic, Nazir, & Marwaha, 2020). Risk factors found to be associated with panic disorder are numerous: stressful life events (financial crisis, interpersonal conflict), family history, childhood trauma, psychological disorders (major depressive disorder, GAD), lower socioeconomic status, and tobacco use (Liu et al., 2015). Some individuals have an increased sensitivity to anxiety and fear and are more susceptible to the effects of trauma, particularly stressful life events. Shim et al., (2016) expanded on the causes and symptoms of panic disorder by examining family relationships and cultural backgrounds. They reported that panic disorder symptoms could originate from anxiety formed from the family of origin and stress caused by family-cultural background (Shim et al., 2016). The majority of patients affected by panic disorder meet the criteria for other psychiatric diagnoses, primarily anxiety or mood disorders (Ogawa et al., 2018). Three systems work singly or in combination to trigger panic: the sympathetic nervous system, the neuroendocrine system, and cognitive processes (see Fig. 27.2). An individual's catastrophic or "what if" thinking can trigger physiologic (somatic symptoms as in the "fight or flight" response), behavioral (avoidant), and affective

CARE PLAN

Name: Sandra Johnson   **Admission Date:** _____

DSM-5 Diagnosis: Panic disorder

Assessment	**Areas of strength**: Patient was managing her role as mother, homemaker, and secretary; was socially active with her friends; is in relatively good health.
	Problems: Fear of dying related to fear of heart attack; unable to leave home; fear of losing her husband; feelings of inadequacy.
Diagnoses	Anxiety: panic related to life stress as evidenced by somatic symptoms and fear of dying.
	Self-esteem disturbance related to feelings of helplessness as evidenced by inability to function.
	Fear related to avoidance as evidenced by difficulty leaving her home.
Outcomes	**Short-term goals**
Date met: _____	Patient will discuss her fears, sense of inadequacy and helplessness, and anger.
Date met: _____	Patient will identify relationship between anxiety and physiologic responses.
Date met: _____	Patient will develop strategies for reducing anxiety, such as relaxation techniques.
Date met: _____	Patient will use problem-solving techniques for life stresses.
	Long-term goals
Date met: _____	Patient will meet with husband and counselor to discuss marital issues.
Date met: _____	Patient will schedule appointment with outpatient therapist for cognitive-behavioral therapy, systematic desensitization, or emotionally focused therapy.
Date met: _____	Patient will identify a schedule for attending a support group.
Planning and Interventions	**Nurse-patient relationship**: Empathy and supportive-acceptance techniques to keep anxiety at a minimum; encourage ventilation of feelings and issues; help patient to identify relationships between stress, anxiety, and physiologic responses; help patient learn adaptive coping strategies.
	Psychopharmacology: Fluoxetine (Prozac) 20 mg every morning.
	Milieu management: Decrease stimuli and provide a quiet, calm atmosphere; monitor anxiety level to prevent escalation; encourage recreational and diversional activities; encourage quiet time if necessary; encourage self-acceptance, meditation, mindfulness techniques, and stress-management groups.
Evaluation	Patient reports having felt less anxious for the past 2 days. Met with husband and counselor.
Referrals	Outpatient appointments for cognitive-behavioral therapy and support group.

(fear) responses. Sensitivity to and vigilance about physiologic symptoms can influence cognitive and neuroendocrine responses (Jurin & Biglbauer, 2018).

Dysregulation of adrenergic receptors—which results in norepinephrine, serotonin, and GABA receptor impairment—causes decreased regulation of the sympathetic nervous system.

PUTTING IT ALL TOGETHER

PSYCHOTHERAPEUTIC MANAGEMENT

Nurse-Patient Relationship

The therapeutic relationship between the nurse and the patient with panic disorder is centered on the same issues and interventions discussed for patients with GAD. Interventions specific for patients experiencing a panic attack are described in the box titled "Key Nursing Interventions for Panic Attack." The rationale for the interventions is to help patients manage the panic attack safely, with as little discomfort as possible. With the nurse's assistance, the patient's anxiety can be reduced to a more manageable level.

The nurse educates patients about panic disorder to reassure them that they are not losing their minds or dying during an attack. Patients experience relief when given information about the disorder, symptoms that are frequently experienced, medications that can relieve symptoms, and effective treatment options. The nurse should help patients realize that attacks are time-limited and that symptoms will abate. Cognitive restructuring helps patients reinterpret and reappraise their beliefs regarding the danger of an event or bodily sensations (Kealy et al., 2017).

Psychopharmacology

SSRIs and SNRIs are most commonly used for the long-term treatment of panic symptoms. Benzodiazepines, such as alprazolam (Xanax) and lorazepam (Ativan), are used for an immediate effect to decrease somatic symptoms until the antidepressant has started working.

The nurse must differentiate symptoms of increased anxiety levels from medication side effects. Anxiety symptoms increase when pertinent issues are addressed, or stressors are present. When symptoms of anxiety remain constant or decrease immediately before the next dose of medication, the symptoms are probably related to the medication. Strategies for anxiety reduction (e.g., deep breathing) might help patients to relax during their panic attacks.

Milieu Management

A holistic method of treating panic disorder involves more physical activities such as walking, basketball, volleyball, or the use of a stationary bicycle, as appropriate, to help decrease tension and anxiety. Other milieu interventions are discussed in the previous section on GAD. CBT plus medication is a first-line treatment for anxious patients; CBT alone has also been found to be effective (Carpenter et al., 2018). CBT works on thoughts and substitutes rational interpretations for the misinterpretation of bodily responses and helps patients to reappraise their beliefs about the danger of an event. Changes in cognition then lead to a decrease in avoidant behavior. CBT helps patients to control their symptoms and improves overall well-being. Computer-assisted or Internet-based CBT (ICBT) is a recommended, cost-effective treatment for panic disorder (Stech et al., 2020). Hovland et al. (2015) found that physical exercise was effective in augmenting the efficacy of ICBT.

AGORAPHOBIA

Agoraphobia is characterized by marked fear or anxiety triggered by real or anticipated exposure to certain situations, such as (1) using public transportation, (2) being in an open space (parking lots, marketplaces, bridges), (3) being in enclosed places (shops, cinemas), (4) being in a crowd, and (5) being outside of the home alone. Individuals with agoraphobia avoid these situations because they are afraid they will be unable to escape, or help will be unavailable to alleviate panic-like symptoms. Agoraphobic situations are endured with intense fear or anxiety, which are out of proportion to the actual danger posed by the situation. The course of agoraphobia is typically chronic and persistent (American Psychiatric Association, 2013).

KEY NURSING INTERVENTIONS

For Panic Attack

1. Stay with the patient who is having a panic attack and acknowledge the patient's discomfort.
2. Maintain a calm style and demeanor.
3. Speak in short, simple sentences and give one direction at a time in a calm tone of voice.
4. If the patient is hyperventilating, provide a brown paper bag and focus on breathing with the patient.
5. Allow patients to pace or cry, which enables the release of tension and energy.
6. Communicate to patients that you are with them and they are not alone.
7. Move or direct patients to a quieter, less stimulating environment. Ask before you touch these patients; touching can increase feelings of panic.
8. Ask patients to express their perceptions or fears about what is happening to them. *Rationale:* To help patients reduce anxiety to a more manageable and comfortable level.
9. Normalize patients' fears related to their physical symptoms.
10. Remind patients that the panic attack episode will be over in about 10 min.

SPECIFIC PHOBIAS

Specific phobias are among the most common psychiatric disorders in children and adolescents; they tend to have an early onset (Oar et al., 2015). Phobias are characterized by marked fear or anxiety in the presence of a specific object or situation (e.g., flying, heights, animals, injections, blood). The feared object or situation provokes immediate fear, which is either avoided or endured with intense anxiety. The fear or anxiety is out of proportion to the actual danger posed by the object or situation. The amount of anxiety experienced varies with proximity to the feared object or situation. Specific phobias typically develop after a traumatic event (such as getting stuck in an elevator) or observing others going through a traumatic event (watching someone almost drown). Specific phobias are commonly experienced disorders (American Psychiatric Association, 2013).

SOCIAL ANXIETY DISORDER

Social anxiety disorder, also known as social phobia, is characterized by marked fear or anxiety of being scrutinized in social situations (i.e., meeting new people, eating at a restaurant, giving a speech). There is a fear of being humiliated or embarrassed by a negative evaluation. The individual is afraid that she will be judged as weak, crazy, stupid, boring, intimidating, or unlikable. In social situations, individuals may fear physical evidence of anxiety such as trembling, sweating, or stumbling over their words. Just thinking about an upcoming social event can produce anticipatory anxiety and dread (American Psychiatric Association, 2013).

Etiology

Research has led to theories stating that specific individual, environmental, family, and biological factors underlie social anxiety disorder. The development of social anxiety disorder (SAD) is oftentimes related to key environmental influences, such as parenting factors, traumatic life events, and aversive social experiences. Particularly in performance-based social situations, an individual fears that he will behave in a way that will be humiliating or embarrassing. The anticipation of future situations is avoided or endured with intense anxiety (Norton & Abbott, 2017). Classical conditioning explains how social anxiety disorders are acquired through a direct negative experience associated with the feared object/situation. For example, a high school prodigy in baseball who is relatively shy and introverted is forced to take center stage in promoting baseball games at school pep rallies. He then goes on to develop social anxiety disorder as an adult. Social and peer-related negative and traumatic events, such as bullying, humiliation, and ostracism, are also considered to be direct conditioning experiences associated with social anxiety disorder. SAD typically has an early onset (median = 13 years of age) and chronic course throughout the lifespan (Norton & Abbott, 2017).

PUTTING IT ALL TOGETHER
PSYCHOTHERAPEUTIC MANAGEMENT
Nurse-Patient Relationship

Patients with phobic disorders, in general, are usually treated on an outpatient basis. If the phobia incapacitates a patient to a severe extent, she might be hospitalized. For example, hospitalization would be indicated if a person who has a phobia about germs is malnourished or dehydrated because he is not eating or drinking. Following are some nursing interventions useful for individuals experiencing phobic disorders:
1. Accept patients and their fears with a noncritical attitude.
2. Provide and involve patients in activities that do not increase anxiety; activities increase involvement rather than promoting avoidance.
3. Help patients with physical safety and comfort needs.
4. Help patients recognize that their behavior is a way of avoiding anxiety.

Psychopharmacology

CBT is the most successful treatment for phobic patients. Systematic desensitization and exposure therapy by trained counselors have been found to be effective for specific phobias. *Clonidine* and *propranolol* may be taken as needed before social engagements to ease the symptoms associated with social anxiety disorder. In addition, SSRIs are used to reduce anxiety and depression if present.

Milieu Management

Individual therapy and goal-setting groups may prove beneficial. It is important to ask patients if they can tolerate groups and other milieu activities or if they prefer individual activities based on their anxiety level. The patient's social interaction can increase as tolerated (Perreault et al., 2014).

OBSESSIVE-COMPULSIVE AND RELATED DISORDERS

According to the *DSM-5*, obsessive-compulsive and related disorders include obsessive-compulsive disorder (OCD), body dysmorphic disorder, hoarding, trichotillomania (hair-pulling), and excoriation (skin-picking).

Obsessive-Compulsive Disorder

OCD is characterized by the presence of obsessions, compulsions, or both. Obsessions are recurrent and persistent thoughts, ideas, impulses, or images that are experienced as intrusive and unwanted (i.e., of contamination, of violent scenes). The performance of compulsions is the individual's attempt to neutralize an obsession with another thought or action. Compulsions or rituals are repetitive behaviors or mental acts that the individual feels driven to perform, such as washing hands, checking, counting, and repeating words. The compulsion is aimed at reducing the anxiety triggered by the obsessions. However, compulsions are typically not connected in a realistic way with the feared thoughts.

Cognitive-behavioral models of OCD have traditionally emphasized the importance of how individuals appraise and/or misinterpret their feared situation. Those who experience OCD may experience catastrophic beliefs that having a thought increases the probability of it becoming a reality. For example, a person who has frequent thoughts of their house being on fire may now misinterpret that they are complicit in their house potentially burning down. This leads to emotional distress and compulsively checking that the stove is off (Aardema et al., 2017).

An important feature of OCD is that the obsessions or compulsions can be so severe that they significantly interfere with the patient's normal routine and are so time-consuming that they interfere with occupational and social functioning. The obsessions and compulsions also interfere with interpersonal relationships because patients are preoccupied with their rituals and magical thinking.

Clinical Example

Joan was found wandering around the hospital in which her son was a patient 3 days after a tornado had destroyed her home and seriously injured her son. She was not injured but complained of nightmares and irritability. She said that she could not bear to see her son because he "just wanted to talk about what happened—things I can't remember." Joan has not been to work since the tornado. She was taken to the crisis unit and diagnosed with and treated for ASD.

In this society, value is placed on performing well in school and at work. Being responsible and perfectionistic is often rewarded by one's boss or by family members. Anyone might be seen as being compulsive at times. However, people generally do not allow their compulsiveness to rule their lives; they are able to maintain a balance between work and play, between role expectations and performance. There is a difference between having characteristics or traits and having an illness. Occasional brooding, rumination, or steadfastness to a task is not usually considered ridiculous or excessively bothersome; these thoughts and feelings do not rule most people's lives.

Body Dysmorphic Disorder

Body dysmorphic disorder is characterized by a preoccupation with perceived flaws in one's physical appearance that are not noticeable to others. The perceived flaws lead the individual to feel ugly, unattractive, abnormal, or deformed.

❓ CRITICAL THINKING QUESTION

1. A patient with OCD washes her hands after each time she touches anything. Her skin is cracked and bleeding. She states to the nurse, "I can't get my hands free of germs." How is this different from the nurse who washes his or her hands before and after each patient contact on a medical-surgical unit?

Preoccupations focus on the outward appearance, such as acne, scars, wrinkles, paleness, nose, hair, teeth, weight, breasts, or lips. Such individuals perform repeated behaviors (mirror checking, excessive surgery) in response to their concerns. The preoccupations are intrusive, unwanted, time-consuming, and difficult to resist or control (American Psychiatric Association, 2013).

Hoarding Disorder

Hoarding disorder is characterized by persistent difficulties in parting with possessions, regardless of their actual value. The difficulty is due to the distress associated with discarding, selling, recycling, or throwing things away. This behavior results in the accumulation of possessions that congest and clutter living areas. For example, family members may be unable to cook in the kitchen, sleep in their beds, or sit in the living room because of a pileup of household items. The main motivation for hoarding is related to the perceived value of the items or strong sentimental attachment to them (American Psychiatric Association, 2013).

Trichotillomania (Hair Pulling)

Trichotillomania is characterized by recurrent pulling out of one's hair, resulting in hair loss in various regions of the body (scalp, eyebrows, eyelids, axillary hair, facial or pubic hair). Repeated attempts to stop are unsuccessful, leading to significant distress, such as feeling a loss of control, embarrassment, and shame. These individuals may attempt to conceal the hair loss by using makeup, scarves, or wigs (American Psychiatric Association, 2013).

Excoriation (Skin Picking)

Excoriation is characterized by recurrent picking at one's own skin, resulting in skin lesions. The most common sites are the face, arms, and hands. Target areas may be healthy skin, pimples, calluses, scabs, or lesions. Individuals pick with their fingernails, tweezers, or pins. Skin picking is preceded by feelings of anxiety or boredom and results in a sense of relief, pleasure, or gratification. Individuals try to conceal tissue damage with makeup or may avoid going out in public (American Psychiatric Association, 2013).

▎ PUTTING IT ALL TOGETHER

PSYCHOTHERAPEUTIC MANAGEMENT

Nurse-Patient Relationship

Basic nursing interventions for hospitalized patients with OCDs are listed in the box titled "Key Nursing Interventions for OCD." Therapeutic work involves the nurse helping to increase patients' abilities to verbalize feelings, solve problems, and make decisions concerning stressors and problems. The nurse focuses on teaching and helping patients develop adaptive coping behaviors to deal with anxiety. Patients need to learn to substitute positive, anxiety-reducing behaviors for obsessions and rituals. Positive behaviors can include physical exercise, such as walking or using a stationary bicycle. Positive coping behaviors are slowly introduced into the patient's schedule, allowing time for rituals as well as normal activities. The nurse supports patients and positively reinforces nonritualistic behavior. Hobbies and social activities are slowly introduced as patients become more able to handle them.

Psychopharmacology

Current treatment strategies for OCD include selective SSRIs and clomipramine, augmented with antipsychotics for OCD cases refractory to medication. Haloperidol, risperidone, olanzapine, quetiapine, or aripiprazole are examples

---

KEY NURSING INTERVENTIONS

For Obsessive-Compulsive Disorder

1. Ensure that basic needs of food, rest, and grooming are met. Patients may be too distracted to attend to these tasks. Reminders and specific directions are usually necessary.
2. Provide patients with time to perform rituals. Patients need to keep anxiety in check. Later, work to decrease the rituals by helping patients set limits, but never take away a ritual, or panic might ensue.
3. Explain expectations, routines, and changes. *Rationale:* To prevent an increase or escalation of anxiety.
4. Be empathic toward patients and be aware of their need to perform rituals. *Rationale:* To convey acceptance and understanding.
5. Assist patients with connecting behaviors and feelings. *Rationale:* To promote the ability to identify and understand feelings.
6. Structure simple activities, games, or tasks for patients. *Rationale:* To help patients focus on alternatives to their thoughts and actions.
7. Reinforce and recognize positive nonritualistic behaviors. *Rationale:* To increase patients' self-esteem and self-worth.

---

of antipsychotics that can be incorporated in the SSRI treatment (Ardic et al., 2017). A response usually occurs at 10 to 12 weeks.

Milieu Management

Historically, some variation of cognitive-behavioral therapy (i.e., exposure and response therapy, mindfulness) has been recommended for OCD and related disorders. There is growing evidence for acceptance and commitment therapy (ACT) that focuses on changing the way the client relates to their thoughts and feelings. CBT focuses on helping individuals create new perspectives, thereby changing the meaning they give to their thoughts. ACT focuses on helping individuals notice and accept their thoughts and feelings without engaging them (Kennedy, 2018). Behavioral techniques such as the "3-minute breathing exercise" allow patients to temporarily stop as opposed to immediately responding to compulsive urges. These techniques increase a patient's ability to tolerate distressing emotions (Fairfax et al., 2014). Repetitive transcranial magnetic

stimulation (RTMS) has been shown to be a robust and promising intervention for patients with severe OCD who have not responded to other treatments (Modirrousta et al., 2015).

OCD is a chronic and impairing illness that predominantly onsets in children and adolescents. Keyes et al., (2018) found that participants commonly reported stressful, and at times traumatic life events in the period before developing OCD. Family-focused CBT has been found to be efficacious for this population. ACT and Attachment-based interventions show promise for the pediatric population (Freeman et al., 2018). Care is always based on the individual needs of patients.

TRAUMA- AND STRESSOR-RELATED DISORDERS

Trauma- and stressor-related disorders include disorders that develop after exposure to a clearly identifiable traumatic event that threatens the self, others, resources, or sense of control or hope. These include PTSD, ASD, and adjustment disorder. An individual's psychological distress is variable after exposure to a traumatic event. The event overwhelms the individual's usual coping strategies. Traumatic stressors that might precipitate the development of these disorders include war, terrorist attack, being a hostage or prisoner of war, torture, disasters, fatalities in fires or accidents, catastrophic illness, rape, and childhood sexual abuse. Examples of more recent events that have the potential for inducing trauma and stressor-related disorders are Hurricane Sandy, the Afghanistan and Iraqi wars, and COVID-19. It is normal for individuals experiencing such traumatic events to feel distressed, intense fear, terror, and a sense of helplessness. In a sense, PTSD and other stressor-related disorders are an adaptive process, designed to help the body respond quickly to traumatic circumstances when they recur (Sherman, 2019). PTSD can also arise from exposure to multiple types of traumatic stressors that are sustained or repeated. Chronic trauma, especially in childhood, leads to the deterioration of emotional and relational capacities resulting in the loss of healthy psychosocial development. An individual's reaction to trauma depends on prior life experiences and psychological factors (Cloitre et al., 2019). See Chapter 33 for additional information about trauma-related disorders.

Posttraumatic Stress Disorder and Acute Stress Disorder

PTSD and ASD are characterized by intense emotional reactions (fear, helplessness, terror) after exposure to a traumatic event (threatened death, serious injury, sexual violence). Witnessing an event as it occurs to others or learning that a traumatic event occurred to a close family member is considered exposure and can lead to PTSD or ASD. ASD is characteristically similar to PTSD except for onset and duration. The diagnosis of ASD is made when an individual has dissociative symptoms *during or immediately after* the distressing event (3 days to 1 month), including amnesia, depersonalization, derealization, decreased awareness of surroundings, numbing, detachment, or lack of emotional response. The diagnosis of PTSD is made based on the same characteristic symptoms that occur *1 month or more after* the trauma. It is common for PTSD to be unrecognized for years—sometimes 10 to 20 years. This delay in recognition is a result, in part, of the major characteristic of both ASD and PTSD—numbing of responsiveness or reduced involvement with the external world. Many individuals may not perceive their symptoms as indicative of PTSD or ASD because they were not victims of a huge catastrophic event such as war (Lee et al., 2017).

Avoidance is an important feature of PTSD and ASD. There is a persistent attempt to avoid situations, activities, and sometimes even people who might trigger memories of the trauma. These efforts include trying to avoid thoughts and feelings related to the event. A constricted or blunted affect or a limitation in the range of feelings can occur. Patients may feel detached or estranged from family and friends. An inability to trust and to love can lead to withdrawal. Patients often lose interest in activities, even activities unrelated to the traumatic event.

Another major characteristic of ASD and PTSD is reexperiencing the traumatic event in some way, which might be in the form of intrusive, unwanted memories; upsetting dreams or nightmares; or suddenly feeling as if the event were recurring (flashbacks). The triggers for episodes being reexperienced might have obvious connections to the trauma or might not resemble the original situation at all. In either case, patients try to avoid all activities and people in an effort to prevent experiencing the flashback.

Clinical Example

Josie is married and has two small children. Before going to bed, she checks to make sure that the front door is locked. She lies down in bed and begins to think that she might have unlocked the door rather than locked it. She can't go to sleep because of her concern, so she gets up to check the door. She lies back down in bed and begins to wonder if she might have unlocked the door rather than locked it.

Other criteria of PTSD and ASD include increased arousal, anxiety, restlessness, irritability, anger, disturbances in sleep, and impairment in memory or concentration. Self-blame may be experienced as survivor guilt and increase the severity of PTSD (Murray, 2018). For example, combat soldiers who survived an attack when others died.

Individuals experiencing posttraumatic symptoms may also develop depression, suicidal ideation, and substance abuse. Individuals with PTSD are at increased risk of attempting suicide (Murray, 2018). These symptoms complicate treatment, especially if PTSD and ASD are undiagnosed and only the other diagnoses are treated.

Personality disorders are associated with ASD and PTSD, particularly if the individual experienced childhood traumatic events. A history of previous traumas—including torture, childhood abuse, rape, and abuse by a partner—leads to an increased risk for PTSD after later traumas. Conversely, events later in life might trigger previously unrecognized PTSD.

PTSD is associated with arrests, unemployment, homelessness, abusiveness, divorce, and paranoia. Mistrust, isolation, abandonment fears, workaholism, focusing on the needs of others, feelings of inadequacy, anger toward God, unresolved grief, and fear of losing control of emotions are also common.

The family members, friends, and coworkers of individuals with PTSD or ASD may also develop problems, becoming "vicarious victims." In some cases, these individuals have experienced the same trauma (e.g., accident, abuse, disaster) and develop symptoms themselves. The family might or might not be able to help their family member with PTSD. The whole family or certain members might need family therapy.

Neurochemical Basis of Acute Stress and Posttraumatic Stress Disorders

Brain structures, neurotransmitters, and the autonomic nervous system are involved in how trauma is processed. During the exposure to trauma, increased heart rate, elevated cortisol levels, and adrenergic overactivity can lead to the development of PTSD. Brain imaging studies indicate that individuals with PTSD have a dysregulated prefrontal cortex and amygdala activity. This leads to an inhibitory and hyperactivity of neuronal pathways that generate exaggerated excitatory reactions, as well as inhibitory responses (Aliev et al., 2020).

A dual-process model of reactivity to chronic trauma associated with PTSD has been explored that includes both desensitization and hypersensitization effects. Desensitization is a process whereby individuals adapt to repeated trauma by suppressing their emotional distress, oftentimes experienced as depression. While these individuals become emotionally numb, their bodies respond to any threats through physiological hypersensitization and hyperarousal. This hypersensitivity and hyperarousal may result in aggression that appears impulsive as the individual attends to incoming information and overreacts to benign, ambiguous, or mild situations. The exaggerated response may be associated with a dysregulated HPA axis. Poor self-regulation leading to dangerous behaviors is also associated with heightened situations in which the self may be negatively judged by others. As impulsive and aggressive behaviors escalate, cognitive desensitization increases leading to normative beliefs about aggressive behaviors, even the use of violence (Gaylord-Harden et al., 2017).

❓ CRITICAL THINKING QUESTION

2. Ron Jenkins's workplace was severely damaged by an explosion. He was found staring at the cars in the parking lot and repeating that he had to find his car and his wife. He was unable to give his address or say where his wife would be at that time of day. He refused to be treated for cuts and bruises until he could find his wife. What interventions would you use at the scene?

Adjustment Disorder

Adjustment disorder is characterized by marked emotional distress resulting from an identifiable stressful life event (e.g., marital breakup, persistent painful illness, job loss, natural disaster). The symptoms develop within 3 months after the stressor, and the reaction is not severe enough to fit the criteria for PTSD. The symptoms or reactions to the stressful circumstance are considered out of proportion to the severity or intensity of the stressor. The acute reaction interferes with functioning but lasts no longer than 6 months *after* the stressor and its consequences have ended. Chronic symptoms might persist more than 6 months if the consequences of the stressor are more enduring, such as a chronic illness or difficulties resulting from a divorce. The major treatment goals are to help the patient recognize the relationship between the stressful situation and current problems and to review and integrate the feelings and memories of the original situation.

▌ PUTTING IT ALL TOGETHER

PSYCHOTHERAPEUTIC MANAGEMENT

It is well known that PTSD is significantly difficult to treat. Symptoms can persist for decades, and the majority of individuals never seek or complete appropriate treatment despite the chronic nature of the disorder (Gurda, 2015). Trauma-focused psychotherapies, including CBT, narrative exposure therapy, present-centered therapy, and couples therapy, have been researched and found effective for PTSD and other trauma-related disorders (Bisson et al., 2019).

However, there are other evidence-based therapies that approach trauma from an experiential perspective. Among the most common are eye movement desensitization and reprocessing (EMDR) therapy and emotionally focused therapy (EFT). Both of these approaches focus on validating the patients' feelings and beliefs and educating them that their physical and emotional symptoms are adaptive responses in the middle of trauma. Current PTSD symptoms are primarily the result of unprocessed memories—the emotions, physical sensations, and beliefs that were experienced at the time the traumatic events occurred. Current situations activate these memories, causing the individuals to be "triggered." EMDR is a practice of stimulating eye movements while processing these emotional memories, causing a transmutation of emotions, beliefs, and somatic responses (Shapiro, 2013).

EFT is an evidenced-based approach efficacious in treating relationship distress that has oftentimes been a direct result of trauma. Within a relationship context, PTSD symptoms associated with trauma are at times activated, exacerbated, and perpetuated. Due to the strong association between interpersonal relationship problems and PTSD, individuals find themselves caught in a vicious cycle of deteriorating relationships and mental health. The goal of EFT is to help couples and family members create safe relationships where the patient can share experiences and talk about triggered emotions without the fear of reprisal. The therapy focuses on changing distressing interactions into positive patterns of relating to one another. As partners and family members create safety by sharing empathy and comfort from one another during difficult times, it becomes easier to regulate PTSD symptoms (Blow et al., 2015).

There are a large number of popular treatments for PTSD that are used to help relieve the distress of patients suffering from this disorder. Yoga, acupuncture, and mindfulness have been found to have some measure of efficacy but need more research documentation (Metcalf et al., 2016; van der Kolk, 2017). Another popular therapy where research is starting to emerge is canine therapy, which is especially popular among war veterans (Epstein et al., 2014).

Nurse-Patient Relationship

The first priority in the nurse's relationship with patients experiencing PTSD or ASD is the development of trust. Because these patients have a tendency to be withdrawn, to feel alienated, and to be suspicious of others, developing trust might be difficult. Seeking help or accepting it when offered is also sometimes difficult for patients. When a patient is aware of the current influence of the trauma, there is often a tendency for him or her to believe that "No one can understand what I've been through unless they have been through it too." The nurse must be nonjudgmental, honest, empathic, and supportive. The nurse can convey the message, "I haven't been through what you have, but the more you tell me, the better I will understand what you have been through and are experiencing." It is important to acknowledge any unfairness or injustices that were part of the trauma. Safety and security are other priorities because of the risk for suicide and aggression. Sleep disturbances must also be addressed to relieve insomnia and nightmares.

These patients must also hear that they are not crazy but are having typical reactions to trauma. Teaching about the dynamics of PTSD or ASD is often appropriate. Depending on the nature of the trauma, the nurse must be prepared to hear stories of atrocities and help patients process the losses and changes that have occurred in their lives as a result of the trauma. Nurses might need help for themselves to avoid vicarious victimization (secondary PTSD), compassion fatigue, or burnout in working with trauma victims in settings such as emergency departments, burn units, and acute psychiatric hospitals.

It might take time for patients to recognize the relationship between their current problems and the original traumatic event. When patients are not initially aware of the connection between the original trauma and current feelings and problems, the nurse should gently clarify these connections as they emerge. Developing a new perspective on the original trauma—which involves clarifying facts, feelings, and values—is not always easy. Patients need significant help in safely verbalizing feelings, particularly anger, that have often been ignored or repressed. Writing in a journal is often helpful. Expressive therapy (art, music, and poetry) can facilitate the externalization of painful emotions that are difficult to verbalize.

As patients struggle through the sometimes lengthy process of reexperiencing, reintegrating, and processing memories of and feelings about traumatic experiences, they need empathy and reassurance that they are safe within the patient-nurse relationship. It is also important to take time-outs as needed. Patients need support as emotional issues such as substance abuse, financial and housing problems, and broken relationships are expressed.

Involving the family as needed helps patients to reestablish relationships that provide support and assistance. Couple or family education and counseling should be recommended. The box titled "Key Nursing Interventions for Posttraumatic Stress Disorder and Acute Stress Disorder" lists additional nursing interventions to use in treating patients with PTSD and ASD.

Psychopharmacology

The choice of medications depends on the primary symptoms the patient is experiencing and the presence of other comorbid disorders. SSRIs are the established medications for PTSD but are ineffective for many patients. Paroxetine and sertraline are the only medications with FDA indications for PTSD (Schneier et al., 2015). TCAs and mono-amine oxidase inhibitors are second-line treatments. Trazodone and prazosin, an adrenergic inhibitor, can help to reduce insomnia and nightmares in some patients (Lipinska et al., 2016).

Benzodiazepines are effective in reducing anxiety, but there are few studies examining their use for PTSD. There is a risk of dependence, especially for patients who are already abusing alcohol or drugs.

Sleep difficulties, particularly insomnia, are known to be the most prevalent symptoms reported by patients with complex PTSD. Sedatives have been found helpful in veterans with PTSD, especially in women compared to men (Rosen et al., 2019).

Clonidine and propranolol can help diminish the peripheral autonomic response associated with fear, anxiety, and nightmares.

Atypical antipsychotics (olanzapine, risperidone, and quetiapine) can be used for severe PTSD or when the patient has a comorbid diagnosis of psychosis or bipolar disorder. These medications might be used for hyperarousal, flashbacks, and nightmares.

Several psychedelics are currently being investigated for the treatment of PTSD: MDMA, ketamine, and cannabis. Psychedelic drugs (sometimes referred to as hallucinogens) are known for inducing a wide range of psychological, cognitive, emotional, and physical effects (Krediet et al., 2020). Psychedelic drugs hold the capacity for inducing an opening of the sense of self, helpful in unlocking the trauma inside (Lijffijt et al., 2019).

Milieu Management

Patients experiencing PTSD or ASD can benefit from many inpatient or outpatient milieu activities. Social activities can be encouraged with an awareness that patients may have a tendency to be suspicious and withdrawn. Recreational and exercise programs can help reduce tension and promote relaxation. Resistance exercise (weightlifting and strength training) has been found to decrease symptoms of PTSD (Whitworth et al., 2019). Group meditation that involves self-compassion may offer benefits to individuals with PTSD, including symptom reduction (Lang et al., 2019). Groups that focus on self-esteem, decision making, assertiveness, anger management, stress management, and relaxation techniques might be useful. Victims of complex trauma might benefit from group meetings that focus on the

---

KEY NURSING INTERVENTIONS
For Posttraumatic Stress Disorder and Acute Stress Disorder

1. Be nonjudgmental and honest; offer empathy and support; acknowledge any unfairness or injustices related to the trauma. *Rationale:* Building trust might be difficult for patients.
2. Assure patients that their feelings and behaviors are typical reactions to complex trauma. *Rationale:* Patients often believe that they are going crazy.
3. Help patients recognize the connections between the trauma experience and their current feelings, behaviors, and problems. *Rationale:* Patients are often unaware of these connections.
4. Help patients evaluate past and present behaviors in the context of the trauma. *Rationale:* Patients often have guilt about past and present behaviors and are judgmental toward themselves.
5. Encourage safe verbalization of feelings, focusing on fear and sadness. *Rationale:* Feelings are or have been repressed or suppressed.
6. Encourage adaptive coping strategies, such as exercise, relaxation techniques, and sleep-promoting strategies. *Rationale:* Patients might have been using maladaptive or dysfunctional coping to avoid dealing with feelings and issues.
7. Encourage patients to establish or reestablish relationships. *Rationale:* Relationships (needed for assistance and support) might have been affected by patients' outbursts or fear of asking for help.

similarities in their reactions and feelings, such as mistrust, helplessness, fear, guilt, numbing, detachment, nightmares, and flashbacks.

Community Resources

CBT and other psychotherapy and self-help groups with others who have experienced the same or a similar trauma are useful. A community might have a Department of Veterans Affairs Hospital or veterans' outreach center for war veterans and their spouses, as well as groups for victims of rape, incest, or torture and their family members. A community might hold meetings for victims after a community disaster or national tragedy. There might also be a victims' assistance program for crime victims. Substance abuse programs or groups might be needed.

CASE STUDY

Craig was 19 years old when he spent a year in Afghanistan as the gunman on a tank. His tank was hit several times during his tour of duty, and one of his buddies was seriously injured. In addition, he witnessed several of his colleagues dying as a result of stepping on improvised explosive devices (IEDs) and many others dying or sustaining injury as a result of getting shot. After returning to the United States, he reentered college and tried to resume a normal life in his hometown. Within 2 years, he met and married a young woman who was just out of high school. Their marriage lasted less than a year. During this time, Craig flunked out of school and spent much of his time playing video games. He was fired from his part-time job for absenteeism and being late for work. He was able to find another job at a local restaurant as a cook. However, occasionally he would become angry, and he developed a habit of hitting the wall with his fist to relieve his pent-up anger. He was fired after several warnings, again related to absenteeism and showing up late. All the while, he never talked about his experiences in Afghanistan with anyone.

Out of work, divorced, and using illegal drugs, Craig was convinced by his family to be evaluated at the Veteran's Administration Hospital. During a series of physician visits, he reported having bouts of depression with suicidal ideation, difficulty focusing and concentrating, flashbacks, nightmares, avoidance behavior, especially during veteran holidays, avoidance of war movies, and angry outbursts. After 9 months of evaluation, Craig was diagnosed with PTSD, major depression, traumatic brain injury, and attention-deficit disorder. He is currently receiving 65% disability pay and outpatient treatment.

SOMATIC SYMPTOM AND RELATED DISORDERS

Somatic symptom and related disorders include the following: (1) somatic symptom disorder, (2) illness anxiety disorder, (3) conversion disorder, and (4) factitious disorder. The major characteristic of somatic symptom and related disorders is that patients have physical symptoms for which there is *no known organic cause or physiologic mechanism*. All of these disorders share a common feature: distressing somatic symptoms associated with abnormal thoughts, feelings, and behaviors in response to these symptoms. Individuals with somatic symptoms are usually encountered in primary acute and other medical (nonpsychiatric) settings (American Psychiatric Association, 2013).

These questions must be asked: What does the process of somatization achieve for individuals? What does it achieve for the 5-year-old who is afraid of leaving his mother to go to kindergarten for the first time? He tells his mother that he is sick and has a stomachache or headache in hopes of avoiding his fears. Mom comforts him and lets him stay home for the day. This is known as primary gain and secondary gain. *Primary gain* refers to the individual's desire to relieve anxiety to feel better and more secure. *Secondary gain* refers to the attention or support the individual derives from others because of illness. These *gain* phenomena immeasurably complicate the treatment of somatic patients.

Somatic Symptom Disorder

Individuals with somatic symptom disorder (previously known as hypochondriasis) have multiple, recurrent, significant somatic symptoms with no evidence of a medical explanation. They tend to have very high levels of worry about their illness, appraising their bodily symptoms as unduly threatening and harmful. The presumption exists that the physical symptoms are connected to psychological factors or conflicts. These patients are not in control of their symptoms, which are unconscious and involuntary. Patients express conflicts through bodily symptoms (primarily pain) and complaints using the defense of somatization. They do not deal with their anxiety or feelings emotionally but displace the anxiety into bodily symptoms. These patients repeatedly see general practitioners seeking medical diagnosis and treatment even though they have been told that there is no known physiologic or organic evidence to explain their symptoms or disability. Medical interventions rarely alleviate the individual's concern. The overconcern with bodily symptoms assumes a central role in the individual's life, impairing social and occupational functioning (American Psychiatric Association, 2013).

Illness Anxiety Disorder

Individuals with illness anxiety disorder are excessively preoccupied with having or acquiring a serious undiagnosed illness (American Psychiatric Association, 2013). If somatic symptoms are present, they are typically mild in intensity. Similar to somatic symptom disorder, a medical evaluation fails to identify a serious medical condition. Such individuals feel substantial anxiety over various types of bodily discomfort (i.e., dizziness, tinnitus, belching)

◎ CARE PLAN

Name: Craig Brown   **Admission Date:** _____

DSM-5 Diagnosis: Posttraumatic stress disorder

Assessment	**Areas of strength**: Patient is intelligent, has a supportive family, and has Department of Veterans Affairs resources.
	Problems: Suicidal ideation, flashbacks, nightmares, outbursts of anger, isolation, difficulty concentrating and focusing.
Diagnoses	Potential for self-directed and other-directed violence related to suicidal ideation and anger outbursts as evidenced by suicidal statements.
	Sleep pattern disturbance related to nightmares, as evidenced by interrupted sleep, increasing irritability.
	Posttrauma response related to war experiences as evidenced by re-experiencing of traumatic events in flashbacks and nightmares.
Outcomes	**Short-term goals**
Date met: _____	Patient will agree to talk to staff if he feels suicidal or aggressive toward others.
Date met: _____	Patient will verbalize feelings of anger and sadness appropriately.
Date met: _____	Patient will share his current experiences with trusted others.
	Long-term goals
Date met: _____	Patient will attend outpatient appointments at the veterans' outreach center and attend co-occurring disorders group.
Planning and Interventions	**Nurse-patient relationship**: Assess and monitor suicidal ideations. Assist patient with identification and verbalization of feelings, especially his sadness and fear. Assist patient in describing current difficulties and experiences.
	Psychopharmacology: Paroxetine (Paxil CR) 20 mg every morning; amphetamine and dextroamphetamine (Adderall XR) 20 mg every morning.
	Milieu management: Co-occurring groups focusing on addiction and anger management, relaxation techniques, social skills, and self-compassion.
Evaluation	Patient verbalizes that he is no longer suicidal. Patient is beginning to verbalize his anger and sadness and the loss of his buddies during wartime and afterward.

---

because they believe that it means they have a serious undiagnosed disease. These individuals become alarmed on hearing about someone else becoming ill or reading a health-related news story. Regardless of medical reassurances, the anxiety is not alleviated and may even be heightened. Preoccupation with an undiagnosed illness results in the individual researching the suspected disease excessively and making it the prominent topic in social interactions among family and friends.

Conversion Disorder (Functional Neurologic Symptom Disorder)

The major feature of conversion disorder is a deficit or alteration in voluntary motor or sensory function that mimics a neurologic or medical condition (American Psychiatric Association, 2013). Conversion disorder is typically associated with psychological or physical stress or trauma. Individuals with this disorder have spontaneous attacks of severe physical disability despite a lack of medical evidence. Motor symptoms that most commonly occur include paralysis, tremors, gait abnormalities, and abnormal limb posturing. Frequent sensory symptoms include altered or absent skin sensation, blindness, or inability to hear. Psychogenic or nonepileptic seizures characterized by

impaired consciousness and generalized limb shaking may occur. Other symptoms may include dysphonia or aphonia (reduced or absent speech volume), dysarthria (altered articulation), globus (lump in the throat), and diplopia. Dissociative symptoms such as depersonalization, derealization, and amnesia may occur during attacks. Symptoms may be transient or persistent. Individuals also may have an attitude of *la belle indifference*, meaning that they express little concern or anxiety about their distressing symptoms. This lack of concern might make it seem that individuals with conversion disorder minimize their illness.

Factitious Disorder

Factitious disorder is characterized by the falsification of medical or psychological signs and symptoms *in oneself or others*. These individuals impose harm on themselves or others by misrepresenting, exaggerating, fabricating, inducing, simulating, or causing signs or symptoms of illness or injury in the absence of obvious external rewards. Behavioral examples of factitious disorder that can lead to excessive medical intervention include adding blood to urine, ingesting warfarin or injecting insulin, and injecting fecal material to produce an abscess or induce sepsis (American Psychiatric Association, 2013).

PUTTING IT ALL TOGETHER

PSYCHOTHERAPEUTIC MANAGEMENT

Nurse-Patient Relationship

The focus of the nurse-patient relationship is to improve patients' overall level of functioning. Patients with somatoform disorders are often unable to identify and express their feelings, needs, and conflicts. The first step is to allow patients to verbalize their feelings in a safe and supportive therapeutic environment.

Patients require time to understand their need for physical symptoms. Awareness and insight slowly develop as patients begin to verbalize their needs. Some patients take longer to develop this awareness and insight. The nurse must convey empathy and reassurance while teaching patients about the connection between emotions and physical symptoms once they become open to such discussions.

The physician or psychiatrist orders tests, a physical examination, and a laboratory workup to assess patients thoroughly for the presence of any physiologic or organic disease or etiology (if this has not been done before). The absence of any relevant medical findings strongly suggests that a somatoform disorder is present, especially if stress and conflicts are present in the patient's life.

The box titled "Key Nursing Interventions for Somatic Disorders" lists nursing interventions used for patients with somatoform disorders.

Psychopharmacology

Antidepressants are the most commonly used medications for somatic disorders. SSRIs, SNRIs, and TCAs are helpful for treating anxiety and depression because of the high incidence of comorbidity of these disorders. In addition, antipsychotics and herbal medication are commonly used. Caution: Patients may be hypersensitive to the side effects of medications owing to the nature of their illness. They may misinterpret the side effects of medications as a symptom of the illness and symptoms of the illness as a side effect of medications (Somashekar et al., 2013).

Milieu Management

CBT and psychodynamic therapy have been found to be effective in the treatment of somatic disorders. These approaches are focused on identifying and expressing emotional issues and connecting them with the patients' physical symptoms (Sharma & Manjula, 2013). In the presence of severe and disabling symptoms, a multidisciplinary approach is essential to keep the focus on self-efficacy rather than medical treatments. An empathetic professional attitude, reflective communication, information, and a cautious, restrained approach to diagnosis are necessary (Roenneberg, Sattel, Schaefert, Henningsen, & Hausteiner-Wiehle, 2019).

Because patients with somatoform disorders are usually over-users of medical care, some hospitals and clinics provide group interventions as part of the medical care. These groups focus on underlying psychosocial needs, not physical needs. When successful, this type of treatment approach can result in decreasing hospital costs while also providing more appropriate patient care. Family therapy is helpful when family conflict is present.

KEY NURSING INTERVENTIONS
For Somatic Disorders

1. Use a sympathetic, professional, and caring approach in communicating with patients. *Rationale:* To decrease secondary gains.
2. Ask patients how they are feeling, and ask them to describe their feelings. *Rationale:* To increase verbalization about feelings (especially negative ones), needs, and anxiety rather than about somatization.
3. Help patients to better understand their feelings and needs. *Rationale:* To help integrate the patient's inner and outer experiences.
4. Use positive reinforcement and set limits when patients focus on physical complaints or make unreasonable demands. *Rationale:* To decrease complaining behavior.
5. Be consistent with patients, and have all requests directed to the primary nurse providing care. *Rationale:* To provide consistency in care.
6. Use diversion by including patients in milieu activities and recreational games. *Rationale:* To decrease rumination about physical complaints.
7. Do not push awareness of or insight into conflicts or problems. *Rationale:* To prevent an increase in anxiety and the need for physical symptoms.

DISSOCIATIVE DISORDERS

Dissociative disorders are characterized by a disruption in consciousness, memory, identity, emotion, perception, body representation, motor control, and behavior (American Psychiatric Association, 2013). The major features of dissociative disorders are depersonalization, derealization, amnesia, numbing, and flashbacks. These disorders are frequently exhibited in the aftermath of trauma and include (1) dissociative amnesia, (2) depersonalization/derealization disorder, and (3) dissociative identity disorder (DID). Dissociative disorders are closely related to trauma and stressor-related disorders. Both PTSD and ASD contain dissociative symptoms (i.e., amnesia, flashbacks, depersonalization).

Dissociation—which is the removal from conscious awareness of painful feelings, memories, thoughts, or aspects of identity—is an unconscious defense mechanism that protects an individual from the emotional pain of experiences or conflicts that have been repressed. This splitting off (removal) helps these individuals to endure and survive intense emotional events or physical pain. Traumatic events such as war, rape, or childhood sexual abuse are closely linked with dissociative episodes.

Dissociative Amnesia

Dissociative amnesia is characterized by the inability to recall important personal information, usually of a traumatic nature (not normal forgetting). The amnesia may be localized, selective, or generalized. Localized amnesia occurs when the

CASE STUDY

William Robinson, 62 years old, started attending a community outpatient day program on June 15 at 9 a.m. He walked into the nurse's office limping, supported by his wife, Harriet. He stated to the nurse that he was experiencing horrible pain in his left leg and foot. Anger and irritability were evident in his voice. During the assessment, Mr. Robinson explained that the pain started suddenly about 7 months earlier. Since that time, he saw numerous physicians to obtain treatment and relief of his pain. The last physician told him that his pain was caused by stress and referred him to a therapist trained to manage somatic-related disorders. The patient stated that he hoped this therapist would know what to do because none of the other health care professionals did.

Mrs. Robinson brought her husband's medications to the day program. The nurse found that a number of analgesics had been prescribed, along with a sleeping medication. Mr. Robinson said that he took what he wanted when he wanted, and it was better than not taking anything at all.

Mrs. Robinson told the nurse that Mr. Robinson needed a lot of help with everything. She had been so physically tired that she had to call their only daughter, Sheila, for assistance. Sheila lives 400 miles away, and they had not seen her for 3 years. Sheila was so concerned about her parents that, a month ago, she had come to help and stayed for 2 weeks.

As the conversation continued, Mrs. Robinson told the nurse that her husband had been in good health except for an occasional cold until about 7 months ago, when he suddenly started to complain about awful pain in his leg and foot. He had never in all his years working for a cabinetmaker experienced anything like this before. Mrs. Robinson did not know why all this pain was occurring now, especially because her husband had retired 9 months earlier. He had been forced to retire early because the company he worked for had not been doing well, and all employees aged 60 and older were ordered to retire. She stated that her husband had never said much about it, and she thought that now they would have time to travel and go on fishing trips, which her husband had always enjoyed. They had gone on many fishing trips as a family while their daughter was growing up and had enjoyed them immensely. Periodically, her husband went fishing with some friends. Since the onset of her husband's pain, however, they had not done anything socially, together, or with friends.

From the time he started the day program, Mr. Robinson refused to do anything but sit in a lounge chair in the community room. He needed much assistance from staff members to walk to the restroom.

Interactions with the nurse centered on his pain and on requests for pain medication. He described his pain in detail and would talk of little else. He requested a wheelchair while at the day program so that he could maneuver around the facility with greater ease. Mr. Robinson was receiving an analgesic for pain and an antidepressant as ordered by his physician.

◎ CARE PLAN

Name: William Robinson   **Admission Date:** _____

DSM-5 Diagnosis: Somatic symptom disorder

Assessment	**Areas of strength**: Patient enjoyed fishing and traveling; had been in good health. Patient's wife is very supportive. Patient had worked for many years.
	Problems: Experiencing pain in his left leg and foot; social functioning has declined; focus with staff is on his pain; secondary gains maintain his sick role.
Diagnoses	Ineffective coping related to anger, as evidenced by complaints of physical pain.
	Chronic pain related to loss of job, as evidenced by inability to verbalize feelings.
	Severe anxiety related to dependency, as evidenced by inability to care for self.
Outcomes	**Short-term goals**
Date met: _____	Patient will verbalize feelings and needs.
Date met: _____	Patient will verbalize underlying anger resulting from early retirement.
Date met: _____	Patient will verbalize awareness about connecting emotions with physical symptoms.
Date met: _____	Patient will develop adaptive coping behaviors.
	Long-term goals
Date met: _____	Patient will assume responsibility for self-care and independent functioning.
Date met: _____	Patient will schedule appointments for joint counseling with his wife.
Date met: _____	Patient will identify plans to socialize with his friends.
Date met: _____	Patient will plan leisure activities.
Planning and Interventions	**Nurse-patient relationship**: Convey interest and support; focus on helping the patient to verbalize feelings and needs related to anxiety, loss, and anger; give positive feedback when the patient focuses on issues other than pain; normalize need for medication; provide psychoeducation on depression.
	Psychopharmacology: Decrease the use of analgesics. Paroxetine (Paxil CR) 20 mg every morning.
	Milieu management: Encourage participation in recreational activities; in sharing his emotions and concerns in an appropriate manner; problem-solving, discharge planning, and social skills groups; diversional occupational therapy.
Evaluation	Patient's focus on pain is decreasing, and he is able to assume self-care activities with little assistance.
Referrals	Appointments for outpatient group therapy and counseling with his wife.

Individual cannot remember what occurred during a specific period of time (e.g., not being able to remember what happened for hours after a bad car accident). The ability to recall only a specific aspect of an event is called *selective amnesia.* Generalized amnesia, a complete loss of memory related to one's life history, is rare; it is seen primarily among combat veterans and sexual assault victims (American Psychiatric Association, 2013). Individuals with generalized amnesia are sometimes found by the police wandering aimlessly while also confused and disoriented. They might be taken to a hospital and be frightened and perplexed.

Depersonalization/Derealization Disorder

Depersonalization/derealization disorder is characterized by persistent or recurrent episodes of depersonalization, derealization, or both in response to overwhelming stress. The essential feature of depersonalization is a feeling of unreality or detachment from oneself. Individuals feel as if they were watching themselves from outside their bodies, an "out of body experience" (American Psychiatric Association, 2013). In addition, such individuals may be detached from their emotions, feeling numb. Bodily sensations are altered (e.g., feeling robotic or lacking control of speech and movement).

Derealization is characterized by a feeling of detachment or unfamiliarity with one's surroundings. Individuals experience perceptual distortions such as blurriness, an altered distance of objects, heightened acuity, or muted sounds. For example, buildings might appear to be leaning, or everything might seem gray and dull. Some individuals report feeling as if they were in a fog, dream, or bubble.

Dissociative Identity Disorder

DID is characterized by (1) the existence of two or more distinct identities or personality states and (2) recurrent episodes of amnesia (American Psychiatric Association, 2013). Alternative personalities ("alters") typically manifest as if another person had taken control, such that the individual begins speaking or acting in a distinctly different way. For example, an alter may seem to be a child, a teenager, or someone of the opposite gender. Alters have distinctive attitudes, emotions, and behaviors. Each personality is different from the others and from the original personality. Each alter has its own name, behavioral traits, memories, emotional characteristics, and social relations. The primary identity might carry the person's name and be depressed, dependent, and guilty, whereas the alternative personalities might be hostile, controlling, and self-destructive. The person may be aware of alters to varying degrees or completely unaware. Such patients can experience memory problems, depersonalization, time loss, voices conversing with each other, somatic symptoms, and suicidality (Bell et al., 2015).

Similar to the other dissociative disorders, DID is a defense against extreme anxiety that is aroused in highly painful and emotionally traumatic situations and is seen most frequently in childhood sexual abuse. DID occurs when a child is so full of pain caused by the trauma that she can no longer integrate the painful experience (Bell et al., 2015). The splitting off of these painful events allows the young person to survive the trauma but leaves an impaired personality with disconnected parts. The alternative personalities have feelings and behaviors associated with the trauma. Dissociated states represent fragments of the person's sense of identity, with different identity states remembering distinct information (Weber, 2007). These states help the person to survive the emotional memories. A shy, quiet woman might have alternative personalities that are promiscuous, flamboyant, childlike, and aggressive. A woman might awaken one morning and find the living room of her apartment littered with toys or strewn with empty alcohol bottles and leftover food. She does not remember what happened because she has amnesia for the span of time when another personality took over or came out. Dissociative fugue is common, where the individual reports that she suddenly found herself at the beach, at work, or in a nightclub with no memory of how she got there.

These patients are admitted to inpatient psychiatric units when they are suicidal or experience hallucinations. Individuals with DID suffer from a variety of psychiatric disorders such as major depression, anxiety disorders, PTSD, relational problems, substance use disorders, borderline personality disorder, and eating disorders (Fox et al., 2013). The array of symptoms that these individuals experience is overwhelming. The safe structure of a hospital setting provides emotional safety and security for the patient when he or she is working with difficult or overwhelming issues.

DID may be described in some cultures as a possession experience. Possession-form identities typically manifest as a "spirit" that has taken control of the individual. For example, the "ghost" of a girl who died years before possesses the individual and speaks and acts as though she were still alive. In some cases, the individual may be "taken over" by a demon or deity, demanding that a relative be punished for a past act. These identities present recurrently, are unwanted and involuntary, and cause significant distress. (Note: Most possession states around the world are normal spiritual practices and do not meet the criteria for DID.)

PUTTING IT ALL TOGETHER

PSYCHOTHERAPEUTIC MANAGEMENT

Nurse-Patient Relationship

The nurse's relationship with individuals experiencing dissociation and amnesia includes interventions to establish trust and support. Patients have physiologic and neurologic workups to rule out organic causes. The nurse assists with gathering data regarding feelings, conflicts, or situations that patients experienced before the dissociative or amnesia state. Patients also might have sessions under hypnosis to gather data about forgotten material. The nurse should slowly help patients deal with anxiety and conflicts in their lives and improve coping skills.

Patients with depersonalization/derealization disorder are not usually found in an inpatient setting unless they have become suicidal, extremely anxious, or depressed. Nurses might work with these patients in outpatient settings.

The treatment goal of DID, ultimately through long-term therapy, occurs in three phases: (1) stabilization and affect regulation, (2) trauma processing, and (3) the promotion of daily functioning. Integration of the personalities or memories occurs by looking at each alter, what memories it has, and what experiences it had. DID survivors are encouraged to strengthen self-awareness through reflection on intrapersonal and interpersonal interactions (Fox et al., 2013). DID patients report that therapy is an emotionally difficult experience that is beneficial to learn grounding techniques and anxiety management (Zeligman et al., 2017). Improving the patients' capacity for emotion regulation is foundational for their recovery. Increased capacity for emotional regulation enables DID patients to tolerate painful emotions, thereby reducing their need to dissociate and compartmentalize into altered states (Brand et al., 2019).

The nurse caring for these patients provides empathy to establish trust because the relationships of these patients with authority figures might have been inconsistent, rigid, and unpredictable. A contract should be initiated for patients' safety to reduce potential self-harm and suicidal behaviors. DID survivors typically respond well to clear nurse-patient boundaries and a structured environment. Compassionate care should include empathy, validation, and acceptance (Jacobson et al., 2015). Management of feelings in a positive, predictable, supportive environment increases trust and promotes healing.

Psychopharmacology

Medication does not eliminate the dissociative disorder itself. If symptoms of anxiety and depression are present, medications may help. For patients with DID, response to medication might be partial; however, each alter's response to medication might be different or inconsistent.

Milieu Management

The nurse assumes an important role in the care of patients who are hospitalized in an inpatient psychiatric unit because of suicidal or recurrent attempts to harm themselves. Provisions for a safe environment and a trusting relationship are basic for helping these patients, who usually have not had trusting relationships with anyone. Assisting with group sessions; providing emotional security, empathy, acceptance, and support; and helping patients cope with daily living all are involved in nursing care.

DID patients have reported significant healing from attending support groups with other DID survivors who understand their experience (Jacobson et al., 2015). Long-term individual therapy with a DID-experienced counselor should be initiated if it is not already occurring. Art therapy is a novel, nonverbal approach that may help patients integrate their emotional nonverbal brain related to childhood abuse and their rational verbal brain related to the adult self as they engage in a journey of self-reflection and even discovery (Sagan, 2019).

Dialectical behavior therapy is a well-known approach utilized when working with DID patients that helps them manage the emotional reactions surrounding issues of childhood physical or sexual abuse. Important therapeutic interventions include working through trauma-based feelings and impulses, skills to regulate affect and promote impulse control, education about the disorder, and adaptive coping strategies (Jacobson et al., 2015). In addition, relaxation, stress management, meditation, and exercise are beneficial.

Before discharge, a safety plan and no-harm contract might be necessary, as well as initiating or continuing a support system for the patient.

❓ CRITICAL THINKING QUESTION

3. A patient with DID is admitted to the inpatient unit because of a suicide attempt. One of the personalities wants to kill the patient, meaning that the patient is suicidal. The patient refuses to sign a no-harm contract. What issues would you expect to help the patient with, including safety precautions?

HIGHLIGHTING THE EVIDENCE

Evidence

Sexual abuse is a strong risk factor in the development of DID. However, not all children who are abused develop psychopathology. New research indicates that the development of DID is best predicted by disorganized attachment and the absence of familial and social support in combination with abuse. Healthy early attachment and solid social support systems contribute to the victim's resiliency and ability to remain psychologically healthy.

Summary

Providing support for children at risk can result in psychological resiliency. Offering social support structures such as mentorship for children in schools is a way of providing role models and support outside the family. Interventions for at-risk expectant mothers and new parents with enduring problems such as substance abuse can promote secure attachment with their child. The child may then be more resilient in the face of trauma.

Modified from Korol, S. (2008). Familial and social support as protective factors against the development of dissociative identity disorder. *Journal of Trauma & Dissociation, 9,* 249.

NEXT-GENERATION NCLEX® EXAMINATION-STYLE CASE STUDY

Scenario: A 50-year-old patient was brought into the emergency department by their spouse after experiencing chest pain early in the evening. The client expressed in a shaky voice, "I'm having a heart attack!", reporting chest pain, shortness of breath, and diaphoresis. An ECG and laboratory values, including a bedside troponin, were normal. While awaiting a consultation with a nurse from the mental health crisis team, the patient begins pacing, is unable to follow basic instructions, and exhibits shallow, rapid breathing, repeatedly asking, "What's happening to me?" It is determined that the patient is likely experiencing a panic attack, and the nurse begins to implement actions to help manage the patient's anxiety level.

Item Type: Multiple Response: Select All That Apply
What action would the nurse take at this time? Select all that apply.

1. Notify the primary care provider of the patient's current emotional state
2. Reassure that other staff will respond if the nurse is out of the room
3. Demonstrate calm behavior when working with the patient
4. Use simple, concise language when providing directions
5. Teach the patient to use relaxing breathing techniques
6. Monitor for signs of suicidal-associated behaviors
7. Utilize therapeutic touch to provide comfort
8. Provide the patient with a safe place to pace
9. Administer PRN anxiolytics as prescribed
10. Provide assurance that the episode will pass

▌ STUDY NOTES

1. Understanding the process of anxiety is key to understanding and intervening therapeutically with patients who have anxiety-related disorders.

2. The patient's anxiety must be reduced to a mild or moderate level before the nurse can work with her or him on problem-solving and adaptive coping.

3. In the category of anxiety-related, obsessive-compulsive, trauma- and stressor-related, somatic, and dissociative disorders, patients feel or directly express symptoms of anxiety.

4. With PTSD, ASD, and adjustment disorder, the goals are to integrate traumatic memories and feelings about the original trauma and to move from victim to survivor status.

5. With somatic-related disorders, anxiety is expressed through physical symptoms.

6. In DID, traumatic experiences are split off (removed) from conscious awareness, which helps patients survive extreme emotional or physical pain.

7. Key nursing interventions include helping patients to process feelings, anxiety, conflicts, and life stressors in an adaptive manner so that they can become independent functioning adults.

REFERENCES

Aardema, F., Wong, S., Audet, J., Melli, G., & Baraby, L. (2019). Reduced fear-of-self is associated with improvement in concerns related to repugnant obsessions in obsessive-compulsive disorders. *British of Clinical Psychology*, 58(3), 327–341. https://doi.org/10.1111/bjc.12214.

Aliev, G., Beeraka, N., Nikolenko, V., Svistunov, A., Rozhnova, T., Svetlana, K., ... & Kirkland, C. (2020). Neurophysiology and psychopathology underlying PTSD and recent insights into the PTSD therapies-A comprehensive review. *Journal of Clinical Medicine*, 9(9). https://doi.org/10.3390/jcm9092951.

American Psychiatric Association. (2013). *Diagnostic and statistical manual of mental disorders* (5th ed.). APA.

Ardic, U., Ercan, E., Kutlu, A., Yuce, D., Ipci, M., & Inci, S. (2017). Successful treatment response with aripiprazole augmentation of SSRIs in refractory obsessive-compulsive disorder in childhood. *Child Psychiatry and Human Development*, 48(5), 699–704. https://doi.org/10.1007/s10578-016-0694-8.

Bell, H., Jacobson, L., Zeligman, M., Fox, J., & Hundley, G. (2015). The role of religious coping and resilience in individuals with dissociative identity disorder. *Counseling and Values*, 60(2), 151–163. https://doi.org/10.1002/cvj.12011.

Bisson, J., Berliner, L., Cloitre, M., Forbes, D., Jensen, T., Lewis, C., ... & Shapiro, F. (2019). The international society for traumatic stress studies new guidelines for the prevention and treatment of posttraumatic stress disorder: Methodology and development process. *Journal of Traumatic Stress*, 32(4), 475–483. https://doi.org/10.1002/jts.22421.

Blow, A. J., Curtis, A. F., Wittenborn, A. K., & Gorman, L. (2015). Relationship problems and military related PTSD: The case for using emotionally focused therapy for couples. *Contemporary Family Therapy: An International Journal*, 37(3), 261–270. https://doi.org/10.1007/s10591-015-9345-7.

Brand, B., Schielke, H., Putnam, K., Putnam, F., Loewenstein, R., Myrick, A., ... Lanius, R. (2019). An online educational program for individuals with dissociative disorder and their clinicians: 1-year and 2-year follow up. *Journal of Traumatic Stress*, 32(1), 156–166. https://doi.org/10.1002/jts.22370.

Butts, C., & Gutierrez, D. (2018). Using acceptance and commitment therapy to (re)conceptualize stress appraisal. *Journal of Mental Health Counseling*, 40(2), 95–112. https://doi.org/10.17744/mehc.40.2.01.

Cackovic, C., Nazir, S., & Marwaha, R. (2020 Nov 29). Panic Disorder Updated. *StatPearls [Internet]*. StatPearls Publishing. https://www.ncbi.nlm.nih.gov/books/NBK430973/.

Carpenter, J., Andrews, L., Witchaft, S., Powers, M., Smits, J., & Hofmann, S. (2018). Cognitive behavioral therapy for anxiety and related disorders: A meta-analysis of randomized placebo-controlled trials. *Depression and Anxiety*, *35*(6), 502–514. https://doi.org/10.1002/da.22728.

Cloitre, M., Hyland, P., Bisson, J., Brewin, C., Roberts, N., Karatzias, T., & Shevlin, M. (2019). ICD-11 posttraumatic stress disorder and complex posttraumatic stress disorder in the United States: A population-based study. *Journal of Traumatic Stress*, *32*(6), 833–842. https://doi.org/10.1002/jts.22454.

Ebberwein, C., Hopper, M., Vedala, R., & Macaluso, M. (2020). When worry is excessive: Easing the burden of GAD. *The Journal of Family Practice*, *69*(7), 357–361. https://pubmed.ncbi.nlm.nih.gov/32936846/.

Epstein, N., Yount, R., Wilson, C., Netting, F., & Quinlan, J. (2014). Service dog training by service members/veterans: A reflection on the need for empirical evidence. *Reflections: Narratives of Professional Helping*, *20*(2), 8–16. https://reflectionsnarrativesofprofessionalhelping.org/index.php/Reflections/article/download/210/1181/.

Fairfax, H., Easey, K., Fletcher, S., & Barfield, J. (2014). Does mindfulness help in the treatment of obsessive compulsive disorder (OCD)? An audit of client experience of an OCD group. *Counselling Psychology Review*, *29*(3), 17–27. https://psycnet.apa.org/record/2014-48807-003.

Fox, J., Bell, H., Jacobson, L., & Hundley, G. (2013). Recovering identity: A qualitative investigation of a survivor of dissociative identity disorder. *Journal of Mental Health Counseling*, *35*(4), 324–341. https://doi.org/10.17744/mehc.35.4.g715qt65qm281117.

Freeman, J., Benito, K., Herren, J., Kemp, J., Sung, J., Georgia, C., … & Garcia, A. (2018). Evidence base update of psychosocial treatments for pediatric obsessive-compulsive disorders: Evaluating, improving, and transporting what works. *Journal of Clinical Child & Adolescent Psychology*, *47*(5), 669–698. https://doi.org/10.1080/15374416.2018.1496443.

Gaylord-Harden, N., Bai, G., & Simic, D. (2017). Examining a dual-process model of desensitization and hypersensitization to community violence in African American male adolescents. *Journal of Traumatic Stress*, *30*(5), 463–471. https://doi.org/10.1002/jts.22220.

Gold, P. W. (2015). The organization of the stress system and its dysregulation in depressive illness. *Molecular Psychiatry*, *20*(1), 32–47. https://doi.org/10.1038/mp.2014.163.

Gurda, K. (2015). Emerging trauma therapies: Critical analysis and discussion of three novel approaches. *Journal of Aggression, Maltreatment & Trauma*, *24*(7), 773–793. https://doi.org/10.1080/10926771.2015.1062445.

Hovland, A., Johansen, H., Sjøbø, T., Vøllestad, J., Nordhus, I. H., Pallesen, S., Havik, O. E., Martinsen, E. W., & Nordgreen, T. (2015). A feasibility study on combining Internet-based cognitive behavior therapy with physical exercise as a treatment for panic disorder–Treatment protocol and preliminary results. *Cognitive Behaviour Therapy*, *44*(4), 275–287. https://doi.org/10.1080/16506073.2015.1022596.

Jacobson, L., Fox, J., Bell, H., Zeligman, M., & Graham, J. (2015). Survivors with dissociative identity disorder: Perspectives on the counseling process. *Journal of Mental Health Counseling*, *37*(4), 308–322. https://doi.org/10.17744/mehc.37.4.03.

Jamieson, J., Crum, A., Goyer, J., Morotta, M., & Akinola, M. (2018). Optimizing stress responses with reappraisal and mindset interventions: An integrated model. *Anxiety, Stress & Coping*, *31*(3), 245–261. https://doi.org/10.1080/10615806.2018.1442615.

Jurin, T., & Biglbauer, S. (2018). Anxiety sensitivity as a predictor of panic disorder symptoms: A prospective 3-year study. *Anxiety, Stress, & Coping*, *31*(4), 365–374. https://doi.org/10.1080/10615806.2018.1453745.

Kealy, D., Goodman, G., & Ogrodniczuk, S. (2017). Psychotherapists' ideals in the treatment of panic disorder: An exploratory study. *Counselling and Psychotherapy Research*, *17*(3), 201–208. https://doi.org/10.1002/capr.12125.

Keltner, N. L., Perry, B. A., & Williams, A. R. (2003). Panic disorder: A tightening vortex of misery. *Perspectives in Psychiatric Care*, *39*(1), 41. https://doi.org/10.1111/j.1744-6163.2003.tb00673.x.

Kennedy, D. (2018). What if I…? *Therapy Today*, *29*(10), 24–28.

Kessler, R. C., Petukhova, M., & Wittchen, H. (2012). Twelve-month and lifetime prevalence and lifetime morbid risk of anxiety and mood disorders in the United States. *International Journal of Methods in Psychiatric Research*, *21*(3), 169. https://doi.org/10.1002/mpr.1359.

Keyes, C., Nolte, L., & Williams, T. (2018). The battle of living with obsessive compulsive disorder: A qualitative study of young people's experiences. *Child and Adolescent Mental Health*, *23*(3), 177–184. https://doi.org/10.1111/camh.12216.

Khalsa, M. K., Greiner-Ferris, J. M., Hofmann, S. G., & Khalsa, S. B. (2015). Yoga-enhanced cognitive behavioral therapy (Y-CBT) for anxiety management: A pilot study. *Clinical Psychology & Psychotherapy*, *22*(4), 364–371. https://doi.org/10.1002/cpp.1902.

Korol, S. (2008). Familial and social support as protective factors against the development of dissociative identity disorder. *Journal of Trauma & Dissociation*, *9*(2), 249. https://doi.org/10.1080/15299730802048744.

Krediet, E., Bostoen, T., Breeksema, J., & Schagen, A. (2020). Reviewing the potential of psychodelics for the treatment of PTSD. *International Journal of Neuropsychopharmacology*, *23*(6), 385–400. https://doi.org/10.1093/ijnp/pyaa018.

Lang, A., Malaktaris, A., Casman, P., Baca, S., Golshan, S., Harrison, T., & Negi, L. (2019). Compassion meditation for posttraumatic stress disorder in veterans: A randomized proof of concept study. *Journal of Traumatic Stress*, *32*(2), 299–309. https://doi.org/10.1002/jts.22397.

Lazarus, R. S. (1966). *Psychological stress and the coping process*. McGraw-Hill.

Lazarus, R. S. (2006). Emotions and interpersonal relationships: Toward a person-centered conceptualization of emotions and coping. *Journal of Personality*, *74*(1), 9. https://doi.org/10.1111/j.1467-6494.2005.00368.x.

Lazarus, R. S., & Folkman, S. (1984). *Stress, appraisal, and coping*. Springer Publishing Company.

Lee, C., Furnham, A., & Merritt, C. (2017). Effects of directness of exposure and trauma type on mental health literacy of PTSD. *Journal of Mental Health*, *26*(3), 257–263. https://doi.org/10.1080/09638237.2016.1276531.

Lijffijt, M., Green, C. E., Balderston, N., Iqbal, T., Atkinson, M., Vo-Le, B., … & Mathew, S. J. (2019). A proof-of-mechanism study to test effects of the NMDA receptor antagonist lanicemine on behavioral sensitization in individuals with symptoms of PTSD. *Frontiers in Psychiatry*, *10*, 846. https://doi.org/10.3389/fpsyt.2019.00846.

Lipinska, G., Baldwin, D. S., & Thomas, K. G. (2016). Pharmacology for sleep disturbances in PTSD. *Human*

Psychopharmacology, Clinical and Experimental, 31(2), 156–163. https://doi.org/10.1002/hup.2522.

Liu, Y., Sareen, J., Bolton, J., & Wang, J. (2015). Development and validation of the risk-prediction algorithm for the recurrence of panic disorder. *Depression and Anxiety, 32*(5), 341–348. https://doi.org/10.1002/da.22359.

Metcalf, O., Varker, T., Forbes, D., Phelps, A., Dell, L., DiBattista, A., … & O'Donnell, M. (2016). Efficacy of fifteen emerging interventions for the treatment of posttraumatic stress disorder: A systematic review. *Journal of Traumatic Stress, 29*(1), 88–92. https://doi.org/10.1002/jts.22070.

Modirrousta, M., Shams, E., Katz, C., Mansouri, B., Moussavi, Z., Sareen, J., & Enns, M. (2015). The efficacy of deep repetitive transcranial magnetic stimulation over the medial prefrontal cortex in obsessive compulsive disorder: Results from an open-label study. *Depression and Anxiety, 32*(6), 445–450. https://doi.org/10.1002/da.22363.

Munir, S., & Takov, V. (2020 Nov 19). Generalized Anxiety Disorder Updated. *StatPearls [Internet].* StatPearls Publishing. https://www.ncbi.nlm.nih.gov/books/NBK441870/.

Murray, H. (2018). Survivor guilt in a posttraumatic stress disorder clinic sample. *Journal of Loss and Trauma, 23*(7), 600–607. https://doi.org/10.1080/15325024.2018.1507965.

Norton, A., & Abbott, M. (2017). The role of environmental factors in the aetiology of social anxiety disorder: A review of the theoretical and empirical literature. *Behaviour Change, 34*(2), 76–97. https://doi.org/10.1017/bec.2017.7.

Oar, E. L., Farrell, L. J., & Ollendick, T. H. (2015). One session treatment for specific phobias: An adaptation for paediatric blood-injection-injury phobia in youth. *Clinical Child and Family Psychology Review, 18*, 340–394. https://doi.org/10.1007/s10567-015-0189-3.

Ogawa, S., Kondo, M., Ino, K., Imai, R., Ii, T., Furukawa, T., & Akechi, T. (2018). Predictors of broad dimensions of psychopathology among patients with panic disorder after cognitive-behavioral therapy. *Hindawi Psychiatry Journal*, 1–6. https://doi.org/10.1155/2018/5183834.

Perreault, M., Julien, D., White, N. D., Bélanger, C., Marchand, A., Katerelos, T., & Milton, D. (2014). Treatment modality preferences and adherence to group treatment for panic disorder with agoraphobia. *Psychiatric Quarterly, 85*, 121–132. https://doi.org/10.1007/s11126-013-9275-1.

Perrone, J., Vickers, M., & Wilkes, L. (2013). Facing adversity: Authentic stories of living and working with panic attacks. *Employee Responsibilities and Rights, 25*, 257–275. https://doi.org/10.1007/s10672-013-9222-1.

Raymond, C., Marin, M., Juster, R., & Lupien, S. (2019). Should we suppress or reappraise our stress? The moderating role of reappraisal on cortisol reactivity and recovery in healthy adults. *Anxiety, Stress, & Coping, 32*(3), 286–297. https://doi.org/10.1080/10615806.2019.1596676.

Roenneberg, C., Sattel, H., Schaefert, R., Henningsen, P., & Hausteiner-Wiehle, C. (2019). Functional somatic symptoms. *Deutsches Ärzteblatt International, 116*(33-34), 553–560. https://doi.org/10.3238/arztebl.2019.0553.

Rosen, R., Cikesh, B., Fang, S., Trachtenberg, F., Seal, K., Magnavita, A., … Keane, T. (2019). Posttraumatic stress disorder severity and insomnia-related sleep disturbances: Longitudinal associations in a large, gender-balanced cohort of combat-exposed veterans. *Journal of Traumatic Stress, 32*(6), 936–945. https://doi.org/10.1002/jts.22462.

Sagan, O. (2019). Art-making and its interface with dissociative identity disorder: No words that didn't fit. *Journal of Creativity in Mental Health, 14*(1), 23–36. https://doi.org/10.1080/15401383.2018.1499062.

Schneier, F. R., Campeas, R., Carcamo, J., Glass, A., Lewis-Fernandez, R., Neria, Y., … & Wall, M. M. (2015). Combined mirtazapine and SSRI treatment of PTSD: A placebo-controlled trial. *Depression and Anxiety, 32*(8), 570–579. https://doi.org/10.1002/da.22384.

Selye, H. (1956). *The stress of life.* McGraw-Hill.

Shahar, B., Bar-Kalifa, E., & Hen-Weissberg, A. (2015). Shame during social interactions predicts subsequent generalized anxiety symptoms: A daily-diary study. *Journal of Social and Clinical Psychology, 34*(10), 827–837. https://doi.org/10.1521/jscp.2015.34.10.827.

Shapiro, F. (2013). The case: Treating Jared through eye movement desensitization and reprocessing therapy. *Journal of Clinical Psychology, 69*(5), 494–496. https://doi.org/10.1002/jclp.21986.

Sharma, M. P., & Manjula, M. (2013). Behavioral and psychological management of somatic symptoms disorder: An overview. *International Review of Psychiatry, 25*(1), 116–124. https://doi.org/10.3109/09540261.2012.746649.

Sherman, C. (2019). The quest to cure PTSD. *Psychology Today, Nov/Dec*, 62–91. https://www.psychologytoday.com/us/articles/201910/the-quest-cure-ptsd.

Shim, D., Lee, D., & Park, T. (2016). Familial, social, and cultural factors influencing panic disorder: Family therapy case of Korean wife and American husband. *The American Journal of Family Therapy, 44*(3), 129–142. https://doi.org/10.1080/01926187.2016.1145085.

Somashekar, B., Jainer, A., & Wuntakal, B. (2013). Psychopharmacotherapy of somatic symptom disorder. *International Review of Psychiatry, 25*(1), 107–115. https://doi.org/10.3109/09540261.2012.729758.

Stech, E., & Grisham, J. (2017). Modifying obsessive-compulsive beliefs about controlling one's thoughts. *Journal of Psychopathology and Behavioral Assessment, 39*, 534–545. https://doi.org/10.1007/s10862-017-9603-0.

Stech, E., Lim, J., Upton, E., & Newby, J. (2020). Internet-delivered cognitive behavioral therapy for panic disorder with or without agoraphobia: A systematic review & meta-analysis. *Cognitive Behaviour Therapy, 49*(4), 270–293. https://doi.org/10.1080/16506073.2019.1628808.

Substance Abuse and Mental Health Services Administration. (n.d.). Results from the 2010 national survey on drug use and health: Summary of national findings. https://www.samhsa.gov/data/sites/default/files/NSDUHNationalFindingsResults2010-web/2k10ResultsRev/NSDUHresultsRev2010.pdf.

van der Kolk, B. A. (2017). *The evolution of trauma treatment.* Jan/Feb: Psychotherapy Networker.

Vasey, M., Chriki, L., & Toh, G. (2017). Cognitive control and anxious arousal in worry and generalized anxiety: An initial test of an integrative model. *Cognitive Therapy Research, 41*(2), 155–169. https://doi.org/10.1007/s10608-016-9809-6.

Weber, S. (2007). Dissociative symptom disorders in advanced nursing practice: Background, treatment, and instrumentation to assess symptoms. *Issues in Mental Health Nursing, 28*(9), 997. https://doi.org/10.1080/01612840701522085.

Whitworth, J., Nosrat, S., SantaBarbara, N., & Ciccolo, J. (2019). Feasibility of resistance exercise for posttraumatic stress and anxiety symptoms: A randomized controlled pilot study. *Journal of Traumatic Stress, 32*(6), 977–984. https://doi.org/10.1002/jts.22464.

Wilson, T. K., & Tripp, J. (2020 Sep 13). Buspirone Updated. *StatPearls [Internet]*. StatPearls Publishing. https://www.ncbi.nlm.nih.gov/books/NBK531477/.

Yaribeygi, H., Panahi, H., Sahraei, H., Johnston, T., & Sahebkar, A. (2017). The impact of stress on body function: A review. *EXCLI Journal, 16*, 1057–1072. https://doi.org/10.17179/excli2017-480.

Zeligman, M., Greene, J., Hundley, G., Graham, J., Spann, S., Bickley, E., & Bloom, Z. (2017). Lived experiences of men with dissociative identity disorder. *Adultspan Journal, 16*(2), 65–79. https://doi.org/10.1002/adsp.12036.

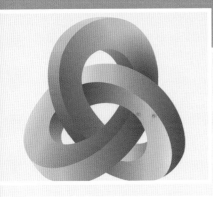

28

Neurocognitive Disorders

Debbie Steele

http://evolve.elsevier.com/Keltner

LEARNING OBJECTIVES

- Describe the biologic and functional changes associated with the most prevalent types of dementia
- Describe the etiologic aspects and behaviors associated with delirium
- Recognize the criteria and terminology for neurocognitive disorders as presented in the *Diagnostic and Statistical Manual of Mental Disorders*, 5th edition (*DSM-5*)
- Differentiate dementia from delirium
- Discuss appropriate pharmacologic interventions for patients with dementia
- Develop a care plan for a patient with dementia
- Develop effective caregiver interventions
- Discuss family issues related to neurocognitive disorders

Neurocognitive disorders are characterized by a deterioration of cognitive functions such as memory and learning. Loss of these fundamental abilities is a common thread in neurocognitive disorders. However, in some cases, these losses may be temporary. This chapter describes the most common neurocognitive disorders that the psychiatric nurse may encounter.

The most common impairments involve memory, orientation, attention, decision making, emotions, language, and motor skills. The sudden or gradual loss of these abilities is a scary experience. Everyday skills, such as identifying common objects or remembering the names of family members, become difficult. Individuals will often use phrases such as "that thing" and "you know what I mean." These individuals may get lost while driving, become unable to do their own banking and shopping, and tend to lose their cell phones. The addition of delusions, hallucinations, and misidentification are particularly frightening.

Neurocognitive disorders are divided into potentially reversible and irreversible types. These disorders can span a few hours (delirium) or many years (dementia). To cloud the diagnostic picture, patients may have more than one cognitive disorder or a coexisting psychiatric illness. For example, elderly hospitalized patients with dementia may develop a superimposed delirium state.

Patients who exhibit a marked change of mental status need to be assessed for a neurocognitive disorder. The *Diagnostic and Statistical Manual of Mental Disorders*, 5th edition (*DSM-5*) (American Psychiatric Association, 2013) provides diagnostic criteria for the following disorders: (1) dementia, (2) major neurocognitive disorder, and (3) mild neurocognitive disorder.

NORM'S NOTES This chapter is so important. There are more and more of us older people, and we are the ones who tend to develop the cognitive disorders discussed in this chapter. Think about it. When you can no longer reason clearly and rationally, the "real" you has been taken. As a kid, I used to wonder if I would rather lose an arm or a leg. Well, kids think about silly stuff. But I know now that I do not want to lose my cognitive functions. Fortunately, our government (run by a bunch of older people) spends a lot of money studying how these conditions can be stopped or reversed. I just want the researchers to hurry.

In dementia research, dozens of diagnostic tools are used, ranging from pen-and-pencil examinations to sophisticated neuroimaging studies. Genetic studies have isolated chromosomes and genes that are related to certain diseases. Since 1993, six different medications to treat Alzheimer disease have reached the market.

DELIRIUM

Delirium is a clinical syndrome characterized by acute fluctuations in attention, cognition, and awareness. The word *delirium* literally means "out of one's furrow," which refers to the dramatic behavioral changes that the person may experience. Some have called delirium "brain failure" because it may represent a variety of causes: a medical condition, medication, substance intoxication or withdrawal, exposure to a toxin, or multiple etiologies (American Psychiatric Association, 2013). The hallmark sign of delirium is its acute onset, which is key because the disorder develops rapidly in most cases. Other signs include a fluctuating level of consciousness, slurred speech, disorientation, and confusion. There are three types of delirium: hyperactive, hypoactive, and mixed. Hyperactive patients are restless and agitated; they may have visual hallucinations and delusions. Such a patient may be able to follow a conversation for a short period, followed by an acute bout of confusion and restlessness. With emotions on edge, the patient may startle easily and become combative. Hypoactive delirium is oftentimes not diagnosed because it mimics symptoms of depression, characterized by lethargy, fatigue, quickly falling back to sleep, and stupor. The patient appears drowsy and sedated, responding slowly to questions, and moving very little. Patients with mixed subtypes have symptoms of both hyperactive and hypoactive delirium. Studies on subtypes of delirium differ on which type is more common; however, hypoactive symptoms are less likely to be documented by health care professionals (FitzGerald, 2018; Lahariya, Grover, Bagga, & Sharma, 2016).

Delirium is a medical emergency that is reversible once the cause is identified. Assessment and treatment of any underlying physical problem or illness should be addressed immediately when delirium symptoms manifest in a patient. The nurse must assess and initiate interventions on patients who are confused, disoriented, and often resistant so as to ensure their safety and provide the best nursing care for them (Phillips, 2013). Safety measures to prevent delirium or shorten its course include making sure the patient is well hydrated, has access to eyeglasses and hearing aids, early ambulation, adequate sleep, and is socially engaged by hospital staff and loved ones (Wallis, 2020). Kolanowski (2018) reported that older adults with dementia are at greatest risk for delirium, with 89% experiencing delirium when hospitalized. "ICU psychosis" is another name for hospital-based delirium. Acute changes in the patient's mental status may be a sign that a serious underlying medical illness exists. Delirium is associated with many physical illnesses, especially pneumonia, myocardial infarction, and urinary tract infection. Toxic response to medications occurs with prescribed and over-the-counter (OTC) medications. For example, drugs with anticholinergic properties can cause delirium, such as diphenhydramine (Benadryl), some tricyclic antidepressants, and benztropine (Cogentin). Other drugs, including lithium and divalproex, may become toxic at lower serum levels than the laboratory reference range indicates. Polypharmacy (four or more medications), allergies, dehydration, electrolyte imbalance, and bowel and bladder function are all associated with the development of delirium (Phillips, 2013). During the initial medication assessment, the nurse should ask the patient or family member about prescription *and* OTC medications. The nurse should ask specifically about cough syrup; dietary supplements; and medications for allergies, pain, and sedation.

Table 28.1 compares dementia and delirium. Delirium is challenging to recognize. Mental health carers may attribute confusion to normal aging or dementia and consequently not respond to it as a medical emergency. Misdiagnosed or unrecognized, delirium leads to delays in medical treatment, increased risk of adverse outcomes, further cognitive decline, and increased morbidity and mortality (Kolanowski, 2018).

Clinical Example: Patient With Delirium

Mrs. Edwards, 64 years old, was found crawling around her bedroom. She thought her husband was plotting to kill her. She found his pistol, took it, and was waiting to shoot him when her daughter found her. At that time, she was taking diphenhydramine in three OTC preparations: a cough syrup, an allergy capsule, and a pill to aid sleep. Discontinuation of these medications resulted in a return to the patient's premorbid level of cognitive function. She did not require any further psychiatric care.

Family members who witness delirium in their elderly loved one may experience distressing negative emotions due to their limited understanding of this phenomenon. Nurses can assist family members by addressing their need for psycho-education and providing appropriate emotional support (Martins et al., 2018).

Clinical Example: Patient With Mild Neurocognitive Disorder

Mrs. Peacock, 72 years old, retired from working as the head librarian in the public library. During her career, she coordinated many regional conferences. Now her daughter sometimes has to remind her to take her medication. She recognizes that she is having memory problems, but she is still able to live independently.

DEMENTIA

The word *dementia*, from the Latin, literally means "out of one's mind." Dementia is commonly understood as a slow deterioration of cognitive abilities that affect learning and memory, complex attention, perception, language, behavior, affect, and motor movements. Dementia is the customary term for major neurocognitive disorders that usually affect older adults. The term neurocognitive disorder is oftentimes preferred for cognitive impairments that affect younger individuals, such as traumatic brain injury (TBI) or HIV infection (American Psychiatric Association, 2013). The common denominator for these disorders is the progressive loss of function in multiple domains.

> **❓ CRITICAL THINKING QUESTIONS**
>
> 1. Why is it important to recognize the difference between dementia and delirium?
> 2. Explain why petting a service dog at a senior center may be therapeutic for a patient with dementia.

Memory loss represents one of the most feared, if not the most feared, aspects of growing older (Higgs & Gilleard, 2017). At the present time, no cure is available for most of the neurocognitive disorders discussed in this section, but medications

TABLE 28.1 Comparison of Dementia and Delirium

Characteristics	Delirium	Dementia
Onset	Occurs quickly, is obvious	Slow, unnoticeable at first
Course	Acute: rapid development, usually hours to days, but can last for months	Chronic: slow development over months and years, with a progressive deterioration spanning 3–10 years until death
Causes	Usually the result of other physical problems (e.g., illness, postsurgical complications, toxins)	Usually the primary disorder, but may be related to other illnesses (e.g., AIDS)
Memory	Short-term memory is impaired when assessed during an interim lucid or clear moment	Short-term memory is lost initially; long-term memory fails slowly
Level of consciousness	Fluctuating level of consciousness; alert at times; sleep is erratic; no pattern	No change; sleep patterns are usually consistent; day-night reversal is common
Thought content	Matches level of consciousness	Normal at first; later may be difficult to assess because of confusion or expressive or receptive aphasia and poverty of content
Thought process	Logical alternating with illogical, depending on the level of consciousness	Logical at first, then loss of abstraction (e.g., understanding a joke); concrete thinking occurs as disease progresses
Speech	May have slurred speech	Normal speech
Perceptual differences	Hallucinations—*visual:* seeing animals or unusual colors; picking at the air; *tactile:* feeling bugs on or under skin	Misidentification: calling one relative another's name—for example, calling a daughter "mama"; hallucinations may occur in the later stage, usually not initially
Mood	Anxiety and fear	Wide range of feelings
Affect	Appears bewildered, frightened	Appearance matches feeling

have been developed, with U.S. Food and Drug Administration (FDA) indications for these diseases. The course of a progressive decline may be slowed and it may even plateau, but ultimately brain disease continues. Alzheimer disease is the most prevalent neurocognitive disorder, comprising 60% to 80% of all patients diagnosed with dementia. Cerebrovascular disease is the second most prevalent neurocognitive disorder. The remaining types of neurocognitive disorders include frontotemporal lobar degeneration (e.g., Pick disease), dementia with Lewy bodies (DLB), Parkinson disease, human immunodeficiency virus (HIV), Huntington disease, traumatic brain injury, and Prion disease (Alzheimer's Association, 2020).

All of the dementia diagnoses are categorized as mild or major neurocognitive disorders. Mild neurocognitive disorder is characterized by a mild to modest cognitive decline (forgetfulness) that does not interfere with activities of daily living (ADLs), such as paying bills and managing medications. Major neurocognitive disorder is characterized by a substantial and significant decline in cognitive function that interferes with independence in everyday activities, requiring assistance with ADLs (American Psychiatric Association, 2013). The criteria for major neurocognitive disorder with specifiers are provided in the box titled "*DSM-5 Criteria for Major Neurocognitive Disorders.*"

DSM-5 CRITERIA

For Major Neurocognitive Disorders

Major Neurocognitive Disorder

A. Evidence of significant cognitive decline from a previous level of performance in one or more cognitive domains (complex attention, executive function, learning and memory, language, perceptual-motor, or social cognition) based on:
   1. Concern of the individual, a knowledgeable informant, or the clinician that there has been a significant decline in cognitive function
   2. A substantial impairment in cognitive performance, preferably documented by standardized neuropsychological testing or—in its absence—another quantified clinical assessment

B. The cognitive deficits interfere with independence in everyday activities (i.e., at a minimum, requiring assistance with complex instrumental ADLs such as paying bills or managing medications).

C. The cognitive deficits do not occur exclusively in the context of a delirium.

D. The cognitive deficits are not better explained by another mental disorder (e.g., major depressive disorder, schizophrenia).
   Specify whether due to:
- Alzheimer disease
- Frontotemporal lobar degeneration
- Dementia with Lewy bodies
- Vascular disease
- Traumatic brain injury
- Substance/medication use
- Human immunodeficiency virus (HIV) infection
- Prion disease
- Parkinson disease
- Huntington disease
- Another medical condition
- Multiple etiologies
- Unspecified

From American Psychiatric Association. (2013). *Diagnostic and statistical manual of mental disorders* (5th ed., pp. 602–603). APA.

Neurocognitive Disorder Due to Alzheimer Disease

Alzheimer disease (AD) is the most common cause of dementia characterized by prevalent memory loss and other cognitive impairment. Mild Neurocognitive Disorder Due to Alzheimer's Disease is the *DSM-5* diagnosis that represents the early stage of AD. Once individuals are no longer able to manage their ADL independently, the appropriate diagnosis is Major Neurocognitive Disorder Due to Alzheimer's Disease. Typically, ADL such as driving and handling finances and medication are affected earlier in the disease than more basic activities such as dressing, toileting, or feeding (Ryd, Nygard, Malinowsky, Ohman, & Kottorp, 2017).

AD affects 5.8 million persons in the United States. The percentage of patients diagnosed with Alzheimer increases with age: 3% of people age 65 to 74, 17% of people age 75 to 84, and 32% of people age 85 and older. Almost two-thirds of Americans with Alzheimer and other neurocognitive disorders are women. The prevailing reason is that women live longer than men on average, and older age is the greatest risk factor for AD. (Alzheimer's, 2020). Alois Alzheimer, a German neurologist, first described a patient with this disease in 1907. He identified the plaques and tangles that are now considered pathognomonic (hallmark signs) for Alzheimer disease. However, the disease did not attract much attention for many years. For example, *Introduction to Psychiatry*, a psychiatric nursing text published in 1948, included only three sentences about Alzheimer disease. None of the other aforementioned dementias were referred to (Biddle & van Sickel, 1948).

According to the Alzheimer's Association (2020), people age 65 and older survive an average of 4 to 8 years after receiving an Alzheimer diagnosis, yet some live with the disease as long as 20 years. In addition, current research is focused on identifying biological changes that precede the onset of cognitive symptoms by as much as 20 years (Milne et al., 2018). This reflects the insidious onset and gradual progression of AD. A person who lives from age 70 to age 80 with Alzheimer will spend an average of 40% of this time in a nursing home during the advanced stage. Alzheimer disease is the sixth leading cause of death in the United States for people 65 years and older (Alzheimer's Association, 2020).

The diagnosis of Alzheimer's Disease should be done by specialists—such as neurologists, neuropsychologists, geriatricians, and geriatric psychiatrists—who assess the patient's medical history, mental status exams, physical and neurological exams, diagnostic tests, and brain imaging (Alzheimer's Association, 2020). AD may be diagnosed by evidence of: (1) a causative genetic mutation from family history or (2) genetic testing. Banner Alzheimer's Institute (2017) recommends the following assessment protocol to accompany cognitive screening: (1) test for thyroid or nutritional deficiencies; (2) magnetic resonance imaging (MRI) and computed tomography (CT) scan to rule out stroke, tumor, or hydrocephalus; and (3) spinal tap or positron emission tomography (PET) scan if needed. Apolipoprotein E (APOE) genotyping is recommended to determine whether the disease is familial. To receive a diagnosis, there must be clear evidence of a decline in memory and learning, as well as a steady, progressive, and gradual decline in cognition (American Psychiatric Association, 2013). There appears to be significant public interest in learning information about one's likelihood of developing Alzheimer's disease, particularly among those with a family history of dementia. The perceived value of attaining this risk information can be used to inform later-life decisions and plan future care (Milne et al., 2018).

Stages of Alzheimer Disease

Alzheimer disease is typically divided into three stages: mild, moderate, and severe. The Mini-Mental State Examination (MMSE) is the most commonly used screening tool for assessing cognitive decline associated with dementia. The MMSE is known to be easy to administer within a short period of time and has high sensitivity and specificity for the detection of cognitive impairment, with sufficient test-retest reliability. The Revised Hasegawa's Dementia Scale (HDS-R) consists of nine simple questions without any performance tasks involved and is useful for patients with impaired visual and motor function (Jeon et al., 2019). The Montreal Cognitive Assessment (MOCA) is also useful in the assessment of Alzheimer disease. This assessment includes the following directions: (1) draw a clock (10 minutes past 11 o'clock); (2) copy a cube; (3) name a picture of a lion, hippopotamus, camel; (4) read a list of words, repeat immediately and after 5 minutes; (5) read a list of digits, letters; (6) subtract 7 starting at 100; (7) identify the similarities between: banana-orange, train-bicycle, watch-ruler; and (8) tell the current date, month, year, day, place, city. The clock-drawing exercise is particularly revealing, as the patient's pictures clearly demonstrate a progressive decline in functioning.

An understanding of the Global Deterioration Scale (GDS) can assist nurses in a quick assessment of patients' level of cognitive function. It is broken down into seven different stages. Stages 1 to 3 are the pre-dementia stages. Stages 4 to 7 are the dementia stages. Beginning in stage 5, patients will require outside assistance. Nurses observe patients' behavioral characteristics and compare them to the GDS to determine patients' level of disease process. Nurses and caregivers can plan appropriate interventions when they make an accurate assessment of a patient's capabilities. The following summary (Bellenir, 2008) was based on the original article titled "The Global Deterioration Scale (GDS)."

Stage 1: No cognitive decline
   Experiences no problems in daily living
Stage 2: Very mild cognitive decline
   Forgets names and locations of objects
   May have trouble finding words
Stage 3: Mild cognitive decline
   Has difficulty traveling to new locations
   Has difficulty handling problems at work

Stage 4: Moderate cognitive decline
   Has difficulty with complex tasks (finances, shopping,
      planning for guests)
Stage 5: Moderately severe cognitive decline
   Needs help to choose clothing
   Needs prompting to bathe
Stage 6: Severe cognitive decline
   Needs help putting on clothing
   Requires assistance bathing; may have a fear of bathing
   Has decreased ability to use the toilet or is incontinent
Stage 7: Very severe cognitive decline
   Vocabulary becomes limited, eventually no or only single
      words are spoken
   Loses ability to walk and sit
   Becomes unable to smile

 CRITICAL THINKING QUESTION

3. How do you explain the difference between dementia and
   Alzheimer disease?

Causes of Alzheimer Disease

Alzheimer disease most likely has multiple etiologies.
Despite decades of research, Alzheimer disease has a complex etiopathogenesis, which presents a major obstacle to the development of effective treatments and prevention strategies. Historically, the main pathological changes observed in brain tissue are amyloid and tau proteins, forming the toxic plaques and neurofibrillary tangles associated with AD. The presence of toxic beta-amyloid and tau proteins are believed to activate immune system cells in the brain, in particular, microglia. Microglia engulfs and destroys toxic cells in the brain. The National Institute on Aging, (2020) reports that chronic inflammation may be caused by the buildup of these glial cells. Normal brain function is also compromised in AD by decreases in the brain's ability to metabolize glucose, its main fuel (Alzheimer's, 2020). Tobore (2019) highlighted that oxidative stress and mitochondria dysfunction are also involved in the pathogenesis and pathophysiology of AD. There is a great deal of interest in the relationship between neurodegenerative disorders such as AD and vascular and metabolic conditions including heart disease, stroke, high blood pressure, diabetes, and obesity. There is also a substantial body of research focused on the association between affective distress/disorders (depression and anxiety) and increased dementia risk (Stewart, 2019). More and more, researchers are suggesting that AD involves a broad variety of etiologies and could be associated with many other disorders (Ferrari et al., 2017).

Neuronal loss. Although the brain typically shrinks to some degree in healthy aging, with AD the shrinkage is significant as a result of neuronal demise. A hallmark sign of AD is the atrophied brain. A normal adult brain weighs approximately 3 lb. The brain of a person with advanced AD may weigh less than half that amount. Neuronal damage and the loss of neuronal connections occur initially in the entorhinal cortex and hippocampus — the parts of the brain involving memory. Later, the cerebral cortex, which is responsible for language, reasoning, and social behavior, is affected. As the atrophy progresses throughout the entire brain, the ability to live and function independently is progressively lost (National Institute on Aging, 2020). Examples of the brain's atrophic changes are shown in Figs. 28.1 through 28.4. The more the brain shrinks, the larger the ventricles become.

The loss of the cholinergic neurons that produce the neurotransmitter acetylcholine has been strongly implicated in AD—so much so that the first class of medications developed specifically for this disease targets this deficiency. The cholinergic system forms the basis of memory acquisition, but that is not all. Many other cognitive aspects are affected as well, such as processing new information and making complex decisions. The ability to understand abstract thought may slowly fade away.

Neurofibrillary tangles. Neurofibrillary tangles are abnormal accumulations of tau proteins that collect inside neurons. The microtubules within neurons help guide nutrients and molecules from the cell body to the axon and dendrites. Tau normally binds to and stabilizes microtubules, helping them work properly. In a brain with Alzheimer disease, extra tau protein gathers, causing the microtubules to collapse. The tau protein fibrils (segments), now separated from the microtubules, start twisting. These twists, known as *neurofibrillary tangles*, block the neuron's transport system, which impedes the synaptic connections between neurons (National Institute on Aging, 2020).

β-Amyloid plaques. The beta-amyloid protein is formed from the breakdown of a larger protein, called amyloid precursor protein (APP). APP is partly inside and partly outside the neuron, "like a toothpick stuck in an orange." As the APP moves outside the cell through the semipermeable membrane, the protein is "sniped" or "cleaved" by enzymes known collectively as *secretases*. Some of the resulting APP pieces are shorter and clump together to form β-amyloid peptide. Several of the β-amyloid peptides (up to a dozen) form oligomers. In the Alzheimer's brain, abnormal levels of these beta-amyloid plaques collect between neurons and disrupt cell function (National Institute on Aging, 2020).

Genetics. A genetic predisposition exists for the development of Alzheimer disease; this is especially true for late-onset AD, with a 60% to 80% risk factor (Casey, 2012). The genetic components of AD are described subsequently.

Alzheimer disease—early onset or young onset. Early-onset AD typically has an autosomal dominant inheritance pattern. These patients are diagnosed in their 30s to mid-60s and have a faster course than patients who develop AD at an older age. The following single-gene mutations have been identified for individuals with early-onset AD:

- Presenilin 2 (PSEN2) on chromosome 1
- Presenilin 1 (PSEN1) on chromosome 14
- Amyloid precursor protein (APP) on chromosome 21

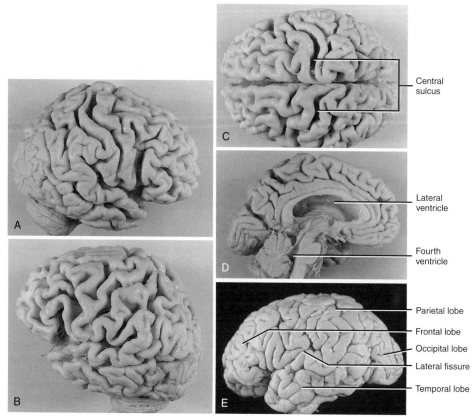

FIG. 28.1 (A) Right side of the brain of a patient with Alzheimer disease. Narrow gyri and larger sulci are shown. (B) Left side of the same brain demonstrates even narrower gyri and larger sulci. (C) Superior view. The central sulcus is very wide. (D) Midsagittal view of the left hemisphere. The greatly enlarged lateral and fourth ventricles are demonstrated. (E) Normal brain. (A–D, Photographs by Berto Tarin, Western University of Health Science. E, Courtesy Dr. Richard E. Powers, University of Alabama at Birmingham Brain Resource Program.)

Mutations in these genes play a role in the breakdown of APP; a part of the process that generates harmful forms of amyloid plaques associated with AD. If only one parent has only one of these abnormal chromosomes, offspring have a 50% chance of developing early-onset AD. Although genetic testing for APOE or other genetic variants is done on family members, it cannot predict the disease with 100% accuracy (National Institute on Aging, 2020).

Clinical Example: Lifting the Curse of Alzheimer

The article discusses families near Medellín, Colombia, who carry a rare genetic mutation called the Paisa mutation, which causes early-onset Alzheimer disease. Familial Alzheimer, as this form of the disease is called, is disturbingly common among 26 extended families and present in more than 20% of the 5000-plus family members. A carrier will most likely get the disease before age 50. Neurologist Francisco Lopera and others are currently conducting a clinical trial of the drug crenezumab (a monoclonal antibody targeting beta amyloid) in Medellín with the families affected by the Paisa mutation to determine the effect of early treatment prior to the presentation of dementia symptoms.

Stir, G. (2015). Lifting the curse of Alzheimer's. *Scientific American, 312*(5), 50–57.

Alzheimer disease—late onset. Researchers have not found a specific gene that directly causes the late onset of AD. However, having a genetic variant of the APOE gene on chromosome 19 is known to increase a person's risk. The APOE gene on chromosome 19 has been linked to the development of β-amyloid plaque seen in AD. The more β-amyloid plaque deposited in the brain, the greater the impairment is thought to be. If one or both parents provide the Apo ε4 gene, the recipient is not only more likely to develop AD but also more likely to develop the disease at an earlier age than an individual without the allele. However, a person who does not inherit the gene for Apo ε4 may also develop the disease (National Institute on Aging, 2020).

Hormones. Research in the area of studying levels of sex hormones and cognitive decline is ongoing (Burke et al., 2019). Is there a correlation between the natural decrease of sex steroid with age and deteriorating cognition? The administration of transdermal estradiol or conjugated estrogen has not demonstrated a statistically significant ability to stop or slow cognitive decline in women.

Nontraditional findings. The traditional roots of AD development have been discussed, but the cause of AD is not without controversy. The *Nun Study*, a longitudinal research study that explored topics related to normal aging and AD, generated new questions. More than 30 years ago, 678 nuns

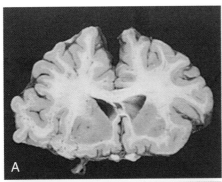

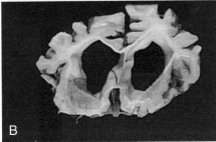

FIG. 28.2 (A) Normal brain. The sulci and gyri are not atrophied. (B) Brain shows the effects of Alzheimer disease. Widened sulci and narrowed gyri are demonstrated. In addition, the lateral ventricles are increased in size because of the decrease in brain mass associated with Alzheimer disease. (Courtesy Dr. Richard E. Powers, University of Alabama at Birmingham Brain Resource Program.)

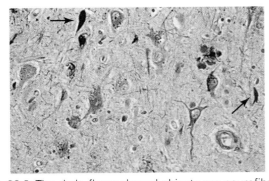

FIG. 28.3 The dark, flame-shaped objects are neurofibrillary tangles—or dead neurons *(arrows)*. Tangles are twisted fibrils inside the neuron that disrupt cellular processes and eventually kill the cell. (Courtesy Dr. Richard E. Powers, University of Alabama at Birmingham Brain Resource Program.)

from the Order of the School Sisters of Notre Dame agreed to undergo physical and mental assessments annually. In addition, each nun volunteered to have her brain autopsied. The sisters of this order had been teachers while they lived. Their contributions would be a great source of future knowledge about AD (Snowdon, 2001). Hundreds of professional articles have been published using this unique data set.

The Nun Study had some unexpected findings. One sister who lived to be more than 100 years old showed no signs of cognitive decline, although her brain autopsy showed an abundance of both plaque and tangle formations. Another

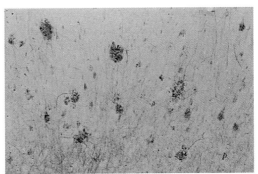

FIG. 28.4 The darker objects are plaques, one of two microscopic findings in Alzheimer disease (the other finding is the tangles; see Fig. 28.3). Plaques can be found in about 50% of individuals older than 70 years; it is the quantity of plaques in relation to the person's age that is significant. (Courtesy Dr. Richard E. Powers, University of Alabama at Birmingham Brain Resource Program.)

nun, who died in her 70s, had profound dementia yet had few tangles and plaques. The Nun Study researchers explored reasons for these unusual findings and concluded that the degree of resistance or cognitive reserve has some effect on the clinical manifestations of AD. Complex use of language and advanced education were two background issues that were isolated in the nuns who had the highest cognitive ability. Also, nuns with a more positive lifetime attitude were found to be in the highest cognitive group (Snowdon, 2001).

Classic Behaviors

Memory loss is most noticeable initially. Impairment of short-term memory usually occurs first. The patient and family may think that this loss is minor because the long-term memory remains intact at first. Long-term memory loss generally follows. Sometimes the patient has a developmental regression. When a female patient confuses her son for her deceased husband, she is most likely remembering the era when her spouse was her son's age. As the regression continues, the patient may think that her children are of school age. Finally, the cries for "Mama" reflect complete memory deterioration and come at the final stages of this disease.

Word-finding difficulty is the easiest problem for the nurse to assess because the nurse likely would be unable to discern short-term memory losses at first. Only people who were with the patient would know what was served for breakfast. The patient often describes an object rather than names it— "the thing you tell time with" for a watch or "hitting the ball over the fence" for a home run. Describing rather than identifying is a common form of aphasia. The two types of aphasia, expressive and receptive, refer to these communication barriers. *Expressive aphasia* means difficulty expressing oneself, as exemplified by problems with word finding. *Receptive aphasia* means that the patient has difficulty understanding what is being said. It is common to have both types of aphasia, which complicates communicating with the patient.

Difficulty concentrating may be subtle at first. Trouble understanding a conversation, comprehending the plot in a book, or following a television program are frequent problems. As the disease progresses, the patient usually no longer finds interest in previous pleasurable activities. The lack of mental stimulation further contributes to cognitive decline. Box 28.1 outlines what is referred to as the "four 'A's of Alzheimer's disease."

One unusual symptom associated with AD is *misinterpreting the environment*. Patients often have visual hallucinations of dead relatives. One patient was found to be routinely preparing meals for visiting family members, all of whom were deceased. Auditory hallucinations may accompany the visual hallucinations—for example, the perceived deceased relative is *speaking* to the patient. Olfactory, tactile, and gustatory hallucinations are the least common types of hallucinations.

Delusions are common. These are misconceptions that have no basis in reality and are often accusatory. Delusions held by patients with AD are very different from those held by patients with psychoses related to chronic mental illnesses (e.g., schizophrenia). Delusions in patients with schizophrenia are typically bizarre and often frightening. Patients with AD have delusions that are based on reality and are not usually fantastical. Common delusions of patients with AD may include the following:

- Thinking that a deceased relative is alive (perhaps the most common)
- Pathologic jealousy about the spouse having an extramarital affair
- Stealing something odd, such as the mortgage papers out of a safe while leaving money in it

The nurse would have to find out if any of these ideas were factual; whether the patient's 85-year-old wife is going out on the town, or the patient's mother is still alive.

Illusions are almost universal and represent a worsening of the disease. An illusion is a misinterpretation of something that really exists. Thinking one's image in a mirror is an intruder or trying to give ice cream to a doll means that the patient really *sees* something other than a self-reflection or an inanimate object.

Somatic preoccupations blended with aphasia produce complaints that may not make sense. Patients may say "my stomach hurts" regardless of the question. Frequent somatic complaints often result in diagnostic testing without clear-cut results.

Misidentification is an example of calling a family member or a friend by another person's name. Family members are often devastated when the patient cannot remember their names. The nurse can educate the family about misidentification and provide emotional support to them as appropriate.

Sundowning is a period of restlessness, agitation, irritability, or confusion that can begin or worsen as daylight begins to fade. The term sundowning describes when this behavior classically occurs but it can continue into the night, making it hard for these patients to fall asleep and stay in bed. As a result, they may have trouble getting enough sleep and may take frequent naps during the day. No definitive cause has been found for sundowning. The causes of sundowning are not well understood. One possibility is that Alzheimer-related brain changes can affect a person's "biological clock," leading to confused sleep-wake cycles and resulting in agitation and other sundowning behaviors (National Institute on Aging, 2020).

Loss of the ability to care for oneself is difficult for all parties. Over time, the patient forgets how to attend to personal

---

BOX 28.1 The Four "A"s of Alzheimer Disease[a] and Adaptive Actions

Agnosia

Impaired ability to recognize or identify familiar objects and people in the absence of a visual or hearing impairment.

- Assess and adapt for visual impairment.
- Do not expect the patient to remember you; introduce yourself.
- Cover mirrors or pictures if they cause distress.
- Name objects and demonstrate their use.
- Keep area free of ingestible hazards (toiletries, chemical cleaning supplies, checkers, buttons, unmonitored medicine).

Aphasia

Language disturbances are exhibited in both expressing and understanding spoken words. Expressive aphasia is the inability to express thoughts in words; receptive aphasia is the inability to understand what is said.

- Assess and adapt for hearing loss.
- Observe and use gestures, tone, and facial expressions.
- Provide help with word finding.
- Restate your understanding of behaviors and word fragments.
- Acknowledge feelings expressed verbally and nonverbally.
- Use simple words and phrases; be concise and organized.

- Allow time for response.
- Listen carefully and encourage with nonverbal praise.
- Use pictures, symbols, and signs.

Amnesia

Inability to learn new information or to recall previously learned information.

- Do not expect the patient to remember you; introduce yourself.
- Do not test the patient's memory unnecessarily.
- Operate in the here and now.
- Provide orientation cues.
- Remember, *you* must adapt when the patient cannot change.
- Compensate for a patient's lost judgment or reasoning.

Apraxia

Inability to carry out motor activities despite intact motor function.

- Assess and adapt for motor weakness and swallowing difficulties.
- Simplify tasks; give step-by-step instructions and time for response.
- Initiate motion for patient with gentle guidance or touch.

[a] May also be present in other cognitive disorders.

care. Incontinence of bowel and bladder and wandering can become unmanageable behaviors. When the behavioral and functional decline reaches this point, the patient usually requires 24-hour care. Incontinence and wandering often mean that the patient can no longer be cared for in the home.

Drugs for Alzheimer Disease

Only six medications have FDA approval for AD. Acetylcholine deficiency is the neurotransmitter problem most often implicated in the disease. The first drug approved for AD targeting acetylcholine deficiency was released over 25 years ago. Tacrine (Cognex) was the first in a class of medications called cholinesterase or acetylcholinesterase (AChE) inhibitors. Donepezil (Aricept), rivastigmine (Exelon), and galantamine (Razadyne, formerly known as Reminyl [name changed in 2005]) followed. All four have FDA indications for mild to moderate AD. These medications in effect boost the level of acetylcholine by preventing its metabolic breakdown. Although these drugs increase the amount of available synaptic acetylcholine, the disease itself continues to progress. In other words, if two patients with equal neurodegeneration were followed clinically for 1 year, one receiving an AChE inhibitor (e.g., donepezil) and one not receiving any medication, they would have approximately equal brain pathology. The patient taking donepezil may function better during the year, but the underlying disease process would continue in both patients. There is much research to be done before treatment of AD is adequate.

Memantine (Namenda) is an agent approved for moderate to severe AD; it is the only approved medication for AD that is not an AChE inhibitor. Memantine works by blocking abnormal signaling by glutamate at the N-methyl-D-aspartate receptor. This blocking effect antagonizes an overactive glutaminergic system, which is believed to be involved in the neurotoxicity seen in AD. This action moderates the symptoms of Alzheimer disease (Lyseng-Williamson & McKeage, 2013). Memantine can be used alone or with an AChE inhibitor.

In 2014, Namzaric, the newest drug approved for AD, came on the market. It is the first and only once-a-day treatment that works in two ways in the brain to help fight the symptoms of moderate to severe AD. It is the first treatment that combines memantine and donepezil. It is indicated for the treatment of moderate to severe dementia. The once-a-day extended-release capsules should be swallowed whole or opened and sprinkled on applesauce, given at bedtime. The patient should start Namzaric extended release only once he or she is stabilized on 10 mg of donepezil daily (Namzaric Prescribing, 2020).

Note to students: In this chapter, we do not make a distinction between AChE and butyrylcholinesterase. We refer to all cholinesterase inhibitors as AChE inhibitors. See Chapter 18 for more detailed information.

All six of the AD medications may be effective, although to caregivers, improvements can be subtle. Prescribers usually start with an AChE inhibitor. Tacrine is rarely used now because of the potential for severe hepatotoxic side effects. Donepezil, rivastigmine, or galantamine is usually started first. Each of these has FDA approval for mild to moderate AD. In addition, donepezil has an indication for severe AD. Convenience in giving medications is always important, but it is particularly so with these patients (Table 28.2).

Patient and family education about these medications poses a perplexing situation. Most medications are prescribed to produce improvements, but there is no evidence that they prevent or slow the underlying disease process in patients with AD (Namzaric Prescribing, 2020). Although the disease continues to progress, AChE inhibitors increase the amount of acetylcholine in the areas of the brain most affected, which may mask the deterioration caused by the disease. For a patient with AD, staying the same (and not regressing) can theoretically be seen as an improvement. However, the illness continues to take its toll on the cholinergic system. The AChE inhibitors have been artificially boosting the acetylcholine in the brain. Stopping the medications can cause a precipitous drop in the patient's cognitive status.

Memantine, by working on glutamate, affects a different neurotransmitter system. Typically it works on behavioral and functional aspects of the disease rather than cognition. Families may want to stop these medications for a variety of reasons. Some cannot accept the idea that the patient is not getting better. Some do not want to delay the inevitable.

TABLE 28.2 Antidementia Drugs

Drug	Typical Daily Dosage	Half-Life (hours)	Protein Binding (%)	Cytochrome P-450 Enzymes	Mechanism of Action
Donepezil (Aricept)	5–10 mg at bedtime	~ 70	~ 95	2D6, 3A4	Cholinesterase inhibitor
Rivastigmine (Exelon)	6–12 mg in two divided doses	~ 2	~ 40	Not metabolized	Cholinesterase inhibitor
Galantamine (Razadyne)	8–12 mg twice a day	~ 6	Insignificant	2D6	Cholinesterase inhibitor
Memantine (Namenda)	20 mg in two divided doses	~ 60–80	~ 45	Not extensively metabolized	NMDA antagonist
Memantine and Donepezil (Namzaric)	28 mg/10 mg at bedtime				NMDA antagonist Cholinesterase inhibitor

NMDA, N-methyl-D-aspartate.

Expense is another consideration for many families. These drugs are expensive. Some pharmaceutical companies have initiated cost-saving programs, including medication samples, vouchers for free medications, and patient-assistance programs.

 CRITICAL THINKING QUESTION

4. How do you explain that patients taking an AChE inhibitor (e.g., donepezil, rivastigmine, or galantamine) may stay the same over a period of 6 months?
Should patients take AChE inhibitors for the rest of their lives?

Clinical Example: Patient With Mild Neurocognitive Disorder Due to Alzheimer Disease

Mrs. Jackson, 72 years old, has had difficulty recalling the names of people in her church for many years. Now, she is having difficulty understanding jokes because she has a diminished ability for abstract thinking. Mrs. Jackson has a type of expressive aphasia called *word-finding difficulty*. She described the choir as "those people who sing at church." Recently, she had a kitchen fire after she turned on her oven, not realizing that she had put her purse in it the day before. Mrs. Jackson has Alzheimer disease.

Neurocognitive Disorder Due to Vascular Disease

The second most prevalent neurocognitive disorder is vascular, which occurs most frequently after age 65 years. The diagnosis of vascular dementia is determined by the presence of cerebrovascular disease, ranging from large vessel stroke to microvascular disease. The presentation of symptoms depends on the severity of the blood vessel damage and the area of the brain affected. Onset may be acute or gradual, with slow or rapid progression depending on the etiology of the vascular infarct. Symptoms of vascular dementia such as disorientation, difficulty speaking or understanding speech, and difficulty walking may have an abrupt onset when large blood vessels are damaged. When microvascular disease occurs, the decline would assume a stepwise pattern or fluctuating deterioration. Memory loss may or may not occur depending on the specific brain areas where blood flow is reduced (Alzheimer's, 2020). The length of time the patient remains at a diminished cognitive level may be days, months, or years, depending on the vascular changes.

The diagnosis of dementia is confirmed by neurocognitive testing that evaluates specific skills such as judgment, planning, problem-solving, reasoning, and memory. An MRI can confirm a recent stroke, or other vascular brain changes whose severity and pattern of affected tissue would be consistent with the degree of impairment documented in the neurocognitive exams. The major risk factors for vascular dementia are hypertension, diabetes mellitus, previous stroke, cardiac arrhythmias, coronary artery disease,

tobacco use, and alcohol or substance use. Treatment focuses on the patient's medical problems and health care issues; it is geared toward interventions designed to minimize the risk factors and subsequently reduce vascular damage to the brain.

Because improving physical health is one treatment for vascular dementia, the Alzheimer Association advocates lifestyle changes that improve overall cardiovascular health. Such changes include improved dietary habits, regular exercise, and control of blood pressure, blood glucose, and cholesterol levels (Alzheimer's Association, 2020).

 CRITICAL THINKING QUESTION

5. Which risk factors for vascular neurocognitive disorder may be modified by the patient or caregiver?

Clinical Example: Patient With Major Neurocognitive Disorder Due to Vascular Disease

Mr. Babb, 76 years old, was hospitalized for depression. During the initial interview, he had difficulty understanding why he was admitted. He did not know the day, date, month, or year; however, he was able to do serial calculations. He had been in an automobile accident a week before admission because he had pulled out into traffic without looking. Mr. Babb has hypertension and diabetes mellitus. He has had two transient ischemic attacks in the last 6 months. Mr. Babb has vascular dementia.

Neurocognitive Disorder Due to Frontotemporal Disease

Frontotemporal neurocognitive disorder is a type of dementia caused by atrophy of the frontal and anterior temporal lobes of the brain. Originally known as Pick disease, the current designation of the disease groups together Pick disease, primary progressive aphasia, and semantic dementia. Pick disease is now a subtype of frontotemporal dementia; it features Pick cells and Pick bodies in the brain. Pick cells are swollen and ballooned neurons. This disease is usually diagnosed when patients are in their 50s or early 60s. The major symptoms of frontotemporal dementia involve progressive development of either (1) changes in behavior, or (2) problems with language. The first type is characterized by dramatic behavioral changes that can be either impulsive (disinhibited) or bored and listless (apathetic). Symptoms may include inappropriate social behavior such as disrobing in public; lack of social tact such as intrusiveness; lack of empathy; easily distracted; lack of insight into the behaviors of oneself and others; hypersexuality; changes in eating habits; agitation or, conversely, blunted emotions; neglect of self care and personal responsibilities; repetitive or compulsive behavior such as hoarding, and anhedonia. The second type features symptoms of language disturbance, including difficulty speaking or understanding speech, often in conjunction with behavioral symptoms. Memory and spatial skills remain intact. Eventually loss of sphincter control occurs. Insight is usually lacking, which may delay medical consultation. There is a strong genetic component to the disease; frontotemporal dementia often runs in families. Neuroimaging (CT or MRI) may show distinct patterns of atrophy in the frontal and anterior temporal lobes. The outcome for individuals with frontotemporal lobe dementia is poor because the disease may progress rapidly, requiring either institutional or 24-hour care (National Institute of Neurological Disorders and Stroke, 2020b).

Clinical Example: Patient With Major Neurocognitive Disorder Due to Frontotemporal Disease

Ms. Brewer, 66 years old, was found nude in the foyer of her assisted-living facility. She had taken her clothes off three times in the past week. Before this occurrence, she had been quite modest. A few days later, she cursed at the housekeeper. Pick disease was diagnosed based on Ms. Brewer's behavior, her relatively good memory, and neuroimaging, which revealed both frontal and anterior temporal lobe atrophy.

Neurocognitive Disorder Due to Parkinson Disease

Parkinson disease (PD) is another devastating neurodegenerative disorder. PD is a common, yet complex movement disorder, diagnosed primarily by the presence of key motor features. PD was first described by James Parkinson in 1817. PD is more prevalent in men than in women; men are about 1.5 times more at risk for PD than women. Symptoms are associated with deterioration of dopaminergic neurons of the substantia nigra pars compacta (SNpc), resulting in loss of dopamine in the ventral mesencephalon of the extrapyramidal system. All the signs of PD are related to motor dysfunction such as a shuffling gait, resting tremors, difficulty in starting or stopping movement, rigidity, and mask-like facial expression (Khan et al., 2019). Most patients present with tremor as the dominant and persistent motor feature, whereas others may never experience tremor. Patients are also affected by a number of different nonmotor features, including cognitive impairment, sleep disturbance, depressed or anxious mood, hallucinations, delusions, and personality changes (Greenland et al., 2018). Language skills are usually maintained. In addition to memory problems, patients with PD have problems with visuospatial skills, attention, and executive functioning. PD is usually diagnosed when patients are in their 50s or 60s, although patients in their 30s, such as the actor Michael J. Fox, have been diagnosed with the disease. Levodopa is a dopamine agonist and is the traditional medication prescribed for treatment of PD. Dopamine agonists are used to treat the motor symptoms associated with PD by stimulating the dopaminergic receptors to release dopamine in the neuronal cells (Khan et al., 2019).

Clinical Example: Patient With Major Neurocognitive Disorder Due to Parkinson Disease

Mr. McGreevy, 72 years old, has had Parkinson disease for 7 years. He has a blunted affect, excessive drooling, and shuffling gait. He was hospitalized a year ago for aspiration pneumonia. Managing his parkinsonian signs was made difficult by frequent visual hallucinations caused by the dopamine component in the levodopa-carbidopa that he took. He had a prescription for an atypical antipsychotic drug to reduce the hallucinations (he and his wife had been told about the FDA "black box" warning that described the greater risk for stroke and its off-label use).

The delicate balance of prescribing a dopaminergic drug for Parkinson disease (dopamine deficiency in the nigrostriatal tract) and a dopamine-blocking antipsychotic medication (excessive dopamine in the mesolimbic tract) may be the most difficult prescribing challenge in psychiatry. The medications are seemingly at cross purposes. One is intended to boost dopamine and the other to reduce its effects. With too much dopamine, the patient may hallucinate; with too little, the patient may become stiff. Do not be surprised if a patient prefers flexibility even if it means having hallucinations. These patients usually can discern that the hallucinations are part of their illness and learn to live with them.

Neurocognitive Disorder With Lewy Bodies

DLB is second only to AD in prevalence. The cardinal features of DLB include cognitive impairment, visual hallucinations, and extrapyramidal signs. Prominent symptoms include (1) fluctuations in attention and alertness, (2) recurrent visual and auditory hallucinations, (3) features of parkinsonism, and (4) rapid-eye-movement (REM) sleep behavior disorder. These patients tend to experience repeated falls, syncope, and unexplained loss of consciousness. Depression and delusions are also common (American Psychiatric Association, 2013).

Lewy bodies are intracellular bodies found in neurons. Originally, Lewy bodies were found only in the substantia nigra and were thought to be associated only with PD. With the availability of better tissue staining methods, Lewy bodies have been found in the cortex as well. A patient can have Lewy bodies in both places, which makes diagnosis a challenge. Clinicians find it difficult to distinguish DLB from AD. DLB tends to be underdiagnosed and misdiagnosed as AD. It is imperative to differentiate the two diseases at the earliest stages because DLB patients may experience severe adverse effects if given neuroleptic drugs to manage their psychotic symptoms, such as visual hallucinations. If an atypical antipsychotic medication is used, the patient and family must be informed of the FDA-imposed black box warnings. In addition, patients with DLB seem to exhibit a faster disease progression (Bonanni et al., 2017).

Clinical Example: Patient With Major Neurocognitive Disorder Due to Lewy Body Dementia

Mr. Wade, 68 years old, started having recurrent visual hallucinations. He has fallen twice as a result of gait disturbance. He slept well at night despite sleeping off and on throughout the day. According to the family, some days he seemed like his old self, and at other times he became easily agitated. When he was given an intramuscular injection of haloperidol during the night, he became progressively more agitated. Based on Mr. Wade's symptoms, diffuse Lewy body dementia was diagnosed.

Fluctuations in behavior and mood are pathognomonic for this disease. Families have a difficult time coping with these changes. One day, the patient may be lucid, and the next day, he may be confused. Because of this waxing and waning, family members sometimes think that the patient is playing tricks, or family members may not believe that the patient has a dementing illness because he may sometimes be clear and not hallucinating. The nurse can help the family understand that all these changes are part of the disease process.

Neurocognitive Disorder Due to Traumatic Brain Injury

TBI is defined as brain trauma that can result in: (1) loss of consciousness, (2) amnesia, (3) disorientation and confusion, or (4) neurologic signs (onset of seizures, hemiparesis, visual field cuts, anosmia). TBI is caused by an impact to the head or rapid movement of the brain (American Psychiatric Association, 2013). Trauma to the head can be sustained from a wide range of events, including falls, motor vehicle crashes, sports injuries, and combat blasts (Peterson & Sanders, 2015). TBI is the leading cause of neurocognitive disturbances in individuals under the age of 45 years. The debilitating effects of head trauma associated with professional football and combat duty have become highly publicized in the past 10 years. In fact, TBI has been identified as the "signature injury" of the Operation Iraqi Freedom/Operation Enduring Freedom conflicts (Godwin et al., 2015). Research done in soldiers has shown that TBI during a deployment was by far the strongest predictor of postdeployment posttraumatic stress disorder (PTSD) symptoms in service members and veterans. The effects of TBI were found to be far more significant than the intensity of combat these veterans experienced (US Department of Veterans Affairs, n.d.).

TBI is classified as a chronic condition rather than an acute injury owing to the enduring nature of the physical, emotional, behavioral, and social manifestations. Disturbances in emotional function include irritability, ready frustration, anxiety, and lability; behavioral disturbances include apathy, suspiciousness, and aggression; physical disturbances include headache, fatigue, sleep disturbances, vertigo, tinnitus, and anosmia; and neurologic symptoms include forgetfulness, seizures, hemiparesis, and cranial nerve deficits. The emotional manifestations of TBI are known to cause extreme distress for the individual as well as within the family system. TBI is often identified as a "family injury" (American Psychiatric Association, 2013; Godwin et al., 2015).

Neurocognitive Disorder Due to Prion Disease

Creutzfeldt-Jakob disease (CJD) is a rare, degenerative, fatal brain disorder. The typical age of onset is approximately 60 years, although it can occur in individuals from the teenage years to late life. There are three major categories of CJD: (1) sporadic, (2) hereditary, and (3) acquired. A variant form of CJD has also been identified, which is the human form of mad cow disease (National Institute of Neurological Disorders and Stroke, 2020a). Until mad cow disease (bovine spongiform encephalopathy) became headline news, little information appeared in the media about CJD. Patients contract this variant after ingesting meat infected with bovine spongiform encephalopathy. Subacute spongiform encephalopathy is the key feature of both mad cow disease and CJD.

On microscopic examination, these brain cells look like sponges, and they are stripped of their intracellular material. The infecting agent is the prion, a protein particle, which is unlike either a bacterium or a virus. CJD is one of at least 12 prion-related diseases, some of which are transmissible from person to person (Walker & Jucker, 2015). A genetic component also exists, but it accounts for 10% or less of patients with CJD. When a genetic component is suspected, the causative agent is a mutation of the tau protein. There are no definitive diagnostic tests that can identify CJD (American Psychiatric Association, 2013; National Institute of Neurological Disorders and Stroke, 2020a). CJD is potentially transferable between people when blood and bodily fluids are present. However, the illness is not contagious by casual contact with the patient. No airborne pathogen is involved either.

Dementia is inevitable and occurs early in the disease. Personality changes, ataxia, seizures, and myoclonic movements may also occur. Impairment of vision and blindness are not unusual. The course is rapid; on average, 90% of patients die within 12 months (National Institute of Neurological Disorders and Stroke, 2020a).

There is no treatment that can cure or control CJD. Current treatment is aimed at symptom alleviation and making the person as comfortable as possible. Opiates are used for pain relief, while clonazepam and sodium valproate may reduce the involuntary muscle jerks. IV fluids and NG feedings may be needed in later stages of the disease. The nurse should focus on anticipatory grief for the family and the patient if he or she is cognitively able. The nurse should also expect that family members will be concerned that they may inherit CJD and will be understandably anxious. Neuronal tissue is extremely contagious. Anyone who may be involved with the brain and cerebrospinal fluid must observe very strict precautions. If an invasive procedure is performed, the physician and staff should be notified of the patient's illness. The funeral home personnel must also be told that the deceased individual had CJD.

Clinical Example: Neurocognitive Disorder Due to Prion Disease

Mrs. Mercer, 65 years old, became openly hostile toward her husband while they were dining out. She had never had outbursts like this before. Her vision was steadily declining, and she was blind within 6 months. She also developed myoclonic jerks that were not controlled with medication. Based on the change in personality, visual impairment, and movement disorder, CJD was diagnosed. Mrs. Mercer died 9 months later. Postmortem examination confirmed the diagnosis.

Neurocognitive Disorder Due to Human Immunodeficiency Virus Infection

Due to the success of HIV treatments, people living with HIV are now living longer and into older age. In addition to being at similar risk of developing dementias as the general ageing population, ageing people with HIV have an increased risk of neurocognitive co-morbidities, in particular, HIV-associated neurocognitive disorder (HAND). HAND is a acronym used to describe a subcortical neurodegenerative disease caused by HIV infection. HAND can impact a range of cognitive functions such as memory lapses, decreased ability to concentrate and comprehend, and impaired motor skills. While most neurocognitive disorders primarily affects individuals over 65 years, HAND will impact a much younger population (Cummins et al., 2018). There is no specific treatment for dementia related to HAND. And because HAND can occur at any age, behavioral and cognitive changes in all patients with HIV and AIDS should alert the nurse that the patient may be developing dementia.

Clinical Example: Major Neurocognitive Disorder Due to Human Immunodeficiency Virus Infection

Mrs. Halston, 36 years old, had HIV unknowingly for 8 years. Her family reported that she had been raped 10 years earlier and that the rapist was HIV-positive. Now Mrs. Halston is agitated, does not eat, and does not sleep well. Six months ago, Mrs. Halston's memory began to fail. Because of the early onset of this cognitive disorder, she had a diagnostic HIV test, which was positive. She died 10 months after receiving her diagnosis.

Alcohol-Induced Neurocognitive Disorder

Excessive alcohol intake over many years can result in cognitive impairment that persists beyond intoxication and acute withdrawal. Two neurologic conditions, known as Wernicke-Korsakoff syndrome, are associated with persistent and excessive alcohol ingestion. The first is Wernicke encephalopathy, and the second is Korsakoff syndrome. Both are attributable to a thiamine deficiency. The alcoholic patient usually has poor eating habits, which is one avenue leading to this deficiency. The other is the alcohol itself, which causes malabsorption problems in the stomach. Wernicke encephalopathy is a medical emergency. The typical triad of symptoms is confusion, ataxia, and abnormal extraocular movements (e.g., nystagmus). Thiamine replacement is crucial. The most effective route of administration is either intramuscular or intravenous because the patient most likely has a malabsorption problem.

Korsakoff syndrome, also known as Korsakoff psychosis, is a more chronic neurologic problem. The major symptom of Korsakoff syndrome is prominent antegrade amnesia and confabulation. The patient has severe difficulty learning new information and forgets rapidly. In response to questions, the patient will attempt to answer by making something up, since he has memory problems. However, this confabulation is done unconsciously. The patient may talk about some very interesting experiences, and the nurse may find out later that none of them really happened. He may also repeat certain comments. In addition to memory loss, the patient may experience fatigue, weakness, apathy, insomnia, and difficulty with concentration.

Thiamine replacement and abstinence from alcohol are urgently indicated. Any chance for improvement hinges on both. If the patient continues to drink alcohol, he is likely to develop liver disease as well as cardiovascular and cerebrovascular disease (American Psychiatric Association, 2013). Most symptoms can be reversed if detected and treated promptly and completely. However, improvement in memory is usually slow and may be incomplete (National Institute of Neurocognitive Disorders and Stroke, 2020 c,d.)

If the patient is too cognitively impaired, he will become unable to process new information and will be unable to benefit from participating in a support group such as Alcoholics Anonymous (AA).

Clinical Example: Alcohol-Induced Neurocognitive Disorder

Mr. Kelly, 75 years old, was admitted to a general hospital for chest pain. He was transferred 3 days later to a geriatric psychiatry unit with altered mental status. Mr. Kelly was unable to speak rationally; he made gestures in the air as if he were having visual hallucinations. His wife said that he did not have a drinking problem, but he did drink wine each evening. After 3 days of abstinence, Mr. Kelly was experiencing delirium related to alcohol withdrawal and was placed on an alcohol withdrawal protocol.

The patient returned to the hospital 2 years later with short-term memory loss. He said that he was in Hawaii when asked where he had been before admission. His wife confirmed that Mr. Kelly had not gone to Hawaii. He was confabulating. He had developed Korsakoff syndrome.

Neurocognitive Disorders Due to Huntington Disease

Huntington disease (HD) is an incurable, progressive, inherited neurocognitive disorder (Parekh et al., 2018). It is transmitted through an autosomal dominant gene that either parent may provide. It takes only one autosomal dominant gene to produce the illness. The patient may not know that he or she has (or will develop) HD before having children. Each offspring of a patient with HD has a 50% chance of inheriting the mutated gene, specifically within a protein called huntingtin. The defective gene causes the cytosine, adenine, and guanine (CAG) building blocks of DNA to repeat more times than normal. HD does not skip generations. It is transmitted through the generations *if and only if* the person has the affected chromosome 4.

This illness is not usually diagnosed until patients are in their 30s or 40s; however, children as young as 2 years old have been diagnosed. Symptoms can last up to 30 years (Parekh et al., 2018). At the present time, more than 30,000 people in the United States have HD, and another 150,000 have a 50% or greater chance of developing the disease. By the time patients are diagnosed with HD, they may already have had children and grandchildren. Each offspring has a 50% chance of inheriting the disease. This does not mean that half of the children will inherit the disease and the other half will not. Regarding the affected chromosome, no children may have inherited it, some may have inherited it, or all may have inherited it.

Cognitive changes are usually the first signs to appear, predating the motor abnormalities by at least 15 years. Initial symptoms include irritability, anxiety, or depressed mood. A mild-tempered person may develop mood swings or start drinking alcohol. Other signs may include apathy, disinhibition, and impulsivity. Early movement symptoms, known as choreiform movements, begin with facial twitches or involuntary limb movement (apraxia), and progress to myoclonus (jerking movements) of all extremities. These involuntary movements include ataxia and postural instability, making walking and balance difficult. Motor impairment eventually affects speech production (dysarthria), where speech becomes very difficult to understand. Dementia may develop before or after the choreiform movements begin. Short-term memory is affected first, followed by long-term memory loss. Eventually, individuals become non-ambulatory, with the added distress of difficulty eating and swallowing. Pneumonia is the predominate cause of death (American Psychiatric Association, 2013; National Institute of Neurological Disorders and Stroke, 2020c,d).

Genetic testing for HD involves a simple laboratory blood sample. Testing must follow rigorous guidelines. Multiple issues are involved; only some of them are listed here. Should individuals at risk be tested before having children, should they decide not to have children, or should they proceed and take the chance that a child will not have HD? HD is treated symptomatically. Tetrabenazine and deuterabenazine can treat both tardive dyskinesia and HD chorea. Antipsychotic drugs may also ease chorea and help to control hallucinations,

delusions, and aggression (National Institute of Neurological Disorders and Stroke, 2020c,d). Threats or violence perpetrated by the person with HD is a primary cause of family stress (Parekh et al., 2018). Counseling is always important with these patients and their families.

Clinical Example: Neurocognitive Disorder Due to Huntington Disease

Mrs. Thompson, a 57-year-old woman with Huntington disease, was admitted to the psychiatric unit for unmanageable behavior. She had severe myoclonus to the extent that she almost fell out of her wheelchair. She could no longer feed herself and was incontinent of bowel and bladder. She no longer recognizes family members and did not know that she was in the hospital. Dementia related to Huntington disease was diagnosed based on Mrs. Thompson's previous diagnosis of Huntington disease and her obvious memory loss.

 CRITICAL THINKING QUESTION

6. Why is genetic counseling essential with a patient who has Huntington disease?

Other Dementias

The most prevalent neurocognitive disorders have been described. Dozens of other illnesses may include dementia. For example, progressive supranuclear palsy, thyroid disease, Wilson disease, neurosyphilis, herpes simplex encephalitis, partial complex status epilepticus, and limbic encephalitis are examples of other types of dementia. Although individual patients have a different presentation of symptoms, all dementias involve cognitive, behavioral, and self-care issues (Casey, 2012).

 CRITICAL THINKING QUESTION

7. Why is it important to know the type of dementia that a patient has?

PUTTING IT ALL TOGETHER

PSYCHOTHERAPEUTIC MANAGEMENT

Nurse-Patient Relationship

Nursing care of patients with "forgetfulness" is challenging. It is common for patients with dementia to progressively experience confusion and "time-shifts." For example, patients may be shifted back to an emotional time in their past when they believe something needs to be resolved or attended to (i.e. call their spouse; visit a sick relative; pick up children from school; go to work). When such beliefs are triggered by patients, nursing staff are in an ethical dilemma about how to respond. At such times, telling the patient the truth (i.e. your spouse or sister is dead) would be received as untrue, confusing, and even shocking. In these kinds of situations, nurses are going to be torn about how to respond, tell the truth or lie. This deception dilemma has long been endemic in dementia care. There have been a number of different ways to respond to patients in such cases: tell a little white lie, humor the patient, bend the truth, or go along with it. Research shows that 96% of care staff use "little white lies" and withholding the truth in their work with dementia patients. If staff felt that telling the truth would cause distress in the patient, they would consider using deception. Turner et al. (2017) found that the hospital staff are reluctant either to tell the truth or to lie to patients. Preferred strategies were to distract the patient or to pass the buck to another staff member.

Some argue that deception by nursing staff is never justified within a person-centered approach. A therapeutic relationship must be genuine, honest, and respectful. An alternative approach is provided by Alter (2012), offering support to the patient by using *validation techniques*. He makes the following suggestions:

- *Accept* the patient's insistence about losing an item, not seeing family members, and so on.
- Do not revert to reality orientation to convince a patient that her father is dead, for example.
- Do not create an untrue reality.
- Attempt to *address the patient's feelings* of fear, sadness, and loss. For example, "Of course you're scared, sad, and/or lonely."
- Use nonthreatening factual words to *build trust*, focusing on questions of who, what, where, when, how. For example, "Who is stealing your shoes?" Do not ask "why" questions.
- *Don't challenge* something that doesn't make sense. Instead, respond to the patient's level of emotional concern. Once he or she feels understood, the patient's distress may be reduced.

❓ CRITICAL THINKING QUESTION

8. Should deception ever be used in the care of patients with Alzheimer disease? Explain your answer.

Communication Strategies

The importance of the nurse-patient relationship cannot be overstated. It is important for the nurse to realize and to help subordinates realize that many cognitively impaired individuals live in the moment. They may be incapable of retrieving the past (memory failure) and unable to contemplate the future. The present is what they have. The nurse must be pleasant and kind, smile, and use good eye contact. The following tips have been used successfully:

- If the patient seems to be confused, validate her emotional state and tell her that you are going to stay with her until she feels better.

- Effective communication starts with nonverbal behavior, so use a kind voice and make eye contact.
- Be positive and stay with pleasant subjects.
- Do not use sarcasm, jokes, and metaphors because the patient's loss of abstract thinking makes understanding these language subtleties almost impossible.
- Recognize that patients may be unable to tell the difference between a real argument and an impassioned discussion. Observing staff members in such a debate can be frightening and confusing to these patients.
- Use short sentences, not complex ones.
- Give directions slowly, one step at a time.
- Do not finish sentences for patients; give them time to finish their thoughts.
- Approach patients from the front in case they have visual or hearing impairment.
- Lots of chatter can be confusing because patients struggle to track one conversation when several are going on around them.

Scheduling Strategies

The way in which a cognitively impaired patient's day is structured is crucial in the plan of care. The nurse should do the following:

- Develop a schedule that provides structure to the day because patients adapt better when they have a predictable routine.
- Focus on patient-centered activities.
- Develop singular activities because multiple activities overwhelm the patient. For example, turn off the television while the patient is putting together a puzzle.
- Provide a group experience with one subject approached at a time. Too much stimulation increases anxiety and may lead to agitation.

Nutritional Strategies

Many patients with cognitive impairment do not want to eat, will not eat, and sometimes cannot eat without great difficulty. Patience and developing a strategy to meet nutritional needs are important. The nurse should consider the following:

- Ensure that patients are eating properly by tailoring dietary needs to the patient. Serve smaller meals several times per day. If too much food is on the plate, the patient may be overwhelmed.
- Finger foods work well for people who will not stay at the table.
- Find out about a patient's favorite foods and provide them as often as possible even if this means spaghetti for breakfast.
- Beverage supplements can provide nutrition when regular food intake decreases.
- If the patient has swallowing difficulties, a consultation with a dietitian is in order. This health care professional can determine if the patient needs a change in beverage consistency or if he or she needs foods that all have the same texture.

Toileting Strategies

Toileting is a big issue. This often is *the* issue that causes families to seek placement outside the home. The nurse should do the following:

- Make sure that the patient does not have an illness that may be affecting toileting.
- Seek to keep the patient comfortable.
- Give meticulous attention to personal hygiene and toileting needs.
- Take the patient to the bathroom every 2 hours to promote continence (incontinence contributes to the formation of decubitus ulcers, as does immobility).

Wandering Strategies

Wandering is the second major reason why families choose to place a loved one in a long-term care facility. The clinical term "wandering" denotes movement that lacks an exact destination, such as lapping, pacing, elopement, and getting lost and is associated with a person who is disoriented and lacks awareness. In long-term care facilities, residents who wander may enter, uninvited into another resident's bedroom. This experience may be frightful, especially if it occurs in the middle of the night and is known to impact both residents' quality of life (MacAndrew et al., 2017). Managing patients who wander involves balancing their right to freedom of movement against the caregiver's moral and legal responsibility to ensure patients' safety (Solomon & Lawlor, 2018).

Many law enforcement agencies have partnered with the Alzheimer's Association "Safe Return" program. These patients wear a "Safe Return" armband that identifies them and provides other personal information. Some families may use a bracelet, necklace, or watch with pertinent emergency information from MedicAlert (call 1-800-ID-ALERT).

Global positioning system (GPS) is a technology that is utilized to mitigate the risks associated with wandering. Devices with GPS allows caregivers to monitor a loved one's geographic location in case they get lost, providing "peace of mind" to family members (Liu, Cruz, Ruptash, Barnard, & Juzwishin, 2017).

Another option is a lanyard—if the patient will keep it on. In this situation, a flash drive can be attached to it. Emergency names, addresses, telephone numbers, allergies, medication lists, names and numbers of physicians, insurance information, and other personal information can be easily stored. The caregiver can keep a duplicate flash drive. The caregiver's flash drive can keep photo and video files of the patient. Because the flash drive can plug into any computer with a universal serial bus (USB) port, instant information can be available to hospitals and the police.

Psychopharmacology

Geriatric patients with cognitive disorders often face the double burden of dealing with a psychiatric diagnosis superimposed on a chronic medical condition. Because of this comorbidity, these individuals are often prescribed many medications. Part of the nurse's role is to ensure that prescribed medications are helping and not harming the patient. Because most drugs used in geriatric psychiatry do not have FDA indications specifically for patients with cognitive disorders, nurses must be particularly vigilant in assessing drug effects.

Some individuals with dementia are prescribed psychotropics to manage aggressive behavior, psychosis, depression, and anxiety. Although psychotropic drugs have been found to cause severe side effects, they continue to be widely prescribed in patients with dementia (Smeets, Gerritsen, Zuidema, Teerenstra, van der Spek, Smalbrugge, & Koopmans, 2018). Because most patients with dementia are older, the dosage of psychotropics should be on the lower dosage range. Nonpharmacological interventions for behavioral and psychological symptoms should always be the first line of treatment utilized for geriatric patients.

Milieu Management

Much is involved in making these patients comfortable. At home or in a specialized care facility, the room temperature and lighting should be at the patient's preference and not that of family or staff. Nursing staff should seek to reduce noxious sounds that may offend or frighten patients. Television may be useful if there is purposeful viewing. For patients in a specialized care facility, it is important to match roommates' personalities when possible.

Memory Aids

Individuals with cognitive disorders may benefit from memory aids. Many patients keep track of appointments on a calendar that has big blocks for each date. Notes are good reminders, but the patient must know to look for them. Directions may be written in large print to instruct patients about how to operate new appliances, such as a new microwave. One patient bought a new television system that required three separate remote controls to operate all the features of the television, cable television box, and DVD player. The daughter made a color photocopy of these remote controls and took it home. When the patient had difficulty turning on his television, finding the right channel, or operating the DVD player, he would call his daughter to talk him through it.

In another example, a patient's son took digital photographs of each of his mother's pills. He then made a daily grid for her with pictures of the real pills placed according to the time of day that she needed to take them.

Pillboxes for the day, week, or month help patients keep their medications sorted out. Some pillboxes have an alarm in them to remind patients when to take their medications. Sometimes, all a patient needs is a telephone reminder to take the medication. Here are some examples of medication errors that could have been prevented:

1. A patient did not know which medication to take, so he took all his blue pills on one day and all his white pills on another.
2. Another patient took both lorazepam prescribed by one physician and Ativan prescribed by another. She did not know that they were chemical equivalents.

If there is any doubt about a patient's ability to take medication, the nurse should ask the patient to demonstrate which medication to take and when.

CARE FOR FAMILY MEMBERS

In preparation for end-of-life issues, it is recommended that as one reaches the age of 65, a dementia directive be completed. The dementia directive gives options for each stage of dementia based on the wishes of the person. There are four options: (1) to prolong my life at all costs, (2) to receive treatment to prolong my life but DNR, (3) to receive treatment in my home or residence, or (4) to receive comfort care only. As the disease progresses, the person has the ability to alter his or her end-of-life choice. Dementia directives assist family members in feeling assured of the wishes of their loved one and alleviates the burden of making difficult end-of-life decisions (Gaster, 2019).

The decision to place a loved one with dementia in a nursing home is known to be particularly difficult for family members. Family caregivers will often make significant personal sacrifices to care for their loved one at home. Caregivers experience exhaustion, deep sorrow, fractured relationships, and apprehension as a result of providing home care 24 hours a day (Clark et al., 2016). Caregiver burden has been widely researched for over 30 years.

Family members will need education and support around issues of end-of-life decisions for advanced dementia. The chronic, progressive cognitive and physical decline associated with Alzheimer disease is compromised in its advanced stage by numerous comorbidities and acute events (i.e., pneumonia). The routine use of advanced technologies, such as artificial nutrition, is considered burdensome in advanced dementia. Aggressive medical care with advanced disease has been shown to be associated with poorer outcomes for both patients and their families.

Therefore, the use of palliative care such as hospice with an emphasis on comfort care is deemed a loving response to the complex needs of the patient with advanced dementia. The clinical and ethical dilemmas of treating disease symptoms in advanced dementia must be sensitively addressed with family members (Reinhart, 2014).

The grief associated with losing a loved one to AD is unique because it is so prolonged. Family members of those with memory loss experience grief that is "the constant yet hidden companion of AD and other related dementias" (Doka, 2004). Family members grieve the loss of the individual with dementia prior to the actual death and then grieve the loss of the loved one when actual death occurs. The phenomenon known as ambiguous loss happens as the loved one is physically present but psychologically absent. The multiple losses experienced over the course of the disease include changes to shared pleasurable activities, the level of physical or emotional intimacy in communication, and roles change (Pote & Wright, 2018). Particularly for spouses, the sadness, longing, and loneliness tend to escalate as the disease worsens. Giving the caregiver and other family members permission to grieve and validating their enormous grieving experience is an essential support that communicates compassion and sensitivity.

CASE STUDY

Roberta Evans, an 81-year-old woman with type 2 diabetes, lived in a retirement community apartment before being admitted to a geropsychiatric unit. A retired high school science teacher, she had been living independently since her husband died 5 years earlier. Her only child, a son, had moved to Texas about a year earlier.

Mrs. Evans drove her car to a local discount store 3 weeks before her admission. Two women approached her in the parking lot and told her that they knew a way to invest her money that would double it overnight. Mrs. Evans went to the bank with them, withdrew $1000, and gave it to them. The women were con artists and disappeared with the money. When her son learned about the scam, instead of calling the retirement community director to report what had happened, he called a friend who lived locally and had him disable his mother's car battery. When Mrs. Evans' car would not start, she started walking out on the busy streets. She never considered that her car could be repaired. Mrs. Evans wandered away from the retirement community 2 weeks later and was found several blocks away. She did not know where she was going and could not remember how to get back to her apartment. A police officer brought her back to the apartment complex's director, who called her son. He flew in from Texas the next morning.

When he visited his mother in her apartment, he saw plates with dried half-eaten food all over the kitchen and living room. He found a plastic bag with her diabetes supplies and prescription in it. Dirty clothes were strewn about the apartment. Her bathtub faucet did not work. He did not know how long it had been since she had bathed, and his mother could not tell him. She agreed to be evaluated for this change in cognitive status, although she thought nothing was wrong. She was admitted to the geriatric psychiatric unit in a university hospital in her town. The multidisciplinary treatment team met the day after Mrs. Evans was admitted to plan her care. Her son did not know what her most recent baseline behavior was because he had only spoken with her over the telephone. He said he could not detect any changes in their telephone conversations. The patient was able to take care of her ADL independently when she had prompts, especially for hygiene and grooming. Mrs. Evans attended all the unit activities and enjoyed being with her peers. However, she needed to be reminded to go to each session. She told the music therapist that she was glad that he had started the music group that day. She did not remember participating in music therapy the week before. Mrs. Evans ate well and slept through the night.

She participated in all the diagnostic testing and did not complain. An MRI scan of her brain showed some atrophy. Electroencephalography showed mild background slowing. A single-photon emission computed tomography (SPECT) scan of her brain demonstrated reduced perfusion in the frontoparietal lobes. Neuropsychological testing showed that she had difficulty with short-term memory as well as visuospatial difficulties. On admission, she scored 23 out of 30 on the Mini-Mental Status Examination. She said, "I don't keep up with these things anymore since I've retired." These findings were consistent with a diagnosis of Alzheimer disease. She was started on an AChE inhibitor.

Before discharge, the geriatric psychiatrist, nurse, and social worker met with the patient and her son to make treatment recommendations. The results of the diagnostic testing were discussed. The patient had asked the team members while she was being evaluated to tell her what was wrong. "I'm not crazy, you know!" she insisted.

The son agreed that it was in his mother's best interest that she be told her diagnosis. The physician told her that she had Alzheimer disease. She said at first, "I don't believe it." Later, she admitted that she had "memory problems, but I do not have Alzheimer's disease." She reluctantly agreed to move to the assisted-living facility in the same retirement community. "I know I need some help with my cooking."

The patient did well in the assisted-living facility. She liked the various activities; in addition, her roommate was a woman who had taught in the same high school as she had. Mrs. Evans seemed to tolerate the AChE inhibitor. She was able to live in the assisted-living facility for 3 more years before she had to move to the nursing home.

◎ CARE PLAN

Name: Roberta Evans   **Admission Date: _____**

DSM-5 Diagnosis: Major neurocognitive disorder due to Alzheimer disease

Assessment	**Areas of strength:** Patient is willing to be evaluated, has good relationships with fellow residents and staff at the retirement community, and has a strong faith.
	Problems: Short-term memory loss, confusion, poor judgment, wandering.
Diagnoses	Acute confusion (got lost).
	Memory impairment (forgot that she had been diagnosed with type 2 diabetes mellitus).
	Impaired judgment (was conned out of $1000).
	Social isolation—relationship with her son; although their relationship is a good one, he lives at a distance.
	Self-care deficits—poor personal hygiene and apartment filth.
	Wandering.
Outcomes	**Short-term goals**
Date met: _____	Patient will have a comprehensive geriatric psychiatric evaluation.
Date met: _____	Patient will be medically stable, especially related to new-onset type 2 diabetes mellitus.
Date met: _____	Patient will participate in group activities.
Date met: _____	Patient and son will meet with multidisciplinary treatment team to discuss diagnosis, patient's progress, and plans for discharge.
	Long-term goals
Date met: _____	Patient will be safe and free of injury (both physical and emotional).
Date met: _____	Patient will be discharged to appropriate level of care.
Date met: _____	Patient will maintain her independence as long as possible, even though she now needs assistance.
Date met: _____	Patient will be introduced to a variety of social activities in which she can participate at her new residence.
Date met: _____	Patient will have medical and psychiatric follow-up scheduled before discharge.
Date met: _____	Patient will have her dignity preserved and her self-esteem enhanced.
Planning and Interventions	**Nurse-patient relationship**
	Explain the process of evaluation and treatment by the nursing staff and the rest of the multidisciplinary treatment team.
	Educate the patient about her recent-onset diabetes mellitus, even though she will have assistance managing her disease.
	Validate the patient's concern that others will think she is "crazy" because of her Alzheimer diagnosis. Normalize her anxiety and concerns.
	Psychopharmacology
	Educate the patient and her son about AChE inhibitors and the specific one she is taking.
	Educate the patient and her son about the oral hypoglycemic agent that she is taking for type 2 diabetes mellitus.
	Monitor for any adverse reactions.
	Milieu management
	Assess and provide the level of care for her activities of daily living associated with bathing, hygiene, and grooming.
	Reorient the patient to her environment at frequent intervals. Ask her if she has any questions or concerns. Respond to questions with simple, short answers. Use a soft, soothing voice to comfort her fears.
Evaluation	Patient will meet her short-term and long-term goals. She will be prepared to move to the assisted-living facility in her retirement community.
	Patient's son has agreed to visit his mother every 3 months and to call her at least once a week. To comply with the Health Insurance Portability and Accountability Act regulations, the patient has signed a release of information so that her son can call the assisted-living facility director with any concerns that he may have.
Referrals	The referral was made to the assisted-living facility in her retirement community about her transfer from her apartment.
	The police department was notified about the scam artists because this had not been done at the time.

NEXT-GENERATION NCLEX® EXAMINATION-STYLE CASE STUDY

Scenario: A 74-year-old client with a history of type II diabetes lived alone and was responsible for all activities of daily living (ADLs). The client had minimal contact with adult children who all live out-of-state but attended church regularly. During home health visits, the nurse began to express concern that the client's blood glucose level was becoming erratic. When questioned about adherence to medication therapy, the client stated "I forget to take my medicine and I eat whenever I'm hungry." The client was admitted for blood glucose management and cognitive evaluation. Neuropsychological testing showed that the client had difficulty with short-term memory and visuospatial difficulties. The Mini-Mental Status Examination produced a score of 23 out of 30. The client was diagnosed with Alzheimer disease (AD) and AChE inhibitor therapy was initiated. It has now been 4 months since the client was transferred to an assisted-living facility. The following findings were noted by the nurse when assessing the client today.

Item Type: Matrix

For each client finding, use an X to indicate whether these assessment findings indicate that nursing interventions over the past 4 months have been Effective (helped to meet expected outcomes), Ineffective (did not help to meet expected outcomes), or Unrelated (not related to the expected outcomes) in meeting goals of care. Only one selection can be made for each client finding.

Assessment Finding	Effective	Ineffective	Unrelated
A1c is 7.6%			
Responds appropriately when given toileting cues			
Experienced a fall resulting in bruising on forearms bilaterally			
Demonstrates pleasure when attending unit activities			
Engages in weekly telephone calls from adult children			
Client's family provides money to cover non-care related expenses			

STUDY NOTES

1. The normal aging process does not include the development of cognitive disorders.

2. On first glance, delirium and dementia share some commonalities. However, in contrast to dementia, delirium can be imminently life-threatening, and treatment for delirium must be started immediately based on the etiology of presenting symptoms.

3. Most types of dementia feature a progressive cognitive deterioration over time. Only a few types are potentially reversible. Normal-pressure hydrocephalus, vitamin B$_{12}$ deficiency, and alcohol-related dementia may be reversed in their early stages. Alzheimer disease, DLB, and vascular dementia—the three types of dementia that account for most of these illnesses—are characterized by chronic deterioration.

4. Alzheimer disease is not a new disease. Alois Alzheimer, a German neurologist, first described a patient with these signs in 1907. Frederic Lewy, also a neurologist and a contemporary of Alzheimer, first described Lewy bodies.

5. Although not a perfect predictor of Alzheimer disease, a person with mild cognitive impairment is more likely to develop Alzheimer disease than a person who has no cognitive impairment.

6. Vascular dementia is caused by mini-strokes. The progression is unpredictable because it depends on the occurrence of another vascular event. The deterioration takes a stepwise progression, meaning that the patient may stay on a plateau for days to years before another ischemic event occurs. Risk factors include hypertension, diabetes mellitus, smoking, and obesity. The reduction of these risk factors may also reduce the likelihood of a subsequent ischemic event.

7. A pathognomonic (hallmark) sign of diffuse Lewy body dementia is the hypersensitivity that the patient demonstrates with antipsychotic medication.

8. A patient with Parkinson disease may also have a dementia and/or depression.

9. Patients with dementia who exhibit disruptive behavior may be delirious, confused, or uncomfortable. Many cannot make their needs known.

10. Nursing care must be patient-focused. Dignity must be preserved, and safety must be maintained. The nurse promotes as much independence for the patient as possible.

11. Genetics play a part in some types of dementia (e.g., Huntington disease is an autosomal dominant transmitted disease). Several chromosomes that are related to Alzheimer disease have been identified. The most prominent ones are chromosomes 1, 14, and 21—which have been linked to familial Alzheimer disease—and the Apo ε4 allele on chromosome 19—which has been linked to β-amyloid plaque.

12. Caregiver burden is a significant stressor felt by caregivers of patients with dementia. Family members need support around their emotional grief and end-of-life decisions.

REFERENCES

Alter, T. (2012). The growth of institutional deception in the treatment of Alzheimer's disease: The case study of Sadie Cohen. *Journal of Social Work Practice, 26*(1), 93–107. https://doi.org/10.1080/02650533.2011.571767.

Alzheimer's, Association. (2020). 2021 Alzheimer's disease facts and figures. https://www.alz.org/media/documents/alzheimers-facts-and-figures.pdf.

American Psychiatric Association. (2013). *Diagnostic and Statistical Manual of Mental Disorders* (5th ed.). APA.

Banner Alzheimer's Institute. (2017). Symptoms and diagnosis. http://www.banneralz.org/patient-family-care/symptoms-and-diagnosis.aspx.

Bellenir, K. (Ed.). (2008). Alzheimer disease sourcebook (4th ed.). Omnigraphics.

Biddle, W., & van Sickel, M. (1948). *Introduction to psychiatry* (2nd ed.). Saunders.

Bonanni, L., Cagnin, A., & Agosta, F. (2017). The Italian dementia with Lewy bodies study group (DLB-SINdem): Toward a standardization of clinical procedures and multicenter cohort studies design. *Neurological Sciences, 38*, 83–91. https://doi.org/10.1007/s10072-016-2713-8.

Burke, S., Hu, T., Fava, N., Li, T., Rodriguez, M., Schuldiner, K., Burgess, A., & Laird, A. (2019). Sex differences in the development of mild cognitive impairment & probable Alzheimer's disease as predicted by hippocampal volume or white matter hyperintensities. *Journal of Women & Aging, 31*(2), 140–164. https://doi.org/10.1080/08952841.2018.1419476.

Casey, G. (2012). Alzheimer's and other dementias. Kai Tiaki. *Nursing New Zealand, 18*(6), 20–24.

Clark, P., et al. (2016). Wellness-based counseling for caregivers of persons with dementia. *Journal of Mental Health Counseling, 38*(3), 263–277. https://doi.org/10.17744/mehc.38.3.06.

Cummins, D., Waters, D., Aggar, C., Crawford, D., Fethney, J., & O'Connor, C. (2018). Voices from Australia - Concerns about HIV associated neurocognitive disorder. *Aids Care, 30*(5), 609–617. https://doi.org/10.1080/09540121.2018.1426826.

Doka, K. (2004). Grief and dementia. In K. Doka (Ed.), *Living with grief: Alzheimer's disease* (pp. 169–195). Hospice Foundation of America.

Ferrari, C., Nacmias, B., & Sorbi, S. (2017). The diagnosis of dementias: A practical tool not to miss rare causes. *Neurological Sciences, 39*, 615–627. https://doi.org/10.1007/s10072-017-3206-0.

FitzGerald, J. (2018). Delirium clinical motor subtypes: A narrative review of the literature and insights from neurobiology. *Aging & Mental Health, 22*(4), 431–443. https://doi.org/10.1080/13607863.2017.1310802.

Gaster, B. (2019). An advanced directive for dementia. *Journal of the American Society on Aging, 3*, 79–82. https://www.evergreenhealth.com/documents/For-Medical-Staff/CME-advance-directive-dementia.pdf.

Godwin, E. E., Lukow, H. R., & Lichiello, S. (2015). Promoting resilience following traumatic brain injury: Application of an interdisciplinary evidence-based model for intervention. *Family Relations, 64*(3), 347–362. https://doi.org/10.1111/fare.12122.

Greenland, J., Williams-Gray, C., & Barker, R. (2018). The clinical heterogeneity of Parkinson's disease and its therapeutic implications. *European Journal of Neuroscience, 49*(3), 328–338. https://doi.org/10.1111/ejn.14094.

Higgs, P., & Gilleard, C. (2017). Ageing, dementia and the social mind: Past, present and future perspectives. *Sociology of Health & Illness, 39*(2), 175–181. https://doi.org/10.1111/1467-9566.12536.

Jeon, D., Ju, H., Jung, D., Kim, S., Moon, J., & Kim, Y. (2019). Usefulness of the University of California San Diego Performance-Based Skills Assessment for the evaluation of cognitive function and activities of daily living function in patients with cognitive impairment. *Aging & Mental Health, 23*(1), 46–52. https://doi.org/10.1080/13607863.2017.1393796.

Khan, A., Akram, M., Daniyal, M., & Zainab, R. (2019). Awareness and current knowledge of Parkinson's disease: A neurogenerative disorder. *International Journal of Neuroscience, 129*(1), 55–93. https://doi.org/10.1080/00207454.2018.1486837.

Kolanowski, A. (2018). Delirium in people living with dementia: A call for global solutions. *Aging & Mental Health, 22*(4), 444–446. https://doi.org/10.1080/13607863.2016.1244805.

Lahariya, S., Grover, S., Bagga, S., & Sharma, A. (2016). Phenomenology of delirium among patients admitted to a coronary care unit. *Nordic Journal of Psychiatry, 70*(8), 626–632. https://doi.org/10.1080/08039488.2016.1194467.

Liu, L., Cruz, A., Ruptash, T., Barnard, S., & Juzwishin, D. (2017). Acceptance of global positioning system (GPS) technology among dementia clients and family caregivers. *Journal of Technology in Human Services, 35*(2), 99–119. https://doi.org/10.1080/15228835.2016.1266724.

Lyseng-Williamson, K. A., & McKeage, K. (2013). Once-daily memantine. *Drugs & Aging, 30*, 51. https://doi.org/10.1007/s40266-012-0041-0.

MacAndrew, M., Fielding, E., Kolanowski, A., O'Reilly, M., & Beattie, E. (2017). Observing wandering-related boundary transgression in people with severe dementia. *Aging & Mental Health, 21*(11), 1197–1205. https://doi.org/10.1080/13607863.2016.1211620.

Martins, S., Pinho, E., & Correia, R. (2018). What effect does delirium have on family and nurses of older adult patients? *Aging & Mental Health, 22*(7), 903–911. https://doi.org/10.1080/13607863.2017.1393794.

Milne, R., Diaz, A., Badger, S., Bunnik, E., & Wells, K. (2018). At, with and beyond risk: Expectations of living with the possibility of future dementia. *Sociology of Health & Illness, 40*(6), 969–987. https://doi.org/10.1111/1467-9566.12731.

Namzaric Prescribing, Information. (2020). http://www.namzarichcp.com/.

National Institute of Neurological Disorders and Stroke. (2020a). Creutzfeldt-Jakob disease information page. https://www.ninds.nih.gov/Disorders/All-Disorders/Creutzfeldt-Jakob-Disease-Information-Page.

National Institute of Neurological Disorders and Stroke. (2020b). Frontotemporal Dementia Information Page https://www.ninds.nih.gov/Disorders/All-Disorders/Frontotemporal-Dementia-Information-Page.

National Institute of Neurological Disorders and Stroke (2020c). Hungtingtons disorder: Hope through research. https://www.ninds.nih.gov/Disorders/All-Disorders/Hungtingtons-Disorder-Information-Page.

National Institute of Neurological Disorders and Stroke (2020d). Huntingtons disease: Hope through research https://www.https://www.ninds.nih.gov/Disorders/All-Disorders/Huntingtons-Disease.

National Institute on Aging. (2020). Causes of Alzheimer's Disease: What happens to the brain in Alzheimer's Disease? https://www.nia.nih.gov/health/what-happens-brain-alzheimers-disease

Parekh, R., Praetorius, R., & Nordberg, A. (2018). Carers' experiences in families impacted by Huntington's disease: A qualitative interpretive meta-synthesis. *British Journal of Social Work, 48*(3), 675–692. https://doi.org/10.1093/bjsw/bcw173.

Peterson, H., & Sanders, S. (2015). Caregiving and traumatic brain injury: Coping with grief and loss. *Health & Social Work, 40*(4), 325–328. https://doi.org/10.1093/hsw/hlv063.

Phillips, L. A. (2013). Delirium in geriatric patients: Identification and prevention. *Medsurg Nursing: Official Journal of the Academy of Medical-Surgical Nurses, 22*(1), 9.

Pote, S., & Wright, S. (2018). Evaluating anticipatory grief as a moderator of life and marital satisfaction for spousal caregivers of individuals with dementia. *Educational Gerontology, 44*(2-3), 196–207. https://doi.org/10.1080/03601277.2018.1438085.

Reinhart, J. P. (2014). Vital conversations with family in the nursing home: Preparation for end-stage dementia care. *Journal of Social Work in the End-of-Life & Palliative Care, 10*(2), 112–126. https://doi.org/10.1080/15524256.2014.906371.

Ryd, C., Nygard, L., Malinowsky, C., Ohman, A., & Kottorp, A. (2017). Can the everyday technology use questionnaire predict overall functional level among older adults with mild cognitive impairment or mild-stage Alzheimer's disease? - A pilot study. *Scandinavian Journal of Caring Sciences, 31*(1), 201–209. https://doi.org/10.1111/scs.12330.

Smeets, C., Gerritsen, D., Zuidema, S., Teerenstra, S., van der Spek, K., Smalbrugge, M., & Koopmans, R. (2018). Psychotropic drug prescription for nursing home residents with dementia: Prevalence and associations with non-resident factors. *Aging & Mental Health, 22*(9), 1239–1246. https://doi.org/10.1080/13607863.2017.1348469.

Snowdon, D. (2001). *Aging with grace: What the Nun Study teaches us about leading longer, healthier, and more meaningful lives.* Bantam Books.

Solomon, O., & Lawlor, M. (2018). Beyond V40.31: Narrative phenomenology of wandering in autism and dementia. *Culture, Medicine, and Psychiatry, 42*, 206–243. https://doi.org/10.1007/s11013-017-9562-7.

Stewart, R. (2019). Anxiety and dementia: Cause or effect? *Acta Psychiatrica Scandinavica, 139*(1), 3–5. https://doi.org/10.1111/acps.12992.

Stir, G. (2015). Lifting the curse of Alzheimer's. *Scientific America, 312*(5), 50–57. https://doi.org/10.1038/scientificamerican0515-50.

Tobore, T. (2019). On the central role of mitochondria dysfunction and oxidative stress in Alzheimer's Disease. *Neurological Sciences, 40*, 1527–1540. https://doi.org/10.1007/s10072-019-03863-x.

Turner, A., Eccles, F., Keady, J., Simpson, J., & Elvish, R. (2017). The use of the truth and deception in dementia care amongst general hospital staff. *Aging & Mental Health, 21*(8), 862–869. https://doi.org/10.1080/13607863.2016.1179261.

US Department of Veterans Affairs. (n.d.) Traumatic brain injury. http://www.research.va.gov/topics/tbi.cfm.

Walker, L., & Jucker, M. (2015). Neurodegenerative disease: Expanding the prior concept. Annual Review of Neurosciences, 38, 87–103. http://doi.org/10.1146/annurev-neuro-071714-033828.

Wallis, C. (2020). Delirium: Taken seriously at last. Scientific American, 322(3), 28.

29

Personality Disorders

Karmie M. Johnson

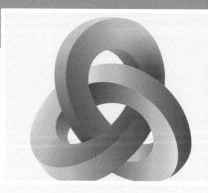

e http://evolve.elsevier.com/Keltner

LEARNING OBJECTIVES

- Recognize characteristics of each personality disorder.
- Describe behaviors of individuals with personality disorders.
- Describe nursing interventions for patients with personality disorders.

- Recognize issues related to the care of patients with personality disorders.

This chapter focuses on patients with personality disorders either hospitalized in the inpatient psychiatric setting or treated in outpatient programs. Except for patients with a borderline personality disorder (BPD), these patients usually are hospitalized not because of their personality disorders but because of other diagnosed mental disorders. Although a patient may present because of another diagnosis, it is important to note that the personality disorder significantly impacts treatment options and their efficacy. Interventions focus primarily on the nurse-patient relationship unique to each personality disorder; however, this chapter does not repeat the general nurse-patient interventions described in Chapter 9. Milieu issues and psychopharmacologic factors are not addressed for each disorder because unique milieu and pharmacologic interventions are not appropriate for all disorders. Medication might be given if a patient has a comorbid diagnosis or if a symptom is severe enough to interfere with functioning, such as severe anxiety or depression.

PERSONALITY

All individuals have personality traits and characteristics that make them unique and interesting human beings. Traits are exhibited in the way individuals think about themselves and others and through behaviors. Although experience varies across environmental, cultural, and social lines, every human possesses expected and persistent facets of behavior and cognition to one extent or another. Because these traits are evident across the diversity of humanity, they can be used to dimensionalize personality (Eaton & Greene, 2018).

There are five pathological or maladaptive personality domains: negative affectivity, detachment, psychoticism, antagonism, and disinhibition (American Psychiatric Association (APA), 2013; Oltmanns & Widiger, 2020). Negative affectivity or neuroticism is associated with negativity and pessimism. People with high negative affectivity might be described as "worriers." An individual who displays an excessive amount of neuroticism has a high probability of having a mental illness, such as anxiety or depression, at some point in their life. Those with high detachment avoid socioemotional experiences and have difficulty or do not like engaging with others. They might be considered "introverts" who prefer a solitary existence with little social interaction and are less influenced by certain types of positive encouragement. The opposite domain would be extraversion. Extraverted people tend to be optimistic, favor interacting with others, and being the life of the party. They are usually responsive to positive reinforcement and enjoy praise for their efforts. Antagonism is an interpersonal personality domain. People who display this domain are often oppositional, easy to anger, and prone to contentious relationships. They think highly of themselves and very little of others. Individuals who are not antagonistic are agreeable, cooperative, and easygoing, sometimes to a fault. The domain of disinhibition describes individuals who are impulsive, disorganized, and prefer immediate gratification. They often have difficulty planning for the future and instead live in the emotional "here-and-now." Disinhibition can be contrasted with conscientiousness, which reflects the level of self-control and focus that an individual has. Conscientious people are responsible, dependable, and take an organized, goal-oriented approach to life and work to achieve their long-term goals. Individuals with difficulties regulating their openness can exhibit psychoticism. Openness is associated with curiosity and imagination, which can be expected when balanced with lucidity. Individuals with too much openness are interested and engaged in various pursuits that may be at odds with the dominant culture in which they live. Others would describe them as odd or "weird" because of the eccentric thoughts and behaviors that they display.

Personality traits are usually ego-syntonic; they are consistent and acceptable to the ego or one's sense of self. Individuals with personality disorders have traits and habits that are fixed and pathological. Individuals with personality disorders exhibit lifelong, inflexible, and dysfunctional patterns of relating and behaving. These dysfunctional patterns and behaviors usually cause distress to others. However, because personality traits are ego-syntonic, individuals with personality disorders might not find their behaviors distressing; they become distressed because of other people's reactions or behaviors toward them. These reactions affect these individuals by causing immense emotional pain and discomfort. Difficulty in managing complicated symptoms and significant impairment in functioning have resulted in increased contact with the mental health system and the use of services. Patients do not usually seek treatment to change their personalities but want help for depression, anxiety, somatic symptoms, alcohol and chemical dependency, and work and personal relationship difficulties. If a patient does present to a provider with a personality complaint, it is usually not of their own accord: "I don't think there's anything wrong with me, but my wife thinks I'm too hard on our kids. What's so bad about having high standards?"

NORM'S NOTES In my opinion, these disorders are the toughest to treat. For instance, people with narcissistic personality disorder can be charming and delightful company, but at their center, they are always scheming and looking out for number one. They tend to be subversive and undermine authority whenever they can. Note that personality disorders were placed on axis II in the fourth edition (text revision) of the *Diagnostic and Statistical Manual of Mental Disorders (DSM-IV-TR)*. The other category of disorders placed under axis II was mental retardation. Why were personality disorders placed there? I will answer that with another question, "How deep does the yellow go in a banana?" Our personalities go to our core. Although *DSM-5* brings some needed changes, I think the *DSM-IV-TR* axis system better reflected the uniqueness of personality disorders better by differentiating these conditions as innately tied in with who we fundamentally are.

Personality disorders (PDs) are differentiated from personality traits. While both may be stable over time and circumstances, personality disorders cause significant impairments in self and interpersonal functionality to the extent that is pathological. For example, compulsive traits are not the same as obsessive-compulsive personality disorder, which is not the same as obsessive-compulsive disorder. Many high-functioning people have compulsive traits, whereas only a few have compulsive personality disorders. Patients benefit from the fact that some nurses might have compulsive traits—for example, rechecking labels, dressings, and drainage tubes. Personality disorders are often associated with other comorbidities such as mood and substance abuse disorders and increased mortality. The interpersonal difficulties that people with personality disorders display can adversely affect the treatment they receive and, therefore, prevent or delay positive outcomes and recovery (Volkert, Gablonski, & Rabung, 2018).

In 2013, the American Psychiatric Association published the fifth edition of the *Diagnostic and Statistical Manual of Mental Disorders*, commonly referred to as the *DSM-5*. The *DSM-5* removed personality disorders from Axis II to Axis I and introduced an alternative model for personality disorders (AMPD) in the "Emerging Measures and Models" section. The AMPD proposes a dimensional approach that combines aspects of the categorical model currently used. The AMPD characterizes impairments across two main criteria: personality functioning and pathologic personality traits. Criterion A requires impairments in personality functioning in self (identity and self-direction) and interpersonal relationships (empathy and intimacy). Criterion B consists of 25 pathological personality traits under the five domains referenced above (American Psychiatric Association APA, 2013). The rest of this chapter will focus on the current model of personality disorders in the *DSM-5*, not the alternative model. While the AMPD is producing a rich body of research on how we view and eventually treat personality disorders (McCabe & Widiger, 2020), most clinicians in a diagnostic setting like hospitals are still using the categorical approach to personality disorder.

DSM-5 criteria for a personality disorder include experiences and behaviors very different from those usually expected in an individual's culture. The individual must have disturbances in two of the following areas: (1) cognition, (2) affect, (3) interpersonal functioning, and (4) impulse control. The enduring pattern of a personality disorder is lifelong, becoming recognizable during adolescence or early adulthood. The personality impairments should be relatively pervasive and stable and not considered normal related to the development and sociocultural environment. For these reasons, most personality disorders, although in evidence, are usually not diagnosed before age 18 (American Psychiatric Association APA, 2013); see the box titled "*DSM-5* Criteria for General Personality Disorder."

For General Personality Disorder

A. An enduring pattern of inner experience and behavior that deviates markedly from the expectations of the individual's culture. This pattern is manifested in two (or more) of the following areas:
 1. Cognition (i.e., ways of perceiving and interpreting self, other people, and events).
 2. Affectivity (i.e., range, intensity, lability, and appropriateness of emotional response).
 3. Interpersonal functioning.
 4. Impulse control.
B. The enduring pattern is inflexible and pervasive across a broad range of personal and social situations.
C. The enduring pattern leads to clinically significant distress or impairment in social, occupational, or other important areas of functioning.
D. The pattern is stable and of long duration, and its onset can be traced back at least to adolescence or early adulthood.
E. The enduring pattern is not better explained as a manifestation or consequence of another mental disorder.
F. The enduring pattern is not attributable to the physiologic effects of a substance (e.g., a drug of abuse, a medication) or another medical condition (e.g., head trauma).

From American Psychiatric Association APA, 2013. *Diagnostic and statistical manual of disorders* (5th ed.). APA.

ETIOLOGY: CONTEMPORARY VIEWS

Historically, the causes of personality disorders were thought to be only psychological in origin based on problems experienced in childhood, growth and development disturbances, reactions to childhood experiences, family, and environmental factors. Current biologic research and neuroimaging studies have produced data that add to our understanding of the psychopathology of some personality disorders. The aggression often seen in personality disorders, particularly Cluster B, has been linked to alterations in the prefrontal cortex; the secretion of cortisol; and the functioning of neurotransmitters, particularly serotonin (Trifu, Tudor, & Radulescu, 2020). Adverse childhood experiences also affect the functioning of the orbitofrontal cortex (OFC) and amygdala circuitry, resulting in increased pathological personality traits of antagonism and disinhibition (Bounoua, Miglin, Spielberg, Johnson, & Sadeh, 2020). Personality disorders may have a shared link with substance use disorders since both conditions have overlapping behavioral and biological pathways (Smith & Cottler, 2020).

Some personality disorders have been studied more than others, particularly borderline and antisocial disorders. Biologic factors alone are not totally responsible for the occurrence of these disorders. The social environment, coupled with psychological vulnerability, strongly influences the individual. Along with biologic factors, the effects of societal changes, a stressful environment, and adverse childhood experiences are important in the genesis of personality disorders.

PERSONALITY DISORDER CLUSTERS

According to the *DSM-5*, personality disorders are grouped into three clusters based on descriptive features. Cluster A (schizoid, schizotypal, and paranoid disorders) is characterized by odd or eccentric behaviors. Cluster B (narcissistic, histrionic, antisocial, and borderline disorders) is characterized by dramatic, emotional, or erratic behaviors associated with increased anger and aggression. Cluster C (dependent, avoidant, and obsessive-compulsive disorders) is characterized by anxious or fearful behaviors. The following box lists these three clusters. As a simplification, they may be remembered as "Odd, Angry, and Anxious."

Cluster A—Odd, Eccentric Behaviors
Paranoid personality disorder
Schizoid personality disorder
Schizotypal personality disorder

Cluster B—Dramatic, Emotional, Erratic Behaviors
Antisocial personality disorder
Borderline personality disorder
Histrionic personality disorder
Narcissistic personality disorder

Cluster C—Anxious, Fearful Behaviors
Avoidant personality disorder
Dependent personality disorder
Obsessive-compulsive disorder

From American Psychiatric Association APA, 2013. *Diagnostic and statistical manual of disorders* (5th ed.). APA.

Prevalence estimates are 5.7% for cluster A disorders, 1.5% for cluster B disorders, and 6% for cluster C disorders. Data from the 2001 to 2002 National Epidemiologic Survey on Alcohol and Related Conditions suggest that 15% of Americans have at least one personality disorder (American Psychiatric Association APA, 2013). A 2020 study on pooled prevalence from 21 different countries estimated 7.8% of the world had a personality disorder, with 3.8% for Cluster A, 2.8% for Cluster B, and 5.0% for Cluster C (Winsper, Bilgin, Thompson, Marwaha, & Chanen, 2020).

CLUSTER A: ODD-ECCENTRIC

PARANOID PERSONALITY DISORDER

Suspiciousness and mistrust of people characterize a person with paranoid PD. These individuals interpret the actions of others as personal threats, which results in an increase in anxiety and the need for defensiveness. They are hypersensitive to other people's motives and feel vulnerable because they think others mistreat them. They hold grudges and are litigious; because they want vindication for any minor slight, they are quick to sue to prove that the fault does not lie with them. Individuals with paranoid PD cannot laugh at themselves and are often humorless, rigid, and guarded. Their fear of confiding in others makes them secretive or scheming. Their speech is logical and goal-directed, although the basis of an argument may well be false because of their suspiciousness. Other symptoms include prejudice and sometimes ideas of reference. These individuals have a blunted affect, so they might appear cold, although they are capable of close relationships with a select few. However, they might also be suspicious and jealous of people close to them. For example, an individual with paranoid PD might unjustifiably believe that his spouse is having an affair.

In contrast to patients with paranoid schizophrenia, people with paranoid PD do not have fixed delusions or hallucinations. While they may accuse their spouse of cheating, once their significant others can reassure them, usually through excessive evidence of fidelity, they may recant their accusations. But because they are so irrationally mistrustful, these suspicions usually reoccur. Transient psychotic symptoms might be precipitated by extreme stress. People with paranoid PD are hospitalized when their behavior is out of control due to a threat perceived as overwhelming or immediate. Because they are quick to respond with anger or rage if they feel threatened, these individuals might be brought to the hospital because of their potential loss of control and potential for violence. Treatment may be court-ordered for these individuals.

Unique Causes

Studies on the unique etiology of paranoid personality disorder are few. Cluster A has long been thought to be related to schizophrenia, but more recent studies indicate that the relationship between paranoid PD and schizophrenia is not as strong as schizotypal PD. Instead, paranoid PD may have a genetic relationship to affective disorder and delusional disorder and is not related to dopaminergic psychosis. As in other personality disorders, childhood trauma has long been a risk factor in paranoid personality disorder, particularly brain trauma. Whether or not a traumatic brain injury results in a neural circuitry alteration or a functional change like hearing loss, which might result in paranoia due to increased difficulty and stress from communicating with others, is an ongoing area of research (Lee, 2017).

Clinical Example

James Sneed is admitted to the hospital accompanied by a female friend. Mr. Sneed states, "My neighbor is taking my land. He built a fence on my property instead of his. He's always trying to put one over on me." The female friend states that James had barricaded himself in his house, surrounded by his collection of shotguns and threatened to "blow away" his neighbor. James then becomes angry with her, accusing, "You would side with him! In fact, I think you bringing me here isn't to help me at all but to get me out of the picture so you two can take everything I've worked for all my life."

SCHIZOID PERSONALITY DISORDER

People with schizoid personalities do not want to be involved in interpersonal or social relationships, including being part of a family or having sexual experiences. These individuals rarely have close friends and appear aloof and indifferent. They might be thought of as loners because of their introversion and detachment. They respond with short answers to questions and do not initiate spontaneous conversation. They work best in isolation where they do not need to engage with others and do not have emotional responses to praise or criticism. Although they are reality-oriented, solitary activities are more gratifying compared with social situations. In the description of these individuals, one might think of another diagnosis: autism spectrum disorder (ASD). Research is still ongoing with both diagnoses, but the shared interpersonal and social interaction deficits may indicate that schizoid PD is a variant of high functioning autism. Schizoid PD remains a separate diagnosis from ASDs because more research is needed to determine the causes behind similar behaviors. People with schizoid PD may not want or desire connection with others, whereas individuals with ASD may want them but have reduced social capabilities and struggle to form relationships (Cook, Zhang, & Constantino, 2020).

If a person with schizoid PD is hospitalized, usually because of another mental disorder, the nurse-patient relationship should focus initially on building trust, followed by the identification and appropriate verbal expression of feelings. At first, the patient might be able to participate only on the fringes of unit activities because they exhibit no need or desire to be with people. Slowly involving such patients in milieu and group activities, if possible, might help to improve their social skills.

SCHIZOTYPAL PERSONALITY DISORDER

Individuals with schizotypal PD appear similar to patients with mild schizophrenia but do not meet enough of the criteria for a diagnosis of psychosis or schizophrenia. These patients have problems in thinking, perceiving, and communicating. Their outward appearance might be eccentric, and their thinking and behavior might be odd; they are sensitive to the behaviors of others, especially rejection and anger, and feel that they are different and do not fit in. Paranoid ideation, ideas of reference, and odd beliefs are the most prevalent and unchangeable criteria for this disorder. People with schizotypal PD often have an inappropriate affect and excessive social anxiety.

When a person with schizotypal PD is hospitalized, interventions offering support, kindness, and gentle suggestions help the patient become involved in activities with others. It is essential for the nurse to help the patient improve interpersonal relationships, social skills, and appropriate behaviors. Social situations are uncomfortable and cause discomfort and anxiety because of the reactions of others to the patient's appearance and behavior. These patients can benefit from socializing experiences if the interactions are carefully orchestrated. Vocational counseling and assistance with job placement increase these patients' opportunities for success.

Unique Causes

Schizotypal PD is viewed as part of the schizophrenia spectrum. Schizotypal PD and schizophrenia share many symptoms, including peculiar speech and appearance, inappropriate affect, and cognitive symptoms such as odd beliefs. Neurobehavioral, neurophysiological, and neuroimaging abnormalities observed in those with schizophrenia are also seen in people with schizotypal PD but to a lesser extent. The differentiating feature between these two disorders is that schizotypal PD has less functional impairment that does not require antipsychotic medication (Apthorp et al., 2019).

PUTTING IT ALL TOGETHER

PSYCHOTHERAPEUTIC MANAGEMENT

Nurse-Patient Relationship

The most important psychotherapeutic task centers on dealing with trust issues. A professional demeanor coupled with honesty and nonintrusiveness helps to develop trust. Clear, simple explanations and requests reduce the patient's feelings of being threatened or controlled. These patients do not tolerate group therapies that expect or involve confrontation or questioning.

CLUSTER B: DRAMATIC-ERRATIC

ANTISOCIAL PERSONALITY DISORDER

The main feature of antisocial personality disorder (ASPD) is a pattern of disregard for the rights of others, which is usually demonstrated by repeated violations of the law. Before the age of 15, these behaviors are diagnosed as conduct disorder. Affected individuals engage in unlawful behavior, such as driving while intoxicated, engaging in domestic violence, or any number of other harmful and illegal activities. They feel no remorse about hurting strangers or even those they claim to love. While they may seem amiable, internally, they have intense insecurity and anger that they tend to assuage by creating chaos and bringing out the worst in others. Lying, cheating, and stealing are common as people with ASPD are often irresponsible and impulsive. Their criminal behavior places them within the judicial and prison systems more than the mental health system. Not all criminals have ASPD, and not every person with ASPD enters the legal system. However, studies show that those with ASPD have a more violent criminal history and enter the judicial system earlier, more often, and spend more time in prison than offenders without ASPD (DeLisi, Drury, & Elbert, 2019).

The diagnosis of ASPD is based on a history of disordered life functioning rather than on mental status. These individuals might experience distress and anxiety because of others' hostility toward them, but they see the problem as being in others and not in themselves. They use others to their advantage and do not assume responsibility for their behaviors. People with ASPD might appear charming and intellectual; they are smooth talkers and deny and rationalize their behavior. Expected anxiety over their predicament is absent. Guilt, sorrow for offenses, or loyalty is nonexistent as if they do not have a conscience.

? CRITICAL THINKING QUESTION

1. A patient with antisocial personality disorder verbally threatens the staff when limits are set on his manipulative behaviors. How would the nurse manage such a patient's threatening behavior?

Unique Causes

Both genetics and the environment are known to influence ASPD development, and it is often difficult to separate the two. While there may be a heritability for ASPD, environmental factors like adverse childhood experiences play a role in the disorder's development and extent of manifestation. Adverse childhood experiences like abuse, neglect, witnessing violence, and an unstable home life contribute to ASPD manifestation, with childhood sexual abuse and physical abuse being the most significant risk factors (DeLisi, Drury, & Elbert, 2019).

Abnormalities in brain functioning are another common finding in ASPD. Brain scans of individuals with ASPD indicate decreased size and functioning of the amygdala, hippocampus, and prefrontal cortex. Changes in physiologic biomarkers are also seen in those with ASPD. Cortisol and norepinephrine, released from the hypothalamic-pituitary-adrenal (HPA) axis and sympathetic nervous system in response to stress, are altered in people with ASPD, as is are serotonin and testosterone, hormones that impact the stress response and influence levels of aggression. Research findings on ASPD include lower basal cortisol levels, decreased cortisol reactivity, increased testosterone levels, reduced serotonin levels, and decreased oxytocin levels (Junewicz & Billick, 2020). The etiology of ASPD is not linear, and research continues to be conducted on the interplay between environment, genetics, brain structure, and connectivity.

PUTTING IT ALL TOGETHER

PSYCHOTHERAPEUTIC MANAGEMENT

Nurse-Patient Relationship

Long-term treatment is necessary if any type of lasting change is to occur. With short-term hospitalization, the nurse can initiate the therapeutic process by setting firm limits. These patients try to manipulate staff and bend rules for their desires and needs. The nurse must be steadfast and consistent in addressing behaviors and enforcing rules and policies. Both on the unit and for the patient's life, consequences of behavior are a point of focus. Helping the patient become aware of consequences is a concrete way to assist the patient in realizing what the results of behaviors are or will be. The patient must learn to be responsible for their behaviors. Pointing out the patient's behaviors' effects on others is also part of the therapeutic process. The patient must begin to understand others' reactions to his behaviors and why people react the way they do. The nurse avoids moralizing and assists the patient in identifying and verbalizing feelings that might reflect anxiety and depression. Membership in a group can help the patient feel accepted as a person, even if the patient's behaviors are unacceptable. Groups of other individuals with this same diagnosis can effectively confront inappropriate and manipulative behavior because these individuals are experts in spotting smooth-talking, rationalizing, and lying. Such groups can be effective in helping antisocial patients. The keys to working with antisocial patients are consistency on the part of the nursing staff and fostering responsibility in the patients.

BORDERLINE PERSONALITY DISORDER

Individuals with BPD display a pattern of unstable relationships, identity or self-image disturbances, and labile affect along with increased impulsivity (American Psychiatric Association APA, 2013). Those with BPD have high emotionality with limited coping skills and often display anger, self-harm, and suicidality. The alterations in their cognition, mood, and behaviors significantly impair functioning. Of all personality disorders, BPD is the most diagnosed and treated, triggering high health care utilization. These patients usually require hospitalization when they are in a crisis or exhibit self-injurious or suicidal behaviors. When they do not require inpatient care, their somatic symptoms may result in numerous physician office visits, telephone calls, and prescriptions (Campbell, Clarke, Massey, & Lakeman, 2020).

Individuals with BPD have an intense fear of abandonment and use self-defeating behaviors to test if those around them will leave them. Identity problems are apparent in such a person, who is uncertain about their self-image and personal values. In a dysfunctional cycle of fear, insecure self-image, and unstable attachments, people with BPD continually set themselves up for disappointment in others and themselves. They often have problems choosing healthy relationships; impulsively engaging in casual attachments in which they alternate between the over idealization and devaluation of others. For example, an individual with BPD quickly and passionately "falls in love" with the "perfect" person. When this person is disappointing or even inappropriate from the beginning, immediately their significant other is "awful" and has no redeeming qualities. The relationship is another validation that they are not worthy of love and that everyone will leave them. Related to their fear of abandonment, these individuals have great difficulty in being alone and experience intense yet brief relationships.

Patients with BPD display identity confusion. Because they have poor self-conceptualization, they are directionless and feel unworthy, unhappy, restless, or empty. Their affect is labile and erratic; their mood can toggle between extreme emotional responses. Although their pervasive mood is usually dysphoric, others can describe them as "moody" or "too intense." *Projective identification* is used to protect the limited self-esteem that they possess. Patients unconsciously project their angry feelings onto others so that they can identify appropriate emotional responses. Although dysfunctional and inappropriate, blaming others helps these patients deal with their feelings, but this defense mechanism has the opposite intended effect; people *do* display an appropriate response and withdraw from the person with BPD, thereby reinforcing feelings of abandonment and rejection. Intense emotional

pain contributes to mood shifts and may result in acting-out behaviors, such as temper tantrums, physical fights, self-mutilation, and suicidal ideation. Impulsivity is exhibited as substance abuse, overspending, promiscuity, compulsive overeating, and unhealthy risk-taking and decision making. The complexity of behaviors associated with BPD can include severe symptoms of posttraumatic stress disorder and dissociative disorder related to a history of abuse and adversity. See Chapters 27 and 36 for related discussions.

The dissociation used during childhood maltreatment/trauma might result in *splitting*, often found in patients with BPD. The defense mechanism of splitting is defined as the inability to view both the self and others as having both good and bad qualities. Patients with BPD use dichotomous all-or-nothing thinking to view themselves and others as either all good or all bad. One minute a person can be on a pedestal and "the greatest thing ever," and as soon as they disappoint, they are "evil" and "the worst." Splitting also extends to patients' views of themselves. When they see themselves in the worst light, patients are prone to self-injurious or impulsive behaviors. Splitting helps the individual avoid the pain and feelings associated with past abuse and adversity and current situations involving threats of rejection or abandonment. Such individuals may also use self-harm to reflect their internal perception of their own "badness" due to their cognitive distortion of splitting. Self-injurious behavior may provide temporary relief from psychological pain and intolerable feelings by shifting the focus to somatic pain and releasing neurohormones, now leading to a physical manifestation of all the patient's psychic inner turmoil. Self-injurious behaviors include cutting, overdosing, hair pulling, and headbanging. Their intense feelings of hopelessness and despair contribute to their suicidality, and their self-harm should never be ignored and interpreted as simple manipulation or attention-seeking. Patients with BPD are at risk for suicide because of their depression, aggression, impulsivity, underestimation of the lethality of their behavior, and the more prolonged and more frequent occurrence of suicidal thoughts. These patients are often unaware of the likelihood of death and misperceive the lethality of their attempts. Comorbid diagnoses of posttraumatic stress disorder and major depression increase the risk of suicide.

Unique Causes

The development of BPD is multifactorial. Heredity, genetics, environmental factors, childhood experiences, and neurologic and biochemical dysfunction contribute to the complexity of BPD.

Historically BPD was thought to arise when people do not achieve mastery in the developmental stage of *separation-individuation*. In this stage, children learn to separate themselves from parental figures (differentiation) and develop their own identities while also learning that they can be independent yet return to their caregivers as needed (rapprochement); the object of emotional stability, usually the mother, is permanent even when they are not visible (object constancy). If this psychological process is not accomplished, children develop into adults who have disturbed self-images and identities, fear abandonment, and use splitting to process their anger and disappointment dysfunctionally. Within a chaotic, unstable childhood, immature psychological development and maladaptive cognitive distortions cause people with BPD to constantly anticipate and expect abandonment and failure.

Research indicates that early trauma and stress related to adverse childhood experiences like emotional abuse alter brain structure and functioning. Studies have shown alterations in brain scans in those with BPD, particularly in the hypothalamus, hippocampus, amygdala, and prefrontal cortex. Excess activation of the hypothalamic-pituitary axis (HPA) results in increased cortisol production, which overactivates the hippocampus, amygdala, and prefrontal cortex and may account for the increased perception of threats, emotional dysregulation, and cognitive dysfunction seen in BPD (Mainali, Rai, & Rutkofsky, 2020).

The diagnosis, assessment, and treatment of BPD owe much to the work of Marsha Linehan (1993) and her biosocial theory, which posits that there are biologic factors like vulnerable temperament along with social and environmental stressors that cause the hyperarousal, hyperactivity, and a slow return to baseline arousal (impaired habituation) that are key features of the emotional dysregulation in BPD. Using her biosocial theory, Linehan created dialectical behavioral therapy (DBT), a highly effective treatment approach based on cognitive-behavioral therapy (CBT). Research continues to refine the biosocial theory and DBT, but there is agreement that both biology and psychosocial factors are implicated in the etiology of BPD (Rios, 2020).

💡 CRITICAL THINKING QUESTION

2. A 22-year-old woman is admitted to the unit with borderline personality disorder and self-injurious behaviors. What are the nurse's priorities in caring for this patient?

PUTTING IT ALL TOGETHER

PSYCHOTHERAPEUTIC MANAGEMENT

Nurse-Patient Relationship

Many nurses consider the treatment of people with BPD a challenge. Due to their increased use of the healthcare system and the false belief by some healthcare providers that BPD is incurable, the diagnosis carries an increased stigma. When people with BPD are in crisis, a brief hospital admission can be beneficial because an inpatient stay acknowledges the patient's distress, provides structure and safety, and allows for a comprehensive outpatient treatment plan with additional resources to be developed. In addition to symptom stabilization by the medical team, nursing interventions like a behavior management plan are also useful.

The use of empathy by the nurse while maintaining clear boundaries is important in establishing a therapeutic relationship with a patient with a diagnosis of BPD. The nurse is not a friend but a health care professional. The nurse acknowledges the reality of the patient's pain; offers support; and empowers and works with the patient to understand, control, and change dysfunctional behaviors. With the nurse's assistance, the patient can learn to identify and verbalize feelings, control negative behaviors, and slowly begin to replace the negative behaviors with more appropriate actions.

The patient is usually hospitalized because of suicidal behavior, self-mutilation, acute personality disorganization, or inability to function. The nurse conducts a suicide assessment and provides a safe environment to decrease the risk of self-harm and contain impulses. The nurse also works with the patient to find less destructive ways to handle anger, rage, and psychic pain. For self-harm behaviors to diminish, the nurse helps the patient identify feelings and verbally express them nonaggressively, which enables the patient to understand that self-harming actions are habitual responses to experiencing painful emotions. Recognizing behavioral and emotional cues can help the patient decrease impulsive and self-harming behaviors. The nurse then discusses with the patient safe, alternative methods to handle feelings. Using a behavioral contract to decrease self-injurious behaviors in inpatient and outpatient settings provides the patient with clear expectations of behavior. Because these patients feel out-of-control and powerless, the nurse can help them recognize that they can choose to harm themselves or choose alternative methods to manage their feelings and reduce anxiety.

CASE STUDY

Sherry Morgan, a 27-year-old woman, is brought to the psychiatric inpatient unit from the emergency department. Both of her wrists have been sutured and are bandaged. She vacillates between being angry and crying. Sherry states, "I know I am bad. I should not have done it. I do not want to die, but I am tired of the hassles. You wouldn't understand." During the admission interview, the nurse finds that Sherry has had three previous admissions to this inpatient unit during the past 8 years. Sherry states that she refuses to return to work because her boss accuses her of bothering the other employees instead of doing her work. She states that her boss is falsely accusing her of using alcohol and drugs and does not accept her reasons for being absent from work. On the morning of admission, she called her outpatient therapist, whom she had not seen in a year and a half; he agreed to see her at 3 P.M. When she called the therapist back at noon and found that he was at lunch, she used her scissors to cut her wrists.

"I used to think he understood me, but now I know he doesn't care." Her parents are on vacation out of state, and her only close friend is busy with a sick child. She had taken some of her mother's Valium, but it did not calm her down. She has averaged only 3–4 h of sleep each night for the past 5 days and has been unable to eat regular meals. Her attempts to clean her parents' house failed. She could not even finish watering her mother's plants. A male acquaintance of 2 weeks was no longer calling her, so she was frequenting several bars and inviting men home. She never heard from these men again, even though she thought that their relationships were sexually satisfying.

Sherry completed 2 years of college and is dressed attractively. She enjoys reading romance novels and has brought five of her favorite books.

Patients can be helped with understanding themselves and their feelings by having them write in a notebook or journal on a daily basis. In sharing the journal with the nurse, the patient understands self and a sense of autonomy and responsibility. This technique can be useful for many patients with BPD.

Patients with BPD who are victims of abuse need to talk about their trauma in a safe environment. The nurse should acknowledge their pain, convey empathy, and normalize their feelings. When patients understand that their current behaviors are linked to past trauma, they can learn to recognize and change dysfunctional actions toward themselves and others. See Chapter 33 for more detailed interventions.

Patients with BPD are often manipulative. Consistency, limit setting, and supportive confrontation are necessary interventions to provide clear expectations regarding patient behaviors. These patients are adept at sidestepping rules, avoiding consequences, and pitting staff members against each other. Enforcing unit rules, providing clear structure, and placing the responsibility for appropriate behaviors on the patient, although vigorously resisted, benefits a patient with BPD. Consistency toward them and others decreases disappointment and the cognitive distortion that the world is "out to get them." Helping the patient develop realistic short-term goals must be part of the treatment plan if the patient's responsibility for self is to increase.

The psychiatric nurse is in a perfect position to help a patient with BPD with the daily give-and-take issues of life that create many problems for such patients. The nurse should work with the patient on the appropriate verbal expression of feelings and be appropriately self-assertive, even if the nurse's ability to be empathic and nonjudgmental is tested by the patient's behaviors. Boundaries are essential for the improvement and care of the patient with BPD, but they must be set with therapeutic communication in mind and be delivered in a calm, professional manner. Individuals with BPD may have a pattern of undermining themselves when a goal is soon to be achieved (American Psychiatric Association APA, 2013). After a therapy session that went well, a patient with BPD may decompensate and regress to previous self-harming or impulsive behaviors. The nurse might feel frustrated and ineffective as a caregiver and blame or withdraw from the patient. It is important to understand that these behaviors are part of a lifelong condition; while such a patient may be making progress, improvement will not happen overnight. However, understanding and working with the patient therapeutically can result in a positive experience for the nurse and be of lasting import to the patient.

Psychopharmacology

There are no medications approved for treating BPD. Instead, psychopharmacology is employed for specific symptoms and may be part of a comprehensive treatment plan. Antidepressants like selective serotonin reuptake inhibitors (SSRIs) decrease symptoms of a depressed mood and reduce hostility. Antipsychotics control cognitive-perceptual symptoms like transitory hallucinations, paranoia, dissociations, lability, and aggression. Mood stabilizers help with affect stability and impulsivity. Pharmacotherapy aids in clearing symptoms so that patients can integrate the self-regulatory processes and techniques that psychotherapy provides (Parker & Naeem, 2019).

◎ CARE PLAN

Name: Sherry Morgan   **Admission Date:** _____
DSM-5 Diagnosis: Major Depressive Disorder; Borderline Personality Disorder

Assessment	**Areas of strength:** Patient is well-groomed, neat, and clean; is intelligent; enjoys reading.
	Problems: Self-mutilating behavior, absence of support system, loss of job, decreased sleeping and eating, irresponsible and impulsive sexual behavior.
Diagnoses	Risk for self-directed violence related to absence of support system and history of cutting wrists
	Defensive coping related to low self-esteem, as evidenced by angry and labile emotions
Outcomes	**Short-term goals**
Date met: _____	Patient will eliminate self-mutilating behavior and appropriately verbalize feelings of anger and sadness.
Date met: _____	Patient will use alternative methods of coping with emotions.
	Long-term goals
Date met: _____	Patient will schedule outpatient appointment and meeting with boss regarding job problems.
Planning and Interventions	**Nurse-patient relationship:** Monitor and set limits on acting-out behaviors. Assist patient with identification and verbalization of feelings. Teach healthy coping behaviors. Discuss fears about accepting responsibility for self and decision-making. Discuss behaviors interfering with job performance.
	Psychopharmacology: Fluoxetine (Prozac) 20 mg every morning; trazodone 150 mg at bedtime.
	Milieu management: Groups focusing on self-esteem, stress and anger management, assertiveness training, social skills, problem-solving skills, and discharge planning.
Evaluation	Patient has not engaged in self-mutilating behavior. Patient is appropriately verbalizing feelings of anger and sadness. Patient has identified and is using two methods of coping with feelings. Patient has a crisis plan when overwhelmed by emotions.
Referrals	Appointment weekly after discharge with therapist at outpatient mental health clinic.

3. Staff members on the unit are frustrated and angry with a patient diagnosed with BPD who is attempting to pit members on the various shifts against each other. They are even beginning to be angry with each other for the inconsistencies in this patient's care. What strategies should the head nurse employ to help the staff and ultimately treat the patient?

Milieu Management

Patients with BPD are viewed as among the most difficult and exasperating patients for nurses to treat, so it is vital that the nurse is aware of any countertransference that may occur. On admission to an inpatient psychiatric unit, a patient with BPD may exhibit a need for attention and affection by contradictory behaviors of manipulation, dependency, or acting out. Frustration on the part of the staff might be seen as rejection. This perception by the patient can lead to increased anger and withdrawal because of fear of abandonment. Under stress, the patient regresses to immature behaviors and is unable to cope with conflict. The patient vacillates between clinging and disengaged behaviors, as demonstrated by wanting the staff to solve all problems or viewing inpatient treatment as unnecessary and meaningless. When progress seems to be occurring, a patient with BPD may suddenly exhibit opposite behaviors, making it seem as if the staff will have to start over. It is vital for nurses to control their emotions and remain professional so that they do not adversely contribute to the patient's distress and undo the slow progress that the patient is making.

Interventions mentioned in the discussion of the nurse-patient relationship regarding firm limits, consistency, and clear structure are essential to the milieu for patients with BPD. The patient's manipulation of other patients must be addressed in a nonjudgmental manner that does not stigmatize the patient and contribute further to their feelings of inadequacy and negativity. Consistent communication among staff members is essential to minimize the patient's attempts to divide and split them. Therapeutic activities that are important for these patients in both inpatient and outpatient settings include assertiveness training, problem-solving, stress management, and anger management.

Referral to self-help groups for alcohol and drug problems, eating disorders, and victimization is also important. Vocational counseling and training are important to foster autonomous and independent functioning. Residential treatment may have to be considered, particularly for patients with chronic self-destructive behaviors.

NARCISSISTIC PERSONALITY DISORDER

People with narcissistic PD have increased interpersonal antagonism, resulting in arrogance, a lack of empathy, a sense of entitlement, and a need for admiration. The key component of narcissistic PD is grandiosity. A patient with

HIGHLIGHTING THE EVIDENCE

Balanced Therapy: How to Avoid Conflict and Help Patients With Borderline Personality Disorder

Description

Dialectical behavioral therapy (DBT) is an evidence-based, comprehensive treatment modality that helps patients with BPD who have problems regulating their emotions and are suicidal. The outpatient model for DBT requires patients to meet weekly in individual psychotherapy and skills training groups. Patients consult with their therapists between sessions by telephone to decrease suicide crisis behaviors, increase behavioral skills, and decrease feelings of conflict and alienation or distance from the therapist.

DBT consists of four stages. In stage 1, patients move from severe behavioral dyscontrol to behavioral control to decrease suicidal and other life-threatening behaviors. Stage 2 consists of moving from desperation to emotional experiencing. In stage 3, patients address problems in living and moving toward happiness/unhappiness. In stage 4, patients move from incompleteness to a capacity for joy and freedom.

Results

In seven randomized controlled trials, DBT was shown to be useful to patients with BPD. In the initial trial by DuBose and Linehan (2005), subjects were assessed every 4 months while in treatment for 1 year and for 1 year afterward. DBT was effective in reducing suicide attempts and self-injury; decreasing premature dropout from therapy; reducing emergency department admission and length of psychiatric hospitalization; and reducing drug use, depression, hopelessness, and anger.

Implications

Nurses trained in DBT can offer patients with BPD effective, evidence-based, comprehensive, and compassionate treatment.

Modified from DuBose, A. P., & Linehan, M. M. (2005). Balanced therapy: How to avoid conflict and help "borderline" patients. *Current Psychiatry, 4*, 12.

narcissistic PD exaggerates their importance and achievements. This grandiosity is rooted in reality but is a distortion or embellishment of the actual situation or accomplishment to make themselves feel important, which is different from the delusions of grandeur found in patients with schizophrenia or bipolar disorders. For example, a man with narcissistic PD might say that he was a star football player in high school and that he could have played in the Super Bowl; he does not tell the nurse that he barely made the second-string on the football team in high school.

The grandiose self-importance of a patient with narcissistic PD is displayed through interpersonal exploitation, lack of empathy, arrogance, intense envy, and a sense of entitlement. These individuals may also superficially seem supportive to others but secretly harbor contempt for the person being helped and manipulate the interaction to reflect their specialness, goodness, or superior capabilities. These patients believe that they are special and unique and harbor fantasies of brilliance and success.

Another less obvious component of narcissistic PD is vulnerability. Individuals with narcissistic PD are intensely troubled when faced with disappointments and threats to their extremely positive self-image. Because no one is perfect, these patients must use maladaptive strategies to manage the constant obstacles and challenges to the unfulfilled or unattainable perfection they see in themselves. A person with vulnerable narcissism might appear nonchalant or indifferent to criticism while hiding feelings of anger, rage, or emptiness. Constant reinforcement from others is needed to boost such a person's self-esteem. These individuals use others selfishly to meet their own needs and to lessen their loneliness and feelings of inadequacy.

Clinical Example
A patient has been admitted to the unit and insists on a private room with a telephone and television because he needs to keep up with the reports on the financial news network. He says he's "not like these other people up here" and that he can't let their problems keep him from his important work. When you are unable to meet his demands, he smugly states, "You wouldn't understand all the big decisions I have to make for others. You're just a nurse."

Unique Causes

There are limited data on etiology, but the available research indicates that cold, overprotective parenting styles may be linked to the development of narcissistic PD (Valashjardi, MacLean, & Charles, 2020).

PUTTING IT ALL TOGETHER

PSYCHOTHERAPEUTIC MANAGEMENT

Nurse-Patient Relationship

A therapeutic nurse-patient relationship may be difficult to achieve, as patients with narcissistic PD feel that they have nothing to learn from the nurse. Careful use of supportive confrontation may point out discrepancies between what the patient says and what exists to increase responsibility for self and reinforce reality. Limit-setting and consistency are used to decrease manipulation and entitlement behaviors. Realistic short-term goals focused on the here and now, not the past (which can be exaggerated) or the future (which can be fantastical), are important to decrease rationalization and to increase responsibility for self. Group therapy provides the opportunity for the patient to see how his behavior affects others and, perhaps for the first time, gives the patient a chance to become involved with the problems of others. The nurse must be careful that the patient with narcissistic PD does not dominate the group.

HISTRIONIC PERSONALITY DISORDER

A person with histrionic PD dramatizes events and draws attention to self. The person is extroverted and thrives on being the center of attention. Behavior is flirty, silly, frivolous, and seductive. They dress provocatively, attempting to appear more youthful to gain as many devotees as they can. Speech is exaggerated and theatrical but lacking in depth and insight. The person is highly excitable and energized, always in a hurry and restless. Overreactions and excessive emotionality to minor events are seen. These behaviors are a way to form quick relationships that lack genuine intimacy. They are notorious name-droppers who regard people they just met as dear friends. They are easily influenced and will reward admirers with a ticket to the show that is their lives. But like an actor passionately reading lines they did not write, the content is not their own, so they have difficulty making decisions when challenged for rationales and can easily become dependent on others. Those with a diagnosis of histrionic PD may use somatic complaints to avoid responsibility and support dependency. Dissociation is a common defense to avoid feelings. Such a patient, while superficially attuned to the moods of others, cannot deal with their feelings.

Unique Causes

The causes of histrionic PD are unknown but are likely a result of many factors, including high emotional responsiveness and the role modeling of histrionic behaviors previously observed in caregivers.

PUTTING IT ALL TOGETHER

PSYCHOTHERAPEUTIC MANAGEMENT

Nurse-Patient Relationship

People with histrionic PD do not generally present for treatment; if they do, it is when their need to be admired has not been fulfilled, leading to an emotional crisis. It is important that nurses be consistent with these patients and provide therapeutic opportunities for the patient to make decisions for themselves. The patient's tendency is to be dependent so that their needs are fulfilled. The nurse should provide positive reinforcement for appropriate behaviors and expressions of feelings that foster independence but strike a blend between encouraging without overvaluing.

CLUSTER C: ANXIOUS-FEARFUL

DEPENDENT PERSONALITY DISORDER

The main characteristic of dependent PD is a "pervasive and excessive need to be taken care of that leads to submissive and clinging behaviors and fears of separation" (American Psychiatric Association APA, 2013). Dependent individuals want others to make daily decisions for them, such as the type of clothes to wear and the type of job to seek. They need direction and reassurance. These individuals feel inferior and cling to others excessively because they are afraid that they will be left alone. Avoiding responsibility and expressing helplessness, the person maintains the need to rely on others. These persons perceive themselves as being unable to function without the help of others. They are willing to perform unpleasant tasks so that others will support them and not disturb the attachment. They are passive and avoid conflict, often staying in dysfunctional relationships because that is better than being alone.

Clinical Example

A patient has been telling the nurse about her alcoholic and abusive husband. She has been married to him for 16 years. She expresses sadness and frustration about her marriage but states, "How could I leave him? Who will take care of me? I could never live alone. He's not perfect, but at least he cares about me." The patient continues to ask the nurse what she should do.

Unique Causes

Biochemical and genetic factors have not been correlated with dependent PD. Psychosocial theories consider culture to be the basis of the development of this disorder.

PUTTING IT ALL TOGETHER

PSYCHOTHERAPEUTIC MANAGEMENT

Nurse-Patient Relationship

The nurse slowly works on decision-making with the patient to increase responsibility for self in daily living. The patient needs assistance with managing anxiety because it will increase as the patient assumes more responsibility for self. Assertiveness is an important area of the nurse's teaching, which enables the patient to state clearly their feelings, needs, and desires. Verbalization of feelings and ways to cope with them are essential.

AVOIDANT PERSONALITY DISORDER

Patients with the avoidant PD fear disapproval and rejection, so they avoid relationships. They are timid, socially uncomfortable, and withdrawn. They feel inadequate and are hypersensitive to criticism. Although they are fearful and shy, patients with avoidant personality disorder desire relationships; however, they need to be certain of being liked before making social contacts. To keep their anxiety at a minimal level, these individuals avoid situations in which they might be disappointed or embarrassed. When interacting with someone, this person sounds uncertain and lacks self-confidence and is afraid to ask questions or speak up in public, withdraws from social support, and conveys helplessness. In contrast with another PD with a similar presentation, in schizoid PD, patients display high levels of social anhedonia; they have no strong desire for relationships. People with avoidant PD have a strong desire for social attachments, but they cannot risk the hurt that may occur with any relationship.

Unique Causes

Few biologic, genetic, and psychological studies have been conducted on avoidant PD, but a combination of genetics,

temperament, childhood environment, and attachment style is part of the development of avoidant PD. Avoidant PD may be associated with social anxiety disorder and could be considered the extreme end of this spectrum (Fariba & Sapra, 2020).

PUTTING IT ALL TOGETHER

PSYCHOTHERAPEUTIC MANAGEMENT

Nurse-Patient Relationship

The nurse helps the patient gradually confront their fears. Discussing the patient's feelings and fears before and after doing something they are afraid to do is essential for the relationship. The nurse supports and directs the patient in accomplishing small goals. Helping the patient to be assertive and develop social skills is necessary. The nurse includes the patient in interactions with others and progresses to small groups as the patient can tolerate them. Because of the patient's anxiety, relaxation techniques are taught to enable the patient to be successful in interactions. The nurse gives positive feedback to the patient for any real success and for any attempts to engage in interactions with others to promote self-esteem.

OBSESSIVE-COMPULSIVE PERSONALITY DISORDER

Individuals with obsessive-compulsive PD are perfectionistic and inflexible. These individuals are overly strict and often set standards for themselves that are too high; their work is never good enough. They are preoccupied with rules, trivial details, and procedures. When others are asked to describe them, the phrase "control freak" might be used. These individuals find it challenging to express warmth or tender emotions. There is little give-and-take in their interactions with others; they are rigid, controlling, and cold. Such a person is serious about all their activities, so having fun or experiencing pleasure is difficult. Because the person is afraid of making mistakes, they can be indecisive or put off decisions until all the facts have been obtained. The person's affect is constricted, and he might speak in a monotone. Because personality traits are ego-syntonic, perfectionism does not disturb these individuals; they see nothing wrong with a rigorous, orderly approach. In contrast, obsessive-compulsive disorder is part of the anxiety spectrum and is *ego-dystonic*; the need to check obsessions compulsively does cause these patients tremendous distress because they recognize the abnormality of their thoughts and behaviors.

Unique Causes

Early parent-child relationships around issues of autonomy, control, and authority might predispose a person to this disorder. Many of the features of obsessive-compulsive PD resemble a "type A" personality and may be present in people at risk for myocardial infarction. There is an association between obsessive-compulsive PD and eating disorders, and their etiologies may be similar (American Psychiatric Association APA, 2013).

PUTTING IT ALL TOGETHER

PSYCHOTHERAPEUTIC MANAGEMENT

Nurse-Patient Relationship

The nurse must support the patient in exploring their feelings and in attempting new experiences and situations. The nurse helps the patient with decision-making and encourages follow-through behavior. Sometimes a need exists to confront the patient's procrastination and intellectualization. The nurse teaches the patient the importance of leisure activities and exploring interests in this area. Because the patient lacks awareness of how they affect others, the patient needs to look at and understand others' views of them. Teaching the patient that they are human and that it is all right to make mistakes helps decrease irrational beliefs about the need to be perfect.

STUDY NOTES

1. Personality traits are enduring approaches to the world expressed in the way a person thinks, feels, and behaves.
2. When personality traits become rigid and dysfunctional and cause distress to self and others, a personality disorder might be diagnosed. Personal discomfort arises primarily from others' reactions to or behaviors toward the person.
3. The odd-eccentric cluster of personality disorders includes the following:
   a. Paranoid, characterized by suspiciousness and mistrust
   b. Schizoid, characterized by no close friends, solitary activities
   c. Schizotypal, characterized by symptoms similar to but less severe than symptoms of schizophrenia
4. The dramatic-erratic cluster of personality disorders includes the following:
   a. Antisocial, characterized by the violation of others' rights without guilt
   b. Borderline, characterized by problems with self-identity, interpersonal relationships, emotional dysregulation, and self-injurious behaviors, an intense fear of abandonment
   c. Narcissistic, characterized by grandiosity, arrogance, and lack of empathy
   d. Histrionic, characterized by dramatic behaviors, attention-seeking, and superficiality
5. The anxious-fearful cluster of personality disorders includes the following:
   a. Dependent, characterized by submissiveness, helplessness, fear of responsibility, and reliance on others for decision making
   b. Avoidant, characterized by no close relationships, timidity, socially withdrawn behavior, and hypersensitivity to criticism
   c. Obsessive-compulsive, characterized by indecisiveness, perfectionism, inflexibility, and difficulty expressing feelings
6. Nursing interventions for individuals with personality disorders help the patient recognize specific behaviors that are distressing to self, others, or both; to manage feelings; and to develop coping behaviors that are less dysfunctional.

REFERENCES

American Psychiatric Association (APA). (2013). *Diagnostic and statistical manual of mental disorders* (5th ed.). Arlington, Virginia: APA.

Apthorp, D., Bolbecker, A. R., Bartolomeo, L. A., O'Donnell, B. F., & Hetrick, W. P. (2019). Postural sway abnormalities in schizotypal personality disorder. *Schizophrenia Bulletin*, 45(3), 512–521. https://doi.org/10.1093/schbul/sby141.

Bounoua, N., Miglin, R., Spielberg, J. M., Johnson, C. L., & Sadeh, N. (2020). Childhood trauma moderates morphometric associations between orbitofrontal cortex and amygdala: Implications for pathological personality traits. *Psychological Medicine*, 1–10. https://doi.org/10.1017/S0033291720004468.

Campbell, K., Clarke, K. A., Massey, D., & Lakeman, R. (2020). Borderline personality disorder: To diagnose or not to diagnose? That is the question. *International Journal of Mental Health Nursing*, 29(5), 972–981. https://doi.org/10.1111/inm.12737.

Cook, M. L., Zhang, Y., & Constantino, J. N. (2020). On the continuity between autistic and schizoid personality disorder trait burden: A prospective study in adolescence. *The Journal of Nervous and Mental Disease*, 208(2), 94–100. https://doi.org/10.1097/NMD.0000000000001105.

DeLisi, M., Drury, A. J., & Elbert, M. J. (2019). The etiology of antisocial personality disorder: The differential roles of adverse childhood experiences and childhood psychopathology. *Comprehensive Psychiatry*, 92, 1–6. https://doi.org/10.1016/j.comppsych.2019.04.001.

DuBose, A. P., & Linehan, M. M. (2005). Balanced therapy: How to avoid conflict and help "borderline" patients. *Current Psychiatry*, 4(4), 13–26. https://cdn.mdedge.com/files/s3fs-public/Document/September-2017/0404CP_Article1.pdf.

Eaton, N. R., & Greene, A. L. (2018). Personality disorders: Community prevalence and socio-demographic correlates. *Current Opinion in Psychology*, 21, 28–32. https://doi.org/10.1016/j.copsyc.2017.09.001.

Fariba, K., & Sapra, A. (2020). Avoidant personality disorder: *StatPearls*. StatPearls Publishing. https://www.ncbi.nlm.nih.gov/books/NBK559325/.

Junewicz, A., & Billick, S. B. (2020). Conduct disorder: Biology and developmental trajectories. *Psychiatric Quarterly, 91*(1), 77–90. https://doi.org/10.1007/s11126-019-09678-5.

Lee, R. (2017). Mistrustful and misunderstood: A review of paranoid personality disorder. *Current Behavioral Neuroscience Reports, 4*(2), 151–165. https://doi.org/10.1007/s40473-017-0116-7.

Linehan, M. M. (1993). *Cognitive-behavioral treatment of borderline personality disorder*. Guilford Press.

Mainali, P., Rai, T., & Rutkofsky, I. H. (2020). From child abuse to developing borderline personality disorder into adulthood: Exploring the neuromorphological and epigenetic pathway. *Cureus, 12*(7), e9474. https://doi.org/10.7759/cureus.9474.

McCabe, G. A., & Widiger, T. A. (2020). A comprehensive comparison of the ICD-11 and DSM-5 section III personality disorder models. *Psychological Assessment, 32*(1), 72–84. https://doi.org/10.1037/pas0000772.

Oltmanns, J. R., & Widiger, T. A. (2020). The five-factor personality inventory for ICD-11: A facet-level assessment of the ICD-11 trait model. *Psychological Assessment, 32*(1), 60–71. https:/doi.org/10.1037/pas0000763.

Parker, J. D., & Naeem, A. (2019). FPIN's help desk answers: Pharmacologic treatment of borderline personality disorder. *American Family Physician, 99*(5).

Rios, E. Y. Z. (2020). Dialectical behavior therapy in the treatment of borderline personality disorder. *Journal of Cognitive-Behavioral Psychotherapy and Research, 9*(2), 148–157. https://doi.org/10.5455/JCBPR.49540.

Smith, N., & Cottler, L. B. (2020). What's old is new again: Updated findings on personality disorders and substance use disorders. *Current Opinion in Psychiatry, 33*(1), 51–56. https://doi.org/10.1097/YCO.0000000000000558. PMID: 31577542.

Trifu, S. C., Tudor, A., & Radulescu, I. (2020). Aggressive behavior in psychiatric patients in relation to hormonal imbalance (Review). *Experimental and Therapeutic Medicine, 20*(4), 3483–3487. https://doi.org/10.3892/etm.2020.8974.

Valashjardi, A., MacLean, R., & Charles, K. (2020). Recollections of parenting styles in the development of narcissism: The role of gender. *Personality and Individual Differences, 167*, 110246. https://doi.org/10.1016/j.paid.2021.110659.

Volkert, J., Gablonski, T. C., & Rabung, S. (2018). Prevalence of personality disorders in the general adult population in Western countries: Systematic review and meta-analysis. *The British Journal of Psychiatry, 213*(6), 709–715. https://doi.org/10.1192/bjp.2018.202.

Winsper, C., Bilgin, A., Thompson, A., Marwaha, S., Chanen, A. M., et al. (2020). The prevalence of personality disorders in the community: A global systematic review and meta-analysis. *The British Journal of Psychiatry, 216*(2), 69–78. https://doi.org/10.1192/bjp.2019.166.

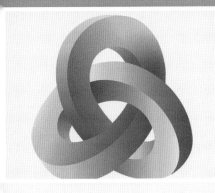

30

Sexual Disorders and Gender Dysphoria

W. Chance Nicholson and Kate Pfeiffer

http://evolve.elsevier.com/

LEARNING OBJECTIVES

- Recognize the importance of the nurse's role in assessing patients' sexual concerns and complications.
- Describe the categories of sexual dysfunctions, paraphilic disorders, and gender dysphoria.
- Identify the issues related to the care of patients or clients with sexual disorders.

- Demonstrate an understanding of the need for referring patients with sexual disorders for further assessment and specialty treatment.

This chapter presents an overview of the sexual disorders, followed by gender dysphoria, as designated by the DSM-5. Sexual disorders are divided into two major categories: *sexual dysfunctions* and *paraphilic disorders*. To understand how sexual health can be disordered, it is important to recognize what constitutes healthy sexual behavior beyond prevention of sexually transmitted illness. Sexual health encompasses the development, knowledge, awareness, and acceptance of one's own behaviors and values around sexuality relative to emotional, physical, mental, and social well-being. Importantly, it involves the choice of intimacy, the communication of and ability to express needs and desires, sexual functionality (i.e., ability to experience desire, arousal, and/or orgasm), and, ultimately, the achievement of healthy sexual satisfaction. It requires intention and accountability for positive, consensual, and safe sexual encounters while creating boundaries free of coercion, discrimination, trauma, and violence. As such, to satisfy the status of healthy sexuality, sexual rights of all persons or subjects must be maintained. *Gender dysphoria*, on the other hand, is not a sexual disorder. It is defined as incongruence of gender, with separate, developmentally appropriate diagnostic criteria for children and adults.

DSM-5 CRITERIA AND TERMINOLOGY

The DSM-5 (American Psychiatric Association, 2013) categorizes sexual dysfunctions as a significant disturbance in a person's ability to respond sexually or to experience sexual pleasure. Paraphilic disorders are characterized by intense sexual urges in conflict with social norms or expectations around sexual activities or preferences.

Gender dysphoria is characterized by a persistent affective/cognitive discontent with one's experienced, expressed, and assigned gender. As with all psychiatric disorders, each must cause clinically significant distress or an impairment of social, personal, and/or occupational function before a diagnosis is warranted.

NORM'S NOTES We will now discuss a topic that evokes a kind of proscriptive curiosity. Sexual disorders come in many varieties, from the inability to participate in healthy sexual activity to atypical, and even illegal behaviors. You probably will not run into these individuals during your clinical rotation, but I think you will find this short chapter interesting.

DSM-5 DIAGNOSES RELATED TO SEXUAL AND GENDER DISORDERS

1. Sexual dysfunctions
2. Paraphilic disorders
3. Gender dysphoria

SEXUAL DYSFUNCTIONS

Sexual dysfunctions are best conceptualized using a quadriphasic human sexual response cycle: (1) desire, (2) arousal, (3) orgasm, and (4) pain. Dysfunctions are classified according to the phase primarily affected. While each of these represent stepwise phases in the sexual response (except pain),

BOX 30.1   Initial Nursing Assessment of Sexual Concerns

1. Describe any difficulties that you have experienced with sexual performance or satisfaction.
2. What are your feelings and concerns about sexuality?
3. How satisfied are you with your sexual relationship?
4. What type of changes would you like to make in your sexual relationship?
5. What type of negative sexual experiences have you had?

it is best to think of them as existing on an interacting spectrum in which dysfunction can occur at or influence multiple phases. For example, if someone is experiencing a delayed or nonexistent orgasm (phase three), then over time, this might also reduce one's desire and/or arousal toward sex (phase one and two).

As part of the admission interview, the nurse assesses each patient for potential or actual problems with sexual functioning. Sexual dysfunction (Box 30.1) lists initial questions that the nurse might use to assess the patient's feelings and concerns about sexuality. Once sexual dysfunction has been identified, it is important for nurses to understand the interactions between biological, psychological, and/or psychosocial etiologies to help guide assessment (Box 30.2).

A thorough medical, psychiatric, and social history should emphasize onset, duration, and situation, as this could help identify the cause. For example, does sexual dysfunction occur in response to highly anxious states? If so, what promotes the anxiety? Did it occur after starting a selective serotonin reuptake inhibitor (SSRI), insulin, or blood pressure

medication? Does it only occur with your spouse/partner? Does it occur during penetration and/or stimulation?

Furthermore, this timeline will help distinguish the subtypes: *lifelong* or *acquired*. Lifelong dysfunction suggests that the issue runs concurrent to sexual activity, while *acquired* dysfunction onsets after a period of normal sexual functioning. Likewise, determining onset helps establish sexual dysfunction specifiers: *generalized* (dysfunction not limited to certain types of stimulation, situations, or partners) or *situational* (dysfunction limited to certain types of stimuli, situations, or partners). The duration of symptoms within the dysfunction must be at least 6 months to be considered a disorder (American Psychiatric Association, 2013).

The experience of sexual dysfunction is often accompanied by compounding distress or interpersonal conflict, which only exacerbates the problem; therefore, treatment and referrals should focus on both the physiologic aspects and the emotional needs of the individual. Table 30.1 provides an overview of sexual disorder classifications and select treatments. Note, as mentioned previously, sexual dysfunction exists on a spectrum; therefore, many of the treatment approaches overlap for each dysfunction type.

? CRITICAL THINKING QUESTION

1. A patient with insulin-dependent diabetes states, "After I leave the hospital, I'm going to use only half of the prescribed insulin because I heard insulin might affect my sexual performance." What are your interventions with this patient?

BOX 30.2   Select Sexual Dysfunction Etiologies

Biological
- Cardiovascular: Hypertension, atherosclerosis, high cholesterol
- Endocrine: Thyroid, pituitary, adrenal gland issues
- Metabolic: Diabetes
- Neurological: Multiple sclerosis, neuropathy, tumor
- Psychiatric: Depression, anxiety, posttraumatic stress disorder
- Skeletal: Spinal cord injuries
- Hormones: Deficient testosterone, estrogen, other androgens
- Reproductive: Infection, menopause, genital trauma, premenstrual syndrome

Psychological and Psychosocial
- Fears or guilt surrounding sex or dysfunction
- Stress
- Sexual abuse or trauma (past or present)
- Marital discord
- Recent divorce
- Occupational changes
- Culture or religious conflict or practices
- Partner context (lack of foreplay, intimacy; sexual dissatisfaction; abusive; health status of partner; infertility)

Substances
- Chronic marijuana use (particularly in females)
- Nicotine
- Alcohol
- Stimulants
- Opioids

Medications
- Antidepressants: SSRIs (e.g., paroxetine, fluoxetine), serotonin norepinephrine reuptake inhibitors (SNRIs) (e.g., venlafaxine), tricyclics, monoamine oxidase inhibitors (MAOIs)
- Sedative-hypnotics: Benzodiazepines (e.g., alprazolam), barbiturates (e.g., phenobarbital)
- Anticonvulsants: Carbamazepine, phenytoin, primidone
- Antihistamines: H_1 (e.g., diphenhydramine) and H_2 antagonists (e.g., cimetidine)
- Parkinson: Anticholinergics (e.g., benztropine)
- Nonsteroidal antiinflammatory drugs (NSAIDs): Propionic acid class (e.g., naproxen)
- Antihypertensives and diuretics: Beta-blockers (e.g., propanolol), calcium-channel blockers (e.g., nifedipine), furosemide
- Birth control: Intramuscular depo provera
- Any medication that binds testosterone

Modified from Brotto, L., Atallah, S., Johnson-Agbakwu, C., et al. (2016). Psychological and interpersonal dimensions of sexual function and dysfunction. *Journal of Sexual Medicine, 13*(4), 538–571; Rew, K. T., & Heidelbaugh, J. J. (2016). Erectile dysfunction. *American Family Physician, 94*(10), 820–827; Shivananda, M. J., & Rao, T. S. (2016). Sexual dysfunction in medical practice. *Current Opinion in Psychiatry, 29*(6), 331–335.

TABLE 30.1 Sexual Disorder Types and Definitions

Sexual Disorder Types and Definitions	Select Psychiatric Treatments
1. **Sexual aversion or hypoactive sexual desire:** Experience anxiety, fear, or disgust around sexual interaction; have little or no interest in sexual activities (decreased libido); more common in women (age not a factor). **Female sexual arousal disorder:** Inhibited response to sexual stimulation; altered arousal perception and lacks vaginal lubrication; increase after menopause.	**Male biomedical:** Correct underlying problem (e.g., medications, depression, low testosterone). No standard pharmacological treatment available but could switch from SSRI or SNRIs to bupropion. **Female biomedical:** Correct underlying cause. Nonhormonal medication called flibanserin ($5\text{-}HT_{1A}$ agonist and $5\text{-}HT_{2A}$ antagonists; also binds $5\text{-}HT_{2B}$, $5\text{-}HT_{2C}$, and D_4 receptors); estrogen vaginal cream; combination of estrogen and progesterone; testosterone (particularly postmenopausal women); bupropion; lubricants. **Male/female therapy:** Cognitive-behavioral therapy; mindfulness; psychosexual and relationship; sex therapy; exercise; sensate focus (i.e., partners taking focus off sex and exploring affection/intimacy).
2. **Erectile dysfunction:** Cannot obtain or maintain an erection sufficient for sexual activity. Affects 10% of men and increases with age.	**Biomedical:** Reduce substance use (e.g., alcohol, nicotine, etc.); phosphodiesterase inhibitors (e.g., sildenafil); testosterone; vascular reconstructive surgery; penile implants; vasodilators (e.g., alprostadil). **Therapy:** Same as noted in section 1.

3. **Male orgasmic disorders:**
 • *Delayed:* Experience a marked delay or absence of orgasm.
 • *Premature* (early): Reaches orgasm within 1 min of vaginal penetration and before desired. Occurs in approximately 25% of men.
    • Mild: Occurs within 30–60 s
    • Moderate: Occurs within 15–30 s
    • Severe: Occurs within 15 s
 Female orgasmic disorders: Anorgasmia—inability to orgasm. Many woman can achieve orgasm via oral, hand, or vibrator, but not from penis.
	Male biomedical: Off-label: buspirone, cyproheptadine, amantadine.
	 Male therapy: Same as above in section 1. Stop-start technique—Partner or individual stimulates male erection, then stops, then repeats.
	 Female therapy: Eros clitoral therapy device; sex therapy; Kegel exercises (strengthen muscles [pubococcygeal] surrounding vagina).

4. **Genito-pelvic pain/penetration:** Genital pain during intercourse. Can be persistent; varies in intensity, burning or sharp; chronic and phobic difficulties with penis, digit, and/or object vaginal penetration despite a desire to do so. For men, pain is in testes/penis (often caused by Peyronie disease); retraction of foreskin.	**Therapy:** Vaginal dilators; systematic desensitization; same as noted previously in section 1.

Modified from Shivananda, M. J., & Rao, T. S. (2016). Sexual dysfunction in medical practice. *Current Opinion in Psychiatry, 29*(6), 331–335; Worsley, R., Miller, K. K., Parish, S. J., & Davis, S. R. (2016). Role of estrogens and estrogen-like compounds in female sexual function and dysfunction. *Journal of Sexual Medicine, 13*(3), 305–316.

PARAPHILIC DISORDERS

Historically, the DSM classified sexual aberrations as "psychopathic personality" and "personality disorder of sociopathic subtype," suggesting that all sexual aberrations were criminal acts (unlawful) and those participating must be psychopaths. The DSM-5 introduced more precise and evidence-based nomenclature, which changes "paraphilia" to a "paraphilic disorder." The term "paraphilia" has now been repurposed to represent a persistent and atypical sexual pattern that *does not* cause distress to the individual. The qualifier "disorder" was added to reflect distress or impairment experienced by the individual, as well as the satisfaction experienced when inflicting personal harm (or risk) to others. This change reflects both scientific and social shifts in our understanding of these conditions as existing within and outside the law. While some behaviors threaten sexual norms and are clinically significant, others simply represent social taboos and do not meet clinical definitions or concerns.

A paraphilic disorder is an intense and chronic sexual arousal related to anything other than a physically normal and mature consenting adult. Importantly, for a disorder to be diagnosed, physically engaging in the paraphilic behavior is not a necessary requirement. Paraphilic disorders involve any behaviors, fantasies, fetishes, and/or urges directed toward an abnormal activity (e.g., nonconsensual voyeurism or exposure of one's genital areas) or target (e.g., animals, children, etc.), regardless of sexual contact. Abnormal activities can be divided into *courtship* disorders (distortions of acceptable human courtship behaviors [e.g., pedophilia]) and *algolagnic* disorders (which involve pain and suffering [e.g., sexual sadism]) (American Psychiatric Association, 2013).

Generally, treatment for severe paraphilic disorders occurs in the forensic setting (e.g., prison, etc.). Outpatient treatment programs and programs for incarcerated individuals also provide information about assessment and treatment, with most research being carried out on convicted sex offenders. In the inpatient setting, nurses might encounter a paraphilic disorder in the context of comorbid disorders such as mood, suicidal ideation, substance-related, anxiety, impulse, and personality (particularly, antisocial). The goal is to treat the underlying condition versus paraphilic disorder. On occasion, individuals with a paraphilic disorder might also seek inpatient admission to reduce criminal sentencing or prosecution. Individuals are unlikely to seek treatment specific to the paraphilic disorder itself due to the legal or social ramifications (First, 2014).

Treatment

The strategy for treating paraphilic disorders involves combining psychotherapeutic and psychopharmacologic approaches. The intensity and duration of treatments are based on severity of paraphilic disorders, degree of distress, or those at the highest risk of perpetration or victimization. At minimum, treatment occurs over a 3- to 5-year period, with many requiring life-long therapies. Cognitive-behavioral therapy (CBT) is considered the gold-standard treatment that focuses on cognitive distortions. In addition, eye movement desensitization and reprocessing (EMDR), empathy and impulse control training, along with biofeedback and neurofeedback therapies are often added as complements. Pharmacological treatments are divided into three categories: (1) SSRIs, (2) antiandrogens, and (3) gonadotrophin-releasing hormone (GnRH) analogs (Box 30.3).

As discussed in this book, SSRIs can cause decreased libido, impair orgasms, and interfere with ejaculation (particularly in higher doses). Pharmacological treatments for sexual dysfunctions take advantage of their $5HT_2$ activation and use these side effects for a therapeutic benefit. Steroidal antiandrogen therapy reduces testosterone levels and is the gold-standard pharmacological treatment for paraphilic disorders, particularly in forensic populations. While research does not support the relationship between paraphilic disorders and increased testosterone, reducing testosterone can result in erectile dysfunction, lower levels of aggression and frequency of masturbation, along with decreased libido and sperm counts, thereby suppressing aberrant sexual behaviors. GnRH analogs target the endocrine system by suppressing the release of the luteinizing hormone, thereby reducing testosterone. Of note, the most recent World Federation of Societies of Biological Psychiatry's guidelines have rated the evidence level of these agents as "C," which suggests minimal scientific support for their use in paraphilic disorders (Tozdan & Briken, 2021). Nonetheless, at present, it is the only treatment available.

Pedophilic Disorders

Pedophilic disorders involve recurrent, intense sexual urges and arousing fantasies involving sexual activity with prepubescent or young adolescents (American Psychiatric Association, 2013). By definition, the victim of pedophilia

---

BOX 30.3 Select Pharmacological Treatments and Action in Paraphilic Disorders

Select-serotonin reuptake inhibitors	Fluoxetine and sertraline: Reduces fantasies and behaviors in pedophilia, fetishism, exhibitionism, and voyeurism
	Paroxetine: Reduces paraphilic fantasies and urges in patients with voyeurisms
	Fluvoxemine: Reduces pedophilic behaviors and possibly compulsive masturbation and exhibitionism
	Escitalopram: Reduces transvestic fetishism (case report)
Steroidal antiandrogens	Medroxyprogesterone acetate: Reduces sexual urges, cravings, and fantasies
	Cyproterone acetate: Reduces sexual fantasies and activity in pedophilia, and compulsive masturbation
Gonadotrophin-releasing hormone analogs	Triptorelin, leuprorelin, and goserelin: Reduces sexual fantasies and behavior in pedophilia

Modified from Tozdan, S., & Briken, P. (2021). Paraphilias: Diagnostics, comorbidities, and treatment. In *Psychiatry and sexual medicine* (pp. 407–416). Springer; Holoyda, B. J., & Kellaher, D. C. (2016). The biological treatment of paraphilic disorders: An updated review. *Current Psychiatry Reports, 18*, 19. https://doi.org/10.1007/s11920-015-0649-y.

---

must be younger than 13 years old, and the individual primarily or exclusively attracted to children must be 16 years old or older, and at least 5 years older than the victim. Pedophilic behavior can be expressed for opposite-sex children, same-sex children, or both. A distinction should also be made between a victim's gender and a perpetrator's sexual orientation. Even if the perpetrator abuses a child of the same sex or gender, the perpetrator's identified sexual orientation toward adults may be heterosexual. Patients with pedophilic disorders bear distinctions from child sexual abusers in that their sexual fixation on children persists over time and is not limited to a crime of opportunity or exploitation. Of note, incest is a specifier in pedophilic disorders. The primary difference here is that the perpetrator and victim are related by blood, marriage (stepparents), or live-in partners.

Typical pedophilic behaviors are peeping (voyeurism), inappropriate touching, masturbating in a child's presence (exhibitionism), and penetration of the mouth, anus, or vagina. In general, these individuals experience their sexual urges as ego-syntonic; and, to syntonically maintain this behavior, rationalization, minimization, normalization, or even delusional ideation can result. Cognitive distortions include denial of any wrongdoing, as well as thinking that he or she is teaching the child about sexuality and giving the child pleasure. To compensate for feelings of powerlessness, these individuals might need to feel power over the victim through control and domination. Some are physically aggressive, while others use less overtly aggressive tactics like coercion. The threat of violence might be used to encourage the victim's silence and/or compliance (First, 2014; Tenbergen et al., 2015).

Persons primarily or exclusively attracted to children might seek occupations that provide easy access to children, such as teaching, working in a daycare center, babysitting, coaching, or scout leadership. A prominent example of this occurred in 2018 when Larry Nassar was convicted and sentenced to 45 to 150 years in prison for first-degree criminal sexual conduct against girls and young women whom he treated as a doctor for the USA Gymnastics national team and Michigan State University. Nassar used his position in the gymnastic community to engage in repetitive illegal and abusive sexual activity disguised as normal medical protocol for over 20 years.

The internet era (particularly social media platforms) brings new challenges to protecting minors from abuse, in terms of both communication access and opportunities to engage with under-aged children. Certain designs of social media sites reinforce voyeuristic, exhibitionistic, and fantasy-based urges by providing continued access to digital photos, interests, and ability to send photos via private, direct messaging. Despite the increased access via the internet, the typical perpetrator of child sexual abuse is likely to be a trusted person in the child's immediate network of family or friends.

The psychological (motivational) and neurobiological domains involved in pedophilic disorders are varied. Antisocial personality disorder and a history of sexual abuse as a child are potential risk factors. Presently, neuroimaging provides the most promising evidence for assessing, classifying, and treating pedophilic disorders. Widespread dysfunctional brain activity involving the frontal, temporal, and parietal areas along with subcortical areas (insula, cingulate gyrus, basal ganglia) are observed in those living with pedophilia. These domains are highly associated with social, emotional, motivational, cognitive, and inhibitory processes. Interestingly, antisocial personality disorders express similar, but functionally different, connectivity patterns. While neuroimaging research is in its infancy, the psychobiological differences identified could help individualize treatment and provide methods for evaluating their effectiveness (Scarpazza et al., 2021). See Box 30.4 for a brief overview of other paraphilic disorders.

Exhibitionistic Disorder

The primary characteristic of exhibitionism is sexual pleasure derived from exposing one's genitals to an unsuspecting stranger. The stereotypical offender is a young man in a raincoat who flashes women while walking down the street. No other sexual activity is attempted. The exhibitionist is stimulated by the effect of shocking or frightening the victim.

BOX 30.4 Sexual Disorders

Paraphilic Disorders

The following paraphilic activities last over a period of 6 months and cause distress or impairment in social, occupational, or other important areas of functioning.

Exhibitionistic Disorder
- Recurrent, intense sexually arousing fantasies, urges, or behaviors involving exposing one's genitals to unsuspecting strangers.

Fetishistic Disorder
- Recurrent, intense sexually arousing fantasies, urges, or behaviors using nonliving objects.

Frotteuristic Disorder
- Recurrent, intense sexually arousing fantasies, urges, or behaviors involving touching and rubbing against a nonconsenting person.

Pedophilic Disorder
- Recurrent, intense sexually arousing fantasies, urges, or behaviors that involve sexual activity with a child or children generally 13 years old or younger.
- The person is at least 16 years old and at least 5 years older than the child or children involved.

Sexual Masochism Disorder
- Recurrent, intense sexually arousing fantasies, urges, or behaviors involving the act of being humiliated, beaten, restrained, or otherwise made to suffer.

Sexual Sadism Disorder
- Recurrent, intense sexually arousing fantasies, urges, or behaviors involving acts in which the psychological or physical suffering of the victim is sexually exciting to the person.

Transvestic Disorder
- Recurrent, intense sexually arousing fantasies, urges, or behaviors involving cross-dressing or dressing as the opposite sex.

Voyeuristic Disorder
- Act of observing an unsuspecting person who is naked, in the process of disrobing, or engaging in sexual activity.

Modified from McManus, M., Hargreaves, P., Rainbow, L., & Alison, L. J. (2013). Paraphilias: Definition, diagnosis and treatment. *F1000Prime Reports, 5*, 36.

Fetishistic Disorder

The primary characteristic of fetishism is sexual pleasure derived from inanimate objects. Common fetish objects are bras, underpants, stockings, and shoes. Less common fetish objects include urine-soaked and feces-smeared items. The individual with fetishism often masturbates while holding or rubbing these items. An individual with fetishism may also have a sexual partner wear the fetish object to increase arousal.

Frotteuristic Disorder

The primary characteristic of frotteurism is sexual pleasure derived from touching or rubbing one's genitals against a nonconsenting individual's body. An individual with frotteurism might also attempt to fondle the person's breasts or genitals. Frotteurism usually occurs in areas of natural opportunity (e.g., subways) or a crowded place in which contact and escape can be accomplished without notice.

Sexual Masochism Disorder

The primary characteristic of sexual masochism is that sexual pleasure is derived from physical or mental abuse or humiliation. These urges and behaviors involve being humiliated, beaten, or otherwise made to suffer. Some sexually masochistic individuals enjoy being urinated or defecated on and might pay prostitutes to do so. Hypoxyphilia or erotic asphyxiation is the act of enhancing sexual arousal by strangulation or some other oxygen-depleting activity. Sexual response is heightened by these activities. People have died in their search for enhanced orgasms.

Sexual Sadism Disorder

The primary characteristic of sexual sadism is sexual pleasure derived from inflicting psychological or physical suffering on another. Partners can be consenting or masochistic. Sadistic behaviors include spanking, whipping, pinching, beating, burning, and restraining. Some sadistic individuals derive great pleasure from torturing or even killing their victims. Sexual sadism affects mostly men and can progress to sadistic rape.

Transvestic Disorder

The primary characteristic of transvestic disorder is sexual arousal derived from cross-dressing or dressing as the opposite sex. This behavior is almost exclusively seen in heterosexual men who continue to identify with the male gender and do not meet criteria for gender dysphoria. The female partner may be unaware of the activity or may help in the selection of clothing. It is important to note that the gender noncomforming clothing choices themselves are not clinically relevant, nor does this diagnosis apply to all individuals who dress outside the expectation of current social norms. Rather, it is the sexual arousal reported by the individual that is associated with distress and/or impairment. This may be associated with difficulty managing behaviors related to the disorder (i.e., dressing secretively, spending large sums of money on clothing, etc.).

Voyeurism

The primary characteristic of voyeurism is sexual arousal derived from observing unsuspecting people who are naked or undressing or who are engaged in sexual activity. Individuals engaging in voyeurism often masturbate during peeping or after returning home. Given the primary distinction of non-consensual viewing, these behaviors are different from viewing consensual pornographic or webcam internet sites displaying naked or sexually engaged persons.

GENDER DYSPHORIA

Gender dysphoria (formerly known as gender identity disorder), and sometimes referred to as *gender incongruence,*

involves feelings of conflict or incompatibility between one's biologic sex (natal) and one's gender identity (see the "*DSM-5* Criteria for Gender Dysphoria" box). As is the case with many psychiatric diagnoses and definitions describing human behavior, these may not capture all the nuance in this evolving field of healthcare; however, understanding evolving language is important. *Sex* refers to the biologic indicators of male and female such as sex chromosomes, sex hormones, and genitalia. *Gender* refers to a spectrum of attitudes, feelings, and behaviors that a given individual or social culture ascribes to a person's biological sex (i.e., a spectrum of masculinity or femininity) (American Psychological Association, 2015). *Gender identity* refers to an inherent sense of being a male, female, or a variety of other expressions of one or more genders (i.e., agender, genderqueer, gender-nonconforming, nonbinary, etc.). Gender identity may or may not correspond to a person's natal sex or primary or secondary sex characteristics; it also involves a confluence of biological, social, and cultural factors. *Gender-nonconforming* and *gender diverse* are terms to describe those individuals who do not follow typical gender norms. Variation in gender identity and expression is not a psychiatric illness; rather, it is a variation in developing and experiencing one's identity in the world. Additionally, not all individuals who experience these variations experience dysphoria.

The presence of *gender dysphoria* indicates an individual's significant subjective distress related to an ascribed gender category; it is more specifically described by developmentally relevant diagnostic criteria in DSM-5, outlined in this chapter. Notably, as gender identity issues have gained increased attention, so too has an increase in gender dysphoria reporting with a prevalence of 0.6% to 1.7% (Zucker, 2017). Gender dysphoria can present as early as age 3 (and as late as adulthood), with behaviors indicative of rejecting stereotypes associated with an assigned natal sex (e.g., clothes, toys, mannerisms, etc.) and a preoccupation with getting rid of primary and secondary sexual characteristics. For youth arriving at puberty, this can be a tumultuous time. In fact, increased rates of depression, anxiety, and suicidal ideation are observed in gender dysphoria (Twist & Graaf, 2019).

Families and health care providers may evaluate the risks and benefits of various medical and psychotherapeutic interventions to address gender dysphoria. Medical or endocrine care interventions exist, such as puberty blockers to delay onset of puberty, cross-sex hormones to bring bodies in line with affirmed gender, and even gender affirming surgery. These interventions are intended to reduce body-related concerns and have been, in some cases, shown to reduce depression, anxiety, and anger surrounding dysphoria. Importantly, studies are equivocal regarding the benefit of reassignment transitions with some suggesting better mental health outcomes and others suggesting worse. Generally, persons with gender dysphoria without significant mental health needs or psychosocial stressors prior to surgery or endocrine treatment respond best to transition therapies (Kaltiala, Heino, Tyolajarvi, & Suomalainen, 2019).

Counseling helps clarify issues surrounding the individual's biological, psychological, emotional, and social concerns and desires. Emotional, medical, surgical, financial, and legal issues are explored, along with the risks involved with treatment and transition. Candidates for gender reassignment or confirmation surgery must be thoroughly assessed for the presence of other primary or comorbid psychiatric disorders (e.g., delusional disorders, autism). Some treatment programs require a written second opinion from another physician or psychologist before proceeding with medical or surgical intervention. Although data exist around characteristics that determine persistence, it is not uncommon for a child to present with gender dysphoria until puberty and then "realign" with their natal sex. It is also not uncommon for this dysphoria to persist past puberty into adulthood (Turban & Ehrensaft, 2018). Given the nuance and lack of objective measures to "confirm" a gender dysphoria diagnosis, and relatively ineffective treatments, early biological interventions and surgical transitions are not without controversy (Claahsen-van der Grinten et al., 2021; Nicholson & McGuinness, 2014). Ultimately, more rigorous and longitudinal studies are needed to understand the risk-benefits of such interventions and long-term outcomes.

Gender diverse and transgender individuals who experience gender dysphoria often represent an underserved population with regards to education, care, and proper referrals and access to treatments (Rafferty et al., 2018). Despite progress in legal protections, policy, public awareness, and treatments, individuals who experience gender dysphoria may face discrimination and stigma that can impact mental health and overall wellbeing. Of priority concern is evidence suggesting that transgender and gender diverse adolescents engage in significantly higher rates of suicide behavior compared with other adolescent populations (Toomey et al., 2018). Therefore, it is very important to provide nursing care oriented towards understanding the patient's experience with compassion, psychoeducation, appropriate referrals, and evidence-based treatment options to children, adolescents, and caregivers alike. Careful evaluation and prudent, participatory decision-making by a multidisciplinary team is necessary and should include both medically informed interventions and psychosocial support.

DSM-5 CRITERIA

Gender Dysphoria

Diagnostic Criteria

Gender Dysphoria in Children

A. A marked incongruence between one's experienced/expressed gender and assigned gender, of at least 6 months' duration, as manifested by at least six of the following (one of which must be Criterion A1):

1. A strong desire to be of the other gender or an insistence that one is the other gender (or some alternative gender different from one's assigned gender).
2. In boys (assigned gender), a strong preference for cross-dressing or simulating female attire; or in girls (assigned gender), a strong preference for wearing only typically masculine clothing and a strong resistance to wearing typically feminine clothing.
3. A strong preference for cross-gender roles in make-believe play or fantasy play.
4. A strong preference for the toys, games, or activities stereotypically used or engaged in by the other gender.
5. A strong preference for playmates of the other gender.
6. In boys (assigned gender), a strong rejection of typically masculine toys, games, and activities and a strong avoidance of rough-and-tumble play; or in girls (assigned gender), a strong rejection of typically feminine toys, games, and activities.
7. A strong dislike of one's sexual anatomy.
8. A strong desire for the primary and/or secondary sex characteristics that match one's experienced gender.

B. The condition is associated with clinically significant distress or impairment in social, school, or other important areas of functioning.

Gender Dysphoria in Adolescents and Adults

A. A marked incongruence between one's experienced/expressed gender and assigned gender, of at least 6 months' duration, as manifested by at least two of the following:

1. A marked incongruence between one's experienced/expressed gender and primary and/or secondary sex characteristics.
2. A strong desire to be rid of one's primary and/or secondary sex characteristics because of a marked incongruence with one's experienced/expressed gender (or in adolescents, a desire to prevent the development of the anticipated secondary sex characteristics).
3. A strong desire for the primary and/or secondary sex characteristics of the other gender.
4. A strong desire to be of the other gender (or some alternative gender different from one's assigned gender).
5. A strong desire to be treated as the other gender (or some alternative gender different from one's assigned gender).
6. A strong conviction that one has the typical feelings and reactions of the other gender (or some alternative gender different from one's assigned gender).

B. The condition is associated with clinically significant distress or impairment in social, occupational, or other important areas of functioning.

Specify if:

With a disorder of sex development (e.g., a congenital adrenogenital disorder such as 255.2 [E25.0] congenital adrenal hyperplasia or 259.50 [E34.50] androgen insensitivity syndrome).

Coding note: Code the disorder of sex development as well as gender dysphoria.

Specify if:

Posttransition: The individual has transitioned to full-time living in the desired gender (with or without legalization of gender change) and has undergone (or is preparing to have) at least one cross-sex medical procedure or treatment regimen—namely, regular cross-sex hormone treatment or gender reassignment surgery confirming the desired gender (e.g., penectomy, vaginoplasty in the natal male; mastectomy or phalloplasty in a natal female).

From American Psychiatric Association. (2013). *Diagnostic and statistical manual of mental disorders* (5th ed., pp. 452–453). APA.

PUTTING IT ALL TOGETHER

PSYCHOTHERAPEUTIC MANAGEMENT

Nurse-Patient Relationship

The nurse must have an accepting, empathic, and non-judgmental approach with patients in order to establish trust and elicit sexual health concerns. This trust is predicated on the nurse's understanding of their own personal feelings and beliefs about sexuality; the nurse must avoid projecting them onto patients. Patients might interpret the nurse's discomfort with sexual issues and sexuality as disapproval of their behaviors or concerns. It is of particular importance to be sensitive to any guilt, shame, self-esteem, or confidence issues expressed during the assessment. The goal is to maintain a supportive, validating, and sensitive environment for individuals seeking treatment. A private area in which to discuss fears or concerns about sexuality and victimization helps patients disclose and discuss their feelings. The nurse discusses options for dealing with sexual issues and problems. Clarification and education might be needed about sexual functioning, effective communication, and healthy relationships. The nurse discusses possible referrals with patients and family members and refers patients to sex therapists, if necessary. Referrals to outpatient treatment programs or therapy groups for specific disorders might be necessary.

Helping patients who have engaged in illegal sexual activity deal with physical and emotional dimensions is necessary. Physical dimensions might include anorexia, insomnia, and weight loss. Emotional dimensions might include guilt, helplessness, shame, and relief about getting caught. Setting limits on how much information the patient discloses in a group setting, especially if other group members might be victims of sexual assault, must be discussed.

The nurse is involved in the planning of patients' care regarding the specific issues and problems that are addressed during an inpatient stay versus issues and problems addressed in outpatient treatment. The nurse also collaborates with interdisciplinary partners to develop treatment plans. While the patient's cultural preferences are always considered, these constructs do not take precedence over the safety of others. While there are certain cultures (e.g., religious or ethnic) that consider pedophilia acceptable, all states have mandatory child abuse reporting statutes. As a nurse, there is a legal obligation to report suspected and actual sexual abuse of children to police or appropriate agencies in accordance with state laws and facility policies. In such cases, an ethics committee should be sought for guidance. Individual, group, and family treatment for pedophilic disorders and support groups for perpetrators and victims might be appropriate.

 CRITICAL THINKING QUESTION

2. What approaches would the nurse use while working with patients with sexual problems?

Milieu Management

Patients with sexual disorders and dysfunctions benefit from support groups dealing with self-esteem, assertiveness, anger management, social and relationship skills, sex education, and stress management. Self-help groups such as Sex Addicts Anonymous can benefit some individuals. The goal of treatment for sexual offenders is relapse prevention and may include CBT, psychopharmacology, family therapy, and specialized groups on education, coping, and social skills training. It is hoped that longitudinal research studies will eventually help determine treatment plans that are effective in reducing recidivism rates.

CASE STUDY

Bill Wood, 62 years old, has been admitted to the inpatient unit. His wife died 2 years earlier; he has one daughter and three grandchildren. Bill is presently employed but has few friends or hobbies. He visits his daughter and grandchildren approximately once a month. He does not date and does not have any female companions. For the past year, he has noticed an increase in sexual fantasies concerning children. He did not act on the fantasies until a week ago when he was babysitting for his youngest grandchild, 8-year-old Stephanie. He admits to fondling Stephanie's breasts but denies other sexual contact with her. Bill states to the nurse, "I never thought I could be capable of such a horrible thing. I deserve to die. I even thought of killing myself."

CARE PLAN

Name: Bill Wood   *Admission Date:*

DSM-5 Diagnosis: Major Depression and Pedophilia

Assessment	**Areas of strength:** Patient is employed, visits daughter and grandchildren, has remorse for contact with child; first offense.
	Problems: Death of wife, few friends, disturbing sexual fantasies, suicidal ideation
Diagnoses	Risk for self-directed violence related to guilt and suicidal ideation
	Sexual dysfunction related to lack of significant other, as evidenced by fondling child
	Social isolation related to lack of social support, as evidenced by loneliness
Outcomes	**Short-term goals**
Date met: .——	Patient will state that he no longer has thoughts of suicide.
Date met: .——	Patient will discuss sexual concerns and needs and methods to satisfy these needs.
	Long-term goals
Date met: .——	Patient will contact support groups and senior citizen organizations.
Date met: .——	Patient will attend outpatient appointment for further assessment and treatment of sexual disorder.
Planning and Interventions	**Nurse-patient relationship:** Instruct patient to approach staff when suicidal thoughts occur. Discuss feelings of guilt, remorse, anger, loneliness, and low self-esteem. Discuss the patient's beliefs and values about sexuality with him. Discuss and help the patient to identify sexual concerns, needs, and methods to satisfy needs.
	Psychopharmacology: Fluoxetine (Prozac) 20 mg q morning.
	Milieu management: Groups focusing on self-esteem, stress and anger management, assertiveness training, social skills, and discharge planning.
Evaluation	Patient reports that he is no longer suicidal.
Referrals	Patient will attend senior citizen activities at his church with a friend. Appointment is scheduled at a sexual disorders clinic.

STUDY NOTES

1. Sexual dysfunctions might occur as the result of psychological, physiologic, and pharmacologic factors.

2. Paraphilic disorders involve sexual activity with objects, children, and consenting or nonconsenting adults that are socially prohibited, unacceptable, or biologically undesirable.

3. Efforts to achieve sexual pleasure do not give individuals the right to violate the rights of others through coercion and control.

4. Currently, cognitive behavioral techniques and the use of antiandrogen medications are effective treatments for paraphilic disorders.

5. Gender dysphoria in adults involves persistent discomfort with one's gender.

6. The nurse's role in the treatment of sexual disorders is primarily one of referral.

REFERENCES

American Psychiatric Association. (2013). *Diagnostic and statistical manual of mental disorders* (5th ed.). APA.

Brotto, L., Atallah, S., Johnson-Agbakwu, C., Rosenbaum, T., Abdo, C., Byers, E. S., … Wylie, K. (2016). Psychological and interpersonal dimensions of sexual function and dysfunction. *The Journal of Sexual Medicine*, 13(4), 538–571. https://doi.org/10.1016/j.jsxm.2016.01.019.

Claahsen-van der Grinten, H., Verhaak, C., Steensma, T., Middelberg, T., Roeffen, J., & Klink, D. (2021). Gender incongruence and gender dysphoria in childhood and adolescence—Current insights in diagnostics, management, and follow-up. *European Journal of Pediatrics*, 180(5), 1349–1357. https://doi.org/10.1007/s00431-020-03906-y.

First. M. B. (2014). DSM-5 and paraphilic disorders. *Journal of American Academy of Psychiatric Law*, 42, 191–201.

Kaltiala, R., Heino, E., Työläjärvi, M., & Suomalainen, L. (2020). Adolescent development and psychosocial functioning after starting cross-sex hormones for gender dysphoria. *Nordic Journal of Psychiatry*, 74(3), 213–219. https://doi.org/10.1080/08039488.2019.1691260.

McManus, M. A., Hargreaves, P., Rainbow, L., & Alison, L. J. (2013). Paraphilias: Definition, diagnosis and treatment. *F1000Prime Reports*, 5, 36. https://doi.org/10.12703/P5-36.

Nicholson, C., & McGuinness, T. M. (2014). Gender dysphoria and children. *Journal of Psychosocial Nursing and Mental Health Service*, 52(8), 27–30. https://doi.org/10.3928/02793695-20140625-01.

Rafferty, J., & Committee on Psychosocial Aspects of Child and Family Health., (2018). Ensuring comprehensive care and support for transgender and gender-diverse children and adolescents. *Pediatrics*, 142(4). https://doi.org/10.1542/peds.2018-2162.

Rew, K. T., & Heidelbaugh, J. J. (2016). Erectile dysfunction. *American Family Physician*, 94(10), 820–827.

Scarpazza, C., Finos, L., Genon, S., Masiero, L., Bortolato, E., Cavaliere, C., … Ciani, A. S. C. (2021). Idiopathic and acquired pedophilia as two distinct disorders: An insight from neuroimaging. *Brain Imaging and Behavior*, 1–12. https://doi.org/10.1007/s11682-020-00442-z.

Shivananda, M. J., & Rao, T. S. (2016). Sexual dysfunction in medical practice. *Current Opinion in Psychiatry, 29*(6), 331–335. https://doi.org/10.1097/YCO.0000000000000281. PMID: 27636599.

Toomey, R. B., Syvertsen, A. K., & Shramko, M. (2018). Transgender adolescent suicide behavior. *Pediatrics, 142*(4), 1–8. https://doi.10.1542/peds/2017-4218.

Tozdan, S., & Briken, P. (2021). Paraphilias: Diagnostics, comorbidities, and treatment. In M. Lew-Starowicz, A. Giraldi, & T. H. C. Krüger (Eds.), *Psychiatry and sexual medicine: A comprehensive guide for clinical practitioners* (pp. 407–416). Springer. https://doi.org/10.1007/978-3-030-52298-8.

Turban, J. L., & Ehrensaft, D. (2018). Research review: Gender identity in youth: Treatment paradigms and controversies. *Journal of Child Psychology and Psychiatry, 59*(12), 1228–1243. https://doi. 10.1111/jcpp.12833.

Worsley, R., Miller, K. K., Parish, S. J., & Davis, S. R. (2016). Role of estrogens and estrogen-like compounds in female sexual function and dysfunction. *The Journal of Sexual Medicine, 13*(3), 305–316. https://doi.org/10.1016/j.jsxm.2015.11.015.

Zucker. K. J. (2017). Epidemiology of gender dysphoria and transgender identity. *Sexual Health, 14,* 404–411. https://doi.org/10.1071/SH17067. PMID: 28838353.

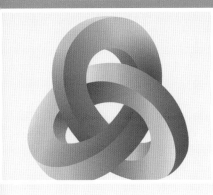

31

Substance Use Disorders

Susanne A. Fogger

A single death is a tragedy; a million deaths is a statistic.

Joseph Stalin

http://evolve.elsevier.com/Keltner

LEARNING OBJECTIVES

- Recognize the personal and societal toll of misuse of alcohol and other substances.
- Recognize *DSM-5* criteria and terminology for substance use disorders with a focus on alcohol use disorder.
- Recognize and describe objective and subjective symptoms of substance use disorders.
- Describe theoretical explanations for the development of substance use disorders.

- Develop a nursing care plan for patients with alcohol use disorder.
- Understand the contributions of nonmedical interventions in substance use recovery.
- Identify evidence-based websites for additional information and teaching material on substance use disorders.

Illicit drug use has taken a heavy toll in the United States. In 2018, 11.7 % of the American population age 12 or older had used an illicit drug in the previous month. This increase is reflected in the recreational use of marijuana in particular (National Center for Health Statistics, 2021).

INTRODUCTION

Humans have used mood-altering substances since the beginning of recorded history. Whether using heroin from Afghanistan, cocaine from Colombia, North American peyote, French wine, prescribed drugs, or a morning cup of Starbucks coffee, humans consistently find ways to alter their moods. Misuse of mind-altering substances can lead to many complications and problems. However, mind-altering drugs often provide therapeutic benefits (e.g., pain relief, decreased anxiety), thus clouding the distinction between therapeutic and abusive use.

It is beyond the scope of this text to cover all types of addictions; however, this chapter provides an overview of the most prevalent chemical substances of misuse. In addition, there are suggestions for additional resources. This chapter will highlight alcohol as one of the most commonly misused substances in the United States. Individual case presentations represent the many individuals who make up the staggering statistics. The effects of drug use (including alcohol) ripple

through our society, touching everyone to some degree and at a cost to the US economy of $600 billion annually. This enormous figure is related to lost work, crime, and health care costs such as treatment for lung cancer and heart disease directly related to substance use (NIDA, 2020, June 3).

Substance Use as a Brain Disorder

All addicting substances and behaviors directly or indirectly affect the dopamine pathways, as dopamine is the primary neurotransmitter associated with the reinforcing effect of the substance. All substances directly or indirectly increase dopamine intracellularly in the brain's limbic regions, including the nucleus accumbens. Drug exposure causes dopamine levels to spike much higher and for a longer time than any natural reward such as food or sex. With repeated use over time, the brain has become accustomed to the effect of the drug-induced dopamine response and no longer responds to natural rewards that also trigger dopamine. While this theory does not fully explain the addiction process, it simplifies concepts that are multi-dimensional and complex.

Drug use can reduce uncomfortable, unpleasant experiences such as stress and anxiety, reinforcing substance abuse. Repeated exposure is thought to alter neurons permanently; although an individual may be free of a substance for years, she or he remains vulnerable to the effects of reexposure.

Substance use disorders are considered chronic diseases because of the remitting nature of the illness. It is helpful to think about substance use disorders as similar to heart failure or diabetes. All are chronic, remitting disorders. Although the person may be in remission, acute crisis and relapse can occur, especially under stress. Keep in mind that the relapse rate for substance use is approximate to other chronic conditions (NIDA, 2005). A helpful way to consider the long-term effect of a substance on the brain is best illustrated by an old Alcoholics Anonymous (AA) saying considering the brain as a cucumber—once exposed (to substances with neuropathways altered) to a chemical and changed into a pickle, it will never be anything but a pickle in the future—"once a pickle, always a pickle."

Prevention measures focused on limiting early exposure to substances may decrease the risks associated with substance use. Adolescents who begin use are especially at risk for substance use disorders. Their frontal lobe, which regulates decision-making and executive function, is not fully developed until their mid-20s. Behaviors prevalent among adolescents—such as risk-taking and impulsiveness—increase the potential for substance use. Substance exposure later in life makes it less likely that the individual will experience the same degree of neuroadaptive changes as their frontal lobe is fully myelinated.

 NORM'S NOTES Substance use disorders are a big problem in the United States, and the issue does not seem to be getting any better. A recent news story highlighted the plight of families devastated by the opioid epidemic. As the story goes, first responders found both parents overdosed on heroin in the front seat of their car, with their children strapped in their car seats in the back. Indeed, this is a big problem in our country.

As a nurse, you will see patients suffering from the consequences of substance use as part of your work. You probably know people personally who have substance-related disorders and have experienced problems associated with use. You might suspect that other people whom you know have a substance-related disorder as well. Your ability to recognize the possibility and to suggest appropriate referrals or interventions might save a home, a family, a friendship, or a life. Friends and acquaintances might turn to you first, as a nurse, when they realize that their substance use has become a problem. We hope that you will take the time to study this information carefully and diligently. The road to recovery begins with the initial assessment.

We have to stop treating addiction as a moral failing and start seeing it for what it is: a chronic disease that must be treated with urgency and compassion.

Dr. Vivek H. Murthy, United States
Surgeon General, 2017

Clinical Example: Back from the brink of self-destruction

Robert had an average childhood and made good grades in school. He grew up in a home with both parents and with other siblings. In other words, Robert had a good start in life. In high school, he was particularly talented in sports and was popular among his peers. He began drinking beer with his baseball teammates when he was 15 years old. After graduating from high school with honors, he went to college on a baseball scholarship. In college, he was known to smoke some marijuana but "never let it get in the way" of his sports or his studies. He was good at hiding his drug use. It never occurred to him that he "had a problem," not even later, when his self-destruction became blatantly apparent to everyone else but Robert.

At first, he stayed out a little too late the night before a big game and had a bad game or two because of his slightly compromised performance. Eventually, he was introduced to cocaine, discovered intravenous use (mainlining), lost his promising sports career, was divorced by his wife, stole from people, lied to his family, tried to kill himself, and spent time in prison. While incarcerated, he realized how self-destructive his drug use had become and vowed to do whatever it took to become and remain drug-free. He reasoned that he had been willing to do a great many things in his search for dope, so he ought to be willing to exert the same amount of energy in his search to break free from its grip. Robert had been hospitalized for detoxification in the past, but he "wasn't ready," he says. When he attended a small treatment group at the county jail, he was ready to listen and learn. At that time, he was in his late 20s.

As of this writing, Robert is in his late 40s. After he cleared up his legal troubles, he earned his bachelor's degree and found a good career in which he advanced. Today he plays baseball in a local community league, is married to a wonderfully supportive spouse, and—most importantly—remains drug-free more than 20 years after he resolved to quit. His life is full of love, hope, and happiness. Robert's life did not get back on track overnight, however. Undoing most of the damage that his drug use caused took several years. Some of the damage that he caused can never be repaired. But he is far better off now than he was before he took steps to deal with his addiction.

What is addiction, and how does it differ from the "normal use" of a substance?

A helpful working definition for drug addiction is:
A chronic relapsing disorder characterized by a compulsive drive to take a drug despite serious adverse consequences, loss of control over intake, and emergence of a negative emotional state during abstinence (Volkow & Koob, 2020).

One way to think about addiction is called the four "C"s of addiction: loss of control, compulsive use, craving, and continued use despite consequences. People who use substances recreationally do not meet these criteria.

A more formal way to examine what addiction is is to review the diagnostic criteria put forth by the American

Psychiatric Association in the *Diagnostic and Statistical Manual of Mental Disorders*, 5th Edition (*DSM-5*).

DSM-5 CRITERIA FOR SUBSTANCE USE DISORDERS

DSM-5 (American Psychiatric Association, 2013) contains a common language for the psychiatric/health care community and specifies criteria for classifications of substance use disorders, substance intoxication, and substance withdrawal. In addition, substance use severity can be defined as mild, moderate, or severe. Criteria include using the substance longer; using more than intended; desiring to cut back; spending a great deal of time seeking, using, and recovering from use; experiencing cravings for the substance; failing to fulfill role obligations; using despite the potential for worsening social or interpersonal problems; giving up important obligations to use; using when it is physically hazardous; and using despite known physical or psychological problems that worsen with use. Additional criteria include tolerance—the need to use more of the substance to obtain the desired effect and not experiencing the same effect if using the same amount as previously. Withdrawal is experiencing physiologic or psychological symptoms when cutting back or stopping use. The individual may use more of the substance or a similar drug to avoid withdrawal symptoms.

The use of substances is recognized as a problem when the effects of use interfere with and disrupt family, work, or social relationships. If these areas of a person's life are adversely affected, the person probably meets the criteria for a substance use disorder. Substances that can be misused fall into several classes: Sedatives-alcohol, barbiturates, and other central nervous system (CNS) depressants, opioids, stimulants, nicotine, and hallucinogens (Table 31.1).

Assessment Strategies for Chemical Dependency

As a component of every assessment, the nurse should inquire about the amount and type of alcohol and other drugs (AODs) used by the patient. In inquiring about prescription medication, the nurse should always ask about the amount the patient actually takes (not simply the amount prescribed, because many people abuse prescription medications as well). Ask simple questions such as, "Do you drink alcohol now and then?" If the person responds positively, follow up with a question about the amount. "On an average week, what is the greatest number of alcohol-containing drinks you have per day?" Then, "How many drinks per week?" The responses can help to determine if the person's alcohol use is in or above the risky level. The nurse should also ask about medical problems associated with AOD use. A helpful link about what heavy drinking looks like may be found here: https://www.rethinkingdrinking.niaaa.nih.gov/How-much-is-too-much/Is-your-drinking-pattern-risky/whats-At-Risk-Or-Heavy-drinking.aspx.

DSM-5 CRITERIA FOR ALCOHOL USE DISORDER IS LISTED BELOW. THE CRITERIA IS THE SAME FOR ANY SUBSTANCE.

Diagnostic Criteria

A. A problematic pattern of alcohol use leading to clinically significant impairment or distress, as manifested by at least two of the following occurring within a 12-month period:
   1. Alcohol is often taken in larger amounts or over a longer period than was intended.
   2. There is a persistent desire or unsuccessful efforts to cut down or control alcohol use.
   3. A great deal of time is spent in activities necessary to obtain alcohol, use alcohol, or recover from its effects.
   4. Craving, or a strong desire or urge to use alcohol.
   5. Recurrent alcohol use resulting in a failure to fulfill major role obligations at work, school, or home.
   6. Continued alcohol use despite having persistent or recurrent social or interpersonal problems caused or exacerbated by the effects of alcohol.
   7. Important social, occupational, or recreational activities are given up or reduced because of alcohol use.
   8. Recurrent alcohol use in situations in which it is physically hazardous.
   9. Alcohol use is continued despite knowledge of having a persistent or recurrent physical or psychological problem that is likely to have been caused or exacerbated by alcohol.

10. Tolerance, as defined by either of the following:
    a. A need for markedly increased amounts of alcohol to achieve intoxication or desired effect.
    b. A markedly diminished effect with continued use of the same amount of alcohol.
11. Withdrawal, as manifested by either of the following:
    a. The characteristic withdrawal syndrome for alcohol (refer to Criteria A and B of the criteria set for alcohol withdrawal, pp. 499–500 of *DSM-5*).
    b. Alcohol (or a closely related substance, such as a benzodiazepine) is taken to relieve or avoid withdrawal symptoms.

Specify If

In early remission: After full criteria for alcohol use disorder were previously met, none of the criteria for alcohol use disorder have been met for at least 3 months but for less than 12 months (with the exception that criterion A4, "Craving, or a strong desire or urge to use alcohol," may be met).

In sustained remission: After full criteria for alcohol use disorder were previously met, none of the criteria for alcohol use disorder have been met at any time during a period of 12 months or longer (with the exception that criterion A4, "Craving, or a strong desire or urge to use alcohol," may be met).

From American Psychiatric Association. (2013). *Diagnostic and statistical manual of mental disorders* (5th ed.). APA.

TABLE 31.1   Drug Information

Class	Examples or Other Names	Withdrawal Syndrome	Withdrawal Treatment	Psychiatric Symptoms During Chronic Use	Overdose Fatal?[a]	Unassisted Withdrawal Fatal?[a]	Overdose Symptoms
CNS depressants	Alcohol, Barbiturates; other depressants	Tremors, sweats, autonomic irritability, seizures, anxiety, irritability, hallucinations, death[a]	Tapering doses of long-acting benzodiazepine, barbiturates	Mood disorder, depression, psychosis, dementia	Yes[a]	Yes[a]	Shallow respiration, clammy skin, dilated pupils, weak and rapid pulse, coma, death
Opioids	Demerol, heroin, morphine, opium, codeine, OxyContin	Lacrimation, runny nose, diaphoresis, chills, muscle aches, n/v, diarrhea, leg spasm, goosebumps	Taper of methadone or buprenorphine, clonidine, supportive medications	Psychosis, mood disorder	Yes	No	Respiratory depression, pulmonary edema, pinpoint pupils, seizures, coma, death
Cannabinoids	Marijuana, hash	Craving, irritability		Psychosis, paranoia	No	No	Hallucinations, paranoia, insomnia, hyperactive
Cocaine	Crack, coke, snow	Anhedonia, craving, irritability, fatigue, mood disorder, anxiety	Dopamine agonists, catecholamine precursors	Psychosis	Yes	No	Delirium, psychosis, violence, tachycardia, hypertension, coma, hyperreflexia, myocardial infarction
Methamphetamine	Oral: speed, meth; smokable: ice, crystal, crank	Dysphoria, fatigue, insomnia	Supportive	Psychosis, mood disorder, anxiety disorder	Yes	No	Delirium, psychosis, violence, tachycardia, hypertension, coma, hyperreflexia
Inhalants	Gasoline, Freon, paint, and others	Mouth ulcers, gastrointestinal problems, anorexia, confusion, headache	Supportive	Psychosis, panic, memory loss	Yes	No	Seizures, coma
Hallucinogens	LSD, psilocybin, PCP	None specific	Supportive	Psychosis, panic	No	No	Seizures, panic, depression

[a]These are generalizations that are typically true.
CNS, Central nervous system; LSD, lysergic acid diethylamide; n/v, nausea, and vomiting; PCP, phencyclidine.

Assessing each patient for risky substance use can help reduce the likelihood of the individual developing worsening consequences. One effective method is called screening, brief intervention, and referral to treatment (SBIRT)—a concept that can help health care providers assess and intervene early, helping patients to make better decisions about the use of substances.

Interview Approaches

Because underreporting can lead to misdiagnosis, it is important that the nurse's manner encourages forthrightness. The nurse should be *matter-of-fact* and *nonjudgmental* while eliciting information that may be shameful to the individual. Gathering accurate information during the interview is a high priority. Use non-stigmatizing language to explore the patient's history as well as current use. It also might be helpful initially to focus more on legally or culturally accepted substances such as caffeine and nicotine. The patient's consumption should be evaluated in detail if the initial assessment data identifies the patient's substance use as high risk. For example, a patient can drink in a risky manner (drinking 12 beers during a football game) but be unaware that such use is considered "hazardous." In addition, using the phrases such as *problems because of drinking* and *using more than intended* is more likely to help the patient link substance use with other problems in their lives.

Diagnostic Tools

There is currently no lab test that can diagnose psychiatric or substance use disorders. A structured clinical interview is the most diagnostic. The interview can be guided by or initiated by a positive screening. Many tools exist for the evaluation of chemical dependency from caffeine to opioid use. Quick screens such as the AUDIT-C, a 3-question screen, can avoid asking unnecessary questions to patients who do not have any issues with alcohol. A positive screen would flag the patient's record for a more in-depth interview. Early identification of problematic use can prevent the development of the disorder, and early diagnosis can mean a better treatment prognosis. Under-recognition of a substance use disorder can lead to unsuspected withdrawal, drug interactions, or both. It is important that the nurse assess all patients for behavioral and physical clues which may identify substance use and misuse. Some screens specific to a population, such as adolescents, may prefer to complete questions on a website or an iPad. Adolescents may be more forthright with their responses, not having to verbally communicate their history of use.

Alcohol Use Disorder Identification Test

The Alcohol Use Disorder Identification Test (AUDIT) is a questionnaire helpful in identifying individuals with hazardous alcohol use or alcohol use disorder. The care provider reviews the questions with the patient and then discusses the significance of the patient's score. Scores above a certain level suggest a substance use disorder. However, a positive screen is not diagnostic. Copies of the questionnaire are available online and can be downloaded and used free of charge (Table 31.2).

CAGE

The CAGE questionnaire is another valid instrument; it comprises four questions related to substance use. It is short and easy to administer. The CAGE is not useful in determining risky drinking, as the questions are written to identify an alcohol use disorder. A positive response to two or more of the questions requires an additional assessment to include a standardized interview for alcohol use disorder. Here are the four CAGE questions:

1. Have you ever felt that you should **cut down** on your drinking? (C)
2. Have you ever found that people were **annoyed** with you on account of your drinking? (A)
3. Have you ever felt bad or **guilty** about your drinking? (G)
4. Have you ever had an **eye-opener** in the morning to steady your nerves or get rid of a hangover? (E)

Many addicted patients do not readily reveal more than what the nurse can already discover by other means. For example, someone referred to treatment because alcohol use has led to problems with the legal system may not share their cocaine or marijuana use until objective testing reveals it. Some patients even deny the use of the substances when confronted with the lab results. Signs and symptoms raising the suspicion of a substance-related disorder might include the following:

Absenteeism, especially after days off
Frequent accidents or injuries
Drowsiness
Slurred speech
Inattention to appearance
Increasing isolation
Frequent secretive disappearances
Tremors
Flushed face
Watery or reddened eyes
Appearing spaced out
Odor of alcohol on the breath or strong mouthwash or breath mint smell
High number of physical complaints
Disappearing prescriptions (raiding the medicine cabinet)

The primary defense mechanisms of an individual addicted to substances are frequently denial and minimization. A person with a substance-related disorder may not recognize the destructive nature of use, although it may be obvious to others. Denial prevents the individual from linking their problems with substance use. The inability to see self-destructive behavior and attitudes, continuing to use despite knowledge of a worsening mental and physical condition, or the inability to link life problems with substance use defines substance use disorders.

Identification and detection from lab work. Urinalysis often provides the most objective measure of recent drug use, although it is important to get confirmational testing on any sample testing positive. False-negative and false-positive results need to be considered before confronting an individual. The nurse can lose the patient's trust if the individual is accused of use before the nurse checks with the lab. Blood and saliva

TABLE 31.2   Screening Instrument: The Alcohol Use Disorders Identification Test (AUDIT)

	0	1	2	3	4	Score
How often do you have a drink containing alcohol?	Never	Monthly or less	2–4 times a month	2–3 times a week	4 or more times a week	
How many drinks containing alcohol do you have on a typical day when you are drinking?	1 or 2	3 or 4	5 or 6	7–9	10 or more	
How often do you have 5 or more drinks on one occasion?	Never	Less than monthly	Monthly	Weekly	Daily or almost daily	
How often during the last year have you found that you were not able to stop drinking once you had started?	Never	Less than monthly	Monthly	Weekly	Daily or almost daily	
How often during the last year have you failed to do what was normally expected of you because of drinking?	Never	Less than monthly	Monthly	Weekly	Daily or almost daily	
How often during the last year have you needed a first drink in the morning to get yourself going after a heavy drinking session?	Never	Less than monthly	Monthly	Weekly	Daily or almost daily	
How often during the last year have you had a feeling of guilt or remorse after drinking?	Never	Less than monthly	Monthly	Weekly	Daily or almost daily	
How often during the last year have you been unable to remember what happened the night before because of your drinking?	Never	Less than monthly	Monthly	Weekly	Daily or almost daily	
Have you or someone else been injured because of your drinking?	No		Yes, but not in the last year		Yes, during the last year	
Has a relative, friend, doctor, or other healthcare worker been concerned about your drinking or suggested you cut down?	No		Yes, but not in the last year		Yes, during the last year	
Total Score						

Instructions to patient: Circle the option that best describes your answer to each question. *Scoring:* Record the score (0, 1, 2, 3, or 4) for each response in the blank box at the end of each line and then add up the total score. The maximum possible is 40. A total score of 8 or more (for men up to age 60) or 4 or more (for women, adolescents, and men over 60) is considered a positive screen. For patients with totals near the cut points, clinicians may wish to examine individual responses to questions and clarify them during the clinical examination.
Reprinted with permission from the World Health Organization. To reflect standard drink sizes in the United States, the number of drinks in question 3 was changed from 6 to 5. In Burchum, J., & Rosenthal, L. (2019). *Lehne's pharmacology for nursing care* (10th ed.). Elsevier.

levels can also detect recent use and trigger treatment protocols. Hair toxicology effectively determines long-term patterns of use but costs more than other methods of detection. Hair toxicology kits available on the retail market enable parents, if they suspect drug use, to test the hair of their children.

Assessment tools can help the nurse to clarify the extent of how substance use has affected the individual's life. Tools help psychiatric nurses to better identify substance misuse as well as a substance use disorder. They provide a common, consistent way to quantify the patient's experience. When working with a psychiatric population, it is an important aspect of any initial assessment to include a review of the person's substance use. About half of all patients with mental illness also have some type of substance use disorder. Patients with both mental illness and substance use disorders are considered to have **co-occurring disorders**. For example, in the United States, a large percentage of smokers with nicotine dependence also have a mental disorder. Having a mental disorder in childhood or adolescence puts the individual at an increased risk for substance use as well as the development of a substance use disorder (NIDA, 2020, May 28). Recognizing that problematic substance use can affect other health conditions such as diabetes and heart disease highlights the importance of the need for all nurses to be skilled in assessing for substance use. The nurse must understand and be skilled in methods for screening, including how to perform a brief intervention that recognizes the patient's readiness for change. The nurse establishes a relationship with the patient and, using motivational interviewing, communicates the importance of the person's active participation in their health care decisions. The nurse provides support, voices discrepancies between behavior and goals, and offers encouragement and educational counseling.

Transtheoretical Model

The transtheoretical model developed by Prochaska and DiClemente (1983) is helpful in working with individuals who have substance use issues or any health-related concern. The model assists the nurse in identifying the individual's readiness to change behaviors that may be harmful or in some way interfering with their life plans. The nurse can determine the individual's current stage of change and support the individual's move toward a healthier lifestyle. The nurse assists in examining relevant factors such as objective data to understand the consequences related to personal choices. When the patient wants to change some part of their lifestyle, the nurse helps the individual frame their goals into a workable plan and follows up during each subsequent visit. The nurse translates laboratory work, identifies an individual's strengths, and gathers evidence concerning milestones toward change. Transtheoretical stages of change are precontemplation, contemplation, preparation, action, maintenance, and relapse.

Precontemplation: The person is not thinking about change in the foreseeable future. They may not recognize the behavior as problematic and are not interested in changing behavior.

Contemplation: The person recognizes the behavior as problematic. They begin to consider the pros and cons of making a change.

Preparation: The person intends to take action and may take small steps toward change.

Action: The person makes specific overt modifications or acquires new healthy behaviors.

Maintenance: The person is able to sustain action and works to prevent relapse to old behaviors.

Relapse: The person recycles from action or maintenance to an earlier stage.

Behavioral changes may not be linear and should be considered as fluid and in flux. An individual may progress or digress at any time. Each issue should be considered separately and uniquely as the behavioral change is in flux, not the individual. For example, the individual may attend Weight Watchers meetings weekly (*action*) yet does not want to stop using alcohol (*precontemplation*). To be successful in reaching a weight loss goal, the patient may have to move to the action phase and decrease their intake of alcohol.

Alcohol and Alcohol Use Disorder

Alcohol misuse is one of the major causes of significant health issues across the world. This chapter will address alcohol in detail because of the enormity of the problem. The cost to the United States is tallied with health problems, lost work hours, a decline in military readiness, family disruption and disintegration, and criminal activities. It has been estimated at the cost of more than $223 billion annually. More than 85.6 % of Americans older than 12 years of age have had a drink of alcohol in their lifetime. Problematically, in 2019, 29.7% of men, 18 and older, and 22.2 % of women engaged in binge drinking in the previous month. An emerging trend is high-intensity drinking, which is defined as consuming alcohol at levels that are two or more times the gender-specific binge

drinking thresholds. Compared to people who do not binge drink, people who engaged in high-intensity drinking were 70 times more likely to have an alcohol-related emergency room visit. Of the 14.5 million people with an Alcohol Use Disorder (AUD) in 2019, only about 7.2 percent of those individuals received any treatment in the previous year, and less than 4% received FDA-approved medication to treat their disorder (SAMHSACenter for Behavioral Health Statistics and, 2019).

AUD ranks as one of the leading causes of death and disability in the United States. These individuals have a premature death rate two to four times higher than individuals who do not drink in excess related to increased risk of cirrhosis of the liver, cardiovascular damage, arrhythmias, and cancer risks, such as breast, mouth, and esophageal cancers.

Etiology

Psychodynamic Theories

Many older psychological theories have attempted to explain substance dependence, such as alcohol use disorder. Alcohol-dependent individuals have often been viewed as those who easily succumbed to the escape that alcohol provides. More recent theories have described people likely to become dependent on alcohol as fearful and with greater feelings of inferiority compared with social drinkers. Over time, the search for an "alcoholic personality" has given way to a multivariate model that incorporates the biopsychosocial components of addiction. Currently, researchers believe that many of the stereotypical characteristics found in alcohol-dependent individuals (e.g., dependency, low self-esteem, passivity, introversion) are the result of, not the cause of, substance use disorders.

Biologic Theories

Heredity as an etiology continues to provide insight into understanding the genesis of alcohol use disorder. Genetic predisposition is considered the most significant piece of information in identifying risk for alcohol use disorder as offspring of people with this addiction are 4 to 10 times more likely to develop alcohol use disorders. One example would be the amount of the enzyme called alcohol dehydrogenase, which breaks alcohol down. The amount of this enzyme an individual produces is often inherited, so some people have more, and some have much less than average. Although studies have indicated different degrees of effect, hereditary explanations at least provide a satisfactory basis for understanding a person's vulnerability to alcohol dependency. As genomic science advances, genetic markers may be able to identify substance use and mental illness vulnerabilities, ideally to prevent these co-occurring disorders (Peng, Wilhelmon, & Eklers, 2021). Other events such as exposure to adverse childhood events (ACEs) can increase the individual's vulnerability to alcohol because of stress-induced neuroplastic changes in the peripheral and central nervous system (Yang et al., 2015). However, predisposition suggests neither fatalism nor determinism. For example, even patients who are genetically predisposed to certain types of cancer can take steps to minimize their risk. Recognizing their familial predisposition to addiction, individuals can avoid the use of alcohol and other addictive substances.

Pharmacokinetics of Alcohol

Absorption

Alcohol, a lipid, is highly water-soluble. It is absorbed partially from the stomach (20%) but mostly from the small intestine (80%). If a person with an empty stomach ingests alcohol, 50% is in the bloodstream within 15 minutes, and peak levels are reached in 40 to 60 minutes (Colyar, 2003). The form of alcohol consumed affects the rate of absorption. Alcohol in beer and wine is absorbed more slowly than alcohol in liquor. This characteristic is related to the dilution ratio; domestic beer contains 4% ethanol; wine, 12% ethanol; and whiskey, 40% to 50% ethanol. Other issues that factor into absorption rates include dehydration, the relationship of drinking to the timing of a fatty meal, and the health of the individual's stomach and small bowel.

Distribution

Ethanol is distributed equally in all body tissues according to water content. Larger individuals (who have greater amounts of body water) can ingest more alcohol than smaller people who have less body water. Because muscle contains more water than fat tissue, men tend to have lower blood alcohol levels than women, even when weight is controlled. Alcohol affects the cerebrum and cerebellum before it affects the spinal cord and other vital centers because the cerebrum and cerebellum contain more water (Fig. 31.1).

Metabolism

Although the rate of absorption largely determines how quickly a person becomes intoxicated, a person's metabolic rate largely determines how long alcohol affects the body. Alcohol is metabolized at a constant amount over time and is proportional to the person's body weight. The metabolism averages to be 1 oz. of pure alcohol over 3 hours in adults (Woodard, 2020). A healthy body can metabolize about 15 mL of alcohol per hour, or roughly the alcohol content in a 12-oz. can of beer or a 4-oz. glass of wine. Individuals who drink alcohol constantly over several years have increased hepatic drug-metabolizing enzymes that hasten alcohol metabolism (metabolic tolerance [pharmacokinetic tolerance]). Hot coffee, sweating it out, and other home remedies do not increase alcohol metabolism, and they do not hasten the sobering-up process. Attempts by scientists to develop a pill to prevent or decrease intoxication have been unsuccessful. In late-stage alcoholism, tolerance decreases because the abused liver can no longer metabolize the alcohol adequately.

The chemical name for alcohol is *ethanol* (CH_3CH_2OH). Alcohol is primarily metabolized in the liver, but 10% is excreted unchanged in the breath, sweat, and urine (see Colyar, 2003). The oxidation process can be described chemically as follows:

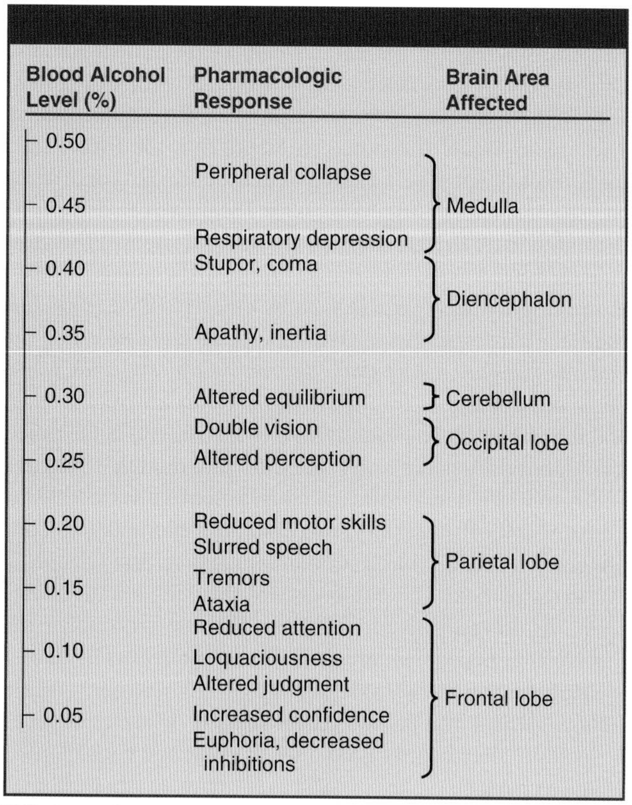

FIG. 31.1 Central nervous system responses at various blood alcohol levels.

Alcohol is converted to **acetaldehyde** (*a toxic molecule*), which is converted to **acetic acid** (*nontoxic*).

At each step of the metabolic process, an enzyme breaks down the chemical and speeds up the reaction. *Alcohol dehydrogenase* breaks down alcohol (CH_3CH_2OH) to acetaldehyde (CH_3CHO) and H_2. The H_2 molecule causes the liver to bypass normal energy sources (H_2 from fat) and to use the H_2 from alcohol. Fat accumulates because it is not being used as a primary energy source; this leads to fatty liver, hyperlipidemia, hepatitis, and ultimately cirrhosis. Acetaldehyde is *toxic* to the body; it compromises normal cell function in the liver. If the metabolism of acetaldehyde is impaired, acetaldehyde accumulates in the liver, causing cell death and necrosis. Acetaldehyde also interferes with vitamin activation. *Aldehyde dehydrogenase* breaks down acetaldehyde to acetic acid (CH_3COOH), which is a harmless substance. One medication, disulfiram, uses this mechanism to make drinking unattractive. When enzymatic action on acetaldehyde is blocked by the aldehyde dehydrogenase blocker, disulfiram (Antabuse), acetaldehyde accumulates, causing severe sickness.

Research confirms the suspicion that women become intoxicated more easily than men, even when studies are controlled for size differences. Frezza and colleagues (1990) discovered that the gastrointestinal tissue of women and of alcohol-dependent men contains little alcohol dehydrogenase. The alcohol dehydrogenase in the gastrointestinal tissue of men who are not dependent on alcohol oxidizes a significant amount of CH_3CH_2OH in the gut before it enters the bloodstream. The inability of women's bodies to undergo this first-pass metabolism accounts for their enhanced vulnerability to alcohol. For example, if a 140-lb. male drinks two drinks in 1 hour, his blood alcohol level will be 0.038. If a 140-lb. female drinks two drinks in 1 hour, her blood alcohol level will be 0.048. Another enzyme system, the cytochrome P-450 2E1 enzyme, breaks down some alcohol. This metabolic pathway becomes more important after chronic heavy alcohol consumption because chronic drinking induces the synthesis of this enzyme. An important adverse effect can develop when someone who has been drinking excessively or chronically uses acetaminophen. Because cytochrome P-450 2E1 metabolizes acetaminophen, and alcohol creates more cytochrome P-450 2E1, more acetaminophen is broken down. The first metabolite of acetaminophen is very toxic and, in some cases, cannot be metabolized to a nontoxic molecule before liver damage occurs.

Blood Alcohol Levels

Blood alcohol levels accurately indicate the amount of ethanol to which the brain is exposed. Behavioral and physiologic effects of alcohol are predictable for most drinkers. For example, at a 0.05% blood alcohol level, most individuals are predictably feeling good and experience disinhibition (i.e., they might do and say things they would typically just think about doing). Ingestion of large amounts of alcohol can raise levels to the acute poisoning range (>0.45 %), which, if not treated, can lead to coma and death.

Tolerance to Alcohol

Tolerance to alcohol is probably related to elevated hepatic enzyme levels (pharmacokinetic tolerance) and to cellular adaptation (pharmacodynamic tolerance). At the point where the normal drinker might be noticeably drunk after 10 to 12 drinks, the long-term drinker with pharmacodynamic tolerance might seem unaffected by drinking the same amount. However, tolerance to the respiratory depressing effects of alcohol does not develop appreciably. Blood alcohol levels just slightly higher than those required to feel intoxicated have resulted in the deaths of long-term pharmacodynamically tolerant drinkers.

Physiologic Effects

Alcohol targets multiple neurotransmitter receptors: glutamate, N-methyl-D-aspartate (NMDA), GABA, 5-hydroxytryptamine 3, and nicotinic acetylcholine receptors. Each of these receptors influences dopamine. A secondary effect—called a "second hit"—occurs when alcohol modulates opioids and endocannabinoids. These neurotransmitters plus dopamine are thought to be responsible for the "rewarding" effect of alcohol. People generally begin consuming alcohol because it causes a reaction they desire. Relaxation, disinhibition, impaired judgment, and fuzzy thinking are initial responses to alcohol ingestion. In many situations, these responses are pleasant. Alcohol is a social lubricant, as it relaxes self-imposed barriers that inhibit sociability. Over time, persistent heavy drinking becomes defensive; that is, the individual often drinks to avoid the effects of many years of drinking. For example, when the initial anxiety-reducing effect wears off, the person will experience more tension and anxiety produced secondary to an early withdrawal state. Then the drinker must consume more alcohol to regain the desired state. This becomes a vicious cycle of use to avoid negative feelings and physical symptoms. Many people with severe alcohol use disorder may be unable to quell the rebound psychomotor upheaval caused by years of alcohol-related CNS irritation and withdrawal. Often individuals who seek treatment for severe alcohol use disorder have anxiety or depression directly related to their substance use.

Central Nervous System Effects

The adverse effects of alcohol can be categorized as central or peripheral. CNS effects are related to sedation and toxicity. As the vital centers become affected, a slowed, stuporous to unconscious mental state develops. Alcohol consumed in large amounts can cause sleep, coma, deep anesthesia, or death. Other common symptoms of intoxication include slurred speech, short retention span, loud talk, and memory deficits. Large amounts of alcohol prevent the hippocampus from recording short-term memory, and blackout occurs. "Blackout" refers to a period during which the drinker functions socially but later has no memory of the experience.

Alcohol is highly toxic, even when a nutritious diet is maintained, causing damage to the brain. Neuronal death is likely related to changes in the sensitivity of NMDA receptors over time (as opposed to the reinforcing effect of NMDA modulation mentioned previously), thus heightening the excitotoxicity potential of glutamate. Brain changes include reduction of brain weight, frontocortical gray matter loss, atrophy, reduction in white matter, hippocampal changes, hypothalamic neuronal loss, and cerebellar neuronal loss (Woodward, 2020).

Acetaldehyde, the first metabolic product of alcohol, increases psychomotor activity in a phenomenon called *alcohol withdrawal syndrome*. While sedation is the predominant effect of alcohol, when the sedative effect wears off, psychomotor activity increases. This state is referred to as a *rebound phenomenon*. As the CNS becomes more irritated, a normal drinker feels sick and irritable (a hangover) but lives through it, perhaps vowing never to go through it again. Heavy, at-risk drinkers and those with AUD may drink again to sedate the psychomotor system. Eventually, a person has to drink increasing amounts to feel normal. A few drinkers reach the point where they cannot drink enough alcohol, and alcoholic tremors, sweating, palpitations, and agitation occur. Although these symptoms usually arise when alcohol ingestion has stopped (blood alcohol level at 0.00) or the CNS irritability of withdrawal may begin when the blood alcohol level decreases, sometimes a drinker may still be legally intoxicated but in withdrawal. (Their "normal" blood alcohol level is at 0.40%, but they go into withdrawal at 0.30%.) Blood pressure and pulse may spike in response to the CNS rebound (Table 31.3).

TABLE 31.3 Withdrawal Estimates From Addictive Drugs

Substances	Length of Acute Detoxification	Common Agents Used for Managing the Withdrawal	Withdrawal Signs and Symptoms
CNS Depressants			
Alcohol	3–5 days Use Clinical Institute Withdrawal Assessment for Alcohol scale (CIWAS) assessment scale	Tapering doses of Librium, Serax, Valium (long-acting benzodiazepine), Vistaril for sleep, rarely—alcohol (cheap but effective) in reducing doses over 3–5 days	Anxiety, sweats, tremors, flushed face, irritability, increased BP, pulse sleeplessness, Severe life-threatening confusion, seizures, delirium
Valium	Slow drug taper, up to 2 weeks or longer depending on the current dose and how long patient has been on the med	Librium, Valium in tapering doses	Anxiety, tremors, insomnia, increased BP, pulse, agitation, muscle twitching, and seizures
Phenobarbital	Slow drug taper, 2–4 weeks or longer	Librium, (long-acting benzodiazepine) phenobarbital	Withdrawal is similar to other CNS depressants with risk of seizure primary concern
Opioids			
Length of withdrawal depends on the opioid as there is considerable difference between a short-acting (dilaudid) and a long-acting opioid such as methadone	3–5 days Use Clinical Opioid Withdrawal Scale (COWS) to assess and monitor withdrawal	Methadone, buprenorphine, other tapering opioids, or non-opioid withdrawal regimen using clonidine and symptomatic comfort measures	Yawning, dilated pupils, gooseflesh, vomiting, diarrhea, runny nose and eyes, sleeplessness, anxiety, irritability, elevated blood pressure and pulse, craving for narcotics
Stimulants			
Amphetamines	3–5 days	Drug intervention usually not required Comfort measures, nutrition, and sleep.	General fatigue, apathy, depression, drowsiness, irritability, paranoia, suicidal ideation
Cocaine	3–5 days	Same as above	Similar to other stimulants
Hallucinogens			
Marijuana	2–3 days (metabolites remain in the body up to 2–3 weeks)	Drug intervention usually not required	Craving for marijuana, general anxiety, and restlessness

BP, Blood pressure; *CNS*, central nervous system.

For chronic AUD, alcohol-induced psychotic disorder (formerly referred to as alcoholic hallucinosis) may manifest as short-lived delusions or hallucinations. This phenomenon may begin 48 hours or so after they have stopped drinking. Most hallucinations are auditory and tend to resolve within 1 week. Frightening voices or sounds may be heard, usually within the context of a clear sensorium.

A potentially life-threatening level of CNS irritability is delirium tremens ("DTs"). In DTs, the body not only invents sensory input but also develops extreme motor agitation. Hallucinations become visual (e.g., the proverbial pink elephants), and the drinker is tremulous and terrified. Tonic-clonic seizures (grand mal seizures) are associated with a high risk of aspiration or death.

A chronic alcohol-related disease is Wernicke-Korsakoff syndrome. This is a mental disorder characterized by amnesia, clouding of consciousness, confabulation (falsification of memory), memory loss, and peripheral neuropathy. This disorder is a result of poor nutrition (specifically inadequate amounts of thiamine and niacin) and the neurotoxic nature of alcohol. To prevent further advancement of the disease, the health care provider gives thiamine as an intramuscular injection as part of a standard protocol for alcohol detoxification in an effort to halt the progression of Wernicke-Korsakoff syndrome.

Peripheral Nervous System Effects

Alcohol effects on the peripheral nervous system (PNS) are varied and cause many physical problems. Cirrhosis and peripheral neuritis are health problems most commonly associated with alcohol. As liver function becomes impaired in the alcohol-dependent person, they are less able to tolerate alcohol. The drinker who once boasted of drinking exploits becomes intoxicated after only a few drinks. The physical consequences of cirrhosis include obstructed blood flow (which leads to portal hypertension, ascites, and possibly esophageal varices), decreased liver cell function, low serum albumin levels, high ammonia and bilirubin serum levels, and clotting problems. High ammonia levels add to the neurotoxic insult to the brain, which can lead to delirium, coma, and death.

Chronic alcohol use can cause painful peripheral neuritis, leaving the person at risk for injury since their limbs are numb. A malabsorption syndrome is caused by irritation of the intestinal lining. This condition seems to affect B vitamins generally and leads to a deficiency of vitamin B1 (thiamine) in particular. Thiamine deficiency contributes to peripheral neuritis. Alcohol is an irritant to mucus membranes; it burns the oral mucosa and prompts the stomach to secrete more hydrochloric acid. The elevated hydrochloric acid and irritation may lead to the formation of gastric ulcers. In addition, individuals with heavy alcohol use can experience gastritis, bleeding, and hemorrhage. This type of ulceration can eventually perforate, creating a life-threatening situation as coagulation factors are abnormal. In addition, chronic alcohol use increases the risk of oral and stomach cancers. The pancreas is affected by alcohol in many ways. Pancreatitis and diabetes are common consequences of alcoholism. Alcohol also has a direct effect on muscle tissue, a condition known as *alcoholic myopathy*. Other organs affected by alcohol include the eyes (loss of peripheral and night vision), the heart (hypertension, enlarged left ventricle), and the reproductive organs. Prolonged drinking shrinks the testicles and decreases testosterone. A failing liver is unable to detoxify female hormones, thus increasing the level of estrogen, compromising male sexual potency. As many men have experienced, alcohol can increase interest in sex but can lead to decreased sexual performance.

Clinical Example: AA saved his life

Anthony is a 36-year-old man with severe alcohol use disorder. Presenting at a local treatment facility, he said, "I just can't keep it up anymore. I have been drinking for 23 years, and my life is falling apart. Everyone I know hates me. I cannot keep a job. No one trusts me. I have to get some help." First, Anthony needed detoxification and went through a 28-day treatment program. He attended AA five times each week and got a sponsor, someone with whom he could confide. From his sponsor, he "learned to live life on life's terms." He also attended an aftercare treatment group three times a week to focus on dealing with his shame. After 108 days of sobriety, Anthony began to think that he was cured and no longer needed his sobriety support system. He began to drink again, and just before he was pulled over for driving under the influence, he managed to throw away the cocaine he had bought.

The consequences of his past lifestyle caught up with Anthony a few months later. As he is considered a habitual offender, he was sentenced to 20 years in prison. After getting the alcohol out of his system and reconnecting with AA, Anthony prepared to go to prison rather than trying to run from his obligations. The AA program teaches responsibility for one's actions and surrender of self-will to a "higher power." Anthony says, "I did it. I don't want to go to prison, but if that's what God has in mind for me because of my foolish decisions, then so be it. Might be there's somebody out there who needs to hear my story. I can share my experience, strength, and hope, and let them know that God is a way maker." These attitudes of surrender of self-will to a higher power are characteristic of 12-step programs and are considered essential to recovery.

Nursing Issues: Treating Users of Alcohol
Overdose

People die as a result of overdoses of alcohol because it depresses the CNS. Vital centers in the brain become anesthetized, compromising breathing and heart rate, and leading to a comatose state or death. People consistently underestimate the potency of alcohol, and deaths have occurred simply because individuals consumed too much. Almost every year, newspapers report the deaths of college students by alcohol poisoning. Although alcohol alone can kill, most overdose-related deaths are the result of combining alcohol with other CNS depressants or an opioid.

Interactions

Alcohol taken with other CNS depressants causes profound CNS depression and can lead to death. For instance, diazepam, which is not lethal when taken alone, has led to death when combined with alcohol. Alcohol should be avoided when a person is taking barbiturates, antipsychotic drugs, antidepressants, benzodiazepines, and other sedatives.

Use by Older Adults

Older adult alcoholics can be divided into the following two groups:
1. Lifelong users
2. Late-onset users responding to stress

Lifelong users tend to have increased physical, cognitive, and emotional problems associated with their drinking. Late-onset alcoholics include individuals who, as they grow older, tend to cope with the many and persistent losses of later life by drinking. If not effectively treated, these individuals can deteriorate rapidly. Luckily, late-onset heavy alcohol users have a robust response when treated.

Alcohol use in older adults is underreported, frequently unrecognized, and rarely treated. As the population of older adults has grown, so have substance-related problems in older adults. Decreased liver function is a product of aging; consequently, older individuals cannot drink much alcohol without becoming inebriated, confused, and sedated. Elderly people with impaired liver function do not metabolize alcohol efficiently and can have a low tolerance for alcohol. The nurse should be particularly watchful for combinations of alcohol with other CNS depressants among patients in this age group.

Withdrawal and Detoxification

Withdrawal from alcohol can be painful, scary, and lethal. As a person abstains from alcohol, they begin to experience CNS irritation caused by alcohol: tremulousness, nervousness, anxiety, anorexia, nausea and vomiting, insomnia and other sleep disturbances, rapid pulse, high blood pressure, profuse perspiration, diarrhea, fever, unsteady gait, difficulty concentrating, exaggerated startle reflex, and a craving for alcohol or other drugs. As withdrawal symptoms become increasingly pronounced, a few individuals can experience hallucinations.

The level of supervision needed during withdrawal depends on the severity of alcoholism. Mild dependence can

CASE STUDY

Mr. Evan Franklin's wife brought the 68-year-old man to treatment after his third DUI offense. He had run off the road and into a neighbor's mailbox. His history was life-long, starting to use alcohol and drugs at age 14. Although neither of his parents drank, his family history was positive as his grandfather died of cirrhosis of the liver and bleeding esophageal varices.

Evan has been in counseling twice in an effort to salvage his previous marriage. After the breakup of that marriage, he lost his business and became extremely depressed. When Evan drank, he became belligerent and, at one point, threatened his ex-wife. He also began gambling in an effort to make quick money.

Evan is willing to enter treatment so that he does not lose his current wife and because he fears the men to whom he owes gambling debts. He knows that he will be safe in the hospital until he can figure out what to do. He does not believe that he has a problem with alcohol, drugs, or gambling. He attributes his misfortunes to the ill will of others. He denies suicidal ideation currently. Evan's blood alcohol level on admission was 0.04%. He used to enjoy hunting and spending time with his wife.

be managed on an outpatient basis. However, severe withdrawal can be life-threatening related to CNS excitation, which causes tachycardia, hypertension, and seizures. Given the high risk of severe withdrawal, patients with severe alcohol use disorder require medical supervision. Withdrawal symptoms are managed with medications that are similar to alcohol in the brain, such as other CNS depressants, to diminish symptoms of withdrawal. At times, when someone who is alcohol-dependent is admitted to the hospital, they may receive alcohol such as beer to prevent alcohol withdrawal because maintaining some alcohol in their system is less stressful than having them go into withdrawal.

Medications Used to Treat Alcohol Withdrawal

Long-acting benzodiazepines such as chlordiazepoxide (Librium), diazepam (Valium), and shorter-acting lorazepam (Ativan) are useful for the treatment of alcohol withdrawal.

The principle behind this treatment is the rapid substitution of the benzodiazepine for the alcohol to suppress withdrawal symptoms stemming from rebound CNS excitation. Benzodiazepines bind to the GABA-benzodiazepine receptor sites, mimicking alcohol's mechanism of action. Withdrawal from severe alcohol use is most acute 24 to 48 hours after cessation of alcohol and is normally complete in 5 days. A gradual tapering of benzodiazepines follows this trajectory with discontinuation after the 5th day. Some clinicians prefer to use barbiturates for alcohol withdrawal, but respiratory depression and safety concerns dissuade most prescribers.

All patients treated for alcohol use disorder, moderate to severe, should be given thiamine supplements as alcohol interferes with B vitamin absorption in the intestine. The provision of thiamine prevents the development of Wernicke's encephalopathy.

CARE PLAN

Name: Evan Franklin   **Admission Date:** _____
DSM-5 Diagnosis: Alcohol Use Disorder, Severe

Assessment	**Areas of strength:** Patient has mild hypertension and denies suicidal ideation, has been in counseling twice previously, and enjoys hunting and doing things with his wife. Values this relationship.
	Problems: Has a family history of long-term use of alcohol and drugs. Denies that alcohol is a problem in his life despite family and occupational problems. Moderate level of depression
Nursing diagnoses	Difficulty coping related to alcohol use and gambling as evidenced by legal and financial issues
	Impaired family process related to alcohol use, potential marriage separation, and financial difficulties
	Depressed mood, low self-esteem related to business loss, and feeling like a failure
Outcomes	**Short-term goals**
Date met: _____	Patient will identify one emotional trigger for use and one coping strategy to manage alcohol cravings.
	Long-term goals
Date met: _____	Patient will remain chemical-free (alcohol or other non-prescribed substances) for monthly testing, assessed through urine screening by his probation officer. Patient will not go to places where he used to gamble. Sign Casino paperwork barring him from the establishments.
Planning and Interventions	**Nurse-patient relationship:** Discuss the natural consequences of his drinking and the need for total abstinence; educate regarding the health consequences of alcohol use, need to take one day at a time; create a concrete plan for recovery; offer hope for long-term recovery; encourage attendance at AA meetings.
	Psychopharmacology: Lexapro 10 mg daily. Encourage stopping smoking, avoid caffeine and sugar; provide multivitamin daily.
	Milieu management: Family treatment; encourage activities of daily living.
Evaluation	According to his probation officer, the patient is sober after 1 month.
Referrals	Refer to AA and make follow-up appointments with addiction counselor/family therapist as well as primary care provider to follow for depression, hypertension and monitor liver functions.

OTHER MEDICATIONS WITH SEVERE WITHDRAWAL POTENTIAL

Barbiturates

The medication class called barbiturates acts to depress the CNS, causing sedation and quieting seizures. Barbiturates were medically prescribed as sedatives in the last half of the 19th century. Barbiturates were initially thought to be safe; however, in 1950, researchers confirmed that barbiturates could produce physical dependence. The primary action of the CNS depressants is to decrease the awareness of and response to sensory stimuli. These medications are effective for seizure disorders, can decrease pain related to severe headaches, and are still in use today despite the risk of addiction and overdose death.

Barbiturate Withdrawal

Barbiturates, along with benzodiazepines and alcohol, have similar withdrawal symptoms, including the risk for life-threatening withdrawal symptoms in unsupervised settings. CNS symptoms usually begin 8 to 12 hours after the last dose. This is called a rebound effect and occurs when the consistent drug level drops. Minor withdrawal symptoms include anxiety, muscle twitching, tremor, progressive weakness, dizziness, distorted visual perception, nausea, vomiting, insomnia, and orthostatic hypotension. Withdrawal symptoms that are more serious include convulsions and delirium. Untreated withdrawal symptoms may not decline in intensity for about 1 week. Safe detoxification requires a cautious and gradual reduction of these drugs. Educating patients about medication such as Fioricet® can help reduce the risk of overuse and withdrawal from sudden cessation.

SUMMARY OF HOW ABUSED DRUGS WORK

Abused Substance	Mechanism of Action
Barbiturates	Increase effect of GABA
Opioids	Mimic endogenous neurotransmitters by stimulating opioid receptors; increase release of dopamine in the nucleus accumbens
Cocaine	Decreases reuptake of dopamine
Amphetamines	Increase release of norepinephrine; enhance dopamine release; block reuptake of dopamine, and retard dopamine reuptake
Methamphetamine	Blocks breakdown of dopamine, enhances its release, and blocks its reuptake
Ecstasy	Increases release of serotonin and dopamine
Marijuana	Stimulates dopamine pathways in the nucleus accumbens
LSD	Binds tightly to 5-HT_{2A} receptors, causing a psychedelic effect

GABA, Gamma-aminobutyric acid; *5-HT$_{2A}$*, 5-hydroxytryptamine 2A; *LSD*, lysergic acid diethylamide.

Benzodiazepines

Benzodiazepines have many legitimate uses and are reviewed in Chapter 17. However, one benzodiazepine, flunitrazepam (Rohypnol; also known as *roofies, rophies, roche, roaches*, and *ruffies*), is known primarily for its criminal potential. Because of its sedative and amnesic effects, flunitrazepam as Rohypnol has been used in date rape on unsuspecting women and men. It was manufactured as a colorless, odorless, and tasteless substance that could be mixed with liquids. Sexual predators slip it easily into the beverage of an unsuspecting person. This drug is not legally available in the United States.

OTHER SUBSTANCES OF MISUSE AND ADDICTION

Opioids (Narcotics)

Opioids include morphine, codeine, heroin, hydromorphone (Dilaudid), methadone (Dolophine), and others. Opioids can be swallowed, smoked, snorted, injected into soft tissue (skin popping), and mainlined (intravenous injection).

It is believed that misinformation about the safety of opioids in the 1990s by drug companies led to overprescribing opioids for pain. With the increased exposure to opioids, more individuals became addicted. As providers began to restrict the use, opioid-dependent people began purchasing heroin as the availability increased. The opioid-dependent person was likely to switch to the cheaper and easier-to-access heroin.

Clinical Example: It started with a toothache

Sam Jones is a 32-year-old maintenance man. He has a history of drinking and using marijuana since junior high school. He began showing a strong preference for opioids after a visit to the dentist to have a tooth extracted. Since that visit, Sam has had several other teeth extracted and has been to the emergency department several times for treatment for one type of intense pain or another. Sam has lost several jobs because of suspected stealing. When confronted, he stated that he was only trying to get people's prescriptions that they "weren't using anyway." Sam recently started injecting drugs and became obviously impaired quickly. After he was found wandering around the apartment complex, confused and slurring his speech, his boss fired him. Still using, he had a motorcycle accident. In the emergency department, his urine drug screen was positive for opioids. Once he had been stabilized medically, he agreed to be evaluated for his substance use, recognizing that he had no control over his drug use. He was diagnosed with severe opioid use disorder and was transferred to the substance use treatment center. Once there, he was tapered off his pain medication, but due to his constant cravings, was started on a low dose of buprenorphine. He will remain in treatment while he works on learning how to cope without resorting to opioid use. Sam has a long way to go with his recovery.

Physiologic Effects

Opioids relieve pain by increasing the pain threshold and by reducing anxiety and fear. These drugs accomplish this by stimulating opioid receptor sites in the brain. Naturally occurring neurotransmitters, or endorphins, produce various responses, including being able to mediate pain and regulate mood by activating opioid receptors. Opioids are endorphin agonists. Users are attracted by the drug's effect on mood (a feeling of euphoria) or just feeling normal when using. Some describe the euphoric mood created by opioids like morphine or heroin as being better than sex. Intravenous heroin delivers a rush (lasting <1 minute) described as similar to a sexual orgasm. After the euphoria, an overall CNS depression occurs. Drowsiness and sleep are common effects. Heroin has a higher abuse potential than morphine and other opioids because it more readily passes the blood-brain barrier. When heroin enters the brain, its chemical structure is changed to that of morphine; it then becomes trapped in the brain, causing a more sustained high. CNS effects of opioids include respiratory depression related to the medullary center, resulting in a decreased sensitivity to carbon dioxide stimulation. PNS effects include constipation; decreased gastric, biliary, and pancreatic secretions; urinary retention; hypotension; and reduced pupil size. Pinpoint pupils (miosis) are a sign of opioid overdose.

Nursing Issues

Overdose

At therapeutic doses prescribed by professionals, opiates are helpful and safe analgesics. However, individuals using recreationally may be opiate-naive and die of an inadvertent overdose. Users who buy drugs off the street cannot be sure of the amount of opioid as illicitly manufactured drugs are not standardized and may be a purer drug than anticipated. In addition, synthetic fentanyl has been mixed with a variety of substances such as heroin, cannabis, or Xanax with deadly results. A narrow window exists between an intoxicating dose and one that is lethal. Concomitant use of other CNS depressants (e.g., alcohol, benzodiazepines) increases the risk of a fatal overdose. A respiratory rate of 12 breaths/min or less is cause for alarm because respiratory depression is the primary cause of death due to opioid use.

Symptoms of overdose—respiratory rate less than 12 breaths/min:

- Person is stuporous and unresponsive.
- Skin is wet and warm.
- Coma develops, accompanied by respiratory depression and hypoxia.
- Skin becomes cold and clammy.
- Pupils dilate.
- Death quickly follows.

Emergency treatment priorities include the provision of an adequate airway and assisted ventilation and administration of a narcotic antagonist intranasally to reverse the effects of opioids.

Narcotic Antagonists: Antidotes to Opioids

Naloxone (Narcan), a narcotic antagonist, is the intervention of choice if opioid overdose is suspected. Naloxone blocks the neuroreceptors affected by opioids and moves the opioid off the reception. The patient responds in a few minutes to an intravenous injection. Respiration improves, and the patient responds consciously. However, as many opioids have a longer-lasting effect than naloxone, it is often necessary to repeat the antagonist to maintain adequate respiration. The nurse who administers naloxone must observe the patient carefully to determine whether an additional antagonist will be needed. If the dose of the antagonist is proportionately higher than the dose of opioids in the system, it is possible to precipitate a narcotic withdrawal or abstinence syndrome. Patients using opiates for chronic pain and opiate-dependent individuals will be in significant pain after reversal of the opiate.

Clinical Example: What they don't know can kill

A hospice team member told the following story. The patient Ben was a 70-year-old man with prostate cancer and painful bone metastases. A nursing concern is maintaining a balance between the need for pain management and the risk of respiratory suppression. Ben had been building a tolerance to his pain medication and required a dose increase (not unusual). His family members were afraid that he was becoming an "addict," so they decided to reduce his medication intake without consulting the physician. Cutting in half and administering a time-release pain pill (synthetic morphine that loses its time-release properties when the capsule is broken), they quickly noticed that he was suddenly unresponsive. Ben was taken to the hospital, and naloxone (Narcan) was administered. Because naloxone blocks the opioid receptor sites, there was no effective pain relief for this man. He was in extreme physical pain because his family had been afraid of the legitimate medical use of the opioid. Additionally, their lack of knowledge about how time-release medications work led to an erratic and potentially fatal dose.

Use by Older Adults

Some older patients may have chronic medical conditions associated with chronic pain, for which long-term narcotic pain medication has been prescribed. Such adults are particularly at risk for decreased pulmonary ventilation associated with opioids.

Opioid Withdrawal and Detoxification

Unassisted withdrawal from alcohol, benzodiazepines, and barbiturates can be fatal, but unassisted withdrawal from opioids is rarely fatal, although often painful. The terms *kicking the habit* and *going cold turkey* come from the leg spasms associated with withdrawal from opioids. Withdrawal symptoms are related to the degree of dependence and the abruptness of the discontinuance. Maximal intensity is reached within 36 to

72 hours, and symptoms subside in about 1 week. Withdrawal symptoms include yawning, rhinorrhea, sweating, chills, piloerection (goosebumps), tremor, restlessness, irritability, leg spasms, bone pain, diarrhea, and vomiting.

Clonidine has been used successfully for withdrawal by relieving some of the autonomic symptoms (e.g., vomiting and diarrhea). However, clonidine does not reduce craving or insomnia. A controlled taper with buprenorphine (Buprenex) or methadone can assist with the pain related to withdrawal. Treatment is primarily symptomatic and supportive.

Methadone

Methadone (Dolophine), although an opioid similar to morphine, is used specifically to prevent withdrawal symptoms; it is also used as an analgesic in conditions associated with severe pain, such as cancer. Methadone is used as an opioid treatment when the person is unable to discontinue opiate use successfully without assistance. Methadone is given orally and is poorly metabolized in the liver. It has a much longer half-life (15 to 30 hours) than morphine (about 2 hours). Because of its long half-life, once-daily dosing is effective and useful for outpatient care. In addition, methadone is used for the management of chronic pain. It has the potential for accidental overdose if misused or used concomitantly with benzodiazepines or other CNS depressants.

Heroin

Heroin is derived from morphine; it was initially believed to be a cure for morphine addiction but proved more addictive by comparison. Heroin can be taken intravenously (its effect is felt within 7 to 8 seconds), smoked, snorted, or mixed with other substances such as cocaine or methamphetamine (speed-ball). Heroin is more potent and lipid-soluble than morphine; therefore, it crosses the blood-brain barrier faster with a more rapid onset.

Clinical Example: Dying from overdose and nobody knew

A 32-year-old mother of two was seen in an emergency department in a medium-sized city. With a history of psychiatric disorders and substance use, she admitted to having ingested a large number of oxycodone (OxyContin) pills along with other CNS depressants. She was alert at times but also displayed slurred speech and psychomotor retardation. After an initial assessment, it was decided that she should be sent to a free-standing psychiatric facility, where she was taken several hours later. On admission, her speech was unintelligible, and her respirations were noted to be slowed (12 per minute) and irregular. A full assessment was deferred. She died as a result of opioid-induced respiratory depression before morning. Because only nurses were involved in the admissions process, those nurses were deemed negligent (although the case was settled out of court).

STIMULANTS

CAFFEINE

Worldwide, this drug is enjoyed by many. It can be found in soda, coffee, and tea, as well as cocoa drinks. Many people feel sluggish if they do not start their day with a cup of coffee. Caffeine increases attention and alertness and decreases fatigue; however, it can also increase anxiety, and when heavy use stops, it results in withdrawal. Excessive use can occur with caffeine intoxication at 300 mg, with symptoms of jitters and an increased heart rate. For example, a 12 oz. Starbucks coffee contains about 250 mg of caffeine. Some types of caffeine drinks have been mixed with alcohol with the misperception that this will override the sedating effect of alcohol. The unfortunate result is that young individuals often can have a potentially fatal amount of alcohol as they continue to ingest more alcohol without being rescued by alcohol's sedating effect and "pass out."

COCAINE

Cocaine is a fine white, odorless powder with a bitter taste that was introduced to Western medicine as an anesthetic in 1858. Sigmund Freud used cocaine and believed it to be a remedy for morphine addiction; he reported on the effects of cocaine in his book *Cocaine Papers*. Coca plants are grown high in the Andes Mountains, and indigenous people chewed coca leaves long before the Spanish explorers arrived. This plant is not cacao, from which we get chocolate, but *coca*. Cocaine was once used in some cola drinks (e.g., Coca-Cola), and advertisements extolled the ability of cola as well as of other brain tonics to refresh. After the Pure Food and Drug Act was passed in 1906, cocaine was eliminated from these beverages. Cocaine (cocaine hydrochloride) and crack (free-base cocaine) are the two forms most commonly used.

Physiologic Effects

Cocaine's exhilarating effect is related to its ability to block dopamine reuptake, particularly in the nucleus accumbens, the pleasure center of the brain. Euphoria, increased mental alertness, increased strength, anorexia, and increased sexual stimulation are initial desired effects. Increased motor activity, tachycardia (up to 200 beats/min), and high blood pressure are PNS effects. CNS effects include deep respirations (from medullary stimulation), euphoria, increased mental alertness, dilated pupils, anorexia, and increased strength. The cocaine user can be loquacious and easily stimulated sexually (libido is increased; ejaculation is retarded). These last characteristics undoubtedly add to the drug's overall appeal. Intense paranoia is common.

Less common reactions are specific hallucinations and delusions. Chronic cocaine users report that they think that bugs are crawling beneath their skin (formication) and that they sense foul smells. Nasal septum perforation has been associated with snorting cocaine; it is the result of extreme vasoconstriction, which impedes blood supply to this area and causes nasal necrosis. Death from cocaine is linked to metabolic and respiratory acidosis and hyperthermia associated with prolonged seizures. Tachyarrhythmias and coronary artery spasms have also led to death. Heart failure or stroke in young adults is often caused by cocaine use.

Routes of Cocaine Use

Cocaine hydrochloride is snorted or injected intravenously but not smoked. Crack (freebase cocaine) is smoked. Cocaine passes the blood-brain barrier quickly, causing an instantaneous high. When administered intravenously (mainlining), cocaine is rapidly metabolized by the liver; the rush, although exhilarating, does not last long. Cocaine exerts both CNS and PNS effects because of its ability to block norepinephrine and dopamine reuptake into presynaptic neurons; it depletes these neurotransmitters in the process.

Crack

Crack is a less expensive way of using cocaine compared with snorting or mainlining, primarily because it is sold in smaller packages. It is produced by a mixture of baking soda and water, heated, hardened, then smoked; it is reported to produce an instantaneous high and almost as instantaneous a crash.

CASE STUDY

Jerry Random (J.R.) is a 25-year-old unemployed carpenter who lives with his aunt. One night he began tearing the house apart; then, he locked himself in the bathroom, yelling that he was going to kill himself. His aunt called the police, who took J.R. to the emergency department of the local hospital. The emergency department examiner noted that J.R. was suicidal and having auditory hallucinations, delusions of persecution, disorganized thinking, anorexia, insomnia, anxiety, and agitation. He had been threatening the police and continued to be extremely agitated, threatening the emergency department personnel. Based on a history provided by his aunt, he was diagnosed with cocaine intoxication. J.R.'s aunt stated that she had been concerned about possible drug use for the last year but had never pursued the issue. J.R. was often belligerent and was told to leave his job until he was able to get "cleaned up." His aunt had noticed items missing but never questioned J.R. about it.

The physician decided to keep J.R. in the emergency department until his thinking cleared and to monitor him for tachycardia, cardiac arrhythmia, and seizure activity. The MD ordered 5 mg of diazepam (Valium) to be administered intravenously every 10 to 15 minutes if needed for seizures and agitation. Also, propranolol (Inderal) could be administered intravenously should the patient experience cardiac arrhythmias. After 4 hours of observation of being medically stable, J.R. was transferred to the psychiatric unit. On arrival, J.R. was noticeably irritable, agitated, and anxious, and he complained of a headache. He continued to have difficulty concentrating and was disorganized in his thoughts.

? CRITICAL THINKING QUESTION

1. Some cocaine users turn to heroin as they grow older. Name a reason why this might occur.

Clinical Example: She would do anything for cocaine

Gladys, a 32-year-old woman with a severe cocaine use disorder, was referred to outpatient treatment through the legal system after being charged with possession. After her second group therapy session, she asked for an individual session with her counselor. She told the counselor that she had been raped a month earlier by other "customers" at the local crack house. Gladys is frightened and embarrassed; her urge to use drugs to escape the emotional pain was strengthened by her traumatic experience at the crack house. Although Gladys says that she has a supportive family, she is further ashamed because she thinks that she is pregnant. In her helplessness, Gladys experienced suicidal ideation and talked about aborting the pregnancy. After she calmed down, Gladys was persuaded to see her physician. She did not return to treatment, no one answered her phone, and there was no response to letters sent to her. Six months later, Gladys called her counselor to say that she put aside her shame and talked with her pastor, her mother, and her 12-year-old daughter. She reports that all is going well, although the baby was stillborn. She has not used since that time.

This explains why crack is considered the most addictive drug. When the user's money is gone, they emotionally crash, often giving way to cocaine-induced depression. The depression induced by neurotransmitter depletion may have the user feel that being dead is less painful than being alive.

AMPHETAMINES AND RELATED DRUGS

Amphetamines, developed in 1887, have legitimate medicinal uses, as in the short-term treatment of obesity as well as in treating attention-deficit/hyperactivity disorder (ADHD) in childhood and narcolepsy. The illicit use of amphetamines and some variants—referred to as *speed, crystal, meth, ice,* or *crank*—is widespread in many areas of the United States. Related drugs include methylphenidate (Ritalin), a drug used in the treatment of ADHD, and 3,4-methylenedioxymethamphetamine (MDMA, or ecstasy). These drugs are often "traded" or sold to high school or college students so that they can achieve improved test performance or remain alert while completing assignments.

Methamphetamine

Methamphetamines were heavily used during World War II, especially by pilots flying long distances or on many missions without rest. In the past 30 years, cheap manufactured drugs from Mexico have flooded the black market. In an effort to thwart homegrown "meth labs," the Combat Meth Act of 2005 restricted the sale of some ingredients for methamphetamine (meth) production. Restrictions of pseudoephedrine and ephedrine have been effective. These drugs are now kept behind the pharmacy counter, with a limitation on the quantity sold to any one person. Methamphetamine (*speed, meth, crystal, crank,* or *ice*) is more attractive than cocaine as it produces a longer high and typically is less expensive (Table 31.4). Meth's length of action is roughly 10 times longer than cocaine (NIDA, 2020, October 14). Methamphetamines can be snorted, swallowed, injected, or smoked, causing an immediate, intense feeling of pleasure, followed by a lasting high. When the high wears off, an equally intense crash occurs. Users become paranoid and may hallucinate or experience violent rages. Long-term use of methamphetamines can cause damage to dopaminergic systems and other brain regions.

Ecstasy

Ecstasy (MDMA; also known as *XTC, E, X, rolls,* or *Adam*) was synthesized in the early 1900s and briefly used sometime later as an adjunct to psychotherapy. Its use seems to be leveling off at about 0.2% of individuals older than 12 years of age, or about 869,000 people in the United States. The average age of first use is 20.3 years (SAMHSA, 2014). Ecstasy is a popular club drug promoted as enhancing closeness to others, affection, and communication abilities. At higher doses, an amphetamine-like stimulation occurs, including euphoria, heightened sexuality, diminished self-consciousness, and disinhibition. Unpleasant amphetamine-type side effects also occur, such as tachycardia, increased blood pressure, anorexia, dry mouth, and teeth grinding.

Physiologic Effects

Amphetamines are indirect-acting sympathomimetics that cause the release of norepinephrine from nerve endings. Amphetamines also block norepinephrine reuptake in

TABLE 31.4 Comparison of Methamphetamine and Cocaine	
Methamphetamine	**Cocaine**
Synthetic	Plant-derived
Smoking produces a high that lasts 8–24 h	Smoking produces high lasting 20–30 min
Half-life, 12 h	Half-life, 1 h
Limited medical use	Can be used as local anesthetic

From NIDA. (2020, October 14.) How is methamphetamine different from other stimulants, such as cocaine?. https://www.drugabuse.gov/publications/research-reports/methamphetamine/how-methamphetamine-different-other-stimulants-such-cocaine.

presynaptic nerve endings. Similar to cocaine, amphetamines also have a profound effect on the pleasure pathway by enhancing dopamine. Amphetamines block dopamine reuptake but also stimulate the excess release of dopamine and retard its enzymatic breakdown. This effect on the dopamine system likely accounts for the addicting effects of amphetamines. The most common side effects of amphetamine use are restlessness, dizziness, agitation, and insomnia. PNS effects are palpitations, tachycardia, and hypertension. Respirations also increase because amphetamines, similar to cocaine, stimulate the medulla. A psychiatric side effect of amphetamine use is amphetamine-induced psychosis. In the emergency department, the psychotic presentation can be indistinguishable from paranoid schizophrenia.

Nursing Issues
Overdose

Cocaine and amphetamine overdoses have resulted in numerous deaths, primarily from cardiac arrhythmias, stroke, and respiratory collapse. Treatment includes induction of vomiting, acidification of the urine, and forced diuresis.

◎ CARE PLAN

Name: Jerry Random   *Admission Date:* _____
DSM-5 Diagnosis: Cocaine Intoxication

Assessment	**Areas of strength:** Patient is young (25 years old); lives with his aunt, who wants him to return home once he is better; previous employer will rehire him if he gets "clean."
	Problems: Suicidal ideation, hallucinations (auditory), delusions that someone wants to kill him, disorganized thoughts, anorexia, insomnia, anxiety (has exaggerated startle reflex), agitation.
Nursing problem	Increased risk for self-directed violence related to substance use and CNS agitation.
	Substance-induced sensory-perceptual alteration related to substance use. CNS agitation results in suicidal ideation, disorganized thinking, hallucinations, and delusions.
	Low body weight, poor nutritional status, body weight below ideal due to cocaine use disorder.
Outcomes	**Short-term goals**
Date met: _____	Patient will not experience physical injury during hospitalization.
Date met: _____	Patient will be as comfortable as possible with minimal symptoms of withdrawal of cocaine.
Date met: _____	Patient will sleep 6–8 hours per night.
Date met: _____	Patient will recognize the consequences of his substance use.
	Long-term goals
Date met: _____	Patient will maintain optimal levels of nutrition and maintain at least 90% of normal weight.
Date met: _____	Patient will attend outpatient Cocaine Anonymous meetings.
Date met: _____	Patient will practice abstinence from psychoactive drugs.
Date met: _____	Patient will verbalize and show some evidence of developing non–drug-using friends.

Continued

◎ **CARE PLAN**—*cont'd*

Planning and Interventions	**Nurse-patient relationship:** Develop a contract with the patient to report to the nurse if suicidal thoughts occur. Establish a relationship with the patient. Provide acceptance-based conversation. Accept the patient as he is. Set limits on behavior and mention inconsistencies. All staff must be consistent. Allow the patient to verbalize anxiety and fear. Teach the patient the effects of drugs on his body through discussion on consequences of use. Guide patient to create personalized recovery plan identifying triggers and relapse plan. **Psychopharmacology:** Haloperidol (Haldol) 5 mg orally every 4 hours as needed for agitation and psychosis; benztropine mesylate (Cogentin) 2 mg orally with first dose of haloperidol on days it is given. Acetaminophen (Tylenol) 2 tablets every 4 hours as needed for headache. Encourage smoking cessation and reduction in caffeine and sugar intake. If patient is nicotine-dependent, offer nicotine patches daily to assist with nicotine withdrawal. **Milieu management:** Provide patient with a quiet room to decrease stimulation and agitation. Provide safe environment, including frequent observation by staff, assessing vital signs every 4 hours while awake. Monitor environment for dangerous objects such as glass, razors, and belts. Offer patient the opportunity to choose foods from the hospital menu. Provide group setting for patient to explore the issues of substance use with other patients and to help the patient recognize that he is not alone in his struggles.
Evaluation	Patient has not experienced significant cocaine withdrawal; appetite is returning with 2-pound weight gain. Sleeping better at night (4–6 hours). Patient has not attempted self-injury and denies suicidal intent. Motivated to change and learn to live without cocaine.
Referrals	Outpatient treatment for aftercare, including Cocaine Anonymous meetings and random urine screens for increased accountability.

Withdrawal and Detoxification

Although cocaine and amphetamines are highly addictive, physical withdrawal is mild. However, psychological withdrawal is severe because the drugs are highly pleasurable, and depletion of monoamines is associated with depression and lethargy. As a rule of thumb, the low of withdrawal is inversely proportional to the high experienced.

HALLUCINOGENS

Hallucinogens, also referred to as *psychotomimetics* or *psychedelics*, cause hallucinations. Hallucinogens are in two basic groups, natural and synthetic. Natural hallucinogenic substances include mescaline (peyote [from cactus]), psilocybin (psilocin [from mushrooms]), and marijuana (*Cannabis sativa*). Synthetic or semisynthetic substances include lysergic acid diethylamide (LSD) and phencyclidine (PCP). In general, hallucinogens can heighten awareness of reality or can cause a terrifying psychosis-like reaction. Users report distortions in body image and a sense of depersonalization.

Cannabis (Marijuana)

Cannabis or marijuana, also known as *pot, weed,* or *grass,* has been cultivated for more than 5000 years. All forms of *Cannabis sativa* (Hash oil, hashish, and tetrahydrocannabinol [THC]) come from the hemp plant and have various concentrations. Cannabis is the most widely used illicit drug in the United States. However, as of 2020, it has been legalized by 20 states for recreational use and legalized for medical purposes in 35 states and territories. College students have increasingly turned to marijuana use with increased problems related to use. It is estimated that 21% of students use marijuana each month (Jordan, Madson, Bravo, Pearson, & The Protective Strategies Study Team, 2020).

Synthetic Cannabinoids

This engineered substance has a higher affinity for cannabinoid receptors than THC, has active metabolites that prolong their duration of action, which, in turn, increases accumulation in the system and increases the potential for toxicity. They are not detectable on routine urine drug screens, and as often, the chemical formulation changes are not controlled or identified by the Drug Enforcement Administration (DEA). Synthetic cannabinoids may be sold as "Spice" or other creative names (Welch, Smith, Malcolm, & Lichtman, 2020).

Metabolism

The active ingredient in cannabis, THC, is changed by the liver into metabolites and stored in fatty tissues. THC can remain in the body for up to 6 weeks after it is smoked. It can be detected in blood and urine from 3 days to about 4 weeks thereafter, depending on the level of use. The effects of smoking marijuana last for 2 to 4 hours. If marijuana is ingested, effects can last as long as 12 hours.

Physiologic Effects

Marijuana produces a sense of well-being, is relaxing, and alters perceptions. Increased hunger (known as the *munchies*) is an effect that makes marijuana useful for anorexic individuals (e.g., patients with cancer who are undergoing chemotherapy). Marijuana's antiemetic properties make it useful for treating nausea and vomiting associated with chemotherapy. Balance and stability are impaired for 8 hours after marijuana use. Short-term memory, decision-making, and concentration are also impaired. Dry mouth, increased heart rate, dilated pupils, conjunctival irritation (i.e., red eyes), and keener sight and hearing are physical responses to marijuana. Marijuana use is thought to be motivational; however, a few individuals react with agitation or aggression.

Other effects associated with the use of cannabis include harmful pulmonary effects (bronchitis), weakening of heart contractions, immunosuppression, and reduction of serum testosterone levels and sperm count. Anxiety, impaired judgment, paranoia, and panic are common reactions to cannabis. Memory is also impaired, owing to THC receptors occupying the hippocampus.

Lysergic Acid Diethylamide

LSD stimulates the nervous system by binding tightly to serotonin receptors (i.e., 5-hydroxytryptamine 2 A); the effects are experienced for up to 12 hours. LSD causes a phenomenon known as *synesthesia*, which is the blending of senses (e.g., smelling a color or tasting a sound). Expectations and environment govern the quality of the LSD trip. LSD causes an increase in blood pressure as well as tachycardia, trembling, and dilated pupils. CNS effects include a sense of unreality, perceptual alterations and distortions, and impaired judgment.

INHALANTS

Inhalants are a "cheap high" favored by adolescent men. Inhalants are absorbed by the transpulmonary route nasally or orally by inhaling the gaseous product. They are used because they are cheap, readily available, and typically legal. Examples include airplane glue, gasoline, rubber cement, polyvinylchloride cement, hair spray, air freshener, spot remover, nail polish remover, paint remover, white-out, keyboard cleaner, and lighter fluid. Gasoline is the most common inhalant. They usually depress the CNS producing the experience of hilarity and cause excitability. Common side

---

Clinical Example: Seeing the meaning of life with LSD

Mary Sky, an 18-year-old high school student, has recently become involved with peers who use various hallucinogenic drugs to help with their spiritual quests. One night Mary attended a ceremony during which she took LSD for the first time. Initially, she experienced anxiety, as the sky became a brilliant blue and particular stars seemed to shine very brightly. Mary soon began smiling a lot, realizing the depth of "this process called life" and that we are all "a part of the stars." This heightened experience continued throughout the evening. By the next day, all that remained was a memory of bliss and insights, but Mary's actual state of consciousness had returned to its usual condition, with all her previous inner conflicts.

---

effects include mouth ulcers, anorexia, confusion, headache, and ataxia. Inhalants are particularly dangerous because the amount inhaled cannot be controlled. Inhalants cross the blood-brain barrier quickly. Deaths from asphyxiation, suffocation, and choking (e.g., on vomit) have occurred. Brain damage has been reported to include frontal lobe, cerebellar, and hippocampal damage, leading to diminished problem solving, ataxic gait, and memory dysfunction, some so severe as to require total nursing care.

Treatment and Related Issues
A Family Illness

All family members are affected in some way by substance use when one member is actively using. The family can benefit from treatment and often fluctuates between enabling (e.g., making excuses, lying for, doing things for) or blaming the addicted member. A point repeatedly verified is that some families are better at coping with a substance-using family member than dealing with a recovered family member. Past behaviors, which may have included deception and resulted in disappointment and loss of respect, may require family members to seek assistance for their own recovery. Family therapy can help families develop new methods of coping. Al-Anon can also help families heal, while the individual with the substance use disorder goes to AA or NA.

Abstinence-Based Treatment

The most common goal of treatment for a chemically dependent person is abstinence from alcohol or drugs. It is believed that a person who is dependent on one substance can easily become dependent on another. The term *cross-dependence* describes this condition. Professionals working with chemically dependent individuals realize their patients' vulnerability and usually refrain from thinking of anyone as cured. Professionals treat a substance use disorder as a chronic, remitting, ongoing, lifelong process during which the person is in recovery while working to remain substance-free. A chronic disease model includes the concept of *recovery*, which indicates a current and dynamic process but also involves the ever-present possibility of relapsing to substance use.

Risk Reduction

When the individual cannot recognize the consequences of their substance use or does not want to be abstinent from a substance, then a risk reduction plan may come into play. Risk reduction looks for the potential for harm and considers how to reduce the risk of use. One example is a person who often drives while intoxicated. In which case, the plan may be no more than three drinks in one period, and if more, do not drive. Call a taxi or an Uber. Most may think that the person should be able to identify that they are not fit to drive, but many people who are heavy drinkers are unaware of how intoxicated they are. Those individuals with alcohol tolerance may be desensitized to the sedating effect of the alcohol.

For a college student whose cannabis use has become problematic, but they want to continue to use recreationally, the nurse may teach Protective Behavioral Strategies for Marijuana. Behaviors can include buying less to use less, using marijuana only with trusted friends, not using marijuana with other substances such as alcohol. Avoid using marijuana before events where cognition is important such as school, work, and time with loved ones (Jordan, Madson, Bravo, Pearson, & The Protective Strategies Study Team, 2020). Harm reduction strategies create planned behaviors that can reduce the risk of use.

PSYCHOTHERAPEUTIC MANAGEMENT

Substance use disorders are highly treatable. However, the success of treatment depends on the patient's motivation, ability to cope with new skill development, and management of the cravings (Box 31.1). The nurse's role in the patient's recovery involves each of the three crucial elements of psychotherapeutic management interventions. Milieu management is a key element for this group of patients. One of the ideal goals of treatment is total abstinence. However, when the individual is not ready to commit to abstinence, risk reduction may be an appropriate goal. This process involves an ongoing relationship with the nurse and reinforcement of the individual's personal goals. When something as significant as alcohol is removed from a person's life, something must take its place. This replacement can take the form of group counseling facilitated by nurses or other professionals or a 12-step program directed by successfully recovering individuals. The concept encourages support and new coping skills; the individual will use less of the substance and therefore not experience the same degree of harm. If the person's use was tied to attempts to manage emotions, new skills could assist in avoiding relapse as a coping method (Table 31.5).

Nurse-Patient Relationship

Authenticity is the most important quality of this relationship. Often seeking treatment is initiated out of a crisis, whereby the nurse can express empathy and provide a safe environment that minimizes anxiety. This is important, especially in the early stages of treatment. Engendering feelings of hope for the future is also necessary as the patient begins to establish new life goals. Nurses working with chemically dependent patients must become skilled at motivational interviewing, pointing out discrepancies, and managing

---

BOX 31.1   Motivation

Whether external coercion is a positive influence on treatment outcome is a matter of disagreement. Participants who voluntarily seek treatment are more invested in their recovery than are those coerced into treatment. Participants who are coerced into treatment might be compliant only while the coercive influence is present and might be compliant only with behaviors specified by the coercive agent. The underlying principle is harm reduction, and some people who are off the drug come to realize what the drug use was costing them. The individual is still vulnerable to unconscious cravings or the negative influence of peers who continue to use.

---

attempts at manipulation. Assisting the substance user to recognize these discrepancies by gentle confrontation can help individuals recognize their own cognitive inconsistencies. While some patients may be defensive, a genuine concern can help overcome this barrier.

As denial is the most predominant defense of an individual dependent on alcohol/drugs, it is important to recognize and treat it appropriately. A group therapy setting seems to provide the best avenue because groups are especially effective in breaking down the denial process. The group is able to point out the disparity between what is believed to be true and what others know to be true. Group support of individuals who share a common goal diminishes isolation and builds a sense of belonging and trust. In addition, as substance use personally affects many nurses, it is important for them to be aware of their feelings and to avoid projecting any negative attitudes onto the patient.

Understanding positive motivators can help in establishing new goals and directions for the patient's life. Therapy can help the patient replace ineffective behaviors with new coping skills, giving them a better chance of getting and staying sober. Nurses aid the recovery process by teaching a variety of skills—including social skills and habits, parenting, family communication, family role responsibilities, and introducing the patient to new leisure activities. The nurse develops a trusting therapeutic relationship with the patient, which requires the rules for treatment to be consistently applied.

Confrontation (Use With Care)

Here are two common examples of confrontation:
1. "You say you have not been drinking (or using drugs), but I can smell alcohol on your breath (or cocaine was detected in your urine sample)."
2. "I hear you saying that you are in treatment because you believe you need help, so help me understand how you see your need, given your absence from treatment all week without a medical excuse."

What seems to be most effective is when the patient's peers provide appropriate confrontation. For example, Lloyd reported to the group that he had not used alcohol in the previous 3 months. Lloyd's peer, Christy, had appropriately used the group for support earlier that session to process her recent relapse episode. Christy was able to confront Lloyd directly about the fact that she had seen him in the same bar the previous weekend.

Personal Responsibility for Recovery

It is important to help the patient learn to foster personal responsibility for recovery. The nurse must cultivate awareness by the patient that he is responsible for change. Although the nurse expresses support and concern, they must not shield the patient from the negative consequences of their addictive behavior.

Milieu Management

All six dimensions of milieu management (see Chapters 1 and 21 to 23) are important in shaping the milieu for an

TABLE 31.5   Principles of Drug Addiction Treatment

1. **Addiction is a complex but treatable disease that affects brain function and behavior**. Drugs of abuse alter brain structure and function, resulting in changes that persist long after drug use has stopped. These persistent changes may explain why those in recovery are at the risk of relapse after prolonged abstinence.

2. **No single treatment is appropriate for everyone**. It is critical to match treatment settings, interventions, and services to each patient's problems and needs.

3. **Treatment must be readily available**. Treatment applicants can be lost if treatment is not immediately available or readily accessible. As with other chronic diseases, the earlier treatment is offered in the disease process, the greater the likelihood of positive outcomes.

4. **Effective treatment must attend to multiple needs of the individual, not solely substance use**. In addition to addressing drug use, treatment must address the individual's medical, psychological, social, vocational, and legal problems.

5. **Remaining in treatment for an adequate time is critical**. Treatment duration is based on individual needs. Most patients require at least 3 months of treatment to significantly reduce or stop drug use. Additional treatment can produce further progress. As with other chronic illnesses, relapses can occur, signaling a need for treatment to be reinstated or adjusted. Programs should include strategies to prevent patients from leaving prematurely.

6. **Individual and/or group counseling and other behavioral therapies are the most common forms of drug abuse treatment**. In therapy, patients address motivation, build skills to resist drug use, replace drug-using activities with constructive and rewarding activities, and improve problem-solving abilities. Behavioral therapy also addresses incentives for abstinence and facilitates interpersonal relationships. Ongoing group therapy and other peer support programs can help maintain abstinence.

7. **Medication can be an important element of treatment, especially when it is combined with counseling and other behavioral therapies**. Methadone, buprenorphine, and naltrexone can support recovery in those with opioid use disorder. Nicotine replacement therapy (e.g., patches, gum), bupropion, and varenicline can support efforts to quit smoking. Disulfiram, naltrexone, and acamprosate can help persons recover from alcohol use disorder.

8. **Because the needs of the individual can change, the plan for treatment and services must be reassessed continually and modified as indicated**. At different times during treatment, a patient may develop a need for medications, medical services, family therapy, parenting instruction, vocational rehabilitation, and social and legal services.

9. **Many individuals with substance use disorder also have co-occurring mental disorders that must be addressed**. Patients presenting with substance use disorders should be assessed for other conditions and treated as indicated.

10. **Medically assisted detoxification is only the first stage of addiction treatment and, by itself, does little to change long-term drug use**. Medical detoxification manages the acute physical symptoms of withdrawal and can serve as a precursor to effective long-term treatment.

11. **Treatment need not be voluntary to be effective**. Sanctions or enticements coming from the family, employer, or criminal justice system can significantly increase treatment entry, retention, and success.

12. **Drug use during treatment must be monitored continuously, as relapses during treatment do occur**. Knowing that drug use is being monitored (e.g., through urinalysis) can help the patient withstand urges to use drugs. Monitoring also can provide early evidence of drug use or lack of medication on board (diversion), thereby allowing timely adjustment of the treatment program.

13. **Treatment programs should provide assessment for HIV/AIDS, hepatitis B and C, tuberculosis, and other infectious diseases, along with counseling to help patients modify risky behaviors**.

HIV/AIDS, Human immunodeficiency virus/acquired immunodeficiency syndrome.
Modified from National Institute on Drug Abuse. (2012). *Principles of drug addiction treatment: A research-based guide* (3rd ed.). (Publication No. 12-4180). National Institutes of Health.

inpatient unit treating patients with a chemical dependency. Some dimensions are significant for outpatient care as well. Safety issues, such as a drug-free environment, are critical. Nurses and others must be vigilant to protect the environment from individuals who might bring substances into the milieu. Any hospital, as well as a psychiatric unit, is at high risk for contraband, as multiple avenues exist for illicit contraband. Other safety issues, such as suicide prevention and thwarting inappropriate sexual behavior, are the responsibility of nursing staff. Effective unit structure maximizes the benefit of the milieu. Norms of expectations for nonviolent behavior, openness, feedback, and the prohibition of nonprescribed drugs are critical to an effective treatment program. As previously noted, confrontation, motivation, and coaching are useful techniques to help individuals in recovery.

Limit-setting is perhaps the most important and most challenged (by patients) milieu management technique. Limit-setting is characterized as providing an environment that protects patients from themselves and from other patients. As part of this process, the nurse must recognize the symptoms of a still actively addicted mind (i.e., mood swings and substance-seeking as well as stubborn, belligerent, violent, and aggressive behavior) and set limits on these behaviors. Urine drug screens are also a dimension of limit-setting because these tests reinforce the no-drug policy. If drugs are found, or there is evidence of use, the patient must be confronted and held accountable. Facilities should have policies in place to guide the management of such behavior.

Balance and environmental modification also play significant roles in a well-managed milieu for chemically dependent patients. Balance is especially important in using the technique of confrontation. Although confrontation is important and therapeutic, in the hands of less skilled staff, it can become little more than a heavy-handed counterpart to the abuse that patients may have experienced in the past. The proper technique requires sensitivity to confront without crushing or totally alienating the patient. Skillful confrontation combines knowledge, empathy, and concern with accurate timing. Nursing and other professional staff need to have good team communication around patient behaviors as well as empathic concerns to keep all informed.

Psychopharmacology

Pharmacological treatment for chemical dependency is becoming increasingly important as the science of addictions progresses. Many of the current available pharmacologic agents for the treatment of substance use disorders are helpful for some and ineffective for others, due in part to individual biologic differences. However, medications offer added support to the recovery process. For example, medication for nicotine dependence, such as varenicline (Chantix), helps smokers to become nicotine-free; yet some people are sensitive to neurochemical changes of the serotonin and nicotine receptors and experience negative mood changes, such as suicidal ideation or extreme irritability. As researchers continue to explore brain function, our understanding of ideal prescribing practices will improve recovery outcomes,

Medications for Alcohol Use Disorder

Naltrexone: decreases the pleasure of drinking. Naltrexone hydrochloride (ReVia) is an opioid receptor antagonist used to treat narcotic dependence and is approved for the treatment of alcohol dependence. This would be the first choice when treating alcoholism. Naltrexone increases abstinence and reduces alcohol craving when used as a part of a comprehensive treatment plan. Naltrexone interferes with opioid functioning, which may compromise the pleasurable effects of alcohol. Naltrexone is also available as an intramuscular injection given on a monthly basis. The medication does not stop the individual from drinking, but it can lengthen the periods of sobriety. However, only about 40% of patients report a response to the anti-craving medication.

Acamprosate: restores chemical balance in the alcoholic brain. Acamprosate is used when abstinence has begun but not while the person is still drinking. Initial reports have suggested that acamprosate enhances abstaining behaviors. It may be used in conjunction with other medications to support recovery. It may also help decrease post-withdrawal anxiety.

Disulfiram: makes drinking painful. Disulfiram is an aversive drug, which means the patient knows that drinking while taking it will make them sick. This medication is not recommended unless the patient is in full awareness of the side effects. Disulfiram inhibits the breakdown of CH_3CHO (acetaldehyde) by the enzyme aldehyde dehydrogenase. Because CH_3CHO is toxic, a person who drinks alcohol while taking disulfiram becomes ill (as evidenced by sweating, flushing of

the neck and face, tachycardia, hypotension, throbbing headache, nausea and vomiting, palpitations, dyspnea, tremor, weakness, or any combination of these effects). Disulfiram and alcohol can also cause arrhythmias, myocardial infarction, cardiac failure, seizures, coma, and death. The unpleasant response to alcohol is intended to help reinforce the alcoholic's efforts to stop drinking alcohol. A patient taking disulfiram must make only one decision a day about drinking: once the pill is taken, the patient dare not drink. A person who is very sensitive to the effects of disulfiram may also have to avoid skin bracers or cologne because alcohol is absorbed through the skin and can trigger a reaction. Disulfiram is most effective in patients with significant motivation for long-term change and who have someone willing to oversee daily medication ingestion.

Medications to Treat Opioid Overdose

Drugs used to treat opioid dependence are divided into agents for withdrawal or opioid overdose and agents for long-term replacement therapy or medication for opioid use disorder or MOUD.

Naloxone. Naloxone is an opioid antagonist which binds to the receptor and displaces and blocks the receptor to other opioids. In case of an opioid overdose, naloxone is given to reverse opioid-induced CNS depression and respiratory arrest. The large number of opioid overdose deaths due to heroin/fentanyl use has mobilized community efforts to provide first responders and patients' families with naloxone kits. These kits have saved the lives of countless individuals when such persons are discovered in time. Although improvement occurs rapidly in a patient who has taken an overdose, the effect of naloxone is time-limited due to its short half-life; therefore, symptoms of opioid overdose may reemerge if the drug has a long half-life. In addition, the very powerful opioids such as synthetic fentanyl may require several doses to reverse the OD.

Medications to Treat Opioid Use Disorder

Methadone. Methadone as a treatment for opioid use disorder has been available since the 1950s. It is dispensed from federally regulated programs that have monitoring systems in place. Methadone has a much longer half-life compared with the prototype opioid morphine, so it can be given in once-daily doses. Benefits include once-a-day dosing to a therapeutic level. Methadone relieves the drug hunger associated with opioid use disorder. When used for opiate treatment, it is given in high doses to cause opioid receptor blockade. This helps prevent the use of other opiates and blocks their benefit should the person attempt to use them with methadone in their system.

Buprenorphine. Buprenorphine is an agonist-antagonist opioid or a partial agonist for the mu receptor and an antagonist for the kappa receptor. This pharmacologic activity seems to reduce the craving for opioids. Two different formulations are available that can prevent illicit opiate use. The first, buprenorphine, can be used for chronic pain management, opiate replacement therapy, or opiate taper for detoxification. The other is a combination of buprenorphine and naloxone, which prevents the individual from achieving the benefit of the injected opiate. Like methadone, only providers qualified to prescribe this medication may treat OUD.

Naltrexone. Naltrexone acts by blocking the opioid receptor preventing the individual from experiencing the desired effect from the opioid. This medication cannot be started until after the person has been free of opioids for 6 to 10 days. Earlier would precipitate withdrawal and can weaken the person's resolve to quit, and they may drop out of recovery to seek an opioid. Naltrexone is highly effective in reducing cravings and prevent relapsing to opioid use. However, the medication must be taken daily to be effective. The long-acting injectable has a better success rate, but the injections can be painful and are quite expensive. This medication treatment is covered by most insurances.

INTERVENTION AND PEER SUPPORT

The best-known treatment for substance use disorders is the peer support programs such as AA and Narcotics Anonymous (NA). These programs use a self-help support-group model made up of fellow users in various stages of recovery.

Philosophically, AA and NA view psychosocial problems as stemming from substance use and generally reject the idea that underlying psychopathology is responsible for the use. AA (more than 1 million members in the United States) has established the 12 steps (Box 31.2), which start with a person admitting personal powerlessness over alcohol and end with the person being available, night or day, to help another alcoholic in need. The popular bumper sticker slogan "Easy does it" reflects a philosophy of taking life one day at a time and avoiding a frenetic lifestyle. AA and NA subscribe to the belief that only total abstinence can free a chemically dependent person from the bondage of alcohol and drugs, as they maintain that "a drug is a drug is a drug," meaning that if someone is addicted to one substance, that person is by definition addicted (at least potentially) to all substances. Although AA has helped many people, it does not appeal to everyone.

Reasons vary, but some find that the spiritual nature of AA is a deterrent, as 8 of the 12 steps have a spiritual perspective. Specifically, the concept of a higher power, the expectation that a person will tell his or her story publicly, of making a searching and fearless moral inventory, and then making amends when needed, are incongruent with some people's belief systems. Others feel this unwillingness to commit as a vestige of substance use. AA continues to be an important treatment alternative for many thousands of individuals with alcoholism.

BOX 31.2 Twelve Steps of Alcoholics Anonymous

1. Admitted we were powerless over alcohol—that our lives had become unmanageable.
2. Came to believe that a power greater than ourselves could restore us to sanity.
3. Made a decision to turn our will and our lives over to the care of God as we understood Him.
4. Made a searching and fearless moral inventory of ourselves.
5. Admitted to God, to ourselves, and to another human being the exact nature of our wrongs.
6. Were entirely ready to have God remove all these defects of character.
7. Humbly asked Him to remove our shortcomings.
8. Made a list of all persons we had harmed and became willing to make amends to them all.
9. Made direct amends to such people wherever possible, except when to do so would injure them or others.
10. Continued to take personal inventory, and when we were wrong, promptly admitted it.
11. Sought through prayer and meditation to improve our conscious contact with God as we understood Him, praying only for knowledge of His will for us and the power to carry that out.
12. Having had a spiritual awakening as the result of these steps, we tried to carry this message to alcoholics and to practice these principles in all our affairs.

The Twelve Steps are reprinted with permission of Alcoholics Anonymous World Services, Inc. Permission to reprint this material does not mean that AA has reviewed or approved the contents of this publication. AA is a program of recovery from alcoholism only—use of the Twelve Steps in connection with programs and activities that are patterned after AA, but that address other problems does not imply otherwise.

A STUDENT'S CLINICAL LOG

I went to the substance treatment meeting the week of November 2. When the two other students and I arrived, we were amazed to see all the teenagers standing in front of the building. As I waited in line to sign in, I heard several of them talking. They were talking about the party they went to last weekend, how they got "messed up," and how they were planning on doing it again the next weekend. They talked about how they hated the substance treatment program and thought it was a waste of their time. I was annoyed by this conversation. If they had that kind of attitude, they did not need to be there. They were wasting their time and money. I should have expected this type of attitude from them. Most of them were there because they had to be there. Some judge thought it was the solution to their problem. I wonder if they were paying for this program or whether others were "throwing their money away." I think most of them viewed this as a social gathering. I wish I did not think this way. I want to believe that these kids want to "get better," but based on their actions, I do not think some of them are ready. They will have to hit rock bottom before they see the error of their ways.

❓ CRITICAL THINKING QUESTION

3. The founders of AA were clear that the recovery process was a spiritual journey. However, we now live in times where most people are reluctant to speak of spiritual matters for fear of offending or of imposing their views on others. Do you think that in our efforts not to offend people, we have deemphasized an important part of psychiatric nursing?

SPECIAL NOTES

The traditional stereotype of an addict or alcoholic is a person at the end-stage disease process. However, all individuals are at risk, and health care providers are often at a higher risk because of chronic stress, physical injuries, and their ready access to medications. Exposure to opioids increases the risk of developing an addiction; therefore, in 2016, the CDC recommended the avoidance of opioids for all but the most intense acute pain.

Addicted Health Care Professionals

Substance use among health care professionals is a particularly difficult problem because it is an ethical violation of the professional's relationship with the patient. Substance use becomes the individual's coping mechanism for managing life demands, with nurses often having easier access than other people to widely abused substances. Health care professionals who divert (take drugs) from patients are particularly scorned by other nurses. As substance use disorders are considered diseases, many states have adopted nonpunitive monitoring programs that give nurses an opportunity to work under strict guidelines while actively participating in a recovery program. Nurses and nursing students who are dependent on substances need treatment and will need monitoring to make sure that they will remain in recovery while continuing to provide care to patients.

Follow-up Care

Follow-up care is essential for preventing relapse as it is common early in the recovery process. Patients and nurses need to be aware that recovery takes time, and learning needed skills is part of recovery. The first few months after completion of a treatment program can be challenging for a chemically dependent person. A relapse prevention plan developed during treatment can help the patient to avoid "triggers." At times, triggers are unconscious, so avoiding people, places, and the localities where they once used is important. The nurse should confirm arrangements for aftercare, outpatient counseling, and self-help support group meetings before discharge. One saying used in support meetings is "H.A.L.T.: Don't get too hungry, angry, lonely, or tired," because any of these mental states increases the chance of poor decision making and reverting back to old habits, thus increasing the risk of using.

This concept is illustrated as being "hangry." Consider the Snickers candy bar commercial of young men playing tag football with an old lady. She falls down and does not get up. A friend hands her a Snickers bar and says, "You're just not yourself when you're hungry." Eating the candy, he is once again a young man.

Clinical Example: The face of addiction: Stealing a patient's meds

Terry is a 39-year-old opioid-dependent registered nurse whose presentation in treatment was precipitated by her employer turning her into the State Board of Nursing. Nursing is Terry's life, and her identity is as a nurse. However, Terry has beliefs that have perpetuated her use. She reports that "it was common to share medication with patients." Terry, at first, documented the administration of the maximum as-needed pain medication in a patient's chart while not always giving that dose to the patient. She rationalized her behaviors, thinking, "I never let one of my patients ever be in pain." She frequently volunteered to be the med nurse and gave her meds like clockwork. Terry's supervisor did not suspect a problem until some narcotics were unaccounted for. Terry believed that she had been careful and would not get caught. However, she was eventually discovered diverting drugs but not because of impaired judgment because of drug use. She had begun to forget to sign out the medication she was taking, and the count was frequently off.

Terry's nursing license was placed on probationary status. Most facilities were unwilling to hire a nurse on probation, as the limitations placed by the board were strict. Terry cannot work the night shift, cannot hold the keys to the narcotics supply, or pass any controlled substances. She must also submit to random drug testing monthly for the duration of her probationary period, which is often 2 years in length. Terry was lucky that her employer recognized that substance use disorders are an illness and require treatment. She was not fired but was reassigned. She entered a treatment program designated by the Board of Nursing as acceptable for nurses in recovery. Like most women, she had hidden her disease until it became severe. In treatment, Terry is learning the importance of self-care, as well as the effects of trauma earlier in her life. Getting out of bed for her is painful each day, but she has been focusing on "one day at a time."

❓ CRITICAL THINKING QUESTION

4. What can you do to help an adolescent avoid substance use?

NEXT-GENERATION NCLEX® EXAMINATION-STYLE CASE STUDY

Identifying Alcohol Use Disorder

Scenario: A 40-year-old client was brought to the emergency department by the police after being involved in an automobile accident. The client sustained a fractured left forearm. Serum blood alcohol level was 0.38%. A family member provided a history that included a previous diagnosis of alcohol use disorder and two hospitalizations for alcohol-related injuries and withdrawal treatment.

Item Type: Extended Multiple Response

In caring for this client, which condition will the nurse attempt to prevent? **Select all that apply**.

Visual hallucinations
Grand mal seizures
Hypertension
Tachycardia
Aspiration
Paranoia
Tremors
Coma

STUDY NOTES

1. Chemical dependency is a major physical and mental health problem in North America, and most nurses, whether they want to or not, will take care of patients with chemical dependencies.

2. Drugs of abuse are categorized into the following basic groups: (1) alcohol, (2) CNS depressants, (3) opioids, (4) CNS stimulants, (5) hallucinogens, and (6) synthetic drugs.

3. *DSM-5* defines substance use disorders as mild, moderate, and severe, depending on the degree of problems related to use. Alcohol represents the leading drug problem in North America; it exacts a high price economically from society and is responsible for much suffering and death.

4. Alcohol causes disinhibition as well as impaired judgment. The primary concern with respect to alcohol overdose is severe and often fatal CNS depression. Withdrawal causes tremors, nausea, vomiting, tachycardia, diaphoresis, seizures, anxiety, and even death if untreated.

5. Prevention of tobacco use in children, adolescents, and young adults is a health priority.

6. Substances that are depressants cause euphoria, disinhibition, and drowsiness. The primary effect of overdose is respiratory depression. Withdrawal from CNS depressants can be life-threatening.

7. Opioids (narcotics) come from the juice of the opium poppy, a natural product, which can be manufactured into morphine, codeine, semisynthetic heroin, and synthetic fentanyl. Opioids can be smoked, taken intravenously, orally, intramuscularly, and subcutaneously (skin popping). Overdose can be fatal, with respiratory depression being the most serious side effect. Withdrawal, although unpleasant (influenza-like symptoms), is not life-threatening.

8. Naloxone is an opioid receptor blocker and is given by first responders in the field to treat the overdose immediately. Naloxone causes opioid abstinence syndrome by blocking the opioid receptors. When someone has overdosed, they may require several doses of intranasal naltrexone before they begin to respond.

9. Stimulants include amphetamines, cocaine, and caffeine. They cause elation, grandiose thinking, talkativeness, sleeplessness, and other less pleasant effects. The primary concerns in the event of overdose are agitation, tachycardia, cardiac arrhythmias, stroke, and convulsions.

10. Hallucinogens include mescaline, marijuana, LSD, and PCP. Hallucinogens cause illusions, hallucinations, diminished ability to perceive time and distance, anxiety, and paranoid thinking. The primary effects of hallucinogenic overdose are intense trips, psychotic reactions, and panic.

11. Treatment is effective, and one of the therapeutic goals for most approaches is abstinence from the substance. If the patient is not ready to quit, the nurse—through motivational interviewing—can help the patient to identify what changes he or she is willing to make to decrease the risk of the substance. This is called risk reduction.

12. Medications such as methadone, buprenorphine, and naltrexone can support recovery and decrease cravings, as well as diminish the effect of the illicit drug should relapse occur.

13. Nursing interventions include motivational interviewing, group work, education, confrontation, boundaries, providing for physical and nutritional needs, and helping the patient become involved in groups such as AA and NA and families with Al-Anon.

14. Health care professionals are at increased risk as they have access to medications that can be diverted for their personal use. Most licensing boards monitor recovery by making sure that individuals in recovery remain abstinent through long-term monitoring programs and ongoing urine drug screening.

REFERENCES

American Psychiatric Association. (2013). *Diagnostic and statistical manual of mental disorders* (5th ed.). APA.

Burchum, J., & Rosenthal, L. (2019). *Lehne's pharmacology for nursing care* (10th ed.). Saunders.

Colyar. M. R. (2003). Testing for drugs of abuse. *Advance for Nurse Practitioners*, 9, 30.

Frezza. M., et al. (1990). High blood alcohol levels in women: The role of decreased gastric alcohol dehydrogenase and first-pass metabolism. *New England Journal of Medicine, 322,* 95–99. https://doi.org/10.1056/NEJM199001113220205.

Jordan, H., Madson, M., Bravo, A., Pearson, M., & The Protective Strategies Study Team. (2020). Post-traumatic stress and marijuana outcomes: The mediating role of marijuana protective behavioral strategies. *Substance Abuse, 41*(3), 375–381. https://doi.org/10.1080/08897077.2019.1635965.

National Center for Health Statistices (2021, March 1). Illicit drug use. https://www.cdc.gov/nchs/fastats/drug-use-illicit.htm.

National Institute on Alcohol Abuse and Alcoholism. (2021, March). Alcohol facts and statsticis. https://www.niaaa.nih.gov/sites/default/files/publications/NIAAA_Alcohol_Facts_and_Stats_1.pdf.

National Institute on Drug Abuse. (2012). Principles of drug addiction treatment: A research-based guide: 12-4180 (3rd ed.). Publication No. https://www.drugabuse.gov/sites/default/files/podat_1.pdf.

NIDA. (2005, June 1). Drug Abuse and Addiction: One of America's Most Challenging Public Health Problems. https://archives.drugabuse.gov/publications/drug-abuse-addiction-one-americas-most-challenging-public-health-problems.

NIDA. (2020, May 28). Part 1: The Connection Between Substance Use Disorders and Mental Illness. https://www.drugabuse.gov/publications/research-reports/common-comorbidities-substance-use-disorders/part-1-connection-between-substance-use-disorders-mental-illness.

NIDA. (2020, June 3). How long does drug addiction treatment usually last? https://www.drugabuse.gov/publications/principles-drug-addiction-treatment-research-based-guide-third-edition/frequently-asked-questions/how-long-does-drug-addiction-treatment-usually-last.

NIDA. (2020, October 14). How is methamphetamine different from other stimulants, such as cocaine? https://www.drugabuse.gov/publications/research-reports/methamphetamine/how-methamphetamine-different-other-stimulants-such-cocaine.

Prochaska, J., & DiClemente, C. (1983). Stages and processes of self-change of smoking: Toward an integrative model of change. *Journal of Consulting and Clinical Psychology, 51,* 390–395. https://doi.org/10.1037//0022-006x.51.3.390.

Peng, Q, Wilhelmsen, K, & Ehlers, C. (2021). Common genetic substrates of alcohol and substance use disorder revealed by pleiotrophy detection against GWAS catalog in two populations. *Journal of Addiction Biology, 26,* e12877. https://doi.org/10.1111/abd.12877.

SAMHSA. (2014). Results from the 2013 national survey on drug use and health: Summary of national findings, NSDUH Series H-48, HHS Publication No. (SMA) 14-4863. SAMHSA.

SAMHSA, Center for Behavioral Health Statistics and Quality. (2019). National Survey on Drug Use and Health. Table 2.32A – Alcohol Use in Lifetime, Past Year, and Past Month and Binge and Heavy Alcohol Use in Past Month among Persons Aged 12 to 20, by Demographic Characteristics: Numbers in Thousands, 2018 and 2019. https://www.samhsa.gov/data/sites/default/files/reports/rpt29394/NSDUHDetailedTabs2019/NSDUHDetTabsSect2pe2019.htm#tab2-32a.

Volkow, N., & Koob, G. (2020). Drug addiction: The neurobiology of motivation gone awry. In A. J. Herron, & T. K. Brennan (Eds.), *American Society of Addiction Medicine (ASAM) essentials of addiction medicine* (3rd. ed, pp. 2). Wolters Kluwer.

Welch, S., Smith, T., Malcolm, R., & Lichtman, A. J. (2020). Pharmaology of cannabinoids. In A. J. Herron, & T. K. Brennan (Eds.), *American Society of Addiction Medicine (ASAM) essentials of addiction medicine* (3rd. Ed, pp. 778–783). Wolters Kluwer.

Woodard. J. (2020). The pharmacology of alcohol. In A. J. Herron, & T. K. Brennan (Eds.), *American Society of Addiction Medicine (ASAM) essentials of addiction medicine* (3rd. ed, pp. 44–49). Wolters Kluwer.

Yang, H., Spence, S., Briggs, R., Rao, V., North, C., Devous, M., et al. (2015). Interaction between early life stress and alcohol dependence on neural stress reactivity. *Addiction Biology, 20,* 523–533. https://doi.org/10.1111/adb.12135. https://www.ncbi.nlm.nih.gov/pmc/articles/PMC4893323/.

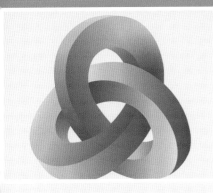

32

Eating Disorders

Joan Grant Keltner

ⓔ http://evolve.elsevier.com/Keltner

LEARNING OBJECTIVES

- Recognize criteria and terminology for eating disorders used in *DSM-5*.
- Recognize and describe objective and subjective symptoms of eating disorders.
- Describe current etiologies for eating disorders.
- Describe treatment issues for professionals who deal with patients with eating disorders.
- Recognize the continuum from dieting to an obvious eating disorder.
- Develop nursing care plans for patients with eating disorders.
- Evaluate the effectiveness of nursing interventions for patients with eating disorders.

Almost 29.0 million people of all ages and genders in the United States have an eating disorder (Deloitte Access Economics, 2020), with an estimated lifetime prevalence of approximately 14.3% in men and 19.7% in women by 40 years of age, with the highest first-time prevalence occurring by age 25 years (i.e., 95%; Ward et al., 2019). Generally, eating disorders have increased by 25% but fewer than one-fourth of those with eating disorders actually seek treatment (Treasure, Duarte, & Schmidt, 2020). Mortality rates also are significant, as eating disorders have the highest mortality rate of any psychiatric disorder. Almost $65 billion are associated with eating disorders, with about $327 billion in reduced well-being (Deloitte Access Economics, 2020). Eating disorders are becoming increasingly prevalent worldwide, especially in women (Galmiche et al., 2019), highlighting the significant challenge for nurses and other healthcare providers.

Hospitalizations have increased by 13% for anorexia nervosa and decreased by 14% for bulimia nervosa (Zhao & Encinosa, 2011). Although hospitalizations for men have increased by 53%, 9 in 10 cases of hospitalizations for eating disorders are still for women. These hospitalizations increased most sharply for children younger than 12 years old (119%), adults 45 to 64 years old (48%), and older adults (38%). Finally, hospitalizations for less common eating disorders, such as pica (an obsession with eating nonedible substances such as clay), increased by 93% (Agency for Healthcare Research and Quality, 2011). Hospitalization data for the United States have not been updated recently but in England, hospital admissions have increased tremendously for ethnic minorities. In comparing 2017–18 and 2019–20

data, the sharpest increase (216%) in hospitalizations was for those with an African background, raising questions regarding whether cultural or racial factors may be contributing to this sharp rise (Guardian News & Media Limited, 2021).

Eating disorders are associated with devastating psychological and physical sequelae (Treasure, Duarte, & Schmidt, 2020). Individuals with eating disorders have higher levels of other mental illnesses (Demmler et al., 2020). Serious secondary conditions include fluid and electrolyte imbalances; cardiac dysrhythmias; nutritional deficiencies or other nutritional, endocrine, or metabolic disorders; menstrual disorders; iron deficiency and anemia; acute renal or liver failure; and convulsions and epilepsy (Treasure, Duarte, & Schmidt, 2020; National Eating Disorders Association, 2018). Other symptoms associated with eating disorders include distractibility, depression, anxiety, anger, sadness, agitation, sleep disturbance, and obsessive-compulsive patterns of behavior (Ulfvebrand et al., 2015).

These disorders affect not only the patient but also family members. Family members commonly report a diversity of feelings, ranging from sadness, guilt, and hopelessness for those with anorexia nervosa and frustration and anger toward those individuals with BN and other eating disorders. Just as important, both patients and families discuss a mismatch of health providers focusing predominantly on physical aspects of eating disorders without an equal focus on associated psychosocial issues and how to obtain more personalized, life-long skills in managing these disorders (Mitrofan et al., 2019). Nurses and other health care professionals have a role in assisting both patients and their families in addressing these feelings and identifying useful treatments for eating disorders.

This chapter focuses on patients with anorexia nervosa and bulimia nervosa, the most common eating disorders. Similarities and differences of these two disorders are highlighted, as well as the continuum of eating behavior from dieting to anorexia, bulimia, and other eating disorders. Binge-eating disorder (BED), other specified feeding and eating disorders (OSFED), and orthorexia nervosa, a significant medical problem not yet recognized by *DSM-5* criteria, will also be discussed.

ANOREXIA NERVOSA

DSM-5 Criteria

A core feature of anorexia nervosa (AN) is a restriction of caloric intake relative to body requirements, which leads to a significantly low body weight. People with anorexia nervosa have an intense fear of gaining weight or of becoming overweight. Individuals with anorexia typically have a fear of "fatness," accompanied by a loss of weight or efforts to avoid gaining weight (American Psychiatric Association [APA], 2013). Although anorectics limit their intake or refuse to eat, they generally do not lose their appetites but rather suppress their appetite in an effort to remain thin or get thinner (Marzola et al., 2020). Anorectics think about food and eating much of the time. They have a disturbance in the way they view their weight or shape, but these two factors are the most important influence on the anorectic's sense of worth. They

might deny that they are dangerously thin or might acknowledge their underweight status but then deny that their condition is problematic (APA, 2013).

NORM'S NOTES When I was a younger psychiatric nurse, it was difficult for me to believe that eating disorders were legitimate mental health concerns. I just could not grasp that someone could not stop purging or could not start eating if they really wanted to. I held that uninformed view until I worked with a few young people who could not stop or not start whatever their particular problem was. I saw how it dominated and, in a few cases, ruined their lives. I can only say this—it is real, and it can be devastating.

While amenorrhea is no longer a diagnostic criterion for anorexia nervosa (APA, 2013), empirical data support that menstrual difficulties or irregularities may occur in this disease. For example, menstruation might cease early in the illness, before significant weight loss has taken place, or menstruation might continue but be irregular and spotty. If menarche has not been reached, menstruation might not begin. One theory for the cause of amenorrhea suggests that lack of nourishment significantly slows pituitary functioning, which is fundamental to the menstrual cycle. A low body mass index (BMI) can result in amenorrhea, with accompanying reduction of hormone levels and inadequate development of secondary sexual characteristics. In anorectic men, low sex

---

DSM-5 CRITERIA FOR ANOREXIA NERVOSA

A. Restrictions of energy intake relative to requirements, leading to a significantly low body weight in the context of age, sex, developmental trajectory, and physical health. Significantly low weight is defined as a weight that is less than minimally normal or, for children and adolescents, less than that minimally expected.

B. Intense fear of gaining weight or becoming fat, or persistent behavior that interferes with weight gain, even though at a significantly low weight.

C. Disturbance in the way in which one's body weight or shape is experienced, undue influence of body weight or shape on self-evaluation, or persistent lack of recognition of the seriousness of the current low body weight.

Coding note: The ICD-9-CM code for anorexia nervosa is 307.1, which is assigned regardless of the subtype. The ICD-10-CM code depends on the subtype (discussed later).

Specify whether:

(F50.01) Restricting type: During the last 3 months, the individual has not engaged in recurrent episodes of binge eating or purging behavior (i.e., self-induced vomiting or the misuse of laxatives, diuretics, or enemas). This subtype describes presentations in which weight loss is accomplished primarily through dieting, fasting, and/or excessive exercise.

(F50.02) Binge-eating/purging type: During the last 3 months, the individual has engaged in recurrent episodes of binge

eating or purging behavior (i.e., self-induced vomiting or the misuse of laxatives, diuretics, or enemas).

Specify if:

In partial remission: After full criteria for anorexia nervosa were previously met, Criterion A (low body weight) has not been met for a sustained period, but either Criterion B (intense fear of gaining weight or becoming fat or behavior that interferes with weight gain) or Criterion C (disturbances in self-perception of weight and shape) is still met.

In full remission: After full criteria for anorexia nervosa were previously met, none of the criteria have been met for a sustained period of time.

Specify current severity:

The minimum level of severity is based, for adults, on current BMI (discussed later) or, for children and adolescents, on BMI percentile. The ranges below are derived from World Health Organization categories for thinness in adults; for children and adolescents, corresponding BMI percentiles should be used. The level of severity may be increased to reflect clinical symptoms, the degree of functional disability, and the need for supervision.

Mild: BMI ≥ 17 kg/m^2

Moderate: BMI 16–16.99 kg/m^2

Severe: BMI 15–15.99 kg/m^2

Extreme: BMI < 15 kg/m^2

From American Psychiatric Association. (2013). *Diagnostic and statistical manual of mental disorders* (5th ed., pp. 338–339). APA.

drive and low testosterone levels might be the equivalent of amenorrhea in female patients (Jagielska et al., 2016; Treasure et al., 2019).

Anorexia affects up to 4.0% of women during their lifetime (Micali et al., 2017). Women account for the majority of reported cases of anorexia nervosa, although anorexia in men appears to be increasing. The age of diagnosis is trending toward younger children before 14 years, yet extends into middle and later adulthood (Jenkins et al., 2020). Initial morbidity and relapse from adolescent episodes are seen in adulthood. Of anorectic patients, 0.51% per year die as a result of their illness, usually through starvation or suicide (Arcelus et al., 2011). The mortality rate of anorexia nervosa is significantly higher than mortality rates from all other diseases (van Hoeken & Hoek, 2020).

Behavior

The onset of anorexia is often insidious because the typical adolescent victim, who is usually female, appears compliant and does not cause problems for others. Because dieting and fad foods are common in adolescence and young adulthood, often no one notices until the young woman has lost a significant amount of weight. A common premorbid personality profile is that of a perfectionistic and introverted girl with self-esteem and peer relationship problems, but patients might also be accomplished and active in school activities (Dufresne et al., 2020; Treasure, Duarte, & Schmidt, 2020). A meta-analysis of eating disorders found that individuals with anorexia nervosa have decision-making deficits, especially during the acute phase of illness, although nutritional status does not affect these skills (Guillaume et al., 2015).

Objective Signs

The most observable behavior of anorexia nervosa is deliberate weight loss in an effort to control weight through changing eating behaviors. Patients with anorexia nervosa are in two groups: the restricters and the vomiters/purgers. The restricters are more often young people in the normal or slightly above normal weight range for height and build before the eating disorder begins. This group views losing weight as more probable if they simply eat less and avoid social situations in which they are expected to eat. Restricters often withdraw to their rooms and avoid family and friends. It is

Clinical Example

Kristin Chambliss, age 15, was in the normal weight range when she joined the school volleyball team with her friends. The first time they donned their uniforms, one of Kristin's friends called her "piano legs." Kristin was horrified and began to diet. In addition, she asked her parents to join the local health club so that she could exercise to keep in shape for the team. Her entire day revolved around participation on the team to the extent that she forfeited all other social involvement. She did not arrive home until after 9 P.M. each night because she went to the health club to exercise after a volleyball game or after practice. Kristin lost 21 lb before anyone verbalized concern.

common for them to be competitive, compulsive, and obsessive about their activities. They might participate in rigid exercise programs to help reduce their weight. Many restricting anorectics become hyperactive to lose weight, becoming highly anxious and unable to relax. They might take early morning walks because of insomnia and a need to burn off calories (Gianini et al., 2016; Mitchell & Peterson, 2020).

Compared with restricters, vomiters/purgers are more often overweight before the eating disorder begins, and their weight tends to fluctuate (Riedlinger et al., 2020). These young women are prone to dangerous methods of weight reduction, such as induction of vomiting or excessive use of laxatives or diuretics. These anorectic patients commonly deny concerns about weight and typically eat normally in social situations. After the meal, they retreat to the nearest bathroom and purge themselves of the consumed food, although the amount is not excessive. Dental problems frequently occur in these patients because the acidic vomitus decays the enamel on their teeth. This group also might be susceptible to times when they uncontrollably eat large amounts of food if unsuccessful in maintaining the severe dietary restriction that they impose on themselves. Purging anorectics are more likely to have histories of behavior problems, substance abuse, and open family conflict than restricting anorectics (Stein et al., 2020). In a longitudinal study spanning 22 years using 100 participants with anorexia nervosa, Franko et al. (2018) indicated that binge eating, purging, and major depressive disorder predicted a lower likelihood of recovery.

Clinical Example

Tina Easterling was always a chubby child. When she was 23 years old, she lost considerable weight by dieting. Shortly thereafter, she began seriously dating and was married. Tina was thrilled with her new look and worked hard to maintain her weight loss, consistently keeping her weight slightly under the ideal for her height. After 2 years of marriage, Tina became pregnant. The thought of gaining weight during her pregnancy upset Tina greatly, and she vowed to herself never to let herself become chubby again. Before long, Tina's physician noticed that she was not gaining weight at her monthly prenatal checkups and asked what she was eating. When she did a food log for the office nurse, her anorectic behavior was revealed.

In a large systematic review of eating patterns and dietary intake of individuals with eating disorders, Dörsam et al. (2019) found similarities in dietary intake when comparing pregnant and non-pregnant women with eating disorders. These women varied, however, in consuming greater amounts of caffeine and artificially sweetened beverages. They also were more likely to be vegetarian and had a higher prevalence of iron deficiency anemia, which potentially can impact fetal development.

Some empirical data suggest that the intake of nutrients is so low in anorectic patients that their bodies try to adjust by using less energy. Consequently, other physiologic processes are affected. Hypotension, bradycardia, and hypothermia are common. The skin is often dry and lanugo might appear. Many patients have delayed gastric emptying, causing them to feel full much longer than most people, and they do not have the normal desire to eat as often as others. They believe that they can get by on one small meal a day. Slower abdominal peristalsis combined with decreased intake leads to constipation, which fuels the use of laxatives, leading to dehydration and giving the anorectic a false sense of decreased weight. Dehydration can lead to irreversible renal damage. Refeeding syndrome, involving severe shifts in fluid and electrolyte levels from extracellular to intracellular spaces in severely emaciated patients, can occur, causing cardiovascular, neurologic, and hematologic complications and death. In severely malnourished individuals, refeeding must be done slowly and under very close supervision to prevent serious problems. Pitting edema occurs in some anorectic patients, most often after attempts to gain weight by eating more food during the refeeding process while in treatment. Noticing the swelling, the patient often becomes anxious about the weight gain, immediately stops eating, and might attempt to counteract the perceived weight gain, further complicating the emaciated condition. In addition, osteopenia or osteoporosis might develop as a consequence of prolonged amenorrhea and malnutrition. Studies have found ventricular dilation, decreases in thickness of the left ventricular wall, alterations in the size of the cardiac chambers, and decreased myocardial oxygen uptake, which can lead to life-threatening cardiac arrhythmias (Reber et al., 2019).

Anorectic patients become preoccupied with food and eating. This preoccupation involves all aspects of life. Patients are often found reading numerous materials on food and dieting and attempting to control family meals because they believe that they are the nutrition authorities in their household. Patients might engage in bizarre behavior regarding food and eating, such as hoarding food or preparing elaborate meals for others but not eating the food they prepare. Elaborate rituals before and during eating might become a compulsion, which adds to the patient's problems and might result in the patient being diagnosed with obsessive-compulsive disorder as well as anorexia (Reber et al., 2019).

Subjective Symptoms

An outstanding feature of anorexia nervosa is the conscious fear that these patients have of losing control over the amount of food eaten, resulting in becoming fat. Patients are concerned about being obese, losing weight, or preventing weight gain. Some patients even say that they would rather be dead than fat. This fear motivates them to begin dieting. The fear might be triggered by an event that seems trivial to others, such as an offhand comment by a friend or relative or one or more events perceived as traumatic by the patient. These patients might feel abandoned or inadequate, which can precipitate an overall feeling of helplessness. They try to combat helplessness by controlling what they can control—how much food they eat and their weight. Much of the patient's energy becomes invested in this effort (Reber et al., 2019).

In addition to problems with eating behavior and weight concern, anorectic individuals have other psychological symptoms known to be consequences of semi-starvation. These patients exhibit depression, irritability, social withdrawal, lessened sex drive, and obsessional symptoms, which are normal symptoms of starvation. In essence, some of an anorectic's bizarre behavior is the result of starvation. These symptoms often diminish with weight gain, but if they do not, the patient might have a comorbid condition, such as obsessive-compulsive disorder, major depression, substance abuse, or a personality disorder (Jagielska et al., 2016; Rothenberg, 2018).

Etiology

Today, most experts agree that eating disorders have multifactorial causes, including biologic, sociocultural, family, cognitive, behavioral, and psychodynamic factors. These factors are discussed in the following sections.

Biologic Factors

Earlier in the 20th century, physiologic disturbances were postulated as causative in anorexia. Currently, researchers believe that the physiologic abnormalities found in anorectic patients are mostly a result of semi-starvation and purging behavior rather than the cause of disordered eating.

An exception might be increased serotonin levels. Studies using positron emission tomography and single photon emission computed tomography with 5-HT-specific radioligands have consistently shown 5-HT_{1A} and 5-HT_{2A} receptor and 5-HT transporter alterations in anorexia nervosa in cortical and limbic structures, which may be related to anxiety, behavioral inhibition, and body image distortions. These disturbances exist both during illness and after recovery. A better understanding of neurobiology is likely to be important for developing specific and more powerful therapies for this disorder. However, the binding potential of the serotonin (5-HT) receptor 1 A (5-HT_{1A}) also is increased in individuals with eating disorders. The neuronal circuits that control the ingestion of food are mainly related to catecholaminergic, serotonergic, and peptidergic systems. However, the use of selective serotonin reuptake inhibitors (SSRIs), which regulate serotonin levels in depressed patients, has not been effective in treating anorexia (Blanchet et al., 2019; Skowron et al., 2020). Another field of study is examining the influence of a biological microbial imbalance in the gut, but this research is still in its infancy (Bulik et al., 2019). Biological aspects involving central and peripheral neurohormonal pathways, endocrine function, as well as the microbiome–gut–brain axis are potential areas of future research. Essentially, the microbiota–gut–brain axis allows bidirectional communication between the central nervous system and the gut-affecting symptoms (Skowron et al., 2020).

Sociocultural Factors

The increased incidence of eating disorders in the 20th century has been recognized as corresponding to an increasingly and unrealistically thin beauty ideal for women—almost a culture of thinness. In addition, American culture has advanced the notion that body weight is a matter of personal choice and that shape can be changed at will. Computer imaging technology has resulted in the enhancement of photos on the Internet in response to the current societal standard of beauty. These images encourage dieting, which is a major predisposing factor to both anorexia nervosa and BN (Batista et al., 2018).

Another factor is the relational need of women, which creates a vulnerability to the opinions of others, particularly during adolescence. American culture stresses the importance of physical attractiveness in obtaining approval; because of the thin beauty ideal, girls begin to experience that thinness leads to approval by others. Lack of approval is interpreted as being caused by a less than ideal body size, which causes girls, in particular, to begin dieting. In examining interventions to prevent anorexia, the greater a repertoire of adolescents' social skills, the greater their protection against developing eating disorders (Batista et al., 2018).

Family Factors

Several studies of identical and fraternal twins have suggested a genetic component to the etiology of anorexia (Duncan et al., 2017). Family environment is known to play a role in the development of eating disorders. Traditional views have supported excessive rigidity and enmeshment in the families of adolescents with eating disorders, with poor communication and satisfaction among family members. Emotional restraint, enmeshed relationships, rigid organization in the family, tight control of child behavior by parents, and avoidance of conflict are other factors. Odd eating habits and an emphasis on appearance and weight by other family members, especially mothers and sisters, have been described. However, the extent to which the observed family problems of anorectics are consequences of the disorder rather than etiologies is still undetermined, and empirical evidence suggests that additional factors are at play (Erriu et al., 2020).

Current research also has challenged these traditional views of family. For example, Fisher and Bushlow (2015) examined whether these traditional views remain true or have changed over time to include a wider range of families of those with anorexia nervosa. Findings indicated that the majority of patients with eating disorders and their parents reported their family styles to be in the healthy range (i.e., regarding connectivity, flexibility, enmeshment, rigidity, chaos, and communication). The one exception to this view was found in depressed individuals who expressed dissatisfaction with their families. While these traditional views may need to be further examined, preliminary evidence suggests that family-based treatment may be useful for younger patients with anorexia nervosa. Empirical data suggest that early treatment and weight gain predict better outcomes, which is obtained in family-based therapy (Davis & Attia, 2019). In a systematic review of studies involving children and adolescents, Couturier et al. (2020) found strong support for use of family therapy, especially if the duration of anorexia is less than 3 years. Current literature supports a multifactorial view of anorexia in which relationships between families and individuals with anorexia nervosa, as well as genetic, psychological, neuroendocrine, and sociocultural factors are investigated (Erriu et al. 2020).

Cognitive and Behavioral Factors

Behavioral theorists have noted that anorectic behavior develops and is maintained as a function of environmental contingencies. Rejecting food and losing weight may be reinforced by positive attention from others. The use of behavioral treatments such as assertiveness training and cognitive restructuring is based on such cognitive factors. A study by Nyman-Carlsson et al. (2020) examined the effectiveness of individual cognitive behavioral therapy and combined family/individual therapy for 78 young adults with anorexia nervosa. Both groups received 60 hours of either cognitive behavioral or family/individual therapy and were reassessed immediately and 18 months after treatment. BMI as well as eating-related and general psychopathology and depressive symptoms were study outcomes. In comparing baseline and posttreatment data, both groups had significant improvements in weight gain and reduced eating and general psychopathology. This study was different in that rates of remission increased at follow-up at 18 months. These findings are substantial given that 70% of participants in the family therapy group completed more than half of the sessions while those assigned to the cognitive behavioral group completed less than half of the sessions. One meta-analysis of adolescents showed that cognitive behavioral therapy improved weight and psychological symptoms. This literature, however, is in its infancy and needs further research in randomized clinical trials (Couturier et al., 2020).

Psychodynamic Factors

Modern psychoanalytic theorists have stressed the role of sexuality in anorexia nervosa. In addition, some clinicians have suggested that eating disorders might be related to an early history of sexual abuse, although systematic reviews indicate that these findings are inconsistent for anorexia nervosa (Monteleone et al., 2020). Some research indicates that childhood sexual abuse seems to be related to increased body shame, which is a risk factor for eating disorders and self-mutilation. In fact, some studies suggest that child sexual abuse is more often perpetrated by a nonstranger and associated with anorexia nervosa with binge-eating behaviors (Micali et al., 2017). In comparing emotional, physical, and sexual abuse, reports of emotional abuse are the most strongly related to emotion regulation difficulties and anorexia symptom severity (Monteleone et al., 2020).

Some researchers have suggested that anorexia involves a regression to a prepubertal state, so that the adolescent does not mature physically or emotionally. Regression is reinforced when the anorectic adolescent's dependency needs are met. The conscious fear of becoming fat is thought to be the symbolic expression of becoming bigger, or growing up—supposedly the real subconscious fear of the anorectic. Other psychoanalytic theorists have suggested that the drive for thinness might be an attempt to reduce the control of an overcontrolling maternal figure, especially for bingeing disorders (Oldershaw et al., 2019).

Another theory has described anorexia nervosa as an obsession with weight stemming from a fear of being out of control because of the lack of a well-defined self. Patients use reaction formation to organize their lives with a set of rules and regulations for everything they do. They experience a tremendous amount of anxiety if their rules are broken and attempt to regain control by tightening the rules and punishing themselves for their failure (Oldershaw et al., 2019).

Experts agree that the causes of anorexia nervosa are multifactorial. Biologic, sociocultural, family, cognitive, behavioral, and psychodynamic factors all might contribute to the disease. Factors contributing to the maintenance of anorexia might differ from factors leading to its development. Today, most research focuses on factors contributing to the onset of dieting. Greater emphasis on factors contributing to the development and maintenance of eating-disordered behavior might result in a better understanding of this disorder and more effective prevention of the disease. Research on adult-onset eating disorders might also prove fruitful, as this phenomenon has been observed more frequently in recent years.

Unfortunately, the efficacy of therapies for anorexia nervosa is limited (van den Berg et al., 2019; Zeeck et al., 2018). For example, in a meta-analysis of 17 randomized clinical trials ($n = 1279$) conducted using a variety of therapies (i.e., family therapy, cognitive behavioral therapy, psychodynamic or psychoanalytic therapy, interpersonal therapy, social skills training, motivational interviewing), no significant differences were found between therapy groups and control treatments (e.g., dietary suggestions, psychoeducational interventions, etc.) receiving usual treatment regarding weight gain, eating disorder pathology, and quality of life. Studies using participants older than 18 years of age were more effective in gaining weight than those studies including adolescents in the sample. Studies that had therapist training to assure quality had greater effects on weight gain and quality of life than those studies without therapist training (van den Berg et al., 2019). Zeeck et al. (2018) found similar results in another meta-analysis of 18 clinical trials ($n = 622$). In this analysis, family-based psychotherapy was primarily used for adolescents and individual psychotherapy was used with adults. These analyses found the two types of psychotherapy to be similar regarding weight and eating behavior. However, adolescents and inpatients gained weight quicker, suggesting the benefit of family therapy. Weaker support was found for other therapies (e.g., multifamily, cognitive behavioral therapy, adolescent-focused therapy, and use of atypical antipsychotics [i.e., olanzapine or aripiprazole]), but they may be reasonable treatment options. As suggested, future research is necessary in examining subgroups of individuals (i.e., adolescents and adults; therapist effectiveness, etc.) to truly examine the effectiveness of different approaches. In summary, the psychotherapies for anorexia nervosa are comparable and provide a moderate outcome for weight gain, eating disorder pathology, and quality of life. As the type of treatment does not appear to predict outcome, it is necessary to consider what other factors might do so (Jansingh et al., 2020). Providing insight, Murray et al., (2019) questioned whether weight gain was the best outcome in determining the effectiveness of psychotherapy treatments.

CRITICAL THINKING QUESTION

1. Some theorists contend that adolescent eating disorders are an expression of emotional distress within the family system. Explain how this might have some validity.

BULIMIA NERVOSA

DSM-5 Criteria

Bulimia nervosa (BN) is characterized by three behaviors: recurrent episodes of binge eating, compensatory behaviors to avoid weight gain, and an evaluation of self that is significantly influenced by body weight and shape. These behaviors must be present an average of at least once per week, for a minimum of 3 months (APA, 2013). BN usually begins in adolescence or early adult life, primarily in women, although it has been diagnosed more often in men than in the past (Udo & Grilo, 2018). Bulimia affects a little over 2.0% of women during their lifetime (Micali et al., 2017). The usual course of the disorder is chronic and intermittent over many years. Most commonly, the binge episodes alternate with periods of restrictive eating, complicating the diagnosis and treatment.

Behavior

The word *bulimia* literally means to have an insatiable appetite. The term is often used to describe massive overeating and is used interchangeably with *binge eating* or *bingeing*. Until recently, BN was considered to be part of anorexia nervosa because many of these patients regularly have binge-eating episodes (Riedlinger et al., 2020). BN is considered a separate disorder, although there is still much overlap between the disorders. The true prevalence of BN is unknown because many patients hide their eating-disordered behaviors. In these patients, diagnosis of other more familiar psychiatric disorders, such as major depression, personality disorder, or post-traumatic stress disorder, may be made. Individuals who seek medical attention (usually for gastrointestinal or menstrual disturbances) could be identified as having bulimia, but the lack of weight loss may blind the treatment provider to the patient's bulimia (Treasure, Duarte, & Schmidt, 2020).

The peak onset of the illness is between the ages of 15 through 19 years (Volpe et al., 2016). The disease may develop after anorexia nervosa or after a period of dieting. The dieting predisposes the individual to binge eating, and purging develops as a means of compensating for calories ingested during the binge in an attempt to prevent weight gain. The individual continues restrictive eating during the disorder, which precipitates binge eating and then purging, perpetuating the cycle.

Clinical Example

Mary Franklin, age 28, was a young professional with an active social life. Although she was approximately 15 lb overweight, Mary used her sense of humor to hide any serious concern she had about her appearance. However, Mary worried that her weight might deny her a highly prized job that she wanted. Before applying for the job at a prestigious banking firm, Mary began dieting and ate less food than her friends did at lunch. However, when she arrived home, Mary felt hungry and secretly raided her refrigerator, making several sandwiches before dinner. Despite feeling guilty over her uncontrolled snacking, Mary ate dinner with her roommate. After dinner, feeling uncomfortably full, Mary retreated to the bathroom and vomited until she felt empty. She vowed to try harder to diet the next day, only to have a similar experience.

DSM-5 CRITERIA FOR BULIMIA NERVOSA

A. Recurrent episodes of binge eating. An episode of binge eating is characterized by both of the following:
1. Eating, in a discrete period of time (e.g., within any 2-h period), an amount of food that is definitely larger than what most individuals would eat in a similar period of time under similar circumstances.
2. A sense of lack of control over eating during the episode (e.g., feeling that one cannot stop eating or control what or how much one is eating).

B. Recurrent inappropriate compensatory behavior in order to prevent weight gain, such as self-induced vomiting; misuse of laxatives, diuretics, or other medications; fasting; or excessive exercise.

C. The binge eating and inappropriate compensatory behaviors both occur, on average, at least once a week for 3 months.

D. Self-evaluation is unduly influenced by body shape and weight.

E. The disturbance does not occur exclusively during episodes of anorexia nervosa.

Specify if:

In partial remission: After full criteria for bulimia nervosa were previously met, some, but not all, of the criteria have been met for a sustained period of time.

In full remission: After full criteria for bulimia nervosa were previously met, none of the criteria have been met for a sustained period of time.

Specify current severity:

The minimum level of severity is based on the frequency of inappropriate compensatory behaviors (see below). The level of severity may be increased to reflect other symptoms and the degree of functional disability.

Mild: An average of 1–3 episodes of inappropriate compensatory behaviors per week.

Moderate: An average of 4–7 episodes of inappropriate compensatory behaviors per week.

Severe: An average of 8–13 episodes of inappropriate compensatory behaviors per week.

Extreme: An average of 14 or more episodes of inappropriate compensatory behaviors per week.

From American Psychiatric Association. (2013). *Diagnostic and statistical manual of mental disorders* (5th ed., p. 345). APA.

It is important to distinguish overeating from binge eating. To meet *DSM-5* diagnostic criteria for a binge episode, the eating behavior must qualify as an "objective bulimic episode." That is, the person consumes an unusually large amount of food in a relatively short period (e.g., several thousand calories in <2 hours). The amount of food eaten is considered by others to be atypically large for the particular situation. In addition, there is a feeling of lack of control over eating during the binge (APA, 2013).

Objective Signs

Most bulimic patients are secretive about their behavior. A variety of foods might be eaten during a binge, but the most common is high-calorie, high-carbohydrate "snack" food easily ingested in a short period of time. Some bulimics visit several different fast-food restaurants or grocery stores during a binge, so that no one knows how much they are eating during an episode. Some patients with bulimia have been caught shoplifting food. Most binges occur during the evening or at night. The number of calories consumed during a binge varies but is considerably more than the recommended daily allowance. There is a tendency to eat rapidly during the binge.

Patients report that their bulimic episodes usually end when they begin to induce vomiting, are physically exhausted, suffer from painful abdominal distention, are interrupted by others, or have run out of food. After a binge, patients promise themselves to adhere to a strict diet and vow never to binge again, only to return to this behavior because they find themselves addicted to the high that they experience when bingeing. Many bulimics resume their usual schedules as if they had never been interrupted. The frequency of binges varies greatly, depending on the patient. Some patients report having several episodes a day; others report losing control two or three times a week.

Medical complications in bulimic patients depend on the form and frequency of purging. Fluid and electrolyte imbalances might result from self-induced vomiting or abuse of laxatives or diuretics; these can include dehydration, hyponatremia, hypochloremia, hypokalemia, and metabolic alkalosis and acidosis. Self-induced vomiting and laxative abuse can cause mechanical irritation and injuries to the gastrointestinal tract. Abuse of laxatives, diuretics, and diet pills can result in addiction. Laxatives can lead to reflex constipation, and both laxatives and diuretics are associated with rebound edema (Riedlinger et al., 2020; Treasure, Duarte, & Schmidt, 2020).

The use of ipecac syrup to induce vomiting is dangerous and can cause fatal cardiomyopathy. Bulimics often have menstrual irregularities or enlarged salivary glands, particularly the parotid glands. Erosion of the dental enamel from chronic vomiting often occurs. The Russell sign, callusing of the knuckles of the fingers used to induce vomiting, is also common. Pancreatitis also has been reported in bulimics (Riedlinger et al., 2020; Treasure, Duarte, & Schmidt, 2020).

Subjective Symptoms

Although most bulimic patients have a normal body weight, they are gravely concerned about their body shape and weight. Loss of control over eating causes them great anxiety and shame, and similar to anorectic patients, they express a fear of becoming fat. Moods vary considerably among bulimic patients. Some bulimics have reported feeling weak before a binge, followed either by continued anxiety or by relief from tension during the binge. Patients have reported feeling anxious, lonely, or bored or uncontrollably craving food before the binge. The anxiety present before the binge is replaced with guilt after the binge. If the anxiety is not relieved after the binge, patients feel angry and agitated and might become depressed, which appears to be common in bulimic patients. The relationship between bulimia and depression might be one in which one causes the other, or there might be independent factors contributing to both disorders. Researchers have found a high rate of mood disorders, particularly depression, in families in which bulimia occurs. About half of bulimic patients have attention deficit/hyperactivity disorder and also exhibit substance abuse, compulsive behavior, and may have multiple sexual partners. Anxiety disorders also occur at a higher-than-normal rate among bulimics. It appears that although pharmacotherapy can be helpful, it should be combined with psychotherapy for the most effective long-term outcome (Treasure, Duarte, & Schmidt, 2020; Wade, 2019).

Most bulimic patients induce vomiting to reduce the fear of becoming fat. Patients might self-induce vomiting by sticking their fingers, a toothbrush, or an eating utensil down their throats; this is a dangerous practice because patients have swallowed objects used to induce vomiting. Over time, vomiting becomes easier and might require only slight abdominal pressure or no physical manipulation at the end of the binge. Some bulimics eat what is known as a *marker* food at the beginning of the binge and then vomit until this food comes back up. This practice is ineffective because food is quickly mixed in the stomach. Although bulimics believe that self-induced vomiting rids them of all binge calories, researchers have determined that only a partial amount of calories consumed can be regurgitated. Abuse of laxatives or diuretics primarily causes fluid loss rather than a reduction in absorbed calories. Diabulimia is deliberate insulin underuse in people with type 1 diabetes for the purpose of controlling their weight (National Eating Disorders Association, 2018).

Etiology

Similar to anorexia, the causes of BN are thought to be multifactorial, with biologic, sociocultural, family, cognitive, behavioral, and psychodynamic contributing factors. Many of the factors thought to precipitate anorexia are also thought to be involved in bulimia. The focus of this discussion is on the proposed causes of bulimia that differ from the causes stated for anorexia.

Biologic Factors

Brain chemistry has been increasingly implicated in studies relating to the cause of eating disorders, with several neuroendocrine and neurotransmitter abnormalities demonstrated in dieters and in individuals demonstrating symptoms of eating disorders. Biologic and genetic factors have also been implicated

in the causes of bulimia and anorexia. Most researchers believe that illness symptoms are related to the physiologic state of the victims and lessen when weight is restored. Abnormalities in peripheral 5-HT uptake (associated with low serotonin levels) are observed in individuals with BN in both acute and recovery stages of illness, suggesting that these findings may be trait features rather than the outcome of abnormal eating patterns (McDonald, 2019; Trace et al., 2013). Findings of fMRI reported by Molina-Ruiz et al. (2020) indicated that individuals with BN had decreased cognitive abilities and prefrontal hyperactivation patterns associated with self-regulatory functions, which correlated with their symptoms. These findings suggest inefficient prefrontal self-regulatory function of BN, which correlates with BN–associated symptoms. A systematic review of studies examining binge eating disorders indicates psychological treatments as first-line interventions, although behavioral and self-help interventions also show some efficacy in patients with lower psychopathological features.

Data are still limited regarding the role of pharmacological treatment. Treatment of bulimia with SSRIs, particularly fluoxetine (Prozac), appears to be helpful whether or not patients have comorbid depression, so it is unknown whether the antidepressant has a direct effect on the bulimia. A meta-analysis ($n = 7515$) supports use of lisdexamfetamine but these studies show small to medium effect sizes, so they must be used in conjunction with other therapies because attrition may be more than that of psychotherapies (Couturier et al., 2020; Hay, 2020; Hilbert et al., 2019). Topiramate augments reductions achieved with cognitive behavioral therapy (CBT) for both binge eating and weight (Himmerich et al., 2021).

Sociocultural Factors

Sociocultural factors are thought to be the same as factors for anorexia nervosa, as noted earlier in this chapter.

Family Factors

As with anorexia nervosa, a heritable component for bulimia has been proposed. Twin studies have found a higher concordance rate for bulimia in identical versus fraternal twins (Silén et al., 2020). In addition, mood disorders and substance abuse disorders are found at a higher rate in the families of bulimics, which might be a result of both biologic and environmental factors. Families of bulimics are seen as having a great deal of conflict, being disorganized, lacking in nurturance, and not being cohesive (Wade, 2019). Observations of family interactions have yielded similar data, lending credence to the idea that the bulimia might be a response to chaos in the family. In contrast, better maternal care appears to be protective against the development of BN (Monteleone et al., 2020).

Cognitive and Behavioral Factors

Fairburn (2005) pioneered work on cognitive behavioral theory for the treatment of BN. According to this theory, bulimia is maintained by cycles of low self-esteem, extreme concerns about body shape and weight, strict dieting, binge eating, and compensatory behavior, which interact and affect each other. Bulimia is maintained by the behaviors of dieting, bingeing, and purging, which are both affected by and contribute to distorted and negative cognitions about the self and the body. This theory has led to the development of successful cognitive behavior therapy programs for BN that target both eating-disordered behaviors and cognitions.

Dakanalis et al. (2015) proposed an enhanced cognitive model that extended the original approach by including four maintenance factors (i.e., interpersonal problems, core low self-esteem, clinical perfectionism, and mood intolerance). In comparing the original approach and enhanced models, the enhanced model explained more eating-disordered behaviors than the original one. More interpersonal problems, clinical perfectionism, and low self-esteem resulted in less dietary restraint through over-evaluation of shape and weight. More interpersonal problems and mood intolerance resulted in more binge eating. Restraint only indirectly affected binge eating via mood intolerance, indicating that factors other than restraint may play a more critical role in the maintenance of binge eating.

In conjunction with pharmacological therapy, a review of empirical data indicates CBT and interpersonal therapy are first- and second-line treatments, respectively, for adults with BN. Both dialectical behavior therapy and integrative cognitive-affective therapy also show promise. In children and adolescents, there is strong support for use of family therapy and CBT may be a reasonable option; however, the number of randomized clinical trials are few (Couturier et al., 2020). In a systematic review and meta-analysis of 42 studies, therapies that include pretreatment motivation provide evidence of patient improvement, supporting the need to include patient engagement in the treatment of eating disorders (Sansfacon et al., 2020). Further trials are recommended using other subgroups, such as ethnic minorities and low-income samples.

Agras et al., (2017) suggest that sophisticated forms of treatment via mobile applications may provide more personalized and efficacious treatments for bulimia. Systematic reviews show that smartphones can be used effectively with children, adolescents, and young adults to self-monitor and treat psychiatric disorders, including eating disorders (Melbye et al., 2020; Tønning, Kessing et al., 2019). In addition, Linardon et al., (2020) found that digital interventions were effective in lessening risk factors and symptoms in patients with eating disorders. Further studies are needed comparing these interventions with face-to-face interventions. Digital delivery is a necessary mode of treatment providing access to care or as an option to a waitlist (Machado & Rodrigues, 2019).

Psychodynamic Factors

Some psychodynamic theorists have placed particular emphasis on ambivalent feelings of self-esteem in bulimics. The binge eating and purging behavior is thought to express the negative thoughts that patients feel toward themselves. On the one hand, patients believe that they are worthy of the nurturing that they lack, and because food is a symbolic form of nurturing, they binge. On the other hand, patients feel unworthy of nurturing, so they purge. Bingeing and purging can also be seen as patients' attempts to numb themselves from the pain in their lives resulting from abuse, neglect, and

trauma. Similar to anorexia nervosa, childhood sexual abuse has a role in binge-/purge-type disorders. Childhood life events and interpersonal sensitivity are known to be associated with all EDs (Wade, 2019).

PUTTING IT ALL TOGETHER

PSYCHOTHERAPEUTIC MANAGEMENT

Psychotherapeutic management for anorexia and bulimia shares many characteristics and has some differences. In this section, the commonalities and differences are highlighted. The psychotherapeutic management of each disorder varies, depending on the period of treatment being considered and whether the focus is on short-term or long-term treatment. For example, when an anorectic patient is hospitalized because of extreme weight loss and its life-threatening physical effects, the focus must be on weight restoration before any treatment dealing with changing the patient's perceptions about his or her body or any long-term goals can be addressed.

COMPARING ANOREXIA AND BULIMIA

Shared Features

Restriction of intake, especially anorectics
Bingeing or overeating at times, especially bulimics
Purging through vomiting, laxatives, or diuretics
Excessive exercise
Extreme concern about appearance
Perfectionistic traits—dissatisfaction with appearance and performance in aspects of life such as work or school
Negative beliefs of self based on appearance
Discomfort in social settings, especially with the opposite gender
Misperception of body size, shape, and level of fat
Low self-esteem

Differentiation of Behaviors

Anorexia	Bulimia
Early onset	Later onset
Very low weight	Normal weight or slightly overweight
Fluid/electrolyte and hormonal imbalances	Fluid and electrolyte imbalance
Constipation if not using laxatives	Gastrointestinal problems related to bingeing and purging

Management of anorexia is geared toward three primary objectives: (1) increasing weight to at least 90% of the average body weight for the patient's height; (2) helping patients reestablish appropriate eating behavior; and (3) increasing self-esteem, so that patients do not need to attain the perfection that they believe thinness provides. The objectives for bulimics are similar but, rather than the need for weight increase, are more likely to focus on stabilizing weight without purging because bulimics are more likely to be of normal weight.

When patients are severely malnourished in anorexia, treatment occurs in a medical environment in which appropriate supplies and equipment, such as intravenous lines and feeding tubes, are readily available for feeding the patient if he or she will not eat voluntarily. Refeeding and weight restoration in the starvation phase of anorexia must be done slowly and carefully, with close monitoring by experts to avoid life-threatening physical complications and possible death. Medical stabilization of the patient is the initial treatment goal. After medical stabilization, treatment with higher calories appears safe under medical supervision (e.g., monitoring electrolytes) using meals alone or combined with nasogastric feedings (Reber et al., 2019). When medical crises are resolved, patients are transferred to a specialized outpatient program, in which effective psychotherapeutic intervention can occur.

In conjunction with pharmacological therapy (Hagan & Walsh, 2020), CBT and interpersonal therapy are first- and second-line treatments, respectively, for adults with BN. Both dialectical behavior therapy and integrative cognitive-affective therapy also show promise. Despite promising therapies, nearly 60% of individuals with BN fail to achieve remission and there are a paucity of randomized clinical trials using adolescents (Hagan & Walsh, 2020). Regarding interventions, empirical data from 30 randomized clinical trials suggest guided self-help may be useful for mild-moderate global eating disorders and binge abstinence (Traviss-Turner et al., 2017).

Nurses might encounter anorectic or bulimic patients on an inpatient basis in a medical or psychiatric unit or on an outpatient basis in a physician's office, clinic, or school. Bulimics are less likely to be encountered in inpatient settings unless their purging has led to medical complications, but these individuals should be hospitalized in the following circumstances: (1) to treat a psychiatric or medical crisis, (2) when respite is needed from a chaotic home life so that the patient can examine his or her living situation more objectively, and (3) if the patient cannot obtain treatment in his or her home community. In any setting, a multidisciplinary treatment approach is crucial. Members of the treatment team should include a physician, nurse, dietitian, and psychotherapist specializing in the treatment of eating disorders. These patients need thorough medical and psychiatric assessment, medical monitoring, nutritional education and counseling, and psychotherapy. Assessment should include use of instruments from self-reporting to more structured interview tools as well as differential diagnosis of other psychiatric conditions, including affective disorders, personality disorders, anxiety disorders such as obsessive-compulsive disorders, and substance abuse or dependence.

Empirical evidence for the effectiveness of family therapy for adolescent anorexia nervosa is strong, with less support for the use of multifamily therapy, CBT, adolescent psychotherapy, and atypical antipsychotics (Couturier et al., 2020). In CBT, findings are controversial, although there are several case studies reporting a decline in binge and purge symptoms. See the accompanying "Highlighting the Evidence" boxes. The first study compares the effectiveness of psychosocial interventions with eating disorders. The remaining three studies highlight the value of family therapy for anorexia nervosa and cognitive behavioral and self-help therapy (via smartphones) for BN.

HIGHLIGHTING THE EVIDENCE

Comparison of Treatment Approaches for Eating Disorders

Description: This study examined the effectiveness of psychosocial interventions in treating eating disorders, examining 101 primary studies and 30 systematic reviews, meta-analysis, and guidelines or narrative reviews of literature. Main outcomes were symptomatic remission, body image issues, cognitive distortions, psychiatric comorbidity, psychosocial functioning, and patient satisfaction.

Results: The cognitive behavioral approach was the most effective treatment for bulimia nervosa, binge eating disorder, and the night eating syndrome. For anorexia nervosa, the family approach was more effective. Other valuable approaches were interpersonal psychotherapy, dialectic behavioral therapy, support therapy, and self-help manuals. Moreover, there were promising preventive and promotional approaches addressing individual, family, and social risk factors which promote the development of positive self-image and self-efficacy.

Implications: Further studies are required to evaluate the influence of multidisciplinary approaches on all eating disorders.

Modified from Costa, M. B., & Melnik, T. (2016). Effectiveness of psychosocial interventions in eating disorders: An overview of Cochrane systematic reviews. *Einstein (Sao Paulo), 14*(2), 235–277. https://doi.org/10.1590/S1679-45082016RW3120.

HIGHLIGHTING THE EVIDENCE

Comparison of Single- and Multifamily Therapy in Adolescents With Anorexia Nervosa

Description: This study was a pragmatic multicenter randomized controlled superiority trial comparing single-family therapy (FT-AN) and multifamily therapy (MFT-AN). A total of 169 adolescents with a diagnosis of anorexia nervosa or eating disorder (restricting type) were enrolled from two outpatient clinics and randomized to two treatment groups. Independent assessors who were blind to treatment groups completed evaluations at baseline, 3 months, 12 months (end of treatment), and 18 months' follow-up.

Results: Both treatment groups showed clinically significant improvements, with just under 60% achieving a good or intermediate outcome (on the Morgan-Russell scales) at the end of treatment in the FT-AN group and more than 75% in the MFT-AN group—a statistically significant benefit in favor of the multifamily intervention (OR = 2.55 95%; CI 1.17, 5.52; *P* = .019). At 18 months' follow-up, there was no significant difference compared with the end of treatment at 12 months. Clinically significant gains in weight were associated with improvements in mood and eating disorder symptomology. Almost half of the patients in FT-AN and nearly 60% of those in the MFT-AN treatment group had started menstruating.

Implications: This study highlights the additional benefits of bringing together groups of families, augmenting the value of family resources and mutual support, leading to improved outcomes.

Modified from Eisler, I., Simic, M., Hodsoll, J., Asen, E., Berelowitz, M., Connan, F., et al. (2016). A pragmatic randomised multi-centre trial of multifamily and single family therapy for adolescent anorexia nervosa. *BMC Psychiatry, 16*(1), 422. https://doi.org/10.1186/s12888-016-1129-6.

Examining If Smartphone-guided Self-help and Cognitive Behavioral Therapy May Work in Individuals With Bulimia Nervosa

Description: The study purpose of this randomized controlled trial was to compare the effectiveness of health coach-delivered smartphone-guided self-help with standard care for adults with binge eating. In this study, 52 weeks of CBT-guided self-help (CBT-GSH) plus a Noom Monitor smartphone app (N = 114) were compared with standard care (e.g., psychiatric services; *N* = 111) among members of an integrated health care system.

Results: Participants who received CBT-GSH plus the Noom Monitor had significantly lower amounts of binge-eating days and higher remission rates (56.7% compared with 30%) at 52 weeks compared with those individuals in standard care. Comparable patterns occurred for other behaviors (e.g., vomiting, laxative use, excessive exercise, eating disorder symptoms, and clinical impairment).

Implications: Results suggest that the use of CBT-GSH, in conjunction with a Noom Monitor via telemedicine by health coaches, are important treatment components for improving binge-eating days, remissions, and associated eating behaviors in individuals with BN.

Modified from Hildebrandt, T., Michaeledes, A., Mayhew, M., Greif, R., Sysko, R., Toro-Ramos, T., & DeBar, L. (2020). Randomized controlled trial comparing health coach-delivered smartphone-guided self-help with standard care for adults with binge eating. *American Journal of Psychiatry, 177*(2), 134–142. https://doi.org/10.1176/appi.ajp.2019.19020184.

Treatment for comorbid diagnoses with psychotherapy and medication enhances the success of treatment for eating disorders. Premorbid physical conditions that should be ruled out include thyroid conditions, bowel disease or other gastrointestinal conditions, pancreatitis, cancer, or the effects of medications. If eating behaviors are caused by one of these conditions, therapeutic effectiveness involves different treatments than if the eating behaviors were solely the result of an eating disorder. About 38% of females and 16% of males with type 1 diabetes have eating disorders, increasing their risk of severe medical complications (e.g., ketoacidosis, retinopathy) and mortality (Hanlan et al., 2013).

Working with anorectic or bulimic patients presents a challenge to the psychotherapeutic team as patients continue their struggle to maintain control. When the treatment team requires weight gain or an end to bingeing and purging, patients perceive themselves as losing control, which triggers unconscious feelings of helplessness and resistance to treatment goals and interventions. Consciously, patients again experience the fear of becoming fat. This fear underlies the need to gain more control, restarting the vicious cycle of disordered eating. Nurses need to explore this fear and help patients find ways to deal with it (Treasure, Duarte, & Schmidt, 2020; Wade, 2019). See the "Tips for Professionals and Families From Persons Recovering From

Comparing Focused and Broad Enhanced Cognitive Behavioral Therapy

Description: This study compared the effectiveness of focused and broad enhanced cognitive behavioral therapy for individuals with bulimia nervosa with comorbid borderline personality (mean age, 25.63 years; standard deviation, 8.13) in a randomized clinical trial. The broad version of Enhanced Cognitive Behavior Therapy (CBT-E) addressed co-occurring problems that lessen treatment response. Fifty participants were randomly assigned to receive either focused CBT-E (CBT-Ef) or broad CBT-E (CBT-Eb) treatment. Participants in both groups received a preparatory 90-min session and 20 50-min sessions. Sessions are conducted twice weekly for the first 4 weeks, weekly through session 16, and biweekly through session 20. Outcomes were assessed at baseline and end of the study and at a 6-month follow-up.

Results: Forty-two percent of participants reported remission from binge eating and purging at the end of the study. Significant changes across symptom domains were observed at termination and at 6-month follow-up. Participants with higher severity showed better ED outcomes in CBT-Eb, whereas those with lower severity showed better outcomes in CBT-Ef. Severity of affective/interpersonal BPD symptoms at baseline predicted negative outcomes overall. Follow-up BPD affective/interpersonal problems were predicted by baseline affective/interpersonal problems and by termination EDE score.

Implications: Results suggest the importance of CBT-E for patients with bulimia nervosa and complex comorbidity. CBT-Ef appears to be more valuable for patients with relatively less severe comorbid borderline personality disorder symptoms while CBT-Eb appears to be more worthwhile for patients with more severe comorbid borderline personality disorder symptoms.

Modified from: Thompson-Brenner, H., Shingleton, R. M., Thompson, D. R., Satir, D. A., Richards, L. K., Pratt, E. M., & Barlow D. H. (2016). Focused vs. broad enhanced cognitive behavioral therapy for bulimia nervosa with comorbid borderline personality: A randomized controlled trial. *International Journal of Eating Disorders, 49*(1), 36–49. https://doi.org/10.1002/eat.22468.

Eating Disorders" box and the "Key Nursing Interventions for Patients With Eating Disorders" box.

Nurse-Patient Relationship

Because most anorectic patients have been forced into treatment by concerned family or friends, developing a therapeutic alliance is a challenge. Patients might believe that the nurse's purpose is simply to make them gain weight, so the nurse is perceived as an enemy, not an ally. Bulimic patients differ from anorectic patients in that bulimics are more likely to want help. They are more likely to enter therapy of their own volition, are eager to please, and so behave in a manner that will lead therapists to like them. However, in trying to please, bulimic patients have a tendency to become manipulative and might conceal the full extent of their problem. The desire to be helped is the greatest strength of bulimic patients. See Chapter 9 for general information about communicating with patients and developing rapport and trust with patients.

Psychopharmacology

No psychopharmacologic agent is approved specifically for anorexia nervosa at the present time. Medication management of anxiety, depression, somatic disturbances, or other comorbid conditions is appropriate and might assist in treatment of the patient's symptoms. Small amounts of anxiolytics might help patients with eating if given just before meals when refeeding is occurring. Anxiolytics can also be used to decrease the anxiety that fuels bingeing and purging in a bulimic patient, although antidepressants are a safer, more effective way to achieve that end. The long-term use of anxiolytics can lead to medication dependence, adding to the patient's problems. The atypical antipsychotic olanzapine (Zyprexa) has been tried to promote weight gain with some success, with its action achieved through growth hormone secretagogue receptor signaling (Couturier et al., 2020).

Other Treatments

In a study comprising 35 females with anorexia nervosa, Clus, Larsen, Lemey, and Berrouiguet (2018) conducted a review of empirical data regarding the use of virtual reality to evaluate and treat patients with eating disorders. Studies used a combination of tools, including audio stimuli, visual kinematics, and visual-tactile stimulation. Analyzing 28 studies, including 8 randomized control trials, empirical data support virtual reality as a promising tool regarding evaluation of eating behaviors and body image distortions. Virtual reality technology also lessened negative emotional responses to either virtual food stimuli or when seeing their body shape. Combining virtual reality modules and CBT was more effective than either virtual reality or CBT alone.

In severe cases of treatment-refractory anorexia nervosa, deep brain stimulation (DBS) is seen as a last resort invasive intervention to prevent death. Martínez et al. (2020) conducted a randomized trial using DBS to either the subcallosal cingulate or nucleus accumbens in eight patients for treatment-refractory anorexia nervosa. In comparing initial and 6-month body mass index, no significant differences were found for participants. However, five of the eight patients achieved an increase in BMI of 10% or more at 6 months and a few (i.e., 3) had less physical activity and laxative and diuretic use. Quality of life also improved. However, nearly 40% of patients had skin complications requiring surgery. These data suggest that DBS may be effective for some patients but further longitudinal studies are required. Following this recommendation, Liu et al. (2020) examined the safety, feasibility, and clinical outcomes of using DBS of the nucleus accumbens in treatment-refractory anorexia nervosa, using 28 women who were followed for 2 years. BMI and mood, anxiety, and obsessive symptoms were measured at 6 and 12 months. No fatalities were noted but 1 patient had rejection of their device, while some (i.e., 22) had mild irritation at the surgical site, which dissipated 3 to 4 days after surgery. Participants had improved outcomes on all measures at 6 months, which were maintained at 2 years. This treatment was more effective for those patients with binge-eating/purging than for restricting anorexia, suggesting that this treatment may be effective and safe as a treatment for patients with restrictive anorexia, but further, larger-scale studies are needed.

TIPS FOR PROFESSIONALS AND FAMILIES FROM PERSONS RECOVERING FROM EATING DISORDERS

- Some patients never binge or purge but control weight with exercise and restriction of intake.
- Some patients do not stop menstruating, although there might be changes in their cycles.
- Depression, anxiety, neglect, and domestic violence might predispose patients to eating disorders or occur concurrently with them. If these conditions or problems are addressed without treating the eating disorder, efforts are likely to fail.
- Patients' concentration on exactness and perfection might lead them to deny their illness by rationalizing that if they do not exhibit *all* the criteria of the disorder, they do not have the disorder.
- Patients might recognize that their body image is distorted but are unable to stop their destructive behavior.
- Not all patients with eating disorders have rituals about eating. They might simply avoid being in situations in which they have to eat in front of others.

When educating adolescents about eating disorders, avoid using films or other graphic materials that might teach the teens more ways to beat the system regarding eating and maintaining healthy weight.

Dishonesty (lying to self and others) is a hallmark of patients with eating disorders. Honesty toward self and others is the key to recovery and relapse prevention.

Watch for the onset of eating disorders at times of major life transition with increased pressure on an individual to fit in or adjust. These times include the move to middle school from elementary school, to high school from junior high or middle school, and graduation from high school with the move to college or a job.

Patients with eating disorders believe that calories are everywhere and go to great lengths to avoid them, including not smelling food or licking stamps for fear calories will be absorbed.

Media images of very thin models and celebrities might be viewed by very young girls as an ideal to be achieved, but most patients use media images of thinness to justify their behavior after the start of the eating disorder rather than motivation to begin their disordered eating.

KEY NURSING INTERVENTIONS

For Patients With Eating Disorders

- Monitor daily caloric intake and electrolyte status while in the hospital; patients should not gain too much weight too quickly.
- Observe patients for signs of purging or other compensation for food consumed.
- Monitor activity level, and encourage appropriate levels of activity for patient.
- Weigh daily while in the hospital but encourage patients to diminish focus on weight after refeeding.
- Plan for a dietitian to meet with patients and families to (1) provide accurate information on nutrition, (2) discuss a realistic and healthy diet, and (3) assist the nurses in monitoring the nutritional intake of the patient (particularly crucial for patients who are diabetic or pregnant).
- Encourage use of therapies or support groups to attain healthy weight and prevent relapse.
- Promote patient decision-making concerning issues other than food.
- Promote positive self-concept and perceptions of body as well as interactions with others.
- Convey warmth and sincerity. Patients must believe that the nurse genuinely understands and cares about their concerns and efforts to overcome their fears about treatment.
- Listen empathically. Although anorectic patients are likely to deny that weight is a problem, they do admit being lonely and tired of compulsively striving to meet unreachable goals. Bulimics are more likely to admit their problems with weight but still feel helpless in addressing them.
- Encourage regular eating patterns.
- Be honest. Patients enter treatment distrustful of everyone. Honesty is essential to developing a trusting relationship with any patient with an eating disorder.
- Set appropriate behavioral limits. Because of control needs, patients are likely to attempt to manipulate the nurse. A clear contract between the nurse and patient helps establish trust and minimize power struggles.
- Assist patients in identifying their positive qualities. Because self-esteem is low, patients need to see concrete evidence of their positive qualities. Improving patients' view of self is a primary objective in recovery.
- Collaborate with patients. To elicit cooperation, engage patients in planning to foster trust and a sense of control, which will diminish their need to maintain control through eating strategies.
- Teach patients about their disorders. Providing accurate information about eating disorders should decrease denial and help patients understand the effects of the disease on their bodies, minds, and emotions.
- Determine the anorectic's ability to be weighed in the early stages of treatment. Often, anorectics need to be weighed with their backs to the scale to help reduce their focus on body weight.
- Help patients understand the effects of the disease on their families, as well as the effect that the family has on them.
- Initiate a behavior modification program with patient input that rewards weight gain or lack of purging with meaningful privileges or rewards. Although the idea of gaining weight is stressful to patients, it is crucial to recovery. When a safe weight is attained, allow patients more control of their own progress and program as long as they do not backslide. Patients must eventually take control of maintaining a safe weight.
- Model and teach appropriate social skills. Acquiring social skills, particularly expressing emotions appropriately, is crucial for patients with eating disorders. Encourage patients to examine their interpersonal relationships and work to decrease their loneliness.
- Help patients identify and express bodily sensations and feelings related to their disorders.
- Identify non–weight-related interests of the patient. Involvement with these interests can reduce anxiety as patients invest their energies in areas not related to eating. Encourage the development of new hobbies and interests that are not food-related.

Treatment with antidepressants, especially SSRIs, has proved helpful in reducing bingeing, purging, and depression in bulimic patients. These drugs have been shown to have a positive effect on associated mood disturbances and preoccupation with shape and weight. Antidepressants appear to be equally effective in both depressed and nondepressed patients with BN. These results suggest that the mechanism of the drug action might not be the antidepressant, but rather the drug might have direct central effects on neurotransmitter systems, particularly serotonin and norepinephrine. However, although antidepressants have beneficial effects in the short term, this improvement does not appear to be maintained over the long term. Significant affect dysregulation and poor impulse control may limit responsiveness. Patients with comorbid impulsive and dysregulated symptoms and behaviors (e.g., self-harming, substance abuse, excessive risk-taking, and reactive, erratic mood shifts) tend to achieve less benefit from antidepressant monotherapy. In general, psychotherapy is recommended before a trial of an antidepressant. Antidepressants are considered when the patient has failed to respond adequately to psychotherapy alone or when there is comorbidity with severe clinical depression (Couturier et al., 2020; Hay, 2020; Hilbert et al., 2019).

Milieu Management

Provide an orientation to the setting to prepare the patient for inpatient or outpatient treatment so that fears are reduced.

Provide a warm, nurturing atmosphere. It is important for patients to feel support to reduce anxiety and increase trust.

Closely observe patients. Avoidance behaviors should be identified to plan appropriate interventions. Common behaviors include hiding food in a paper napkin to be discarded later, leaving bread crusts on the plate and discarding the rest, discarding food into plants or out the window, spilling food while eating so that it cannot be determined how much the patient really ate, and holding food in the mouth to be discarded when the patient brushes his or her teeth. Respond to such behaviors with nonjudgmental limits, conveying understanding of weight gain fears.

Encourage the patient to approach a team member if feeling the need to purge. Expression of feelings reduces anxiety and helps patients discover alternatives to restricting food or vomiting.

Involve the patient's family in treatment, when appropriate. If the family denies the problem or is not supportive of treatment, the family might need to be temporarily excluded from the treatment team. If parents, particularly of minors, provide emotional support, treatment efforts have a greater chance of success. Families must understand the disorder and its treatment. Family therapy and family education are crucial components for helping adolescents with eating disorders in both short-term and long-term treatment.

Respond with consistency. The behavioral program or treatment regimen implemented must be constantly adhered to by the entire staff to diminish patient manipulation and avoid sabotage of treatment.

Encourage participation in art, recreation, and other types of therapy. These modalities teach patients alternative ways to express their feelings and provide activities other than focusing on food and dieting.

Involve a dietitian in the treatment plan who can teach proper nutrition while providing patients with an opportunity to select menus. Increase caloric intake gradually to increase patient cooperation in the weight gain program, maintain patient safety, and avoid the medical risks in adding weight too quickly. Encourage compliance with planned schedules for meals and snacks. Regularization of eating prevents the precipitation of binge eating resulting from dieting or restrictive eating practices. Encourage all patients to follow the advice of dietitians regarding normalization of eating.

Encourage patient attendance at group therapy sessions. Providing an opportunity for patients to participate in a group with peers helps them see that they are not alone in having difficulty expressing feelings and dealing with developmental issues. Nurse-led support groups encourage patients to share issues, feelings, and fears.

Recommend follow-up psychotherapeutic groups and support groups for patients and their families and individual psychotherapy for patients with a qualified therapist. These sessions are particularly beneficial after significant weight gain and after discharge from a treatment program. Patients might relapse or die because of lack of appropriate outpatient follow-up or might attempt suicide. A comprehensive continuum of care provides the best option for relapse prevention in view of the chronic nature of the disease.

Treatment in various settings from outpatient to day treatment and inpatient treatment for the most physically compromised patients has been attempted, but research has not shown any clear difference in results related to the treatment

CASE STUDY

Sarah Hodge, a 17-year-old girl, was brought to the hospital by her parents and outpatient therapist, whom she had been seeing weekly for 1 month. Sarah and the therapist had a contract of a 2-lb weight gain every week, but Sarah had continued to lose weight. On admission, she was 5 feet 5 inches tall and weighed 86 lb. Sarah strongly opposed her hospitalization and denied she had a problem.

Sarah is the youngest of three daughters, ages 27, 24, and 17, a late addition to her middle-class family. Sarah's parents admitted that she had been steadily losing weight for the last 6 months. At first, Sarah's parents believed that she was just dieting, but when they began to see her ribs and vertebrae through her nightgown, they became gravely concerned.

Sarah was recently named recipient of a college scholarship. She has been active in school activities and was well-liked by her teachers because of her hard work. Although she appeared to have many friends, Sarah claimed that she had only one real friend, another anorectic.

Sarah said that her obsession with weight began approximately 6 months ago, when the family went to visit the oldest daughter, whom Sarah idolized. One afternoon, the three sisters went berry picking, and the oldest daughter told Sarah, "Don't eat all the berries, or you'll grow into a real chub!" Sarah interpreted this to mean that her sister thought that she was fat. She became obsessed with food and became a vegetarian. She adopted the role of planning menus and educating the family on proper nutrition. When her mother attempted to intervene, Sarah screamed that she knew what she was doing and was tired of being treated like a baby. If her mother attempted further control over Sarah's eating behavior, Sarah refused to eat at all. The situation at home deteriorated until there was little communication between family members and Sarah. She engaged in irrational rituals and lost 30 lb. When Sarah began to look very thin, they persuaded her to seek help, although she continued to lose weight during outpatient therapy.

Sarah is a likable girl. The other adolescents in the hospital were attracted to her and wanted to be her friend. However, they noticed Sarah's odd eating habits, such as mixing cornflakes in vanilla pudding and pouring cranberry juice over cereals. At first, she resisted eating meals and snacks, but she complied when faced with tube feeding to replace what she refused to eat. Sarah always dressed in baggy overalls and wore oversized sweaters. When other patients asked Sarah if she felt cold, she quietly told them that she did not want them to stare at her fat body, a comment that tended to put off her peers.

During break times, Sarah was found writing morbid poetry, which contained subtle suicidal messages. She preferred to be alone and became irritable and rude when asked to participate in group therapy sessions. Sarah tried to be as compliant as she thought others wanted her to be; however, the lack of control that she experienced in the hospital added to her anxiety and discomfort and fueled her feelings of being alone in the world.

setting. A stepped care approach might be useful, in which patients first participate in a simple treatment, such as guided self-help or a psychoeducational group with their families, and then, if they do not respond, are referred for cognitive behavior therapy. Patients who do not improve with therapy can be referred for a more intensive form of treatment, such as interpersonal psychotherapy, partial or full hospitalization, and possibly antidepressant medication.

EATING DISORDERS IN MEN

The lifetime prevalence of eating disorders are approximately 14% in men (Ward et al., 2019), and various studies suggest the risk of mortality for males is higher than it is for females (Iwajomo et al., 2020). Although 9 out of 10 cases of eating disorders were women, cases in men increased by 53% (Zhao & Encinosa, 2011).

Identification of men with partial and full syndromes of eating disorders has increased the number of men diagnosed with eating disorders. Although diagnoses, etiologies,

and treatment of men and women with eating disorders are similar, there appear to be differences in risk factors, clinical presentation, comorbidity, and consequences (Raevuori et al., 2014). Some research indicates men are more likely than women to have a history of obesity before the onset of symptoms of an eating disorder and to have a later onset and higher initial BMI before engaging in disordered eating (Scheffers et al., 2017). Other studies suggest a higher percentage of comorbidities (i.e., generalized anxiety disorder) in males with binge eating disorder (Ulfvebrand et al., 2015). However, a more recent systematic review showed men and women with bulimia are more similar than different regarding their weight and associated comorbidities (Guerdjikova, Mori, Casuto, & McElroy, 2019).

Treatment for men with eating disorders is similar to that for women. From a psychotherapeutic management standpoint, the following three areas need particular focus with men:

1. The excessive attention that adolescent boys can place on attaining a masculine physique and its effect on their body image

---

⊚ CARE PLAN

Name: Sarah Hodge   **Admission Date:** _____
DSM-5 Diagnosis: Anorexia Nervosa

Assessment	**Areas of strength:** Intelligence; past achievements; likableness; past healthy interpersonal relationships; good personal hygiene; some insight into reasons for hospitalization; family support
	Problems: Low weight, disturbed body image, low self-esteem, depression, lack of accurate knowledge regarding nutrition, avoidant behavior
Diagnoses	Imbalanced nutrition; less than body requirements, related to not eating enough nutrients, as evidenced by continued weight loss and inappropriate eating habits
	Disturbance in body image, related to feeling fat when actually underweight, as evidenced by inappropriate dress and comments about how fat she is
	Disturbance in self-esteem, related to fear of becoming fat and repulsive, as evidenced by suicidal messages in poetry and by social withdrawal
	Knowledge deficit in proper nutrition, related to fear of being fat, as evidenced by odd eating habits and refusal to eat certain foods
Outcomes	**Short-term goals**
Date met: _____	Patient will gain 1 lb per week.
Date met: _____	Patient will identify two positive qualities about herself.
Date met: _____	Patient will discuss fears of losing control.
	Long-term goals
Date met: _____	Patient will gain at least 20 lb within 6 months.
Date met: _____	Patient will verbalize knowledge of illness and proper nutrition.
Date met: _____	Patient will identify at least three alternative coping mechanisms to use when feeling out of control.
Date met: _____	Patient will verbalize increased comfort in relating to peers.
Planning and Interventions	**Nurse-patient relationship:** Establish a contract to meet with the patient daily to discuss feelings; express concern for the patient; encourage verbalization of feelings about depression and lack of control; encourage patient to identify positive qualities about herself.
	Milieu management: Encourage patient to attend meals and sit with peers; encourage participation in group therapy to discuss feelings with peers and normalize her experience; encourage patient to share positive qualities of herself with peers; maintain consistency of unit rules and ensure that patient is adhering to them.
Evaluation	Patient gained 2 lb in the first 10 days of hospitalization; attended all unit activities; attended individual therapy with nurse therapist, and stated one positive thing about herself.
Referrals	Patient has been given information about an eating disorder support group in her community and a person to contact regarding group attendance after discharge. Patient encouraged to continue individual and family therapy.

2. Dietary habits to promote health, fitness, and muscle mass without using disordered eating patterns

3. The expression of feelings and the exploration of any underlying sexual identity concerns

Although most adolescents with eating disorders have difficulty expressing their feelings, boys seem to have more difficulty than girls. A therapeutic relationship can be especially instrumental in the recovery of these young men, especially regarding family dynamics that encourage interdependence, without excessive conflict and control.

> ### ❓ CRITICAL THINKING QUESTION
>
> 2. A 17-year-old boy remarks to you that he feels too fat and is afraid that he will not be able to "make weight" for wrestling. You do not observe that the patient is overweight. How do you begin to assess whether the patient has an eating disorder?

BINGE-EATING DISORDER

Binge-eating disorder (BED) is a newer diagnosis found in the *DSM-5*. BED is characterized by recurrent episodes of binge eating during a discrete period of time (within a 2-hour period), associated with a lack of control. The binge-eating episodes involve the individual rapidly eating large amounts of food, feeling uncomfortably full, eating alone, and feeling disgusted—at least once a week for 3 months. BED shares many criteria of BN (lack of control over intake, patient distress, and guilt over bingeing) but without the regular compensation for excess intake through purging or excessive exercise. As a consequence, individuals with BED tend to be overweight or obese. Binge eating occurs in children, adolescents, and college-age individuals and is associated with increases in psychological symptoms (APA, 2013). Empirical data suggest that neurobiological, familial, and genetic factors influence the risk of this disorder. Often women have a chronic history of low mood, anxiety, steady weight gain or a history of "yo-yo" dieting habits, sleep problems, impaired concentration, and anhedonia, or an impaired ability to feel pleasure. Therefore, treatment for depressive symptoms is very important (Guerdjikova et al., 2019).

In a review of 48 randomized clinical trials and other studies regarding BED and major outcomes, second-generation antidepressants, topiramate (an anticonvulsant), and lisdexamfetamine (a stimulant) were superior to placebo in obtaining abstinence and lessening binge episodes and/or binge days and eating-related obsessions and compulsions. Second-generation antidepressants reduced depression while topiramate and lisdexamfetamine resulted in weight reduction in individuals who were overweight or obese. Therapist-led, partially therapist-led, and guided self-help CBT were superior to placebo in attaining abstinence and reducing binge frequency but were ineffective for reducing weight or depression (Agency for Healthcare Research and Quality, 2015).

Reporting similar findings in a more recent systematic review, Brownley et al. (2016) examined the benefits and harms of psychological and pharmacologic therapies for adults with BED, reviewing nine waitlist-controlled psychological trials and 25 placebo-controlled trials. Therapist-led CBT, lisdexamfetamine, and second-generation antidepressants decreased binge-eating frequency and increased binge-eating abstinence, lessened binge-eating-related obsessions and compulsions, reduced symptoms of depression, and reduce related psychopathology. Second-generation antidepressants reduced depression while topiramate and lisdexamfetamine dimesylate (LDX) resulted in weight reduction in individuals who were overweight or obese.

In mild cases with no significant psychiatric comorbidities, psychotherapy alone (e.g., cognitive behavior, interpersonal, and perhaps dialectical therapy) or with self-help tools are the first line of treatment for lessening binge-eating symptoms, and related psychopathology. Psychoeducation also is valuable. In more severe cases, medications either alone or with psychotherapy are options. LDX is approved for treatment of moderate to severe BED in adults. Other medications include antiepileptic drugs, antiobesity drugs, and those approved for attention-deficit/hyperactivity disorder (ADHD), improving binge-eating habits in randomized control trials. However, those who took both LDX and ADHD medication had a significantly higher risk of adverse symptoms, so side effects must be monitored closely (Guerdjikova et al., 2019).

Orthorexia Nervosa

While not classified as an official diagnosis in either the *DSM-5* manual or International Classification of Diseases-10, health professionals are describing orthorexia nervosa as a problem in individuals with a compulsive fixation on healthy eating and an unbending adherence to diet rules. While eating nutritious foods is a desirable trait, these individuals focus extensively on only eating "healthy" food, causing physiological and psychological harm. Impaired social behaviors and social relationships are common (Kalra, Kapoor, & Jacob, 2020; National Eating Disorders Association, 2018). This condition overlaps with that of anorexia nervosa and avoidant/restrictive food intake disorder. Common clinical manifestations include obsessively checking food labels and methods for producing and manufacturing foods, weighing whether ingredients are healthy for them to eat. These individuals also compulsively eliminate many food group items (e.g., all/most sugar and other carbohydrates, meat and animal products, dairy, etc.) and are unable to eat foods other than a very select food list. An excessive amount of energy is spent thinking about foods to be served at upcoming events and these individuals experience extreme distress when foods that they deem "healthy" are unavailable to them. Often, they spend an elaborate amount of time reading materials about "healthy" foods. Because orthorexia nervosa involves these individuals limiting the amount and variety of foods that they allow themselves to eat, malnutrition is a common concern

(Kalra *et al.* 2020; National Eating Disorders Association, 2018). Health professionals commonly treat this disorder as a form of either anorexia or obsessive-compulsive disorder, with the goal of increasing the types of foods eaten and gradually introducing the intake of anxiety-provoking or feared foods. Restoring weight to normal parameters is another goal (Kalra *et al.* 2020; National Eating Disorders Association, 2018).

WEB RESOURCES

The following websites represent a small sampling of available resources for professionals, patients, and families. Nurses should evaluate the appropriateness of web resources as with all other resources before giving them to patients and families.

There is a disturbing phenomenon on the Internet known as *pro anorexia* (pro ana) and *pro bulimia* (pro mia) websites, bulletin boards, and chat rooms hosted by individuals with eating disorders and proclaiming anorexia and bulimia as lifestyle choices rather than life-threatening illnesses. These sites offer tips on how to be the "best anorectic" or "best bulimic" and often feature alarming pictures of individuals with the disorders in a macabre competition of thinness. The web addresses of these sites are often passed from patient to patient, making them very difficult to track and control.

National Eating Disorders Association
http://www.nationaleatingdisorders.org
The National Eating Disorders Association (NEDA) is the leading nonprofit organization in the United States that supports individuals and families affected by eating disorders. NEDA was formed in 2001, when Eating Disorders Awareness & Prevention (EDAP) joined forces with the American Anorexia Bulimia Association (AABA)—merging the largest and longest standing eating disorders prevention and advocacy organizations in the world.

National Association of Anorexia and Associated Disorders
http://www.anad.org
This site is sponsored and maintained by the Association of Anorexia and Associated Disorders (ANAD), the oldest national nonprofit organization devoted to helping patients with eating disorders and their families through providing networking, support groups, and advocacy for patients and their families. Current efforts are directed at monitoring and advocating against media references that portray eating disorders as funny and that the organization believes are dangerous and demeaning.

Eating Disorders Referral and Information Center
http://www.edreferral.com
This site is sponsored and maintained by the International Eating Disorders Referral Organization, a nonprofit organization. The website contains much information and many links to other resources, as well as referrals worldwide to caregivers experienced in treating eating disorders.

Binge Eating Disorder Association
https://www.eatingdisorderhope.com/information/help-overcome-eating-disorders/beda
The Binge Eating Disorder Association (BEDA) is a national organization focusing on providing leadership, recognition, prevention, and treatment of BED and associated weight stigma. Through outreach, education, and advocacy, BEDA facilitates increased awareness, proper diagnosis, and treatment of BED.

Academy for Eating Disorders
http://www.aedweb.org
The Academy for Eating Disorders (AED) is the international source for state-of-the-art information in the field of eating disorders. The organization is a global, multidisciplinary, professional association committed to leadership in eating disorder research, education, treatment, and prevention. AED advocates for the field on behalf of patients, the public, and eating disorder professionals.

Something Fishy Website on Eating Disorders
http://www.something-fishy.org/
This site serves as a clearinghouse for eating disorder resources and information. It provides discussion forums for people with eating disorders and another forum for loved ones of individuals with eating disorders and proclaims itself as pro recovery.

Eating Disorder Hope
http://www.eatingdisorderhope.com
This site offers education, support, and inspiration to eating disorder sufferers; their loved ones; and eating disorder treatment providers. Resources include articles on eating disorder treatment options, support groups, and recovery tools.

STUDY NOTES

1. Anorexia nervosa is characterized by a refusal to maintain body weight at or above a minimally normal weight for age and height, an intense fear of becoming fat, a distorted body image, and amenorrhea or irregular menstrual cycles in women and low testosterone levels in men.

2. Anorectic dieters might begin their illness in a normal weight range but then isolate themselves socially from others, become competitive concerning weight loss, and exercise excessively.

3. Bulimia is characterized by episodes of binge eating, a feeling of lack of control over eating, use of compensatory behavior, and an overconcern with body shape and weight. Depression commonly coexists with bulimia.

4. Anorectic and bulimic patients experience a variety of physiologic problems that can lead to death. Personality and emotional changes are also evident in these patients, which might result from the eating disorder or might be a contributing factor in its genesis.

5. The causes of eating disorders are thought to be multifactorial, including biologic, sociocultural, familial, cognitive, behavioral, and psychodynamic factors.

6. Family therapy and cognitive behavior therapy have the most research support in the treatment of eating disorders.

7. The incidence of eating disorders in men is increasing, with similarities in presentation and treatment to those in women with eating disorders, although eating disorders in men seem to manifest at a later age than in women.

8. Nursing interventions with patients with eating disorders require caring, supportive relationships; limit setting; a behavior modification program; and a consistent milieu. Family involvement, individual psychotherapy, and group therapy are also essential.

9. Hospitalization with a structured milieu and antidepressant medications might be needed if weight decreases below what is appropriate for the patient's height or if medical complications related to the patient's condition are present.

REFERENCES

Agency for Healthcare Research and Quality. (2011). Hospitalizations for eating disorders declined, but big increase seen in pica disorder. https://archive.ahrq.gov/news/newsroom/news-and-numbers/090811.html.

Agency for Healthcare Research and Quality. (2015). Comparative effectiveness review: Management and outcomes of binge-eating disorder (#160). https://effectivehealthcare.ahrq.gov/sites/default/files/pdf/binge-eating_research.pdf.

Agras, W. S., Fitzsimmons, E. E., & Wilfley, D. E. (2017). Evolution of cognitive-behavioral therapy for eating disorders. *Behaviour Research and Therapy, 88*, 26–36. https://doi.org/10.1016/j.brat.2016.09.004.

American Psychiatric Association. (2013). *Diagnostic and statistical manual of mental disorders* (5th ed.). APA.

Arcelus, J., et al. (2011). Mortality rates in patients with anorexia nervosa and other eating disorders. A meta-analysis of 36 studies. *Archives of General Psychiatry, 68*, 724. https://doi.org/10.1001/archgenpsychiatry.2011.74.

Batista, M., Žigić Antić, L., Žaja, O., Jakovina, T., & Begovac, I. (2018). Predictors of eating disorder risk in anorexia nervosa adolescents. *Acta Clinical Croatica, 57*(3), 399–410. https://doi.org/10.20471/acc.2018.57.03.01.

Blanchet, C., Guillaume, S., Bat-Pitault, F., Carles, M., Clarke, J., Dodin, V., … Godart, N. (2019). Medication in AN: A multidisciplinary overview of meta-analyses and systematic reviews. *Journal of Clinical Medicine, 8*(2), 278. https://doi.org/10.3390/jcm8020278.

Brownley, K. A., et al. (2016). Binge-eating disorder in adults: A systematic review and meta-analysis. *Annals of Internal Medicine, 165*(6), 409–420. https://doi.org/10.7326/M15-2455.

Bulik, C. M., Flatt, R., Abbaspour, A., & Carroll, I. (2019). Reconceptualizing anorexia nervosa. *Psychiatry and Clinical Neurosciences, 73*(9), 518–525. https://doi.org/10.1111/pcn.12857.

Clus, D., Larsen, M. E., Lemey, C., & Berrouiguet, S. (2018). The use of virtual reality in patients with eating disorders: Systematic review. *Journal of Medical Internet Research, 20*(4), e157. https://doi.org/10.2196/jmir.7898.

Costa, M. B., & Melnik, T. (2016). Effectiveness of psychosocial interventions in eating disorders: An overview of Cochrane systematic reviews. *Einstein (Sao Paulo), 14*(2), 235–277. https://doi.org/10.1590/S1679-45082016RW3120.

Couturier, J., Isserlin, L., Norris, M., Spettigue, W., Brouwers, M., Kimber, M., … Pilon, D. (2020). Canadian practice guidelines for the treatment of children and adolescents with eating disorders. *Journal of Eating Disorders*(8), 4. https://doi.org/10.1186/s40337-020-0277-8.

Dakanalis, A., Giuseppe, C., Calogero, R., Zanetti, M., Gaudio, S., Caccialanza, R., … Clerici, M. (2015). Testing the cognitive-behavioural maintenance models across DSM-5 bulimic-type eating disorder diagnostic groups: A multi-centre study. *European Archives of Psychiatry and Clinical Neuroscience, 265*, 663–676. https://doi.org/10.1007/s00406-014-0560-2.

Davis, L. E., & Attia, E. (2019). Recent advances in therapies for eating disorders. *F1000 Research, 8*, 1–9. https://www.ncbi.nlm.nih.gov/pmc/articles/PMC6764116/pdf/f1000research-8-21775.pdf.

Demmler, J. C., Brophy, S. T., Marchant, A., John, A., & Tan, J. O. (2020). Shining the light on eating disorders, incidence, prognosis and profiling of patients in primary and secondary care: National data linkage study. *The British Journal of Psychiatry, 216*(2), 105–112. https://doi.org/10.1192/bjp.2019.153.

Deloitte Access Economics. (2020, June). The social and economic cost of eating disorders in the United States of America: A report for the strategic training initiative for the prevention of eating disorders and the Academy for Eating Disorders. https://cdn1.sph.harvard.edu/wp-content/uploads/sites/1267/2020/07/Social-Economic-Cost-of-Eating-Disorders-in-US.pdf.

Dörsam, A. F., Preißl, H., Micali, N., Lörcher, S. B., Zipfel, S., & Giel, K. E. (2019). The impact of maternal eating disorders on dietary intake and eating patterns during pregnancy: A systematic review. *Nutrients, 11*(4), 840. https://doi.org/10.3390/nu11040840.

Duncan, L., Yilmaz, Z., Gaspar, H., Walters, R., Goldstein, J., Anttila, V., … Bulik, C. M. (2017). Significant locus and metabolic genetic correlations revealed in genome-wide association study of anorexia nervosa. *American Journal of Psychiatry, 174*(9), 850–858. https://doi.org/10.1176/appi.ajp.2017.16121402.

Dufresne, L., Bussières, E. L., Bédard, A., Gingras, N., Blanchette-Sarrasin, A., & Bégin, C. (2020). Personality traits in adolescents with eating disorder: A meta-analytic review. *International Eating Disorders, 53*(2), 157–173. https://doi.org/10.1002/eat.23183.

Eisler, I., Simic, M., Hodsoll, J., Asen, E., Berelowitz, M., Connan, F., … Landau, S. (2016). A pragmatic randomised multi-centre trial of multifamily and single family therapy for adolescent anorexia nervosa. *BMC Psychiatry, 16*(1), 422. https://doi.org/10.1186/s12888-016-1129-6.

Erriu, M., Cimino, S., & Cerniglia, L. (2020). The role of family relationships in eating disorders in adolescents: A narrative review. *Behavioral Sciences (Basel), 10*(4), 71. https://doi.org/10.3390/bs10040071.

Fairburn, C. G. (2005). Evidence-based treatment of anorexia nervosa. *International Journal of Eating Disorders, 37*, S26–S30. https://doi.org/10.1002/eat.20112.

Fisher, M., & Bushlow, M. (2015). Perceptions of family styles by adolescents with eating disorders and their parents. *International Journal of Adolesent Medicine & Health, 27*, 443–449. https://doi.org/10.1515/ijamh-2014-0058.

Franko, D. L., Tabri, N., Keshaviah, A., Murray, H. B., Herzog, D. B., Thomas, J. J., … Eddy, K. T. (2018). Predictors of long-term recovery in anorexia nervosa and bulimia nervosa: Data from a 22-year longitudinal study. *Journal of Psychiatric Research, 96*, 183–188. https://doi.org/10.1016/j.jpsychires.2017.10.008.

Galmiche, M., Déchelotte, P., Lambert, G., & Tavolacci, M. P. (2019). Prevalence of eating disorders over the 2000–2018 period: A systematic literature review. *The American Journal of Clinical Nutrition, 109*(5), 1402–1413. https://doi.org/10.1093/ajcn/nqy342.

Gianini, L. M., et al. (2016). The reinforcing effect of exercise in anorexia nervosa: Clinical correlates and relationship to outcome. *Eating Disorders, 24*(5), 412–423. https://doi.org/10.1080/10640266.2016.1198204.

Guardian News & Media Limited (2021) NHS hospital admissions for eating disorders rise among ethnic minorities. https://www.theguardian.com/society/2020/oct/18/nhs-hospital-admissions-eating-disorders-rise-among-ethnic-minorities.

Guerdjikova, A. I., Mori, N., Casuto, L. S., & McElroy, S. L. (2019). Update on binge eating disorder. *Medical Clinics of Noth America, 103*(4), 669–680. https://doi.org/10.1016/j.mcna.2019.02.003.

Guillaume, S., Gorwood, P., Jollant, F., Van den, Eynde, F., Courtet, P., & Richard-Devantoy, S. (2015). Impaired decision-making in symptomatic anorexia and bulimia nervosa patients: A meta-analysis. *Psychological Medicine, 45*(16), 3377–3391. https://doi.org/10.1017/S003329171500152X.

Hagan, K. E., & Walsh, B. T. (2020). State of the art: The therapeutic approaches to bulimia nervosa. *Clinical Therapeutics, S0149-2918*(20), 30483–30485. https://doi.org/10.1016/j.clinthera.2020.10.01.

Hanlan, M. E., et al. (2013). Eating disorders and disordered eating in Type 1 diabetes: Prevalence, screening, and treatment options. *Current Diabetes Reports, 13*, 909–916. https://doi.org/10.1007/s11892-013-0418-4.

Hay, P. (2020). Current approach to eating disorders: A clinical update. *Internal Medicine Journal, 50*(1), 24–29. https://doi.org/10.1111/imj.14691.

Hilbert, A., Petroff, D., Herpertz, S., Pietrowsky, R., Tuschen-Caffier, B., Vocks, S., & Schmidt, R. (2019). Meta-analysis of the efficacy of psychological and medical treatments for binge-eating disorder. *Journal of Consulting and Clinical Psychology, 87*(1), 91–105. https://doi.org/10.1037/ccp0000358.

Hildebrandt, T., Michaeledes, A., Mayhew, M., Greif, R., Sysko, R., Toro-Ramos, T., & DeBar, L. (2020). Randomized controlled trial comparing health coach-delivered smartphone-guided self-help with standard care for adults with binge eating. *American Journal of Psychiatry, 177*(2), 134–142. https://doi.org/10.1176/appi.ajp.2019.19020184.

Himmerich, H., Kan, C., Au, K., & Treasure, J. (2021). Pharmacological treatment of eating disorders, comorbid mental health problems, malnutrition and physical health consequences. *Pharmacology & Therapeutics, 217*, 107667. https://doi.org/10.1016/j.pharmthera.2020.107667.

Iwajomo, T., Bondy, S. J., de Oliveira, C., Colton, P., Trottier, K., & Kurdyak, P. (2020). Excess mortality associated with eating disorders: Population-based cohort study. *British Journal of Psychiatry, 29*, 1–7. https://doi.org/10.1192/bjp.2020.197.

Jagielska, G. W., Przedlacki, J., Bartoszewicz, Z., & Racicka, E. (2016). Bone mineralization disorders as a complication of anorexia nervosa—Etiology, prevalence, course and treatment. *Psychiatria Polska, 50*(3), 509–520. https://doi.org/10.12740/PP/59289.

Jansingh, A., Danner, U. N., Hoek, H. W., & van Elburg, A. A. (2020). Developments in the psychological treatment of anorexia nervosa and their implications for daily practice. *Current Opinion in Psychiatry, 33*(6), 534–541. https://doi.org/10.1097/YCO.0000000000000642.

Jenkins, Z. M., Chait, L. M., Cistullo, L., & Castle, D. J. (2020). A comparison of eating disorder symptomatology, psychological distress and psychosocial function between early, typical and later onset anorexia nervosa. *Journal of Eating Disorders, 8*(1), 56. https://doi.org/10.1186/s40337-020-00337-w.

Kalra, S., Kapoor, N., & Jacob, J. (2020). Orthorexia nervosa. *Journal of Pakistan Medical Association, 70*(7), 1282–1284. PMID: 32799294.

Linardon, J., Shatte, A., Messer, M., Firth, J., & Fuller-Tyszkiewicz, M. J. (2020). E-mental health interventions for the treatment and prevention of eating disorders: An updated systematic review and meta-analysis. *Journal of Consulting and Clinicl Psychology, 88*(11), 994–1007. https://doi.org/10.1037/ccp0000575.

Liu, W., Zhan, S., Li, D., Lin, Z., Zhang, C., Wang, T., … Sun, (2020). Deep brain stimulation of the nucleus accumbens for treatment-refractory anorexia nervosa: A long-term follow-up study. *Brain Stimulation, 13*(3), 643–649. https://doi.org/10.1016/j.brs.2020.02.004.

Machado, P. P. P., & Rodrigues, T. F. (2019). Treatment delivery strategies for eating disorders. *Current Opinion in Psychiatry, 32*(6), 498–503. https://doi.org/10.1097/YCO.0000000000000542.

Martínez, G. V., Justicia, A., Salgado, P., Ginés, J. M., Guardiola, R., Cedrón, C., … Pérez, P. (2020). A randomized trial of deep brain stimulation to the subcallosal cingulate and nucleus accumbens in patients with treatment-refractory, chronic, and severe anorexia nervosa: Initial results at 6 months of follow up. *Journal of Clinical Medicine, 9*(6), 1946. https://doi.org/10.3390/jcm9061946.

Marzola, E., Cavallo, F., Pradella, P., Brustolin, A., & Abbate-Daga, G. (2020). A tasting experiment comparing food and nutritional supplement in anorexia nervosa. *Appetite, 1*(155), 104789. https://doi.org/10.1016/j.appet.2020.104789.

McDonald, S. (2019). Understanding the genetics and epigenetics of bulimia nervosa/bulimia spectrum disorder and comorbid borderline personality disorder (BN/BSD-BPD): A systematic review. *Eating and Weight Disorders, 24*(5), 799–814. https://doi.org/10.1007/s40519-019-00688-7.

Melbye, S., Kessing, L. V., Bardram, J. E., & Faurholt-Jepsen, M. (2020). Smartphone-based self-monitoring, treatment, and automatically generated data in children, adolescents, and young adults with psychiatric disorders: Systematic review. *JMIR Mental Health, 7*(10), e17453. https://doi.org/10.2196/17453.

Micali, N., Martini, M. G., Thomas, J. J., Eddy, K. T., Kothari, R., Russell, E., … Treasure, J. (2017). Lifetime and 12-month prevalence of eating disorders amongst women in mid-life: A population-based study of diagnoses and risk factors. *BMC Medicine, 15*(1), 12. https://doi.org/10.1186/s12916-016-0766-4.

Mitchell, J. E., & Peterson, C. B. (2020). Anorexia nervosa. *New England Journal of Medicine, 382*(14), 1343–1351. https://doi.org/10.1056/NEJMcp1803175.

Mitrofan, O., Petkova, H., Janssens, A., Kelly, J., Edwards, E., Nicholls, D., … Byford, S. (2019). Care experiences of young people with eating disorders and their parents: Qualitative study. *British Journal of Psychiatry Open, 5*(e6), 1–8. https://doi.org/10.1192/bjo.2018.78.

Molina-Ruiz, R., Garcia-Saiz, T., Looi, J. C. L., Virgili, E. V., Zamorano, M. R., de Anita Tejado, L., … Diaz-Marsá, M. (2020). Neural mechanisms in eating behaviors: A pilot fMRI study of emotional processing. *Psychiatry Investigation, 17*(3), 225–236. https://doi.org/10.30773/pi.2019.0038.

Monteleone, A. M., Ruzzi, V., Patriciello, G., Pellegrino, F., Cascino, G., Castellini, G., … Maj, M. (2020). Parental bonding, childhood maltreatment and eating disorder psychopathology: An investigation of their interactions. *Eating and Weight Disorders, 25*(3), 577–589. https://doi.org/10.1007/s40519-019-00649-0.

Murray, S. B., Quintana, D. S., Loeb, K. L., Griffiths, S., & Le Grange, D. (2019). Treatment outcomes for anorexia nervosa: A systematic review and meta-analysis of randomized controlled trials. *Psychological Medicine, 49*(4), 535–544. https://doi.org/10.1017/S0033291718002088.

National Eating Disorders Association (2018). What are eating disorders? Health consequences. https://www.nationaleatingdisorders.org/health-consequences-eating-disorders.

Nyman-Carlsson, E., Norring, C., Engström, I., Gustafsson, S. A., Lindberg, K., Paulson-Karlsson, G., & Nevonen, L. (2020). Individual cognitive behavioral therapy and combined family/individual therapy for young adults with anorexia nervosa: A randomized controlled trial. *Psychotherapy Research, 30*(8), 1011–1025. https://doi.org/10.1080/10503307.2019.1686190.

Oldershaw, A., Startup, H., & Lavender, T. (2019). Anorexia nervosa and a lost emotional self: A psychological formulation of the development, maintenance, and treatment of anorexia nervosa. *Frontiers in Psychology, 10*, 219. https://doi.org/10.3389/fpsyg.2019.00219.

Raevuori, A., Keski-Rahkonen, A., & Hoek, H. (2014). A review of eating disorders in males. *Current Opinion in Psychiatry, 27*(6), 426–430. https://doi.org/10.1097/YCO.0000000000000113.

Reber, E., Friedli, N., Vasiloglou, M. F., Schuetz, P., & Stanga, Z. J. (2019). Management of refeeding syndrome in medical inpatients. *Journal of Clinical Medicine, 8*(12), 2202. https://doi.org/10.3390/jcm8122202.

Riedlinger, C., Schmidt, G., Weiland, A., Stengel, A., Giel, K. E., Zipfel, S., … Mack, I. (2020). Which symptoms, complaints and complications of the gastrointestinal tract occur in patients with eating disorders? A systematic review and quantitative analysis. *Frontiers in Psychiatry, 11*, 195. https://doi.org/10.3389/fpsyt.2020.00195.

Rothenberg, A. (2018). October 10. Anorexia nervosa is a modern obsessive-compulsive disorder. *Psychology Today.* https://www.psychologytoday.com/us/blog/creative-explorations/201810/anorexia-nervosa-is-modern-obsessive-compulsive-disorder.

Sansfacon, J., Booij, L., Gauvin, L., Fletcher, E., Islam, F., Israel, M., & Steiger, H. (2020). Pretreatment motivation and therapy outcomes in eating disorders: A systematic review and meta-analysis. *International Journal of Eating Disorders, 53*(12), 1879–1900. https://doi.org/10.1002/eat.23376.

Scheffers, M., van Busschbachab, J. T., Bosschera, R. J., Aertsb, L. C., Wiersmab, D., & Schoeversc, R. A. (2017). Body image in patients with mental disorders: Characteristics, associations with diagnosis and treatment outcome. *Comprehensive Psychiatry, 74*, 53–60. https://doi.org/10.1016/j.comppsych.2017.01.004.

Silén, Y., Sipilä, P. N., Raevuori, A., Mustelin, L., Marttunen, M., Kaprio, J., & Keski-Rahkonen, A. (2020). DSM-5 eating disorders among adolescents and young adults in Finland: A public health concern. *International Journal of Eating Disorders, 53*(5), 520–531. https://doi.org/10.1002/eat.23236.

Skowron, K., Kurnik-Łucka, M., Dadański, E., Bętkowska-Korpała, B., & Gil, K. (2020). Backstage of eating disorder—about the biological mechanisms behind the symptoms of anorexia nervosa. *Nutrients, 12*(9), 2604. https://doi.org/10.3390/nu12092604.

Stein, D., Keller, S., Ifergan, I. S., Shilton, T., Toledano, A., Pelleg, M. T., & Witztum, E. (2020). Extreme risk-taking behaviors in patients with eating disorders. *Front Psychiatry, 11*, 89. https://doi.org/10.3389/fpsyt.2020.00089.

Thompson-Brenner. H., et al. (2016). Focused vs. broad enhanced cognitive behavioral therapy for bulimia nervosa with comorbid borderline personality: A randomized controlled trial. *International Journal of Eating Disorders, 49*(1), 36–49. https://doi.org/10.1002/eat.22468.

Tønning, M. L., Kessing, L. V., Bardram, J. E., & Faurholt-Jepsen, M. (2019). Methodological challenges in randomized controlled trials on smartphone-based treatment in psychiatry: Systematic review. *Journal of Medical Internet Research, 21*(10), e15362. https://doi.org/10.2196/15362.

Traviss-Turner, G. D., West, R. M., & Hill, A. J. (2017). Guided self-help for eating disorders: A systematic review and metaregression. *European Eating Disorders Review, 25*(3), 148–164. https://doi.org/10.1002/erv.2507.

Trace, S., Baker, J., Penas-Lledo, E., & Bulik, C. (2013). The genetics of eating disorders. *Annual Review of Clinical Psychology, 9*, 589. https://doi.org/10.1146/annurev-clinpsy-050212-185546.

Treasure, J, Duarte, D, & Schmidt, U (2020). Eating disorders. *Lancet, 395*(10227), 899–911. https://doi.org/10.1016/S0140-6736(20)30059-3.

Ulfvebrand, S., Birgegård, A., Norring, C., Hogdahl, L., & von Hausswolff-Juhlin, Y. (2015). Psychiatric comorbidity in women and men with eating disorders: Results from a large clinical database. *Psychiatry Research, 230*(2), 294–299. https://doi.org/10.1016/j.psychres.2015.09.008.

Udo, T., & Grilo, C. M. (2018). Prevalence and correlates of DSM-5 eating disorders in nationally representative sample of United States adults. *Biological Psychiary, 84*(5), 345–354. https://doi.org/10.1016/j.biopsych.2018.03.014.

van den Berg, E., Houtzager, L., de Vos, J., Daemen, I., Katsaragaki, G., Karyotaki, E., … Dekker, J. (2019). Meta-analysis on the efficacy of psychological treatments for anorexia nervosa. *European Eating Disorders Review, 27*(4), 331–351. https://doi.org/10.1002/erv.2683.

van Hoeken, D., & Hoek, H. W. (2020). Review of the burden of eating disorders: Mortality, disability, costs, quality of life, and family burden. *Current Opinion in Psychiatry, 33*(6), 521–527. https://doi.org/10.1097/YCO.0000000000000641.

Volpe, U., Tortorella, A., Manchia, M., Monteleoneae, A. M., Umberto, A., & Monteleoneae, P. (2016). Eating disorders: What age at onset? *Psychiatry Research, 238*, 225–227. https://doi.org/10.1016/j.psychres.2016.02.048.

Wade, T. D. (2019). Recent research on bulimia nervosa. *Psychiatric Clinics of North America, 42*(1), 21–32. https://doi.org/10.1016/j.psc.2018.10.002.

Ward, Z. J., Rodriguez, P., Wright, D. R., Austin, S. B., & Long, M. W. (2019). Estimation of eating disorders prevalence by age and associations with mortality in a simulated nationally representative US Cohort. *JAMA Network Open, 2*(10). https://doi.org/10.1001/jamanetworkopen.2019.12925. e1912925-e1912925.

Zeeck, A., Herpertz-Dahlmann, B., Friederich, H. C., Brockmeyer, T., Resmark, G., Hagenah, U., … Hartmann, A. (2018). Psychotherapeutic treatment for anorexia nervosa: A systematic review and network meta-analysis. *Frontiers in Psychiatry, 9*, 158. https://doi.org/10.3389/fpsyt.2018.00158.

Zhao, Y., & Encinosa, W. (2011). *Update on hospitalizations for eating disorders, 1999 to 2009. HCUP statistical brief #120.* Rockville, MD: Agency for Healthcare Research and Quality. http://www.hcup-us.ahrq.gov/reports/statbriefs/sb120.pdf.

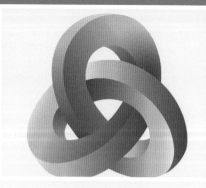

33

Survivors of Violence and Trauma

Debbie Steele

http://evolve.elsevier.com/Keltner

LEARNING OBJECTIVES

- Recognize the seriousness of violence and trauma in the United States.
- Describe the emotional reactions of terrorism, torture, ritual abuse, mind control, human trafficking, rape and sexual assault, childhood sexual abuse, and partner abuse.
- Recognize the dynamics involved in interpersonal violence crimes.

- Analyze the way in which the cycle of violence inhibits individuals from leaving abusive relationships.
- Identify the needs of victims of violence and trauma.
- Describe strategies for facilitating the transition from victim to survivor of violence or trauma.
- Develop a nursing care plan for survivors of violence and trauma.

The victimization of any individual by another creates serious mental health, social, community, and legal problems. Violence in all forms is prevalent in all societies. Nurses, regardless of their areas of practice, will come into contact with the victims—as inpatients, outpatients, home care patients, emergency care patients, parents of patients, friends, and relatives. Although victims are typically seen initially for physical injuries, their psychological and emotional needs require attention both short-term and long-term.

Forensic nursing (including sexual assault nurse examiners [SANEs]) is a vital aspect of the holistic care of victims and perpetrators of violent crimes and their families. This care includes obtaining clinical histories, documenting evidence including photographs of injuries, and carrying out quality nursing interventions in a holistic care framework, which includes consideration of all the medicolegal aspects of the patient's problems (Meunier-Sham, Cross, & Zuniga, 2013). The rights of the alleged perpetrators of crime, suspects, and victims must be protected so that the legal cases are not jeopardized.

This chapter focuses on victims of violence, beginning with an overview of trauma, followed by an in-depth look at terrorism, torture, ritual abuse, human trafficking (HT), rape survivors, adult survivors of childhood sexual abuse (CSA), and individuals abused by their partners. The short-term and long-term reactions of victims described in this

chapter are generally true for both male and female victims; however, men sometimes have a more difficult time admitting to and dealing with their emotional victimization than do women.

> **NORM'S NOTES** If ever there was a timely topic, this is it. I read notes weekly, and a high number of adult patients were abused as children—sexually or physically or both. Sometimes the behavior of some child pornographers is so barbaric that newscasters refuse to describe them on the air. The victims, when they survive such abuse, are potentially scarred for life. How in the world do they ever learn to trust again? Whatever your views on capital punishment, I have no mercy in my heart for these people (mostly men). The Bible says, "But whoso shall offend one of these little ones…, it were better for him that a millstone were hanged about his neck, and that he were drowned in the depth of the sea." AMEN!

TRAUMA

Trauma can be defined as the perception of imminent threat to one's person or livelihood that results in the subjective experience of feeling "afraid and alone" (Helsel, 2015).

Bessell van der Kolk (2015), a prominent trauma researcher, describes trauma as being more than an event that took place sometime in the past; it is also the imprint left by that experience in one's mind, brain, and body. Van der Kolk reports that more than half the people who seek psychiatric care have been assaulted, abandoned, neglected, raped, or witnessed violence. Trauma usually has an interpersonal aspect; most people are traumatized in the context of close relationships. Child abuse and family violence are traumatic events that frequently occur at the hands of people who are supposed to provide love and security.

The Centers for Disease Control and Prevention (CDC) and Kaiser Permanente conducted a large-scale research study known as the Adverse Childhood Experiences (ACE) Study. The researchers reported that traumatic life experiences during childhood and adolescents are common occurrences, more common than expected. ACE were defined as childhood exposure to the following: (1) emotional abuse, (2) physical abuse, (3) sexual abuse, (4) violent treatment of mother/stepmother, (5) mental illness in the family, (6) criminal behavior in the household, and (7) substance abuse in the family. Exposure to these adverse childhood events was found to produce chronic anxiety, anger, and depression in children (Felitti et al., 1998).

Development trauma disorder is a proposed *Diagnostic and Statistical Manual of Mental Disorders (DSM)-5* category that describes the outcome of complex childhood trauma associated with the previously mentioned adverse events but adds the following: parental divorce and/or incarceration, dating violence, gang-related violence, school shootings, bullying, war-related crimes, and drug-related crimes. Intentional acts by others that threaten the life or bodily integrity of children or their primary caregivers in the form of complex trauma have severe adverse effects on the children's neurologic and relational development. Children and adolescents can potentially fit the criteria of poly-victimization: those who endure disruption in their primary caregiving relationships while also experiencing chronic familial and community violence. All too often, love is in short supply, danger abounds, and attempts to survive take the form of pervasive emotional dysregulation associated with mental disorders such as depression, anxiety, and posttraumatic stress disorder (PTSD) (Spinazzola et al., 2018).

The incidence of trauma prior to and during emerging adulthood (ages 18 to 25 years) is 74% (Sharp et al., 2017). The following traumatic events are particularly prevalent among emerging adults: dating violence, sexual assault, homicide, robbery, physical assault, motor vehicle accidents, and suicide attempts. Because 50% of adolescents report exposure to adverse childhood events, almost half of emerging adults will experience poly-victimization (Woo & Brown, 2013). Exposure to multiple traumatic events exerts a greater negative impact on the severity of posttraumatic outcomes compared with a single trauma occurrence (Ogle, Rubin, & Siegler, 2014). This population has unique support systems that are not available to children, namely, increased autonomy from family members and stronger connections in social and romantic relationships (Sharp et al., 2017).

Adults who have been exposed to trauma have reported marked disparities in functioning, including strained family relationships, unemployment, and vulnerability to co-occurring mental health disorders (Lenz & Lancaster, 2017). Exposure to trauma of greater severity, as measured by proximity, duration, or frequency, is associated with greater impairments. The more severe traumas of adulthood include physical assaults, warzone exposure, sexual assaults, death, and illness (Ogle et al., 2014).

The effects of trauma on the elderly are difficult to distinguish for a number of reasons. The normal aspects of aging such as sleep disturbances, social isolation, and withdrawal may actually be cumulative symptoms of trauma. In addition, alcohol misuse may be misinterpreted as a normal part of aging. Common traumatic events that occur in later life include death of a spouse or close other, retirement, chronic pain, cognitive impairment, and other experiences associated with aging. Hiskey and McPherson (2013) reported that many elderly patients uphold the motto of "that's just life," which reduces help-seeking such that the effects of trauma remain undisclosed, undiagnosed, and untreated. In addition, mental health services may be seen as stigmatizing and foreign to their self-concept of aging, leaving them to suffer in silence.

VIOLENCE

Violence causes more than 1.6 million deaths every year worldwide. However, most individuals survive violence, left with permanent physical and emotional scars. From infants to the elderly, violence affects people of all ages (CDC, n.d.).

Not all violence involves physical injury and threat to life, yet all crimes involve emotional despair and trauma. Violence undermines foundations formed in the early stages of human development, regardless of the victim's age when the trauma occurred (see Chapter 7). Most importantly, there is a loss of *trust*, not only in the perpetrator but also to some degree in all other individuals. The inability to trust others leads to a sense of vulnerability and lack of safety in one's life, relationships, and environment. As a result, victims will develop anxiety and fear in certain areas of their lives that resemble the trauma that they experienced in vivo. Subsequently, they will be easily triggered by similar events and appear to others as overreactors. However, their hyperarousal is considered normal based on the trauma that they endured.

Emotional reactions to violence and trauma vary greatly according to the individual, his or her resources, past history, the situation, and the meaning of the event to that person. Common emotional reactions include denial, fear, anxiety, anger, powerlessness, and depression. A sense of failure and guilt frequently occurs; victims wonder what they did to cause the violence and how they might have prevented or stopped it. Victims usually feel ashamed and unworthy as well as contaminated or dirty, whether or not they were physically touched by the perpetrator. Fantasies of revenge or a wish for legal retribution are typical. The relationships of victims to family and friends can be disturbed in part because of the loss of trust but also because of the response of others. Caring individuals often imply that the victim was responsible for the violence with questions such as the following: "Why were you there alone at night?" "Why were you carrying so much cash?" "Why didn't you install that burglar alarm?" The victim might feel alienated and isolated. Hospital personnel, the police, and the legal system might also unwittingly convey what could be called a "blame the victim" attitude in their manner of questioning and in focusing only on the facts, without any emotional support or empathy. Long-term effects of violence may result in prolonged stress, PTSD, depression, anxiety, substance abuse, and suicidality.

Recovery From Violence and Trauma

Many models have been formulated about the process of recovery from traumas such as crimes and disasters. Most researchers agree that the duration and severity of the trauma, the victim's resources, and the nature of help available during and immediately after the crime or trauma influence recovery. Typically, three stages of recovery are defined: (1) initial disorganization (impact), (2) a struggle to adapt (recoil), and (3) reconstruction (reorganization). The brief summary here is derived from the views of Foa (2005), Lacy and Benedek (2003), and Tynhurst (1951). The stages are not clearly separated, and the readjustment process is not smooth. Vacillation among the stages might occur, and recovery might take months or years, especially if revictimization or secondary victimization (from involvement with the criminal justice system) continues after the crime.

Impact

The initial reaction to a single-event trauma usually lasts a few minutes to a few days. Common responses are shock, denial, disbelief, and confusion. There might be paralyzing fear, hysteria, horror, anger, rage, shame, guilt, a sense of helplessness and vulnerability, physiologic responses, and disturbed sleeping and eating. These reactions might occur for a longer time when the trauma is ongoing, such as harassment or stalking. Some victims react less visibly or in a delayed manner; they look calm, organized, and rational, and they take all the necessary actions initially needed. Later, the other reactions might occur. Occasionally the victim's reaction might include dissociative symptoms (amnesia, depersonalization, numbing, detachment), intrusive memories (nightmares, flashbacks), and severe anxiety. These symptoms might indicate that the victim is experiencing acute stress disorder (see Chapter 27).

Recoil

In the recoil stage, victims begin the struggle to adapt. The immediate danger might be over, but a great deal of emotional distress remains. In the beginning of this phase, there are periods in which victims look and act normal and are able to carry out daily routines at home and at work. Activity helps to suppress fears, anger, and sadness. Later in this phase, there may or may not be a desire to talk about all the details of and

feelings about the trauma ("What happened?"). Victims often need support, and some may become temporarily dependent. Fantasies of revenge for the crime are natural during this stage. In the weeks and months after the trauma, victims gradually become aware of the impact that the event has had on their lives.

Reorganization

Reorganization might take months or years to accomplish. Although the trauma is not forgotten, the anxiety, fear, and anger diminish, and victims reconstruct their lives. The beginning of this phase includes making sense of what happened and why ("Why me?"); attributing blame to self, others, or both; justifying one's own actions at the time and later ("Why did I act the way I did then and since then?"); and regaining a sense of control and self-protection. Grief over losses resolves slowly. Lingering nightmares, frustrations, and disillusionment might occur; however, these subside as survivors become reengaged in life and activities.

Even with satisfactory recovery, survivors sense that they and their lives are, and always will be, different as a result of the crime ("What if it happens again?"). Moving to victor status is the goal for individuals experiencing trauma, which can be accomplished by integrating the memories of the trauma and moving on in life with restored functioning, a sense of safety and security, healthy relationships and self-image, and a sense of purpose in life.

PUTTING IT ALL TOGETHER

PSYCHOTHERAPEUTIC MANAGEMENT

Nurse-Patient Relationship

Although trust, empathy, emotional support, and a willingness to listen are important in all stages of recovery, specialized care is needed in each stage. During the *impact stage*, the focus is on the survivor's need for physical safety and emotional security. Reassurance, protection from further harm, and sometimes medical care are needed. Survivors might need clear, simple directions on what to do, where to go, and what to avoid. It is crucial that nurses avoid accusations (blaming), intimidation, unnecessary intrusions, and invasion of privacy. In most instances, crisis intervention occurs face-to-face at the scene of the trauma or in the emergency department. For survivors who are superficially calm and in control, the crisis intervention might be needed a few hours or days later, when the impact of the trauma reality hits. Phone numbers for crisis centers or walk-in services can be given to survivors before they leave the police interview at the scene or the emergency department.

During the *recoil stage*, survivors need validation of their self-worth and rights. Referrals can be made to a victim's assistance program and for legal, insurance, or financial assistance if needed. Family and friends are important sources of support during the episodes of emotional turmoil in the recoil phase; counseling might also be beneficial. During the struggle to adjust, support groups with other survivors can be useful. Whether the group is of short duration (6 to 8 weeks) or ongoing, and whether the group is professionally led or peer-led, there is value in receiving information, encouragement, and companionship from others "who have been there."

During the *reorganization stage*, most survivors are able to recover and grow with supportive assistance. Long-term counseling is sometimes needed to overcome anxiety, phobias, depression, suicidal ideation, or other posttraumatic symptoms. It is uncommon for survivors to need hospitalization beyond initial medical care. Exceptions are survivors who are unable to function or meet their basic needs and individuals who become suicidal.

Psychopharmacology

Survivors of violence and trauma may benefit from antianxiety agents (benzodiazepines), prescribed occasionally for short-term use to decrease anxiety, and trazodone (Desyrel) to facilitate sleep.

Milieu Management

Many communities have temporary or ongoing groups for survivors of divorce, death of a loved one, sudden infant death syndrome, rape, incest, and physical and emotional abuse, as well as for people affected by suicide or homicide, mass murders, torture, and abduction of children.

TERRORISM

Nature of the Problem

September 11, 2001, is the day that awakened the United States to the realities of terrorism and its unpredictability and devastation. Before this day, terrorism was a news story about terrible acts in foreign countries. Terrorism can be perpetrated under the justification of military, political, social, cultural, or religious reasons. Acts of terrorism can involve plane crashes, bombings, military warfare, biologic and chemical agents, trained or programmed assassins, and suicide/homicide bombers. Terrorism rarely affects only a single individual; victimization can involve thousands who have been injured or killed in a single event. The victims of terrorism include people who were injured or killed; police, fire, and rescue personnel; businesses and their employees; friends and families of all the victims; and potentially anyone who witnessed the tragedy vicariously (in-person or through the media).

Effects

Terrorism can have more devastating results than natural disasters or major accidents because terrorism is not only perpetrated by humans, but it is also not accidental. The purpose of terrorism is not fully understood but results in terror, death, and/or injury to targeted groups. The trauma of terrorism is more pervasive, long-lasting, and severe than other violent crimes. Survivors typically experience some degree of grief and mourning and acute or posttraumatic stress symptoms, which are expected reactions to a horrifying event

(Zawahir & Scudder, 2012). Box 33.1 lists typical reactions to terrorism. The event might also trigger memories of previous traumatic experiences.

Recovery

Most individuals recover with the support of loved ones, coworkers, and friends; memorial or religious services and community meetings; sleep, stress management techniques, relaxation techniques, and physical activities; and a return to normal activities.

A major goal of recovery is to regain a sense of trust, safety, and security, while acknowledging that future terrorist attacks are possible. Depending on the severity and duration of the trauma experienced, recovery may be lengthier and more complicated. On a larger scale, cities and hospitals continue to update their disaster plans in preparation of terrorist attacks, biologic and chemical warfare, large-scale bombings, and other disasters. For most cities, efforts have been made to improve citywide, coordinated plans among police, fire, and rescue agencies; hospitals and mental health facilities; and local, state, and federal emergency management

---

BOX 33.1 Specific Responses Resulting From Terrorism, Serial Ritual Abuse, and Human Trafficking

Shock, disbelief, fear, anxiety, powerlessness
Insecurity, guilt, shame, spiritual distress
Unresponsiveness, dissociation, numbness
Decreased concentration, confusion
Panic, terror, sense of violation, anger, rage
Aggression, fantasies of revenge, impulsiveness
Helplessness, hopelessness, despair
Suicidal or homicidal ideation, self-mutilation
Mistrust, suspiciousness, paranoia, alienation
Estrangement, withdrawal, isolation
Fatigue, insomnia, nightmares, flashbacks
Memory disturbances, amnesia
Hyperarousal, stress sensitivity, startle response
Denial, repression, suppression, intellectualization
Body kinesthetic memories, psychosomatic symptoms
Extreme passivity, loss of self-esteem
Depression, prolonged grieving, substance abuse, posttraumatic stress disorder (PTSD)
Sexual dysfunction, eating disorders, anxiety disorders
Labile emotions, personality changes

Modified from Anorexia Nervosa and Associated Disorders. (2002). *Anorexia nervosa and associated disorders (Indianapolis Chapter of ANAD): Personal interviews.* ANAD; Cole, H. (2009). Human trafficking: Implications for the role of the advanced practice forensic nurse. *Journal of the American Psychiatric Nurses Association, 14,* 6; Lacy, T. J., & Benedek, D. M. (2003). Terrorism and weapons of mass destruction: Managing the behavioral reaction in primary care. *Southern Medical Journal, 96,* 394; Sarson, J., & MacDonald, L. (2009). *Behavioural harms: Enforced and survival tactics in ritual abuse-torture.* Presented at the Thirty-first SALIS Conference; van der Kolk, B. (2015). *The body keeps the score: Brain, mind & body in the healing of trauma.* Penguin Books.

administrations. Psychiatric nurses and mental health personnel are included in the planning.

RITUAL ABUSE AND HUMAN TRAFFICKING

Nature of the Problem

Ritual abuse and HT are crimes that are committed underground; they occur in the shadows of society and are difficult to detect (Rajaram & Tidbell, 2018). Knowledge about the prevalence, psychological effects, and treatment of ritual abuse and HT has grown exponentially within the past 25 years. Ritual abuse can be defined as organized sexual, physical, and psychological abuse that is systemic and may be sustained over a long period. It involves the use of rituals with multiple abusers. Ritual abuse involves the use of programming that induces extreme physical, emotional, and/or psychological pain. These malevolent acts are perpetrated by a trusted family member, gangs, cults (satanic or nonsatanic), hate groups, organized crime, work/sex trade traffickers, or military-political organizations (Matthew & Barron, 2015). Abusers rely on coercion, lies, and tricks to control their victims' thinking and behavior. Victims are subjected to a pattern of submission that includes tactics to frighten, humiliate, isolate, degrade, exploit, and control them (Stark, 2012). Repeated victimization as a result of ritual abuse and HT results in long-term traumatic effects including PTSD, substance use, developmental delays, health, and hygiene challenges; they also are known to negatively affect interpersonal skills (Hardy et al., 2020; Stark, 2019).

HT is defined as control over another person for the purposes of exploitation, including sexual exploitation, forced labor, slavery, servitude, and the removal of organs (Campana & Varese, 2016). It involves the transportation and harboring of individuals for profit, estimated to be no less than $32 billion a year (de Chesnay, 2013; Newby & McGuinness, 2012). Risk factors associated with HT include poverty, young age, limited education, homelessness, lack of family support, history of physical, emotional, and sexual abuse, living in high-crime areas, and experiencing family violence (Schwarz et al., 2016). Women and children, especially those who have experienced multiple adverse events, are particularly vulnerable (Reid et al., 2017).

HT is a global human rights concern impacting unknown numbers of victims worldwide. The causes of HT and child sexual exploitation are complex and include discrimination, inequality, poverty, inefficient legal systems, and sexual entitlement among perpetrators (Tsai, Lim, & Nhanh, 2020). The Victims of Trafficking and Violence Protection Act of 2000 is the cornerstone of anti-HT legislation in the United States; it is now known as the Trafficking Victims Protection Act (Schwarz, 2019). The Super Bowl event has been described as "the single largest HT incident in the U.S."

Tactics

Recruitment into HT may begin as offers of money (to the victims or their families who sell the individual), a promise of a "better life," deceptions, threats, coercion, force, or kidnapping. Ongoing coercive tactics can include torture such as using hot irons, electric shock, submersion, suffocation, large doses of drugs/alcohol, beatings, physical restraint, confinement in cramped or buried containers, watching or forced participation in others' torture/killings, gang rape, sexual and physical mutilation, being tied or hung in the air, being photographed during the abuse, starvation, and sensory and sleep deprivation (Crane, 2013; Schwartz, 2011).

Effects

Common physical outcomes of ritual abuse and HT are injuries to the head (including traumatic brain injury), teeth, and genitals; infections, sexually transmitted diseases, malnutrition, poor hygiene, reproductive problems, bone fractures/dislocations, scars, burns, pain, chronic headaches, and forced pregnancies/abortions (Campana & Varese, 2016; Hoerrner, 2013; Lapp & Overman, 2013; Newby & McGuinness, 2012). The emotional effects are longer lasting and include a sense of violation, dehumanization, humiliation, horror, shame and guilt, emotional dysregulation, and betrayal. Trauma-specific fears (e.g., small dark spaces or nudity); hypersexuality; and obsessions with rituals, magic, or devils are common. Victims might have been forced or programmed to commit crimes against others. They might talk about topics—such as the Greek alphabet, sex trade, "Dr. Black," "Dr. White," white slavery, witchcraft, drinking blood, satanic rituals and holidays, and the *Satanic Bible*—that do not make sense to professionals (Shurter, 2012). Other specific responses resulting from ritual abuse and HT are listed in Box 33.1.

There is much controversy about assigning psychiatric diagnoses (e.g., PTSD, adjustment disorder, major depression, anxiety disorders, dissociative identity disorder, or other dissociative disorders) to victims who are having *typical* reactions to *horrific* crimes (de Chesnay, 2013; Lapp & Overman, 2013). Labeling a person who has experienced complex trauma with a mental illness diagnosis may be construed as another form of victimization, stigmatization, and discounting of the validity of reports of these crimes. Some professionals even view PTSD as insufficient for acknowledging the catastrophic effects experienced by victims and their families. The Salvation Army and the U.S. Department of Health and Human Services have developed guides for identifying and assessing victims of HT. Another resource is *The Crime of Human Trafficking* (Anonymous n.d.).

Recovery

Because ritual abuse and HT tend to be ongoing, the *impact* stage of recovery persists but might wax and wane over the years. In the *recoil* stage, adaptation is difficult because of the severity of the emotional distress that remains after these crimes end. Trauma-informed care needs to be integrated from the first interaction with providers and for the duration of all therapeutic relationships (McGuire, 2019). Although evidence-based treatment such as trauma-focused cognitive behavioral therapy, dialectical behavior therapy, eye movement desensitization and reprocessing (EMDR), and multisystemic therapy (Görg et al., 2019) are useful in helping these survivors *reorganize* their lives, this stage is likely to be prolonged, with more relapses during other life crises. In particular, individuals may experience dissociation, which is characterized as an individual's compartmentalizing of a fearful experience, as a life-long defense mechanism (McGuire, 2019).

Aftercare services are needed for those exiting a life of victimization. "After" they have been rescued, the victims need trauma-responsive care. They need highly individualized care that emphasizes safety, security, and compassion. The focus is on providing practical help, as well as hope and healing to those devastated by complex trauma. A shelter or recovery program is needed to ensure basic necessities, emotional support, and critical legal services (criminal, civil, immigration, or other legal proceedings). Advocacy is needed to ensure access to services and to provide supportive counseling that emphasizes validation, normalization, and sensitivity. Major goals for recovery include the following:

1. Understanding self-destructive behaviors (self-mutilation, suicide attempts, substance abuse, and manipulation)
2. Acknowledging one's thoughts, feelings, and behaviors as "normal reactions to abnormal situations"
3. Understanding one's intense emotions, especially anxiety, guilt, anger, rage, and desire for revenge
4. Becoming aware of suppressed or repressed thoughts and feelings, positive emotions, and body memories and reactions
5. Allowing oneself to grieve for the tremendous losses experienced
6. Processing and integrating the memories of the experiences, often from the least to the most bizarre experiences (as in the recovery from PTSD and the integration of multiple personalities)
7. Developing healthy relationships with family, friends, and the community
8. Developing boundaries, a sense of privacy, self-awareness, and empathy
9. Using complementary or alternative medicine and spiritual practices that are helpful
10. Developing occupational and community living skills that lead to economic and social interdependence
11. Becoming aware of new perspectives in life and a desire to live in light of the past
12. Gaining a sense of hope, personal power, and control over oneself and one's life

PUTTING IT ALL TOGETHER
PSYCHOTHERAPEUTIC MANAGEMENT

Nurse-Patient Relationship

Nurses working with individuals who have experienced ritual abuse and HT should provide a person-centered approach that is strengths-based and collaborative. Conveying acceptance, care, and support; ensuring confidentiality; and believing what is being described are crucial if survivors are going to trust the nurse enough to discuss their experiences. Survivors must have time and space to process the issues at their own pace and within their own cultural framework.

Initial care typically involves meeting practical needs such as food, clothing, medical and dental care, transportation, physical safety, reunification, and protection. Treatment of physical injuries may be needed by dentists, plastic surgeons, gynecologists, neurologists, endocrinologists, or gastroenterologists. Survivors may also require support and protection while they are involved with the criminal justice system when their perpetrators are being investigated and prosecuted. Foreign-born survivors may require the use of translators and may face immigration charges and deportation.

A priority of care involves the meeting of the survivors' emotional needs. Individual counseling, group therapy, psychoeducation, and safety planning are all essential elements targeting feelings of betrayal, abuse, terror, powerlessness, hopelessness, and deprivation (Johnson, 2012). Survivors of sexual abuse are often afraid of disclosing their experiences because they fear the reactions of others. Given time to establish trust, survivors are presented the opportunity to confide in someone, to put words to their experiences, and to share what is difficult to talk about with a caring other. If disclosures are met with belief, validation, lack of blame, and an accepting attitude, survivors can effectively put their hurt into words, enhancing psychological healing over time (Rudolfsson & Tidefors, 2015).

Psychopharmacology

Using medication for treating survivors is highly controversial, especially because drugs were often a part of the abuse as it occurred. Sometimes medications used in treating PTSD are helpful, especially selective serotonin reuptake inhibitors.

Milieu Management

Safe houses are needed for survivors once they move beyond the initial crisis situation. They need to be involved in a transitional recovery program that provides them with skills to reenter and function in normal life. These programs need to include intensive psychotherapy and job and life skills. Psychological support also needs to be provided to the survivors' friends and family members to educate them about the survivors' trauma and to provide them with the tools to deal with the ups and downs bound to happen down the road (Rajaram et al., 2018). Peer-led support groups can be useful for survivors with similar experiences and needs. Nurses and survivors of HT can access information and resources from the national hotline (888-373-7888) of the U.S. Department of Health and Human Services or The Trafficking in Persons and Worker Exploitation Task Force (888-428-7581).

Individuals who are survivors of ritual abuse and HT are resilient and persevering. The following autobiographers have written their own personal stories:
Family torture: David Pelzer, Richard Pelzer, deJoly LaBrier
Fundamentalist/religious/polygamous cults: Jenna Hill, Brent Jeffs, Carolyn Jessop, Flora Jessop, Elissa Wall
Military-political/satanic RA and MC: Carol Rutz, David Shurter, Kathleen Sullivan

RAPE AND SEXUAL ASSAULT

Nature of the Problem

Sexual assault or rape occurs when the sexual act is both unwanted and coerced, meaning that victims perceive they could not have stopped it (Ford, 2018). Rape and sexual assault remain major crimes committed throughout the world. Valid statistics are unavailable for sexual assault and rape because of a lack of reporting. Many victims of rape are concerned that they will not be believed or may face blame or retaliation or that the justice system will not be able to prosecute (Lankford, 2016). This is especially true for male victims of sexual assault (Hawkins et al., 2019).

It is estimated that rape among women is between 14% and 16% (Wilson & Scarpa, 2015). In the U.S. military, 1% of active-duty men and nearly 5% of active-duty women are victims of sexual assault each year (Rosellini et al., 2017). College students are at increased risk of rape; Muehlenhard and associates (2017) found that one in five women on college campuses has been sexually assaulted. Women who are violated within the context of intimate partner rape are at increased risk when they are trying to leave their partner to seek safety (Weldon, 2016). Older adults are vulnerable at home and in extended care facilities, especially if they have medical conditions, a physical or mental disability, or dementia (any of which might result in their reports being discounted by caregivers, family, and officials). Sexual violence is also used as a weapon of war, experienced as rape, gang rapes, sexual slavery, forced marriage, and forced impregnation (Bamidele, 2017). Based on this information, it becomes apparent that the majority of sexual assaults are committed by a nonstranger, perpetrated by a family member, friend, neighbor, or acquaintance. Unfortunately, some police and prosecutors view stranger rape as more "winnable" over against acquaintance or date rape. Date or acquaintance rape might be complicated by the use of amnesiacs (date rape drugs), other drugs, and alcohol, which interfere with remembering the rape.

In general, rape is defined as unwanted, nonconsensual, or forced vaginal, oral, or anal intercourse (Wilson & Scarpa, 2015). Any other form of forced sexual contact (from touch to mutilation) is considered sexual assault. Despite sexual contact, it is generally acknowledged that sexual violence is not sexually motivated but involves a fear tactic to prevent rejection (Weldon, 2016), or a need to immobilize, dominate, and humiliate the victim (Bamidele, 2017).

Effects

Similar to other crime victims, the rape victim experiences extreme fear and despair, as well as severe violation. There may be internal and external bodily injuries, along with the fear that the perpetrator will return to rape again. Some victims may experience episodes of wishing they had died. The traumatic memories of the rape usually include specific tastes, smells, sounds, and sights associated with the assault. These memories and the powerlessness, loss of control, fear, shame, guilt, humiliation, rage, and feelings of being contaminated or dirty might be overwhelming. A typical reaction of the victim is the wish to regain a sense of control and retreat to a safe place, take a thorough shower, and destroy any damaged belongings. However, these actions would destroy most of the evidence that is required if the victim decides to report the rape and prosecute. Avoiding medical attention also places victims at risk for acquired immunodeficiency syndrome (AIDS), hepatitis B infection, sexually transmitted diseases, pregnancy, and improper healing of any physical injuries (Marchetti, 2012). Beyond the injuries, there are long-term physical and mental health complications, including sexual dysfunction, human papillomavirus infections, depression, anxiety, substance abuse, dissociative disorders, eating disorders, suicidality, and PTSD (Munro-Kramer et al., 2017).

Recovery

Despite an outward appearance of calm composure and a denial at times of the need for help (as in silent or delayed reactions), the rape survivor needs assistance, information, and support. It might not be until the survivor begins the up-and-down struggle of the *recoil* stage that the losses, anger, and needs are recognized. In an emergency department, collecting evidence, taking away clothes, and other procedures might be a priority for staff, but for the survivor it may be experienced as further intrusion and violation. To staff, survivors might seem resistant and uncooperative as they struggle to protect themselves and regain a sense of control. Box 33.2 lists some of the needs and rights of rape survivors.

Many communities have developed specialized services for rape survivors within clinics or emergency departments. SANEs have skills in collecting forensic evidence while

---

BOX 33.2 Needs and Rights of Rape Survivors

1. Crisis intervention—information, counseling, and referrals
2. Help with basic needs—housing, transportation, child care, safety
3. Medical information and care—information about pregnancy prevention, testing for sexually transmitted diseases, follow-up care, and counseling
4. Advocacy for whatever choices are made about reporting or prosecuting
5. Protection of rights—to privacy, confidentiality, gentleness, sensitivity, and explanations of procedures and tests (trauma-informed care)
6. Protection of rights—to refuse collection of evidence, to determine who will and will not be present during examinations, to get copies of all medical and legal reports, and to apply for reimbursement through victim's compensation
7. Fairness, information, and protection of legal rights during investigations, hearings, and trial, including not being asked about prior sexual experiences with anyone other than the suspect or defendant
8. Reasonable protection against further harm—escorts to court, restraining order, additional patrols, relocation if necessary

providing empathy, support, and information (Jackson, 2011). Nurses also can encourage the beginning of the recovery process by challenging any rape myths stated by the survivor, such as, "I should have fought him off" or "I shouldn't have been drinking" (Annan, 2011).

Specialized rape services have information packets prepared for rape survivors and staff in hospitals, counseling centers, and other crisis areas. Survivors can be encouraged to keep the information sheets and phone numbers of resources for later use. A victim who appears temporarily composed and calm and denies the need for help should be especially encouraged to take materials home. A SANE might also call a sexual assault advocate, an advocate from a victim's assistance program, or a rape crisis counselor to initiate contact with the survivor (Jackson, 2011).

In the *recoil* stage, most survivors begin to react to the significant effect that rape has had on their lives. Fear and mistrust are major issues. Survivors might be afraid to leave the one place they designate as safe. They may experience difficulty with intimacy, especially within sexual relationships. If the rape occurred in their residence, survivors might move or at least make safety-related changes to prevent recurrence, or they might ask for someone to stay with them at night for a while. Being alone and unprotected is usually frightening, especially when nightmares and traumatic memories occur. Survivors need affirmation that they are worthwhile individuals, with dignity and rights. They need to know that their despair is natural, especially around the violation of person and privacy, the humiliation, and the sense of powerlessness. Survivors often question whether they might have fought harder during the attack. Survival is paramount; if the victim survived the rape, he or she did exactly what was necessary to stay alive. Progress in the reorganization stage is not linear but cyclical, especially as new situations trigger memories of the rape. Survivors might avoid situations where they could reexperience the trauma (Tambling, 2012) (e.g., gynecologic exams and intercourse). Revictimization is sure to occur during the victim's police and court experiences (Jordan, 2013). The goals of recovery from rape and sexual assault are the same as the goals for all survivors of crime. Rape survivors will need acceptance, time, and patience as they regain safety in sexual functioning and intimate relationships.

PUTTING IT ALL TOGETHER
PSYCHOTHERAPEUTIC MANAGEMENT
Nurse-Patient Relationship

The rape or sexual assault survivor needs continual empathy, support, and an opportunity to process the events and manage the intense feelings as well as to regain a sense of psychological and physical safety. Although it is time-intensive and energy-consuming, the best approach in collecting evidence and providing nursing care is to move slowly and supportively at the individual survivor's pace and to give rationales for and descriptions of procedures and referrals. Nurses can

be particularly helpful to rape survivors. Male and especially female survivors tend to feel safer with a woman and might refuse to talk to a man, especially alone. The presence of a SANE or sexual assault advocate during examinations and interrogations can be reassuring. Survivors might or might not choose to have a friend or family member stay with them for additional support or stay with them when they get home.

Crisis intervention is the most appropriate approach during the impact stage. Short-term counseling and a rape support group can be beneficial during the recoil stage. However, not all survivors will respond in the same way, needing the same interventions. Individualized care is recommended, paying careful attention to the woman's narrative (Jordan, 2013). Long-term counseling might be needed during the reorganization stage, especially if the survivor decides to prosecute the perpetrator. A lengthy legal process can be retraumatizing because of having to relive the events and emotions, and the survivor is treated as a criminal during cross-examinations in many trial situations. On the other hand, conviction and imprisonment of the perpetrator can help survivors feel vindicated, compensated, and safer in their environments.

If the symptoms of rape trauma do not gradually diminish and if reorganization of lifestyle does not seem to occur, the survivor needs to be assessed for and helped with any co-occurring disorders such as PTSD, anxiety, depression, and substance use.

Psychopharmacology

Although rarely prescribed to rape survivors, benzodiazepines to reduce anxiety and enhance sleep might be used on a temporary basis. Alternatively, an antidepressant taken at bedtime (especially trazodone) might be ordered if symptoms of depression exist with sleep disturbances.

Milieu Management

Referral can be made to a rape support group or center, which encourages the expression of anger, guilt, and shame, building confidence, trust, and a sense of safety. Support groups are sometimes available for relatives, especially partners or parents of the rape survivor to help them deal with the trauma. Also available are the Rape, Abuse and Incest National Network (RAINN); National Sexual Assault Hotline (800-656-HOPE); and the National Sexual Assault On-line Hotline (http://rainn.org).

Clinical Example

A case of rape: A 24-year-old woman called a rape crisis line complaining of anxiety at work, not sleeping, fear of being out at night, overwhelming anger, and feeling dirty and ashamed. For several weeks she thought that a coworker was watching her. Last Friday, as she was leaving work late, the coworker pushed her into her car and raped her. She did not report the rape and hid in her apartment all weekend. She forced herself to go to work on Monday. The man acted friendly toward her, as if nothing had happened.

ADULT SURVIVORS OF CHILDHOOD SEXUAL ABUSE

Nature of the Problem

When children are sexually victimized, they are profoundly affected in short-term and long-lasting ways. Recent research has consistently shown that females are more than twice as likely as males to experience childhood sexual abuse (CSA) (Kozak et al., 2018). It is likely that the Internet is compounding the problem. CSA experiences such as child pornography, CSA (by nonrelatives), and incest (by relatives) are destructive for two major reasons: (1) the crimes usually are not one-time occurrences, and (2) the perpetrators may be known and trusted. These crimes are common, but more are getting attention (e.g., victims of Jerry Sandusky at Penn State, Catholic priests, and child actors in California). The number of children who have been sexually abused and never reported it, even when they became adults, is unknown.

CSA involves voyeurism and exhibitionism, which can lead to intercourse and/or molestation and always involve a younger victim who is not capable of giving consent to the older, more powerful perpetrator. Male perpetrators are commonly fathers, uncles, stepfathers, older brothers, cousins, grandfathers, neighbors, scout leaders, camp counselors, coaches, and religious leaders. Less frequently, the perpetrators are women—mothers, older sisters, other relatives, daycare workers, teachers, coaches, neighbors, and babysitters. Perpetrators tend to choose either male or female victims, so there can be male-to-male, male-to-female, female-to-male, and female-to-female abuse. Perpetrators and victims are from every social, cultural, ethnic, and economic group.

Children can experience severe sexual abuse, including early age of onset, invasive sexual acts, and the use of perpetrator force. They also experience other forms of childhood maltreatment and adversity, including parental conflict, neglect, and physical and emotional abuse (Ressel et al., 2018). Although sexual abuse can be violent, it often is not. Coercion is possible because of the victim's dependent, trusting, or loving relationship with the perpetrator. The victim is urged to maintain the secret with various threats, such as the following: the victim will be taken away from the family; the perpetrator will be put in a mental hospital or jail; the parents will divorce; the other parent will get sick; there will be no abuse of siblings if the victim is compliant; love will be withdrawn; no one would believe the victim anyway; or there will be physical abuse if the victim does not comply. Even when no physical violence takes place, victims usually fear that it will occur if they resist the perpetrator. Factors such as family conflicts or disorganization, witnessing violence, parental loss, parental mental illness, economic instability, secrecy and communication difficulties, substance abuse, and other forms of abuse and neglect seem to correlate with sexual abuse.

Although disclosure enables these children to access support and protection, it may be difficult for them for a variety of reasons: (1) fear of what will happen to them and the perpetrator; (2) fear that they will not be believed; (3) age-related interpretations of the abuse such as shame and guilt; (4) lack of an opportunity to tell; (5) concern for safety of self and others based on threats by the perpetrator; and (6) conflicted feelings toward the perpetrator. These variables provide insight into the unique thought processes that children experience when considering disclosure. In fact, children typically consider in detail the ramifications of their disclosure prior to sharing their abuse experience (Morrison et al., 2018).

Even if the young victims want to disclose the abuse, it is difficult for them because they lack the words and concepts to describe the event. An emotional reaction of fear, pain, and confusion usually occurs but not a moral, ethical, or legal concept of right or wrong. Most victims who, as children, tried to tell a parent or other adult were met with disbelief, denial, or pressure to retract their accusations. It is difficult for a parent to believe that the partner whom they love or a respected member of the family or community is capable of sexually abusing a child. Some children are made to feel special by the perpetrator by the extra attention they receive. A sense of acceptance comes from pleasing the adult and receiving a degree of (distorted) affection. It should be noted that all children make bids for attention and affection. Even if they are cute, coy, or flirtatious, these bids should not be viewed as seductive. Perpetrations of sexual abuse misinterpret the child's behavior to meet their own needs and should always be held responsible for the crime.

Effects of Childhood Sexual Abuse
On the Child

Childhood maltreatment accounts for approximately 45% of the risk factors associated with the development of childhood-onset psychopathology. Children depend on caregivers to reach and maintain emotional homeostasis. When they are sexually violated by their caregivers, they may find themselves dysregulated and unable to trust and depend on others. Confused, these child victims act out in ways to cope with this innate sense of loss. In addition, these children are more likely to engage in violent and impulsive behavior in response to their shame, powerlessness, and blame. Both males and females have been found to cope with their trauma by acting out. However, male victims exhibit violent and delinquent behaviors more frequently than their female counterparts. Females are more likely to internalize feelings of shame and guilt related to sexual victimization. In addition, victims tend to be overly helpful, quickly taking care of others' needs to the exclusion of their own personal needs, an effect of emotional numbing and repression. These findings highlight how CSA victims attempt to cope with the emotional dysregulation that is a consequence of their trauma (Kozak et al., 2018). Other adverse effects are disturbed growth and development issues such as sleep and eating disturbances, enuresis, anxiety, depression, overactive fantasy life, masturbation, sexualized play, sexual aggression, poor impulse control, cruelty to animals, spiritual distress, somatization, alienation, fear, shame, self-blame, self-destructive behaviors, running away, and truancy.

Clinical Example

Trauma-informed caregivers can learn to support a child who is violent and acting out by seeking to understand and respond to the root causes of the behavior as overwhelming emotions that have been triggered. Rather than the child attempting to self-regulate, he or she can be provided with an opportunity to experience coregulation with a trusted other.

On the Adolescent

As adolescents, sexual abuse victims exhibit additional adverse effects such as impulsivity, abuse of others, cruelty to animals, self-destructive behaviors, self-mutilation, eating disorders, suicide attempts, running away, truancy, delinquency, substance abuse, spiritual distress, sexual acting out, prostitution, early pregnancy, and early marriage. Regression, depression, depersonalization, dissociation, manipulation, low self-esteem, impaired social skills, thought and memory disturbances, self-neglect, aimlessness, and withdrawal are also common. Due to high-risk behavior, CSA survivors are also more likely than the general population to be physically and sexually assaulted in adolescence and later in life.

Adolescents might have fantasies of revenge and wish for the perpetrator's death. The anger toward the perpetrator and other adults (for not protecting them) approaches rage but may not be directly expressed. Victims might not even be aware of the reason for their rage, shame, guilt, confusion, sense of alienation, and isolation and might not realize that their acting-out behaviors are related to the abuse.

On the Adult

The process of surviving CSA and becoming an adult is similar to a delayed PTSD response: repression of memories (even nonsexual ones), followed by a breakthrough of unwanted, intrusive memories. The memories might begin as nightmares, kinesthetic sensations (e.g., flinching or vaginal pain when touched by a partner in the same way as the perpetrator), or flashbacks. The memories might return gradually, in pieces, or in a sudden, overwhelming flood. In general, survivors should not be encouraged to remember the abuse. However, dealing with any presenting memories is appropriate by a qualified mental health clinician.

On the surface, adult survivors might look relatively uninjured because of denial, dissociation, amnesia, emotional numbing, or repression. They enter counseling for manifestations of the abuse rather than for the incest or sexual abuse itself. The list of typical reactions in Box 33.3 can be used as a checklist to identify the issues to be addressed in counseling. Survivors who see this list typically express amazement (that so much has resulted from the sexual abuse) and relief (that they can finally make sense of their "craziness"). Up to this point, survivors might tend to deny or minimize the relationship of the sexual abuse to any of their current problems. It becomes evident to survivors that the event has disturbed

their entire growth and development process and has set them up for subsequent distressing relationships (Waite et al., 2010).

Overwhelming painful emotions can induce thoughts of suicide to escape the despair, to die with the secret, to avoid conflict with family members, to stop feeling "crazy," and to end the nightmares and flashbacks that are so frightening. Self-harm or mutilation, which serves to replace the emotional pain with physical pain, is a common way of dealing with the sadness, loss, rage, and abandonment. Survivors describe the following various patterns of their self-mutilation (Cerdorian, 2005; Isaacs, 2011; Williams & Bydalek, 2009):

1. When feeling overwhelmed, they inflict harm as a cry for help when they believe that no one is listening or cares.
2. When emotions build up, they go numb or dissociate and have to inflict pain to make sure that they can still feel.
3. When they are feeling unreal (depersonalization), they draw blood to make sure that they are alive.
4. They cause physical pain as a distraction to their emotional pain.
5. They punish themselves when they are feeling self-loathing, guilt, shame, or fear.
6. They use the mutilation as a way of avoiding suicide.
7. They use the mutilation to relieve the anger or rage toward self and others.
8. They might use the mutilation as an attempt to manipulate others.
9. The mutilation might become chronic and addictive, especially if it produces a high (related to the release of endogenous opiates/endorphins).

Self-mutilation might become a chronic pattern of coping with emotional pain.

Alcohol and drugs are often used to avoid or numb the pain and memories and to bring fleeting pleasure that is otherwise elusive. Food might also provide brief pleasure or fill emptiness inside (bingeing) but leads to feeling bloated and guilty and a need to purge. Although sex may not be particularly enjoyable, it can bring relief from loneliness, temporary attention, affection, and approval. Sexual encounters also might trigger traumatic flashbacks, anxiety, fear, shame, disgust, or a sense of helplessness. Healthy adult relationships and sexual intimacy are difficult because of problems in trusting anyone and the history of linking abuse and love. Survivors may have boundary issues, trouble setting limits with others, and difficulty with asking for what they really need (Sigurdardottir et al., 2016). Victims also tend to be caretakers, rescuers, and/or needy.

The reactions of survivors to their trauma (see Box 33.3) are often labeled as clinical symptoms. Those who have experienced trauma will typically be diagnosed with one or more of the following mental disorders: major depression, PTSD, substance use disorder, eating disorder, panic disorder, somatic disorder, dissociative disorder (including dissociative identity disorder), bipolar disorder, schizophrenia, or impulse-control disorder. Personality disorder diagnoses are commonly borderline, narcissistic, histrionic, avoidant, and dependent.

BOX 33.3   Adult Manifestations of Childhood Sexual Abuse

Memory disturbances
  Amnesia about abuse
  Memory gaps about childhood
  Inability to think straight
Keeping secrets
Relationship issues
  Difficulty connecting with others
  Fear of men or fear of women
  Difficulty trusting others and their motives
  Fear of intimacy, inability to maintain intimacy
  Fear of abandonment and rejection
  Difficulty giving and receiving affection
  Feeling alienated from others
  Fear of being used, abused
  Difficulty knowing when to say yes and when to say no
  Difficulty with parenting
  Entering abusive relationships
Body symptoms
  Vague and transient pains
  Memories of physical pain
  Chronic pain or migraine headaches
  Gagging, nausea, vomiting
  Unpleasant sensation when touched
  Distorted body image
  Self-conscious about body
  Overly conscious of appearance
Anger issues
  Fear of expressing anger
  Holding anger in
  Difficulty crying
  Fantasies of revenge
  Feeling violent, full of rage
  Fear of violence
  Homicidal thoughts
Anxiety issues
  Easily startled, inability to relax
  Fear of being attacked, exposed
  Hypervigilance
  Feeling like a frightened child
  Fear of the dark
  Panic attacks, phobias, agoraphobia
Addiction issues
  Alcohol or drug use or dependence
  Compulsive spending
Intrusive thoughts and memories
  Intense nightmares, unwanted thoughts
  Flashbacks—feeling, seeing, smelling, tasting, hearing

Detachment issues
  Feeling numb, unreal
  Disconnected from feelings
  Feeling as if there are "personalities" inside
  "Out-of-body" experiences (dissociation)
Control issues
  Fear of authority, rules
  Need to be in control
  Feeling out of control
  Fear of being vulnerable
  Ambivalent about being taken care of
  Letting others be in control or trying to control others
  Allowing children to be abused
Identity issues
  Confusion about identity or roles
  Negative self-image
  Need to be perfect or perfectly bad
  Underachievement or overachievement
  Need to be totally competent
Sexual issues
  Concealing sexual feelings, feeling nonsexual
  Discomfort with sexual touching
  Lack of orgasms, sexual dysfunction
  Confusion about sexuality, gender identity
  Feeling "dirty," contaminated
  Trading sex for favors
  Promiscuity, prostitution
  Wondering if one is gay
Self-punishment
  Suicidal thoughts, attempts
  Wanting to die or to be dead
  Self-mutilation
  Compulsive eating or dieting
  Bingeing, purging
Other feelings
  Guilt, shame
  Fear of abandonment
  Feeling stuck
  Feeling like a failure
  Chronic dissatisfaction
  Frozen emotions
  Lack of a sense of humor
  Feeling inadequate
  Feeling walled in or "crazy"

Receiving a diagnosis may become a major problem not only because of the stigma and blaming the victim but also because the diagnosis often becomes the focus of treatment rather than the underlying issues; this is especially true when the symptoms of CSA are labeled as a diagnosis of borderline personality disorder instead of an issue of insecure attachments. Lack of appropriate treatment carries a major risk not only for adult survivors but also for their children, especially if the survivors are still in a stage of repression.

Evidence has suggested that survivors who go untreated or are improperly treated reexperience dysfunctional, disorganized families, in which there is neglect and abuse of their children. With their own denial, repression, amnesia, or other coping mechanisms, survivors and/or their partners might sexually abuse their children, grandchildren, nieces, nephews, and others. Examples of incest have surfaced within three and four generations of a family. Breaking this cycle is crucial.

Clinical Example

A man rapes his own daughter: Jan Lester, 30 years old, was admitted to a psychiatric unit as a result of suicidal ideations and 12 superficial cuts on her wrists. She began having nightmares 9 months ago about being awakened at night as a child with someone on top of her. During the nightmares, she would wake up crying with strange body sensations, gagging, pressure on her chest, and vaginal pain. As the nightmares and memories became more complete and vivid, she realized that her father had frequently had sex with her while her mother was asleep. As her father's 50th birthday approached, she felt as if she could not tolerate going to his party. She wanted to be dead but was unable to force herself to cut her wrists more deeply. She felt trapped and longed for relief.

Recovery

Recovery from CSA or incest is similar to recovery from other sexual crimes. The memories and emotions are strong, painful, and confusing. When a child's sense of self and identity is shattered by CSA, personality changes will emerge that reflect the relational trauma. The sexual abuse experience has a profound negative effect on the way that a child views themselves and their world. Although recovery should be highly individualized, there are common patterns within the narrative of survivors. One critical element is making meaning of one's trauma: (1) accepting and understanding the impact of the sexual abuse on the survivor's view of self and others, (2) modifying old self-beliefs and self-views, and (3) restoring congruency. Wright and Gabriel (2018) suggest that psychological interventions should not only focus on symptom reduction but also promote an integration of the survivor's sense of self. Development of a secure sense of connection with caring people is vital to recovery. Jeong and Cha (2019) found that CSA survivors may prefer empathetic peer support from other survivors who truly understand their stories and can share their pain. However, ongoing professional counseling may be necessary to assist survivors in exploring and making sense of their horrific experiences.

Women with a CSA history are at increased risk for problematic sexual health outcomes including revictimization, sexually transmitted infections, and sexual dysfunction (Bird et al., 2017). Survivors of CSA often experience high levels of sexual distress in their adult romantic relationships (MacIntosh, 2017). Considering the potential sexual dysfunctions associated with CSA, disclosure toward a partner becomes necessary. However, survivors may be afraid of their partner's response. Hoping for support and emotional validation, the survivor instead may have their disclosure met by blaming the survivor, not wanting to talk about the abuse, treating the survivor differently, or egocentric responses. Positive responses from romantic partners will serve to appease their fears and reduce shame, guilt, and isolation. Negative responses, such as silence and rejection, from partners may be experienced as retraumatization by the survivor,

eliciting anger and regret (Gauthier et al., 2019). Couples counseling may be necessary as sexual issues present themselves within the romantic relationship.

The overall goals of recovery are safety and security; rebuilding trust; improved self-worth and self-acceptance; forgiveness of self and others; adaptive coping with life and its stresses; self-compassion; the capacity for intimate relationships; understanding of a full range of affect such as anxiety, anger, shame, guilt, and fear; dissociation; and the prevention of suicide, self-mutilation, and sexual abuse of future generations. Although individuals who experience CSA face many challenges, not all demonstrate significant impairment later in life; some demonstrate healthy adjustment years after their abuse and may even experience posttraumatic growth, recovering, and thriving beyond the trauma (Nelson et al., 2019).

PUTTING IT ALL TOGETHER

PSYCHOTHERAPEUTIC MANAGEMENT

Nurse-Patient Relationship

Much depends on the ability of the nurse to develop a trusting relationship with the survivor quickly. Empathy, active support, compassion, warmth, and being nonjudgmental are crucial. Survivors need to be calmly and matter-of-factly asked about CSA, because they are not likely to reveal it spontaneously. The old and perhaps current coercions to keep the secret remain strong in the minds of survivors; they need to feel safe about confidentiality and the nurse's acceptance before disclosure can occur. How much detail is revealed and how soon depend in part on the nurse's ability to be receptive to the experiences without being critical of the perpetrator, of other adults in the family, or of the survivor's loyalty to them. The survivor needs to be reassured that all the emotions (positive, negative, and ambivalent) are valid and that exploring them is important for healing. It is usually helpful for survivors to be reminded periodically that they were not responsible for and did not deserve the sexual abuse, that they are not to be blamed, that they were not in control of the situation, and that the way they coped in the past was the best they could do at the time. Cognitive behavioral approaches and psychoeducation about the dynamics of sexual abuse and reassurances about recovery can be useful in correcting faulty perceptions about the abuse, decreasing self-blame and guilt, and instilling hope for the future despite the inability to change the past. (See the "Key Nursing Interventions for Survivors of Childhood Abuse" box.)

Mentally and emotionally reexperiencing traumatic memories and emotions is disturbing; only periodic, small doses might be tolerable. It is helpful to remind survivors that they went through the abuse alone but do not have to remember it alone. If traumatic flashbacks or dissociation occurs, it is important to bring the survivors back to the present by reminding them where they are now and that the nurse is with them. The nurse and survivors should monitor their

KEY NURSING INTERVENTIONS

For Survivors of Childhood Abuse

- Contract for safety and control of impulses to harm self or others.
- Set limits on self-destructive or self-harm patterns.
- Establish a trusting and supportive environment.
- Validate distressing feelings and reactions as normal.
- Ask permission before touching survivors.
- Reinforce that recovery is possible, even if it is difficult.
- Educate about the dynamics of abuse and the recovery process.
- Assist survivors in understanding current behaviors as reflections of survival strategies used in childhood.
- Facilitate reevaluation of the sexual abuse and its effects but without pressure or excessive rumination.
- Encourage coping choices that are in survivors' best interests.
- Discuss safeguarding other children if the perpetrator still poses a risk.
- Support choices about future disclosures, confrontation, or reporting.
- Be aware that family members and others might feel split loyalty and engage in dysfunctional roles and interaction patterns.
- Decrease feelings of isolation, shame, and stigma.
- Encourage self-acceptance and self-compassion.
- Facilitate acknowledgment, forgiveness, and love for the child within.
- Teach and encourage emotionally focused techniques.
- Facilitate the transfer of responsibility and anger to the perpetrator, but set limits on acting out fantasies of revenge.
- Foster appropriate boundaries with family members and others.
- Help to find meaning in the experience and mourning of all the losses (grieving is a very painful experience).
- Facilitate the cycle from victim to survivor status (reexperiencing and integrating the positive, negative, and ambivalent feelings and memories).
- Facilitate reexperiencing and reworking of maturational tasks that were missed or experienced prematurely.
- Educate about life skills, communication skills, coping skills, decision making, conflict resolution, boundary setting, friendship, intimacy, sexuality, and parenting.
- Refer to outpatient counseling and appropriate support groups.

safety and tolerance of the process to prevent becoming overwhelmed. An important consideration for the nurse and survivor to discuss is the mandatory reporting of child abuse if younger children are currently victims of abuse by the same perpetrators. This type of reporting is understandably difficult for both the nurse and the survivor but needs to be carefully and directly addressed.

When survivors are in outpatient counseling, it is important to consider priorities in each counseling session. Current crises and problems need to be addressed (instead of the sexual abuse) as they arise. This aspect is also critical for self-destructive behaviors that are increased because of counseling, such as suicidal ideation, self-mutilation, and substance abuse. Hospitalization might be necessary if the crisis is severe. Staff should avoid use of restraints that could cause retraumatization. Although survivors view recovery as frightening and painful, they also experience relief that they are making progress.

Psychopharmacology

Medications are not always needed or desirable for adult survivors of CSA, especially if substance abuse is a problem or potential problem. Medications should be given according to the *DSM-5* diagnoses such as major depressive disorder or generalized anxiety disorder. An antidepressant such as trazodone might be used if the depressive symptoms are interfering with sleep. Benzodiazepines or clonidine might be given on a short-term basis. Occasionally, low doses of risperidone, aripiprazole (Abilify), prazosin, quetiapine, or topiramate (Topamax) are given for persistent and severely disturbing nightmares, flashbacks, and agitation (Ripol, 2012).

Milieu Management

On an outpatient basis and during any brief hospitalizations, trauma-informed care and cognitive behavioral and affect management groups can be a useful adjunct to nursing care (Kreidler & Einsporn, 2012). If available, a short-term or ongoing sexual abuse or incest recovery group is beneficial. Some self-help groups include Incest Survivors Anonymous, Survivors of Sexual Abuse, and Daughters and Sons United. Parents United (for the nonperpetrator parent) can be suggested, if appropriate. The perpetrator might also be referred to counseling. Couple therapy should be encouraged for survivors of CSA and their intimate partners related to communication issues, sexual distress, or marital satisfaction (Nielsen et al., 2018).

Other groups that might be recommended, depending on the symptoms and needs of the survivor, are Co-dependency Anonymous, Adult Children of Alcoholics, and Alcoholics or Narcotics Anonymous. Survivors might also be directed to classes or short-term groups that address issues such as decision making, problem solving, communication or relationship skills, conflict resolution, anger management, parenting skills, and human sexuality.

❓ CRITICAL THINKING QUESTION

1. You are working with a patient who was sexually abused as a child by her father. The father insists on visiting his daughter and telling you about her history of emotional problems and lying about the family. What is your approach in working with the father?

PARTNER ABUSE

Nature of the Problem

Exposure to intimate partner violence (IPV) is a traumatic event. Over the past 40 years, IPV has evolved from a social ill to a socially unacceptable crime (Messing et al., 2015). A woman is beaten every 9 seconds in the United States; approximately 2 million are injured in a year (Solnit, 2013). It is estimated that 1 in 3 women and 1 in 4 men have experienced rape, physical violence, and/or stalking by an intimate partner during their lifetime (Stennis et al., 2015). Intimate partner abuse (IPA) is implicated in 30% of female and 5% of male homicide deaths (Gaman et al., 2017). IPA and IPV are at least as prevalent in lesbian, gay, bisexual, and transgender (LGBT) relationships as they are in heterosexual ones. However, the issues, needs, and challenges associated with IPV are complex in all relationships (Gaman et al., 2017).

IPV is also known as domestic violence, partner/spousal abuse, or battery. Different types of abuse occur between partners in romantic (i.e., dating, cohabitating, married) relationships. IPV is characterized by chronic patterns of physically and emotionally abusive intimidation, coercion, and control directed by one partner against the other (Regan & Durvasula, 2015). Hostile exchanges include:

- Physical abuse—pushing, hitting, choking
- Sexual abuse—forced sexual activity
- Emotional abuse—name calling, insults, yelling, humiliation
- Economic abuse—controlling finances, preventing a partner from getting a job
- Coercion and threats—threatening to harm or leave the partner
- Intimidation—destroying the partner's possessions/property; harming the partner's pet
- Social isolation—monitoring or limiting the partner's social contacts/activities
- Denial—minimizing the abuse; blaming the partner for the abuse

Studies have shown that partner abuse crosses all social, racial, cultural, and economic classes, including both homosexual and heterosexual relationships. However, the majority of cases involve younger couples (20 s to 30 s) living in lower socioeconomic conditions. Partners who have prior exposure to domestic violence and childhood abuse are more likely to repeat the abuse cycle. For example, men who witnessed interparental violence and/or were abused as children are more likely to be violent toward their partners. Likewise, women who witnessed interparental violence and/or were abused as children are more likely to experience partner abuse. Although the majority of perpetrators are male and the majority of victims are female, male victims experience the same physical and psychological outcomes as their female counterparts. Oftentimes, IPV is precipitated by alcohol and/or drug use (Regan & Durvasula, 2015).

Effects

Most experts acknowledge the development of helplessness, hopelessness, isolation, and resignation in response to ongoing emotional and physical abuse. Abused individuals report that they fear and hate the abuse. However, these same individuals fear and hate the reality of being alone without their beloved partner. Box 33.4 lists common reasons why individuals endure long-term abuse. A widely accepted view of why individuals endure abuse is the cycle of violence (Box 33.5). The Theory of Attachment can be helpful in understanding the abuse cycle. A pattern of protests (attacking, defending, demanding, and withdrawing) occurs when partners feel emotional distress during times of conflict. These harmful interactions can escalate to the point of violence (see Attachment Theory in Chapter 7). After the violence has occurred and the partners separate for a period of time, the honeymoon stage begins: the loving side of the abusive partner is experienced, and the abused partner is relieved by the lack of tension in the relationship. The abused report thinking that they can help their partners overcome their problems and violent behaviors. The cycle of escalation is a powerful force that keeps partners stuck in painful interactional patterns even when friends and family members try to convince the abused to leave.

BOX 33.4 Why Women Stay as Long as They Do

Situational Factors
- Economic dependence; lack of job skills
- Fear of greater physical danger to themselves and their children if they attempt to leave or have partner arrested
- Fear of emotional damage to children because of being without a father
- Fear of losing custody of children
- Lack of alternative housing
- Social isolation; lack of support from family or friends
- Lack of information regarding alternatives
- Fear of involvement in court processes
- Fear of retaliation from partner or partner's family

Emotional Factors
- Fear of being alone
- Being in a state of denial and living a secret
- Personal embarrassment and protecting the image of husband and family
- Insecurity and lack of emotional support
- Guilt about failure of marriage or relationship
- Fear that partner is unable to survive alone
- Belief that partner is sick and needs her help
- Belief that partner will change
- Fear of being alone and feeling overwhelmed

Cultural Factors
- Knowing that batterers are not held accountable for their violent actions
- Believing that the abuse is her fault
- Being raised to be passive and submissive
- Developing survival skills instead of relationship skills
- Recognizing that the legal system is a male-dominated system

Plus: She Still Loves Him

Modified from Julian Center Shelter, Indianapolis, IN, and Task Force on Families in Crisis, Nashville, TN.

BOX 33.5   Cycle of Violence

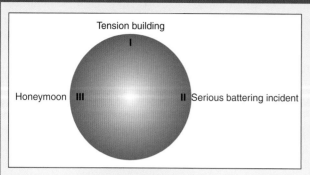

Man

I. Tension Building

He has excessively high expectations of her.
He blames her for anything that goes wrong.
He does not try to control his behaviors.
He is aware of his inappropriate behaviors but does not admit it.
Verbal and minor physical abuse increase.
Afraid that she will leave, he gets more possessive to keep her captive.
He gets frantic and more controlling.
He interprets her withdrawal as rejection.

II. Serious Battering Incident

The trigger event is an internal or external event or substance.
The battering usually occurs in private.
He will threaten more harm if she tries to get help (police, medical).
He tries to justify his behaviors but does not understand what happens.
He minimizes the severity of the abuse.
His stress is relieved.

III. Honeymoon

He is loving, charming, begging for forgiveness, making promises.
He truly believes that he will never abuse again.
He feels that he taught her a lesson and she will not act up again.
He preys on her guilt to keep her trapped.

Woman

I. Tension Building

She is nurturing, compliant, tries to please him.
She denies the seriousness of their problems.
She feels she can control his behaviors.
She tries to alter his behavior to stay safe.
She tries to prevent his anger.
She blames external factors—alcohol, work.
She takes minor abuse but does not feel she deserves it.
She gets scared and tries to hide (withdrawal).
She might call for help as the tension becomes unbearable.

II. Serious Battering Incident

In cases of long-term battering, she might provoke it just to get it over with.
She might call for help if she is afraid of being killed.
Her initial reaction is shock, disbelief, and denial.
Fearing more abuse if police come, she might plead for them not to arrest him.
She is anxious, ashamed, humiliated, sleepless, fatigued, depressed.
She does not seek help for injuries for a day or more and lies about the cause of injuries.

III. Honeymoon

She sees his loving behaviors as the real person and tries to make up.
She wants to believe that the abuse will never happen again.
She feels that if she stays, he will get help; the thought of leaving makes her afraid.
She believes in the permanency of the relationship.

Modified from Gerard, M. (2000). Domestic violence: How to screen and intervene. *RN, 63*, 52; McFarlane, J., Malecha, A., Gist, J., Watson, K., Batten, E., Hall, I., & Smith, S. (2004). Increasing the safety-promoting behaviors of abused women. *American Journal of Nursing, 104*, 40; Walker, L. (1979). *The battered woman.* Harper & Row.

Survivors often report nightmares, flashbacks, recurrent fears of more violence, emotional detachment, numbness, startle response, sleep problems, guilt, impaired concentration, and hypervigilance. Similar to patients with PTSD, battered men and women show typical reactions to a chronic trauma, not symptoms of psychopathology.

According to survivors, it is unlikely that abused individuals will leave their partners until they realize that the cycle is not going to stop and they have the emotional support to leave and a safe place to go. Fearing that the next beating might be fatal, finding that their partners are physically or sexually abusing their children, and realizing that their children are learning to be abusive are incentives for a planned separation.

Recovery

Immediately preceding, during, or after a serious battering incident, victims are frightened and likely to call the police or a crisis service agency for help. It is common knowledge in most states in America that if police are called for an incident involving domestic violence, someone is going to be arrested. For the police, it is just a matter of who it will be. The intended goal is to separate the partners to stop the conflict and provide immediate safety. Getting victims and their children to a shelter or other safe place, if they will go, may be necessary when immediate danger is present. If injuries have occurred, victims should be encouraged to go to an emergency department. In any case, crisis workers, shelter workers, or nurses can begin the important process of assessing and providing information that can interrupt the cycle of abuse. Even if the survivors are not yet ready to separate from their partners, they can be given an easily concealed card with telephone numbers of police, prosecutors, crisis services, victims' assistance, shelters, and support groups. If contact is only by phone or if they are worried that the abusers will find the card, they can be asked to write down the phone numbers on the back of a picture in their wallets or be told to call 911. Survivors can also be given ideas for developing a safety or escape plan, such as packing a bag with medicines and clothes for them and their children, house and car keys, money, a cell phone, and important phone numbers and papers (e.g., bank account numbers, birth certificates, social security numbers, medical insurance cards, no contact/protective orders). They should also be informed of the protections afforded by legal statutes, protective orders, and antistalking laws. Long-term goals for survivors of partner abuse are to develop a sense of safety and security within healthy support systems.

PUTTING IT ALL TOGETHER

PSYCHOTHERAPEUTIC MANAGEMENT

Nurse-Patient Relationship

Because most abused individuals seek help for their injuries and somatic symptoms at least once, nurses can be instrumental in offering information and assistance. Nurses in emergency departments, clinics, physicians' offices, psychiatric facilities, and community health agencies need to be educated on IPV and know how to recognize a survivor, make an assessment, offer support, and make a referral to available services (Trevillion et al., 2012). Some common cues to abuse are listed in Box 33.6. The assessment process is often difficult because survivors fear disclosure, are embarrassed about the situation, and desire to be treated quickly and leave, and sometimes the abusers are present. It is important to interview the victim privately and with sensitivity, empathy, and compassion. Box 33.7 lists other responses that survivors consider helpful.

The most crucial information to document in an initial contact includes the following:

1. Identity and current location of the abuser
2. Location and safety of any children
3. Length and frequency of abuse
4. Types of abuse (physical, psychological, sexual, financial) and use of weapons
5. Types and locations of injuries (photographs and body maps are preferred)
6. Availability of weapons at the place of residence
7. Use and abuse of substances and medications by victim and abuser
8. Active and passive suicidal ideation (with or without a plan or a wish to be dead)
9. Types of service desired (police, legal, shelter, crisis counseling, knowledgeable clergy, social service agencies, transportation)
10. Referrals made

Even if the initial contact is brief, it is important to convey to survivors that they are not alone in their abuse and that there are people who are willing and able to help when they are ready. The nurse must convey to survivors that they are important and have dignity and worth. These individuals need acknowledgment of their mental and physical exhaustion, fears, and ambivalence about the abuser, separating, and their wish to help the abuser as well as themselves. It is difficult for nurses and all professionals to accept that survivors cannot be pushed, rushed, or coerced into separating from the abuser before they are ready. Survivors can be encouraged to enter couples/family counseling and individual counseling.

BOX 33.6 Common Cues to Partner Abuse

- Repeated, vague symptoms or illnesses that are not confirmed by tests, such as backache, abdominal pain, indigestion, headaches, hyperventilation, anxiety, insomnia, fatigue, anorexia, heart palpitations
- Unexplained injuries or injuries with unlikely explanations and embarrassment about them
- Hidden injuries in areas concealed by clothes or visible on physical or x-ray examination only—for example, head and neck injuries, internal injuries, genital injuries, scars, burns, joint pain or dislocations, numbness, hearing problems, or bald spots
- Injuries with recognizable marks such as from a belt, iron, raised ring, teeth, fingertips, cigarette, gun, or knife
- Multiple fractures or bruises in various stages of healing
- Jumpiness or flinching in the presence of the abuser
- Substance abuse and suicidal thoughts or attempts
- Attempts to conceal fear of the abuser
- Continual efforts to keep the abuser from getting angry
- Denial of any problems in the relationship
- Lack of relationships with family or friends
- Isolation or confinement to home
- Guilt, depression, anxiety, low self-esteem, sense of failure, concealed anger
- Continual justification of own actions and whereabouts of the abuser
- Continual justification of the abuser's actions in public; excusing or rationalizing the behaviors
- Believing in family unity at all costs and in traditional stereotypes
- Believing in managing alone, even when help is offered
- An oversolicitous abuser who does not want to leave the victim alone with hospital or agency staff or even with family and friends

Modified from Carretta, C. M. (2008). Domestic violence: A worldwide exploitation. *Journal of Psychosocial Nursing and Mental Health Services, 46,* 3; Merrell, J. (2001). Social support for victims of domestic violence. *Journal of Psychosocial Nursing and Mental Health Services, 39,* 30.

BOX 33.7 Helpful Responses to Partner Abuse

- Be nonjudgmental, objective, and nonthreatening.
- Ask directly if abuse is occurring.
- Acknowledge the seriousness of the abuse.
- Assist the victim in assessing strengths.
- Encourage the use of personal resources.
- Give the victim a list of resources—shelters, financial aid, police, and legal assistance.
- Allow victim to choose own options.
- Offer names of relevant support groups.
- Help victim to develop a safety or escape plan.
- Do not disbelieve or blame the victim.
- Do not get angry with the victim.
- Do not refuse to help if the victim is not ready to separate from the abuser.
- Do not push the victim to separate from the abuser before ready.

When abused women/men do separate from their partner, they should expect escalation of behaviors. Survivors frequently need long-term counseling and social services to recover, especially if the abuser is unwilling to participate in couples' counseling or an abusers' program (often a court-ordered program of group education and counseling lasting ≥26 weeks). Nursing interventions for survivors (individually or in groups, using cognitive behavioral and trauma-informed care techniques) generally focus on the following:

1. Monitoring safety from partner abuse and preventing suicide
2. Reiterating information about the cycle of violence
3. Building self-esteem, confidence, interdependence, and sense of hope
4. Sharing of feelings, especially anger, fear, betrayal, and loneliness
5. Decreasing shame, guilt, embarrassment, manipulation, isolation, and dependency
6. Confirming personal and legal rights
7. Teaching techniques for stress management, communication, conflict resolution, and assertiveness
8. Teaching parenting skills such as responding to their children's emotional needs
9. Building a new, improved support system
10. Setting goals and specific plans for the immediate future
11. Resolving grief

Referrals might also be needed for job counseling or training, legal assistance, financial aid, child care, and permanent housing. At any stage during working with survivors, brief hospitalization might be needed because of injuries, suicidality, self-mutilation, or substance abuse.

❓ CRITICAL THINKING QUESTION

2. Your coworker is sharing with you that she is thinking about separating from her husband because of his drinking and long-term emotional abuse toward her. She expresses a fear that he might try to kill her and fears raising her two children alone. What information would you offer her?

Psychopharmacology

Often-prescribed medications are antidepressants, benzodiazepines, and hypnotics. These medications might be prescribed if the survivor's symptoms of depression, anxiety, sleeplessness, nightmares, or flashbacks are severe. Continual assessment is needed to determine when medications are no longer needed to prevent abuse and addiction.

Milieu Management

The following groups in inpatient, outpatient, and community settings may be relevant for survivors: domestic violence, healthy boundaries, job skills, relationship issues, and stress management. Substance abuse groups should be recommended if necessary. The National Domestic Violence Hotline is also available (800-799-SAFE) and online at www.ndvh.org.

❓ CRITICAL THINKING QUESTION

3. As an emergency department nurse, you are treating a 19-year-old male victim who was tortured and raped by a local gang. The victim refuses to give any details or to identify members of the gang. Describe what information you would give him about being a victim and the benefits of follow-up counseling.

CASE STUDY

Rachael Benton, a 26-year-old survivor of incest by her father, is married to Richard. She has an 8-year-old child, Matthew; Richard has three boys, Robert, James, and Daniel, ages 11, 8, and 7, who live with them. Angela, age 5, was born after Rachael and Richard were married. Matthew was removed from the home after being abused by Robert, his oldest stepbrother. Rachael sought help by attending a battered women's group.

Rachael's situation was difficult to resolve. Because of heavy drinking, Richard was missing work and changing jobs frequently. His income declined and was sporadic, but expenses did not decline. Without insurance, Rachael's repeated treatment of menstrual irregularities, back pain, chronic and severe headaches, and diarrhea were not paid for. She avoided treatment for bruises, a superficial knife wound, head cuts, and contusions. Richard repeatedly punched her stomach during a pregnancy, causing a miscarriage.

When Richard raped her, Rachael realized that she needed a safety plan for herself and the children. As Rachael became more assertive and vocal, Richard demanded that she stay home, bought a shotgun to convince her to stay, and took the starter off the car. He rode to work with coworkers. Rachael had not adopted Richard's boys, so she could not take them with her. She was afraid that his verbal abuse of them would turn to physical violence when she left. Richard knew about all the places she thought of going.

It took 4 months to develop, coordinate, and implement arrangements so that Rachael and Angela felt safe leaving Richard. Neighbors, friends, and teachers were warned of the potential abuse of the boys and given the phone number for anonymous reporting of child abuse. Rachael's mother rented her a small trailer in a rural town and obtained forms for Aid to Families With Dependent Children. Rachael secretly and gradually packed clothes and important documents in the trunk of a group member's car.

One night Richard got drunk, beat Rachael, and tried to rape her again. She fought him off and waited until he passed out. The group member with the packed car drove her to the new trailer. As expected, Richard got his shotgun and went to every friend of Rachael's, but none knew where she was. He drove to Rachael's mother's home, and she called the sheriff when his car pulled into the driveway. Richard was put in custody by the sheriff's department. Within a week, Daniel's teacher filed a child abuse report due to bruises found on him. Within 2 weeks, the boys were removed from the home and returned to their biological mother.

Rachael has received proper medical treatment and feels healthier. She is now divorced, is attending a job-training program, and maintains her secret location. She feels safe and attends family counseling once a month with her two children. She attends a support group for battered women once a week.

◎ CARE PLAN

Name: Rachael Benton   *Admission Date:* _____

DSM-5 Diagnosis: Spouse Violence, Physical, Sexual, Psychological

Assessment	**Areas of strength:** Patient is bright, articulate, and capable of problem solving; her mother and one friend are willing to help; patient is developing trust in her group meetings and beginning to process her feelings and rights.
	Problems: Lack of safe housing and employment; inability to remove husband's children from the house and fear he will abuse them; fear of increased abuse of her, even death, if she tries to leave; severe headaches.
Diagnoses	Decisional conflict related to dysfunctional marriage, as evidenced by attendance in a battered women's support group
	Posttrauma syndrome related to previous sexual, physical, emotional, and economic abuse, as evidenced by physical wounds, fear, and emotional trauma
	Fear (of leaving husband) related to potential abuse of sons, as evidenced by reluctance to leave without stepsons
Outcomes	**Short-term goals**
Date met: _____	Patient will remove bullets from gun; design an escape plan.
Date met: _____	Patient will verbalize confidence in developing and carrying out safety plan; confirm housing in rural county.
	Long-term goals
Date met: _____	Patient will enroll in job-training program.
Date met: _____	Patient will obtain legal assistance.
Date met: _____	Patient will seek medical treatment for chronic health problems.
Planning and Interventions	**Nurse-patient relationship:** Listen nonjudgmentally and empathically; accept behaviors related to secrecy and self-protection; avoid negative talk about spouse; locate resources for training, finances, counseling, and medical care in rural county.
	Psychopharmacology: Trazodone (Desyrel) 50 mg at bedtime to alleviate moderate depression and improve sleep; ibuprofen as needed for severe headaches.
	Milieu management: Encourage continuing in local support group and family counseling; continue assessment of safety of patient and children.
Evaluation	Patient has moved to rural county and attending support group; is receiving family counseling and medical care. Husband's children were removed and placed with their biologic mother.
Referrals	Has an appointment with a job-training program in rural county.

▌ STUDY NOTES

1. Not all crimes involve physical violence and injury; however, all crimes involve emotional violation and injury. Victims lose a sense of the ability to control their own lives and lose trust in others.

2. Progression through the stages of recovery from a crime might take years. Crisis intervention and group meetings with other survivors can facilitate recovery.

3. In assisting survivors, sensitivity to their needs is crucial to build trust and create a sense of safety and security.

4. Information about counseling resources and support groups can be given to the survivors of any crime/trauma for later use, even if there is an initial denial of the need for help.

5. The reexperiencing and working through of any trauma/crime memories is a painful, lengthy, and sometimes sporadic process that requires intense support and empathy.

6. Adult survivors of childhood sexual abuse might repress memories for years as a result of the emotional turmoil and sense of being betrayed by the abuser and others.

7. Adult survivors of childhood sexual abuse typically enter counseling for a variety of overt problems, unaware of how these are related to childhood trauma.

8. The theory of attachment; the cycle of violence; and other situational, emotional, and cultural factors help explain why survivors stay in abusive relationships.

9. Abuse victims are most amenable to crisis intervention and referrals for needed services immediately preceding or at the beginning of a serious battering incident.

10. Patience, support, and information are critical aspects of nursing interventions with all survivors.

REFERENCES

Annan, S. L. (2011). "It's not just a job. This is where we live. This is our backyard": The experiences of expert legal and advocate providers with sexually assaulted women in rural areas. *Journal of the American Psychiatric Nurses Association, 17*(2), 139–147. https://doi.org/10.1177/1078390311401024.

Anonymous. (n.d.). The Crime of Human Trafficking: A Law Enforcement Guide to Identification and Investigation. http://www.theiacp.org/portals/0/pdfs/CompleteHTGuide.pdf.

Anorexia Nervosa and Associated Disorders. (2002). *Anorexia nervosa and associated disorders (Indianapolis Chapter of ANAD): Personal interviews.* ANAD.

Bamidele, O. (2017). War, sex and justice: Barriers to gender justice in post-conflict Liberia. *International Journal of Criminal Justice Sciences, 12*(1), 69–82. https://doi.org/10.5281/zenodo.345708.

Bird, E., Gilmore, A., Stappenbeck, C., Heiman, J., Davis, K., Norris, J., & George, G. (2017). Women's sex-related dissociation: The effects of alcohol intoxication, attentional control instructions, and history of childhood sexual abuse. *Journal of Sex & Marital Therapy, 43*(2), 121–131. https://doi.org/10.1080/0092623X.2015.1124304.

Campana, P., & Varese, F. (2016). Exploitation in human trafficking and smuggling. *European Journal of Criminal Policy and Research, 22*, 89–105. https://doi.org/10.1007/s10610-015-9286-6.

Carretta, C. M. (2008). Domestic violence: A worldwide exploration. *Journal of Psychosocial Nursing and Mental Health Services, 46*(3), 26–35. https://www.researchgate.net/publication/5436952_Domestic_violence_a_worldwide_exploration

Cerdorian, K. (2005). The needs of adolescent girls who self-harm. *Journal of Psychosocial Nursing and Mental Health Services, 43*, 40. https://doi.org/10.3928/02793695-20050801-13.

Cole, H. (2009). Human trafficking: Implications for the role of the advanced practice forensic nurse. *Journal of the American Psychiatric Nurses Association, 14*(6), 462–470. https://doi.org/10.1177/1078390308325763.

Crane, P. (2013). A human trafficking toolkit for nursing intervention. In M. De Chesnay (Ed.), *Sex trafficking: A clinical guide for nurses* (pp. 167–182). Springer Publishing Company.

de Chesnay, M. (2013). Sex trafficking as a new pandemic. In M. De Chesnay (Ed.), *Sex trafficking: A clinical guide for nurses* (pp. 3–22). Springer Publishing Company.

de Chesnay, M., et al. (2013). First-person accounts of illnesses and injuries sustained while trafficked. In M. De Chesnay (Ed.), *Sex trafficking: A clinical guide for nurses.* Springer Publishing Company.

Felitti, V., Anda, R. F., Nordenberg, D., Williamson, D. F., Spitz, A. M., Edwards, V., … Marks, J. S. (1998). Relationship of childhood abuse and household dysfunction to many of the leading causes of death in adults. The Adverse Childhood Experiences (ACE) Study. *American Journal of Preventive Medicine, 14*(4), 245–258. https://doi.org/10.1016/s0749-3797(98)00017-8.

Foa, E. B. (2005). The psychological aftermath of Hurricane Katrina. *Medscape Psychiatry & Mental Health, 8*, 1.

Ford, J. (2018). Heterosexual men's accounts of unwanted sex "going with the flow": How college men's experiences of unwanted sex are produced by gendered interactional pressures. *Social Forces, 96*(3), 1303–1324. https://doi.org/10.1093/sf/sox066.

Gaman, A., McAfee, S., Homel, P., & Jacob, T. (2017). Understanding patterns of intimate partner abuse in male-male, male-female, and female-female couples. *Psychiatric Quarterly, 88*, 335–347. https://doi.org/10.1007/s11126-016-9450-2.

Gauthier, L., Vaillancourt-Morel, M., Rellini, A., & Godbout, N. (2019). The risk of telling: A dyadic perspective on romantic partners' responses to childhood sexual abuse disclosure and their associations with sexual and relationship satisfaction. *Journal of Marriage and Family Therapy, 45*(3), 480–493. https://doi.org/10.1111/jmft.12345.

Gerard, M. (2000). Domestic violence: How to screen and intervene. *RN, 63*(12), 52.

Görg, N., Böhnke, J., Priebe, K., Rausch, S., Wekenmann, S., Ludäscher, P., … Kleindienst, N. (2019). Changes in trauma-related emotions following treatment with dialectical behavioral therapy for posttraumatic stress disorder after childhood abuse. *Journal of Traumatic Stress, 32*(5), 764–773. https://doi.org/10.1002/jts.22440.

Hardy, V., Locklear, A., & Crable, A. (2020). Commercial sexual exploitation of adolescents: Gender-specific and trauma-informed care implications. *Journal of Social Work Values & Ethics, 17*(1), 55–62. https://jswve.org/download/2020-1/articles-17-1/Commercial-sexual-exploitation-of-adolescents.pdf

Hawkins, L., Mullet, N., Brown, C., Eggleston, D., & Gardenhire, J. (2019). All survivors have the right to heal: A #metoomen content analysis. *Journal of Feminist Family Therapy, 31*(2–3), 78–99. https://doi.org/10.1080/08952833.2019.1633840.

Helsel, P. (2015). Witnessing the body's response to trauma: Resistance, ritual, and nervous system activation. *Pastoral Psychology, 64*, 681–693. https://doi.org/10.1007/s11089-014-0628-y.

Hiskey, S., & McPherson, S. (2013). That's just life: Older adult constructs of trauma. *Aging & Mental Health, 17*(6), 689–696. https://doi.org/10.1080/13607863.2013.765832.

Hoerrner, M. (2013). Working with law enforcement. In M. De Chesnay (Ed.), *Sex trafficking: A clinical guide for nurses* (pp. 63–72). Springer Publishing Company.

Isaacs, M. M. (2011). Therapist's page. *Many Voices, 23*, 6.

Jackson, J. (2011). The evolving role of the forensic nurse. *American Nurse Today, 6*, 11.

Jeong, S., & Cha, C. (2019). Healing from childhood sexual abuse: A meta-synthesis of qualitative studies. *Journal of Child Sexual Abuse, 28*(4), 383–399. https://doi.org/10.1080/10538712.2019.1574945.

Johnson, B. (2012). Aftercare for survivors of human trafficking. *Social Work & Christianity, 39*(4), 370–389.

Jordan, J. (2013). From victim to survivor – and from survivor to victim: Reconceptualizing the survivor journey. *Sexual Abuse in Australia & New Zealand, 5*(2), 48–52. https://search.informit.org/doi/10.3316/INFORMIT.832896370790754

Kozak, R., Gushwa, M., & Cadet, T. (2018). Victimization and violence: An exploration of the relationship between child sexual abuse, violence, and delinquency. *Journal of Child Sexual Abuse, 27*(6), 699–717. https://doi.org/10.1080/10538712.2018.1474412.

Kreidler, M., & Einsporn, R. (2012). A comparative study of therapy duration for survivors of childhood sexual abuse. *Journal of Psychosocial Nursing and Mental Health Services, 50*(4), 26–32. https://doi.org/10.3928/02793695-20120306-02.

Lacy, T. J., & Benedek, D. M. (2003). Terrorism and weapons of mass destruction: Managing the behavioral reaction in primary care. *Southern Medical Journal, 96*(4), 394. https://doi.org/10.1097/01.SMJ.0000054783.69453.79.

Lankford, A. (2016). Are there reasons for optimism in the battle against sexual assault? *Sociology Compass, 10*(1), 38–47. https://doi.org/10.1111/soc4.12341.

Lapp, C. A., & Overman, N. (2013). Mental health perspectives on care of human trafficking victims within our borders. In M. De Chesnay (Ed.), *Sex trafficking: A clinical guide for nurses* (pp. 305–320). Springer Publishing Company.

Lenz, S., & Lancaster, C. (2017). A mixed-methods evaluation of intensive trauma-focused programming. *Journal of Counseling & Development, 95*(1), 24–34. https://doi.org/10.1002/jcad.12114.

MacIntosh, H. (2017). Dyadic traumatic reenactment: An integration of psychoanalytic approaches to working with negative interaction cycles in couple therapy with childhood sexual abuse survivors. *Journal of Clinical Social Work, 45*, 344–353. https://doi.org/10.1007/s10615-016-0607-0.

Marchetti, C. A. (2012). Regret and police reporting among individuals who have experienced sexual assault. *Journal of the American Psychiatric Nurses Association, 18*(1), 32–39. https://doi.org/10.1177/1078390311431889.

Matthew, L., & Barron, I. (2015). Participatory action research on help-seeking behaviors of self-defined rituals. *Journal of Child Sexual Abuse, 24*(4), 429–443. https://doi.org/10.1080/10538712.2015.1029104.

McFarlane, J., Malecha, A., Gist, J., Watson, K., Batten, E., Hall, I., & Smith, S. (2004). Increasing the safety-promoting behaviors of abused women. *American Journal of Nursing, 104*(3), 40. https://doi.org/10.1097/00000446-200403000-00019.

McGuire, K. (2019). The embodiment of complex trauma in domestic minor sex trafficking victims and the dangers of misidentification. *Journal of Human Behavior in the Social Environment, 29*(4), 535–547. https://doi.org/10.1080/10911359.2018.1543630.

Merrell, J. (2001). Social support for victims of domestic violence. *Journal of Psychosocial Nursing and Mental Health Services, 39*, 30. https://doi.org/10.3928/0279-3695-20011101-14.

Messing, J., Ward-Lasher, A., Thaller, J., & Bagwell-Gray, M. E. (2015). The state of intimate partner violence intervention progress and continuing challenges. *Social Work, 60*(4), 305–313. https://doi.org/10.1093/sw/swv027.

Meunier-Sham, J., Cross, T., & Zuniga, T. (2013). Assessment of childhood sexual assault & trauma: The seven pillars of quality care in a statewide pediatric sexual assault nurse examiner program. *Journal of Child Sexual Abuse, 22*(7), 777–795. https://doi.org/10.1080/10538712.2013.830665.

Morrison, S., Bruce, C., & Wilson, S. (2018). Children's disclosure of sexual abuse: A systematic review of qualitative research exploring barriers and facilitators. *Journal of Child Sexual Abuse, 27*(2), 176–194. https://doi.org/10.1080/10538712.2018.1425943.

Muehlenhard, C., Peterson, Z., Humphreys, T., & Jozkowski, K. (2017). Evaluating the one-in-five statistic: Women's risk of sexual assault while in college. *Journal of Sex Research, 54*(4–5), 549–576. https://doi.org/10.1080/00224499.2017.1295014.

Munro-Kramer, M., Dulin, A., & Gaither, C. (2017). What survivors want: Understanding the needs of sexual assault survivors. *Journal of American College Health, 65*(5), 297–305. https://doi.org/10.1080/07448481.2017.1312409.

Nelson, K., Hagedorn, B., & Lambie, G. (2019). Influence of attachment style on sexual abuse survivors' posttraumatic growth. *Journal of Counseling & Development, 97*(3), 227–237. https://doi.org/10.1002/jcad.12263.

Newby, A., & McGuinness, T. M. (2012). Human trafficking: What psychiatric nurses should know to help children and adolescents. *Journal of Psychosocial Nursing and Mental Health Services, 50*(4), 21–24. https://doi.org/10.3928/02793695-20120307-03.

Nielsen, B., Wind, G., Tjørnhøj-Thomsen, T., & Martinsen, B. (2018). A scoping review of challenges in adult intimate relationships after childhood sexual abuse. *Journal of Child Sexual Abuse, 27*(6), 718–728. https://doi.org/10.1080/10538712.2018.1491915.

Ogle, C., Rubin, D., & Siegler, I. (2014). Cumulative exposure to traumatic events in older adults. *Aging & Mental Health, 18*(3), 316–325. https://doi.org/10.1080/13607863.2013.832730.

Rajaram, S., & Tidball, S. (2018). Survivor's voices—Complex needs of sex trafficking survivors in the Midwest. *Behavioral Medicine, 44*(3), 189–198. https://doi.org/10.1080/08964289.2017.1399101.

Regan, P., & Durvasula, R. (2015). A brief review of intimate partner violence in the United States: Nature, correlates and proposed preventative measures. *Interpersona: An International Journal on Personal Relationships, 9*(2), 127–134. https://doi.org/10.5964/ijpr.v9i2.186.

Reid, J., et al. (2017). Human trafficking of minors and childhood adversity in Florida. *American Journal of Public Health, 107*(2), 306–311. https://doi.org/10.2105/AJPH.2016.303564.

Ressel, M., Lyons, J., & Romano, E. (2018). Abuse characteristics, multiple victimisation and resilence among young adult males with histories of childhood sexual abuse. *Child Abuse Review, 27*(3), 239–253. https://doi.org/10.1002/car.2508.

Ripol, L.H. (2012). Clinical Psychopharmacology, January 29. http://www.medscape.com.

Rosellini, A., Street, A., & Kessleret, R. (2017). Sexual assault victimization and the mental health treatment, suicide attempts, and career outcomes among women in the U.S. Army. *American Journal of Public Health, 107*(5), 732–739. https://doi.org/10.2105/AJPH.2017.303693.

Rudolfsson, L., & Tidefors, I. (2015). The struggles of victims of sexual abuse who seek pastoral care. *Pastoral Psychology, 64*, 453–467. https://doi.org/10.1007/s11089-014-0638-9.

Sarson, J., & MacDonald, L. (2009, May 8). Behavioural harms: Enforced and survival tactics in ritual abuse-torture, Presented at the Thirty-First SALIS Conference. Halifax, Nova Scotia, Canada.

Schwartz, J. (2011). Introduction. In O. B. Epstein, J. Schwartz, & R. W. Schwartz (Eds.), *Ritual abuse and mind control: The manipulation of attachment needs* (pp. xiii–xvii). Karnac Books.

Schwarz, C., Unruh, E., Cronin, K., Evans-Simpson, S., Britton, H., & Ramaswamy, M. (2016). Human trafficking identification and service provision in the medical and social service sectors. *Health & Human Rights: An International Journal, 18*(1), 181–191.

Schwarz, C. (2019). Human trafficking and meaning making: The role of definitions in antitrafficking frontline work. *Social Service Review, 93*, 484–523. https://doi.org/10.1086/705237.

Sharp, K., Schwartz, L., Barnes, S., Jamison, L., Miller-Graff, L., & Howell, L. (2017). Differential influence of social support in emerging adulthood across sources of support and profiles of interpersonal and non-interpersonal potentially traumatic experiences. *Journal of Aggression, Maltreatment & Trauma, 26*(7), 736–755. https://doi.org/10.1080/10926771.2017.1289999.

Shurter, D. (2012). *Rabbit hole: A Satanic Ritual Abuse Survivor's Story*. Consider It Creative.

Sigurdardottir, S., Halldorsdottir, S., Bender, S. S., & Agnarsdottir, G. (2016). Personal resurrection: Female childhood sexual abuse survivors' experience of the wellness-program. *Scandinavian Journal of Caring Sciences, 30*(1), 175–186. https://doi.org/10.1111/scs.12238.

Solnit, R. (2013, January 24). Violence against women. *The Huffington Post*. http://www.huffingtonpost.com/rebecca-solnit/violence-against-women_b_254194.

Spinazzola, J., van der Kolk, B., & Ford, J. (2018). When nowhere is safe: Interpersonal trauma and attachment adversity as antecedents of posttraumatic stress disorder and developmental trauma disorder. *Journal of Traumatic Stress, 31*(5), 631–642. https://doi.org/10.1002/jts.22320.

Stark, C. (2019). Ritual abuse and developmental trauma: Application of the triphasic model of trauma treatment in the case of "Sarah". *International Journal of Cultic Studies, 10*, 41–51.

Stark, E. (2012). Looking beyond domestic violence: Policing coercive control. *Journal of Police Crisis Negotiations, 12*(2), 199–217. https://doi.org/10.1080/15332586.2012.725016.

Stennis, K., Fischle, H., Bent-Goodley, T., Purnell, K., & Williamset, H. (2015). The development of culturally competent intimate partner violence interventions – S.T.A.R.T. Implications for competency-based social work practice. *Social Work & Christianity, 42*(1), 96–109.

Tambling, R. (2012). Solution-oriented therapy for survivors of sexual assault and their partners. *Contemporary Family Therapy: An International Journal, 34*, 391–401. https://doi.org/10.1007/s10591-012-9200-z.

Trevillion, K., Hughes, B., & Howard, L. (2012). The response of mental services to domestic violence: A qualitative study of service users' and professionals' experiences. *Journal of the American Psychiatric Nurses Association, 18*(6), 326–336. https://doi.org/10.1177/1078390312459747.

Tsai, L., Lim, V., & Nhanh, C. (2020). "I feel like we are people who have never known each other before": The experiences of survivors of human trafficking and sexual exploitation transitioning from shelters to life in the community. *Forum/Qualitative Social Research, 21*(1). https://doi.org/10.17169/fqs-21.1.3259.

Tynhurst, J. S. (1951). Individual reactions to community disaster: The natural history of psychiatric phenomena. *American Journal of Psychiatry, 107*, 764. https://doi.org/10.1176/ajp.107.10.764.

van der Kolk, B. (2015). *The body keeps the score: Brain, mind & body in the healing of trauma*. Penguin Books.

Waite, R., Gerrity, P., & Arango, R. (2010). Assessment for and response to adverse childhood experiences. *Journal of Psychosocial Nursing and Mental Health Services, 48*(12), 51–61. https://doi.org/10.3928/02793695-20100930-03.

Walker, L. (1979). *The battered woman*. Harper & Row.

Weldon, S. (2016). Implicit theories in intimate partner violence sex offenders: An interpretative phenomenological analysis. *Journal of Family Violence, 31*, 289–302. https://doi.org/10.1007/s10896-015-9774-y.

Williams, K. A., & Bydalek, K. (2009). Self-mutilation: The cutting truth. *American Nurse Today, 4*, 8.

Wilson, L., & Scarpa, A. (2015). Unacknowledged rape: The influences of child sexual abuse and personality traits. *Journal of Child Sexual Abuse, 24*(8), 975–990. https://doi.org/10.1080/10538712.2015.1082002.

Woo, C., & Brown, E. (2013). Role of meaning in the prediction of depressive symptoms among trauma-exposed & nontrauma-exposed emerging adults. *Journal of Clinical Psychology, 69*(12), 1269–1283. https://doi.org/10.1002/jclp.22002.

Wright, C., & Gabriel, L. (2018). Perspectives of adult survivors of child sexual abuse: An exploration of the adjustments to self-structure through meaning-making in therapy. *Journal of Child Sexual Abuse, 27*(6), 663–681. https://doi.org/10.1080/10538712.2018.1496961.

Zawahir, N., & Scudder, L. (2012, January 26). PTSD: Principles of diagnosis and treatment. http://www.medscape.org.

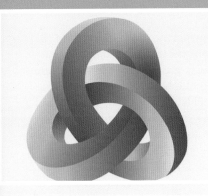

34

Children and Adolescents

Jonathan S. Dowben, Peter C. Kowalski

ⓔ http://evolve.elsevier.com/Keltner

LEARNING OBJECTIVES

- Describe the major categories of child and adolescent psychiatric disorders.
- Identify the relative frequency of serious psychiatric disorders in children and adolescents.
- Identify genetic and environmental factors associated with the development of psychiatric disorders.

- Describe the symptoms of selected child and adolescent psychiatric disorders.
- Identify principles of nursing intervention with child and adolescent psychiatric patients.

The major diagnostic categories that can occur in childhood and adolescence are discussed in this chapter. These include attention-deficit/hyperactivity disorder (ADHD), oppositional defiant disorder (ODD), conduct disorder, depression, disruptive mood dysregulation disorder (DMDD), bipolar disorder (BPD), anxiety type disorders, and autism spectrum disorder (ASD). The phenomenon of bullying is also reviewed. In addition to the above disorders, intellectual disabilities, learning disorders, suicidality, posttraumatic stress disorder (PTSD), tic disorders, and eating disorders are briefly mentioned. Also, the impact of COVID-19 on children's mental health, online relationships and social isolation, pathological computer use, and transgenderism will be discussed. Substance use disorders and addictions, early-onset schizophrenia and psychotic disorder, reactive attachment disorder, gender dysphoria and nonconformity, psychiatric aspects of chronic physical disorders, extreme cases of aggression and violence, and psychiatric emergencies are best left to more in-depth discussion in subsequent courses.

Children are our future. Few things are more upsetting for a parent than a child with a health problem. Many parents tend to readily accept a child's health difficulty when it is attributable to physical illness or injury. An emotional health problem which may be due in part to family genetics and/or exacerbated by adverse family circumstances, including divorce, inconsistent parenting, unsafe home environment, or maternal substance abuse during pregnancy, may be hard for many parents to accept. Children, like adults, often have comorbid emotional health concerns. Vulnerability to psychiatric disorders is a complex interaction between genetic,

biologic, and environmental factors, as is poignantly exemplified in the vignette of Sam, who has a history that is not that uncommon for many youngsters who are seen in outpatient clinic settings.

Some children are more resilient when exposed to early environmental adversities, such as family emotional and/or physical health concerns, parental addiction, poverty, poor educational opportunities, or placement in foster care, while other children will do less well, and will continue to have problematic if not tragic lives as adults. The concept of resilience accounts for why all vulnerable children do not develop mental disorders (Geschwind et al., 2010). Both individual and family factors work together to create resilience, including a more easy-going temperament, the ability to form supportive relationships with peers and adults, family resources, and emotional intelligence (the capacity to delay gratification and understand other people's signals) (Miller-Lewis et al., 2013). Adverse childhood experiences tend to shape mental health into adulthood. Childhood adversities such as parental mental illness, addiction, criminality, and physical and sexual abuse are known to be strongly associated with later psychiatric disorders (Green et al., 2010). Multiple hardships increase the risk; about 45% of all childhood-onset psychiatric disorders are associated with the presence of multiple childhood adversities (Green et al., 2010). The onset of other mental disorders later in life is also associated with childhood adversities. The presence of multiple childhood hardships is also associated with more adult physical health problems and earlier death. Conversely, a childhood free of trauma and abuse is associated with greater overall physical and mental health. An example of how the effects

SAM'S STORY

Sam, a 10-year-old male third grader, is irritable, "moody," and prone to fighting with peers at school and in after-school care. He is frequently aggressive toward his three siblings and half-siblings. His family's dogs and cat avoid him, as Sam tends to "play roughly" with them and has harmed them in the past. Sam was brought to the outpatient clinic on an emergent basis because earlier in the day his mother was asked to pick him up from school after he had turned over many desks and chairs in his classroom, resulting in the destruction of many of his classmates' possessions and school projects. Sam claimed that he did this because his teacher had made him angry when she asked him about some missing assignments. Sam performs poorly in school, receives speech therapy for difficulties with word pronunciation, and has been diagnosed with a reading disorder per psychoeducational testing that he received through his school.

Sam is in basic good physical health, but does have some motor tics, including tendencies to blink his eyes and make repetitive lip smacking and arm flinching movements, particularly when he is under stress. He still tends to wet the bed at night, so it is awkward for him to visit overnight with friends or relatives. Sam has been diagnosed with ADHD and ODD by his family physician, in addition to having a motor tic disorder and nocturnal enuresis (bedwetting). Sam's parents are divorced and his mother struggles to balance her employment with serving as primary caregiver for Sam and his siblings. Sam's father, who provides little economic support for Sam and his older brother, lives 400 miles away, and last had contact with Sam by telephone more than a year ago. His father is a high school dropout, has been diagnosed with Borderline Personality Disorder, and has an extensive history of substance abuse, including marijuana, methamphetamines, and alcohol. He had been diagnosed with ADHD and motor and vocal tics as a child. Sam's mother is currently receiving pharmacotherapy for depression and anxiety. She reported childhood symptoms consistent with ADHD as a child, although she was never diagnosed with ADHD. She also reported difficulties with bedwetting until she was 12 years old. Sam's extensive maternal and paternal family history of mental health concerns includes mood and anxiety disorders, substance abuse, ADHD, and learning difficulties. Sam has not been physically or sexually abused, but he did witness his father beating his mother on multiple occasions as a young child. His parents grew up in a poor neighborhood, met, and married as teenagers. Sam's two younger siblings are a product of a non-marital relationship that his mother had with a man who also physically abused her in Sam's presence.

CRITICAL THINKING QUESTION

1. What additional information would help you understand this case (hint: prenatal history)? Maternal smoking and adversity have been established as risk factors for ADHD (Pliszka, 2016). What possible diagnoses may best describe Sam's situation? What are some interventions that might help Sam and his family?

of trauma persist into young adulthood is illustrated in the accompanying box. Increasing numbers of grandparents are raising children when parents are unable to provide care (Engstrom, 2012). Growing numbers of children are biracial and multiethnic (Rosenblatt, 2013). Gay, lesbian, and transgender parents are also increasingly involved in raising children. It was claimed that children in gender-variant families fare as well as those raised with traditional heterosexual parents (Biblarz & Savci, 2010; Green, 2012). Further review of this research contradicted this assertion, as 26 of the 59 studies on same-sex parenting had no heterosexual comparison groups (Marks, 2012). According to Biblarz & Savci, 2010, the parents alone provided subjective judgments as data, and knew the purpose of the study, leading to social desirability bias.

The recent emergence of gender dysphoria or transgenderism as it relates to younger children deserves wider exploration. In spite of wider acceptance of puberty blocking in early stages of puberty, very little is known about the physical and emotional effects of this experiment in later life. Self-reports of gender identity in adolescents and young adults suggest that only 0.17% to 1.3% of adolescents and young adults identify as transgender (Connolly, Zervos, Barone, Johnson, & Joseph, 2016; Zucker, 2017). In a Swedish nationwide long-term follow-up study of adults who have legal and medical sexual reassignment, psychiatric morbidity, suicide attempts, and suicide mortality remained elevated even after these interventions (Dhejne et al., 2011). Based on prospective follow-up studies from childhood to adolescence, for approximately 80% of children who meet the criteria for gender dysphoria, symptoms of gender dysphoria recede with puberty (Ristori & Steensma, 2016). Gender identity is fluid and changes over the course of development. Biomedical transition to lifelong and irreparable physiological changes without adequate knowledge of need and consequences is unwise in spite of the current social and political climate.

The emergence of severe acute respiratory syndrome coronavirus 2 (SARS-CoV-2) from Wuhan, China in December 2019 led to a worldwide pandemic which has and will have lasting effects on children's mental health. Among the current manifestations are increases in depression and suicides, anxiety, substance and alcohol use, and PTSD and other trauma-related disorders (Brown et al., 2020; Cénat & Dalexis, 2020; Guessoum et al., 2020). Younger children show more dependency, separation anxiety, inattentiveness, disturbed sleep, and poor appetite. Many of them are at greater risk of experiencing multiple traumas such as physical, sexual, and psychological violence; emotional neglect; exposure to parental violence; social isolation; alcoholism; drug addiction; and mental illness of a parent, as well as food insecurity. Because of the disruption of education and physical and social activities, boredom and diminished affect have set in. The long-term effects of over 1 year's substitution of online classes are at present unclear, but difficulties in re-engaging in normal schoolwork have already emerged after re-entry into normal classrooms. Older adolescents have become increasingly anxious over the postponement of athletic events and delays in taking qualifying examinations for college and post-high school vocational training. Internet overuse has been associated with a rise in cyberbullying (see section "Bullying" below). Because of lack of contact with school and other authorities, children and adolescents have had less opportunity to report domestic violence, abuse, and neglect. Because of reduced contact with specialized teachers and therapists, parents have had to cope with a loss of structure and routine with their special needs children. Regression, temper outbursts, and conflicts and aggression toward family members have risen. Children with obsessive compulsive disorder (OCD) may have been greatly affected considering issues over contamination, hoarding, and getting sick. Suicide rates have risen for everyone. Youth suicide was already at a record high before the pandemic. It is the second leading cause of death for 10- to 24-year-olds.

Nurses should be alert to behavioral changes during and after the pandemic: more isolation; changes in sleeping or eating; crying episodes; increased conflicts and irritability; substance and alcohol use; restlessness or agitation; unexplained headache, stomachache, or other somatization symptoms; decrease in school performance; worsened hygiene and appearance; sad or depressed affect; reports of feeling hopeless and worthless or of feeling down or depressed; and statements that suggest that life is not worth living anymore, death fantasies, and particularly thoughts of suicide.

Pathological computer use has been described by many terms such as Internet Addiction Disorder or Compulsive Internet Use. In an appendix, *DSM-5* includes Internet Gaming Disorder as a potential new diagnosis. It is defined as the excessive use of computers or other devices that provide the user access to the Internet, for example, tablets and smartphones, for online activities to the extent that they profoundly compromise daily life activities and responsibilities. In 2014, Wallace (2014) identified the following symptoms associated with IGD: overwhelming preoccupation with online activities to an extent that leads to impairment or distress; inability to limit time spent on the Internet; loss of other interests; the need to spend increasing time on the Internet; unsuccessful attempt to quit Internet use; use of the Internet to improve or escape aversive conditions such as stress, unfavorable duties, and dysphoric mood; and withdrawal symptoms when the Internet is no longer available. Depression and low self-esteem are risk factors for this condition. Other developments include social isolation and the use of social media as proxy for real-life personal relationships. Online environments are often designed with powerful reinforcements like variable ratio (the number of responses needed for a reward varies) and partial reinforcement schedules (also referred to as intermittent reinforcement, whereby the person does not get reinforced every time they perform the desired behavior). These ensure high, steady, and persistent rate of play, to keep children and adolescents playing and to sell in-game products for extraordinary profit for game developers. Treatment approaches vary, ranging from cognitive behavioral therapies and counseling to the use of drugs normally used to treat conditions such as ADHD or depression. Alarm clocks and specific goal setting for controlling Internet use are also promising tools. Solid research on effective treatment is still lacking and clinicians are relying on techniques used to treat other addictions.

COMMON PSYCHIATRIC DISORDERS IN CHILDREN AND ADOLESCENTS

Attention-Deficit/Hyperactivity Disorder

ADHD is a disorder marked by an enduring pattern of inattention and/or hyperactivity-impulsivity that interferes with functioning or development (NIMH, n.d. ADHD). It is often comorbid with other prominent mental health disorders, such as ODD, conduct disorder, anxiety disorders, including obsessive-compulsive disorder (OCD), major depressive disorder, bipolar disorder, tic disorder, Tourette's, and substance use disorders. Children who have ADHD frequently have difficulties with performance in the academic setting, may have one or more specific learning disorders, and may have enuresis. The hallmark symptoms of ADHD are prominent and persistent (6 months or longer) difficulties with diminished attention, motor hyperactivity, and impulsivity. Some individuals may manifest all three hallmark symptoms, while others may only have difficulties with inattention or hyperactive and impulsive type symptoms. Often, symptoms of hyperactivity and impulsivity may diminish in outward observation by others as an individual grows and matures. ADHD symptoms must be present by at least the age of 12 and impact social, academic, and/or occupational performance functioning in two or more distinct settings to a significant degree, and are not better explained by another mental health disorder in order for this diagnosis to be made (American Psychiatric Association, 2013).

ADHD is probably the most common childhood psychiatric disorder. The worldwide prevalence rate of ADHD is estimated to be from 5% to 29% (Posner et al., 2020). According to the Centers for Disease Control and Prevention (CDC), 10.2% of all U.S. children 5 to 17 years of age (14.1% of boys and 6.2% of girls) were diagnosed with ADHD in 2012–14 (Centers for Disease Control and Prevention, 2017). The 2011 National Survey of Children's Health performed telephone interviews of nearly 100,000 parents. Medication use increased by 28% from 2003 to 2011. In 2007, fewer than half of children were taking medication. The increase in medication use reflects growing recognition and treatment of the disorder (Visser et al., 2014).

A variety of ADHD rating scales exist, including the widely used, downloadable National Institute for Children's Health Quality (NICHQ) Vanderbilt Assessment Scale, which is a screening instrument not only for ADHD (children ages 6 to 12), but also for the comorbid emotional concerns of ODD, conduct disorder, anxiety, and depression. There are two separate versions of the Vanderbilt Assessment Scale, one for parents and the other for teachers, so that the impact of ADHD symptoms on performance in two different settings, home and school, may be assessed. Treatment for ADHD often involves parent education; the involvement of school in terms of extra assistance, modifications, or other accommodations in teaching and testing when appropriate; and the appropriate use of medication. Nonpharmacologic interventions are often useful in managing symptoms. Some examples include frequent breaks, verbal or written feedback on a regular basis, consistent and immediate consequences for unacceptable behaviors, and daily visual reminders that prioritize assignments and schedules (Mason & Joshi, 2018).

Clinical Example: Attention-deficit/hyperactivity disorder

Kyle is an 8-year-old boy with a diagnosis of ADHD. He is in the second grade and presents to the psychiatric nurse practitioner for follow-up care. He lives with both of his biological parents and two older siblings, a brother, age 14, and a sister, age 16. Both his mother and older brother have been diagnosed with ADHD and are known to respond well to stimulant medications for treatment of their own ADHD symptoms. Kyle was initially referred to the clinic per the recommendation of his school psychologist. Kyle was fidgety, could not sit still for long, often talked out of turn in class, and performed academically well below what his standardized test scores predicted. He was initially prescribed a methylphenidate long-acting 10 mg (Ritalin LA) capsule in the morning, and after 2 months his dose of Ritalin LA was increased to a 20 mg capsule in the morning for treatment of continued ADHD symptoms.

During their third clinic visit, Kyle's father stated, "He's doing somewhat better in terms of his grades, but he continues to have difficulty sitting still in school and at the dinner table at home. We get frequent emails from his teacher reporting that while Kyle is friendly and well liked, he tends to be the 'class clown' and continues to bother the other students when they are trying to complete their assignments." Kyle's grades dramatically improved after his school made an accommodation to administer testing in a distraction-free area and a behavior modification plan in coordination with his parents. Kyle was then able to earn frequent small rewards when he behaved well at home and school. For the past month, Kyle has been receiving regular tutoring which has improved his retention and learning. His family also displays prominently posted weekly reminders of school assignments and chores at home. For residual hyperactivity and impulsivity at home, he started an adjunctive non-stimulant medication, guanfacine extended release 1 mg daily (Intuniv). Kyle's father contacted the clinic a month later and reported that Kyle has improved with the combination of Ritalin LA and Intuniv daily. Kyle was proud to be asked by his teacher and school principal to make the morning school broadcast because of his improvements.

Oppositional Defiant Disorder and Conduct Disorder

ODD in children and adolescents is defined as a pattern of the following angry/irritable mood symptoms: (1) often loses temper, (2) often touchy or easily annoyed, (3) often angry and resentful, (4) often argumentative/defiant, (5) often argues with adults, (6) often actively defies or refuses to comply with requests from authority figures or rules, (7) often deliberately annoys others, (8) often blames others for his or her mistakes, misbehavior, or vindictiveness, and (9) has been spiteful or vindictive at least twice within the past 6 months. ODD is confirmed when four or more of the preceding symptoms are present for at least 6 months when interacting with at least one individual who is not a sibling (American Psychiatric Association, 2013). As previously mentioned, ODD is a frequent comorbid disorder with ADHD, but may also occur without ADHD being present. Youngsters who have ODD are at risk of having or developing comorbid anxiety or depression symptoms or conduct disorder.

Conduct disorder, which tends to be much more prevalent in males as compared to females, involves a persistent and repetitive pattern of behavior in which the basic rights of others or age-appropriate societal norms or rules are violated. An individual with conduct disorder typically manifests three or more of the following 15 behavioral criteria in four of the following categories: (1) Aggression toward people or animals *(bullying; fighting; has used a weapon that could cause harm [e.g., bat, bottle, knife or gun]; cruelty to people; cruelty to animals; has stolen while confronting a victim [e.g., mugging, purse snatching or armed robbery]; has forced someone to engage in sex activity);* (2) Destruction of property *(deliberate fire setting with the intent to cause serious damage; deliberate destruction of property not involving the use of fire);* (3) Deceitfulness or theft *(has broken into someone's home, building, or car; lies to obtain goods, favors, or avoid obligations; has stolen items of nontrivial value without confronting a victim, [e.g., by shoplifting]);* (4) Serious violation of rules *(often stays out at night, despite parental prohibitions, beginning before the age of 13; has run away from home overnight at least twice when living in parental or parental surrogate home, or once without returning after a lengthy period of time; is often truant from school beginning before the age of 13)* (American Psychiatric Association, 2013). Individuals with conduct disorder are at an increased risk of developing significant substance use difficulties and antisocial personality disorder.

Depression

Both unipolar and bipolar depression occur often in children. The total number of teenagers who reported depressive symptoms increased 59% between 2007 and 2017. The rate of growth was faster for teen girls (66%) than for boys (44%) (Geiger & Davis, 2019). Girls are more likely to rely on close emotional communication and responsiveness as a source of self-definition; extreme concern about social evaluations by others may contribute to higher rates of depressive symptoms in girls. Higher rates of depression and anxiety also occur in women.

Similar to adults, youth with major depression may experience feelings of helplessness, hopelessness, low energy, and social withdrawal. The hallmark symptom of depression for younger children is frequent irritability. Suicidal ideation is prevalent in depressed children and youth, and suicide is the third leading cause of death among adolescents (Thapar et al., 2012). Rates of suicide by youth continue to increase, and Internet bullying has been associated with increased risk of suicide (John et al., 2018).

Clinical Example: Depression and a burgeoning eating disorder

"I've been depressed since I lost my boyfriend, and my mom thought I should see someone." Sara is a 17-year-old high school junior who presents with complaints of depression. Her mother accompanies her to see the nurse. Sara states that she has been doing poorly in school. She had been a straight "A" honor roll student and member of the varsity tennis team prior to her losing her boyfriend 6 months ago, but now she is receiving "Ds" and "Fs" and quit the tennis team. Sara states that she finds it difficult to concentrate and focus on her schoolwork. However, Sara's mother indicates that Sara has been creating color-coded charts detailing the foods that she has eaten and her caloric intake at every meal since the week of her breakup. A review of medical records from the patient's PCM indicates that Sara has lost 30 pounds over the past half year and her BMI has dropped from 22 to 15, which is underweight. She is also experiencing amenorrhea. Her mother also reports periods of extreme sullenness and tendencies to isolate herself, which is not characteristic of Sara. Mother has heard Sara "throw up" in the bathroom following many evening meals for the past month or so. According to her mother, Sara's problems started about 1 year ago when she started dating a popular 18-year-old high school senior varsity football player and track star named Tobey, and became sexually active with him. When Sara discovered 6 months ago that Tobey had cheated on her and had gone out with her best friend, Cassie, a thin, attractive, and popular girl on the cheerleader squad whom she had known since sixth grade, Sara became depressed. She began fervently dieting and playing tennis or working out at the gym for up to 3h every day in an attempt to win back Tobey. But he had moved on, and she had also lost her best friend in whom she had previously confided her love for Tobey and intimate details of their sexual activities. The nurse initiated Sara on fluoxetine (Prozac), and over several weeks increased her dose of Prozac up to 40 mg po qam in order to treat both symptoms of depression and a burgeoning eating disorder. She also placed a consult to a nutritionist with some expertise in working with primary care physicians in managing patients with eating disorders.

❓ CRITICAL THINKING QUESTION

2. If your child had a mental health problem that required hospitalization, what questions would you ask of the staff? What would you look for in the environment? What would be reasonable treatment goals as determined mutually by parents and members of the treatment team?

Bipolar Disorder and Disruptive Mood Dysregulation Disorder

Bipolar disorder (BPD) in childhood is characterized by extreme changes in mood and behavior. In the manic phase, children feel very happy or "up" and are much more energetic and active than usual. In the depressive phase, children feel very sad or "down" and are much less active than usual. The mood changes in BPD are accompanied by changes in sleep, energy level, and the ability to think clearly. The extreme changes in mood can make it hard for young people to perform well in school or to get along with friends and family members (NIMH, n.d. Bipolar disorder in children and youth). BPD in children differs from the adult type in that irritability is a more prominent symptom. As children mature, approaching the later teen years, bipolar symptoms begin to conform more to symptoms experienced by adults. Mood instability, temper tantrums, and impulsivity may gradually morph into grandiosity, hypersexuality, and intrusive behavior.

Clinical Example: Bipolar disorder

Ian is a 10-year-old boy who was admitted to the hospital because he says that "If I can't have friends, I would rather be dead." He has trouble getting along with peers at school, yet frequently worries about "people not liking" him and "not having any friends." He has prominent difficulties with paying attention and has greater difficulties than all the other children in his class with staying in his seat and not talking. He is a fourth grader and has been involved in frequent fights at school. He is impulsive and also engages in frequent reckless and risk-taking behaviors, such as climbing out of his bedroom window and dancing on the roof of the two-story family home. He sleeps very little at night and has been known to stay up for 36h without obtaining any sleep at all. He has recently endorsed that he often sees a vampire with "bloody teeth," which he believes may be his deceased paternal grandfather, stare at him in his bedroom window; particularly on those occasions he has gone with little or no sleep. He was brought to the hospital by the sheriff's department after he had gotten into a major physical altercation at school for which police were summoned. Ian currently lives with his biologic mother and a 12-year-old half-sister. He has no contact with his biologic father, who has a history of BPD and schizophrenia. After a thorough workup, Ian is given a diagnosis of ADHD and BPD.

The clinical example featuring Ian depicts what is often observed clinically: BPD and ADHD may look alike and overlap in presentation. Ian was given a diagnosis of both ADHD and BPD. There are also symptoms that suggest depression (he would rather be dead) and anxiety (worrying about people not liking him and having no friends). Because of this array of symptoms, numerous medications might be considered. In Ian's case, his nurse practitioner prescribed a drug for impulse control (clonidine), a drug for ADHD (methylphenidate [Concerta]), a drug for mood instability (oxcarbazepine [Trileptal]), and a drug for aggression and unrealistic thinking (risperidone [Risperdal]). Although this medication regimen is well meaning and may be exactly the combination that is needed, it can also cause Ian other problems. For example, in a child with BPD, drugs to elevate a depressed mood or to control hyperactivity might have paradoxical responses and result in extreme irritability, mania, or even psychotic-type symptoms. In other words, antidepressants can cause the expression of BPD (McNamara et al., 2012). It has also been shown, at least anecdotally, that when a child does not respond to stimulants and antidepressants and when combined with a family history of bipolar illness, as in Ian's case, the clinician should consider BPD as the primary cause.

The diagnosis of disruptive mood dysregulation disorder (DMDD) was established in *DSM-5* to help account for youngsters who are very irritable or angry much of the day, nearly every day, and who have severe recurrent temper outbursts that may be manifested verbally and/or physically and who do not meet criteria for having major depression or BPD. The diagnosis of DMDD may not be made for the first time in children younger than age 6 or teenagers older than 18. Onset of DMDD symptoms must take place prior to age 10. Persistent manic or hypomanic symptoms preclude the diagnosis of DMDD. The diagnosis of ODD may not be made in youngsters with DMDD (American Psychiatric Association, 2013). However, the diagnosis of DMDD may co-occur with the diagnosis of ADHD, conduct disorder, and even a substance use disorder.

 CRITICAL THINKING QUESTION

3. Many people are very concerned about the increased numbers of children and adolescents diagnosed with ADHD and pediatric BPD and debate potential causes. These concerns/debates are as current as the morning paper. What explanations seem to make most sense to you?

Anxiety Disorders

Anxiety disorders are among the most common psychiatric disorders in children and adolescents. The lifetime prevalence of any anxiety disorder in children and adolescents is between 15% and 32% (Essau & Gabbidon, 2013). Childhood-onset anxiety disorders foreshadow adult anxiety disorders (Rockhill et al., 2010) and are thought to be caused by genetic and environmental factors. Pediatric OCD involves recurring thoughts (obsessions) and repetitive ritualistic behaviors (compulsions) in an effort to decrease anxiety. Perfectionism, intolerance for uncertainty, and overestimation of threats are cognitive beliefs that perpetuate OCD (Jacob & Storch, 2013). Pediatric OCD is often associated with other tic disorders (i.e., Tourette's), depression, and ADHD.

Symptoms of PTSD in children are similar to the symptoms in adults and include nightmares, intrusive memories, and hypervigilance (Wu et al., 2010). PTSD can be caused by a single traumatic event, such as an automobile accident, or long-term sexual/physical/emotional abuse, either as the victim of abuse or as a helpless bystander witnessing the abuse of a parent or another family member. *Therefore, a child who observed repeated beatings of his mother should be evaluated for PTSD.* The greater the magnitude of the stressor, the more likely the child will develop PTSD. For example, a child who has experienced a major natural disaster in which the child's life was in danger and home and family members were lost has a substantial risk for developing PTSD.

Other anxiety disorders, such as separation anxiety disorder, social anxiety disorder, and panic disorder, all may appear in childhood. Anxiety disorders are underdiagnosed and undertreated in children (Walkup, 2017). Harsh parenting, stressful life events, and a genetic predisposition increase vulnerability to anxiety disorders.

Clinical Example: Anxiety and panic disorder

"I'm having a lot of anxiety and an upset stomach every day I'm at school. I feel so uncomfortable in class sometimes that I can't breathe and have even fainted. I can't go to any of the sports events at my school because there are too many people, and I might faint. My heart keeps racing, particularly when I have to answer a question in class." Becky is a 17-year-old girl who has panic attacks and anxiety. She reports being this way since she was in third grade when her mother deployed to Afghanistan, and she was cared for by her maternal aunt. In the past, her anxiety has been manageable and did not greatly impair her ability to function at school up until she entered sixth grade, began menstruating, and was bullied by some "mean girls" at school. She is now a senior and has done well enough to remain on the honor roll. Until recently, Becky's panic attacks occurred about once per month. Recently the attacks have increased in frequency and intensity and are occurring two to three times per week, sometimes requiring Becky to leave school. Becky reports that she worries about everything. She cannot sit still. Her legs seldom stop shaking, and she changes positions nonstop. Occasionally, when meeting with the nurse practitioner at the outpatient clinic, she cannot even remain in her seat. She is up and down, pacing back and forth. She says, "Sometimes staying in my seat, especially when other people are looking at me drives me crazy." She states that sometimes getting up and moving seems like a matter of life and death to her. Her panic symptoms include sweating, a choking feeling, a racing heart, a feeling of tightness in her chest, a fear that she will "lose control or even die." Sometimes she "can't breathe" and senses tingling in her body. She will only go to the grocery store after 11 P.M., just before it closes at midnight, because that is when it is least crowded. She is no longer able to take the bus to school, and relies on being dropped off by her mother, and taking a cab home if a friend can't give her a ride. She worries about causing an accident and so will not sign up to take driver's education. Becky's nurse practitioner recently diagnosed her with Panic Disorder and Agoraphobia (now separate conditions as defined by the *DSM-5*). Becky had been previously diagnosed with Separation Anxiety Disorder when she was younger. The nurse practitioner prescribes sertraline (Zoloft) 25 mg/day for 2 weeks, with an increase to 50 mg/day thereafter. Emotionally focused therapy (EFT) was also recommended.

Autism Spectrum Disorder

Significant changes occurred in the definition of autism when *DSM-5* was published in 2013 and Autism Spectrum Disorder became the overarching diagnosis, which included autistic disorder, Asperger disorder, and pervasive developmental disorder not otherwise specified. The updated criteria that must be met for the *DSM-5* are as follows: (a) persistent deficits in social communication and interaction across multiple contexts; (b) restricted and repetitive behaviors, interests, or activities; (c) symptoms must be present early in childhood (but may be delayed to a later age when social demands exceed the limits of the patient); and (d) symptoms cause significant impairment in social, occupational, or other areas of current functioning. The severity of symptoms in social communication and restricted interests/repetitive behaviors is to be designated in terms of the level of support that a patient needs: Level 1—requiring support; Level 2—requiring substantial support; and Level 3—requiring very substantial support. The following additional specifiers are to also be given when applicable: with or without accompanying intellectual impairment; with or without accompanying language impairment; associated with a known medical or genetic condition or environmental factor; and associated with another neurodevelopmental, mental, or behavior disorder (American Psychiatric Association, 2013). Commonly occurring comorbid disorders with ASD include ADHD, depression, and anxiety. It is also fairly common for a patient with ASD to also have a seizure disorder.

As of March 2018, the CDC estimated the prevalence of ASD as 1 in 57 for school-aged children. ASD occurs much more frequently in males than females. In recent years there has been an increase noted in the prevalence of ASD. Whether this increase could be due in part to better assessment methods, changing diagnostic criteria, or other factors is a subject for debate. ASD has historically been associated with genetic causes or nongenetic causes such as the MMR immunization. But a recent trend also shows an increasing interest in potential environmental triggers to understand the elusive disorder more so than ever before (Gyawali & Patra, 2019).

Clinical Example: Autism spectrum disorder

Eddy is a 10-year-old boy with moderate ASD. He was initially diagnosed with ASD at the age of 3. Eddy's mother recalls that she experienced her pregnancy with Eddy to be different and to have felt something was "not quite right" as compared with her other two pregnancies with Eddy's two older siblings, ages 12 and 14. Eddy has limited face-to-face gaze. His speech is somewhat awkward, and he sometimes utters some words, phrases, or sounds repetitively, much like a parrot. He tends to flap his hands when stressed. He likes to collect toy planes, and frequently lines them up and becomes upset if his planes are moved. There are only four food items that he will eat, and all are crunchy: chicken nuggets, potato chips, Honeycrisp apples, and uncooked carrots. He has some difficulties sleeping through the night and does not like changes in his customary routines. Certain textures bother him, such that when he was younger he refused to touch or use toilet paper when he defecated and screamed when touched by water. In addition to ASD, Eddy has been diagnosed with having a mild intellectual disability and ADHD due to prominent difficulties that he has with maintaining attention, motoric hyperactivity, and tendencies to be impulsive. He has been making improvements in terms of being around other children, including his siblings, and interacting with new people whom he meets since the family has been involved in Emotionally Focused Family Therapy. Parental training that includes emotional attunement is helpful to him when he becomes upset, screams, and throw fits. In addition, his parents can prepare him beforehand when subtle changes in routine take place at home, such as his siblings having a friend over to play. Eddy also now looks forward to attending school each day, as it has become part of his daily routine.

? CRITICAL THINKING QUESTION

4. As noted, the idea that childhood immunizations (MMR) may have caused autism has not been supported by research findings. However, many parents believe that these immunizations were the culprit and refuse inoculations for their other children. What is the scientific evidence on this issue? How would you discuss the need for immunizations with parents who fear that immunizations might lead to autism?

BULLYING

Who hasn't heard of bullying? Most of us have seen it happen, known someone who has been bullied, or even been bullied ourselves as children. *(Hopefully, not one of us was a bully.)* The study of bullying began after three boys who had been targeted by bullies committed suicide in Norway in 1983. Olweus (1993) was commissioned by the Norwegian government to study the trend of bullying, and during his research, he found that 20% of Norwegian children had been bullied. Since he completed his work, many other studies have been published, leading to a better understanding of the prevalence, etiology, and potential remediation of bullying behavior. However, bullying has increased in magnitude, and with the ever-present Internet, bullying can occur any time of the day or night.

Bullying can be defined as the repeated negative actions of one or more individuals toward a victim. Bullying usually entails a systematic abuse of power involving repetition, harm, and unequal power. Playful teasing, one-time aggression, and joking are not bullying; the crucial elements of bullying are that it is intentionally cruel and unprovoked. Surprisingly, bullies can have friends and followers, and bullying can become a social activity. Youth who are being bullied often visit the school nurse's office because of somatic symptoms, and the bullying goes unrecognized unless the nurse understands its devastating impact. Complaints of bullying made to school authorities are often few, and the true number of incidents is likely underreported.

Verbal bullying is the most frequent type of bullying, with name calling and derogatory remarks being most common. Racial and gender slurs are often components of the verbal assaults. *Slander* (defined as malicious, untrue statements) and *name calling* are the most common bullying methods. *Relational bullying* involves shunning and ignoring the victim. The goal is to disrupt shared relationships between peers and is more common among girls than boys. Because of its indirect nature, relational bullying may go unrecognized by parents and teachers. The victim experiences isolation and humiliation.

Physical bullying can range from slight shoving to burns and broken bones. An obvious physical attack at school usually is addressed by a principal, but physical bullying also occurs after school in other locales. The U.S. Secret Service investigated 37 acts of targeted school violence (including Columbine in 1999) and found that three-quarters of the attackers (29) had been physically bullied, attacked, or injured by others (usually just before the shooting incidents; Vossekuil, Fein, Reddy, Borum, & Modzcleski, 2004). Some cases involved chronic, severe bullying in which the threats directly contributed to the decision to target the school and demand revenge. In witness statements from one incident, "schoolmates alleged that nearly every child in the school at some point had thrown the attacker against a locker, tripped him in the hall, held his head under water in the pool, or thrown things at him" (Vossekuil, Fein, Reddy, Borum, & Modzcleski, 2004, p. 21).

Cyberbullying is the newest type of bullying and currently receives the most media attention. It can be defined as any form of abusive behavior in cyberspace (Ioannou et al., 2018). Prevalence rates of cyberbullying indicate that upwards of 72% of middle and high school youth are affected in the United States (Selkie et al., 2016). These messages may take the form of private text messages or e-mails being forwarded; pictures being posted without permission (especially unbecoming or embarrassing photos); and rumors being spread via e-mails, text messages, or social networking websites. Facebook and other social networking websites have exponentially grown; tens of millions of Internet users visit these websites daily. Previously contained in the hallways of schools, bullying has become omnipresent and promises to become an even greater threat to the emotional well-being of youth. Cyberbullying has been found to be associated with physical and mental health problems including depression, suicidality, substance use, and somatic symptoms. The media has taken notice of cyberbullying more recently because of the increase in suicidal thoughts, attempts, and completions that have occurred as the result of electronic bullying activity (Selkie et al, 2016).

Although bullying can never be totally prevented, nurses can take action by understanding that bullying can be a regular occurrence. In addition, nurses can take a stand against bullying. Although some schools say they have a "zero tolerance policy for bullying," the policy may refer only to physical aggression and not to more subtle relational- and cyber-bullying. Nurses can and should educate teachers, administrators, and parents about the realities (frequency and types) of bullying because it can happen in any school setting, does untold damage, and ultimately may result in violence and even suicide.

Clinical Example: Bullied to death
Bullied student kills herself leaping from I-65 overpass
Jemison, Alabama

The father of a Jemison teen who took her life by jumping from an interstate overpass in Chilton County said the family is devastated by the loss and the belief that bullying may have led to her suicide.

"I'm just so sad, you wouldn't believe," Jim Moore said. "We knew she had been picked on some, but we thought it had been dealt with."

Alex Moore, a sophomore at Jemison High School, leaped onto Interstate 65 from a bridge near her home just before 7 A.M. Wednesday. She was pronounced dead on the scene, said Chilton County Coroner Randall M. Yeargen.

She had walked to the overpass after her parents went to work. A Christian, Alex left a note saying she was going to see Jesus.

Moore said his 15-year-old daughter was sometimes teased about her appearance, mainly her weight.

By Carol Robinson, news staff writer, *Birmingham News,* Friday, May 14, 2010, p. 1C.

PSYCHOTHERAPEUTIC MANAGEMENT

This chapter has provided glimpses into some of the mental health issues confronted by children and adolescents and their families. The nurse, as with other patients, has three tools: the relationship with the patient and family (Me), medications (Meds), and the environment (Milieu). A general overview of these tools is provided.

Nurse-Patient Relationship for Patients and Families—Me

When nurses work with children who receive psychiatric care and their families, an important goal is mental health literacy. Ignorance abounds when it comes to psychiatric disorders in children; often parents feel stigmatized by the experience of seeking help for their child's mental illness. These children are not just overly energetic youth who test their parental limits. For the most severely mentally ill children, some parents have made the difficult decision to temporarily or permanently terminate their parental rights. The gradual closing of child/adolescent psychiatric services and general unavailability of care in recent decades have led to child welfare authorities becoming custodians of many youth with serious psychiatric disorders. Many inpatient and residential mental health services have been closed in the past 20 years. Steep decreases in the reimbursement for residential treatment for children have led to these closures. Where residential facilities remain, they serve the most seriously mentally ill youth with public funds supporting the treatment costs. The trend toward psychotropic medications for youth as the primary treatment strategy has caused a shift toward medication-based outpatient treatment as a cost-containment strategy. In some locales, there is a 9-month wait for a medication evaluation.

Psychopharmacology—Meds

Psychopharmacology is not the only intervention for mental disorders of childhood, but it remains a major avenue utilized with most of these patients. Relatively few drug trials have focused on neuropsychiatric disorders in children, and the trials that do exist provide evidence for only a fraction of available drugs used for treatment of these conditions (Murthy, Mandl, & Bourgeois, 2013). This chapter is not meant to substitute for a textbook dedicated to child and adolescent psychiatric nursing, so the student is referred to such a specialty book for very specific information. The medication discussion that follows is meant to provide general information for students who may work with child and adolescent psychiatric patients during their psychiatric nursing clinical rotation. Box 34.1 presents a basic philosophy of care. When dealing with this age group, it is important to be conservative in one's approach to medications. Box 34.2 reinforces the need to work with families and adult caregivers.

Drugs for Depression

SAMHSA's 2017 National Survey on Drug Use and Health reviewed treatment received within the past year by U.S. adolescents ages 12 to 17 with Major Depressive Episode.

It is best to limit the number of psychiatric medications prescribed as much as is reasonably possible, in order both to increase the likelihood of patient compliance and to decrease the likelihood of medication interactions and side effects. When possible, the prescriber should make only one change in medication at a time, whether the goal is to add a new medication, to change the amount or frequency of an existing medication, or to discontinue an existing medication. Prescribing medication can be likened to cooking. Much like the skilled cook, the experienced prescriber may successfully fine-tune the recipe with a slight modification, but the wholesale alteration of a recipe often proves to be disastrous.

An important component of psychopharmacologic treatment of children and adolescents is engagement of the adult caregiving team. Unlike adult patients, children and adolescents are not expected to have unsupervised access to prescription medicines. Parents, guardians, and other trusted adults often become involved in taking care of the child or adolescent, and perhaps no one is more invested in the patient's treatment than the family. Family members can be powerful allies in attempting to monitor and treat a child's mental disorder, but they may also become significant roadblocks to success. Roadblocks can be erected directly or in more indirect, passive-aggressive ways. Family members can be very instrumental in recording symptoms and in tracking symptom frequency, intensity, type, and duration.

In 2017, an estimated 2.3 million adolescents ages 12 to 17 in the United States had at least one Major Depressive Episode with severe impairment. This number represented 9.4% of the U.S. population ages 12 to 17. Among adolescents with Major Depressive Episode, approximately 70.77% had *severe* impairment. Treatment types received in 2017 included health professional only, medication only, and combined health professional and medication. An estimated 19.6% received care by a health professional alone, and another 17.9% received combined care by a health professional and medication treatment. Treatment with medication alone was least common (2.4%). *Approximately 60.1% of adolescents with Major Depressive Episode did not receive treatment.*

Many medications are available for the treatment of Major Depressive Disorder for adults (see Chapter 15). Only a few are approved for use in children and adolescents. The only drug approved by the U.S. Food and Drug Administration (FDA) for treatment of depression for children younger than 12 years old is fluoxetine (Prozac), which is approved for age 8 and above. Escitalopram (Lexapro) has been approved for treatment of depression for children age 12 years old and above. The following antidepressant medications have received approval for treatment of OCD in children:

fluoxetine (Prozac), age 7 and above; sertraline (Zoloft), age 6 and above; fluvoxamine (Luvox), age 8 and above; and clomipramine (Anafranil), age 10 and above. In addition, the antidepressant duloxetine (Cymbalta) has received approval for treatment of generalized anxiety disorder for children age 7 and older. Some of these categories of antidepressant medications are discussed briefly.

Selective serotonin reuptake inhibitors. Selective serotonin reuptake inhibitors (SSRIs) are frequently used in children and adolescents. These agents increase serotonin within the synaptic cleft over time with a resultant antidepressant effect. SSRIs include fluoxetine (Prozac), sertraline (Zoloft), paroxetine (Paxil), fluvoxamine (Luvox), citalopram (Celexa), and escitalopram (Lexapro). Fluoxetine, sertraline, and fluvoxamine have been approved to treat OCD in children, and fluoxetine has been approved to treat depression in children older than 8 years of age. As with many medications for many different conditions, drugs are often prescribed for children and adolescents off-label without FDA approval.

SSRIs can cause side effects. Although the effects are rare, children, teenagers, and young adults under 25 may experience an increase in suicidal thoughts or behavior when taking antidepressants, especially in the first few weeks after starting or when the dose is changed. This warning from the FDA indicates that patients of all ages taking antidepressants should be watched closely, especially during the first few weeks of treatment. SSRIs should be dosed in children in small amounts in the earliest phases of treatment to avoid emergent agitation. See Chapter 15 for more information on SSRIs and other antidepressants.

Tricyclic antidepressants. Tricyclic antidepressants (TCAs) have been used for decades, are inexpensive, and have multiple uses for various conditions and symptoms, including depression, anxiety, ADHD, and nocturnal enuresis. Their use has been surpassed by SSRIs because of their potential risk of fatal overdose, but also because of lapsed exclusivity patents and the extensive marketing of SSRIs. TCAs are as effective as other antidepressant classes. They may produce side effects such as dry mouth, fatigue, dizziness, sweating, weight gain, urinary retention, tremor, tachycardia, and agitation. *Because all TCAs may affect cardiac conduction, baseline cardiograms should be taken and repeated on a scheduled basis afterward.* TCAs are susceptible to drug-drug interactions and changes in serum levels. The use of serum levels helps guide dosing to achieve therapeutic goals without incurring toxicity.

Drugs for Bipolar Disorder and Disruptive Mood Dysregulation Disorder

Many drugs are available for treating BPD in children and adolescents. The medication management goals with BPD are to stabilize mood symptoms by employing antipsychotic and/or other mood stabilizing medications and to treat related symptoms, such as poor sleep. Chapter 16 provides an adult-focused review of the basic drugs used to treat this disorder.

Only four of the atypical antipsychotic medications have been approved by the FDA for treatment of BPD, manic or mixed: aripiprazole (Abilify), quetiapine (Seroquel), and risperidone (Risperdal), for ages 10 to 17, and olanzapine (Zyprexa), for ages 13 to 17 (National Center for Biotechnology Information [NCBI], 2017). Lithium has been approved for adolescents age 12 and above but its use is limited because of long-term kidney effects. Oxcarbazepine (Trileptal), valproic acid (Depakote), and other non-antipsychotic mood stabilizing agents are frequently prescribed off-label for treatment of BPD. The evidence that these medications are safe and effective in children and adolescents is more limited than in adults.

Similarly, antipsychotic and other mood stabilizing medications are used for treatment of DMDD in order to target mood and related disruptive-type behaviors. An antidepressant medication is often added for treatment of depressive symptoms.

Drugs for Anxiety Disorders

Antidepressants typically are good choices for anxiety in children and adolescents. Some SSRIs are particularly beneficial in treating OCD and Separation Anxiety Disorder. The nonbenzodiazepine buspirone (BuSpar) has been found to reduce anxiety in some young patients. The use of benzodiazepine medications for treatment of anxiety for children and teenagers is typically discouraged, given that difficulties are experienced with habituation, tolerance, and even diversion when this type of medication is prescribed.

Drugs for Attention-Deficit/Hyperactivity Disorder

The first-line medication to treat ADHD are two classes of psychostimulants: (1) methylphenidate (Ritalin), long-acting methylphenidate (Concerta), dexmethylphenidate (Focalin), and (2) dextroamphetamine with covalently attached amino acid lysine—lisdexamfetamine [Vyvanse]), plain dextroamphetamine (Dexedrine), and a mixed amphetamine salts mixture (Adderall). These medications improve attention and decrease hyperactivity by improving signal pathways within the brain. Attention and reward are enhanced by dopaminergic and noradrenergic input. By activating these neurotransmitters, presumably underused pathways to attend, concentrate, control impulsive thoughts, and control emotions are opened up. Some children and adolescents respond preferentially and are more susceptible to side effects of one class versus the other, so trials comparing the two in individuals are often warranted.

Other agents are used to treat symptoms associated with ADHD. Alpha-2 agonists that modulate noradrenaline include clonidine (Catapres, Kapvay) or guanfacine (Tenex, Intuniv). As seen in the case of Kyle earlier in the chapter, clonidine is prescribed to help control impulsive behavior. Noradrenergic reuptake inhibitors also enhance noradrenaline input and include atomoxetine (Strattera), TCAs like nortriptyline and imipramine, bupropion (Wellbutrin), and the newly released viloxazine (Qelbree).

Drugs for Autism Spectrum Disorder

There is no specific pharmacotherapy for ASD. Several medications have been used to treat ancillary symptoms of autism—symptoms that emerge from stresses and frustrations caused by ASD, such as anxiety, depression, and agitation. These include antidepressants, mood stabilizers, antianxiety medications, alpha-2 agonists, and stimulants. Atypical antipsychotics are commonly used in ASD. These drugs block both dopamine and serotonin receptors. This dual action provides a more manageable side effect profile than typical antipsychotics. These include aripiprazole (Abilify), risperidone (Risperdal), olanzapine (Zyprexa), quetiapine (Seroquel), and ziprasidone (Geodon). Atypical antipsychotics are used for psychotic thinking, aggressive behaviors, tantrums, tics, and various self-injurious behaviors. Abilify is FDA-approved for the treatment of irritability associated with ASD, for ages 6 to 17, and Risperdal has similar FDA approval, for ages 5 to 16 (NCBI, 2017). The dosage of these agents tends to be generally low. Typical antipsychotics can be used occasionally for aggressive behavior when other approaches have failed. Chapter 14 provides a thorough review of antipsychotic drugs.

Environmental Issues—Milieu

There are many environmental issues confronting psychiatric nurses, patients, and families. Some issues are more relevant for an autistic child than for a depressed adolescent. The following are some general guidelines first covered in Chapter 1 and again in Chapter 20: safety, structure, norms, limit setting, and balance.

Safety

There is no other nursing responsibility more important than safety. Think about it for just a moment and you will agree. A family entrusts their child into your care and expects that you will, above all, "do no harm." Safety concerns include physical safety such as protecting the patient from aggressive peers, harmful objects (e.g., sharps, glass items, plastic bags), and incompetent medication administration. Safety also means protecting the patient from psychological harm (e.g., ridicule, verbal abuse, or harassment). Finally—and this subject is so terrible it is difficult to broach—patients must be protected from predation by staff. Background checks are mandatory for people working with vulnerable children and adolescents.

Structure

Structure can mean the layout of the physical environment or the organization of the treatment plan. For an inpatient setting, how the unit is designed can add a therapeutic element to the patient's care. Furnishings, color selection, areas for privacy, areas for visiting, visibility of nursing staff, and visibility of patients by nurses should be carefully considered when developing the environment for children and adolescent patients. Structure and safety issues overlap. An environment where patients can get away and not be noticed is poorly designed. A well-organized treatment approach is important too. Without being overly rigid, nurses and other staff members should do what they indicate they will do when they indicate they will do it. Even when patients resist, it is therapeutic to provide the structure of doing what is supposed to be done when it is routinely expected to occur.

Norms

Norms are expectations of behavior. For example, norms of nonviolence, cleanliness, participation in chores, and participation in therapeutic activities are minimal expectations on an inpatient unit. Although some patients might resist, it is therapeutic to establish norms and enforce them. For patients who are coming from chaotic home environments, the ability to count on adults to be consistent can be enormously beneficial.

Limit Setting

Limit setting means putting "limits" on certain kinds of behaviors. In particular, acting-out behavior, self-destructive conduct, aggressiveness toward others, and inappropriate sexual actions are behaviors that are off limits on an inpatient unit. Other behaviors that might need to be limited are use of phones and texting, choice of visitors or "friends," and seclusive behaviors. Often limit setting takes the form of rules of behavior. It is important that rules be clearly communicated. No one at any age wants to be held accountable for violating an unknown rule. Some nominal levels of behavior should be expected, and nurses should not get bogged down in attempting to outline every possible deed that is unacceptable. Some adolescent patients can be particularly adept at splitting hairs. In such cases, it is probably better not to "argue" and still enforce the commonly accepted rule.

Balance

Balance involves "balancing" between dependence and independence. Part of maturing is the ability to make decisions for oneself. Achieving full independence is never the end goal; rather, appropriate interdependence is a therapeutic goal. A 2-year-old child often brushes away a parent's hand and says, "I do it." It is innate to want to do things by yourself for yourself. The nurse must also balance a specific patient's needs (rights) with the needs and rights of another patient. Perhaps an example we can all identify with can better illustrate this point. You have the right to listen to any kind of music you want to listen to. However, do you have the right to

play it so loudly that I cannot hear the music I have the right to listen to? As simple as this illustration is, it conveys another aspect of balance that the nurse attempts to achieve.

CONCLUSION

Having a child with a significant mental disorder changes the family—sometimes forever. The impact that the child has on the family is not neutral: some families grow stronger, whereas others disintegrate. A simple pleasure such as going out for dinner may not be able to transpire, or if it does, only with great planning and trepidation. Johnny might explode or have a tantrum. One couple reported these challenges during a coast-to-coast flight with their 5-year-old autistic son. They had overestimated their ability to control his behavior. Shortly after takeoff, the boy had a "meltdown." He was screaming, jumping, and flapping, and the parents had nothing at their disposal to calm him. The boy's behavior ruined the flight for many people. Some passengers were sympathetic, but others accused the couple of poor parenting. One person suggested she might sue because a dress was stained. The couple never attempted another flight with their son.

In Box 34.3 are listed some websites that provide useful information for professionals, patients, and families.

STUDY NOTES

1. Psychiatric disorders in children and adolescents are caused by an interaction of genetic, biologic, and environmental factors.
2. Resilience is the ability to encounter negative factors successfully and emerge mentally healthy.
3. Common psychiatric disorders of children and adolescents include ADHD, ODD, conduct disorder, depression, anxiety, BPD, DMDD, and ASD.
4. ADHD is probably the most common pediatric behavioral disorder. Psychostimulants are most frequently used to treat children with ADHD.
5. Symptoms of ASD include poor social skills; impaired verbal and nonverbal communication; and restricted, repetitive, and stereotypical behavior, interests, and activities.
6. Psychotherapeutic management, in which the nurse manages the nurse-patient relationship, psychopharmacologic intervention, and the environment, remains the best strategy to treat the child or adolescent holistically.

REFERENCES

American Psychiatric Association. (2013). *Diagnostic and statistical manual of mental disorders* (5th ed.). APA.

Biblarz, T., & Savci, E. (2010). Lesbian, gay, bi-sexual and transgender families. *Journal of Marriage and Family*, 72(3), 480–497. https://doi.org/10.1111/j.1741-3737.2010.00714.x.

Brown, S., Doom, J., Lechuga-Peña, S., Watamura, S., & Koppels, T. (2020). Stress and parenting during the global COVID-19 pandemic. *Child Abuse & Neglect*, 110(Pt 2), 104699. https://doi.org/10.1016/j.chiabu.2020.104699.

Cénat, J., & Dalexis, R. (2020). The complex trauma spectrum during the Covid-19 pandemic: A threat for children and adolescents' physical and mental health. *Psychiatric Research*, 293, 113473. https://doi.org/10.1016/j.psychres.2020.113473.

Centers for Disease Control and Prevention. (2017). Attention deficit hyperactivity disorder (ADHD). https://www.cdc.gov/nchs/fastats/adhd.html.

Connolly, M., Zervos, M., Barone, C., Johnson, C., & Joseph, C. (2016). The mental health of transgender youth: Advances in understanding. *Journal of Adolescent Health*, 59(5), 489–495. https://doi.org/10.1016/j.jadohealth.2016.06.012.

Dhejne, C., Lichenstein, P., Boman, M., Johansson, A., Långström, N., & Landén, M. (2011). Long-term follow-up of transsexual persons undergoing sex reassignment surgery: Cohort study in Sweden. *PLoS One*, 6(2). https://doi.org/10.1371/journal.pone.0016885.

Engstrom, M. (2012). Family processes in kinship care. In R. Walsh (Ed.), *Normal family processes* (4th ed., pp. 196–221). Guilford.

Essau, C. A., & Gabbidon, J. (2013). Epidemiology comorbidity and mental health service utilization. In C. A. Essau & T. H. Ollendick (Eds.), *The Wiley-Blackwell handbook of treatment of childhood and adolescent anxiety* (pp. 23–42). Wiley-Blackwell.

Geiger, A., & Davis, L. (2019, July 12). *A growing number of American teenagers-particularly girls-are facing depression.* Pew Research Center. https://www.pewresearch.org/fact-tank/2019/07/12/a-growing-number-of-american-teenagers-particularly-girls-are-facing-depression/.

Geschwind, N., Peeters, F., Jacobs, N., Delespaul, P., Derom, C., Thiery, E., … Wichers, M. (2010). Meeting risk with resilience: High daily life reward experience preserves mental health. *Acta Psychiatrica Scandinavica*, 122(2), 129–138. https://doi.org/10.1111/j.1600-0447.2009.01525.x.

Green, J. G., McLaughlin, K. A., Berglund, P. A., Gruber, M. J., Sampson, N. A., Zaslavsky, A. M., & Kessler, R. C. (2010). Childhood adversities and adult psychiatric disorders in the national comorbidity survey replication I: Associations with first onset of DSM-IV disorders. *Archives of General Psychiatry*, 67(2), 113. https://doi.org/10.1001/archgenpsychiatry.2009.186.

Green, R. J. (2012). Gay and lesbian couples and families. In R. Walsh (Ed.), *Normal family processes* (4th ed., pp. 172–195). Guilford.

Guessoum, S. B., Lachal, J., Radjack, R., Carretier, E., Minassian, S., Benoit, L., & Moro, M. R. (2020). Adolescent psychiatric disorders during the COVID-19 pandemic and lockdown. *Psychiatry Research*, 291. https://doi.org/10.1016/j.psychres.2020.113264.

Gyawali, S., & Patra, B. (2019). Autism spectrum disorder: Trends in research exploring ediopathogenesis. *Psychiatry and Clinical Neurosciences*, 73(8), 466–475. https://doi.org/10.1111/pcn.12860.

Ioannou, A., Blackburn, J., Stringhini, G., Cristofaro, E., Kourtellis, N., & Sirivianos, M. (2018). From risk factors to detection and intervention: A practical proposal for future work on cyberbullying. *Behaviour & Information Technology*, 37(3). https://doi.org/10.1080/0144929X.2018.1432688.

Jacob, M., & Storch, E. (2013). Pediatric obsessive-compulsive disorder: A review for nursing professionals. *Journal of Child and Adolescent Psychiatric Nursing*, 26(2), 138. https://doi.org/10.1111/jcap.12029.

John, A., Glendenning, A.…Hawton, K. (2018). Self-harm, suicidal behaviours, and cyberbullying in children and young people: Systematic review. *Journal of Medical Internet Research*, 20(4), e129. https://doi.org/10.2196/jmir.9044.

Marks, L. (2012). Same-sex parenting and children's outcomes: A closer examination of the American psychological association's brief on lesbian and gay parenting. *Social Science Research*, 41(4), 735–751. https://doi.org/10.1016/j.ssresearch.2012.03.006.

Mason, E., & Joshi, K. (2018). Nonpharmacologic strategies for helping children with ADHD. *Current Psychiatry*, 17, 42–46.

McNamara, R. K., Strawn, J. R., Chang, K. D., & DelBello, M. P. (2012). Interventions for youth at high risk for bipolar disorder and schizophrenia. *Child and Adolescent Psychiatric Clinics of North America*, 21(4), 739–751. https://doi.org/10.1016/j.chc.2012.07.009.

Miller-Lewis, L., Searle, A., & Hedley, D. (2013a). Resource factors for mental health resilience in early childhood: An analysis with multiple methodologies. *Child and Adolescent Psychiatry and Mental Health*, 22, 6–22.

Murthy, S., Mandl, K., & Bourgeois, F. (2013). Analysis of pediatric clinical drug trials for neuropsychiatric conditions. *Pediatrics*, 131(6), 1125–1131. https://www.ncbi.nlm.nih.gov/pmc/articles/PMC4074660/.

National Center for Biotechnology Information. (2017). Tables of FDA-approved indications for first- and second-generation antipsychotics. https://www.ncbi.nlm.nih.gov/books/NBK84656/.

NIMH. (n.d.). Attention-Deficit/Hyperactivity Disorder. https://www.nimh.nih.gov/health/topics/attention-deficit-hyperactivity-disorder-adhd/.

NIMH. (n.d.). Bipolar Disorder in Children and Teens. https://www.nimh.nih.gov/health/publications/bipolar-in-children-and-teens/.

Olweus, D. (1993). *Bullying at school: What we know and what we can do.* Blackwell.

Pliszka, S. R. (2016). Attention-deficit hyperactivity disorder across the lifespan. *Focus*, 14(1), 46–53. https://doi.org/10.1176/appi.focus.20150022.

Posner, J., Polanczyk, G. V., & Sonuga-Barke, E. (2020). Attention-deficit hyperactivity disorder. *Lancet*, 395(10222), 450–462. https://doi.org/10.1016/S0140-6736(19)33004-1.

Ristori, J., & Steensma, T. (2016). Gender dysphoria in childhood. *International Review of Psychiatry*, 28(1), 13–20. https://doi.org/10.3109/09540261.2015.1115754.

Robinson, C. (2010, May 14). *Birmingham News*, p. 1C.

Rockhill, C., Kodish, I., DiBattisto, C., Macias, M., Varley, C., & Ryan, S. (2010). Anxiety disorders in children and adolescents. *Current Problems in Pediatric and Adolescent Health Care*, 40(4), 66. https://doi.org/10.1016/j.cppeds.2010.02.002.

Rosenblatt, P. (2013). Family grief in cross-cultural perspective. *Family Science*, 4(1), 12–19. https://www.ncbi.nlm.nih.gov/books/NBK84656/.

Selkie, E., Fales, J., & Moreno, M. (2016). Cyberbullying prevalence among United States middle and high school aged adolescents: A systematic review and quality assessment. *The Journal of Adolescent Health, 58*(2), 125–133. https://doi.org/10.1016/j.jadohealth.2015.09.026.

Thapar, A., Collishaw, S., Pine, D. S., & Thapar, A. K. (2012). Depression in adolescence. *Lancet, 379*(9820), 1056–1067. https://doi.org/10.1016/S0140-6736(11)60871-4.

Visser, S., Danielson, M., & Blumberg, S. (2014). Trends in the parent-report of health care provider diagnosed and medicated ADHD: United States, 2003-2011. *Journal of the American Academy of Child and Adolescent Psychiatry, 53*(1), 34–46. https://www2.ed.gov/admins/lead/safety/preventingattacksreport.pdf.

Vossekuil, B., Fein, R., Reddy, M., Borum, R., & Modzcleski, W. (2004). The final report and findings of the Safe School Initiative: Implications for the prevention of school attacks in the United States. United States Secret Service and United States Department of Education. https://www2.ed.gov/admins/lead/safety/preventingattacksreport.pdf.

Walkup, J. T. (2017). Generalized anxiety disorder, social phobia, separation anxiety, obsessive compulsive disorder, and movement disorders. Presentation given at AACAP by Douglas B. Hansen, MD, 42nd Annual Review Course, March 18, 2017, New Orleans, LA.

Wallace, P. (2014). Internet addiction disorder and youth. *EMBO Reports, 15*(1), 12–16. https://doi.org/10.1002/embr.38222.

Wu, P., Bird, H. R., Liu, X., Duarte, C. S., Fuller, C., Fan, B., & Canino, G. J. (2010). Trauma, posttraumatic stress symptoms, and alcohol-use initiation in children. *Journal of Studies on Alcohol and Drugs, 71*(3), 326–334. https://doi.org/10.15288/jsad.2010.71.326.

Zucker, K. (2017). Epidemiology of gender dysphoria and transgender identity. *Sex Health, 14*(5), 404–411. https://doi.org/10.1071/SH17067.

35

Older Adults

Joan Grant Keltner

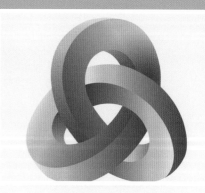

 http://evolve.elsevier.com/Keltner

LEARNING OBJECTIVES

- Describe the barriers to mental health care that exist for older adults.
- Describe the various treatment options and care settings available to older adults.
- Identify the unique variations in symptoms of mental disorders evidenced by older adults.
- Identify major substance use issues in older adults.
- Recognize pharmacokinetic and pharmacodynamic changes in older adults that affect pharmacotherapy.
- Perform a psychological assessment on an older adult.
- State therapeutic goals for older adults.

INTRODUCTION

The number of adults aged 65 and older was more than 54 million in 2019 (US Census Bureau, Population Division, 2020a) and by 2050, the population who are this age will reach 1.6 billion (Roberts, Ogunwole, Blakeslee, & Rabe, 2018). An estimated 25.4% of these adults experience a mental disorder (National Institutte for Mental Illness, 2021). This number includes individuals who experience mental disorders for the first time in late life, as well as individuals whose early-onset psychiatric disorders persist as chronic or recurrent conditions. Mental disorders in older adults might have a clear biochemical basis or might be a reaction to stressors that commonly occur in late adulthood.

Rapid growth in the older population is fueling interest in issues surrounding mental health and aging, with 6.5 million people aged 85 years and older in 2018, which is projected to increase to 14.4 million by 2040, placing a significantly greater number of people at risk for mental disorders, particularly cognitive disorders (Administration for Community Living, 2020b). Box 35.1 provides an overview of the prevalence rates of selected psychiatric diagnoses in older adults. The personal and economic consequences of mental disorders in this rapidly expanding cohort require heightened attention to the special mental health needs of older adults.

Modern American culture, which tends to celebrate youth, has placed little emphasis on understanding old age. This bias has contributed to insufficient knowledge about mental health disorders in the older population and public policies that adversely affect access to care. Research results have increased the ability of health care providers to differentiate illness from normal aging and to identify differences between the clinical presentation and course of mental disorders in older adults and other age groups. Government agencies have joined together to investigate factors that influence older adults. A better understanding of the complex interplay of physical health, social factors, and emotional well-being in older adults is leading to mental health strategies tailored for the special needs of this group.

⚡ CRITICAL THINKING QUESTION

1. Think of the last patient older than age 65 for whom you cared during a medical-surgical clinical rotation. What factors could have placed the patient at risk for depression? If you noted any signs of depression, what actions were in the plan of care?

 NORM'S NOTES The geriatric population, people older than 65, is growing rapidly. There are more and more older people and more of their mental health problems for the health care system to deal with. Sometimes older people in need of mental health care had the same problems during their younger years and have simply grown older. However, others are growing older in a society in which work defines the person, and they may no longer be working. In fact, older people who are working tend to be those who have more advanced degrees and higher incomes (Edleson, 2019). Unfortunately, many older people with mental disorders find themselves without purpose (i.e., no job to do) and alone. I get depressed just thinking about it.

BOX 35.1 One-Year Prevalence Rates for Selected Psychiatric Diagnoses in Older Adults[a]

Psychiatric Diagnosis	Prevalence (%)
Any anxiety disorder	11.4
Generalized anxiety disorder	2.8
Posttraumatic stress disorder	3.5
Specific phobia	5.8
Social phobia	1.5
Panic disorder	1.4
Any mood disorder	6.8
Major depression	5.6
Dysthymia	0.9
Any personality disorder	14.5
Schizoid	2.2
Obsessive-compulsive disorder	6.5
Paranoid	2.3
Narcissistic	3.91
Schizotypal	2.4
Any drug abuse/dependence	0.4
Any substance use disorders	3.8
Alcohol abuse/dependence	3.5
Nicotine dependence	9.29

[a]From a nationally representative sample of 12,312 individuals, age 55 and older.
Modified from Reynolds, K. (2015). Prevalence of psychiatric disorders in U.S. older adults: Findings from a nationally representative survey. *World Psychiatry, 14*(1), 74–81. https://doi.org/10.1002/wps.20193; US Department of Health and Human Services. (1999). *Mental health: A report of the Surgeon General.* U.S. Department of Health and Human Services, Substance Abuse and Mental Health Services Administration, Center for Mental Health Services, National Institutes of Health, National Institute of Mental Health. http://profiles.nlm.nih.gov/ps/access/NNBBHS.pdf.

Nurses involved in the care of older adults should be familiar with prevention, detection, and treatment strategies for mental disorders throughout the continuum of care. This chapter presents an overview of mental health issues in older adults that differ from those of other age groups. Stressors, policy issues, barriers to mental health care, and common mental disorders occurring in older adults are discussed, along with assessment and psychotherapeutic management. Cognitive disorders, which account for some of the most frequently occurring mental disorders in older adults, are discussed in Chapter 28.

Barriers
Patient Barriers

Attitudes of older adults themselves serve as a barrier to seeking mental health care. Patients and families who subscribe to stereotypes about normal aging might delay seeking care if they believe that conditions such as depression or memory loss are a normal part of aging. In addition, older individuals might be reluctant to seek psychiatric care because admitting to mental health problems is seen as a weakness and is more stigmatizing than it might be for a younger person.

Seeking psychiatric care might also represent a loss of control and elicit fear of institutionalization. When outside help is required, people who grew up in an era that emphasized self-reliance are more likely to rely on family, friends, and other informal supports than on mental health professionals, who are often viewed with skepticism. Unfortunately, while empirical data emphasize the essential role of family members, this support often is lacking for older adults with mental illnesses. Patients and their caregivers face financial issues and inadequate transportation in accessing services. Poor communication among providers, social services, and patients, compounded by patient health literacy issues, serve as significant barriers (Valaitis et al., 2020).

Provider Barriers

Older adults are more likely to receive care from primary care physicians than from geriatric specialty providers. Despite the rapid growth in the population aged 65 years and older and recognition of their unique needs, geriatric specialists are scarce. As a result, patients often face prolonged wait times and a lack of programs that meet eligibility criteria to address older adults' needs (Valaitis et al., 2020). Nurses and other health care providers who are not attuned to the complexities of geriatric care might miss opportunities to identify mental health disorders or predisposing factors.

Accurate assessment and diagnosis require familiarity with diagnostic tools, such as the Geriatric Depression Scale. Individuals working with older adults must recognize that mental disorders might be expressed through somatic complaints and that symptoms of comorbid physical problems might compound the difficulty of diagnosing a mental disorder. Ageism, the negative stereotyping and devaluation of people solely because of their age, is also a significant barrier. Ageism includes the stereotypical view that mental health problems are part of the aging process. To serve older adults effectively, professionals must be attentive to their biases and stereotypes and increase their geriatric-specific knowledge.

System-Economic Barriers

Funding issues, along with a lack of collaboration and coordination among primary care, mental health, and aging services providers, thwart the provision and receipt of adequate mental health care for older adults. Frustration caused by the complex navigation required for health and social services and inconsistent assessments among providers and older adults may result in conflicting pathways of care and delays in delivery of care (Valaitis et al., 2020). The cost of mental health care also has been a major disincentive to providers and older adults who might otherwise seek psychiatric assistance.

In the last few years, legislative efforts have addressed parity in mental health coverage with the Domenici-Wellstone amendment and the Patient Protection and Affordable Care Act (ACA).

The ACA includes reforms for addressing high-cost, complex, vulnerable patient populations, such as older adults with mental health problems. These reforms include (1) accountable care organizations, (2) patient-centered medical homes, (3) support for health information technology and telehealth, and (4) other initiatives. The ACA also covered provisions of the Mental Health Parity and Addiction Equity Act, so that more health insurance plans must offer mental health benefits which are comparable with medical and surgical benefits (Mental Health America, 2021b). This legislation is not without challenges, including no or reduced expansion of Medicaid in some states. Major difficulties for low-income seniors are medication affordability and compliance. One strength in legislation is the clarification of references of mental health in the 2016 Older Americans Act (OAA) Reauthorization Act to include "behavioral health," which includes substance abuse and suicide prevention. In support of these goals, the Supporting Older Americans Act of 2020 reauthorizes these programs for 5 years and provides amendments to lessen barriers to the aging network (Administration for Community Living, 2020a). In addressing crises, the Federal Communications Commission (FCC) now designates 988 as the new three-digit number for the National Suicide Prevention Lifeline. Differing from 911 in which staff may not be trained to assist individuals in acute mental crises, staff are trained in answering calls from individuals at risk for suicide and mental health and substance use emergencies. Effective by July 2022, all telecommunications companies must make these accommodations to allow individuals to access the National Suicide Prevention Lifeline using the 988 dialing code. As of early 2021, the FCC is still taking comments and deciding how to handle text (Mental Health America, 2021a).

❓ CRITICAL THINKING QUESTION

2. Many older adults have no insurance coverage to offset the high cost of prescription medications. How might this affect treatment goals?

CONTINUUM OF CARE

Because of the prevalence and profound negative consequences of mental disorders in late life, nurses who encounter older adults in any setting should consider their physical, social, and emotional needs. Whenever possible, factors that place older adults at risk for mental disorders or problems stemming from mental illness should be identified, and plans should be developed to meet the needs of these persons.

Prevention

A balance of physical, social, spiritual, and emotional functioning contributes to mental health. Many of the changes that accompany advancing age affect this balance, increasing vulnerability of older adults to mental disorders. A primary stressful event (e.g., broken hip [physical]) might lead to secondary stressors (e.g., emotional isolation). Acute and chronic health problems might lead to dependence, relocation, isolation, and financial hardship. A closer examination of these consequences might prove enlightening.

Dependence: Loss of independence, even temporarily, is terribly threatening to an older person because having to rely on others might signal a continued dependency.

Relocation: Moving from familiar surroundings to a new environment is also threatening. To many older individuals, familiar surroundings represent a connection to all that is important in life, and the related changes could be overwhelming for some individuals.

Isolation: Most older individuals have fewer meaningful connections than they had earlier in life. Death, a mobile society, and estrangements are only a few reasons for this reality. Health care–related isolation can be particularly devastating for some older adults.

Financial hardship: Although many older individuals are financially secure, a significant number find unexpected medical expenses to be difficult or impossible to meet on a fixed income. Most older adults have little, if any, ability to increase their income to meet additional unplanned expenses.

The COVID-19 pandemic has negatively compounded many of these factors, affecting the mental well-being of older adults. Independence is significantly impaired because of efforts to prevent the spread of the infection. Limiting contacts with family and friends causes isolation and a loss of familiarity that provides meaningful connections within their environment. Many older adults who were previously working have had to stop or limit these activities to decrease their chance of becoming ill. Often, older adults are not skilled in using technology to work or visit with their mental health providers (D'cruz & Banerjee, 2020; De Pue et al., 2021).

Adaptive Mechanisms: Meaning, Control, Support

Losses common in later years of life are listed in Box 35.2 and often precede the onset of mental disorders in older adults. Despite changes in function and physical well-being, most older adults adjust well and express a high degree of satisfaction with life (Federal Interagency Forum on Aging-Related Statistics, 2020). Exposure and adaptation to stressors vary with each older adult's economic and social resources, physical status, ethnicity, gender, and life experiences. Successful adaptation is enhanced by the ability to give *meaning* to experiences. Part of this process is comparing problems with what is experienced and expected by others who are the same

---

BOX 35.2 Losses That Occur More Frequently Among Older Adults

Loss of health
Loss of loved ones
Loss of hearing and vision
Loss of status
Loss of work
Loss of income
Loss of friends
Loss of cognitive skills
Loss of home and community
Loss of mobility (physical abilities; driving privileges)

age. Health declines with age, with 81% of older adults ages 65 to 74 reporting their health as good or better. At age 85 and older, 68% of people report their health as good or better (Federal Interagency Forum on Aging-Related Statistics, 2020). As one sage older adult noted, at some point, simply being alive can be seen as a sign of good health. This coping skill is especially helpful when the stressor, such as a chronic health problem, is not easily modified.

Another adaptive mechanism that helps older adults cope with stressful events is the use of mastery—the sense of an ability to exercise *control* over circumstances. Adequate planning for the social and financial implications of retirement significantly affects adjustment to this major life change. Nurses can reinforce mastery by encouraging the older person's participation in care decisions.

Support systems (family, friends, spiritual communities, and private and government organizations) are valuable sources of emotional support and aid and are important predictors of physical and mental health and delay institutionalization. Measures that contribute to physical health and promote social functioning are important components of preventing mental disorders in older adults. Improved health care and programs developed to target needs of older adults have resulted in declines in rates of disability and poverty, which are key indicators of well-being in older adults (National Association of Area Agencies on Aging, 2020).

Caregiver Training and Transportation

Specific legislation has led to funding programs to meet the special needs of an aging population. The 2016 OAA reauthorized programs for FY 2017 through FY 2019 and included provisions to protect vulnerable elders by strengthening screening and prevention programs. One example is the National Aging Network and Transportation Assistance program, which was established to address transportation needs. Lack of transportation is a factor in isolation and is a barrier to accessing health care. Nurses play a key role in illness prevention by providing information about mental health and available resources at sites where older adults are likely to visit. The OAA also clarifies current law that older adults caring for adult children with disabilities are eligible to participate in the National Family Caregiver Support Program. These new definitions allow this support program to serve older-relative caregivers, including people who are age 55 or older and parents of individuals with disabilities (Administration for Community Living, 2020a). The U.S. Patient Protection and Affordable Care Act Balancing Incentive Program also provides for caregiver support for older adults with mental illness. To illustrate, in a cohort study using over 38,000 participants utilizing the program, caregivers reported an increase in daily caregiving and overall better caregiver well-being. Unfortunately, those caregivers of lower educational level and socioeconomic status benefitted less, potentially related to other stressors such as housing insecurity, geographic isolation, health literacy, and transportation challenges (Anastos-Wallen, Werner, and Chatterjee, 2020). Unfortunately, future nondefense

discretionary program budget cuts are proposed, which may affect the availability and accessibility of other services such as transportation for older Americans (National Association of Area Agencies on Aging, 2020). However, the National Aging and Disability Transportation Center (2021a,b) supports assisted and volunteer transportation services for the older adult.

? CRITICAL THINKING QUESTION

3. If you have had the opportunity to meet the caregiver of an older adult with a mental disorder, were both the patient and the caregiver participants involved in decision making? Did the caregiver treat the patient in the way that you would want to be treated in that situation? Describe both the positive and the negative aspects of nurse-patient-caregiver interactions.

Detection

Measures that promote early detection of mental disorders in older adults include increasing public awareness of mental health issues, encouraging collaboration among service providers, and providing education for health professionals. Public education that emphasizes symptoms of mental disorders and treatment options does much to dispel the myths and stigma surrounding mental illness and empowers older adults to seek treatment. Some programs have been established to enhance community involvement. Public service workers such as grocery clerks, postal employees, and public utility workers are recruited and trained to identify and report vulnerable older adults to significant others. Nurses in all settings can contribute to early detection by assessing and reporting stressors and symptoms. Healthy IDEAS, an initiative aimed at identifying depression and empowering activities for older adults, is an evidence-based program that integrates depression awareness and management into existing case management services provided to older adults. The focus of this program is to ensure availability of the help that older adults need to manage symptoms of depression and live full lives.

Treatment Sites

Federal legislation has strongly influenced the care of older adults who have mental disorders. The Community Mental Health Act of 1963 initiated deinstitutionalization, resulting in a large number of individuals with serious mental illness (SMI) being discharged from state and county mental hospitals to less restrictive settings. Many discharged older adults were placed in nursing homes where inappropriate and inadequate care, including excessive use of physical and chemical restraints, led to the passage of the Nursing Home Reform Act, which was part of the Omnibus Budget Reconciliation Act (OBRA) of 1987. This legislation set stringent limits on the use of physical restraints and established guidelines for psychotropic drug use that regulate drug selection, dosing, and duration of treatment.

In addition, to prevent nursing home placement for individuals who need psychiatric care in hospital or community programs, OBRA requires preadmission screening for all individuals with suspected mental disorders. Nursing home residents whose only need for nursing care stemmed from mental disorders were to be discharged. Nonetheless, many institutionalized older people with SMI continue to live in nursing homes. Many of these residents do not receive adequate psychiatric treatment and are at risk for therapeutic neglect because of a lack of mental health training for nursing home staff (Donald & Stajduhar, 2020).

Most older adults with SMI live in the community. From 2014 to 2017, the number of community mental health centers (CMHCs) decreased by 14% nationally, with a concurrent increase in suicide of 9.7%, indicating that this increase may be potentially related to the decline in CMHCs (Hung et al., 2020). At the present time, only a small percentage of community mental health centers have staff or services that target the needs of older adults, and primary care physicians are ill prepared and typically too rushed to treat mental disorders adequately. Donald and Stajduhar (2020) identified those with SMI as a vulnerable population with multifaceted needs that often are not adequately addressed by the healthcare system. The services needed to help community-based older adults with SMI include the following:

1. Mental health outreach programs
2. Adult day services
3. Respite care and caregiver programs
4. Support groups
5. Self-help groups

Conclusions

State governments should avoid the declining number of CMHCs and the services that these facilities provide, which may be an important component of suicide prevention efforts.

PSYCHOPATHOLOGY IN OLDER ADULTS

Unit V of this text provides an in-depth review of diagnostic classifications. This section is meant to supplement that information by detailing unique information on the presentation, course, and treatment of mental disorders in older adults. It is important for nurses in all practice areas to note that treating older adults with mental disorders benefits overall health by improving functional ability and collaboration with health care instructions.

DEPRESSION

The prevalence of a major depressive episode is 4.7% in those age 50 and older (National Alliance on Mental Health [NAMI], 2019). Those at greater risk for depressive symptoms are individuals 55 years and older, with a prevalence ranging from 10% to 16%. Depressive symptoms are greatest for those who are women, ages 80 and older (Federal Interagency Forum on Aging-Related Statistics, 2020). Unfortunately, depressive symptoms are a measure of general and mental well-being among older adults and these individuals are at greater risk for physical and functional disabilities and often utilize more health care resources.

For most, depression has occurred during much of life. For others, depression has a first onset in later life—even persons in their 80s and 90s. Depression in older persons is closely associated with dependency and disability, and it causes great suffering for the individual and the family (NAMI, 2019). As in other age groups, depression in older adults might result from psychosocial stress, biochemical changes, comorbid medical conditions, pharmaceutical agents, or a combination of factors. The effects of depression extend beyond well-known and emotionally distressing symptoms such as sadness, worthlessness, hopelessness, helplessness, fear, shame, and guilt. Less obvious effects include diminished social, cognitive, and physical functioning, as well as increased mortality.

Incidence

Table 35.1 details the prevalence of late-life depression and the increased risk for women over men. Clinically relevant depressive symptoms are present in 9% of men and 13% of women age 65 and older. The percentage is 14% for all adults age 85 and older (Federal Interagency Forum on Aging-Related Statistics, 2020). Of clinical relevance is that depression occurs concurrently with other serious illnesses of older adults, such as heart disease, cerebrovascular accident, diabetes, cancer, and Parkinson disease. Approximately 1% to 15% of community-dwelling older adults, 13.5% of older people who require home health care, and 11.5% of older adults who are hospitalized are clinically depressed (Centers for Disease Control and Prevention [CDC], 2021).

Presentation

Depression in older adults frequently does not align neatly with current *DSM-5* criteria, and many depressive symptoms can be attributed to physical causes in individuals with comorbid medical illnesses such as chronic pain, prior depression, or traumatic brain injury (CDC, 2021). Older adults are more likely to present with memory disturbance

TABLE 35.1 Percentage of Noninstitutionalized Persons, Age 65 and Older, With Clinically Relevant Depressive Symptoms (2014)			
Age (Years)	Total (%)	Men (%)	Women (%)
65–69	10.0	8.0	12.0
70–74	11.0	10.0	12.0
75–79	11.0	8.0	14.0
80–84	13.0	10.0	16.0
≥85	14.0	11.0	16.0

From Federal Interagency Forum on Aging-Related Statistics. (2020). Older Americans 2020: Key indicators of well-being. Federal Interagency Forum on aging-related statistics. U.S. Government Printing Office. https://agingstats.gov/docs/LatestReport/OA20_508_10142020.pdf.

or somatic complaints than with the feelings associated with depression for which younger patients seek care. Older adults also might lack the range of vocabulary that younger individuals commonly possess to describe emotions. Rather than expressions of sadness, diminished self-esteem, irritability, or apathy, for example, older adults are more likely to complain of having the blues or feeling worthless. Also, cultural competence demands that professionals recognize differences in expression common to ethnic and cultural subgroups within the older population. For example, Jang et al. (2021) found that among Korean immigrant older adults, loneliness and social isolation significantly contributed to cognitive impairment. In contrast, participation in social activities contributes to increased physical and psychosocial well-being (Choi et al., 2020).

For nurses working with older adults, a deeper understanding of how loneliness may contribute to the development of depression, a diminished quality of life, or cognitive decline is important. In a sample of Chinese immigrant older adults, those who participated in a peer intervention reported less loneliness and depressive symptoms, fewer barriers to participating in social activities, and better life satisfaction and happiness than those not participating in the peer intervention (Lai et al., 2020). In an integrative review of risk factors for loneliness using individuals from various countries (e.g., Finland, England, Germany, United States, Sweden, Israel, Netherlands, Canada), most relevant factors were being unmarried/partnered or experiencing the loss of a partner, limited social activity and network, lower self-perceived health status, and either a depression/depressed mood or greater depression (Dahlberg, McKee, Frank, & Naseer, 2021). In an integrative review, factors associated with the most effective interventions to reduce social isolation and loneliness were adaptability, a community development approach, and productive engagement. However, the impact of the COVID-19 pandemic has certainly changed the ability to perform these activities out of a regard for assuring safety of older adults and their families. Further research also is needed to provide more robust data regarding essential components and theoretical understandings of interventions that lessen social isolation and loneliness (Gardiner et al., 2016). Advocating for routine assessments of depression and loneliness in older adults could lead to the development of interventions that would serve as a primary prevention for depression. Another complicating factor in the occurrence of depression in elders is that only a minority receives treatment. Therefore, continuing studies of barriers and opportunities for recognition and access to services is imperative.

In addition to diagnostic barriers already discussed, the connection between medical conditions and depression complicates a diagnosis. The clinician should consider conditions such as cerebrovascular disease in a first episode of depression occurring in a person older than 60 years of age. It is difficult to determine whether or not common physical indicators of depression in older adults, including weight loss, fatigue, insomnia, constipation, and multiple vague aches and pains, are the result of a mood disorder or symptoms of a medical problem. The *DSM-5* diagnosis of "mood disorder due to a general medical condition" can be given when mood symptoms are a direct physiologic consequence of medical conditions.

Although depression is caused by a medical illness in some cases, depression causes physiologic changes that enhance susceptibility to disease in other cases. People with depression are at a significantly greater risk for development of cardiovascular disease, diabetes, stroke, and Alzheimer disease. Research also suggests that people with depression are at a greater risk for osteoporosis when compared with individuals without depression. Reasons for the higher risk of these diseases are probably due to multiple reasons. For example, depression adversely affects endocrine, neurologic, and immune processes by increasing sympathetic tone, decreasing vagal tone, and causing immunosuppression. People with depression are more likely to smoke, drink alcohol excessively, be physically inactive, and have poorer eating habits than people who are not depressed. Individuals who are depressed may have less access to preventive medical care. These individuals also may have more difficulty caring for their health by seeking care, taking prescribed medications, eating well, and exercising (National Institute of Mental Health, 2021).

Impact of COVID-19 on Depressive Symptoms in Older Adults

Evidence strongly suggests that the COVID-19 shelter-in-place orders implemented in April 2020 may have a negative impact on older adults' mental well-being (De Pue et al., 2021). Potential risk factors include a greater risk of disease and death during the pandemic, along with the threat of insecurity, loneliness, isolation, and frailty. Cognitive and sensory impairments and limited access to adequate health care resources add to this burden (D'cruz & Banerjee, 2020). Depression is significantly related to lower activity levels, sleep quality, wellbeing, and cognitive functioning (De Pue et al., 2021). In one study, older adults reported greater depression and loneliness when compared to their mental health before the pandemic. In other words, loneliness was associated with greater levels of depression for older adults who felt closer to their social networks during the pandemic. Conversely, those who were less close to their social networks experienced more depression, regardless of loneliness levels (Krendl & Perry, 2021). Neuropsychiatric symptoms occurred and even worsened in individuals both with and without dementia, with delirium, agitation, and apathy occurring most often, especially in those with dementia. These symptoms were felt to occur as a result of the pandemic and the extended social isolation (Manca et al., 2020). These studies emphasize the need for interventions that address this enforced social isolation in older adults. This provides an opportunity for clinical and community-based organizations to change the processes and modalities for delivering services and programs to older adults. Strategies include the integration of brief and action-oriented screenings to identify individuals at risk. Telephonic engagement and support, with appropriate referrals for older adults who are exhibiting physical and psychosocial needs, are useful. Using older adults as peer volunteers to offer some of this support to older adults during the pandemic is promising (Smith et al., 2020).

Depression or Dementia?

Because of shared cognitive symptoms of depression and dementia, misdiagnosis of dementia occurs frequently. Depression that mimics dementia is termed *pseudodementia*. Shared symptoms include poor memory, disorientation, poor judgment, and agitation or psychomotor retardation. In addition to psychological tests, nursing observations can be critical to correcting a misdiagnosis. Nurses should assess for higher functioning than would be expected in dementia and can look for a downcast mood, which can help distinguish depression from the blander effect of true dementia. Differentiating these disorders is important for treatment because depression is highly treatable. Psychotic depression might also be confused with cognitive or other psychiatric disorders. When depression occurs for the first time after age 60, delusions are more common than with early-onset depression. Delusions of persecution or of having an incurable illness and nihilistic delusions are more frequent than delusions associated with guilt (Agüera-Ortiz et al., 2020). However, hallucinations are an uncommon feature of psychotic depression. Many older adults with psychotic depression might ruminate, express suspiciousness, and voice multiple physical complaints. Psychotic depression is often resistant to traditional antidepressant medications and psychotherapy. As a result, electroconvulsive therapy (ECT) may be used in treatment.

Electroconvulsive Therapy

ECT is often the treatment of choice for severe depression in older adults, especially individuals who are poor candidates for drug therapy or who have failed to respond to other treatments. ECT offers a rapid response that is necessary when patients are suicidal or in danger of medical crisis. The safety and efficacy of ECT have been demonstrated for older adults, although ECT is associated with potential cardiovascular and cognitive side effects. The decision-making process of older adults electing to receive ECT is highly individualized and relates to these potential complications, costs, and the stigma of mental illness. However, there have been significant advances in the safety of ECT, including improvements in anesthesia to minimize medical complications, ECT devices that include electroencephalography (EEG) monitoring of the seizure, and modification of ECT techniques to increase safety and lessen these potential cognitive complications (e.g., electrode placement away from temporal lobes; McDonald, 2016). In older adults, ECT is an essential therapy for treatment-resistant depression, depression with psychotic features, and in severe agitation and aggression in individuals with dementia. During the COVID-19 pandemic restrictions, a decrease of the use of ECT has resulted in greater negative outcomes such as greater agitation in older adults. Sharing among practitioners who deliver this valuable treatment are essential in meeting the needs of older patients while lessening transmission risks associated with this important therapy (Lapid et al., 2020).

Suicide

Older Americans are disproportionately more likely to die by suicide, the most serious consequence of missed or undertreated depression. Suicide is preventable and needs to be addressed in older adults. Adults aged 65 years and older compose 17.0% of the U.S. population suicide deaths (US Census Bureau, 2020b), of which older adults with a known mental illness accounted for 14.2% of these deaths. Common illnesses associated with suicide are depression/dysthymia, anxiety, and bipolar disorder. Current research also indicates that physical illness is a strong risk factor for older adults committing suicide (Kim et al., 2020). Gender differences also are found in suicide, in that 84% of males do not have a mental illness while 69% of women do have a mental illness (CDC, 2018). Perhaps these lower rates in those with a mental illness relate to important assessment and intervention for individuals at risk for suicide. Notably, suicides are particularly high among those 45 to 64 years of age (38.2 suicides per 100,000 people) and for older, white males, aged 65 to 74 years (30.7 suicides per 100,000 people). In fact, the rate of suicide in the oldest group of white males (ages 75+) is significantly higher (46.2 suicides per 100,000 people). Considering the occurrence of suicide in the general population to be at a rate of about 14.0 per 100,000, the older adult rate is higher. Table 35.2 shows that the incidence of suicide increases with age and that white men age 75 and older have the highest rate of all. Suicidal gestures and impulsiveness, common among young adults, are rare in older adults. In older adults, attempts are usually not a cry for help; rather, they are a serious suicide warning. To underscore this point, older people tend to select highly lethal methods for suicide. For example, firearms are the most common method of suicide by both men and women aged 65 years and older (Curtin, 2019; US Census Bureau, 2020b).

TABLE 35.2 Rate of Suicide Among Older Adults Per 100,000

Population Group	Female Suicide Rate per 100,000	Male Suicide Rate per 100,000
45–64 years old	9.7	30.1
65–74 years old	6.2	26.2
75 years and older	4.0	39.7
White men 75 years and older	46.2	
Average rate across the life span	14.0	

Modified from Curtin, S. C. (2019). Suicide rates for females and males by race and ethnicity: United States, 1999 and 2017. https://www.cdc.gov/nchs/data/hestat/suicide/rates_1999_2017.htm.

BOX 35.3   Predictors of Suicide Risk in Older Adults

Age > 65 years
Male sex
White
Chronic or uncontrolled pain
Bereavement
Unmarried (single, widowed, divorced)
Social isolation
Retirement
Financial difficulty
Hopelessness or helplessness
Alcohol or drug abuse
History of previous attempt
Major depressive disorder, particularly psychotic depression or depression caused by a general medical condition

The rate of suicide might be even higher than reported because statistics do not include what is known as *chronic suicide*. This term characterizes death caused by slower, less obvious means than the abrupt acts usually associated with suicide. Refusing to eat, inconsistent medication usage, excessive alcohol intake, and physical risk taking might result in deaths that are not recorded as suicides. Depression is a strong predictor of patients' decisions to support euthanasia or forego life-sustaining treatment (Julião et al., 2021). Suicide does not always arise from depression. For some individuals who face life-threatening illness, suicide is the ultimate means of exercising control over a situation. There are differences between ethnic groups in the methods employed in deliberate self-harm. Social and cultural backgrounds also play a part in structuring cognitive patterns and problem-solving mechanisms that may influence the expression of any of the risk factors identified in Box 35.3. Literature also suggests that symptoms of depression are significantly associated with death ideation in older adults experiencing feelings of perceived burdensomeness. Loneliness and hopelessness are also important factors to consider when assessing death ideation in older adults (Harmer, Lee, Duong, & Saadabadi, 2020).

Active suicidal ideations are present when individuals have a conscious desire to inflict self-harming behaviors and death is their desire. In contrast, passive suicidal ideations occur when individuals have a general desire to die but have no plan for killing themselves. Health professionals may mistakenly believe that passive suicidal ideations are less important than active suicidal ideations, but this belief is untrue. In a very large sample ($n > 85,000$) comparing odds ratios to predict suicide attempts, data showed no difference between reported passive and active suicidal ideations. However, older patients are more likely to sanction passive suicidal ideations, and most are successful on their first attempt. When compared to younger adults, older suicide victims also have less clinical evidence of maladaptive personalities, and the majority did not meet the threshold for a psychiatric diagnosis.

Hence, assessing for both active and passive suicidal ideations is essential in older adults with mental illnesses.

Research data showed that approximately 20 veterans died per day from suicide between 2001 and 2014. Around 65% of these suicides occurred in veterans 50 years of age and older. In 2014, veterans represented 8.5% of the U.S. population but characterized 18% of adult suicides. In the same year, female veterans had an age-adjusted suicide rate 2.4 times higher than that of adult civilian women. In addressing this significant problem, the Veterans Administration has launched aggressive prevention measures such as greater use of telemental and phone health services, creation of a toll-free crisis hotline, improved staffing and case management, use of predictive models to identify veterans at risk for suicide, and creation of new partnerships with community-based mental health organizations. However, achieving access to care to lessen the risk of suicide in veterans may be challenging because only 8.5 million out of an estimated 21.6 million U.S. veterans are actually enrolled in Veterans Affairs (VA) health care (US Department of Veterans Affairs, 2016).

Suicide prevention begins with the detection of risk (see Box 35.3). It is important for nurses to listen to the themes of conversation and observe for signs that might signal suicidal risk or thoughts. Particular attention should be given to older individuals who are beginning to recover from depression because as energy returns, the risk of suicide increases. Intent might be signaled by a new preoccupation with religious issues, giving away possessions, changing a will, or other new behaviors. People might feel ashamed to voice ideas of self-harm plainly, so if negative statements or behaviors are detected, it is essential to ask directly about any intentions. The notion that these discussions can exacerbate suicidal thought is a myth.

Clinical Example: Despondency related to loss

Mr. Nelson is an 86-year-old African American who has outlived two wives. Mr. Nelson has remained sexually active into his 80s, but within the last 2 years he has had difficulty attaining an erection. Mr. Nelson relates that a younger woman (mid-50s) recently asked about spending the night. She did, and Mr. Nelson was unable to perform sexually. He said, "I'm just no good anymore." Mr. Nelson said he was embarrassed by his sexual dysfunction. He states that he has had thoughts of suicide but would not act on them. He promises the nurse that he will call if he has an urge to harm himself.

Clinical Example: I'd be better off dead

Mr. Timchuk is a 77-year-old Pacific Islander with chronic obstructive pulmonary disease. He has great difficulty doing any physical activity. Mr. Timchuk is very despondent over his condition, and there is little hope that he will improve. Although he has not verbalized a desire to "end it all," he states that he "would be better off dead." The nurse understands that he is at great risk for self-harm.

MANIC EPISODES

Manic symptoms in older adults might be associated with bipolar disorder, medical and neurologic conditions, substance abuse, or medication. In older adults, bipolar disorder accounts for 6.0% of mood disorders, most often as a recurrence of an existing disorder. Late-onset bipolar disorder is defined as bipolar disorder in which symptoms first occur after age 40. Differences between early-onset and late-onset bipolar disorder suggest that they might be different types of manic-depressive illness. Late-onset bipolar disorder is generally less severe, with fewer and milder manic symptoms compared with early-onset bipolar disorder. Features might include grandiosity or irritability, disorientation, and euphoria. A substantial proportion of new-onset manic symptoms in older adults is associated with cerebral disorders or injuries and might run a bipolar course, with intervening periods of euthymia. Because of self-reported cognitive complaints in elderly patients with bipolar disorder, an evaluation of cognitive functioning in such patients is an important part of treatment (Dols & Beekman, 2020). Nursing interventions must address the negative impact of agitation and distractibility on self-care and self-protection in older adults.

Clinical Example: Evicted

The local police department's community service officer brought Ms. Ellington, a 72-year-old white woman, to the hospital. She was found sitting outside a homeless shelter surrounded by boxes of personal belongings, drinking orange juice that had a strong odor of alcohol. She wore tight animal-print leggings, a transparent blouse, and thigh-high white boots. A decorated wide-brimmed hat covered her sparse, flame-red hair. On admission, Ms. Ellington was cursing loudly and threw her dentures at the first staff person who approached. Although she was well known to the staff, Ms. Ellington claimed that she was a Hollywood star who had been kicked out of her own mansion by friends, robbed of identification, and shipped to this city where she would be unknown. According to police, she had been evicted from several shelters for disruptive behavior. An empty bottle of lithium and an unfilled prescription for more lithium were found in her purse.

PSYCHOTIC DISORDERS

Psychotic disorders, characterized by delusions, hallucinations, disordered thoughts, bizarre behavior, or other evidence of impaired reality testing, are among the most severe psychiatric disorders. Symptoms often contribute to the institutionalization of older adults. Active psychosis is as disabling as quadriplegia on the disability component of the disability-adjusted life-years measure. Nurses should be familiar with the numerous physical conditions and medications associated with psychosis in older adults. A comprehensive assessment, including the nature and content of delusions and hallucinations, can facilitate identification of reversible causes and contribute to the accurate diagnosis necessary for determining the most effective course of treatment.

Schizophrenia

Schizophrenia is ranked as the third leading cause of disability in individuals age 60 and older (Cohen, 2015), yet empirical literature about older individuals with schizophrenia is sparse. Two generations are now living with schizophrenia—those who are called young-old, between the ages of 55 and 74 years, and those who are named old-old, aged 75 years and older (Cohen, 2015; Häfner, 2019).

Literature commonly indicates that late-onset schizophrenia first occurs after 40 years of age. Most important characteristics for assessing a schizophrenic episode in an older person are hallucinations, delusions, and a history of a psychotic disorder. Patients with late-onset psychosis are more likely than their counterparts with earlier onset to present with bizarre, systematized and persecutory delusions; visual, tactile, and olfactory hallucinations; and accusatory or abusive auditory hallucinations. Disorganization and negative symptoms (withdrawal, apathy, and anhedonia) are less prominent than in early-onset psychosis. Most individuals in whom schizophrenia is diagnosed late in life have abnormal premorbid personality traits but are more likely to have better employment and marital histories compared with persons with early-onset schizophrenia (Cohen, 2015; Häfner, 2019; Ramasamy & Bharath, 2017).

However, while individuals with these symptoms may certainly meet criteria for a diagnosis of schizophrenia, attempts to classify schizophrenia into early-late- and very-late-onset subtypes should be tempered with the recognition that comorbid medical and neurologic diagnoses can contribute to psychotic symptoms in later life (Häfner, 2019). In fact, Talaslahti et al. (2015), in comparing earlier (younger than 60 years of age) to very late-onset (60 years of age or older) schizophrenia, stated that higher mortality rates in those with very late onset were explained primarily by physical comorbidities and accidents.

For many individuals, late-onset schizophrenia marks the beginning of a chronic disorder with periods of remission and symptom recurrence. The insidious deterioration of personality and social adjustment characteristic of early-onset schizophrenia also occurs; however, cognitive declines are no faster in older noninstitutionalized patients with schizophrenia than in normal comparison subjects. In all age groups, antipsychotic medications are an effective treatment for many of the positive symptoms, especially when coupled with a structured environment (milieu), including social skills training and supportive nurse-patient interactions. Research documenting the long-term course of schizophrenia is extremely limited; however, many patients with chronic schizophrenia reach late life despite the high mortality associated with chronic early-onset schizophrenia. Data in later life show that schizophrenia consists of fluctuations in symptoms and level of functioning that require different treatment approaches. Pathways to improvement and recovery in this population exist and should be targeted toward specific outcomes rather than using a specific approach to address several outcomes. Furthermore, outcomes for those with schizophrenia should incorporate a life-span perspective that moves along a continuum from illness to functional recovery to successful ageing (Cohen, 2015).

In examining how sex, age, and other risk factors influence the incidence and course of illness, Häfner (2019) reported that schizophrenia is found along life's continuum. The lifetime risk seems to be the same for both sexes, except for the lower incidence in premenopausal women that results from the negative effect of estrogen on dopamine receptors. Symptoms typically re-emerge post-menopause, and depression is the most frequent symptom in the long-term course. In a rare systematic review and meta-analysis of the effect of age on long-term clinical and psychosocial outcomes of schizophrenia, individuals diagnosed at a younger age have more hospitalizations, negative symptoms, and relapses and less promising social and employment functioning. However, these significant relationships were small and less clinically important than previously thought. These data suggest that duration of illness may potentially explain the association between age at onset and less optimal outcomes (Immonen et al., 2017).

Hazardous lifestyle choices, suboptimal access to health care, poor compliance with treatments, and greater severity of medical comorbidities may all contribute to increased mortality. Men with a past diagnosis of schizophrenia spectrum disorders show excess mortality from infections, cardiovascular diseases, chronic respiratory diseases, substance-induced or mental disorders, and diseases of the nervous system. Cigarette smoking, excessive weight, and alcohol appear to be contributing factors to mortality. The increase of movement disorders and metabolic syndrome (weight gain, obesity, hyperglycemia, and hypertriglyceridemia) in older patients treated with traditional antipsychotics complicates medical management, increases the degree of disability associated with the disorder, and contributes to the high cost of services for older adult patients with schizophrenia. Unlike young adults, older people will visit their primary care physician at least once a year, offering health professionals an opportunity to intervene in order to minimize the harms associated with severe mental disorders (Meesters et al., 2016).

Older patients with schizophrenia, especially individuals who return to the community after long-term institutionalization, may have significant deficits in daily living skills and lack the social networks important to successful adaptation. Similar to what has been reported in younger patients, psychological and social needs appear to be underserviced in the elderly who experience schizophrenia. Chapter 14 in this book provides an overview of antipsychotic agents used to treat schizophrenia along with warnings/cautions to use with the elderly. There is a black box warning for using dementia-related psychotic drugs in elderly patients because of the increased risk for death.

Clinical Example: Just can't get along

Ms. Yu is a 68-year-old Asian American brought to the hospital by her sister, with whom she lives. She accuses her sister of forcing her into the hospital so that the sister can steal her money and car. The sister can recall no recent major stressor or signs of physical illness. She states that Ms. Yu has no history of psychiatric symptoms but has always been a "loner." Despite obtaining a college degree, she had a stormy employment history because she was "unable to get along" with coworkers. She also was unable to sustain a long-term relationship with any man whom she dated. Ms. Yu's appearance is evidence of her inattention to dress and grooming. Although she is cooperative with the examination, her mood is dysphoric, and she has a flat affect. She admits to auditory hallucinations, particularly voices of people whom she knows, often conversing with each other. The voices tell her that they will steal from her, and they sometimes tell her to hurt herself. A complete evaluation resulted in a diagnosis of schizophrenia. The geropsychiatrist ordered olanzapine (Zyprexa) 2.5 mg at bedtime.

Paranoid Thinking

Paranoid symptoms are common in older adults. Delusions are generally chronic and well systematized and, unless associated with dementia or delirium, are not associated with memory loss, disorientation, or diminished cognitive function. The content often involves persecution, jealousy (e.g., infidelity), or unusual situations that might conceivably occur in real life. It is important to investigate actual facts before labeling beliefs as delusional because patients might relate bizarre tales that have a basis in reality. Because physicality is compromised with age, paranoid thinking often emerges as a defense mechanism against a potentially hostile environment. Walking to the corner store in some neighborhoods might be perilous for older individuals because they are less

Clinical Example: A cruel hoax

Mrs. Justice is an 81-year-old African American who was referred to the community mental health center by her primary care physician for treatment of psychosis. The neatly attired and spry woman tearfully relates that "haunts" have been breaking into her house at night, stealing money and other possessions. She sees the ghostly apparitions at least once a month, and when they appear, they speak to her, most often saying, "You stay out of the way, old woman, or we'll get you!" Before initiating pharmacologic intervention, a nurse practitioner conducted a home visit and found Mrs. Justice's home in disarray. Broken windows, gaps where kitchen appliances had been removed, and other findings led the nurse to request a police investigation. On the first night of their home surveillance, police arrested two young men dressed in white sheets who were hiding behind high shrubbery in front of the house. Interventions that were social rather than pharmacologic were instituted. This actual case is an example of how cultural awareness and careful investigation prevented subsequent inappropriate diagnosis and treatment.

able than younger people to fend off aggressors. A retreat into an environment that the fearful older adult can control results in increasing isolation. Although the threat might be based on reality, the resulting isolation and decrease in external stimuli, along with suspicious behaviors, can lead to paranoid thinking. Vasiliadis et al. (2021) also proposes other factors contributing to paranoid thinking, such as socioeconomic status (e.g., widowhood) and health issues (e.g., hearing loss).

ANXIETY DISORDERS

Anxiety disorders along with depression are the most prevalent of the mental disorders in older adults, affecting approximately 30% of adults at some point in their lives (American Psychiatric Association, 2021). Little research has specifically addressed anxiety symptoms and syndromes in older adults, perhaps because epidemiologic data have revealed lower rates of anxiety disorders in community-dwelling older adults compared with younger groups. As with other mental disorders, the majority of anxiety disorders do not begin in later life but are a recurrence or worsening of a preexisting condition, with more of these diagnoses occurring in females rather than in males (Anxiety & Depression Association of America, 2021). Approximately 27% of individuals 45 to 59 years old have an anxiety disorder, decreasing to 9.0% at age 60 and older (National Mental Health Institute, 2017). Available data regarding specific anxiety disorders in older adults found that social phobia was lower among adults aged 50 years or older (0.3%) than among adults aged 26 to 49 (1.2%). Generalized anxiety disorder was more than twice as common among adults aged 26 to 49 (2.5%) years than among those aged 50 years and older (1.2%). Those aged 50 years and older who had a specific phobia, agoraphobia, posttraumatic stress disorder, and obsessive-compulsive and related disorders were similar to those who were aged 18 to 25 and 26 to 49 years (Karg et al., 2014). Cognitive, behavioral, somatic, and physiologic symptoms are similar to those of other age groups.

Many older adults have symptoms of anxiety that fail to meet diagnostic criteria for an anxiety disorder. Two anxiety disorders defined in the *DSM* might be overrepresented in older adults. "Anxiety due to a general medical condition" is a commonly used diagnosis resulting from the frequency of anxiety related to cardiovascular, endocrine, respiratory, and neurologic disorders in this age group. "Substance/medication-induced anxiety disorder" might be present in 10% of community-dwelling older adults and 30% of nursing home residents, a consequence of substance abuse and dependence as well as toxicity from prescription drugs, such as benzodiazepines. Unfortunately, exposure can lead to delirium and falls with subsequent fractures (Hofmann, 2013).

SUBSTANCE USE

Substance use and dependence place older adults at tremendous risk of negative physical, psychological, and social consequences that often go undetected. There are approximately 43.1 million people ages 65 and over who live in the United States. The rate of substance dependence or abuse for males is greater than the rate for females (10.7% vs. 5.7%) and lower among adults aged 45 to 64 (6%) and 65 and older (2.3%). Marijuana use, prescription drugs used nonmedically, and different illicit drugs such as cocaine or heroin were also noted as being used by older adults. For example, marijuana use among adults aged 45 to 64 and 65 years and older are 14.0% and 5.1%, respectively (US Department of Health and Human Services, 2020). Alcohol and medication misuse together has been estimated to affect up to 19% of older Americans. About 25% of older adults use prescription psychoactive medications that have a potential to be misused and abused.

Alcohol Abuse and Dependence

Alcohol abuse and dependence also is a problem for many older adults. Approximately 40% of adults aged 65 and older drink alcohol (National Institute on Alcohol Abuse and Alcoholism, 2020). While alcohol use disorder is lower among adults aged 45 to 64 (4.8%) and 65 or older (2.0%; US Department of Health and Human Services, 2020), a significant number of these individuals drink daily. For example, using pooled data, the National Health Interview Survey (National Center for Health Statistics, 2014) describes the drinking patterns of those aged 60 or older. Of those who reported drinking during the year before the survey, 50% of men and 39% of the women were almost daily drinkers. Almost 6.0% of all men and 0.9% of all women aged over 60 reported binge drinking once a month or more. In an analysis using 135,440 participants age 65 years and older from across the world, current alcohol drinking was positively associated with better health status among older adults, and past alcohol drinking was inversely related with health status. Hence, changes in health status from drinking alcohol occur over time and warrant interventions to lessen consumption (Tyrovolas et al., 2020).

Along with assessment of the quantity of alcohol consumed, physiologic changes that occur with aging, medications, and certain conditions (e.g., cognitive disorders) that intensify effects of alcohol must be considered. Older adults show greater central nervous system sensitivity to alcohol than younger drinkers, so adverse effects on cognition and coordination are more pronounced by comparison. Even if older adults do not increase their level of alcohol consumption compared to earlier years, their bodies react as if they were drinking more. As people age, their bodies work more slowly to clear medications and alcohol. Alcohol can cause adverse reactions to many prescription and over-the-counter (OTC) medications.

Alcohol abuse and dependence might occur for the first time in late life or might represent an unresolved problem from earlier life. More men than women approach late life with problem drinking; although men represent most older adults who abuse alcohol, late-onset alcohol abuse is more common in women than in men. Numerous risk factors have been identified for late-onset problematic drinking. The presence of chronic medical disorders and sleep disturbances might lead some older adults to self-medicate with alcohol to control pain or induce sleep. Some isolated older adults or older adults with excessive free time use drinking to combat boredom or loneliness. Individuals who have lost a spouse are particularly at risk (Butt et al., 2020; Joo et al., 2016).

Problematic alcohol use in older adults is often minimized or undetected by health care providers. Recognition may be difficult because of challenges in recognizing alcohol abuse secondary to the aging process itself. Disorientation, forgetfulness, hoarding, inadequate diet, and neglect of personal appearance all may be attributed to the aging process but are also symptomatic of alcohol misuse. Older adults often underreport alcohol consumption as a result of impaired recall, guilt, or shame. Social stigma is especially strong in older women, who are more likely than men to drink secretly at home and make efforts to conceal their drinking behavior. Screening tools such as the CAGE (Cut Down, Annoyed, Guilty, and Eye Opener) questionnaire and the Geriatric Michigan Alcohol Screening Test (G-MAST) can assist in identification of at-risk drinkers and should be included in health assessments of older adults. It is important to ask questions about alcohol consumption and its effects on life.

Nurses should also be attuned to the possibility of alcohol as a contributing factor in many problems seen in older medical and psychiatric patients. Problem drinkers generally have more health-related complaints than their peers, and older women are particularly susceptible to the toxic effects of alcohol. Withdrawal symptoms might be the first indication of alcohol dependence. Alcohol withdrawal includes a broad spectrum of symptoms, and although the severity of withdrawal symptoms is not appreciably different across age groups, physiologic changes and comorbid physical conditions place older adults at an increased risk. Nurses have a significant role in the management of alcohol withdrawal (Box 35.4).

Various interventions are available to support continued abstinence after withdrawal. For some late-onset drinkers, education and abstinence advice are effective. For other drinkers, including long-term alcohol abusers, formal structured programs are necessary. Greatest success is achieved when the program is geared specifically for older adults. Programs for older adults emphasize peer bonding and shared reminiscing in addition to cognitive behavioral training that addresses themes such as self-efficacy, self-esteem, and relapse prevention strategies. Whenever possible, it is of paramount importance to address factors that initially led to problem drinking.

Drug Misuse and Abuse

Problems may result from the overuse, misuse, and dependency on prescription and OTC medications by older adults. Individuals aged 65 years and older also account for greater than one-third of total outpatient spending on prescription medications in the United States. Older patients are more likely to be prescribed long-term and multiple prescriptions, which could lead to the improper use of medications. Chronic aches and pains from osteoarthritis, aging, and other disorders also make older individuals at risk for misuse of pain medications, with women having a higher use than men. Most frequently used medications were opioids and benzodiazepines. The use of these medications is also linked to falls (Haddad et al., 2019) and an increased risk of suicidal ideations in older adults (Schepis et al., 2019). Clinicians encountering older adult patients at-risk for or engaged in prescription medication misuse also should screen for suicidality.

Psychoactive, mood-changing drugs have the potential for misuse, abuse, or dependency. Box 35.5 provides guidelines for the use of psychotropic drugs in older adults. Benzodiazepines, used for the treatment of anxiety and insomnia, are of particular concern because they are frequently prescribed at inappropriately high doses and for excessive periods (Gerlach et al., 2018). This practice might lead to tolerance, physiologic dependence, and psychological dependence. Adult men are two to three times more likely than women to develop drug abuse/dependence disorders. These differences between men and women may relate to (1) biological responses to the drug, (2) drug dependence progression, and (3) comorbid psychiatric diagnoses.).

BOX 35.4 Nursing Care of Alcohol Withdrawal Syndrome in Older Adults

Assess withdrawal symptoms.
Assess vital signs.
Educate about withdrawal process.
Assist with activities of daily living.
Reduce environmental stimuli.
Supplement diet to meet nutritional needs.
Reorient patient.
Provide relaxation exercises.

BOX 35.5 Guidelines for Psychotropic Drug Use in Older Adults

Initial Dose (Start Low-Go Slow)
- Usually one-third to one-half of dose used for younger adults is effective.
- Start with a small dose and gradually increase until therapeutic effect or adverse side effects occur.

Daily Dosage
- Use the smallest dose that produces relief.
- Simplify dosing schedule.

Individualization
- Monitor blood levels when possible.
- Consider effects of other drugs and conditions.
- Partial symptom relief might be the most judicious and realistic goal.

Discontinuation
- Gradually taper off psychotropic drugs.
- If patients can manage without drug therapy, they should be allowed to do so.

Variable usage of prescribed drugs is a significant problem, exacerbated by poor vision and hearing, physical deficits, confusion, mental disorders, and inadequate instructions. Drug costs and packaging should also be considered as factors that impede optimal usage. Further complicating the situation, older adults might add several OTC agents, combine medications with alcohol, or take medication prescribed for others without notifying their prescriber. Many older adults see multiple providers, each of whom might prescribe drugs without reliable information about medications that the others have prescribed. Confusion caused by generic and trade names can result in older adults taking the same medication under two names at the same time. Polypharmacy is common, so the nurse should be aware of potential complications and encourage patients to show the nurse all medications for cataloging. Drug regimens should be simplified and carefully explained, verbally and in writing.

CRITICAL THINKING QUESTION

4. Do nurses at the facility where you have clinical rotations routinely include the same questions for alcohol and other drugs in their assessments of older adults as they do for younger adults? Do you feel comfortable asking your patients questions about alcohol or drug use?

ASSESSMENT OF OLDER ADULTS WITH MENTAL DISORDERS

Mental disorders are not isolated phenomena in older adults. Comprehensive psychosocial and physical assessments are required to determine factors that influence the older adult's level of function. Family members or other caregivers, who often play a pivotal role in the function of older adults, should be included in the assessment process whenever possible. The goals of the initial assessment and subsequent reassessments are to collect accurate information, identify problems and assets, plan interventions, predict outcomes, and measure changes over time. Because of the amount and depth of information needed, the nurse often works collaboratively with the health care team to complete the assessment in collaboration with the patient and caregivers and develops goals and methods for care. Strategies to facilitate effective communication are found in Box 35.6.

PSYCHOSOCIAL ASSESSMENT

A wealth of clinical data can be obtained by listening to the stories that many older adults love to tell. Listening not only conveys a sense of appreciation for the individual's contributions across the life span but also provides the patient a nonthreatening means of communicating pertinent information. The nurse should listen carefully during these conversations for persistent themes, such as guilt, stress, grief, fear, or despair. By accepting expressed fears and concerns, the nurse

BOX 35.6 Enhancing Communication With Older Adults

Considerations	Nursing Implications
Slowed information processing	Do not rush; allow adequate time for questions to be answered.
	Use common words and short sentences.
	Avoid unnecessary interruptions.
Establishment of rapport	Offer a handshake; if appropriate culturally, physically acceptable (not painful).
	Make eye contact.
	Position at equal or lower level than patient while remaining in view.
	Address by title and last name unless asked to use another name.
Hearing deficits	Use a calm, clear voice.
	Articulate words clearly.
	Face patient when speaking.
	Adjust volume of speech to patient's need; do not shout.
	Ensure use of hearing aid or amplifier.
	Use complementary nonverbal strategies (e.g., facial expressions, gestures).
Visual deficits	Provide adequate nonglare lighting.
	Ensure use of corrective lens.
Competing stimuli	Minimize background noise.
	Avoid times when patient is excessively tired, is in pain, is hungry, or has toileting needs.
	Provide privacy.
Education level	Match vocabulary to patient's level of use.
Decreased physical tolerance	Avoid overtiring.

assures the patient that these expressions will not result in rejection. Box 35.7 lists information to obtain during the initial assessment.

Caregivers should be included in the assessment process. Not only can they provide information to clarify or expand on that given by the patient, but also their perspective of problems is important for inclusion in a plan of care. Family members might be embarrassed to contradict information given by the patient in a joint interview. Because assessing family interaction is important, time should be spent interviewing the patient and family members both separately and together.

PHYSICAL ASSESSMENT

Throughout this chapter, the connection between physical conditions and mental disorders has been stressed. A complete physical examination is an essential component in the assessment of any older adult presenting with symptoms of mental disorders. The examination techniques for each

BOX 35.7 Initial Assessment Information

Demographics (age, marital status)
Spiritual and cultural values
Personal and family history
History of legal difficulties
Economic status and sources of income
Education and work history
Lifestyle and perception of current life situation
Current living arrangements
Interests, pleasures, and activities
Friendship and social interactions
Sexual functioning
Medical information and history
Prescription and over-the-counter drugs
Alcohol, tobacco, and other chemical use
Cognitive, behavioral, and emotional status
Goals and plans for the future

BOX 35.8 Functional Assessment

Activities of Daily Living	Instrumental Activities of Daily Living
Bathing	Preparing meals
Dressing	Shopping
Eating	Managing money
Transferring	Using the telephone
Walking	Toileting
Doing housework	Taking medication

subsystem do not differ substantially from the examination of younger adults. Adaptations for decreased mobility and obvious impairments must be made. Careful attention to every subsystem is required because in older adults examination might reveal abnormalities in a system not suggested by the presenting symptoms. For example, subtle hearing loss can result in bizarre or incorrect responses, leading to erroneous assumptions about psychopathologic conditions. The nurse should use all senses during the examination, attending to the patient's visual presentation, odors, voice tone, and content. Blood tests, electroencephalography, and neuroimaging studies might be ordered to identify conditions that contribute to symptoms of mental disorders.

Special attention should be given to defining how physical problems interfere with the patient's functional ability. Older adults assign a great value to independence, and loss of independence can contribute to lower self-esteem and declines in mental health. The loss of key abilities might result in shame and frustration. Older adults who are dependent on others might resent the idea that others have to provide care and might believe that they have become a burden. The resulting anger can be directed internally and result in depression or withdrawal, or it might be directed at caregivers. Assessment of activities of daily living (ADLs) and instrumental activities of daily living (IADLs) provides a measure of the older adult's functional ability and guides the selection of interventions and services to meet identified needs. Box 35.8 identifies some of the variables for both ADLs and IADLs. Patients and sometimes their families are often unable or unwilling to describe functional difficulties because of the threat to established patterns of lifestyle and interactions. According to the Administration on Aging (2020), approximately 19% of those who are age 45 to 64 years and 50% of those who are age 75 years and older have difficulty with physical functioning, 95% of institutionalized Medicare beneficiaries had difficulties with one or more ADLs, and 81.0% experience difficulty with three or more ADLs. Observing task performance and

carefully listening both to the patient and to collateral sources (e.g., family or caregiver) as they describe daily activities might provide a more accurate picture of functional ability than direct questioning.

The physical examination should be used as an opportunity to assess for signs of abuse or neglect. Each state has laws that specify reporting requirements for intentional abuse, neglect, and exploitation of older adults. Laws also cover endangerment resulting from mental disorders. Chapter 3 discusses some legal issues that might stem from abuse or neglect.

PSYCHOTHERAPEUTIC MANAGEMENT

Nurse-Patient Relationship

Ageist attitudes, intergenerational differences, communication deficits, and the multiple problems of older adults can pose significant obstacles to developing a therapeutic nurse-patient relationship. Nurses who are aware of their own feelings and reactions are able to focus on patients and their significant others in a therapeutic manner. By empathizing with the patient and caregivers and focusing on the patient's needs, the nurse can assist patients and their families to manage the activities and demands of daily living and improve the overall quality of both physical and mental health.

Communication

Communicating a sense of unconditional acceptance of the patient might be the most important intervention that the nurse can provide. Spending time with the patient beyond that required for tasks such as medication administration and ADLs communicates an appreciation for the patient as a person of worth. Providing opportunities for the patient to participate in care decisions and to control the sequence of events, such as allowing the patient to choose when to bathe, enhances self-esteem, self-worth, and decision-making skills. The nurse must be aware of problems and unspoken needs and incorporate them into the plan of care.

Realistic Goals

Establishing short-term and long-term goals is important for nurses and patients. Discussions should be held with patients to stress the importance of goal setting. ADLs often can be a challenge, and developing a schedule of the day's

Case Study

Ms. Othelia Thatcher, 78 years old, with a 10-year history of severe depression, has been hospitalized twice in the last 2 years. She received a series of ECT treatments during each stay, with the last treatment given 11 months ago. Ms. Thatcher's cousin, a woman about 60 years old, brought the patient to the hospital emergency department this morning. The cousin described a gradual worsening of depressive symptoms over the past few months and says that Ms. Thatcher seems to need ECT approximately once a year. About 6 or 7 months after a course of ECT has been completed, the patient "goes bad again."

Ms. Thatcher complains of erratic sleep patterns and decreased appetite. She will not eat unless her cousin spoon-feeds her. The cousin reports that after a series of ECT, the patient is "easier to live with," plays with children, takes care of herself, helps with household tasks, and will "eat anything not nailed down."

The cousin estimates that the patient's depression began in the 1990s when "her only son, to whom she was very devoted," abandoned Ms. Thatcher to the welfare of the state and sold all her furniture. This occurred after the patient's extended hospitalization for treatment of pneumonia and a urinary tract infection. Since that time, Ms. Thatcher had reportedly lived in five different boarding homes before her cousin took her to the hospital 3 years ago.

The cousin states that Ms. Thatcher has never verbalized suicidal or homicidal thoughts, but she has a basically "paranoid view of life." The cousin cannot recall Ms. Thatcher ever having hallucinations.

---

activities with goals can help patients make decisions and cope with demands. Simple decisions might be difficult for older adults with mental disorders. Reducing the options available before allowing the patient choices can diminish frustration. For example, when it is time to dress, the nurse might restrict the choices of attire to two rather than offering an entire closet of options. The caregiver must be gentle and supportive because additional time might be needed to achieve goals. Caregivers who base care decisions on the goal of restoring the patient to maximal independent function are likely to resist the urge to save time and energy by taking over tasks. Nurses should provide information on self-care and disease management at a pace that facilitates understanding. Patience, positive reinforcement, and consistency by the nurse benefit the patient.

Psychopharmacology

Unit III contains a detailed overview of medications used in psychiatric care. Therefore, that information is not repeated here. However, two important aspects of aging that affect these medications are discussed: pharmacokinetic changes and pharmacodynamic changes.

Pharmacokinetic Changes in Older Adults

Polypharmacy, physiologic changes, and comorbid physical disorders combine to increase the risk of unexpected drug effects in older adults. The negative impact of typical side effects is also exacerbated. Age-related changes that affect drug absorption, distribution, metabolism, and elimination are listed in Table 35.3 (Maher et al., 2021). Knowledge of *pharmacokinetics* is important, particularly when elderly patients take multiple drugs. For example, antacids might delay absorption; proximal loop and potassium-sparing diuretics affect lithium excretion. Knowledge of drugs' characteristics and their site and mechanism of action is important to understanding the sensitivity that older adults' exhibit. For example, antipsychotic medications that act by blocking dopamine receptors have an increased likelihood of causing extrapyramidal side effects (EPSEs) in older adults who already have diminished dopamine concentrations. Nurses must observe and report expected therapeutic and adverse medication reactions and plan interventions to minimize the negative consequences of drug therapy.

Absorption. In general, the percentage of oral dose absorbed by older patients typically does not change with age. However, the rate of absorption may be slowed because of delayed gastric emptying and decreased splanchnic blood flow, which results in delayed drug responses. Gastric acidity also is reduced in older adults, which may alter drug absorption of some drugs (Maher et al., 2021).

Distribution. Four primary factors may alter drug distribution in older adults: (1) increased percentage of body fat, (2) reduced percentage of lean body mass and (3) total body water, and (4) decreased serum albumin concentration. The increased body fat serves as a storage depot for lipid-soluble drugs resulting in decreased drug plasma levels and responses. As a result of the reduced lean body mass and total body water, water-soluble drugs (e.g., ethanol) become distributed in smaller volumes than in younger adults. Therefore increased drug concentrations cause their effects to be more pronounced. Although serum albumin levels are only slightly lower in healthy adults, they are significantly lower in individuals who are malnourished. The low serum levels result in reduced sites for protein binding of drugs and cause increased free drug levels in the body. As a result, drug effects become more pronounced (Maher et al., 2021).

Metabolism. Rates of drug metabolism lessen with age as a result of reduced hepatic blood flow and liver mass and decreased activity of some hepatic enzymes. Because liver function is decreased, the half-life of some drugs may be increased with prolonged drug responses. Responses to drugs that normally undergo extensive first-pass metabolism may be enhanced because fewer drugs are inactivated prior to entering the systemic circulation. Unfortunately, the degree of decline in drug metabolism varies greatly among individuals, making drug responses uncertain in specific patients (Maher et al., 2021).

Excretion. Renal function and renal drug excretion progressively decline, beginning in young adulthood. Drug

TABLE 35.3   Age-Related Changes: Effects on Pharmacokinetics

Physiologic Change	Effects	Special Considerations
↑ Gastric pH ↓ Absorptive surface area ↓ Splanchnic blood flow ↓ Gastrointestinal motility ↓ Gastric emptying	Absorption	Delayed absorption of oral medication Acid drugs more rapidly absorbed than base drugs
↑ Body fat	Distribution	Extended half-life of lipid-soluble drugs, which accumulate in adipose tissue (e.g., barbiturates, phenothiazines, benzodiazepines, phenytoin, TCAs)
↓ Lean body mass ↓ Total body water ↓ Serum albumin		↓Total plasma albumin = ↓ binding sites for protein-bound drugs, resulting in increased amount of free or active drug
↓ Cardiac output ↓ Hepatic blood flow ↓ Hepatic mass	Metabolism	Multiple drugs competing for same enzyme—might ↓ liver metabolism
↓ Hepatic enzyme activity		High degree of genetic variability in available hepatic enzymes
↓ Renal blood flow	Excretion	Creatinine clearance—can be reduced despite normal serum creatinine levels because of ↓ lean body weight and ↓ creatinine production
↓ Glomerular filtration rate ↓ Creatinine production ↓ Creatinine clearance ↓ Tubular secretion ↓ Number of nephrons		Reduction in renal clearance—might reduce dose requirements

TCAs, Tricyclic antidepressants.

Modified from Maher, D., Ailabouni, N., Mangoni, A. A., Wiese, M. D., & Reeve, E. (2021). Alterations in drug disposition in older adults: A focus on geriatric syndromes. *Expert Opinion on Drug Metabolism & Toxicology, 17*(1), 41–52. https://doi.org/10.1080/17425255.2021.1839413.

accumulation secondary to decreased renal excretion is the primary reason for adverse drug reactions in older adult. Reduced renal function occurs from decreased renal blood flow, glomerular filtration rate, active tubular secretion, and number of nephrons. Therefore, in caring for older individuals who are taking drugs eliminated primarily by the kidneys, renal function should be assessed by nurses. In older adults, creatinine clearance rather than serum creatinine levels should be assessed. Creatinine fails to reflect kidney function in older adults because the source of creatinine, lean muscle mass, declines along with renal function. In fact, creatinine levels may be normal even though renal function may be significantly impaired (Maher et al., 2021).

Pharmacodynamic Changes in Older Adults

While changes in receptor properties may cause altered sensitivity to some drugs, pharmacodynamic empirical data are very limited. Supporting the hypothesis of altered pharmacodynamics is the observation that agents are less effective in older than in younger adults, even when these agents are present in the same concentrations. Reasons for the reduced effectiveness may be due to a lower number of receptors or changes in drug-receptor interactions. Other drugs produce more intense effects in older adults, suggesting either a higher number of receptors, increased affinity, or both. For example, the elderly are particularly vulnerable to more intense reactions to anticholinergic drugs, and many psychotropic medications (e.g., some antidepressants, some antipsychotics) have this property as a side effect. Unfortunately, our knowledge of

pharmacodynamics changes in older adults is limited to a few drug families (Maher et al., 2021).

Milieu Management

Nurses responsible for older adults with mental disorders in inpatient or day care settings have a therapeutic responsibility to facilitate optimal function. Attention to all elements of the milieu can increase psychological functioning and prevent the deterioration resulting from withdrawal and disuse of skills that has been well documented in institutionalized older adults.

Normalizing the Environment

Effective milieu management changes the quality of life in institutional environments by working with residents to normalize the environment as much as possible. The traditional associations of home involve control over people who come and go as well as control of personal spaces, furnishings, and accessories. Furniture, at a height that facilitates independent mobility, can be placed in conversational groupings. Common rooms are best equipped with large-print books, games with large print and pieces, and stimulating pictures. Individual rooms can be deinstitutionalized by encouraging residents to use their own bedspreads, family pictures, favorite calendars, and other personal items. This same strategy, even in acute care settings, has the added benefit of providing orientation cues. It is important to remember privacy needs and respect personal space. Environmental adaptations that promote safety and independence for older adults are listed in Table 35.4.

◎ CARE PLAN

Name: Ms. Othelia Thatcher   Admission Date: _____
DSM-5 **Diagnosis: Major depression**

Assessment	**Areas of strength:** Patient is willing to be treated; is cooperative, has a good support system (cousin very concerned and wants patient back in home).
Problems: Withdrawn, decreased interest in interactions and activities, decreased self-esteem, decreased energy, hopelessness, poor judgment.
Diagnoses	Ineffective coping, disturbed sleep pattern, dysfunctional grief (son's behavior, loss of contact, and loss of home and belongings), imbalanced nutrition; less than body requirements, impaired social interaction, self-care deficits
Outcomes
Date met: _____
Date met: _____
Date met: _____

Date met: _____
Date met: _____
Date met: _____
Date met: _____ | **Short-term goals**
Patient can maintain safety.
Patient can express feelings verbally.
Patient will have increased energy for self-care.
Long-term goals
Patient will initiate and respond to social interactions.
Patient will be able to talk about anger and disappointment related to son.
Patient will have an increase in self-concept.
Patient will maintain independence although living in cousin's home. |
| **Planning and Interventions** | **Nurse-patient relationship:** Convey concern and acceptance, encourage expression of feelings, encourage interactions with others as tolerated, help patient explore anger with son.
Psychopharmacology: fluoxetine (Prozac) 20 mg every morning; risperidone (Risperdal) 0.5 mg q12h; docusate sodium 100 mg twice a day (prophylactic)
Milieu management: Provide adequate nutrition and hydration. Monitor patient for safety issues. Keep patient around others (not alone in her room) as much as is reasonable. Keep naps short to facilitate sleep at night. |
| **Evaluation** | Patient expressed feelings of anger at being abandoned by son. Activity level increased. Able to perform activities of daily living independently. Minimal confusion after electroconvulsive therapy. Medication maintained. Patient will be discharged to return to cousin's home. |
| **Referrals** | Schedule visit with home health nurse for follow-up care. Schedule appointment with outpatient program coordinator within 7 days. |

TABLE 35.4   Environmental Adaptation

Considerations	Interventions
Decreased ability to distinguish colors	Use high-contrast colors in vivid hues
Mobility impairments	Ensure nonslip floor surfaces
Provide adequate, nonglare lighting
Ensure well-fitting footwear
Provide chairs and toilets at comfortable height with armrests or handrails
Avoid placing rolling tables where patients might attempt to use them for stability
Provide shower stools, nonskid tub guards, and grab bars
Provide ambulation rails
Remove obstacles, clutter, and spills promptly
Inability to read	Mark spaces with pictures or universal symbols
Decreased thermoregulation	Ensure comfortable temperature
Observe for signs of hypothermia or hyperthermia
Provide sweaters, blankets
Ensure safe water temperature

Controlling Aggression

Controlling aggression is a major component of maintaining individual and environmental safety. Violent or agitated behavior might be the result of poor frustration tolerance, ineffective coping strategies, impulsivity, or real or imagined threats to personal space. Nurses must look at the environment and develop strategies to minimize precipitating factors. Careful attention should be paid to the potential for background stimuli such as constant music or television to cause distress. Physical and chemical restraints to control behavior have numerous negative consequences, and alternative interventions should be attempted before use. Managing environmental stimuli, providing productive outlets for energy, and practicing redirection and diversion are important for reducing outbursts.

Tailoring Activities

Therapeutic approaches should be based on the concept that all individuals have a need for human contact, social participation, and meaningful activity to maintain function. Individual and group interactions and activities should be planned to foster the greatest degree of independence and develop interpersonal and communication skills. Various activities can be tailored to match individual levels of physical and psychological function. Animal-assisted interventions help fulfill patients' needs to give and receive affection through supervised sessions of holding, stroking, and playing with specially screened animals. In fact, these interventions are efficient in improving anxiety, depressive symptoms, apathy, loneliness, and quality of life in residents of long-term care facilities with mental illness (Chang et al., 2021). Exercise therapy, tailored to all needs, including the needs of patients with limited physical ability, provides outlets for the excess energy of anxiety and provides stimulation and socialization opportunities. Music is also an effective way to make contact with patients. Songbooks, hymnals, and various forms of music via technology offer an array of choices familiar to older adults, who often enjoy sing-alongs or simply listening to familiar and comfortable tunes. In fact, community singing in groups appears to significantly affect quality of life, potentially serving as a therapeutic intervention to maintain and enhance the mental health of older people (Corvo, Skingley, & Clift, 2020). Nurturing and tending to plants can enhance physical function, relieve tension, and provide a sense of responsibility and accomplishment. These therapeutic activities and others are important opportunities to provide patients with positive experiences and help them attain realistic goals.

Valuing the Person Through Reminiscence

Reminiscence is the process of recalling past experiences, which provides the listener with insight into the patient's history and perspective. Patients can benefit from multiple dimensions of reminiscence, including clarifying their sense of self, connecting with others, providing instruction, restructuring recalled events, recalling previously used problem-solving strategies, and bringing closure and calmness in death preparation. In fact, in a systematic review, group-based reminiscence therapy was effective in reducing depression and in improving self-esteem, psychological well-being, and happiness (Tam et al., 2021).

STUDY NOTES

1. Despite the increase in the population of individuals aged 65 years and older, this group experiences major barriers to obtaining quality mental health care because of issues such as ageism, their own attitudes, lack of transportation, and cost of care.

2. Depression is a common mental disorder among older adults, but it is often overlooked, misdiagnosed, and inadequately treated.

3. Symptoms of other illnesses might mask depression because older adults might be preoccupied with physical rather than emotional symptoms.

4. Age-related life events, losses, changes, and physical decline are associated with the onset of depression.

5. The nurse-patient relationship focuses on helping patients achieve their highest level of functioning. Caregivers, when available, should be included in planning strategies to manage the activities and demands of daily living.

6. Adequate nutrition, socialization, and achievement of small realistic goals in ADLs help reduce anxiety and maintain or restore psychological functioning.

7. Use of medications in older adults involves risks associated with polypharmacy, variable usage, and altered pharmacokinetics.

8. Recommended agents for treating depression in older adults include selective serotonin reuptake inhibitors (SSRIs), bupropion, and trazodone.

9. When treating psychotic disorders, atypical antipsychotics are usually prescribed. If an older traditional agent is to be used, haloperidol is the most often used agent because of fewer antiadrenergic and anticholinergic effects.

10. Benzodiazepines using phase II metabolism (e.g., lorazepam and oxazepam), SSRIs, and nonbenzodiazepine anxiety agents are prescribed most often for older adults.

11. ECT can be an effective treatment for older adults with depression.

12. Milieu management in the care of older adults includes special attention to normalization, controlling aggression, specifically tailoring activities, and valuing the person through reminiscence.

REFERENCES

Administration for Community Living. (2020a). 2016 Older Americans Act (OAA). https://acl.gov/about-acl/authorizing-statutes/older-americans-act.

Administration for Community Living. (2020b). 2019 profile of older Americans. https://acl.gov/sites/default/files/Aging%20and%20Disability%20in%20America/2019ProfileOlderAmericans508.pdf.

Administration on Aging. (2020). 2019 profile of older Americans. https://acl.gov/sites/default/files/Aging%20and%20Disability%20in%20America/2019ProfileOlderAmericans508.pdf.

Agüera-Ortiz, L., Claver-Martín, M. D., Franco-Fernández, M. D., López-Álvarez, J., Martín-Carrasco, M., Ramos-García, M. I., & Sánchez-Pérez, M. (2020). Depression in the elderly. Consensus statement of the Spanish Psychogeriatric Association. *Frontiers in Psychiatry, 11*, 380. https://doi.org/10.3389/fpsyt.2020.00380.

American Psychiatric Association. (2021). What are anxiety disorders? https://www.psychiatry.org/patients-families/anxiety-disorders/what-are-anxiety-disorders.

Anastos-Wallen, R., Werner, R. M., & Chatterjee, P. (2020). Prevalence of informal caregiving in states participating in the US Patient Protection and Affordable Care Act Balancing Incentive Program, 2011-2018. *JAMA Network Open, 3*(12), e2025833. https://doi.org/10.1001/jamanetworkopen.2020.25833.

Anxiety and Depression Association of America (2021). Generalized anxiety disorder (GAD). https://adaa.org/understanding-anxiety/generalized-anxiety-disorder-gad.

Butt, P. R., White-Campbell, M., Canham, S., Johnston, A. D., Indome, E. O., Purcell, B., Tung, J., & Van Bussel, L. (2020). Canadian guidelines on alcohol use disorder among older adults. *Canadian Geriatrics Journal*, 23(1), 143–148. https://doi.org/10.5770/cgj.23.425.

Centers for Disease Control and Prevention (CDC). (2021). Depression is not a normal part of growing older. https://www.cdc.gov/aging/depression/index.html.

Centers for Disease Control and Prevention (CDC) (2018). Vital signs: Suicide rising across the US. https://www.cdc.gov/vitalsigns/pdf/vs-0618-suicide-H.pdf.

Chang, S. J., Lee, J., An, H., Hong, W. H., & Lee, J. Y. (2021). Animal-assisted therapy as an intervention for older adults: A systematic review and meta-analysis to guide evidence-based practice. *Worldviews on Evidence-based Nursing*, 18(1), 60–67. https://doi.org/10.1111/wvn.12484.

Choi, J., Yang, K., Chu, S. H., Youm, Y., Kim, H. C., Park, Y. R., & Son, Y. J. (2020). Social activities and health-related quality of life in rural older adults in South Korea: A 4-year longitudinal analysis. *International Journal of Environmental Research and Public Health*, 17(15), 5553. https://doi.org/10.3390/ijerph17155553.

Cohen, C. I. (2015). New perspectives on schizophrenia in later life: Implications for treatment, policy, and research. *Lancet Psychiatry*, 2, 340–350. https://doi.org/10.1016/S2215-0366(15)00003-6.

Corvo, E., Skingley, A., & Clift, S. (2020). Community singing, wellbeing and older people: Implementing and evaluating an English singing for health intervention in Rome. *Perspecives in Public Health*, 140(5), 263–269. https://doi.org/10.1177/1757913920925834.

Curtin, S. C. (2019). Suicide rates for females and males by race and ethnicity: United States, 1999 and 2017. https://www.cdc.gov/nchs/data/hestat/suicide/rates_1999_2017.htm.

Dahlberg, L., McKee, K. J., Frank, A., & Naseer, M. (2021). A systematic review of longitudinal risk factors for loneliness in older adults. *Aging & Mental Health*, Februrary 10, 1–25. https://doi.org/10.1080/13607863.2021.1876638. Advance online publication.

D'cruz, M., & Banerjee, D. (2020). 'An invisible human rights crisis': The marginalization of older adults during the COVID-19 pandemic – An advocacy review. *Psychiatry Research*, 292, 113369. https://doi.org/10.1016/j.psychres.2020.113369.

Dols, A., & Beekman, A. (2020). Older age bipolar disorder. *Clinics in Geriatric Medicine*, 36(2), 281–296. https://doi.org/10.1016/j.cger.2019.11.008.

Donald, E. E., & Stajduhar, K. I. (2020). A scoping review of palliative care for persons with severe persistent mental illness. *Palliative & Supportive Care*, 17(4), 479–487. https://doi.org/10.1017/S1478951519000087.

De Pue, S., Gillebert, C., Dierckx, E., Vanderhasselt, M., De Raedt, R., & Van den Bussche, E. (2021). The impact of the COVID-19 pandemic on wellbeing and cognitive functioning of older adults. *Scientific Reports*, 11, 4636. https://doi.org/10.1038/s41598-021-84127-7.

Edleson, H. (2019). More Americans working past 65. https://www.aarp.org/work/employers/info-2019/americans-working-past-65.html.

Federal Interagency Forum on Aging-Related Statistics. (2020). *Older Americans 2020: Key indicators of well-being. Federal Interagency Forum on aging-related statistics.* US Government Printing Office. https://agingstats.gov/docs/LatestReport/OA20_508_10142020.pdf.

Gardiner, C., Geldenhuys, G., & Gott, M. (2016). Interventions to reduce social isolation and loneliness among older people: An integrative review. *Health & Social Care in the Community*, 26(2), 147–157. https://doi.org/10.1111/hsc.12367.

Gerlach, L. B., Wiechers, I. R., Donovan, T., & Maust, D. T. (2018). Prescription benzodiazepine use among older adults: A critical review. *Harvard Review of Psychiatry*, 26(5), 264–273. https://doi.org/10.1097/HRP.0000000000000190.

Haddad, Y. K., Luo, F., Karani, M. V., Marcum, Z. A., & Lee, R. (2019). Psychoactive medication use among older community-dwelling Americans. *Journal of the American Pharmacists Association*, 59(5), 686–690. https://doi.org/10.1016/j.japh.2019.05.001.

Häfner, H. (2019). From onset and prodromal stage to a life-long course of schizophrenia and its symptom dimensions: How sex, age, and other risk factors influence incidence and course of illness. *Psychiatry Journal*, 2019, 9804836. https://doi.org/10.1155/2019/9804836.

Harmer, B., Lee, S., Duong, T. V. H., & Saadabadi, A. Suicidal ideation. [Updated 2020 Nov 23]. In StatPearls [Internet]. StatPearls Publishing. https://www.ncbi.nlm.nih.gov/books/NBK565877/#_NBK565877_pubdet_.

Hofmann, W. (2013). Benzodiazepines in geriatrics. *Zeitschrift fur Gerontolgie und Geriatrie*, 4, 769–776. https://doi.org/10.1007/s00391-013-0551-3. quiz 776.

Hung, P., Busch, S. H., Shih, Y., McGregor, A. J., & Shiyi Wang, S. (2020). Changes in community mental health services availability and suicide mortality in the US: A retrospective study. *BMC Psychiatry*, 20, 188. https://doi.org/10.1186/s12888-020-02607-y.

Immonen, J., Jääskeläinen, E., Korpela, H., & Miettunen, J. (2017). Age at onset and the outcomes of schizophrenia: A systematic review and meta-analysis. *Early Intervention in Psychiatry*, 11(6), 453–460. https://doi.org/10.1111/eip.12412.

Jang, Y., Choi, E. Y., Park, N. S., Chiriboga, D. A., Duan, L., & Kim, M. T. (2021). Cognitive health risks posed by social isolation and loneliness in older Korean Americans. *BMC Geriatrics*, 21, 123. https://doi.org/10.1186/s12877-021-02066-4.

Joo, S. H., Wang, S., Kim, T., Seo, H., Jeong, J., Han, J., & Hong, S. (2016). Factors associated with suicide completion: A comparison between suicide attempters and completers. *Asia Pac Psychiatry*, 8(1), 80–86. https://doi.org/10.1111/appy.12216.

Julião, M., Chochinov, H. M., Samorinha, C., Soares, D. D. S., & Antunes, B. J. (2021). Prevalence and factors associated with will-to-live in patients with advanced disease: Results from a Portuguese retrospective study. *Pain and Symptom Management*, S0885-3924(21). https://doi.org/10.1016/j.jpainsymman.2021.02.018. 00207-4.

Karg, R. S., Bose, J., Batts, K. R., Forman-Hoffman, V. L., Liao, D., Hirsch, E., …, Hedden, S. L. (2014). Past year mental disorders among adults in the United States: Results from the 2008–2012 mental health surveillance study. CBHSQ Data Review. Substance Abuse and Mental Health Services Administration (US).

Kim, S. H., Kim, H. J., Oh, S. H., & Cha, K. (2020). Analysis of attempted suicide episodes presenting to the emergency department: Comparison of young, middle aged and older people. *International Journal of Mental Health Systems*, 14, 46. https://doi.org/10.1186/s13033-020-00378-3.

Krendl, A. C., & Perry, B. L. (2021). The impact of sheltering in place during the COVID-19 pandemic on older adults' social and mental well-being. *Journal of Gerontology B Psychological*

Sciences, 76(2), e53–e58. https://doi.org/10.1093/geronb/gbaa110.

Lai, D., Li, J., & Ou, C. (2020). Effectiveness of a peer-based intervention on loneliness and social isolation of older Chinese immigrants in Canada: A randomized controlled trial. BMC Geriatrics, 20, 356. https://doi.org/10.1186/s12877-020-01756-9.

Lapid, M. I., Seiner, S., Heintz, H., Hermida, A. P., Nykamp, L., Sanghani, S. N., … Forester, B. P. (2020). Electroconvulsive therapy practice changes in older individuals due to COVID-19: Expert consensus statement. American Journal of Geriatric Psychiatry, 28(11), 1133–1145. https://doi.org/10.1016/j.jagp.2020.08.001.

Maher, D., Ailabouni, N., Mangoni, A. A., Wiese, M. D., & Reeve, E. (2021). Alterations in drug disposition in older adults: A focus on geriatric syndromes. Expert Opinion on Drug Metabolism & Toxicology, 17(1), 41–52. https://doi.org/10.1080/17425255.2021.1839413.

Manca, R., De Marco, M., & Venneri, A. (2020). The impact of COVID-19 infection and enforced prolonged social isolation on neuropsychiatric symptoms in older adults with and without dementia: A review. Frontiers in Psychiatry, 11, 585540. https://doi.org/10.3389/fpsyt.2020.585540.

McDonald, W. M. (2016). Neuromodulation treatments for geriatric mood and cognitive disorders. American Journal of Geriatric Psychiatry, 24, 1130–1141. https://doi.org/10.1016/j.jagp.2016.08.014.

Meesters, P. D., Comijs, H. C., Smit, J. H., Eikelenboom, P., de Haan, L., Beekman, A. T., & Stek, M. L. (2016). Mortality and its determinants in late-life schizophrenia: A 5-year prospective study in a Dutch catchment area. American Journal of Geriatric Psychiatry, 24(4), 272–277. https://doi.org/10.1016/j.jagp.2015.09.003.

Mental Health America. (2021a). FAQ for understanding 988 and how it can help with behavioral health crises. https://mhanational.org/sites/default/files/FAQ%20with%20vibrant%20FINAL%20COPY.pdf.

Mental Health America. (2021b). Position statement 71: Health care reform. https://www.mhanational.org/issues/position-statement-71-health-care-reform.

National Aging and Disability Transportation Center. (2021a). Transportation: Aging & disability. https://www.nadtc.org/about/transportation-aging-disability/.

National Aging and Disability Transportation Center. (2021b). Older adults and transportation. https://www.nadtc.org/about/transportation-aging-disability/unique-issues-related-to-older-adults-and-transportation/.

National Alliance on Mental Illness (NAMI). (2019). Major depression. http://www.nami.org.

National Association of Area Agencies on Aging. (2020). 2020 policy priorities. https://www.n4a.org/files/n4a_2020PolicyPriorities_Web%20(1).pdf.

National Center for Health Statistics. (2014). Summary health statistics for U.S. adults: National health interview survey, 2012. Author.

National Institute of Mental Health. (2021). Major depression. https://www.nimh.nih.gov/health/statistics/major-depression.shtml.

National Institutte for Mental Illness. (2021). Mental llness. https://www.nimh.nih.gov/health/statistics/mental-illness.shtml.

National Institute on Alcohol Abuse and Alcoholism. (2020). Older adults. https://www.niaaa.nih.gov/alcohol-health/special-populations-co-occurring-disorders/older-adults.

National Mental Health Institute. (2017). Any anxiety disorder. https://www.nimh.nih.gov/health/statistics/any-anxiety-disorder.shtml.

Ramasamy, S., & Bharath, S. (2017). Clinical characteristics of patients with non-affective, non-organic, late onset psychosis. Asian Journal of Psychiatry, 25, 74–78. https://doi.org/10.1016/j.ajp.2016.10.017.

Reynolds, K. (2015). Prevalence of psychiatric disorders in U.S. older adults: Findings from a nationally representative survey. World Psychiatry, 14(1), 74–81. https://doi.org/10.1002/wps.20193.

Roberts, A. W., Ogunwole, S. U., Blakeslee, L., & Rabe, M. A. (2018). https://www.census.gov/library/publications/2018/acs/acs-38.html.

Schepis, T. S., Simoni-Wastila, L., & McCabe, S. E. (2019). Prescription opioid and benzodiazepine misuse is associated with suicidal ideation in older adults. International Journal of Geriatric Psychiatry, 34(1), 122–129. https://doi.org/10.1002/gps.4999.

Smith, M. L., Steinman, L. E., & Casey, E. A. (2020). Combatting social isolation among older adults in a time of physical distancing: The COVID-19 social connectivity paradox. Frontiers in Public Health, 8, 403. https://doi.org/10.3389/fpubh.2020.00403.

Talaslahti, T., et al. (2015). Patients with very-late-onset schizophrenia-like psychosis have higher mortality rates than elderly patients with earlier onset schizophrenia. International Journal of Geriatric Psychiatry, 30, 453–459. https://doi.org/10.1002/ gps.4159.

Tam, W., Poon, S., Mahendran, R., Kua, E., & Wu, X. (2021). The effectiveness of reminiscence-based intervention on improving psychological well-being in cognitively intact older adults: A systematic review and meta-analysis. International Journal of Nursing Studies, 114, 103847. https://doi.org/10.1016/j.ijnurstu.2020.103847.

Tyrovolas, S., Panaretos, D., Daskalopoulou, C., Gine-Vazquez, I., Niubo, A. S., Olaya, B., … Panagiotakos, D. (2020). Alcohol drinking and health in ageing: A global scale analysis of older individual data through the harmonised dataset of ATHLOS. Nutrients, 12(6), 1746. https://doi.org/10.3390/nu12061746.

US Census Bureau, Population Division. (2020a). Annual estimates of the resident population for selected age groups by sex for the United States: April 1, 2010 to July 1, 2019.

US Census Bureau (2020b). NCHS - Injury mortality: United States. https://data.cdc.gov/d/vc9m-u7tv/visualization.

US Department of Health and Human Services. (1999). Mental health: A report of the Surgeon General. Rockville, MD: US Department of Health and Human Services, Substance Abuse and Mental Health Services Administration, Center for Mental Health Services, National Institutes of Health, National Institute of Mental Health. http://profiles.nlm.nih.gov/ps/access/NNBBHS.pdf.

US Department of Health and Human Services. (2020). Substance Abuse and Mental Health Services Administration, Substance Abuse and Mental Health Services Administration. Behavioral Health Barometer: United States, Volume 6: Indicators as measured through the 2019 national survey on drug use and health and the national survey of substance abuse treatment services. HHS Publication No. PEP20-07-02-001. https://www.samhsa.gov/data/sites/default/files/reports/rpt32815/National-BH-Barometer_Volume6.pdf.

US Department of Veterans Affairs. Office of Suicide Prevention. (2016). Suicide among veterans and other Americans 2001–2014. https://www.mentalhealth.va.gov/docs/2016suicidedatareport.pdf.

Valaitis, R., Cleghorn, L., Ploeg, J., Risdon, C., Mangin, D., Dolovich, L., … Chung, H. (2020). Disconnected relationships between primary care and community-based health and social services and system navigation for older adults: A qualitative descriptive study. BMC Family Practice, 21, 69. https://doi.org/10.1186/s12875-020-01143-8.

Vasiliadis, H. M., Gournellis, R., Efstathiou, V., Stefanis, N., Kosmidis, M. H., Yannakoulia, M., … Scarmeas, N. (2021). The factors associated with the presence of psychotic symptoms in the HELIAD Greek community study of older adults. Aging & Mental Health, January, 20, 1–10. https://doi.org/10.1080/13607863.2021.1871882.

36

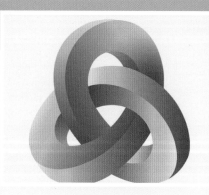

Soldiers and Veterans

Randy L. Moore and Nanci A. Swan Claus

 http://evolve.elsevier.com/Keltner

LEARNING OBJECTIVES

- Recognize the criteria and terminology used in the *Diagnostic and Statistical Manual of Mental Disorders*, 5th edition (*DSM-5*) for posttraumatic stress disorder (PTSD).
- Describe the primary symptoms of PTSD.
- Describe the neurologic alterations associated with PTSD.

- Explain the mechanism of damage-causing traumatic brain injury (TBI).
- Identify criteria for TBI.
- Describe neurologic alterations associated with TBI.
- Identify treatment options for patients with PTSD and TBI.

And there went out another horse that was red: and power was given to him that sat thereon to take peace from the earth, and that they should kill one another….

Revelation 6:4

Many Americans have seen the movie *Saving Private Ryan*. In this movie, viewers were plunged into the horrors of war almost before they could start munching on their popcorn. Up until the 1960s, Hollywood glossed over such brutal realities. Men were shot, staggered a step or two, and then fell—to die quickly, quietly, and often without a trace of blood. Beginning in the late 1960s, movie directors became intent on *realism*. Whether or not cinematic realism is healthy is deserving of careful debate. That discussion aside, *Saving Private Ryan*, winner of five Academy Awards, eliminated all illusions of a clean kill. In the early scenes of the movie, the realistic carnage at the D-Day landing created visceral reactions in most moviegoers. Young men were seen blown asunder with legs no longer attached to bodies and heads rendered unrecognizable. Screams of the dying mixed with cries of "momma" caused all but the most steeled to turn their heads or close their eyes. Many in the audience wondered if such inhuman destruction of other humans was possible. And if so, could anyone survive such brutality and ever be the same?

American soldiers today are subject to such mayhem. In these all-too-frequent scenarios, often only pieces of human flesh can be retrieved, with identification of the dead not always possible. However, more likely for our servicemen is the potential to be injured or killed by an improvised explosive device (IED) carefully hidden along some isolated desert highway. The moviegoers' question remains relevant for mental health providers and for Americans in general: "Can anyone witness such carnage and just pick up their lives where he or she left off?" The answer for many soldiers is a resounding "no."

Readers of this chapter may find themselves in harm's way, although more likely, they may find themselves caring for the survivors. This care can occur close to the point of impact or more remotely after the resulting symptoms have fully developed. Bombings are no longer attacks that occur in faraway lands and are viewed only in the news. On April 15, 2013, a bombing occurred at the end of the Boston Marathon that killed three people and injured another 264. Additionally, mass shootings appear on the nightly news too frequently. The last five major (10+ deaths) mass shootings in the United States as of this writing are recorded here: Boulder, Colorado shooting, 2021–10 deaths and 2 injured; El Paso, Texas, 2019–23 deaths and 23 injured; Virginia Beach shooting, 2019–12 deaths and 4 injured; Stoneman Douglas High School shooting in Parkland, Florida, 2018–17 deaths and 17 injured; Pittsburgh, PA synagogue shooting, 2018–11 deaths and 6 injured. And there are more that can be added, included Santa Fe (TX) high school and Thousand Oaks (CA), to name just a few more.

These examples are provided to express the reality that we face.

Soldiers who are exposed to combat are changed people. The challenge is to ensure that the changes are in a positive direction. Unfortunately, this is not always the case. Two overarching war-caused conditions emerged as soldiers returned from duty in Iraq and Afghanistan: posttraumatic stress disorder (PTSD) and the signature wound of war, traumatic brain injury (TBI). This chapter addresses these two related diagnostic injuries because nurses, particularly psychiatric nurses, will be providing care for these veterans. The accompanying case of a soldier on his second tour of duty in Iraq is typical of the experiences and symptoms associated with PTSD.

 NORM'S NOTES Most people in our nation honor our military and veteran population and remember their families around Memorial Day and Veterans Day. One could argue that keeping these patriots in the forefront of our minds should be occurring daily. After all these years, brothers, sisters, friends, and neighbors still remember. An Army psychiatrist killed 13 people at Fort Hood, Texas. During his trial, someone suggested that he suffered from PTSD. Not true! That kind of sloppy thinking is exactly what the editors of the *DSM* have clarified. Hearing about a battle is not the same as being in a battle. Go figure! This is a serious chapter about men and women who have risked their lives for their country and who have been injured doing so.

OVERVIEW

Since October 2001, more than 2.5 million U.S. troops have deployed to Operations Iraqi Freedom (OIF) and Enduring Freedom (OEF) in Iraq and Afghanistan (U.S.News.com, 2020). Several thousand more have served in Syria. More than 6800 U.S. soldiers have died, and another 52,000 have been injured (U.S. DoD Casualty Status, 2021). One-third of these returning service members have mental health issues, and the Institute of Medicine (2013) data reveal that 4% to 20% of these men and women have PTSD.

Many soldiers have served their time in "hell" only to be redeployed, as happened to Specialist Gomez in the case study. Others have had their tours extended, a particularly demoralizing order when plans to return home were dashed by decision-makers thousands of miles away. In a RAND Corporation report (2008) of roughly 2000 servicemen randomly selected from across the United States, it was found that most had been exposed to trauma, 50% reported having had a friend killed or seriously wounded in battle, almost 50% had seen dead or seriously injured civilians, and 10% reported being injured to the point of needing hospitalization. This RAND report concluded that 31% of all returning servicemen from the war zone met the criteria for PTSD, or TBI, or depression: 12% met the criteria for TBI: more than 7% of those diagnosed with mild TBI had an overlap of PTSD or depression (Tanev, 2014). Converting these percentages into numbers showed that about 300,000 soldiers were experiencing PTSD, and 320,000 may have experienced TBI. In a large study of OIF and OEF veterans (289,328 soldiers) using the Veterans Healthcare Administration services, Seal and colleagues (2009) found that 37% had a mental health diagnosis, with 22% having PTSD. There is a significant concern of underreporting because of the stigma associated with certain "labels."

The military mission in Iraq ended in December 2011 and in Afghanistan in December 2014. Hundreds of thousands of service members have redeployed to home. Although some continue their service to the United States, many have completed their obligated service and returned to their civilian lives. Although statistics can be mind-numbing, nurses should always be aware that these are real people with real hopes and real dreams, with real families praying for their safe return. These military and veteran patients will be receiving health care from nurses reading this book. Around 6 million of the 22 million U.S. veterans in our nation receive any portion of their health care in Veterans Affairs medical centers. It is projected that by 2024 there will be a decline in veterans to 17.4 million, with only 5.9 million receiving VA healthcare, revealing that the majority of veterans are receiving and will continue to receive their healthcare at civilian medical centers (Farmer et al., 2016).

Case Study

Posttraumatic Stress Disorder

Posttraumatic Stress Disorder Specialist Gomez, a 22-year-old infantryman, was brought to Combat Stress Control after an incident in which he was found by hospital staff "choking" a middle-aged civilian Iraqi man who was convalescing on the same hospital ward at an Air Force hospital in northern Iraq. At that time, Specialist Gomez was serving his second combat tour and had just been injured in the fifth IED explosion that he had personally experienced as a member of a five-man team out on patrol in their Bradley Fighting Vehicle. One team member was killed outright. Another team member subsequently died of the injuries that he sustained. Two other team members sustained major injuries, including severed limbs. Specialist Gomez was not sure why he survived and sustained only minor contusions and ruptured eardrums.

In his initial interview at Combat Stress Control, he described "flashbacks" that he was having of the recent explosion, even though he was also having difficulty remembering certain events. He had been in the Air Force Theater Hospital for 2 days. He had asked hospital staff to move him to a different ward because he was afraid that he might injure someone because of the anger, rage, and guilt (at being alive) that he was experiencing. He related how he was having great difficulty in distinguishing who was or was not "the enemy." Bed space was limited at the hospital, and he could not be moved to another area.

On his return home 4 months later, Specialist Gomez sought a referral to the mental health clinic at his army base because he was constantly irritable and having difficulties in his relationship with his fiancée, with whom he was living. She was upset with his tendency to become easily startled "by the smallest thing" and his inability to relax and not be on guard all the time. She felt that he was not the same man with whom she had fallen in love and was displeased with his being constantly moody and distant. He was no longer excited about the plans to marry and start a family, which they had made before his most recent deployment.

Specialist Gomez also described difficulties that he was having in going to sleep and staying asleep. He stated that he seldom slept for more than 2 or 3 hours, even after drinking a fifth of liquor. Also, he realized that there was nothing he could do to stop the combat-related nightmares that he experienced on a nightly basis. He was having intrusive thoughts of his combat experiences many times per day, but he also was having some difficulty remembering certain events and places he had been while in Iraq. He was avoiding most social events, including a unit cookout, because the smell of grilling hamburgers reminded him of the burning flesh that he had smelled while in Iraq.

<table>
<tr><td colspan="2">**AMERICAN DEATHS IN WAR**</td></tr>
<tr><td>U.S. troop deaths: Iraq and Afghanistan</td><td>>6,800</td></tr>
<tr><td>U.S. service member injuries</td><td>>52,000</td></tr>
<tr><td>**Previous U.S. war deaths (by war):**</td><td></td></tr>
<tr><td>Civil War</td><td>>620,000</td></tr>
<tr><td>World War II</td><td>>406,900</td></tr>
<tr><td>Korean War</td><td>>6,000</td></tr>
<tr><td>Vietnam War</td><td>> 58,000</td></tr>
</table>

Data from Military Factory. (n.d.). *American deaths through history: From the war of independence to Operation Enduring Freedom— Blood spilled from sea to shining sea.* https://www.militaryfactory.com/american_war_deaths.asp.

POSTTRAUMATIC STRESS DISORDER

The constellation of symptoms that comprise PTSD has existed under many names for as long as men have fought. During the American Civil War, it was known as *"soldier's heart."* In World War I, *"shell shock,"* and during World War II, *"battle fatigue."* PTSD is a relatively recent term. It was coined about 40 years ago in recognition of the symptom complex manifested by Vietnam War veterans. PTSD first appeared in the third edition of the *DSM*, published in 1980. From there, the term trickled into professional publications with perhaps the first medical and nursing articles printed in 1980 (Horowitz et al., 1980) and 1983 (Keltner et al., 1983), respectively. Today the term *PTSD* is widely understood and employed in dialogue in the United States as the impact of war has stressed families, pressured health care agencies, and affected the national equilibrium.

The term *PTSD* is worth examining. First, the *DSM* considers it a "disorder," a mental diagnosis that is distinct from other mental disorders. Second, it is expressed as "stress"—stress caused by the experience of "trauma." Finally, "post" suggests that the reaction occurs after the exposure to trauma and can be delayed for years before surfacing. The *DSM-5* has also restricted the use of the diagnosis. Criterion A1 focuses on the event—it must involve actual or threatened death or serious injury or threaten the physical integrity of the person or others. Criterion A2 focuses on the person's response—horror, helplessness, or fear. Table 36.1 provides specific criteria as established by the American Psychiatric Association; italicized examples come from the case of Specialist Gomez presented earlier in the chapter.

<table>
<tr><td>**POSTTRAUMATIC STRESS DISORDER RISK FACTORS**</td></tr>
<tr><td>Experiencing intense or long-lasting trauma</td></tr>
<tr><td>Experiencing other trauma earlier in life</td></tr>
<tr><td>Having other mental health problems, including anxiety or depression</td></tr>
<tr><td>Lacking a good support system of family or friends</td></tr>
<tr><td>Having first-degree relatives with mental health problems, including PTSD</td></tr>
<tr><td>Abuse or neglect as a child</td></tr>
<tr><td>Having a job with exposure to traumatic events</td></tr>
<tr><td>*PTSD*, Posttraumatic stress disorder.</td></tr>
</table>

Adapted from https://www.mayoclinic.org/diseases-conditions/posttraumatic-stress-disorder/diagnosis-treatment/drc-20355973 and used with permission of Mayo Foundation for Medical Education and Research, all rights reserved.

TABLE 36.1   Major Symptoms of Posttraumatic Stress Disorder

1. Reexperiencing
   - Recurrence and intrusive thoughts—*"intrusive thoughts of his combat experiences many times"*
   - Recurring dreams
   - Flashbacks
   - Psychological distress related to symbols/remembrance of event—*"anger, rage, and guilt"*
   - Physiologic distress related to symbols/remembrance of event
2. Avoidance
   - Avoidance of trauma-related thoughts
   - Avoidance of trauma-related activities—*"avoiding most social events … burning flesh"*
   - Amnesia for trauma—*"difficulty remembering certain events and places"*
   - Feeling detached or estranged—*"constantly moody and distant"*
   - Restricted affect—*"not the same man"*
   - Sense of foreshortened future—*"no longer excited about plans they had made"*
3. Hyperarousal
   - Insomnia—*"difficulties in going to sleep and staying asleep"*
   - Irritability—*"beginning to choke a middle-aged civilian Iraqi"*
   - Difficulty concentrating
   - Hypervigilance—*"inability to relax and not be on guard all the time"*
   - Exaggerated startle reflex—*"she was upset about his tendencies to become easily startled"*

Note: Italicized text relates to the case of Specialist Gomez (Keltner & Dowben, 2007).
Modified from National Institute of Mental Health. (n.d.). *Posttraumatic stress disorder.* http://www.nimh.nih.gov/health/topics/post-traumatic-stress-disorder-ptsd/index.shtml.

Primary Symptoms of Posttraumatic Stress Disorder

The primary symptoms of PTSD are psychological: the reexperience of trauma, avoidance of trauma-reminding phenomena, and hyperarousal.

Reexperiencing a traumatic event comes in several forms. The event might be replayed over and over *(recurrence)*, or it might inject itself into an otherwise non–trauma-related stream of thought. The latter is referred to as *thought intrusion*. Other manifestations of reexperiencing include troubled sleep. *Repetitive dreams* that replay the event or some distortion of the event render the soldier unable to find escape even in sleep. *Flashbacks* (dissociative reactions) take reexperiencing to yet another level. During flashbacks, the veteran relives the event while awake. Soldiers suggest that for a short period of time, they think they are back in the battle environment. During this period, some may demonstrate reflex behaviors that approximate behaviors expected on the battlefield.

Avoidance is another cardinal symptom of PTSD. Soldiers who experience this symptom *avoid trauma-related thoughts* and *avoid activities* that are trauma-related or reminiscent of the traumatic event. Just as flashbacks can be psychological extensions of repetitive dreams, soldiers with PTSD may go beyond thought avoidance to actual *amnesia* for the event in question. Although avoiding trauma-related activities reflects a conscious problem-solving effort to prevent discomfort, some individuals extend that avoidance psychologically with feelings of *detachment* or *estrangement*. This feeling of unreality can be meaningfully construed as an attempt to avoid pain. These negative alterations in mood and cognition can also include persistent and exaggerated negative beliefs, a negative emotional state, and the inability to experience positive emotions.

Hyperarousal is the third cardinal symptom diagnostic of PTSD. Such soldiers can be on edge or *hypervigilant*. They scan the environment for threats and often overreact to stimuli or exhibit an *exaggerated startle reflex*. For example, many veterans have described diving for safety after hearing a car backfire. Being continuously on guard is exhausting, yet because they are on guard, sleep escapes them, and *insomnia* develops. Researchers note that veterans with PTSD and obstructive sleep apnea (OSA) had decreases in nightmare distress/frequency when using prolonged continuous positive airway pressure (CPAP) (El-Solh et al., 2017). Self-destructive or reckless behavior can occur, including alcohol/drug abuse (43%), driving while impaired (29%), gambling (25%), and aggression (23%) (Lusk et al., 2017). Finally, hypervigilance, overreaction, and lack of sleep take their toll, leaving the soldier tired and *irritable*. Tired, irritable, hypervigilant, and easily startled people are difficult to live with. Marriages and relationships that survive deployment often break up under the strain of this emotional rollercoaster. The stress that family members feel related to a combat veteran who is experiencing PTSD can be described as secondary traumatization. Numbing, arousal, and anger are predictive of family distress. The family members must also be targeted for improving their psychological well-being. Finally, few employers are willing to maintain the employment of a person with acute PTSD.

Symptom Delay

Pai, Suris, & North, 2017 note a variety of reasons why symptom delay can occur. This is described as "delayed expression." This is where the full diagnostic criteria are not met until at least 6 months after an event, although onset and some symptom expression may be immediate. Reasons for this delayed expression may include:

1. *Posttraumatic* may literally be true in that it may take time for the traumas to surface.
2. The stigma of a mental illness may cause some to "fight" the symptoms or to self-medicate (e.g., with alcohol) until doing so no longer works.
3. Physical or other mental health problems may obscure PTSD.

Comorbidities

PTSD is easily accompanied by other mental health disorders, including depression, anxiety, or substance abuse.

Older veterans with PTSD tend to have comorbid depression, whereas younger soldiers tend to have drug and alcohol abuse comorbidity. Psychiatric manifestations resulting from head injuries during war can be predicted based on the age of the soldier. Stated another way, age at the time of neural insult has a high reliability in predicting the kind of psychiatric problem that emerges after injury. Correlations have also been identified between PTSD and dementia (Rafferty, Cawkill, Stevelink, Greenberg, & Greenberg, 2018; Roughead et al., 2017) and Parkinson disease (Chan et al., 2017).

Neurologic Alterations Associated With Posttraumatic Stress Disorder

PTSD is not just a psychological problem. Distinguishable neuroanatomic and neurochemical changes seem to be linked with this disorder. Following is a brief review of these neural alterations.

Neuroanatomic Changes in Posttraumatic Stress Disorder

Soldiers with PTSD are thought to experience changes in the prefrontal cortex and various limbic structures (i.e., amygdala and hippocampus). Although much research has focused on discovering neuroanatomic alterations via various brain scanning technologies—including computed tomography (CT), magnetic resonance imaging (MRI), functional MRI (fMRI), and positron emission tomography (PET)—for the purposes of this brief discussion such changes are reduced to this: individuals with PTSD tend to have reduced volume in key brain areas (Bromis, Calem, Reindeera, Williams, & Kempton, 2018). A recurring theme in these studies is an alteration in the function of the amygdala, which comprises nuclei deep in the temporal lobe that are responsible for memory, decision making, and emotional reactions. Ousdal et al. (2020) demonstrated exaggerated amygdala responses to general negative stimuli in brains affected with PTSD—essentially dissociated hyperresponsivity. The prefrontal cortex is the center of inhibition, sometimes referred to as the "chief executive officer (CEO)" of the brain, responsible for cognitive analysis and abstract thought; it is the part of the brain that says "keep that thought to yourself" or "I probably shouldn't have sex with this person." Brain research suggests that this area does not reach maturation until 25 years of age. The effective prefrontal cortex inhibits the amygdala as well, so that most of us do not overreact to every loud noise or punch someone just because they startle us. It is suggested that this ability to mute stimuli is diminished in brains with PTSD because of a compromised prefrontal cortex (Selemon et al., 2019). The hippocampus, responsible for memory/learning and contextualization (ability to put an event in context), is also affected. These investigators further noted that this reduction in hippocampal volume has been replicated four times in the published literature, with volume reductions reaching 26%. If one is more "on guard" because of diminished inhibition of the emotion center (i.e., amygdala) and has a diminished ability to contextualize life occurrences ("this is a safe area," "this place is not safe"), a recipe for disaster lurks. Stated another way, impaired amygdala function opens the opportunity for overreaction, whereas impaired hippocampal function compounds that tendency with an inability to "read" the environment correctly.

Neurochemical Changes in Posttraumatic Stress Disorder

Two biochemical systems are affected by large doses of stress: the sympathetic nervous system (SNS) and the corticotropin-releasing hormone (CRH) system. These two systems work synergistically, with the SNS providing the body with the energy demanded by the stressor and the CRH system providing the body with the tools required to contain the stress reaction. The CRH neurons are predominantly located in the paraventricular nucleus of the hypothalamus. Tracts extend to the anterior pituitary gland, and when CRH is released, it results in the liberation of adrenocorticotropic hormone (ACTH). On reaching the adrenal cortex, ACTH causes the discharge of the glucocorticoid cortisol into the systemic circulation. This stimulation by ACTH also activates the release of epinephrine and norepinephrine from the adrenal medulla. When abundant epinephrine and norepinephrine are released, as occurs during stress, this activates the SNS, with subsequent stimulation of the adrenal medulla, which releases even more norepinephrine/epinephrine.

Adaptive physiologic responses to stress include increases in glucose, heart rate, blood pressure, and respiratory rate. Elevated cortisol, norepinephrine, and epinephrine increase alertness and vigilance and also diminish interest in sex. Although all of these elevations are adaptive at times, prolonged elevations, which can occur during combat, may result in a system that is continually "turned on," morphing alertness into hyperalertness with insomnia and vigilance into hypervigilance. Finally, prolonged elevations of cortisol are associated with accelerated apoptosis (programmed cell death) of hippocampal neurons—the very structures needed to achieve adaptive responses (Selemon et al., 2019).

Treatment for Posttraumatic Stress Disorder

Psychotherapy is used either alone or in combination with drugs. Different types of psychotherapy include cognitive therapy, behavioral therapy, and eye movement desensitization and reprocessing. Cognitive-behavioral therapy, including prolonged exposure and cognitive processing therapy, is generally considered first-line. Selective serotonin reuptake inhibitors (SSRIs), including sertraline and paroxetine, are approved by the U.S. Food and Drug Administration (FDA) for the treatment of PTSD. Drug therapy may include a short course of antipsychotics or antianxiety medications if clinically indicated. Note, however, that the long-term use

of benzodiazepines is contraindicated. Prazosin is FDA-approved as an antihypertensive and works by blocking the brain's response to norepinephrine. It has a well-documented off-label use to help reduce nightmares associated with PTSD by working on the postsynaptic alpha receptors, resulting in decreased norepinephrine effects. A growing number of nonpharmacologic evidence-based adjuvant therapies are showing further PTSD symptom reduction (Fogger et al., 2016).

Posttraumatic Stress Disorder Resilience Factors

Although countries will continue to find ways to send their young men and women into harm's way, considerable work is being done to discover what might be protective factors. Some of these include social support, coping self-efficacy (the belief that "you can do it"), and hope, including optimism and expecting the positive (Martin-Soelch & Schnyder, 2019). The U.S. Army has recognized the importance of trying to prepare soldiers for the atrocities that they will see; it has therefore developed Resiliency Training, including institutional, operational, and family modules, as well as military resilience trainer and facilitator modules. Although this training will not prove to be a magic bullet, it will insert one more tool into the toolkit of the warriors who are sent into harm's way. The Navy and Marine Corps version is called the Stress Resilience Training System, and the Air Force has Trauma and Resiliency Training Seminars.

DSM-5 DIFFERENTIAL DIAGNOSIS LIST

Posttraumatic stress disorder (PTSD)
Adjustment disorder
Acute stress disorder
Anxiety disorder
Obsessive-compulsive disorder
Major depressive disorder
Personality disorder
Dissociative disorder
Conversion disorder
Psychotic disorder
Traumatic brain injury

Data from American Psychiatric Association. (2013). *Diagnostic and statistical manual of mental disorders* (5th ed.). APA.

TRAUMATIC BRAIN INJURY

According to the United States Department of Defense (DoD), there have been greater than 6600 military casualties during OIF/OEF (U.S. Department of Defense Casualty Status, 2021). In contrast to previous wars, a predominance of deaths and injuries were directly linked to explosions, particularly blast injuries. Improvements in battle armor, emergency care on the battlefield, and the use of helmets have saved soldiers who would most surely have died in previous conflicts; however, this improved protection has had an unforeseen consequence—a tremendous increase in the number of soldiers with TBI. The Traumatic Brain Injury Center of Excellence (TBICoE) reports greater than 430,000 soldiers with TBI worldwide, ranging from mild to penetrating injuries, with the largest population being those who served in the Army (Health.mil, n.d.). The majority of TBIs are classified as mild or moderate. TBI has been designated as the signature wound or injury or invisible injury of the most recent wars. Although an overall improvement in body protection has been achieved, the head is still vulnerable to explosive blasts of air. A soldier with TBI often has not been touched by anything other than the force of the blast. Because mild TBI often is not associated with an obvious wound, or the soldier may have other wounds that take priority (e.g., a hemorrhaging leg wound), TBI may be completely overlooked. Many of these soldiers have been sent back to the battlefield because no injury was detectable.

Defining Traumatic Brain Injury

When a soldier is said to have experienced a TBI, typically, a mild TBI or concussion has occurred. These are defined as closed head injuries caused by blunt trauma or acceleration/deceleration (blast) forces. There is not a penetrating or open head injury. Mild TBI is defined as loss of consciousness for less than 30 minutes, with posttraumatic amnesia lasting less than 24 hours. A CT scan is not typically indicated for these injuries; however, if a CT scan were performed on these soldiers, the results would be normal. Moderate TBI is defined as a confused or disoriented state lasting more than 24 hours or loss of consciousness for more than 30 minutes but less than 24 hours. Severe TBI is characterized by confusion/disorientation/loss of consciousness lasting more than 24 hours or memory loss for more than a week. Penetrating TBI is a head injury that involves damage to the scalp, skull, and dura mater caused by either low- (knife) or high-velocity projectiles (bullets).

The blasts that cause TBIs often come from IEDs. In such cases, a blast of air hits a person in a wave of pressure, and a lowering of the pressure occurs as the blast wave passes. Additionally, just as a tidal wave also rushes back to sea, a reversal of air pressure back toward the victim occurs. This increase, decrease, and then increase of pressure has an injurious impact on the brain and is directly related to the force of the initial explosion. All of the pressures and intensities are magnified when soldiers are in vehicles or buildings in which the blast wave can "bounce" around. Most soldiers with a mild TBI recover within days to weeks. Overt symptoms subside within a year in 85% or more of affected soldiers (Zeitzer & Brooks, 2008). Persistent concussive symptoms (PCS), such as headaches and dizziness, may last up to 9 months after injury.

Case Study

Traumatic Brain Injury

Traumatic brain injury Joe Johnson is a 43-year-old African American veteran who achieved the rank of E-6. He joined the Alabama National Guard as a young man in order to supplement his income. As a "weekend warrior," he was able to obtain a good civilian job. Because it was a civil service position, he enjoyed support for his part-time military career that some Guard members and reservists do not have.

Similar to many once-per-month soldiers, Mr. Johnson never anticipated being activated and sent to war. Although it is made clear from day one that activation is a risk, many generations of these soldiers have never been seriously threatened by this life-changing order.

Mr. Johnson was activated and eventually sent to Iraq. In his 9 months there, his unit experienced more than 35 IED attacks. He escaped serious injury in all but one of these attacks, although fellow unit members were seriously wounded or killed. He recounts standing by helplessly as a young soldier from home bled to death because the medics were unable to stem the hemorrhaging of blood. This and other traumatic stressors gave rise to Johnson's PTSD. His final IED experience tossed his Humvee into the air, rendering him unconscious and amnesic for the event. He was discharged from the military with diagnoses of PTSD and TBI.

Mr. Johnson presented to the advanced practice registered nurse with the following complaints: memory loss, memory problems, irritability, cognitive difficulties (e.g., "I ain't as sharp as I used to be"), fatigue, anxiety, attention impairment, and deficient word finding. He also admitted that he would like to "rip off the head" of a man who he believes is picking on him. When asked if he had worked with this person before activation, he responds, "Yeah, but we didn't have no problem then." When Mr. Johnson was asked if he had taken into account that he might have changed too, he appeared dumbfounded by the consideration. In addition to these symptoms and concerns, Mr. Johnson admitted to all of the classic PTSD symptoms: reexperiencing, avoidance, and hyperarousal.

Primary Symptoms of Traumatic Brain Injury

Symptoms of TBI can be divided into three categories: somatic, neurocognitive function/concentration difficulties, and emotional/behavioral issues. Somatic or physical symptoms include complaints of headaches, tinnitus, blurred vision, and insomnia. Neurocognitive/concentration issues include memory, lack of attention, decreased speed of processing thoughts/expression, and inability to focus. Emotional/behavioral issues include irritability, depression, anxiety, and inability to control behavior (Summerall, 2019; Koebli et al., 2020). Perhaps the most exasperating experience for family and friends is the victim's inability to recognize these deficiencies. Table 36.2 lists symptoms and syndromes associated with TBI. Table 36.3 lists prevalence and incidence rates for selected psychiatric disorders associated with more severe TBIs.

TABLE 36.2   Symptoms and Syndromes Associated With Mild Traumatic Brain Injury

Cognitive	Physical	Emotional and Behavioral
Attention problems	Appetite changes	Aggression
Executive dysfunction	Fatigue	Alcohol abuse
Planning	Headaches	Avolition
Abstract reasoning	Loss of urinary control	Attention-deficit/hyperactivity disorder
Problem solving	Pain	Decreased affective oscillation
Insight, judgment	Decreased libido	Disinhibition
Impaired judgment and decision making	Seizures	Irritability
Impaired self-awareness	Sensitivity to light	Major depression
Memory problems	Sleep disturbances	Posttraumatic stress disorder (PTSD)
Working memory problems	Weight changes	Psychosis
Word-finding difficulties	Vertigo	
	Visual impairment	

Modified from Cooke, B., &. Keltner, N. (2008). Traumatic brain injury: War related. *Perspectives in Psychiatric Care, 43,* 223; Kim et al. (2007). Neuropsychiatric complications of traumatic brain injury: A critical review of the literature (a report of the ANPA Committee on research). *Journal of Neuropsychiatry and Clinical Neurosciences, 19,* 106; Mathiasm, J. L., & Wheaton, P. (2006). Changes in attention and information-processing speed following severe traumatic brain injury (TBI). *Brain Injury, 20,* 569; Zeitzer, M. B., & Brooks, J. M. (2008). In the line of fire: Traumatic brain injury among Iraq war veterans. *AAOHN Journal, 56,* 347.

TABLE 36.3   Posttraumatic Brain Injury Psychiatric Disorders Associated With Brain Injury

Psychiatric Disorder	Incidence (%)	Prevalence (%)
Post-TBI psychosis	20	Unknown
Post-TBI depression	15–33	18–61
Post-TBI mania	9	1–22
Post-TBI PTSD	13–27	3–59

Note: Kim and colleagues reviewed approximately 32 studies to support these findings. *PTSD,* Posttraumatic stress disorder; *TBI,* traumatic brain injury.
Modified from Cooke, B., &. Keltner, N. (2008). Traumatic brain injury: War related. *Perspectives in Psychiatric Care, 43,* 223; Kim, E., Lauterbach, E. C., Reeve, A., et al. (2007). Neuropsychiatric complications of traumatic brain injury: A critical review of the literature (a report of the ANPA Committee on research). *Journal of Neuropsychiatry and Clinical Neurosciences, 19,* 106.

Neurologic Alterations Associated With Traumatic Brain Injury

As with PTSD, TBI is not just a psychological problem. Changes, although subtle at times and apparently not as long-lasting, can be determined in brains with TBI as well. Following is a brief review of what is known or suspected about the neurologic consequences of exposure to explosions and other blunt trauma to the head.

Neuroanatomic Changes in Traumatic Brain Injury

TBI has a complex pathophysiology involving mechanical injury to neurons, glia, and vessels at the time of the initial injury, followed by a secondary injury that may take weeks to months to recover. Both primary and secondary injury damages both white and gray matter that results in loss of homeostasis, impaired mitochondrial function, damage to vessels, and inflammation (Mohamadpour et al., 2019). As more sophisticated technologies such as MRI and PET scans are used, long-term patterns of brain alteration have been noted. These changes tend to be subtle, requiring a different level of imaging than typically provided by CT and MRI. A technique called diffusion tensor imaging (DTI), a form of MRI, provides this level of visualization. DTI is able to produce neural tract images. Magnetoencephalography, a non-invasive functional imaging technique, measures brainwaves to identify injured gray matter. This device has been used in conjunction with DTI, which measures damage in white matter, to determine potential TBI (Huang et al., 2009). In TBIs, the acceleration and deceleration forces cause a shearing of axons, resulting in injury (Zeitzer & Brooks, 2008). These injuries can be so microscopic that only the most sophisticated imaging technologies can reveal and measure them. Symptomatic white matter changes can be noted on DTI in patients with mild TBI that are very similar to white matter abnormalities seen in patients with early Alzheimer dementia (Fakhran et al., 2013). Axonal injuries include tearing of axons, disconnection of axons, microhemorrhages in the frontal and temporal lobes, and hippocampal axonal and hemorrhagic damage (Vasterling et al., 2009).

Neurochemical Changes in Traumatic Brain Injury

Ng & Lee, 2019 have described a biphasic model of neurochemical changes in TBI: an acute phase followed by a chronic phase. During the acute phase, the neural insult causes the activation of large amounts of glutamate. Glutamate, the most abundant excitatory neurotransmitter in the brain, increases neuron firing. This excessive firing of neurons, known as excitotoxity, causes the nonprogrammed death of neurons.

Neuronal death enhances the axonal injury noted in the previous section. The hippocampus is particularly sensitive to these developments. The acute phase, with its increased levels of excitatory transmitters and neuron destruction, is followed by the chronic phase. In this phase—related to the loss of neurons—the synthesis of catecholamine and acetylcholine declines. In keeping with current models of psychopathology, a decrease in catecholamine would contribute to disturbances in affect, whereas a reduction in acetylcholine would foster cognitive deficits.

TREATING POSTTRAUMATIC STRESS DISORDER AND TRAUMATIC BRAIN INJURY

One question surrounding PTSD and TBI is whether a person can have both related to the same trauma. A major consideration for answering this question with a "no" is the fact that core symptoms for PTSD—such as reexperiencing, thought intrusion, flashbacks, and avoidance—are all based on "remembering" the trauma. A core symptom of TBI is amnesia for the event. Straightforward reasoning would suggest that one cannot reexperience, have flashbacks of, or avoid something that one cannot remember. That logic aside, the consensus of opinion is that PTSD and TBI can and do coexist. MacDonald and colleagues (2014) discovered that soldiers who were exposed to blast injuries (TBI) had worse headaches and more severe PTSD than non–blast-exposed controls, intimating that soldiers who had been involved in a blast injury were more likely to experience TBI and PTSD. This combination diagnosis is now referred to as "postdeployment multisymptom disorder" (Uomoto, 2012), and anecdotal reports suggest an even higher comorbidity. Following are treatment considerations for both diagnoses.

Treating Posttraumatic Stress Disorder

The goals of treating PTSD include the following (Davidson, 2006; Dowben et al., 2007):
Reducing primary symptoms (see Table 36.1)
Improving functioning
Strengthening resilience
Relieving comorbid symptoms
Preventing relapse

Antidepressants, particularly SSRIs, are very effective for treating the symptoms of PTSD. SSRIs not only have proven effectiveness for core symptoms but are also beneficial for the comorbid expression of depression and anxiety (Vieweg et al., 2006). Venlafaxine and mirtazapine are agents that can be used when SSRIs fail—with the added property of causing a reduced incidence of sexual side effects.

Antipsychotics and mood stabilizers are frequently prescribed. Antipsychotics can be used to supplement SSRIs (Davis et al., 2006) or for overt psychotic symptoms. Individuals with PTSD may present with both psychosis and subsyndromal symptoms. Because many of these individuals experience mood fluctuations and irritability, medications muting the intensity of these behaviors are important. Drugs such as divalproex and carbamazepine are prescribed in these situations.

Research supports a strong association between interpersonal relationship problems and PTSD, often leaving service members caught in vicious cycles of deteriorating relationships on top of their mental health problems. Emotionally Focused Couples Therapy is an evidence-based intervention that is ideally suited when working with couples as they face PTSD (Blow et al., 2015).

Treating Traumatic Brain Injury

To provide the best care for patients, the VA has established two valuable resources: The U.S. Defense and Veteran's Brain Injury Center and the Polytrauma/TBI System of Care. The Polytrauma/TBI System of Care, which includes 4 Polytrauma Rehabilitation Centers, was formed by the VA to provide comprehensive care for patients with multiple traumatic injuries, including TBI, musculoskeletal, neurological, and psychological (Summerall, 2019). These centers are able to evaluate and provide specialized care for patients who require more long-term care than local facilities. In November 2006, the U.S. Defense and Veterans Brain Injury Center organized a panel that developed clinical practice guidelines for the treatment of TBI. The clinical practice guidelines consisted of an algorithm for the diagnosis and treatment of TBI. These guidelines, last updated in 2016, are currently being revised.

Pharmacotherapy of TBI presents another variable. The very nature of TBI indicates an alteration in brain function. This pathology adds a dimension to the drug response that may not occur in the general population. One soldier might respond in an expected manner, whereas another might respond in a different way. Because of this variance in sensitivity, it is important to start with a low dose of medication and adjust it as needed. However, some patients do not respond to normal dosage, again presumably related to TBI. The conundrum of being on guard for hypersensitive patients while possibly treating a drug-resistant patient can make finding the right drug at the right dosage a long and tedious process for the patient, clinician, and family members. Mohamadpour et al. (2019) indicated the importance of a therapeutic time window to improve the efficacy of TBI treatment.

Treatment for TBI is typically symptom-based and individualized. These patients may need medication for pain, depression, seizures, irritability, anxiety, insomnia, and focus issues.

Nonopioid pain medications are more beneficial for these patients without causing behavioral or addiction potential. The use of selective serotonin reuptake inhibitors (SSRIs), such as sertraline, has had great success in the treatment of depression in this population (Rabinowitz & Watanabe, 2020). Antiseizure medications such as topiramate and levetiracetam are frequently prescribed for seizure prevention and also decreased headache symptoms (Baig et al., 2020).

Methylphenidate, a mixed dopaminergic and noradrenergic medication, and amantadine have been used to treat attention and focus issues (Rabinowitz & Watanabe, 2020). Medications with sedating effects, such as risperidone, trazodone, and mirtazapine, have been used for sleep disturbance with great success, as well as neuropathic pain and headaches (Baig et al., 2020). The use of antihistamines, such as hydroxyzine, has been used for breakthrough anxiety; however, the use of benzodiazepines may worsen focus and memory complaints (Baig et al., 2020).

There are alternatives and augmented psychological therapies for this population. Trauma-focused therapies, such as cognitive-behavioral therapy, have become standards of care for patients with depression and anxiety related to a TBI (Ponsford et al., 2020). This study found that after completing multiple therapy sessions, there was a reduction in anxiety and depression in patients with TBIs.

Family Considerations

Soldiers come from families and go back to families. As with most serious medical and psychiatric conditions, it is the family that is typically left to care for their loved one. After the military command makes its visit and medals are pinned on the soldier, the family must pick up the pieces of a life changed by war. Families have a critical role in the care of their loved ones and need available resources. Box 36.1 has been carefully referenced for the best evidence-based approach for family education. A careful reading and rereading of this box will be beneficial to every nurse.

NORM'S NOTES War is as old as humanity. I finished nursing school in the mid-1960s. Back in the day, it took about 6 weeks to learn if you had passed the state nursing examination. I found out in a matter of days. Why? The army had my tests graded by hand, and within a week of taking my state boards, I had a license and a letter from the U.S. Army. I was to be a soldier. Why? Vietnam! Although I was never shot at, I took care of many soldiers whose lives would never be the same. War leaves lasting memories. Fast forward 40 years—Randy Moore served a tour in Iraq. He also has firsthand knowledge of the traumas of war. Men and women remained ravaged by war. Family emotions endure a crucible. This chapter closes the book, and rightly so. Maybe it is the last thing you should think about as you finish the course. Men and women continue to die, or are traumatized daily, as they carry out their duty to protect and defend the United States. As a nation and as health care professionals, we must learn to do a better job of providing mental health care to these individuals. Why? Because if we have learned anything from previous wars, it is this: Unless we learn to deal with these issues now, we will have to deal with them later.

? CRITICAL THINKING QUESTIONS

1. Many nurses in the United States were/are against the wars in Iraq and Afghanistan. Do you think they should voice their reservations to veterans with PTSD and TBI?
2. It was discussed that some people believe PTSD and TBIs to be mutually exclusive phenomena. Can you make an argument to support or negate this view?

BOX 36.1 Family Caregiving and Traumatic Brain Injury

Caregiver Problems and Needs	Potential Interventions or Strategies for Caregiver Problems
Cognitive and behavioral impairments of people with TBI	Encourage or develop programs to increase family and social support of caregivers or family members
Judgment- and safety-related concerns regarding travel and finances for people with TBI	Offer problem-solving skill training programs for caregivers or family members
Need more information about physical, cognitive, medical, and behavioral status and prognosis of people with TBI	Offer programs to improve coping skills of caregivers or family members
Lack of information regarding how to access outpatient and community-based services and how to navigate the health care system effectively to meet the needs of a loved one with TBI	Provide information regarding physical, cognitive, medical, and behavioral status and prognosis of people with TBI
Lack of free time to meet caregivers' needs	Develop programs that improve socialization of caregivers or family members
Decreased initiative, emotional withdrawal, and fatigue in people with TBI	Identify marital counseling sources
Physical impairment and dependency in people with TBI	Community-based programs conducted by interdisciplinary professionals to assist in setting shared goals and formulating priorities for rehabilitation
Social isolation of people with TBI, leading to caregivers' isolation	Encourage web-based family treatment programs to enhance family problem solving and reduce behavioral and social problems of people with TBI (i.e., NAMI meetings)
Negative impact on caregivers' physical health	Assist with physical, emotional, financial, domestic, transportation, and respite support networks
Marital discord	Encourage Emotionally Focused Couples Therapy
Family discord	Develop materials regarding how to access outpatient and community-based services, particularly family counseling referrals

TBI, Traumatic brain injury.

STUDY NOTES

1. American soldiers are exposed to great carnage, and that exposure cannot help but leave a lasting impression.
2. Two major disabilities associated with the wars in Iraq and Afghanistan are PTSD and TBI.
3. The primary symptoms of PTSD are reexperiencing, avoidance, and hyperarousal.
4. Many soldiers with PTSD also have a comorbid disorder, such as TBI, substance abuse, anxiety, and depression.
5. Significant neurochemical changes (e.g., chronic overactivity of the sympathetic nervous system and the corticotropin-releasing system) are a direct result of the traumatic stress that soldiers experience in war.
6. TBIs are called the signature wounds of recent wars and are directly linked to exposure to explosions.
7. Often, a soldier with TBI was hit "only" by a blast of air.
8. The diagnosis of TBI typically refers to what has historically been identified as a mild concussion.
9. The overarching categories of TBI symptoms are cognitive, physical, and emotional/behavioral. Amnesia is a key symptom.
10. Neurochemically, TBI causes elevations of glutamate, resulting in overfiring of neurons.
11. Both PTSD and TBI are treated with psychotropic medications based on symptoms (e.g., antidepressants for symptoms of depression).
12. Cognitive behavioral therapy and emotionally focused couples therapy are evidence-based approaches to treat PTSD and TBI.
13. "After the military command makes its visit and medals are pinned on soldiers, it is the family that will pick up the pieces of a life changed by war."

REFERENCES

American Psychiatric Association. (2013). *Diagnostic and statistical manual of mental disorders* (5th ed.). APA.

Baig, M., Meraj, A., & Tapia, R. (2020). Development of a practice tool for primary care providers: Medication management of posttraumatic stress disorder in veterans with mild traumatic brain injury. *Psychiatric Quarterly, 91*(4), 1465–1478. https://doi.org/10.1007/s11126-020-09767-w.

Blow, A., Curtis, A., Wittenborn, A., & Gorman, L. (2015). Relationship problems and military related PTSD: The case for using Emotionally Focused Therapy for couples. *Contemporary Family Therapy, 37*, 261–270. https://doi.org/10.1007/s10591-015-9345-7.

Bromis, K., Calem, M., Reindeera, A., Williams, S., & Kempton, M. (2018). Meta-analysis of 89 structural MRI studies in posttraumatic stress disorder and comparison with major depressive disorder. *The American Journal of Psychiatry, 175*(10). https://doi.org/10.1176/appi.ajp.2018.17111199.

Chan, Y., Bai, Y., Hsu, J., Huang, K., Su, T., Li, C., Lin, W., et al. (2017). Post-traumatic stress disorder and risk of Parkinson disease: A nationwide longitudinal study. *The American Journal of Geriatric Psychiatry: Official Journal of the American Association for Geriatric Psychiatry, 25*(8), 917–923. https://doi.org/10.1016/j.jagp.2017.03.012.

Cooke, B. B., & Keltner, N. L. (2008). Traumatic brain injury—War related: Part II. *Perspectives in Psychiatric Care, 44*(1), 54. https://doi.org/10.1111/j.1744-6163.2008.00148.x.

Davidson, J. R. (2006). Pharmacologic treatment of acute and chronic stress following trauma: 2006. *The Journal of Clinical Psychiatry, 67*(Suppl. 2), 34.

Davis, L., Frazier, E., Williford, R., & Newell, J. (2006). Long-term pharmacotherapy for post-traumatic stress disorder. *CNS Drugs, 20*(6), 465. https://doi.org/10.2165/00023210-200620060-00003.

Dowben, J. S., Grant, J. S., & Keltner, N. L. (2007). Psychobiological substrates of posttraumatic stress disorder: Part II. *Perspectives in Psychiatric Care, 43*(3), 146. https://doi.org/10.1111/j.1744-6163.2007.00124.x.

El-Solh, A., Vermont, L., Homish, G., & Kufel, T. (2017). The effect of continuous positive airway pressure on post-traumatic stress disorder symptoms in veterans with post-traumatic stress disorder and obstructive sleep apnea: A prospective study. *Sleep Medicine, 33*, 145–150. https://doi.org/10.1016/j.sleep.2016.12.025.

Fakhran, S., Yaeger, K., & Alhilali, L. (2013). Symptomatic white matter changes in mild traumatic brain injury resemble pathologic feature of early Alzheimer dementia. *Radiology, 269*(1), 249. https://doi.org/10.1148/radiol.13122343.

Farmer, C., Hosek, S., & Adamson, D. (2016). Balancing demand and supply for veterans' health care: A summary of three RAND assessments conducted under the Veterans Choice Act. *RAND Health Quarterly, 6*(1), 12. 2016 Jun 20.

Fogger, S., Moore, R., & Pickett, L. (2016). Posttraumatic stress disorder and veterans: Finding hope and supporting healing. *The Journal for Nurse Practitioners, 12*(9), 598–604. https://doi.org/10.1016/j.nurpra.2016.07.014.

Health.mil. (n.d.). DoD TBI Worldwide Numbers. https://www.health.mil/About-MHS/OASDHA/Defense-Health-Agency/Research-and-Development/Traumatic-Brain-Injury-Center-of-Excellence/DOD-TBI-Worldwide-Numbers.

Horowitz, M., Wilner, N., Kaltreider, N., & Alvarez, W. (1980). Signs and symptoms of posttraumatic stress disorder. *Archives of General Psychiatry, 37*(1), 85. https://doi.org/10.1001/archpsyc.1980.01780140087010.

Huang, M., Theilmann, R., Robb, A. … Lee, R. (2009). Integrated imaging approach with MEG and DTI to detect mild traumatic brain injury in military and civilian patients. *Journal of Neurotrauma, 26*(8), 1213. https://doi.org/10.1089/neu.2008.0672.

Institute of Medicine. (2013). Returning home from Iraq and Afghanistan: Assessment of readjustment needs of veterans, service members, and their families. https://doi.org/10.17226/13499.

Keltner, N. L., Doggett, R., & Johnson, R. (1983). For the Viet Nam veteran the war goes on. *Perspectives in Psychiatric Care, 21*(3), 108. https://doi.org/10.1111/j.1744-6163.1983.tb00184.x.

Keltner, N. L., & Dowben, J. S. (2007). Psychobiological substrates of posttraumatic stress disorder: Part I. *Perspectives in Psychiatric Care, 43*(2), 97. https://doi.org/10.1111/j.1744-6163.2007.00117.x.

Kim, E., Lauterbach, E., Reeve, A. … Lauterbach, E. (2007). Neuropsychiatric complications of traumatic brain injury:

A critical review of the literature (a report of the ANPA Committee on research). *Journal of Neuropsychiatry and Clinical Neurosciences, 19*, 106. https://doi.org/10.1176/jnp.2007.19.2.106.

Koebli, J., Balasubramanian, V., & Zipp, G. (2020). An exploration of higher-level language comprehension deficits and factors influencing them following blast TBI in US veterans. *Brain Injury, 34*(5), 630–641. https://doi.org/10.1080/02699052.2020.1725845.

Lusk, J. D., Sadeh, N., Wolf, E. J., & Miller, M. W. (2017). Reckless self-destructive behavior and PTSD in veterans: The mediating role of new adverse events. *Journal of Traumatic Stress, 30*(3). https://doi.org/10.1002/jts.22182.

MacDonald, C. L., Johnson, A. M., Wierzechowski, L. … Brody, D. L. (2014). Prospectively assessed clinical outcomes in concussive blast vs nonblast traumatic brain injury among evacuated US military personnel. *JAMA Neurology, 71*(8), 994–1002. https://doi.org/10.1001/jamaneurol.2014.1114.

Martin-Solech, C., & Schnyder, U. (2019). Editorial: Resilience and vulnerability factors in response to stress. *Frontiers in Psychiatry* https://doi.org/10.3389/fpsyt.2019.00732.

Mayo Clinic (2018). Post-Traumatic Stress Disorder. https://www.mayoclinic.org/diseases-conditions/post-traumatic-stress-disorder/diagnosis-treatment/drc-20355973.

Mohamadpour, M., Whitney, K., & Bergold, P. J. (2019). The importance of therapeutic time window in the treatment of traumatic brain injury. *Frontiers in Neuroscience, 13*, 7. https://doi.org/10.3389/fnins.2019.00007.

National Institute of Mental Health. (n.d.). Post-traumatic stress disorder. http://www.nimh.nih.gov/health/topics/post-traumatic-stress-disorder-ptsd/index.shtml.

Ng, S., & Lee, A. (2019). Traumatic brain injuries: Pathophysiology and potential therapeutic targets. *Frontiers in Cellular Neuroscience*. https://doi.org/10.3389/fncel.2019.00528.

Ousdal, O., Milde, A., Hafstad, G. … Hugdahl, K. (2020). The Association of PTSD symptom severity with amygdala nuclei volumes in traumatized youths. *Translational Psychiatry, 10*, 288. https://www.nature.com/articles/s41398-020-00974-4.

Pai, A., Suris, A., & North, C. (2017). Posttraumatic stress disorder in the DSM-5: Controversy, change, and conceptual considerations. *Behavioral Sciences, 7*(1). https://doi.org/10.3390/bs7010007.

Ponsford, J., Lee, N. K., Wong, D. … O'Donnell, M. L. (2020). Factors associated with response to adapted cognitive behavioral therapy for anxiety and depression following traumatic brain injury. *The Journal of Head Trauma Rehabilitation, 35*(2), 117–126. https://doi.org/10.1097/HTR.0000000000000510.

Rabinowitz, A. R., & Watanabe, T. K. (2020). Pharmacotherapy for treatment of cognitive and neuropsychiatric symptoms after mTBI. *The Journal of Head Trauma Rehabilitation, 35*(1), 76–83. https://doi.org/10.1097/HTR.0000000000000537.

Rafferty, L., Cawkill, P., Stevelink, S., Greenberg, K., & Greenberg, N. (2018). Dementia, post-traumatic stress disorder and major depressive disorder: A review of the mental health risk factors for dementia in the military veteran population. *Psychological Medicine, 48*(9), 1400–1409. https://doi.org/10.1017%2FS0033291717001386.

Roughead, E., Pratt, N., Kalisch Ellett, L., Ramsay, E., Barratt, J., Morris, P., & Killer, G. (2017). Posttraumatic stress disorder, antipsychotic use and risk of dementia in veterans. *Journal of the American Geriatrics Society, 65*(7). https://doi.org/10.1111/jgs.14837.

Selemon, L., Young, K., Cruz, D., & Williamson, D. (2019). Frontal lobe circuitry in posttraumatic stress disorder. *Chronic Stress, 3*, 1–17. https://doi.org/10.1177/2470547019850166.

Summerall, E.L. (2019). Traumatic brain injury and PTSD: Focus on veterans. https://www.ptsd.va.gov/professional/treat/cooccurring/tbi_ptsd_vets.asp.

Tanev, K., Pentel, K., Kredlow, M., & Charney, M. (2014). PTSD and TBI co-morbidity: Scope, clinical presentation, and treatment option. *Brain Injury, 28*(3). https://doi.org/10.3109/02699052.2013.873821.

Uomoto, J. M. (2012). Best practices in veteran traumatic brain injury care. *The Journal of Head Trauma Rehabilitation, 27*(4), 241. https://doi.org/10.1097/HTR.0b013e31825ee26a.

U.S. Department of Defense Casualty Status. (2021). www.defense.gov/casualty.pdf.

U.S.News.com (2020). https://www.usnews.com/news/elections/articles/2020-01-09/after-recent-deployments-how-many-us-troops-are-in-the-middle-east.

Vasterling, J., Verfaellie, M., & Sullivan, K. (2009). Mild traumatic brain injury and posttraumatic stress disorder in returning veterans: Perspectives from cognitive neuroscience. *Clinical Psychology Review, 29*, 674–684. https://doi.org/10.1016/j.cpr.2009.08.004.

Vieweg, W., Julius, D., & Fernandez, A., et al. (2006). Posttraumatic stress disorder: Clinical features, pathophysiology, and treatment. *The American Journal of Medicine, 119*, 383–390. https://doi.org/10.1016/j.amjmed.2005.09.027.

Zeitzer, M., & Brooks, J. (2008). In the line of fire: Traumatic brain injury among Iraq War veterans. *AAOHN Journal: Official Journal of the American Association of Occupational Health Nurses, 56*(8), 347–353. https://doi.org/10.3928/08910162-20080801-03.

GLOSSARY

A

absence seizure A type of generalized seizure in which there is an abrupt loss of consciousness (usually lasting <10 seconds); these seizures are nonconvulsive in nature and might not be noticed by others.

abstinence syndrome Physical signs and symptoms that occur when the addictive substance is reduced or withheld; also referred to as *withdrawal*.

abstract thinking The ability to find meaning in proverbs; the ability to conceptualize.

abuse Excessive use of a substance that differs from societal norms and causes clinically significant impairment.

acceptance The allowance of respect of individuality.

acetylcholine (ACh) A neurotransmitter synthesized by choline acetyltransferase from acetyl coenzyme A and choline. It is found in the peripheral nervous system at the myoneural junction; in the autonomic ganglia for parasympathetic or sympathetic systems; and in the parasympathetic postganglionic synapses, including cranial nerves III, VII, IX, and X. Acetylcholine is found in the spinal cord, basal ganglia, and numerous sites within the cerebral cortex. Cortical ACh is synthesized primarily in the nucleus basalis of Meynert and in the septal area near the hypothalamus.

acrophobia Fear of high places.

active listening Verbal and nonverbal skills used by the examiner to demonstrate interest and concern to the patient.

acupressure Use of pressure to restore balance by stimulating meridians.

acupuncture Ancient Chinese health practice that involves puncturing the skin with hair-thin needles at particular locations on the patient's body called *acupuncture points*; believed to help reduce pain or change a body function. Sometimes the needles are twirled, giving a slight electric charge.

acute stress disorder The development of characteristic anxiety, dissociation, and other symptoms that occur within 1 month after exposure to an extreme traumatic stressor.

addiction Repeated involvement with a substance or activity that leads to pleasure but is associated with substantial harm.

adverse childhood experiences Distressful experiences that occur before the age of 18, including abuse, household dysfunction, and other environmental stressors.

advocacy Negotiating with others to develop, improve, and provide services for a patient.

affect Emotional range attached to ideas; outwardly demonstrated; feeling, mood, or emotional tone.
  appropriate a. Emotional tone in harmony with the accompanying idea, thought, or verbalization.
  blunted a. Disturbance manifested by a severe reduction in the intensity of affect.

flat a. Absence or near-absence of any signs of affective expression.
inappropriate a. Incongruence between the emotional feeling tone and the idea, thought, or speech accompanying it.
labile a. Rapid changes in emotional tone related to external stimuli.

aggression Forceful verbal or physical action—that is, the motor counterpart of anger, rage, or hostility.

agitation Anxiety associated with severe motor restlessness.

agnosia Difficulty in recognizing familiar objects; a symptom of organic brain disease.

agnostic One who is uncertain about whether there is a god (Greek *a*, no; *gnosis*, knowledge).

agonist In pharmacology, a substance that acts with, enhances, or potentiates a specific receptor type.

agoraphobia Fear of being in a place or situation in which escape might be difficult or embarrassing, or in which help might be unavailable in case of a panic attack.

agranulocytosis A significant decrease in white blood cell count, which can have serious or lethal consequences. Clozapine can cause agranulocytosis.

agraphia Loss of the ability to write.

AIDS dementia complex Dementia attributed to HIV infection.

akathisia Motor restlessness, generally expressed as the inability to sit still, caused by the dopamine blockade by certain types of neuroleptic medications; an extrapyramidal side effect (EPSE).

alcoholic Individual whose compulsive use of alcohol causes problems at home, at work, or socially, and who continues to use alcohol despite these adverse consequences.

Alcoholics Anonymous (AA) Self-help organization that uses a 12-step program to assist alcoholics to achieve and maintain sobriety; Al-Anon assists the spouses of alcoholics; Alateen assists the teenage children of alcoholics.

alertness Awareness and attentiveness to surroundings.

alternative therapy Broad range of healing philosophies and approaches that mainstream Western medicine does not commonly use, accept, study, understand, or make available.

Alzheimer disease More correctly referred to as neurocognitive disorder due to Alzheimer disease. The most common type of dementia. Characteristic symptoms are amnesia, aphasia, apraxia, and agnosia; cognitive mental disorder resulting in dementia that is related to a progressive deterioration of brain tissue due to plaques and neurofibrillary tangles.

ambivalence Opposing impulses or feelings directed toward the same person or object at the same time.

amenorrhea Absence of menstruation.

amnesia Partial or total inability to recall past information.
  anterograde a. Recent memory loss, as in the early stages of Alzheimer disease.
  global a. Total memory loss, as in advanced stages of Alzheimer disease.
  retrograde a. Remote memory loss, as in later stages of Alzheimer disease.
  short-term a. Memory loss observed in alcoholic blackouts (for example).

amygdala Cluster of nuclei in the medial temporal lobe responsible for the response and memory of emotions.

anergia Absence of energy caused by changes in brain chemistry, anatomy, or both.

anger An emotional response to the perception of a frustration of desires or threat to one's needs.

anhedonia Loss of pleasure in activities or interests previously enjoyed; a symptom noted in mood disorders and schizophrenia.

anorexia nervosa Disorder characterized by a refusal to eat over a long period, resulting in emaciation, disturbance in body image, and intense fear of becoming fat.

Antabuse (disulfiram) Drug given to alcoholics that blocks the breakdown of acetaldehyde, producing nausea, vomiting, dizziness, flushing, and tachycardia if alcohol is consumed.

antagonist In pharmacology, a substance that blocks a receptor.

anterior commissure White matter tract that connects the olfactory structures bilaterally as well as the temporal lobes and the amygdala.

anticholinergic effect Effect caused by drugs that block ACh receptors. Common anticholinergic effects include dry mouth, blurred vision, constipation, and urinary hesitancy.

antisocial personality Personality disorder with the essential feature of a pervasive pattern of blatant disregard for social norms.

anxiety Nonspecific, unpleasant feeling of discomfort, with physiologic and psychological symptoms that generally result from a perception of a threat to safety and security.

anxiety disorders Patterns of symptoms and behaviors in which anxiety is either the primary disturbance or a secondary problem that is recognized when the primary symptoms are removed.

anxiolytic Antianxiety drug.

apathy Lack of feeling, interest, or emotion; indifference that is occasionally a mechanism for avoiding intense emotion.

aphasia Difficulty in searching for words.
  motor a. Impaired speech as a result of an organic brain disorder in which understanding remains.
  nominal a. Difficulty in finding the correct words in their appropriate sequence.
  sensory a. Loss of ability to comprehend the meaning of words.

appropriate Suitable or fitting for a particular person, purpose, occasion, or situation, such as appropriate affect, response, or attire.

497

apraxia Inability to perform previously known, purposeful, skilled activities in the absence of loss of motor function.

assault Legally, any behavior that physically or verbally presents an immediate threat of physical or emotional injury to another individual.

assertiveness Direct expression of feelings and needs in a way that respects the rights of others and self.

asylum (1) Place of safety or sanctuary; a refuge; (2) institution for the care of the mentally ill; often associated with mistreatment and callousness.

attachment A strong emotional connection within relationships displayed by acts of comfort, nurturance, and caregiving.

attachment theory The need for infants to attach to consistent caregivers to attain a secure base to explore the world; lack of secure attachment is believed to contribute to emotional disorders in childhood and beyond.

attention-deficit/hyperactivity disorder (ADHD) Relatively common disorder of childhood onset characterized by inattention, impulsiveness, and overactivity.

attitude Pattern of mental views and feelings accumulated through past experiences and affected by present stimuli; a manner, disposition, tendency, or orientation with regard to a person or situation.

atypical depression Subtype of depression occurring more often in younger individuals; expressed by atypical symptoms—for example, increased appetite, weight gain, hypersomnia.

autism (1) As defined by Dr. Bleuler in 1908, a preoccupation with self without concern for external reality; a self-made private world of the individual with schizophrenia; (2) As defined by Dr. Kanner in 1943, a disorder of markedly abnormal or impaired development in social interactions and communication, present from early childhood and characterized by difficulty in communicating and forming relationships with other people and in using language and abstract concepts.

autonomic nervous system Division of the peripheral nervous system that is involuntary and innervates the viscera, heart, blood vessels, smooth muscle, and glands; divided into the parasympathetic (craniosacral) and sympathetic (thoracolumbar) systems.

avolition Lack of motivation.

axon Long process from the neuronal cell body that transmits impulses away from the cell.

B

basal ganglia Large nuclei, including the caudate nucleus, putamen, and globus pallidus, which are responsible for modulating voluntary movement.

battery Touching of another person, of his or her clothes, or anything else attached to the person without consent.

behavior Any observable, recordable, and measurable movement, response, or act of an individual (verbal and nonverbal).

behavior therapy Therapeutic approach that helps the patient modify behavior by changing old patterns of behavior.

binge eating Eating an unusually large amount of food in a relatively short period of time.

biofeedback The use of a machine to communicate physical changes; used to train a person to reduce anxiety and modify behavioral responses.

biologic variations Physical differences between individuals or differences in body structure, skin color, other visible characteristics, enzymatic and genetic variations, electrocardiographic patterns, susceptibility to disease, nutritional preferences and deficiencies, and psychological characteristics.

bipolar disorder Mood disorder characterized by at least one episode of mania, with or without a history of depression.

biracial Individual who crosses two racial and cultural groups.

bizarre Markedly unusual in appearance, thought, style, character, or behavior; absurd.

blackout Period in which a drinker functions socially but of which the drinker has no memory.

blocking Unconscious interruption in train of thought.

blood-brain barrier Guards the brain from fluctuations in body chemistry; regulates the amount and speed with which substances in the blood enter the brain.

borderline personality disorder Personality disorder with the essential feature of a pervasive pattern of unstable interpersonal relationships and mood related to the fear of abandonment.

bradykinesia Slow or retarded movement.

brainstem Vital structure that carries all information to and from the cerebral cortex and spinal cord; responsible for respiration, its function is essential for life. Consists of the midbrain, pons, and medulla.

bulimia Compulsive binge eating accompanied by purging and an overconcern with body shape and weight; characterized by an insatiable craving for food, resulting in episodes of continuous eating and often followed by purging, depression, and self-deprivation.

bulimia nervosa Disorder characterized by binge eating, compensatory behavior, and overconcern with body shape and weight.

bureaucracy Excessive rules and structure that get in the way of efficient, responsive, and creative nursing care solutions.

burnout Spiraling process of decreased effectiveness.

C

case management Collaborative process for meeting health needs through the use of a variety of services in a cost-effective manner.

catalepsy State of unconsciousness in which immobility is constantly maintained.

catatonia Immobility as a result of psychological causes.

catatonic behavior Characterized by muscular rigidity and lack of response to the environment; may alternate from rigidity to hyperactivity.

catecholamines Derived from the amino acid tyrosine, these substances include dopamine, norepinephrine, and epinephrine. Subcategory of the monoamines, which also include serotonin and histamine. Catecholamines and their synthesis products are widely distributed in the central and peripheral nervous systems.

caudate Basal ganglia nucleus that protrudes into the anterior horn of the lateral ventricle.

cerebral cortex Narrow ribbon of gray matter that lies on the surface of the cerebrum. The gray matter lies on top of the white matter. The reverse is true in the spinal cord.

child abuse Harmful physical, emotional, sexual, or verbal behavior inflicted on a child.

cholinergics Substances that stimulate the cholinergic system. In the peripheral nervous system, cholinergic drugs constrict the pupil, increase the production of saliva and respiratory secretions, slow the heart, and increase gastrointestinal peristalsis and urinary output.

chorea Greek term for "dance." The choreas are demonstrated as hyperkinetic disorders characterized by involuntary, unpredictable, and random movements of the trunk, head, face, and limbs.

chromosome The self-replicating genetic structure of cells containing the cellular DNA that bears in its nucleotide sequence the linear array of genes. Eukaryotic genomes (such as humans have) consist of many chromosomes whose DNA is associated with different types of proteins.

circumstantiality A disturbed pattern of speech and thought process in which a person gives an excessive amount of detail (circumstances) that appears irrelevant, particularly seen in schizophrenia and OCD.

cirrhosis Disease of the liver; characterized by the development of scar tissue in the liver. The person most likely to develop cirrhosis is a middle-aged man with chronic alcoholism.

civil law The part of the legal system concerned with the legal rights and duties of private persons. Civil lawsuits can recapture monetary loss from professionals who have been guilty of false imprisonment, defamation of character, assault and battery, or negligence.

clang associations Speech pattern characterized by words similar in sound but not in meaning that rhyme; noted in types of schizophrenia.

clarification Communication skill that helps define a patient's responses through the use of direct questions.

claustrophobia Fear of enclosed places.

clinical supervision Formal meeting among psychiatric nursing peers to examine attitudes, reactions, and conflicts with patients on the unit and to find new ways of approaching patient problems.

clonic State in which rigidity and relaxation succeed each other.

closed-ended questions Questions that generally elicit a "yes" or "no" response. Useful in gathering factual data.

codependency An interdependent relationship promoted by the need to be emotionally close; sometimes used to describe an imbalanced relationship where addiction is enabled.

cognition   Act or process of knowing and perceiving.

cognitive disorders   Disorders that affect consciousness, memory, and other thought processes.

cognitive dissonance   A state that arises when two opposing beliefs exist at the same time.

cognitive processes   Processes that pertain to perception, judgment, memory, and reasoning.

coma   State of depressed consciousness wherein even extreme stimulation of the reticular activating system does not elicit a response.

command hallucinations   Hallucinations that tell the patient to take some specific action, such as to kill himself or herself or someone else.

common law/case law   Applied to the body of principles that has evolved and continues to evolve and expand from judicial decisions that arise during the trial of actual court cases; law based on the outcome of cases.

communication   Process that is the matrix for thought and relationships among all people, regardless of cultural heritage.

community meeting   Meeting that is held in the therapeutic milieu and in which joint problem solving by community members is encouraged.

community mental health   Application of the principles of psychiatric care to communities and groups of people. The goal of this effort is to maintain health, prevent mental illness when possible, and if treatment is indicated, treat the individual closer to his or her support systems.

community worldview   Community needs and concerns are more important than individual ones. Quiet, respectful communication is valued, as well as meditation and reading as a learning style.

comorbidity   Simultaneous existence of medical and psychiatric problems, each complicating the other.

compassion   A deep awareness and expressed understanding for another's suffering.

complementary therapy   Same as *alternative therapy*, but denotes therapy used as an adjunct to, rather than as a replacement for, conventional treatment.

comprehension   Capacity to perceive and understand.

compulsion   Uncontrollable impulse to perform an act or ritual repeatedly; may be in response to an obsession (unwilled, persistent thought), as in obsessive-compulsive disorder. The act or ritual serves to decrease anxiety. Examples include hand washing, cleaning, and checking (e.g., checking to see whether a door is locked).

concrete communication   Inability to think and communicate abstractly.

concrete thinking   Use of literal meaning without ability to consider abstract meaning (e.g., "Don't cry over spilled milk" might be interpreted as meaning, "Okay, I'll cry over the sink.")

confabulation   Unconscious filling of gaps in memory with imagined or untrue experiences that the person believes but have no basis in reality.

confidentiality   Treating the information about and from patients in a private manner; information about patients is confidential and requires patient approval before disclosure.

confused state   Bewildered, perplexed, or unclear. The type and degree of confusion should be specified.

congruence   Accordant states. An example is mood congruence, in which the person's visible emotional state correlates with his or her mood or feeling state.

consciousness   State of awareness.

conservator   Guardian; a legally appointed person who controls the affairs of a gravely disabled person, including the right to consent to or refuse psychiatric treatment.

consultant-liaison nurse   Psychiatric mental health nurse who provides expert consultation for patients and staff in other areas of the hospital agency.

consumer   Person in treatment for psychiatric services.

continuum of care   Levels of care through which an individual can move, depending on his or her needs at a given point in time.

contralateral   Opposite side of the body.

conversion   Process by which a psychological event, an idea, a memory, or an impulse is represented by a bodily change or symptom, such as blindness or paralysis.

coping mechanism   Any effort directed at stress management.

corporate compliance   Health care providers' responsibility to comply with governmental laws and regulations.

corpus callosum   Major connecting and communicating pathway between the brain hemispheres.

cortisol   Glucocorticoid hormone found in the adrenal cortex that is involved in carbohydrate and protein metabolism; levels in the blood tend to increase in response to stress.

creed   Set formula that states the religious and spiritual beliefs of a community of faith (Latin, *credo*, I trust, believe).

criminal law   Part of the legal system concerned with crime that is defined in state and federal statutes.

crisis   A discrete period of severe emotional disorganization following a major stressful event (e.g., divorce, job loss).

cultural awareness   Process whereby the nurse acknowledges his or her cultural biases and recognizes that other individuals, groups, or communities have their unique cultural similarities and differences.

cultural competence   Process whereby the nurse has developed cultural awareness, knowledge, and skills to promote effective and quality health care for patients.

cultural diversity   Variety of cultural groupings; might include age, gender, socioeconomic status, religion, race, and ethnicity.

cultural negotiation   Nurse's ability to work within a patient's cultural belief system to develop culturally appropriate interventions.

cultural preservation   Nurse's ability to acknowledge, value, and accept a patient's cultural beliefs.

cultural repatterning   Nurse's ability to incorporate cultural preservation and negotiation to identify patient needs, develop expected outcomes, and evaluate outcome plans.

cultural values   Unique, individual expressions of beliefs related to culture that have been accepted as appropriate over time for persons in that culture.

culturally diverse nursing care   Modification of nursing approaches to provide culturally competent care.

culture   The internal and external manifestations of beliefs, values, and norms of an individual, group, or community that are used as premises for daily life and functioning.

cupping   Alternative cultural or medical treatment that uses a small glass or cup to conduct the moxibustion treatment.

custodial care   Process of caring for hygienic and nutritional needs in an institution but not providing treatment for a mental disorder.

cyclothymia   Chronic mood disturbance of at least 2 years' duration involving numerous hypomanic episodes and numerous periods of dysphoria. Does not meet the criteria for a manic episode or major depression.

D

deinstitutionalization   Shift in treatment location from large public hospitals to community settings.

delirium   Disorder with alterations in consciousness and changes in cognition, usually caused by a general medical condition or substances. Typically delirium develops over a short period and is treatable; usually a reversible, bewildered state of clouded consciousness, generally accompanied by restlessness, disorientation, and fear. It may include periods of hallucinations.

delusion   Fixed, false belief, inconsistent with the person's intelligence and culture; unamenable to reason.

  bizarre d.   Absurd belief.

  nihilistic d.   False belief that the self, part of the self, or another object has ceased to exist.

  paranoid d.   Oversuspiciousness leading to persecutory delusions.

  persecution d.   False belief that one is being persecuted.

  reference d.   False belief that the behavior of others in the environment refers to oneself; derived from ideas of reference in which one wrongly believes that he or she is being talked about.

  somatic d.   False belief involving functioning of one's body.

dementia   Disorder that causes pronounced memory and cognitive disturbances. Typically dementias are gradual in onset and progressive in course.

dendrites   Projections (branches) from the neuron that transmit impulses to the cell body where they eventually trigger nerve impulses.

denial   Avoidance of disagreeable realities or threats by ignoring or refusing to recognize them; an unconscious defense mechanism that might or might not be adaptive.

deoxyribonucleic acid (DNA) Molecule, primarily located in the nucleus of the cell, that encodes genetic information.

dependence State in which a person must take a usual or an increasing dose of a drug to prevent the onset of abstinence symptoms, withdrawal, or both.

depersonalization Feeling of unreality or strangeness related to oneself, body parts, bodily functions, or external environment (out-of-body experience).

depression Lowered or saddened mood state.

derailment Gradual or sudden deviation in train of thought, without thought-blocking.

derealization Distortion of spatial relationships so that the environment becomes distorted or unfamiliar.

devaluation Criticism of others that defends against one's own feelings of inadequacy.

dexamethasone suppression test (DST) Diagnostic test for clinical depression that measures the function of the hypothalamic-pituitary-adrenal (HPA) axis.

diencephalon Posterior part of the forebrain; includes the thalamus, hypothalamus, epithalamus, and metathalamus.

disinhibition State in which a person is unable to suppress urges or statements that might be socially unacceptable (e.g., telling a dirty joke in an inappropriate situation).

disoriented Disturbance in orientation of time, place, person, or situation.

displacement Shift of emotion from an object or a person who incites the emotion to a less threatening source; an unconscious defense mechanism that might or might not be adaptive.

dissociation (1) Removal from conscious awareness of painful feelings, memories, thoughts, or aspects of identity; (2) splitting or separation of any group of mental or behavioral processes from the rest of the person's consciousness or identity.

distractibility Inability to concentrate attention.

dopamine Brain neurotransmitter that influences muscle movement and emotions. The dopamine theory states that individuals with schizophrenia might have too much dopamine, which might account for their sensoriperceptual alterations.

double bind Conflicting demands by significant individuals in a person's life. The person cannot meet both demands, so he or she is doomed to failure.

dysarthria Difficulty in articulation.

dyskinesia Disturbed coordination and motor activity, usually producing a jerky motion; an EPSE of neuroleptic medications related to their effect on dopamine receptors. (See also *tardive dyskinesia*.)

dyslexia Difficulty in reading.

dysphagia Difficulty in swallowing.

dysphoria Sadness that is similar to, but less severe than, that demonstrated in major depression.

dysthymia Clinical syndrome similar to, but less severe than, that demonstrated in major depressive disorder. Chronic mood disturbance involving a depressed mood for at least 2 years, more days than not.

dystonia Rigidity in muscles that control posture, gait, or ocular movement; an EPSE of neuroleptic medications that block dopamine.

E

echolalia Speech pattern characterized by repeating the words of one person by another; noted in types of schizophrenia.

echopraxia Imitation of the body position of another.

electroconvulsive therapy (ECT) Form of somatic therapy that uses electrically induced seizures to relieve a person's intractable depressive symptoms.

emotion Complex feeling state with psychological, somatic, and behavioral components related to affect and mood.

emotional dysregulation An emotional response that is outside what society considers a "normal" response; also referred to as labile mood or mood swings.

emotionally focused therapy Counseling approach that is attachment-based and focused on the role that emotions play within relationship issues. Techniques include emotional validation, responsiveness, and engagement.

emotional trauma Psychological damage resulting from very stressful events/interactions that disturb one's sense of security, making a person feel helpless and vulnerable.

empathy Objective understanding of how patients feel or how they see their situations.

enkephalins Widely distributed opioid-like neuropeptides that are part of the endorphin family; mediate pain perception, taste, olfaction, arousal, emotional behavior, vision, hearing, neurohormone secretion, motor coordination, and water balance.

environmental control Ability of an individual to control nature by planning activities and tasks to assist in maintaining optimal balance in life.

epidemiology Study of the frequency and distribution of disease conditions in the population.

epilepsy Disorder of the central nervous system (CNS) in which the major symptom is a seizure. The seizure is caused by a temporary disturbance of brain impulses.

ethnicity Characteristic of a group whose members share a common social and cultural heritage passed on to each successive generation.

ethnocentrism Acknowledging and valuing one's own culture only.

ethnopharmacology Study of pharmacogenetic, pharmacodynamic, and pharmacokinetic influences based on different ethnic, racial, and cultural groups.

etiology Study of the causes of diseases, including both direct and predisposing factors.

euphoria Sense of elation or well-being; elevation of mood; complete lack of tension; most notable in the manic/hypomanic phase of bipolar disorder.

euthymia Normal, homeostatic mood state.

existentialism Philosophy that emphasizes the individual's ability and responsibility to make one's existence meaningful by making choices in the face of life's deep pain and uncertainty.

expansive mood Elevated, unrestrained expression of feelings.

extrapyramidal side effects (EPSEs) Involuntary muscle movements resulting from the effects of neuroleptic drugs on the extrapyramidal system; cause a dopamine blockade that creates a dopamine-ACh imbalance. EPSEs include akathisia, akinesia, dystonia, drug-induced parkinsonism, and neuroleptic malignant syndrome.

extrapyramidal system Outside the pyramidal (voluntary) tract; coordinates involuntary movements.

eye contact Occasional glancing into a person's eyes to demonstrate interest during an interaction.

F

faith Traditionally, the creed that one follows within one's religious community, but the term can be used more broadly to describe one's total life view, religiously based or not.

family system Field of influence exerted on one another by family members because of their complex interaction.

fear Anxiety as a result of consciously recognized and realistic danger.

feedback Articulation of one's perception of what another person has said or meant. This process requires at least two people.

flashbacks Cognitive, emotional, and physical reexperiencing of traumatic events.

flight of ideas Speech pattern demonstrated by a rapid transition from topic to topic, frequently without completing any of the preceding ideas; prominent in manic states.

free association In a therapeutic context, saying anything that comes to mind.

fugue Period of dissociation with memory loss.

G

gamma-aminobutyric acid (GABA) Inhibitory amino acid neurotransmitter formed during the citric acid cycle from its precursor, glutamic acid. GABA receptors are widely distributed in the CNS and produce neuronal hyperpolarization through an influx of chloride ions. Drugs that increase the GABA level reduce anxiety and seizures.

gender identity disorder A profound discomfort with one's own gender and a strong and persistent identification with the opposite gender.

general leads Interactive skills that facilitate the communication process by encouraging the patient to continue.

generalized seizure Seizure that involves both hemispheres of the brain at the onset of the seizure. Consciousness is usually impaired.

genes The fundamental physical and functional units of heredity; located in a sequence of nucleotides in a particular position on a particular chromosome. There are about 30,000 different human genes.

genetic vulnerability (1) Tendency to inherent traits, behaviors, and biologic characteristics of one's ancestors; (2) predisposition that increases the risk of exhibiting a psychiatric disorder.

global memory loss Total memory loss, as in advanced stages of Alzheimer disease.

globus pallidus Gray matter structure located medial to the putamen. This portion of the basal ganglia is smaller and triangular in shape; subdivided into the globus pallidus externa and globus pallidus interna.

glutamate Major excitatory transmitter in the CNS with receptors throughout the brain. Glutamate stimulation of *N*-methyl-D-aspartate (NMDA)–activated channels permits excessive inflow of calcium ions and production of free radicals, which might cause neuronal death.

grand mal seizure Type of generalized seizure in which there is loss of consciousness and convulsions; most frequently known as epilepsy by laypersons.

gravely disabled Describes a person who is unable to provide food, clothing, or shelter for himself or herself because of a mental illness.

gray matter Composed of the cell bodies and dendrites of neurons.

grimacing Contortion of facial muscles; might be an EPSE.

gyri Convolutions of gray matter on the cerebrum.

H

half-life The amount of time it takes the body to metabolize and excrete a drug; can range from minutes to weeks.

hallucination False sensory perceptions not associated with real external stimuli; might involve any of the five senses: auditory, visual, olfactory, gustatory, or tactile.

auditory h. "Hearing voices" or noises that others do not hear. Most prevalent in schizophrenia. The sounds might be perceived as thoughts or voices coming from any type of transmitter or from the patient's mind; might be condemning and accusatory or complimentary and encouraging. It is critical that the examiner be aware that the messages might be directing the patient toward harming self or others, so the message content cannot be ignored.

tactile h. False sensory perception on the skin or scalp. Common in alcohol withdrawal. Hallucinations might also be an effect of certain types of drugs, such as amphetamines, hallucinogens, and cannabis.

visual h. "Seeing things" that others do not see. May be associated with organic conditions.

herbaceutical Plant or plant part that produces and contains chemical substances that act on the body.

here and now focus Assisting patients to understand how their current emotions and behaviors influence daily living.

holistic Pertaining to totality or the whole person (holistic care).

homeless Without a home. Homeless individuals, including whole families, might live on the street exclusively or might make use of community shelters, halfway houses, cheap hotels, or board-and-care homes.

homeopathy Unconventional Western medicine system based on the principle that "like cures like" (i.e., that the same substance in large doses produces the symptoms of an illness and in very minute doses cures it). Homeopathic physicians believe that the more dilute the remedy, the greater its potency. Homeopathic practitioners use small doses of specially prepared plant extracts and minerals to stimulate the body's defense mechanisms and healing processes to treat illness.

hostile Feeling intense anger and resentment, exhibited by destructive behavior.

hot or cold treatments Cultural-medical approaches to maintaining or returning a person to a state of wellness. These approaches do not refer to the temperature of a treatment but to the fact that a specific, defined approach is appropriate for each state of wellness or illness.

human immunodeficiency infection Spectrum of illness caused by HIV that ranges from acutely or chronically HIV-infected adults to infants in the neonatal period.

human immunodeficiency virus (HIV) Virus that has been isolated and recognized as the causative agent of acquired immunodeficiency syndrome (AIDS). HIV is classified as a lentivirus in a subgroup of the retroviruses.

human immunodeficiency virus, type 1 (HIV-1) Retrovirus identified as the cause of AIDS.

humanist Individual who emphasizes people, rather than other parts of the observable world or religion.

Huntington disease Genetically transmitted disease that includes motor and cognitive changes.

hydrotherapy Use of water (wet sheet packs, 2- to 10-hour baths) for psychotherapeutic purposes.

hyperactivity (hyperkinesis) Restless, aggressive, often destructive activity; prominent in manic states.

hypersomnia Increased and prolonged sleeping.

hypoactivity (hypokinesis) Decreased activity or retardation (psychomotor retardation); slowing of psychological and physical functions.

hypomania Clinical syndrome similar to, but less severe than, that demonstrated in a full-blown manic episode.

hypothalamus Group of nuclei in the diencephalon that influences eating behavior, temperature regulation, emotional expression, and autonomic system. Dopaminergic neurons in the hypothalamus control lactation.

I

idealization Defense mechanism characterized by viewing others as perfect; exalting others.

ideas of reference Belief that some events have a special meaning (e.g., people laughing are perceived as laughing at the patient).

idiopathic Without known cause.

illogical (thinking) Contains erroneous conclusions or internal contradictions (irrational thoughts).

illusion Misinterpretation of a sensory input; observed in alcoholic withdrawal and delirious states.

impaired parent Parent whose nurturing capabilities are compromised or absent, related to psychiatric or substance abuse disorders.

incidence The rate at which a certain condition occurs, such as the number of new cases of a specific mental disorder occurring during a certain period.

individual responsibility Owning one's tasks, needs, feelings, and thoughts, and taking action to address these responsibilities and needs.

informed consent Providing the patient with information about a specific treatment, including its benefits, side effects, and possible risks, which will enable the patient to make a competent and voluntary decision.

insight Recognition of motivational sources behind one's thoughts, actions, or behavior.

insomnia Inability to sleep or disrupted sleep patterns.

intellectual functioning Individual's general fund of knowledge, orientation, memory, mastery of simple mathematical equations, and capacity for abstract thinking.

intellectualization An (unconscious) defense mechanism; a process of thinking excessively about the philosophical or theoretical basis of a subject to the extent that anxiety-provoking issues are avoided.

internal capsule Broad band of myelinated fibers that separate the lentiform nuclei from the caudate nucleus and thalamus. Corticospinal (motor or pyramidal) tracts travel through the internal capsule, cerebral peduncles, and cerebral pyramids into the spinal cord, where they constitute the lateral corticospinal pathway. Damage to any of these structures can result in hemiparesis or hemiplegia.

involuntary commitment Commitment status in which a person who has the legal capacity to consent to mental health treatment refuses to do so and is involuntarily detained for treatment by the state.

ipsilateral Same side of body.

irrational beliefs Beliefs that are not logical but that influence feelings and behaviors.

J

judgment and comprehension Ability to understand, recall, mobilize, and integrate constructively previous learning in new situations.

K

Korsakoff psychosis Organic mental disorder with memory loss related to chronic and excessive alcohol abuse.

Kraepelin German psychiatrist who initiated a classification system for psychiatry in 1896. He used the term *dementia praecox*.

L

labile Mood, affect, or behavior that is subject to frequent, extreme, or unpredictable changes.

least restrictive alternative Environment that provides the necessary treatment requirements in the least restrictive setting possible. For example, a hospital setting is more restrictive than a board-and-care setting. If the board-and-care setting provides the necessary treatment requirements for a person, that environment represents the least restrictive alternative.

lentiform nuclei Putamen and globus pallidus of the basal ganglia.

lesion Injury to tissue.

Lewy bodies Eosinophilic cytoplasmic inclusions seen in neuromelanin-containing neurons in Parkinson disease or dementia.

ligand An ion, a molecule, or a molecular group that binds to another chemical entity to form a larger complex.

limited or special power of attorney Written document in which one person, the principal, authorizes another person, the attorney-in-fact, to act on the principal's behalf. In a limited power of attorney, the attorney-in-fact is granted only powers specifically defined in the document.

limit setting Holding individuals to established norms with the intent of assisting them to function more constructively.

lipid solubility Ability of a substance to dissolve in fat.

lithium Element or salt used in the treatment and prevention of manic episodes.

locus ceruleus Small nucleus ("blue spot") in the pontine tegmentum whose neurons are the major source of norepinephrine in the brain; present bilaterally.

loose association Pattern of speech in which a person's ideas slip off track onto another idea that is completely unrelated or only slightly related.

M

magical thinking Belief that thoughts, words, or actions can cause or prevent an occurrence by some magical means.

malingering Deliberate feigning of an illness for the purpose of secondary gain.

malpractice Negligence by a professional; a civil action that can be brought against a nurse if he or she has breached a standard of care that a reasonably prudent nurse would meet.

managed care Health care system that arranges the relationship among payers, providers, and consumers; monitors and influences the behavior of the mental health providers and the outcomes of care and reimburses for services.

mania Disordered mental state of extreme excitement, hyperactivity, euphoria, and hyperverbal behavior.

medially Toward the midline.

medulla Approximately 3 cm long; the most caudal portion of the brainstem. Controls respiration and supplies innervation to the tongue and palate.

melancholic depression Subgroup generally seen in older individuals, often misdiagnosed as dementia. Depression usually worse in the morning; early morning awakening, psycho-motor retardation or agitation, excessive or inappropriate guilt, and significant anorexia or weight loss are symptoms of melancholia.

memory Function by which information stored in the brain is later recalled to the conscious mind.

meninges Outer lining of the CNS composed of the dura mater, arachnoid, and pia mater.

mental disability Lack of intelligence so great that it interferes with social and occupational performance.

mental disorder A clinically significant behavioral or psychological syndrome or pattern associated with present distress or disability.

mental status examination (MSE) Record of current findings that includes a description of a patient's appearance, behavior, motor activity, speech, alertness, mood, cognition, intelligence, reactions, views, and attitudes.

meridian Lines in a body that are representative of psychological or physical body functions. Cultural healers stimulate meridians and release harmful toxins or illness-producing spirits through the use of alternative treatment approaches such as moxibustion, cupping, coining, or skin scraping.

mesocortical tract Dopaminergic tract that projects from the ventral tegmental area near the substantia nigra to the neocortex, particularly the prefrontal cortex; involved in motivation, planning, behavior, attention, and social behavior.

mesolimbic tract Catecholaminergic neuronal tract (mostly dopaminergic) with cell bodies located in the ventral tegmental area of the midbrain and axons that project to the hippocampus, entorhinal cortex, amygdala, anterior cingulate gyrus, nucleus accumbens, and other limbic regions.

metabolic tolerance Process that occurs when the body is more efficient at metabolizing a substance.

midbrain Most rostral division of the brainstem. It contains important structures such as the cerebral aqueduct, superior and inferior colliculi, red nuclei, substantia nigra, cerebral peduncles, and oculomotor and trochlear cranial nerve nuclei.

milieu Environment or setting.

milieu management Purposeful manipulation of the environment to promote a therapeutic atmosphere.

milieu therapy Use of the environment to promote optimal functioning in a group or individual.

minority Social, religious, ethnic, occupational, or other group that constitutes less than a numeric majority of the population.

model of care Philosophy of causative and curative factors of mental illness that drives the nature of the care activities offered.

monoamine Category of neurotransmitters that contain one amino group and are derived from amino acids. Subcategories of monoamines include the catecholamines (dopamine, norepinephrine, epinephrine), which are derived from tyrosine, and the indolamine serotonin, which is derived from tryptophan.

Histamine is categorized as a monoamine but is biochemically different. Monoamine-synthesizing neurons are primarily found in the brainstem but have a wide net of influence because of the ubiquitous distribution of their axonal projections.

monoamine oxidase Enzyme that metabolizes monoamines such as dopamine, norepinephrine, and serotonin.

monoamine oxidase inhibitors (MAOIs) Antidepressant drugs that increase the bioavailability of certain neurotransmitters by interfering with their metabolism.

mood Individual's internal state of mind that is exhibited through feelings and emotions.

mood disorder Diagnostic category in *DSM-5* that includes depressive disorders and bipolar disorders.

moxibustion Alternative cultural medical treatment approach that uses moxa and heat to release illness-producing spirits from the body, mind, or spirit.

mutism Refusal or inability to speak.

N

NANDA North American Nursing Diagnosis Association.

narcissism Extreme self-centeredness and self-absorption; narcissistic personality disorder is characterized by a tendency to exploit others and lack of empathy.

narcotherapy Induction of a state of sedation by intravenous administration of sedatives (e.g., amobarbital) or stimulants (e.g., methylphenidate).

National Alliance on Mental Illness A grassroots mental health organization that is dedicated to building hope in people with mental illness, advocating for access to services, treatment, support, and research.

National Institute of Mental Health Government organization in the National Institutes of Health concerned with mental health issues in the United States.

nature argument Proposes that a specific mental disorder is caused by biologic factors (e.g., neurotransmitter irregularities, pathoanatomy) rather than by psychodynamic factors (e.g., related to upbringing, life events, or other stressors).

naturopathic physician Alternative care practitioner who holds a doctor of naturopathy (ND) degree.

naturopathy Discipline that views disease as a manifestation of alterations in the processes by which the body naturally heals itself and emphasizes health restoration rather than disease treatment. Naturopathic physicians use an array of healing practices that include diet and clinical nutrition; homeopathy; acupuncture; herbal medicine; hydrotherapy (use of water in a range of temperatures and methods of applications); spinal and soft tissue manipulation; physical therapies involving electric currents; ultrasound and light therapies; therapeutic counseling; and pharmacology.

negativism Motiveless resistance to all instruction.

negligence Failure to do that which a reasonably prudent and careful person would do under the circumstances or doing what a reasonable and prudent person would not do.

neologism Speech pattern characterized by the production of unknown words; noted in some types of schizophrenia.

neurocognitive disorders Class of disorders of mental functioning caused either by permanent brain damage or by temporary brain dysfunction. Memory, cognition, emotions, and motivation are affected.

neurofibrillary tangle Mass of abnormal filamentous material located within the cell body of neurons; occur in several brain disorders, including Alzheimer disease, and are composed of cytoskeletal components.

neuroleptic Antipsychotic medication.

neuron Nerve cell.

neurotransmitter Chemical found in the nervous system (e.g., norepinephrine, serotonin, dopamine) that facilitates the transmission of nerve impulses across synapses between neurons.

nihilistic ideas Thoughts of nonexistence and hopelessness.

N-methyl-D-aspartate (NMDA) receptor Glutamate receptor that is the primary mechanism for controlling synaptic plasticity and memory function; thought to be present in all or almost all neurons in the CNS.

nonviolence Solving conflictual situations by methods other than verbal or physical aggression.

norepinephrine Catecholamine neurotransmitter that is primarily synthesized in neurons of the locus coeruleus in the pons. Deficiencies of norepinephrine are linked to depression.

norepinephrine and dopamine reuptake inhibitors (NDRIs) Class of antidepressants; the only antidepressants that primarily block the reuptake of dopamine.

norm Expected behavior for a given therapeutic setting.

nucleus accumbens This nucleus is adjacent to the medial and ventral portions of the caudate and putamen. The neurons in this nucleus project to both the globus pallidus and the substantia nigra, a major component of the "reward pathway."

nucleus basalis of Meynert Located bilaterally, directly beneath the anterior commissure, the major brain site for the production of ACh fibers from this nucleus project diffusely to the cerebral cortex.

nurse-patient interaction Purposeful use of the relationship between the patient and nurse for achieving patient treatment goals.

nursing diagnosis Statement that describes a patient's potential or actual problem or response to illness treatable by nurses.

nurture argument Proposes that a specific mental disorder is caused by psychodynamic factors (e.g., related to upbringing, interactions, life events, or other stressors) rather than by biologic factors (e.g., neurotransmitter irregularities, pathoanatomy).

O

obesity Abnormal increase in the proportion of fat cells, mainly in the viscera and subcutaneous tissues of the body.

objectivity Process of remaining open, unbiased, and emotionally separate from a patient.

obsession Pathologic persistence of an unwilled thought, feeling, or impulse to the extent that it cannot be eliminated from consciousness by logical effort.

obsessive-compulsive disorder Disorder in which recurrent obsessions (thoughts) alternate with compulsions (behaviors) in an effort to decrease anxiety.

occupational therapy Uses the activities of daily living to help people with mental disabilities achieve maximum functioning and independence at home and in the workplace.

oculogyric crisis Involuntary tonic muscle spasms of the eye. The eyes usually roll upward in a fixed stare. This frightening dystonic reaction is caused by antipsychotic drugs.

olfactory Pertaining to the sense of smell.

open-ended statement Statement that elicits further exploration of the patient's problem by encouraging communication; can also be in the form of a question.

openness Atmosphere in which people are free to express their thoughts and feelings without fear of ridicule or censure.

open posture Relaxed yet attentive position with arms uncrossed; enhances patient's trust in the examiner.

orientation Conscious awareness of person, place, time, and situation.

P

panic State of extreme, acute, intense anxiety, accompanied by disorganization of thoughts and ability to function.

paranoia Extreme suspiciousness of others and their actions.

paranoid thinking Oversuspicious thinking when a person feels threatened, even when there is no evidence; also described as delusions.

parkinsonism Cause (e.g., brain injury, antipsychotic drugs, carbon monoxide) of parkinsonism symptoms is known or suspected.

parkinsonism symptoms Masked facies, muscle rigidity, and shuffling gait. Symptoms are common in patients taking neuroleptic drugs; EPSEs are related to dopamine blockade.

partial seizure Usually involves one hemisphere of the brain at the onset of the seizure.

pedophilia Intense sexual arousal or desire and acts, fantasies, or other stimuli involving children.

perception Awareness of objects and relationships that follows stimulation of peripheral sense organs.

perseveration Pattern of speech characterized by repetition of the same word or idea in response to different questions.

personal control Exerting limits on one's own impulses to act in a manner that is consistent with one's best interests, treatment goals, or personal needs.

personality disorder Exaggerated, inflexible, and pervasive behavior patterns destructive to the individual and others.

pervasive developmental disorder (PDD) Any one of several conditions characterized by multiple social and cognitive delays.

petit mal seizure A variant of seizure that involves brief, sudden lapses in attention, characterized by three spikes per second and a wave pattern on electroencephalogram.

pharmacodynamic tolerance Tolerance seen when higher blood levels are required to produce a given effect.

phobia Exaggerated, pathologic fear of some specific type of stimulus or situation.

phobic disorder Severe phobic behavior patterns that render the individual dysfunctional. Avoidance of the feared object or situation serves to assuage anxiety.

physical or emotional security Feeling safe from emotional, verbal, and physical assault.

postpartum depression Subtype of depression in the postpartum period occurring 30 days or less after childbirth.

posttraumatic stress disorder (PTSD) Development of characteristic symptoms (e.g., intense fear, helplessness, reexperiencing of events) after exposure to an extreme traumatic stressor.

preconscious Memories that can be recalled to consciousness with some effort.

precursor Something that precedes. For example, tyrosine is a precursor to dopamine in the synthesis of dopamine in the body.

premorbid State before onset of a disorder.

prevalence Estimate of the frequency of a disease condition in the population (e.g., ADHD affects 5% of children).

primary appraisal Initial judgment that an individual makes about an event.

primary gain Relief or expression of anxiety through symptoms of a disorder.

privacy Allowance of physical and emotional space for self and others.

probable cause Sufficient credible facts that would induce a reasonably intelligent and prudent person to believe that a cause of action exists.

process recording Written record of an encounter with a patient that is as nearly verbatim as possible, including both verbal and nonverbal behaviors of the nurse and the patient.

professional chaplain Also known as a spiritual care professional; one who has extensive postgraduate clinical training to offer spiritual care within a health care organization.

projective identification Defense mechanism characterized by projection of qualities on to another that are unacceptable to the self.

psychiatric rehabilitation Promotion of the patient's highest level of functioning in the least restrictive environment.

psychoeducation Strategy of teaching patients and families about disorders, treatments, coping techniques, and resources, based on the observation that people can be more effective participants in their own care if they have knowledge.

psychomotor retardation Markedly slowed speech and body movements.

psychopathology Study of underlying processes, both biologic and psychosocial, that lead to mental disorders.

psychosis Inability to recognize reality, complicated by severe thought disturbances (e.g., hallucinations, delusions) and the inability to relate to others.

psychosocial adversity Environmental conditions such as poverty, unemployment, or overcrowded living conditions that do not support the optimal development of a child.

psychotherapeutic management Model for nursing care that balances the three primary intervention models used by psychiatric nurses: therapeutic nurse-patient relationship, psychopharmacology, and milieu management.

psychotropic drugs Medications used in the treatment of mental illness.

purge Compensation for calories consumed by self-induced vomiting, laxative abuse, diuretics, or enemas.

pyramidal system Motor system for voluntary movement.

R

race Breeding population that primarily mates within itself.

raphe nuclei Nuclei located along the midline of the brainstem (*raphe*, seam). Serotonin is synthesized from these cells.

reappraisal Evaluation made after new or additional information has been received.

receptor A specialized area on a nerve membrane, blood vessel, or muscle that receives the chemical stimulation to activate or inhibit normal actions of nerves, blood vessels, or muscles.

recovery Defined by the Substance Abuse and Mental Health Services Administration as "a process of change through which individuals improve their health and wellness, live a self-directed life, and strive to reach their full potential."

recreational therapist Assists patients in finding leisure interests so that they can learn to balance work and play.

relational worldview Perception of the world grounded in the belief in spirituality and the significance of relationships and interactions among individuals.

religion Defined structures, rituals, beliefs, and values through which communities frequently address spiritual concerns.

religiosity Preoccupation with religious ideas or content.

resiliency Capability to withstand stressors without permanent dysfunction or developmental delay.

respect for the individual Acknowledgment and allowance of the rights of others to be unique.

restraint Physical control of a patient to prevent injury to the patient, staff, and other patients.

reuptake Physiologic process that occurs when a neurotransmitter is taken up into the presynaptic neuron after having been released into the synapse. Some psychotropic drugs are designed to prevent the reuptake of a specific neurotransmitter to increase the synaptic presence of that neurotransmitter.

rigidity Assumption of a stiff, inflexible posture.

S

schizophrenia Syndrome, illness, or mental health disorder characterized by hallucinations, delusions, or both. Symptoms generally reflect a progressive deterioration and disorganization of the individual's personality structure, affect, and cognition.

seasonal affective disorder (SAD) Subtype of depression occurring in late autumn or winter and lasting until spring.

seclusion Process of placing a patient alone in a specially designed room for protection and close observation.

secondary gain Attention and support received from others while ill.

selective serotonin-norepinephrine reuptake inhibitors (SNRIs) Class of antidepressants; block the reuptake of serotonin and norepinephrine. At higher doses, the reuptake of dopamine is also inhibited.

selective serotonin reuptake inhibitors (SSRIs) Class of antidepressants; potent blockers of serotonin reuptake, increasing the level of serotonin in the synapse.

self-mutilation The intentional act of tissue destruction to one's own body with the purpose of shifting overwhelming emotional pain to physical pain.

serotonin (5-HT) Monoamine neurotransmitter from the indolamine family. It is derived from the amino acid tryptophan.

shuffling gait (parkinsonian gait) Style of walking typically demonstrated by individuals whose dopamine stores have been blocked or depleted as a result of Parkinson disease or antipsychotic medications.

smudging Common sacred rite of purification and cleansing practiced by many Native American nations. It includes the burning of cedar and sage for the purpose of fanning smoke with an eagle feather over or near the patient. It is seen as purifying the spirit and preparing the patient for a difficult spiritual journey such as illness or death and is also used for other spiritual rituals.

socialization skills Skills necessary for negotiating daily interpersonal issues (e.g., acknowledging responsibility for one's behavior, using eye contact appropriately, interacting with others for purposes of sharing and support).

social organization Culture around particular units, such as family, racial, or ethnic groups; religious groups; and community or social groups.

social skills group Group that helps psychiatric patients learn, practice, and develop skills for dealing with people in social situations.

somatic therapy Therapeutic approach that uses physiologic or physical interventions to effect behavioral changes. For example, ECT is a somatic treatment.

somatization Conversion of mental states or experiences into bodily symptoms; associated with anxiety.

soul Nonphysical, transcendent part of human beings involving their mind and will.

space Refers to distance and intimacy needs of culturally unique individuals in human interaction.

spirituality Awareness of relationships with all creation, an appreciation of presence and purpose that goes beyond the five senses and the physical world; includes a sense of meaning and belonging. It is often inclusive of religion.

splitting Inability to integrate good and bad aspects of self and others; person views self and others as all good or all bad.

status epilepticus Repetitive seizures; usually refers to repetitive grand mal seizures.

statutory law Written law emanating from a legislative body; written by state and federal legislative authorities and passed in accordance with state and federal law.

steady state Desired state in anticonvulsant and other therapies, when the serum concentration of the drug is consistent and is maintained at a therapeutic level.

stereotyping Assumption that all people in similar cultural, racial, ethnic, or other groups think and act alike.

stereotypy Continuous repetition of speech or physical activities.

stressor Stimulus perceived by the individual or the organism as challenging, threatening, or damaging.

striatum Basal ganglia that include the caudate and putamen.

substance-induced mood disorder Disorder that results from the disturbance or alteration of a person's mood caused by the ingestion of a prescribed or nonprescribed drug or medication or by exposure to a toxic substance.

substantia nigra Literally "black substance;" a pigmented area of the midbrain where dopamine is synthesized.

substrate The material or substance on which an enzyme acts.

suicidal ideation Individual's thinking about and inclination toward self-injury or self-destruction.

suicidal plan Specific method designed to inflict self-injury or self-destruction as verbalized by an individual.

suicide Self-inflicted death.

sulcus Groove separating gyri. Deep sulci are referred to as fissures.

synapse Microscopic space between two neurons.

T

tangentiality Train of thought wanders from topic to topic; inability to have goal-directed associations of thought; never gets to desired goal.

tardive dyskinesia Extrapyramidal syndrome that usually emerges late in the course of long-term antipsychotic drug therapy; includes grimacing, buccolingual movements, and dystonia (impaired muscle tonus); might be irreversible.

terror State of extreme fear.

therapeutic In the psychotherapeutic management model, the communication of respect, a desire to help, and understanding to another person. Understanding includes knowledge of mental mechanisms, coping strategies, and stressors. Active listening is a crucial component of being therapeutic.

therapeutic communication Interactive verbal and nonverbal strategies that focus on the needs of the patient and facilitate a goal-directed, patient-oriented communication process.

therapeutic listening Listening that is focused on the patient and obtains therapeutically useful information about the patient.

therapeutic milieu Treatment environment managed in such a way that the environment itself is therapeutic.

therapy Means, usually with words, to cure or manage the course of another person's mental disorder. Nurses who practice psychotherapy are trained in a specific therapy model (e.g., psychoanalysis, experiential, cognitive therapy).

thought disorder Thinking characterized by loose associations, neologisms, and illogical constructs and conclusions.

time Either a physical quantity measured by a clock or patterns and orientations that relate to social processes.

tolerance Need for increasing amounts of a substance to achieve the same effects.

transference Unconscious emotional reaction to a current situation that is based on previous experiences.

traumatic brain injury (TBI) A brain injury or simply head injury that occurs when a sudden trauma causes damage to the brain.

tricyclic antidepressants (TCAs) Antidepressants that block the reuptake of norepinephrine and serotonin into the presynaptic neuron.

tuberoinfundibular tract Dopaminergic system with neurons in the arcuate nucleus of the hypothalamus that project to the pituitary stalk; controls the secretion of prolactin.

tyramine Substance derived from the amino acid tyrosine and found in many common foods, such as aged cheeses, yogurt, and avocados. Tyramine-rich foods can cause a hypertensive crisis in a person being treated with MAOIs.

tyrosine Amino acid that is the precursor to dopamine.

U

unconscious Memories, conflicts, experiences, and materials that have been repressed and cannot be recalled at will.

undoing Defense mechanism by which a person symbolically acts out to reverse a previously committed act or thought; a common ritual in obsessive-compulsive disorder.

unit norm Expected behavior for a given therapeutic setting.

unnatural cause of illness Belief that outside forces such as a spell or a hex being cast on the sick person are the cause or the source of illness or disease.

V

validation Process of acknowledging an individual's emotional experience.

vascular dementia Results from the interruption of blood flow to the brain, which causes anoxia, ischemia, and subsequent infarction.

ventral tegmental area (VTA) Located in the midbrain, this region is dorsomedial to the substantia nigra and ventral to the red nuclei. The nuclei in this area produce dopamine. The efferent pathways from the VTA include the mesocortical and mesolimbic tracts.

ventricle System of connected brain cavities that are filled with cerebrospinal fluid, including the lateral ventricles (in the central portion of the telencephalon), the third ventricle (which runs between the thalami), the fourth ventricle (in the pons and medulla), and the connecting cerebral aqueduct (in the midbrain).

vesicle Storage sac at the synaptic terminal.

voluntary commitment Situation whereby the patient or his or her conservator or guardian requests psychiatric treatment and signs an application for that treatment. This person is also free to sign himself or herself out of the hospital.

W

Wernicke area Sophisticated auditory association cortex located within the planum temporale that interprets spoken language.

Wernicke encephalopathy Confusion and ophthalmoplegia caused by thiamine deficiency; most common in alcoholics. It results in necrosis and hemorrhage in the mammillary bodies and periventricular structures of the brainstem.

Western medicine Conventional clinicians use this term to describe the medicine practiced by the holders of Doctor of Medicine (MD) or Doctor of Osteopathy (DO) degrees, some of whom might also practice complementary and alternative medicine. Other terms for conventional medicine are allopathic medicine, regular medicine, mainstream medicine, and biomedicine.

white matter Substance in the brain composed of myelinated neuronal axons.

withdrawal (1) Act of turning away in response to an emotional threat; (2) physiologic response to cessation of an addictive substance.

word salad Speech pattern characterized by an incoherent mixture of words or phrases.

INDEX

Page numbers followed by *f* indicate figures, *t* indicate tables, and *b* indicate boxes.